Physiology in Childbearing

Physiology in Childbearing with Anatomy and Related Biosciences

EDITION 5

Edited by

Jean Rankin, PhD, MMedical Science, PGCert LTHE, BSc (Hons), RN, RSCN, RM

Professor Maternal, Child & Family (retired)
UK Advance Higher Education National Teaching Fellow

ELSEVIER

First edition © 1999, Harcourt Brace and Company Limited
Second edition 2005
Third edition 2010
Fourth edition 2017

Notices

Practitioners and researchers must always rely on their own experience and knowledge in evaluating and using any information, methods, compounds or experiments described herein. Because of rapid advances in the medical sciences, in particular, independent verification of diagnoses and drug dosages should be made. To the fullest extent of the law, no responsibility is assumed by Elsevier, authors, editors or contributors for any injury and/or damage to persons or property as a matter of products liability, negligence or otherwise, or from any use or operation of any methods, products, instructions, or ideas contained in the material herein.

ISBN: 978-0-323-93053-6

Content Strategist: Andrae Akeh
Content Project Manager: Taranpreet Kaur/Suthichana Tharmapalan
Design: Miles Hitchen
Marketing Manager: Deborah Watkins

Printed in India

Last digit is the print number: 9 8 7 6 5 4 3 2 1

Working together
to grow libraries in
developing countries

www.elsevier.com • www.bookaid.org

Contents

Section 4B: Puerperium—The Mother

Preface

It is my privilege to accept editorship of the fifth edition of *Physiology in Childbearing with Anatomy and Related Biosciences*. The new edition has welcomed input from a range of authors reflecting the diverse context of midwifery practice and education. This specialist input will enable students, midwifery practitioners and others caring for women during childbearing to base their decision-making on detailed knowledge from a wide range of experts in their field.

As midwives and educators, the authors and coauthors are aware of the increasing need for an in-depth understanding of the physiological processes of childbearing and the wider application of biological sciences to midwifery practice. Acquiring this knowledge and understanding will support the early recognition of pathology which in turn can prevent morbidity and mortality. The aims of this fifth edition are to:

- Provide a biological science-based textbook for basic and postbasic students and practitioners of normal and abnormal midwifery.
- Differentiate between the nonpregnant body systems and the unique and dramatic anatomical, physical and physiological changes that occur during and following pregnancy.
- Enable an understanding of physiology and other biosciences applied to childbearing to ensure safe, efficient and evidence-informed practice.
- Recognize and act on situations where the woman becomes seriously unwell or deal with emergency maternal and neonatal emergencies.
- Integrate knowledge of applied biosciences within the social and health context of pregnancy and childbearing.
- Contribute to the safety-related aspects of childbearing women, mothers and babies.
- Highlight the important role of the psychological, cultural and social aspects of reproduction and how they may affect the physiological wellbeing of women in their reproductive years as well as childbearing individuals.

Childbearing is a normal biological function that brings about profound anatomical and physiological changes in body systems. The changes may occasionally lead to complications and pathological situations. It is imperative for midwives to understand how the systems normally function so they can recognize abnormal situations. This knowledge and understanding of the body systems and physiological processes is essential to underpin safe midwifery practice.

An understanding of the embryological development of each system also helps students and midwives to appreciate problems arising in the neonate. For these reasons, a system-wise approach is used throughout the textbook. Allied biosciences include anatomy, biochemistry, behavioural biology, embryology, evolution, ecology, genetics, microbiology, pharmacology and pathophysiology. There is evidence of the rapid advances in the field of genetics, with implications for diagnosis and treatment of diseases with a genetic basis.

Preparation for this edition focused on finding out the preferred learning styles for students and midwives. This was a key priority given the recent unprecedented COVID-19 pandemic and its profound impact on both midwifery teaching and practice in the short and long terms. Viewpoints were invited from many students, midwives and educationalists across the practice and education sectors. This insight did not highlight a single preferred learning style, but rather a range of different styles depending on the nature of the content and topic area. Brief sections of information were preferred over lengthy narratives. The consensus tended to support the preference for concise summaries of key points and 'easy-to-interpret' figures and tables. The main points at the ends of chapters were found to be helpful. Taking these findings into account, the authors revised their specialist chapters accordingly and, where relevant, repackaged the content into shorter narrative sections, tables, information textboxes and clinical application boxes. At the time of editing, the content was aligned with the relevant available evidence and guidance from key documents and websites. These included the Royal College of Obstetricians and Gynaecologists (RCOG), the National Institute for Health and Care Excellence (NICE) guidelines, MBR-RACE-UK (Mothers and Babies: Reducing Risk through Audit and Confidential Enquiries), the World Health Organization (WHO), Cochrane reviews, and UNICEF. As the main focus of this textbook is on physiology and related biosciences, an outline of the clinical management is provided where required. For further information and management guidelines, the reader is referred to appropriate national and international literature and reports. Relevant chapters have been reviewed, updated and reduced to take account of advancing technology, with the reader being referred to online illustrations and more in-depth specialist textbooks. The overall presentation is enhanced with the introduction of full-colour figures.

The book remains divided into four sections. Section 1 covers the preconception aspects of childbearing and relevant biosciences, anatomical and biological foundation information such as basic biochemistry, cellular structures and regulation of genes. The anatomy and physiology of the male and female reproductive systems are detailed and the chapters on fertility control and infertility have been updated and repackaged. The chapter on preconception care includes wide environmental and lifestyle issues so that the practitioner can select appropriate advice for both the general public and for prospective parents and others seeking specific information.

Section 2 is divided into three parts. Section 2A is concerned with the development and growth of the fetus, placenta and membranes. The embryology chapters were reviewed for relevance to the contemporary reader. These are detailed in an easy-to-follow style over three more concise chapters. Problems associated with fetal health, growth and development are covered. Section 2B is about the physiological adaptation of the woman's body to pregnancy. Each system is described in the nonpregnant state, providing students and midwives a detailed foundation of the anatomy and physiology before pregnancy occurs. This is followed by the many dramatic alterations brought about by pregnancy and their significance to health. Section 2C covers key risk factors and pathological states in pregnancy, including COVID-19. Each disorder and its management is discussed.

Section 3 is divided into two parts. Section 3A is about normal labour and discusses the management that arises from an understanding of related physiology. These chapters include the onset of labour, each of the three stages of labour and one devoted to the aspect related to pain relief in labour. Section 3B is concerned with abnormal labour. Detailed action in alignment with guidance from the RCOG is provided in a concise and logical way. The final chapter in this section has been expanded to include the care of acutely unwell women.

Section 4 is divided into two parts and considers the mother and baby in the puerperium. Section 4A is about the neonate: two chapters examine the normal neonate and adaptation to extrauterine life, and four chapters explore common neonatal disorders and outline their management. Section 4B includes chapters on the breast and breastfeeding in alignment with the UNICEF guidelines, the physiological changes in the puerperium and the pathological conditions that may affect women. The final chapter focuses on the development of mother–infant relationships in terms of biological theory and how this knowledge can be integrated into everyday midwifery practice to promote attachment and bonding through positive parenting.

People involved in the childbearing process, parenting and care of newborns encompass individuals from a range of backgrounds. This includes individuals from different cultures and ethnicities, with different life perspectives and experiences. This edition refers to childbearing women, mothers, fathers, partners, parents and families. For sensitive issues, such as the language used around lactation and breastfeeding, students and midwives are provided references to further reading. It is acknowledged that language and terminology is constantly evolving. This edition aims to represent all individuals involved in reproduction, pregnancy, birth, puerperium, newborn care and parenting.

It is hoped that readers will find that the revised content and format of this textbook supports their learning needs. In doing so, further knowledge and understanding of the physiological processes underpinning childbearing practices will enhance their care for all involved.

Jean Rankin
Professor Maternal, Child & Family (retired)
UK Advance Higher Education National Teaching Fellow

Contributors

Aishah Ahmad, BSc(Hons), MSc, PhD, PGCert, RM, Advance HE (Fellow)
Senior Lecturer in Midwifery, School of Allied Health and Midwifery, University of Wolverhampton, UK

Dawn Cameron, BSc, MSc, PhD, PGCert LTHE, RM, RN
Senior Lecturer (Midwifery), Lead Midwife for Education, School of Health and Life Sciences, University of the West of Scotland, Lanarkshire, UK

Suzanne Crozier, DBA, MSc, BA(Hons), Cert Ed, ADM, RM, RGN, SFHEA
Associate Professor (Midwifery), School Quality Enhancement Lead & Acting School Head of Teaching & Learning, School of Health and Social Care, Edinburgh Napier University, Edinburgh, UK

Lorna D. Davies, BSc(Hons), MA, PhD, RN, RM
Associate Professor (Midwifery), Otago Polytechnic, Te Pukenga, Dunedin, New Zealand

Frankie Fair, BSc, BMedSci, MSc, RM
Research Fellow, Centre for Applied Health and Social Care Research (CARe), Sheffield Hallam University, Sheffield, UK

Yvonne Greig, BSc, MSc, Professional Doctorate, RM, RN
Midwifery Lecturer / Co-lead for Interprofessional Education, School of Health and Social Care, Edinburgh Napier University, Edinburgh, UK

Lyz Howie, BSc, MM, PhD, PGC TLHE, RM, RGN, Advance HE (Senior Fellow)
Lecturer (Midwifery), School of Health and Life Sciences, University of the West of Scotland, Lanarkshire, UK

Sonya MacVicar, BA(Hons), MSc, PhD, RN, RM, Advance HE (Fellow)
Associate Professor (Neonatal Health), School of Health and Social Care, Edinburgh Napier University, Edinburgh, UK

Lynsay Matthews, MBChB, MSc, PhD, PGCert LTHE
Lecturer, Public Health, School of Health and Life Sciences, University of the West of Scotland, Lanarkshire, Scotland, Honorary Research Fellow, Institute of Applied Health Research, University of Birmingham, UK

Thomas McEwan, FRCM, BSc, MSc, PGCert (TLHE), PGDip (ANNP), RM, TCH, Advance HE (Senior Fellow)
Head of Programme & Principal Educator, NHS Education for Scotland, Edinburgh, UK

Shona Montgomery, BSc, MSc, ADM, RM, RGN, Advance HE (Senior Fellow)
Midwife Lecturer / Programme Lead, School of Health & Social Care, Edinburgh Napier University, Edinburgh, UK

Gail Norris, BSc, MSc, PhD, RM, RGN, Advance HE (Senior Fellow)
Associate Professor of Midwifery, Head of International, School of Health and Social Care, Edinburgh Napier University, Edinburgh, UK

Maria Pollard, MM, EdD, RM, RGN, Advance HE (Senior Fellow)
Deputy Director Nursing, Midwifery & Allied Health Professionals. Lead Midwife, NHS Education for Scotland, Edinburgh, UK

Jean Rankin, BSc(Hons), MMedSci, PhD, PG Cert TLHE, RN, RM, RSCN
Advance HE (National Teaching Fellow), Professor Maternal, Child & Family (retired), UK

Elizabeth Smith, QN, BN, PhD, RN, RM, HV
Community Infant Feeding Nurse, NHS Ayrshire & Arran, Breastfeeding Advocacy Lead for Scotland (secondment), Scotland

Hora Soltani, FRCM, BSc, MMedSci, PhD, PGDip, PGCert, RM
Professor in Maternal and Infant Health, Centre for Applied Health and Social Care Research (CARe), Sheffield Hallam University, Sheffield, UK

Jean Watson, BSc, MSc, PhD, PG Cert TLHE, RM, RGN, Advance HE (Senior Fellow)
Midwifery Lecturer and Depute Lead Midwife for Education (retired), School of Health, Nursing and Midwifery, University of the West of Scotland, Lanarkshire, UK

Acknowledgements

The editor would like to thank all contributors for their commitment and invaluable input to this fifth edition. This acknowledgement is extended to the first editor, the late Dot Stables, and previous authors who contributed to earlier editions and provided the foundation for subsequent versions.

Appreciation is also extended to the team at Elsevier, Suthichana, Taranpreet and Andrae for their culmination of the final textbook – this was no mean feat! Suthichana, thank you for your unstinting patience, tolerance and professional guidance to make this edition possible.

Thanks to the student midwives and colleagues in practice and education who were helpful in providing feedback and suggestions for this edition. Special thanks and acknowledgement must be extended to two authors, Dr Lynsay Matthews and Tom McEwan. Their commitment and willingness to share expertise in their specialist areas was appreciated and this made a significant contribution to the editorial process.

Illustration Acknowledgements

The editor and publisher are grateful for permission to reproduce the following illustrations:

Figures 1.1, 3.7, 4.11, 21.3, 22.2, 27.5, 27.6, 28.1, 28.2, 29.4, 29.5: Waugh, A., Grant, A., 2018. Ross and Wilson Anatomy and Physiology in Health and Illness, thirteenth ed. Elsevier, Edinburgh.

Figures 2.1, 18.9: Coad, S., Dunstall, M., 2011. Anatomy and Physiology for Midwives, third ed. Elsevier.

Figures 2.2, 2.6, 5.2, 16.6, 17.2–17.5, 17.9, 17.10, 18.2, 18.5, 19.2, 19.7, 20.1, 23.2, 25.1, 28.4, 28.5: Waugh, A., Grant, A., 2014. Ross and Wilson Anatomy and Physiology in Health and Illness, twelfth ed. Elsevier, Edinburgh.

Figures 2.4, 3.2, 4.4, 9.2, 9.5, 15.5, 16.1, 16.3-16.5, 17.6-17.8, 17.11, 18.1, 18.3, 18.4, 18.6, 18.7, 19.4, 19.8, 19.9, 21.1, 21.2, 21.4–21.8, 22.1, 22.3, 22.4, 24.1, 24.2, 25.3, 25.4, 26.2 - 26.4, 26.6–26.10, 26.12, 27.4, 30.1, 35.1: Hinchliff, S.M., Montague, S.E., 1990. Physiology for Nursing Practice. Baillière Tindall, London.

Figures 2.8, 3.1, 3.3, 3.5, 4.1, 4.2, 4.5, 4.10, 5.1: Coad, S., Pedley, K., Dunstall, M., 2019. Anatomy and Physiology for Midwives, fourth ed. Elsevier.

Figure 2.9: Watson, R., 2011. Anatomy and Physiology for Nurses, thirteenth ed. Elsevier, Edinburgh.

Figures 3.6, 4.3, 4.713.5, 13.6, 15.3, 24.3–24.6, 24.8–24.11, 24.13-24.18, 25.5, 25.6, 25.9, 25.10, 31.1, 31.2, 31.4–31.9, 37.6–37.8, 38.5, 38.7, 38.8, 40.3, 40.4, 40.7, 42.1, 42.3–42.6, 43.2, 43.5–43.7, 43.9, 44.2, 45.2–45.4, 53.2–53.4, 56.1, 56.2: Henderson, C., Macdonald, S. (Eds.), 2004. Mayes' Midwifery: A Textbook for Midwives, thirteeth ed. Elsevier, Edinburgh.

Figures 3.8, 26.2: Hinchliff, S.M., Montague, S.E., Watson, R., 1996. Physiology for Nursing Practice, second ed. Baillière Tindall, London.

Figure 4.6: Drake, R,L., Vogl, A.W., Mitchell, A.W.M., 2020. Gray's Anatomy for Students, fourth ed. Elsevier, Philadelphia.

Figure 4.8: Studd, J.W.W. (Ed.), 1989. Progress in Obstetrics and Gynaecology, vol. 7. Churchill Livingstone.

Figure 4.9: Blackburn, S.T., 2003. Maternal, Fetal and Neonatal Physiology: A Clinical Perspective. Saunders, Elsevier.

Figures 36.4: Johnson, M.H., 2013. Essential Reproduction, seventh ed. Wiley Blackwell, Oxford.

Figures 6.9, 14.1, 14.2, 24.7, 37.1, 37.2, 37.5, 37.9, 37.10, 37.13–37.16, 39.12, 40.5, 43.1, 50.2, 50.4, 50.5: Macdonald, S., Magill-Cuerden, J. (Eds.), 2011. Mayes' Midwifery: A Textbook for Midwives, fourteenth ed. Baillière Tindall, Edinburgh.

Figure 6.6: Reproduced courtesy of Durbin PLC; www.durbin.co.uk.

Figures 6.7, 6.8: Cowper, A., Young, C., 1989. Family Planning – Fundamentals for Health Professionals. Springer US. (Originally published by Chapman and Hall in 1989).

Figures 9.1, 9.11–9.13, 12.7, 12.9, 13.1, 13.2, 13.8, 48.1–48.3: Moore, K.L., 1989. Before We Are Born: Basic Embryology and Birth Defects, third ed. Saunders, Philadelphia.

Figures 9.3, 9.8, 9.9, 9.10, 9.14, 10.1, 10.3–10.6, 11.3–11.5, 12.1, 12.2, 12.3, 13.7, 51.1–51.5, 51.7, 51.8: Fitzgerald, M.J.T., Fitzgerald, M., 1994. Human Embryology. Baillière Tindall, London.

Figures 9.4, 9.6, 9.7: Chiras, D.D., 1991. Human Biology. West Publishing Co., Burlington, MA. www.jblearning.com. Reprinted with permission.

Figure 11.2: Moore, K.L., Persaud, T.V.N., Torchia, M.G., 2020. The Developing Human, eleventh ed. Elsevier.

Figure 12.4: Moore, K.L., Persaud, T.V.N., 1998. Before We Are Born: Basic Embryology and Birth Defects, fifth ed. Saunders, Philadelphia.

Figures 12.5, 12.10, 12.11: Macdonald, S, Magill-Cuerden, J. (Eds.), 2011. Mayes' Midwifery: A Textbook for Midwives, fourteenth ed. Elsevier, Edinburgh.

Figures 12.6, 49.1: Blackburn, S.T., Loper, D.I., 1992. Maternal, Fetal and Neonatal Physiology: A Clinical Perspective. Saunders, Elsevier.

Figures 12.8, 12.12, 12.13, 25.7, 25.8, 41.1, 55.1, 55.3B: Marshall, J.E., Raynor, M.D. (Eds.), 2020. Myles Textbook for Midwives, seventeenth ed. Elsevier, Edinburgh.

Figure 12.14: Wallenberg, H.C.S., 1977. The amniotic fluid, water and electrolyte homeostasis. J. Perinatal Medicine 5,193.

Figures 15.1, 15.2, 15.6, 51.9-51.12, 52.1, 53.1, 53.5, 53.6: Kelnar, C., Harvey, D., Simpson, C., 1995. The Sick Newborn Baby. Baillière Tindall, London.

Figure 15.4: Carlson, B.M., 2014. Human Embryology and Developmental Biology, fifth ed. Elsevier Mosby, Philadelphia.

Figure 16.2: Jones, S., Martin, R., Pilbeam, D., 1994. The Cambridge Encyclopaedia of Human Evolution. Cambridge University Press, Cambridge.

Figure 16.7: Lund, C.J., Donovan, J.C., 1967. Blood volume during pregnancy. Significance of plasma and red cell volumes. Am. J. Obstet. Gynecol. 98(3), 394–403.

Figure 16.8: Hytten, F., Chamberlain, G. (Eds.), 1991. Clinical Physiology in Obstetrics. Blackwell Science, Inc.

Figure 16.9: Rosso, P. 1990. Lipid metabolism. In: Nutrition and Metabolism in Pregnancy. Mother and Fetus, pp 47–58. Oxford University Press, Oxford.

Figures 17.1: Montague, S.E., Watson, R., Herbert, R., 2005. Physiology for Nursing Practice, third ed. Elsevier, Edinburgh.

Figure 17.12: Pipkin Broughton, F., 2013. Physiological changes in pregnancy. In: Symonds, I., Arulkumaran, S. (Eds.), Essential Obstetrics and Gynaecology, fifth ed. Churchill Livingstone, Elsevier, London.

Figure 18.8: de Swiet, M., 1991. The cardiovascular system. In: Hytten, F., Chamberlain, G. (Eds.), Clinical Physiology in Obstetrics, second ed. Blackwell Scientific, Oxford.

Figures 19.1, 19.3, 19.5, 19.6, 37.4, 38.2, 38.3, 38.6, 40.1, 40.2, 43.8, 43.10, 44.1, 44.3, 47.1, 47.4, 53.7, 53.8, 54.1 (courtesy of Liz Ellis), 55.1, 55.3A: Marshall, J.E., Raynor, M.D. (Eds.), 2014. Myles Textbook for Midwives, sixteenth ed. Elsevier, Edinburgh.

Figure 23.1: Public Health England, 2016.

Figure 25.2: Huszar, G., Roberts, J.M., 1982. Biology and pharmacology of the myometrium and labor: regulation at the cellular and molecular levels. Am. J. Obstet. Gynecol. 142,225–237.

Figures 26.5, 26.9, 26.11, 27.2, 27.3,: Fitzgerald, M.T.J., 1996. Neuroanatomy. Saunders, Philadelphia.

Figures 30.2, 30.3: Knight, M., Bunch, K., Patel, R., Shakespeare, J., Kotnis, R., Kenyon, S., Kurinczuk, J.J. (Eds.), 2022 on behalf of MBRRACE-UK. Saving Lives, Improving Mothers' Care Core Report – Lessons Learned to Inform Maternity Care from the UK and Ireland Confidential Enquiries into Maternal Deaths and Morbidity 2018–20. National Perinatal Epidemiology Unit, University of Oxford, Oxford.

Figure 36.1: Norwitz, E.R., Lye, S.J., 2009. Biology of parturition. In: Creasy, R.K., Resnik, R., Iams, J.D. et al (Eds.), Creasy & Resnik's Maternal-Fetal Medicine: Principles and Practice, sixth ed. Saunders Elsevier, Philadelphia.

Figures 36.2, 36.3: Kamel, R.M., 2010. The onset of human parturition. Arch. Gynecol. Obstet. 281, 975–982.

Figures 37.17, 37.25, 46.1–46.3: Gauge, S., 2011. CTG Made Easy, fourth ed. Elsevier, Edinburgh.

Figures 37.18–37.24: Courtesy of Sonicaid, Abingdon, Oxon.

Figures 39.9, 39.10: Johnson, R., Taylor, W., 2011. Skills for Midwifery Practice, third ed. Elsevier Churchill Livingstone, Edinburgh.

Figure 42.2: Clay, L.S., Criss, K., Jackson, U.C., 1993. External cephalic version. J Nurse-Midwif. 38(2), 72S-79S.

Figure 43.3: Beischer, N.A., Mackay, E.V., 1986. Obstetrics and the Newborn. Baillière Tindall, London.

Figures 44.4, 44.5: Fraser, D.M., Cooper, M.A., 2009. Myles' Textbook for Midwives, fifteenth ed. Elsevier, Edinburgh.

Figure 45.1: Winter, C., Crofts, J., Laxton, C., et al., 2018. PROMPT (PRactical Obstetric Multi-professional Training) Course Manual, third ed. RCOG Press, London.

Figure 45.5: McCance, K.L., Huether, S.E., 2014. Pathophysiology: the Biologic Basis for Disease in Adults and Children, seventh ed. Mosby.

Figure 46.5, 47.7, 47.8, 47.9: Reproduced with the kind permission of Resuscitation Council UK.

Figure 47.2: Arulkumaran, S., Robson M.S. (Eds.), 2020. Munro Kerr's Operative Obstetrics, thirteenth ed. Elsevier, Edinburgh.

Figure 47.10: Nutbeam, T., Daniels, R., on behalf of the UK Sepsis Trust. Available at https://sepsistrust.org/professional-resources/our-nice-clinical-tools/. Accessed 11th August 2023.

Figure 51.6: Reproduced from Société Française de Cardiologie, Jean-Yves Artigou, Jean-Jacques Monsuez et al., Cardiologie et maladies vasculaires, 1st edition. © 2020. Elsevier Masson SAS. All rights reserved.

Figures 52.2, 52.3: Bennett, V.R., Brown, L., 1993. Myles' Textbook for Midwives. Churchill Livingstone, Edinburgh.

Figure 53.9: McKee-Garrett, T., 2019. Delivery room emergencies due to birth injuries. Semin. Fetal. Neonatal. Med. 24(6), 101047.

Figure 54.2: Pollard, M., 2011. Evidence-Based Care for Breastfeeding Mothers: A Resource for Midwives and Allied Healthcare Professionals. Routledge, London. Reproduced with permission of Taylor & Francis Group through PLSclear.

Figures 54.3, 54.4: Lawrence, R.A., Lawrence, R.M., 2005. Breastfeeding: A Guide for the Medical Profession, eighth ed. Elsevier, Philadelphia.

Figures 55.2, 55.6: Off to a good start, 2020. Public Health Scotland.

Figure 57.3: Reprinted with permission from Elsevier (The Lancet), 2019, Volume 394, Issue 10216, Pages 2219-2236).

'Wisdom is not a product of schooling but of the lifelong attempt to acquire it.'
Albert Einstein

To all student midwives – the future of our profession and the safe care of everyone involved in childbearing and newborn care are in your hands. Remember – *knowledge has no end, it only has a beginning.*
To my bright and intelligent grandchildren, Lucy, John, Zoe, Fia and Sadie – continue to learn by remaining *curious and inquisitive.*

Preconception

Physiology in Childbearing aims to facilitate an understanding of physiology and other biosciences applied to childbearing ensuring practice is informed, effective and safe. In this first section, basic knowledge is provided to underpin the more complex content of the remaining chapters. Chapter 1 introduces basic biochemistry and is a reference base for those with no previous knowledge of the subject. Chapter 2 examines the nature of the cell and its interactions with other cells. Chapter 3 is about the structure and function of the gene, the advances made and its practical applications. Chapters 4 and 5 present the anatomy of the female and male reproductive systems. Chapters 6 and 7 examine the issues of fertility control and infertility. Chapter 8 is about preconception care and examines wide issues such as environment and lifestyle so that the practitioner can select appropriate advice both for the public and for prospective parents seeking specific information.

1

Basic Biochemistry

JEAN RANKIN

CHAPTER CONTENTS

Introduction

Chemistry is concerned with the scientific study of elements and how they react when combined or in contact with each other. **Organic chemistry** is based on **carbon compounds** whose molecules are central to the structure and function of all living organisms. This chapter provides fundamental information about the chemical nature of the human body and its metabolic processes.

Energy

The production, storage and release of **energy** are all essential to living cells, which need a constant supply of energy to function and reproduce. This energy is acquired from the breakdown of food molecules, particularly sugars. The two main types of energy are **kinetic** and **potential.** Kinetic energy is the energy of movement and includes **thermal** (heat) energy. Potential, or stored, energy is more relevant to biological systems. **Glucose** stores potential energy and is broken down continuously to perform work (Hall & Hall, 2020). **Adenosine triphosphate** is important in energy release (Chapter 23).

Catabolic reactions (breakdown of cell products) release large quantities of energy, whereas **anabolic reactions** (such as the manufacture of proteins) require energy. Cells must have a balance between energy-producing and energy-demanding processes (Hall & Hall, 2020). All forms of energy are interchangeable and can be expressed in the same unit of measurement. The **SI unit** (International System of Units) for measuring energy is the **joule** (J) or kilojoule (kJ): 1 kJ = 4.2 **calories**.

The Chemistry of Living Organisms

Atoms

Living organisms are made up of **chemical elements**. Over 100 elements are known, with each having their own symbol. These elements form a **periodic table** depending on the characteristics of each element. Elements consist of particles called **atoms,** which are the smallest indivisible part of an element that still retains its chemical and physical properties. Atoms are constructed from three subatomic particles: **neutrons, protons** and **electrons** (Crowe & Bradshaw, 2021). The **central nucleus** of the atom is made up of neutrons and protons of similar mass, and the very small electrons are arranged in **orbital shells** surrounding the nucleus. Fig. 1.1 illustrates this for three elements: hydrogen, oxygen and sodium.

The formation of particles within the atom is maintained by minute **electrical charges.** The neutrons of the nucleus carry no charge, protons carry a positive charge and electrons carry a negative charge. The number of protons is equal to the number of electrons so that most atoms are uncharged.

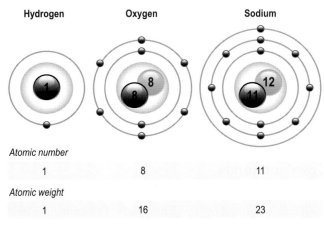

Hydrogen	Oxygen	Sodium

Atomic number

1	8	11

Atomic weight

1	16	23

• **Fig. 1.1** The atomic structure of hydrogen, oxygen and sodium.

TABLE 1.1	Values for the Most Common Elements that Make Up 99% of Living Matter				
Element	Atomic Number	Number of Protons	Number of Neutrons	Mass Number	Atomic Mass
Hydrogen	1	1	0	1	1
Carbon	6	6	6	12	12
Nitrogen	7	7	7	14	14
Oxygen	8	8	8	16	16
Sodium	11	11	12	23	23
Phosphorus	15	15	16	31	31
Calcium	20	20	20	40	40

Each element has a different number of electrons and protons which give it its **atomic number.** Neutrons are heavy and contribute to the **mass** of the element. The number of neutrons and protons together give the element its **mass number.** This determines the atomic mass (**atomic weight**) of an element. Table 1.1 gives values for the most common elements which make up 99% of living matter.

Radioactive Atoms

There can be variation in the number of neutrons present in the nucleus of an atom. This leads to **isotopes** of the element with different forms and different mass numbers. In some isotopes, the presence of extra neutrons causes them to be unstable. They will break down into a more stable configuration (**decay**) during which they radiate energy and atomic particles. This is **radioactivity,** and the isotopes are radioactive. Radioactive stable isotopes are successfully used in medical diagnosis and treatment (Cooper, 2019).

Molecules

Atoms are formed into **molecules** by **chemical bonds**. There are two types of chemical bonds: the strong, stable **covalent bond** (hard to disrupt) and the weaker, less stable **non-covalent bond.** The making and breaking of these bonds are associated with energy changes; the more stable the bond, the greater the thermal energy is needed to disrupt it. These bonds are formed by electrons that can be donated, received or shared by atoms. One bond is formed by one electron, but some atoms have more than one electron that is free to form bonds. The number of available electrons is called the **valency** of the atom. For example, hydrogen has a valency of 1 and carbon has a valency of 4.

Covalent Bonds

When atoms are joined together by sharing electrons, a molecule is formed by covalent bonds. The atoms are held closely together because electrons in their outermost shells move in orbitals that are shared by both atoms. Some atoms require more than one electron to form a bond with another

atom. Bonds may be single, such as in a molecule of hydrogen gas, or double, as in a molecule of oxygen gas. Complex molecules are formed by linkage of different atoms depending on their valency. Molecules can be represented as a molecular formula or structure (Table 1.2).

When more than two atoms form covalent bonds with a central atom, the bonds form a regular structure held in shape by electrical forces. The bonds are always orientated at right angles to each other. The rigid structures formed are necessary for the structure and function of large biological molecules such as proteins and nucleic acids. The molecular mass of a substance can be calculated by adding together the mass of each of its component atoms. Examples are shown in Table 1.3.

Non-covalent Bonds

Many of the bonds maintaining the complex structures of large molecules are not covalent. The three-dimensional structures are stabilized by much weaker forces called *non-covalent bonds.* Only small amounts of energy are released in their formation. There are four main types: the **ionic bond,** the **hydrogen bond,** the **van der Waals interaction** and the **hydrophobic bond.**

Ionic Bonds (Electrovalent Bonds)

In ionic bonds, electrons are not shared by atoms but are donated from one atom to another. The number of ionic bonds that can be formed is dictated by valency. Atoms of metallic elements such as sodium, calcium and iron lose electrons readily. The loss or gain of an electron is called **ionization** and the atom becomes an ion. Electrons carry a negative charge so the atoms that lose an electron become positively charged **cations** such as sodium; this is shown by the addition of a plus sign to the chemical symbol, Na^+. The atom that receives the electron becomes negatively charged and is known as an **anion**; this is shown by the addition of a minus sign, for example chlorine, Cl^-. An atom or molecule that has lost or gained an electron is said to be **polarized**.

Most ionic compounds are soluble in water because a large amount of energy is set free when ions bind to water molecules. Oppositely charged ions are shielded from each

TABLE 1.2   Examples of Molecules

Atomic Element	Valency	Compound	Molecular Formula	Molecular Structure	Bond Type
H	1	Hydrogen gas	H_2	H — H	Single
O	2	Oxygen gas	O_2	O = O	Double
O	2	Water	H_2O	H H $\backslash$ / O	Single
N	3	Nitrogen gas	N_2	N ≡ N	Triple
N	3	Ammonia	NH_3	H—N with H and H	Single
C	4	Carbon dioxide	CO_2	O = C = O	Double
C	4	Methane	CH_4	H H / C / H H	Single
P	5	Phosphoric acid	H_3PO_4	OH | HO—P=O | OH	Single and double

TABLE 1.3   The Molecular Masses of Common Chemical Compounds

Molecular Formula	Calculation	Molecular Mass
H_2	1 + 1	2
O_2	16 + 16	32
H_2O	1 + 1 + 16	18
N_2	14 + 14	28
NH_3	1 + 1 + 1 + 14	17
CO_2	12 + 16 + 16	44
C_2H_5OH (ethanol)	12 + 12 + 1 + 1 + 1 + 1 + 1 + 16 + 1	46
$C_6H_{12}O_6$ (glucose)	$(12 \times 6) + (1 \times 12) + (16 \times 6)$	180

other by the water and do not usually recombine. Molecules with opposite polar bonds (**dipoles**) easily form hydrogen bonds so they attract water molecules. These polar molecules are called **hydrophilic** (water-loving) molecules. Cations are attracted to anions, giving rise to compounds called **salts.** For example, when sodium donates an electron to chlorine, a well-known salt—**sodium chloride**—is formed:

$$Na^+ + CL^- \rightarrow NaCl$$

In this form, the salt is crystalline and consists of a rigid lattice structure, but if dissolved in water, the salt dissociates into free ions which disperse in the solution. The role of **fluids, solutes, acids, bases** and **hydrogen ion concentration** in systemic function is discussed in Chapter 20.

Hydrogen Bonding

Besides covalent and ionic bonds, a weak bond can occur between molecules. Normally a hydrogen atom forms a covalent bond with only one other atom. However, molecules containing hydrogen atoms can also form an additional bond. This occurs because they are attracted to each other by a weak **electropositive** charge left on the hydrogen atom when it is drawn to an **electronegative** atom with which it is associating. Hydrogen is the **donor atom,** and the electronegative atom is the **acceptor atom**.

A good example is the association of oxygen and hydrogen to form water. Although the water molecule is electronically neutral, the positive and negative charges are not distributed uniformly. This ability of hydrogen to create weak bonds is essential for the formation of **helical structures,** as in the double helix of **deoxyribonucleic acid** (DNA) (see Chapter 3).

The van der Waals Interaction

When two atoms closely approach each other, an attractive force called a **van der Waals interaction** (named after a Dutch physicist) is produced. Transient dipoles are created, and that of one atom disturbs the electrons of the other atom, creating a dipole. There is weak attraction between the two dipoles. The bond formed is weaker than a hydrogen bond (Abali et al., 2021).

Both polar and non-polar molecules form this type of bond. If the van der Waals attraction between the two atoms balances the repulsion between their electron clouds, the atoms stay in van der Waals contact. Distance is essential in forming this contact, and each type of atom has a van der Waals radius at which it is in van der Waals contact with other atoms. These radii are very important in biological systems, especially when the precise shapes of two large molecules complement each other, giving many van der Waals contacts. Examples are **antigen–antibody interactions** (Chapter 29) and bonds between **enzymes** and their **substrates** (Chapter 23).

Hydrophobic Interactions

Non-polar molecules contain neither ions nor dipolar bonds. They are insoluble in water and are hydrophobic. The covalent bonds between two carbon atoms or between carbon and hydrogen atoms are the most common non-polar bonds in biological systems. That is why the **hydrocarbons** (Abali et al., 2021) found in cell membranes are almost insoluble in water. A hydrophobic interaction is not a separate type of bonding force. It results from the energy needed to insert a non-polar molecule into water. The non-polar molecule cannot form hydrogen bonds and distorts the structure of water to make a cage around it. Non-polar molecules bind together comfortably using van der Waals interactions.

Chemical Equilibrium

Local environmental conditions such as concentration, temperature and pressure will affect the rate at which a chemical reaction occurs and the extent to which it proceeds. When two **reactants** come together, their individual concentrations determine the formation of a product. As the concentrations decrease, so does the reaction rate. Some of the products will begin to reverse the process, re-forming the reactants.

Eventually the forward and reverse reactions become equal. At this point a chemical mixture is said to be in dynamic **chemical equilibrium**. The **equilibrium constant** (K) defines the ratio of the concentrations of reactants at equilibrium. The presence of a **catalyst** (a substance that aids or speeds up a chemical reaction without being changed itself) may facilitate any reaction.

Composition of the Human Body

About two-thirds of the human body is made up of water. The other third is composed of six main elements, of which carbon is the most important because it readily combines with other carbon atoms to form larger molecules and traces of other elements. Table 1.4 lists the common elements that make up the basic substances of the human body. The

TABLE 1.4	Elements Found in the Human Body	
Element	**Atomic Symbol**	**Approximate Weight (%)**
Oxygen	O	65
Carbon	C	18
Hydrogen	H	10
Nitrogen	N	3
Calcium	Ca	2
Phosphorus	P	1
		TOTAL = 99%
Potassium	K	0.35
Sulphur	S	0.25
Sodium	Na	0.15
Chlorine	Cl	0.15
		TOTAL = 0.9%
Magnesium	Mg	Trace
Iron	Fe	Trace
Zinc	Zn	Trace
Copper	Cu	Trace
Iodine	I	Trace
Manganese	Mn	Trace
Chromium	Cr	Trace
Molybdenum	Mo	Trace
Cobalt	Co	Trace
Selenium	Se	Trace
		TOTAL = 0.1%

chemical elements come together in various combinations to form thousands of components of living tissue. Knowledge of **biochemistry** is essential to the understanding of **physiological processes** such as nutrition, respiration and metabolism. The basic substances such as **carbohydrates** (sugars), **lipids** (fats and oils) and **proteins** are discussed in appropriate chapters.

Proteins are organized in **polymers** and are formed from long chains of small molecules called **monomers**. Other examples of polymers are plant substances such as starch and cellulose. Other essential substances are nucleic acids such as DNA.

Chemical Reactions in the Body

Non-covalent bonds are not as stable as covalent bonds, a feature that is essential to the working of the body. Non-covalent bonds allow complex biological compounds to change during chemical reactions without the need for large amounts of energy. Most chemical reactions in the

TABLE 1.5	Types of Chemical Reactions that Occur During Metabolism	
Type	**Reaction**	**Typical Processes**
Condensation	Combining molecules with the elimination of water	Formation of glycoside, ester and peptide bonds
Hydrolysis	Splitting a molecule with the addition of water	Digestion of carbohydrates, triglycerides and proteins
Dehydration	Removal of water from a molecule	Carbohydrate and fatty acid metabolism
Hydration	Incorporation of water into a molecule	Carbohydrate and fatty acid metabolism
Oxidation	Removal of hydrogen (or electrons)	Conversion of alcohols to aldehydes
Reduction	Addition of hydrogen (or electrons)	Biosynthesis of fatty acids
Carboxylation	Incorporation of carbon dioxide	Carbohydrate synthesis
Decarboxylation	Elimination of carbon dioxide	Fermentation, amine formation
Amination	Incorporation of amino group ($-NH_3$)	Amino acid biosynthesis
Deamination	Elimination of ammonia	Amino acid degradation
Methylation	Incorporation of methyl group ($-CH_3$)	Synthesis of DNA and adrenaline
Demethylation	Removal of methyl group	Amino acid degradation

body require the use of **enzymes** and their associated **cofactors** to act as catalysts. The types of chemical reactions found during metabolic processes are summarized in Table 1.5.

Main Points

- Atoms form compounds by using chemical bonds. There are two kinds: strong, stable covalent bonds and weaker, less stable, non-covalent bonds. Greater thermal energy is required to disrupt stable bonds.
- Covalent bonds are formed by electrons donated, received or shared by atoms. A molecule is formed when two or more atoms share electrons.
- Ionic bonds are also involved in forming compounds. In these bonds, electrons are donated from one atom to another. The loss or gain of an electron is called *ionization,* and the atom becomes an ion.

- Atoms losing an electron become positively charged cations. The atom receiving an electron becomes a negatively charged anion. Cations are attracted to anions, producing salts.
- Weak hydrogen bonds are essential for the formation of helical structures such as DNA.
- When two atoms closely approach each other, a van der Waals interaction is produced and transient dipoles are created.
- The human body is made up of two-thirds water and one-third of main elements—carbon, oxygen, hydrogen, nitrogen, phosphorus and calcium—and traces of other elements.

Grant, A., Waugh, A., 2018. Ross & Wilson Anatomy and Physiology in Health and Illness, thirteenth ed. Elsevier, London.

Chapter 2 provides an excellent summary of physiological chemistry underpinning processes in the human body.

References

Abali, E.E., Cline, S.D., Viselli, S.M., Franklin, D.S., 2021. Biochemistry, eighth ed. Wolters Kluwer Health, Philadelphia.

Cooper, G.M., 2019. The Cell: A Molecular Approach, eighth ed. International Sinauer, Oxford University Press, Oxford.

Crowe, J., Bradshaw, T., 2021. Chemistry for Biosciences: The Essential Concepts, fourth ed. Open University Press, Oxford.

Hall, J.E., Hall, M.E., 2020. Guyton and Hall Textbook of Medical Physiology, fourteenth ed. Elsevier, Philadelphia.

Annotated recommended reading

Reece, J.B., Urry, L.A., Cain, M.L., et al., 2014. Campbell Biology, Introduction to Chemistry for Biology Students, tenth ed. Benjamin Cummings, San Francisco.

This is a comprehensive textbook that looks at each biochemical structure in more depth for the interested reader. There is a related chapter on cell structure with a paragraph on each organelle, proteins, DNA, enzymes and antibodies and on all the metabolic processes.

2

The Cell – Its Structures and Function

JEAN RANKIN

CHAPTER CONTENTS

This chapter provides a comprehensive introduction into the structure and function of the range of cells in the human body. This includes key cell components and organelles, shape, size, organization and cell division and replication.

Physical Characteristics of Human Cells

Living species are made up of a diverse range of **cells** which are small, membrane-bound units filled with a concentrated aqueous solution of carefully balanced chemicals and **organelles** (Fig. 2.1). Although they share a common origin, cells show considerable morphological diversity which has evolved to support the functional adaptation and survival of a specific organism. **Eukaryotic cells** are distinguished from **prokaryotic cells** by their membrane-bound nucleus and organelles. Cell survival depends on their specific intracellular biochemistry which supports their **metabolism** and **homeostasis.** All nucleated mature cells can create copies of themselves by replication and division, which ensures the survival of their **genetic lineage**. The morphological uniqueness and specialized functions are governed by complex **genetic activity**. Over 200 different cell types in the human body are assembled into tissue types such as **epithelia, connective tissue, muscle,** conducting **neural tissue,** non-conducting **neuroglia** and **osteocytes.** The function of different cell types is preserved through communication and co-ordination.

A typical human (mammalian) cell averages 10 μm in diameter (Coad, Pedley & Dunstall, 2019). Light and electron microscopy can reveal structural details as small as a few nanometres. This enables cell biologists to identify complex cellular ultrastructures necessary for microstructural and functional integrity. Cells and their microstructural components are sustained, repaired or replaced, when required, by genetic expression and selective assimilation of matter from the **extracellular compartment** (Alberts et al., 2019).

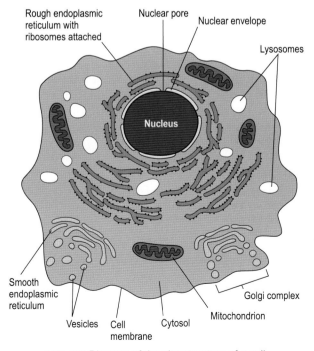

• **Fig. 2.1** Diagram of the ultrastructure of a cell.

Cell Size and Shape

During the stages of cell development, cells differentiate, modify their structure and activities and appropriately aggregate to form specific tissues, organs and systems. Fundamental to these processes are genetic and biochemical controls and communication. Knowledge of the size and appearance of different cells indicates how their morphological and functional features contribute to the whole body (see Box 2.1).

The cell's external appearance depends on its functions, interactions with other cells, external environment and the internal structures masterminding cell activities. Cellular dimensions and metabolic activities are also partly determined by the rate of **substrate diffusion** across highly selective **plasma membranes** (Kierszenbaum, 2021). The plasma membrane permits rapid diffusion of substrates in both directions over short distances of up to 50 μm. As cells increase in size, their mass outstrips their surface area, changing their shape to an irregular or elongated structure (as seen in many neurons). This larger size sustains efficient substrate transport and diffusion, particularly as many physiological processes depend on cellular surface area such as diffusion of gases, ions and nutrient transport.

An increase in cell mass can be problematic. Nuclear control of the **cytoplasm** and plasma membrane becomes more difficult the farther the cell periphery is from the nucleus. This can be overcome with increasing the surface area by either folding the plasma membrane and forming **microvilli,** or other surface protrusions, or flattening the entire body of the cell. Alternatively, nuclear control in larger cells can be enhanced by the presence of multiple nuclei.

Cytoskeleton and Cell Motility

The **cytoskeleton** is a complex network of specialized proteins, organized into filaments and microtubules, extending throughout the cytoplasm. This highly dynamic structure reorganizes continuously as the cell changes shape, divides and responds to its environment. It is responsible for cellular movement such as cell crawling, the beating of cilia, muscle contraction, migration of **phagocytic leucocytes** from blood to a site of tissue injury, or in response to pathogens and changes in cell shape in the developing embryo. The cytoskeleton also provides the machinery for intracellular movement, such as the transport of organelles within the cytoplasm (Alberts et al., 2019).

Motility is also observed in the tip(s) of developing dendrites and axons as they grow in response to local conditions and migrate to their synaptic targets. **Fibroblasts,** during early embryonic development, tissue repair and remodelling, provide a good example of cell migration when they secrete **collagen** which is essential for the development of the extracellular matrix. As the fibroblasts interact with collagen by means of adhesion plaques, they exert traction on the cell matrix. The diverse activities of the cytoskeleton depend on three types of protein filaments: actin filaments, microtubules and the intermediate filaments.

All cells display varying degrees of **motility.** This augments their shape and position and facilitates the best conditions for cellular homeostasis by moving the cytoplasm, specific organelles or vesicles from one part of the cell to another. Whilst the exact molecular mechanisms involved in cell motility are unknown, it is unlikely that a single organelle or cytoskeletal component can be responsible for such complex processes (Alberts et al., 2019). The following interrelated processes are thought to be essential:

1. Cell motility is dependent on adenosine triphosphate (ATP).
2. Cells define their own motility.
3. Cells define their leading edge, which the remainder of the cells crawl towards using traction and adhesions as points for anchorage.
4. Microtubules, intermediate and actin filaments unify the cytoskeleton, forming a mechanical structure that resists external forces on the migrating cells.

Biochemical and micro-anatomical environments modulate the speed and direction of cell motility.

Epithelial Cells

Epithelial cells are derived from the three embryonic germ layers: the **ectoderm,** the **endoderm** and the **mesoderm** (Alberts et al., 2019):

- Ectoderm contributes to the development of epithelia. It is the basis for the epidermis, breast glandular tissue, cornea and the junctional zones of the buccal cavity and anal canal.
- Endoderm forms the epithelial lining of the alimentary canal and its glands, most of the respiratory tract and the distal tract of the urogenital tract.
- Mesoderm gives rise to the epithelium-like cells lining internal cavities such as the pericardium, pleural and peritoneal cavities, and the lining of blood vessels and lymph vessels.

In general, epithelial cells form sheets which line the inner and outer body surfaces and provide a covering for the body and its internal organs. Epithelial cells serve as selective barriers, facilitating or preventing the transfer of substrates across the surfaces which they cover. Some epithelia, such as the skin, protect underlying tissue from dehydration and chemical or mechanical injury. Endocrine and exocrine

---

• BOX 2.1 Examples of Size and Appearance of Cells

Small Cells

- Resting **lymphocytes** (average diameter 6 μm).
- **Erythrocytes** (between 7.5 and 9.0 μm in diameter).
- **Columnar epithelial cells** (20 μm tall and 10 μm wide).

Larger Cells

- Bone marrow **megakaryocytes** (average diameter 200 μm).
- Mature **ova** (diameter ≥80 μm).
  The oocyte, the largest human cell, can be seen with the naked eye. The follicular cells surrounding the oocyte have a more typical human cell size. The sperm cell is one of the smallest human cells (Coad, Pedley & Dunstall, 2019).

glands are formed from epithelial tissue. Other epithelia act as sensory surfaces, a function best illustrated by neural tissue.

Classification of Epithelia

The polygonal, diverse shape of epithelial cells is partly determined by their cytoplasmic contents and partly by pressure and the functional demands of the surrounding tissue (Kierszenbaum, 2021). The conventional classification of the epithelia takes into consideration their structural and functional characteristics (Table 2.1).

Complex Structures Derived from the Epithelium

Complex organ structures derived from epithelia retain familiar cellular complex characteristics; for instance, the capacity of the liver or the placenta to absorb, secrete and transport a diversity of substrates. Similarly, the diverse forms of neural tissue are functional modifications of epithelia. Most neural tissue, differentiated into conducting and non-conducting cells, provides a complex network for processing and managing information by signal transduction.

Cellular Organization

The cell is the fundamental unit of structure and function of all living organisms. A typical cell includes a single nucleus, cytoplasm and a cellular boundary known as the **plasma membrane,** the most common cell feature (Alberts et al., 2019). The different substances making up the cell are collectively known as **cytoplasm** or **protoplasm.** Predominantly, these are composed of water, electrolytes, proteins, lipids and carbohydrates, all of which play crucial roles in shaping the cell and its organelles. These include the cell membrane, the nuclear membrane, the endoplasmic reticulum, Golgi apparatus, mitochondria, lysosomes and centrioles. Table 2.2 summarizes these cell components, structure and function.

The Plasma Membrane

An appropriate plasma membrane is crucial to the survival and function of each cell. It encloses the cellular contents,

TABLE 2.1 Classification of Epithelium

Cell	Structure	Functional Characteristics
Simple epithelium	Single layers of cells on basal lamina (filamentous proteins and proteoglycans). Subdivided by shape—columnar, cuboidal, pseudostratified or squamous. Small cells—low volume, few organelles, low metabolic activity. Highly metabolic cells, secretory cells—tall, cuboidal or columnar with abundant mitochondria and endoplasmic reticulum.	Capable of special functions. Form cilia, microvilli, secretory vacuoles or sensory features.
Stratified squamous epithelium	Superficial cells—thin, fattened, interlocking, polygonal cells. Constantly replaced by regenerating basal layers.	Thinness facilitates diffusion of gases/water. Role in active transport (many endocytic vesicles). Critical positions—lining of the lung alveoli, the glomeruli and the thin segments of the loop of Henle.
Cuboidal and columnar epithelium	Cylindrical cells in regular rows. Free surfaces have microvilli. Columnar cells in gall bladder have a brush border.	Absorption role in small intestine (water and nutrients).
	Ciliated columnar epithelium (e.g., respiratory tract and lining fallopian tubes).	Essential brush-border surface for concentration and storage of bile.
	Large cuboidal cells in convoluted segments of nephrons (brush borders).	Facilitate selective reabsorption in nephron.
Transitional epithelium	Characteristic feature—thickness, formed by arrangement of 4–6 cells held together by desmosomes (filamentous structures). Cells flatten when stretched (no change in position). Most cells attached to basal lamina form a basal structure (appear cuboidal and uninucleate when relaxed). At surface, cells progressively fuse to become larger (sometimes binucleate, polyploid cells with plasma membrane with glycoprotein particles).	Two roles: Facilitates expansion and contraction, stretching without losing structural integrity. Provides impermeable lining for organs with toxic metabolic end-products (e.g., urea and uric acid and high concentration of salts). Forms an impermeable lining in genitourinary tract.

TABLE 2.2 Cell Components, Structure and Function

Component	Structure	Function
Cell (plasma) membrane (crucial to cell survival)	Composed of phospholipid bilayer with various protein structures (e.g., hormone receptors, ion channels and antigen markers; see Box 2.2).	Acts as a differential permeable membrane between cell and immediate environment.
Nucleus (ultimate cell control centre)	Largest organelle (2–10 μm). Nucleus bound by membrane. Outer nuclear membrane continuous with rough endothelial reticulum (RER). Nucleus—several thousand pores (openings) for movement of substances. Nuclei contain large quantities of DNA (thread-like structures, chromatin). Other structures include gel-like nucleoplasm and the nucleoli; the latter—site of ribosomal ribonucleic acid (rRNA) synthesis.	Holds genetic blueprint for cell nuclear genome—determines characteristics of proteins and enzymes in cytoplasm and controls cytoplasmic activities and cellular reproduction. Membrane porosity permits movement of messenger RNA into cytoplasm and entry of enzymes and histones into nucleus during DNA replication.
Endoplasmic reticulum (ER)	Network of specialized membranous structures, continuous with the nuclear membrane—makes up 50% of cell volume. Two distinct membrane types: rough (granular) and smooth (agranular) ER (see Box 2.3).	Functionally both the RER and the smooth endothelial reticulum (SER) are highly dynamic, permitting bidirectional traffic of small substrate-filled vesicles to and from the Golgi apparatus and performing several functions. RER—biosynthesis of protein and lipid in reconstruction of all organelles. SER—involved in lipid/steroid synthesis and regulation of intracellular Ca^{2+} levels.
Mitochondria	In cytoplasm of mature cells. Distinctive structure reflects the complex nature of their function. Organelles (average length 1–2 μm; width 0.1–0.5 μm) are spherical rod-like structures surrounded by a folded inner membrane and a smooth outer membrane (see Box 2.4).	Chemical processes in the formation of adenosine triphosphate (ATP). The cristae—site of oxidative phosphorylation and electron transfer chain of aerobic respiration (Fig. 2.4; Box 2.4). Krebs cycle (or tricarboxylic acid cycle) and the oxidation of fatty acids take place within matrix.
Golgi apparatus	A mass of membrane-bound sacs situated close to the nucleus and close to the centrosomes. Golgi apparatus consists of four or more stacked thin, flat vesicles consisting of an entry point (or *cis* face) and an exit (or *trans* face) (Fig. 2.4).	Modifies proteins from RER and sorts them into secretory vesicles.
Lysosomes	Cell-specific vesicular organelles dispersed throughout the cytoplasm (average 250–750 nm). Spherical or oval organelles enclosed by a single membrane. Contain 40 types of hydrolytic enzymes, synthesized in ER, transported through the Golgi apparatus to lysosomes for storage of granules until needed (Alberts et al., 2019).	Principal sites for intracellular digestion of materials from extracellular environment. Digestive/hydrolytic enzymes act as 'cellular stomach' degrading (i.e., hydrolysing) unwanted intracellular substances (e.g., proteins to amino acid; glycogen to glucose). Removes damaged structures and foreign particles (e.g., bacteria).
Peroxisomes	Formed by budding off from SER (averages 0.15–0.5 μm). All contain oxidases capable of catalysing many reactions, including the oxidation of long-chain saturated fatty acids.	Destroy reactive oxygen species and protect cell. Oxidizes numerous toxic substances. Involved in cholesterol metabolism, gluconeogenesis within hepatocytes.
Cytoskeleton	Filamentous network.	Involved in maintaining cell shape and motility.

defines cellular boundaries and maintains the essential biochemical differences between the cytosol and the extracellular environment. Plasma membranes are dynamic structures capable of considerable adaptation. This is due to the ability of most of their molecules to move about within the plane of the plasma membranes (Box 2.2).

Cytoplasm and its Organelles

Every living cell uses complex communication pathways to sustain its specific microstructures and functional competence. **Eukaryotic cells** (nucleated) use a diverse range of internal processes supported by elaborate internal membrane machinery and complex arrangements of cell-specific organelles within the cytoplasm.

Cytoplasm accounts for almost half of the cell volume. Due to its high protein content (20% by weight), cytoplasm appears more gel-like than an aqueous solution. This creates an environment that suspends small molecular structures, large particles and organelles. Organic and inorganic ions dissolve in this gel-like cytoplasm, where fat globules, glycogen granules, ribosomes and secretory granules are also dispersed. The most

The plasma membrane encloses cellular contents, defines cellular boundaries and maintains essential biochemical differences between the cytosol and the extracellular environment. It is a dynamic structure capable of considerable adaptation due to the ability of most molecules to move about within the plane of the membrane.

The Lipid Bilayer

The plasma membrane (Fig. 2.2) consists of a complex lipid bilayer interspersed by a range of protein molecules. The lipid bilayer is composed almost entirely of fatty acids, made up of phospholipids and cholesterol (Alberts et al., 2019). Phospholipids, small molecules from fatty acids and glycerol, have a head (electrically charged) and hydrophilic (meaning *water-loving*) and a hydrophobic (meaning *water-hating*) tail with no charge (Waugh & Grant, 2018).

The phospholipid bilayer (5–7 nm thick) is arranged like a sandwich (Fig. 2.2) with the hydrophilic heads aligned on the outer surfaces of the membrane and the hydrophobic tails forming a central water-repelling layer (Waugh & Grant, 2018). This lipid bilayer is highly permeable to lipid-soluble substances, such as hormones, corticosteroids, alcohol, oxygen and carbon dioxide but is relatively impermeable to most water-soluble molecules such as inorganic ions and glucose.

Plasma membrane fluidity is important to survival of cellular infrastructure and capacity of the membrane to sustain selective transport processes and enzyme activities. However, these complex membrane functions are dependent on the presence within the lipid bilayer of cholesterol, glycolipids and glycoproteins. Cholesterol molecules stabilize the lipid bilayer rendering it less deformable, reducing its permeability to small water-soluble molecules and preventing the hydrocarbon chains from crystallizing and damaging plasma membrane functional integrity. Glycolipids and glycoproteins act as receptors for extracellular biochemical products (Alberts et al., 2019).

The Membrane Proteins

Proteins are suspended within or are found on the surface of the membrane (averages 50% of its total membrane mass). Because protein molecules are larger than lipid molecules, there are fewer of them than lipid molecules in most plasma membranes. They perform several functions, including:

- Acting as receptors (specific recognition sites) for hormones and other chemical messengers.
- Transmembrane proteins form channels filled with water. This allows the passage of substances (e.g., electrolytes and non-lipid-soluble molecules).
- Some are involved in pumps that transport substances across the membrane.
- Branched carbohydrate molecules attached to the outside of some membrane protein molecules give the cell its immunological identity.
- Some are enzymes.

The quantities and types of plasma membrane proteins vary in keeping with cellular functions (Alberts et al., 2019). For instance, the neural **myelin membrane** serves mainly as an electrical insulation for nerve cell axons; consequently, less than 25% of the membrane mass consists of protein. Conversely, **mitochondrial membranes** involved in energy transduction consist of approximately 75% protein.

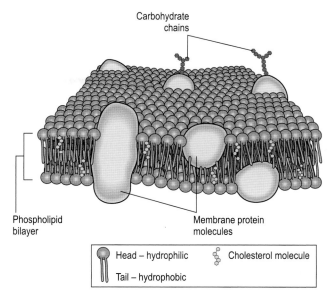

Carbohydrate chains

Phospholipid bilayer

Membrane protein molecules

Head – hydrophilic   Cholesterol molecule

Tail – hydrophobic

• **Fig. 2.2** Diagram of the fluid mosaic model of cell membrane structure

important organelles contained within the cytoplasm are the endoplasmic reticulum (Box 2.3), the Golgi apparatus, mitochondria (Box 2.4), lysosomes and peroxisomes (Table 2.2).

Concept of Selective Permeability

Selective permeability of the plasma membrane facilitates free passage of some gases such as oxygen and water but restricts the movement of larger ions such as sodium, potassium, calcium, chloride and bicarbonate to their specific protein channels. These channels open or close to regulate transmembrane ion traffic, and most integral proteins form **pores** through which the water-soluble substances **diffuse** passively (such as ions). The selective passage of many other substances of larger molecular weight, such as glucose and amino acids, is also limited to protein channels, most of which are ion- or substrate-specific. This contrasts with lipid-soluble substances, such as steroid hormones, which diffuse unhindered through the lipid portion of the plasma membranes.

Cells also take up larger molecules and transport them into other cellular regions by **endocytosis.** This involves the invagination of small segments of plasma membrane to create **vacuoles** or **endocytic vesicles.** In addition, many cells ingest extracellular fluid in large endocytic structures named **macropinosomes**. By contrast, the extrusion of organic molecules such as **thyroxine** and **acetylcholine** is achieved by **exocytic vesicles** which fuse with plasma membrane, releasing their content to the cell's exterior.

Plasma membrane excitability and ion transport processes for the movement of substances across the plasma membrane are detailed in Box 2.5.

The Nucleolus (Nucleoli)

The nucleolus is the most prominent nuclear subdomain. Most mammalian nuclei have 1–5 nucleoli. These appear as

• BOX 2.3 Endoplasmic Reticulum (ER)

These specialized reticular membranes form a barrier between the cytosol and the reticular lumen, mediating the selective transport of molecules between the relevant intracellular compartments (Fig. 2.3).

One difference between **rough ER** (RER) and **smooth ER** (SER) is the association of ribosomes on the cytoplasmic surface of the RER. In addition, RER interacts with the nuclear lamina and chromatin. By contrast, the SER is composed of more tubular elements, is ribosome-free and is commonly located at some distance from the nucleus (Konieczny, Roterman-Konieczna & Spolnik, 2014).

RER has a central role in biosynthesis of protein and lipid used in the reconstruction of all organelles, including the Golgi apparatus and nuclear and plasma membranes. The synthesis of membrane lipids, such as steroids, phospholipids and triglycerides, occurs within both the RER and SER.

SER shows cell-specific functions. For example, its roles in hepatocytes are dedicated to enzyme pathways, including the cytochrome P-450 enzymes involved in drug metabolism, whilst it facilitates steroid synthesis in endocrine cells. By contrast, it acts as a reservoir for calcium in skeletal and cardiac muscle cells (where it is known as the *sarcoplasmic reticulum*), controlling calcium release into the cytoplasm to support muscle contraction and taking it up again, thus facilitating muscle relaxation.

The cytoplasm holds at least two separate groups of **ribosomes** which play critical roles in protein synthesis for that specific cell.

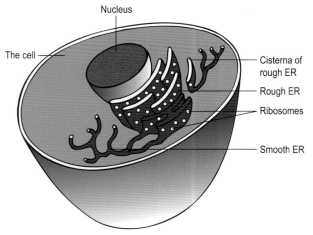

• **Fig. 2.3** **The endoplasmic reticulum (ER).** The rough ER and smooth ER with their connections are illustrated.

Labels: Nucleus; The cell; Cisterna of rough ER; Rough ER; Ribosomes; Smooth ER

dense structures visible within the nucleus during the cell's interphase, although their size, shape and number depend on the activity relative to the cell cycle. Unlike most organelles, nucleoli do not appear to have a limiting membrane. They have four distinct regions:

1. A fibrillar centre containing DNA that is not being transcribed.
2. A dense fibrillar core containing RNA in a process of transcription.
3. A granular region where the maturing ribosomal particles are assembled.

• BOX 2.4 Mitochondria

Mitochondria are found in the cytoplasm of most mature cells. They have their own double-stranded circular DNA replicating before mitochondrial division. The human mitochondrial genome consists of 16,569 nucleotide pairs (see Chapter 3) which encode only 13 mitochondrial membrane proteins, two ribosomal RNAs and just enough transfer RNA (tRNA) to translate these genes. Mitochondria usually contain multiple copies of their genome, a possible factor facilitating rapid growth and division that typically occur in highly metabolically active cells. Despite the mitochondrial numbers in each cell, their DNA makes up less than 1% of the total cellular DNA (Konieczny, Roterman-Konieczna & Spolnik, 2014).

The mitochondrion has an outer and an inner membrane, creating two compartments. The outer membrane contains a major integral protein, **porin,** forming membrane channels to facilitate diffusion of substrates (<50,000 D), including metabolites required for **adenosine triphosphate** (ATP) synthesis (Konieczny, Roterman-Konieczna & Spolnik, 2014). The highly impermeable inner membrane is arranged into folds known as **cristae,** which considerably increase the surface area, an important feature of mitochondria as the power centres of the cell (see Fig. 2.4). The inner membrane consists of 75% protein, which may be significant in supporting the mitochondrial respiratory chain, ATP synthesis and the transport of oxidative phosphorylation substrates in and out of the mitochondria. Because mitochondria provide cells with energy by reducing oxygen and converting **adenosine diphosphate** (ADP) and phosphate to ATP (Chapter 23), in their absence or malfunction, cells would be unable to extract energy from nutrients and oxygen, and cellular functions would cease.

The innermost cavity of the mitochondria is filled with a matrix containing large quantities of dissolved enzymes, which are necessary for extraction of energy from nutrients. These enzymes function in association with oxidative enzymes, providing the mechanism for oxidation of nutrients, liberation of energy and formation of carbon dioxide and water. Importantly, the liberated energy is used to synthesize high-energy ATP, which is transported out of the mitochondria into the cytoplasm to support cellular activities. Increased cellular ATP requirements may be responsible for inducing mitochondrial self-replication. Given that a mitochondrion usually contains multiple copies of its own genome, its efficient replication before division is an important mechanism cells use to ensure that their metabolic and energy demands are met. As the mitochondrial genome mutates at a rate 10-fold greater than nuclear DNA does (Nussbaum et al., 2015), mitochondrial dysfunction may result in human disorders such as epilepsy, neuropathy and myopathy. Many of these disorders can be attributed to mutations in genes for mitochondrial protein encoded by both mitochondrial and nuclear DNA.

4. A nuclear matrix which may participate in the organization of the nucleolus.

Typically, the nucleoli usually contain large quantities of RNA and proteins like those found in the ribosomes. The proteins appear to be fundamental to the production and assembly of ribosomes as complex macromolecular structures. The functions of many other nucleolar proteins are unknown and yet to be discovered, although it is now suggested that nucleoli may be involved in other biological processes.

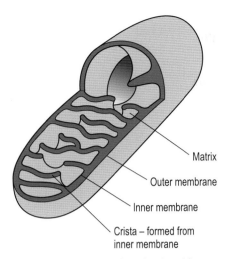

Matrix

Outer membrane

Inner membrane

Crista – formed from
inner membrane

• **Fig. 2.4** Diagram of a mitochondrion.

Cell Division

Controlled cell division is vital to human reproduction, tissue growth and repair, efficient functioning of the immune defence mechanisms and countless other processes. The cycle of cell division is one of the most fundamental processes by which multicellular species replace ageing cells or those lost during programmed cell death (**apoptosis**). To facilitate this, the body must be capable of programmed synthesis and maturation of millions of new cells simply to maintain its status quo. In cases of ill health, trauma or surgery, loss and corresponding replacement of new cells are fundamental to successful healing and recovery. Conversely, when natural cell division is halted or compromised, then the individual may suffer the consequences of rapid and extensive irreparable cell damage and destruction. One key example is the exposure to a large dose of ionizing radiation.

Although details of the cell cycle may vary, certain behavioural requirements of all cells are universal. In the first instance, cells have to co-ordinate various events in the cycle. For example, they must avoid entering mitosis or meiosis until such time as the chromosomes have been replicated. Failure to comply with this requirement can result in cells lacking a particular chromosome, an aberration which may give rise to cancer at a later stage (Turnpenny & Ellard, 2017).

Nucleotide Structure of DNA

All cell nuclei, except for mature erythrocytes, contain large amounts of **DNA**. Within its structure, DNA holds the genetic information required for directing all aspects of embryogenesis, growth, development, metabolism, reproduction and apoptosis. The term '**double helix**' aptly describes the appearance of double-stranded DNA that winds around itself like a twisted ladder (Fig. 2.7). Each strand of DNA is made up of repeating-unit nucleotides referred to as building blocks. The DNA nucleotides are molecules containing three components:

1) Phosphoric acid.
2) *Deoxyribose* (a pentose sugar with five carbon atoms).
3) Four nitrogenous bases: two purines – adenine (A) and guanine (G), and two pyrimidines – cytosine (C) and thymine (T).

Different genes have different sequences of these four nucleotides to code for different biological functions. The nucleotides attach to each other (A with T, and G with C) to form chemical bonds called base pairs, which connect the two DNA strands. Given that there are four types of nucleotides, the number of possible sequences in a DNA strand is enormous.

The double-helix shape allows for DNA replication and protein synthesis to occur by unwinding of the twisted strands. In these processes, the twisted DNA unwinds and opens to allow a copy of the DNA to be made. In DNA replication, the double helix unwinds, and each separated strand is used to synthesize a new strand (further detailed in Chapter 3).

Mitosis and the Cell Cycle

Cells with nuclei have 46 chromosomes and divide by mitosis (Fig. 2.8), a process resulting in two new genetically identical daughter cells (Waugh & Grant, 2018). As most cells also double their mass and duplicate all their cytoplasmic organelles in each cell cycle, co-ordination of the many complex cytoplasmic and nuclear processes is fundamental.

The duration of the cell cycle (Fig. 2.9) varies greatly from one cell type to another (Alberts et al., 2019). However, a standard does prevail to ensure that cell cycles for all dividing cells follow distinct phases: **interphase, mitosis** and **cytokinesis.** Mitosis is the critical process of nuclear division. Because cells require time to grow and mature before they can divide, the standard cell cycle is long, extending to 12 hours or more in fast-growing mammalian tissue. In most cells the mitotic phase takes about an hour – only a small fraction of the total cell cycle time.

- A cell performs all its normal functions during **interphase** and, if necessary, prepares itself for division by facilitating DNA replication. The interphase is the longest phase of the cell cycle, extending from one mitotic phase to the next. It consists of three distinct phases: the **G**$_1$ or **gap1** phase, the **S** or **synthesis phase** and the **G**$_2$ or gap2 phase. During the G$_1$ phase, the cells monitor their internal environment and their size. When the time is appropriate, decisive steps are taken to commit the cells to DNA replication, which occurs in the S phase of the cell cycle. The subsequent G$_2$ phase provides a safety gap ensuring that DNA replication is complete before mitosis.
- During mitosis, the nuclear membrane breaks down and the nuclear contents condense, forming visible chromosomes. This is a continuous process involving four distinct phases: **prophase, metaphase, anaphase** and **telophase** (Fig. 2.8).
  - During **prophase**, the replicated chromatin becomes tightly coiled. Each of the 46 chromosomes

• BOX 2.5 Plasma Membrane Excitability and Ion Transport

The hydrophobic interior of the plasma membrane acts as a barrier to the passage of most polar molecules. This barrier allows required solutes to be maintained in cytoplasm and within each intracellular membrane-bound organelle at vastly different concentrations to those found in extracellular fluid. Cells selectively transfer water-soluble molecules across their membranes, thereby obtaining essential nutrients, excreting metabolic waste products and regulating intracellular ion concentrations (Fig. 2.5).

Two specialized transmembrane proteins transporting inorganic ions and small water-soluble organic molecules across the lipid bilayer are **ion channels** (**channel proteins**) and **carrier proteins**. Carrier proteins are coupled to an energy source facilitating active transport of substrates across the membrane and against a concentration gradient of that substrate. In contrast, channel proteins form a narrow hydrophilic pore, allowing the passive movement of small inorganic ions across the lipid bilayer.

By generating ionic concentration differences across the lipid bilayer, cell membranes store **potential energy** in the form of **electrochemical gradients** which drive many transport processes, convey electric signals in excitable cells and generate adenosine triphosphate (ATP) in mitochondria. In contrast, smaller and more lipid-soluble molecules diffuse more rapidly across the lipid bilayer. Similarly, small non-polar molecules (e.g., oxygen and carbon dioxide) readily dissolve in the lipid bilayers and diffuse rapidly across them. Water and urea cross rapidly, whereas glycerol, a larger molecule, diffuses less rapidly. Diffusion of the more complex glucose molecules is carrier-dependent.

The lipid bilayers are impermeable to charged molecules (ions) no matter how small they are; their charge and high degree of hydration prevent them from entering the hydrocarbon phase of the bilayer. Therefore, ionic transfer is dependent on ion-specific channels that form a continuous pathway across the plasma membrane. Ion-specific channels facilitate passive diffusion of hydrophilic solutes across the cell membrane without coming into direct contact with the hydrophobic lipid bilayer. Because most channel proteins are ion species-specific, they play a crucial role in determining ion diffusion efficiency. The advantage of ion channels over carrier proteins is that more than 1 million ions can pass through an open channel each second, a rate 1000 times greater than any carrier protein.

Ion Channels

Two key properties distinguish ion channels from single aqueous pores (Alberts et al., 2019):

i. They show ion selectivity, permitting some inorganic ions to pass but not others.
ii. More importantly, ion channels are not continuously open, but use 'gates' that open briefly, usually in response to a specific stimulus closing again once the intracellular electrogradient for a particular ion species has been reached.

The main types of stimuli that cause ion channels to open are **changes in voltage** across the membrane (voltage-gated channels), **mechanical stress** (mechanically gated channels) or the binding of a **ligand** to **specific receptors** (ligand-gated channels). The ligand acts as an extracellular mediator, a neurotransmitter or as an intracellular mediator such as a nucleotide.

Ion channels are responsible for the electrical excitability of muscle cells and the mediation of electrical signalling in neurons. However, they are not restricted to electrically excitable cells and are present in all cell membranes, facilitating diffusion of their specific ion species to maintain the required intracellular electrochemical gradient. The most common forms are those ion channels permeable mainly to potassium ions, making the plasma membrane much more permeable to potassium than to any other ion. Potassium is critical in maintaining cell membrane potential and the voltage difference across plasma membranes.

Carrier Proteins

In contrast, carrier proteins, which facilitate selective transport of substrates across the plasma membranes, bind their specific solutes and then undergo a series of conformational changes to transfer these solutes across the plasma membranes. Each carrier protein has one or more **binding sites** for its substrates permitting full saturation of the carrier sites. When all binding sites are occupied, the rate of transport across the plasma membrane is maximal. However, solute binding can be blocked by competitive inhibitors occupying the same binding sites.

Generally, carrier proteins are classified according to their functional capacity: some are **uniporters** and other more complex proteins are **coupled transporters,** where the transport of one solute depends on the simultaneous transfer of a second solute in the same direction (**symport**) or in the opposite direction (**antiport**). For example, the take-up of glucose from extracellular fluid, where its concentration is high relative to that in the cytosol, is achieved by passive transport by glucose carriers operating as uniporters. Intestinal and kidney epithelial cells take up glucose from the lumen of the intestine and the nephron filtrate, respectively. In both instances the low concentration of glucose in the epithelial cells creates a favourable concentration gradient for the influx of glucose along with sodium.

The Sodium–Potassium Pump

Potassium ion concentration is typically 10–20 times higher in cytoplasm than in extracellular fluid, whereas the reverse is true of sodium ions. Although ion channels play a crucial role in maintaining these differences, fine-tuning of these concentrations is achieved by the highly dynamic **sodium–potassium pumps**. These appear to operate as antiporters, actively pumping sodium out of the cell and potassium into the cell against their steep electrochemical gradients. The sodium gradient produced by these pumps regulates cell volume through its osmotic effects, a mechanism also exploited in the transportation of sugars and amino acids into cells (Fig. 2.6).

Almost one-third of a cell's energy is consumed in fuelling the sodium–potassium pumps. ATP is the primary energy required by the sodium–potassium pumps. Its supply is facilitated by ATPase, which hydrolyses the ATP molecule, thereby releasing its stored energy (Alberts et al., 2019).

The sodium–potassium pump is a large molecule with binding sites for sodium and ATP on its cytoplasmic surface and a binding site for potassium on its external surface. During the pumping cycle, the molecule is reversibly phosphorylated and dephosphorylated. The sodium–potassium pump drives three positively charged ions out of the cell for every two ions it pumps into the cell. This creates an electrical potential with the inside surface of the plasma membrane negative to the outside surface. By controlling the solute concentration inside the cell, the sodium–potassium pump regulates the osmotic forces that influence cell expansion and dehydration.

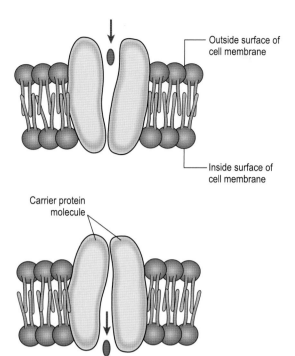

• **Fig. 2.5** Specialized protein carrier molecules involved in facilitated diffusion and active transport.

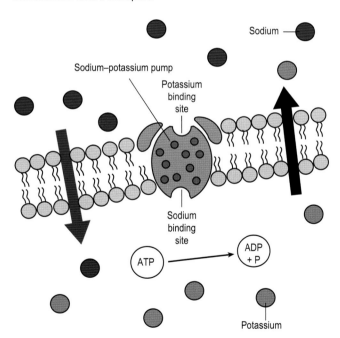

• **Fig. 2.6** Operation of the sodium–potassium pump. Three sodium ions are moved out of the cell, and two potassium ions are moved into the cell. The energy is provided by hydrolysis of one molecule of ATP.

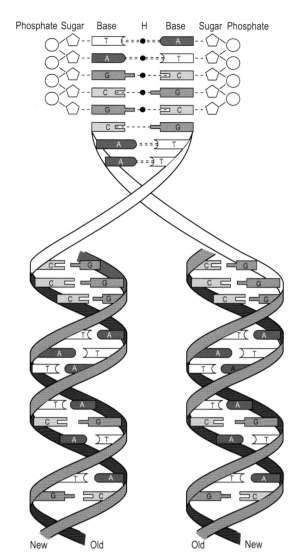

• **Fig. 2.7** The replication of DNA showing the unwinding of the double helix and the formation of new strands with complementary base pairs.

- In **metaphase**, chromatids align on the centre of the mitotic spindle, attached by their centromeres.
- In **anaphase**, the centromeres separate. One of each pair of sisters (now called chromosomes again) migrates to each end of the spindle as the microtubules forming the spindle contract.
- In **telophase**, the mitotic spindle disappears, the chromosomes uncoil and the nuclear envelope re-forms.

Following telophase, the cell membrane contracts and gradually divides into two identical daughter cells by a process commonly known as **cytokinesis.** This is the critical point of the mitotic phase terminating the end of the cell cycle.

In conditions that favour growth, the total protein content of a cell increases continuously throughout the cell cycle (Alberts et al., 2019). Similarly, RNA synthesis continues at a steady rate, except during the mitotic phase when the chromosomes are too condensed to permit **transcription** (Chapter 3). Whilst cell cycles vary, certain behavioural

(chromatids at this stage) is paired with its copy in a double-chromosome unit. The two chromatids are joined together at the centromere. The mitotic apparatus appears, consisting of two centrioles separated by the mitotic spindle. The spindle is formed from microtubules and will eventually separate the chromosomes. The centrioles migrate, one to each end of the cell, and the nuclear envelope disappears.

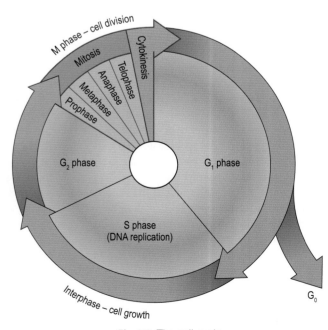

PROPHASE
DNA of chromosome replicates so chromosome appears as pair of chromatids

— Chromatid
— Centromere
— Nuclear envelope

METAPHASE
Nuclear envelope disappears Chromosomes line up at equator

— Centriole
— Spindle fibres

ANAPHASE
Spindle threads shorten so chromosomes are drawn to opposite ends of the cell

— Position of cleavage furrow

TELOPHASE
Two nuclear envelopes form around chromosomes and cell divides into two

— Nuclear envelope

• **Fig. 2.8** Stages of mitosis.

• **Fig. 2.9** The cell cycle.

requirements of all cells are universal; for instance, they must avoid entering mitosis or meiosis until all chromosomes are replicated. Failure to comply with this requirement can result in cells with certain chromosomal aberrations, which may give rise to cancer at a later stage (Alberts et al., 2019).

Meiosis

Meiosis (meaning 'diminution') is a special kind of nuclear division in which the chromosome complement is halved (Coad, Pedley & Dunstall, 2019). Meiosis involves two nuclear divisions rather than one (Fig. 2.10). Except for the **sex chromosomes** (different in males and females), a **diploid nucleus** contains two similar versions of each of the **autosomes** (alike in males and females). One set of these chromosomes is paternal, and one set is maternal in origin.

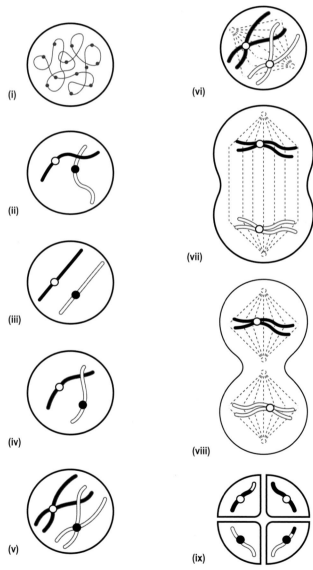

• **Fig. 2.10** The stages of meiosis. Only one chromosome pair is shown for clarity. (i) Interphase. (ii) Prophase I: leptotene. (iii) Zygotene. (iv) Pachytene. (v) Diplotene. (vi) Metaphase I. (vii) Anaphase I. (viii) Telophase I. (ix) Second meiotic division.

These two sets of chromosomes are known as **homologues.** In most cells, the homologues maintain a separate existence as independent chromosomes.

Consequently, a mature **haploid gamete** produced by the divisions of a diploid cell during meiosis contains half the original number of chromosomes. Only one chromosome from each homologous pair is present, ensuring that either the maternal or the paternal copy of each gene, but not both, is present. Clearly, this specific requirement makes an extra demand on the processes governing cell division. Mechanisms have evolved permitting the additional sorting of the chromosomes. This involves the homologues recognizing each other and becoming physically paired before lining up on the mitotic spindle. Pairing of the maternal and paternal copy of each chromosome is unique to meiosis.

It is probably only after DNA replication has been completed that the special feature of meiosis becomes evident. The duplicated homologous pairs form a structure containing four chromatids. This close proximity allows genetic recombination to occur where a fragment of a maternal chromatid is exchanged for a corresponding fragment of a homologous paternal chromatid.

Main Points

- Cells are the fundamental units of life.
- The morphological and functional features of cells are governed by genetic blueprints contained in their nuclei and mitochondria.
- Cells permit selective but rapid diffusion of substrates to ensure metabolic needs are easily sustained.
- In larger cells, the surface area is increased to generate a larger area for selective transport and diffusion.
- Cell motility is influenced by metabolic demands and environmental factors such as tissue injury.
- Ectoderm, endoderm and mesoderm all contribute to the formation and development of different cells in the body.
- Epithelial cells are classified according to morphological and functional characteristics. Each epithelial cell type is identified by size, shape, cell volume and density. Examples include simple epithelia, stratified, columnar, cuboidal and transitional.
- A typical human cell is about 10 μm in diameter. The oocyte (about 100 μm in diameter) is the largest cell and the sperm cell is one of the smallest human cells.
- The plasma membrane is the unique feature of the cell. It consists of a complex lipid bilayer interspersed by a range of protein molecules.
- Selective permeability of the plasma membrane facilitates free passage of gases and water but restricts the movement of larger ions to their specific protein channels.
- Cytoplasm acts as a reservoir for the suspension of small molecular structures, large particles and organelles such as the endoplasmic reticulum, the Golgi apparatus, mitochondria, lysosomes and peroxisomes.
- The endoplasmic reticulum plays a central role in lipid and protein biosynthesis.
- Lysosomes are filled with a granular protein aggregate which constitutes necessary digestive enzymes.
- Mitochondria are self-replicating, contain their own DNA and generate ATP, a form of energy essential to normal cellular function.
- The nucleus is the largest structure of the cell, containing large quantities of DNA.
- DNA holds the cell's genetic blueprint.
- Controlled cell division is vital to human reproduction, tissue growth, repair and other processes.
- Mitosis is the process resulting in two new genetically identical daughter cells.
- Meiosis leads to gamete formation where the chromosome numbers are halved. After exchanging genetic material, one of each pair of homologous chromosomes is represented in the mature gamete.

References

Alberts, B., Hopkin, K., Bray, D., Hopkin, K., Roberts, K., Raff, K., et al., 2019. Essential Cell Biology, fifth ed. W.W. Norton & Company, New York.

Coad, J., Pedley, K., Dunstall, M., 2019. Anatomy and Physiology for Midwives, fourth ed. Elsevier, London.

Kierszenbaum, A.L., 2021. Basic structure and function of cells. In: Standstring, S. (Ed.), Gray's Anatomy: The Anatomical Basis for Clinical Practice, forty second ed. Elsevier, London.

Konieczny, L., Roterman-Konieczna, I., Spolnik, P., 2014. Systems Biology: Functional Strategies of Living Organisms. Springer, New York.

Nussbaum, R.L., McInnes, R.R., Huntington, F.W., 2015. Thompson & Thompson Genetics in Medicine, eighth ed. Saunders Elsevier, London.

Turnpenny, P.D., Ellard, S., 2017. Emery's Elements of Medical Genetics, fifteenth ed. Elsevier, London.

Waugh, A., Grant, A., 2018. Ross & Wilson Anatomy and Physiology in Health and Illness, thirteenth ed. Elsevier, London.

Annotated recommended reading

Tortora, G.J., Neilson, M., 2019. Principles of Human Anatomy, fourteenth ed. Wiley, Jefferson City.

This textbook provides an in-depth description of human anatomy. The section on the 'cell' is in more detail and presented with excellent illustrations of cell division and replication.

Waugh, A., Grant, A., 2018. Ross & Wilson Anatomy and Physiology in Health and Illness, thirteenth ed. Elsevier, London.

This is a comprehensive textbook for interested learners in this area. It provides a detailed and 'easy to read' section on cells in the body in relation to their structure, role and function.

3

Structure, Organization and Regulation of Genes

JEAN RANKIN

Life is dependent on the ability of cells to store, retrieve and translate the genetic instructions to make and maintain a living organism. This chapter covers a range of key factors such as the composition of deoxyribose nucleic acid (DNA) and the double-helix structure of DNA, chromosomes and genes, and patterns of inheritance, including some inherited condition and chromosomal defects.

Introduction

In recent decades, major advances in the science of genetics have made a significant contribution to knowledge and understanding in the maintenance of living organisms. **Genomics** is the study of the human genome (Alberts et al., 2019). The **genetic basis** is now confirmed for many aspects of human disease leading to the search for diagnosis and treatments. The international **Human Genome Project** (1991–2000) was aptly recognized as one of the greatest feats of exploration in research history (genome.gov/human-genome-project). This project sequenced and mapped all human genes (together known as the genome). This had ground-breaking results leading to the ability to read nature's complete genetic blueprint for building a human being.

Major concerns were raised about the ethical, legal and social implications of human genome mapping and how this newfound knowledge could be used to discriminate against people. The public and governments found it difficult to understand the implications of this scientific breakthrough as industries became established based on **recombinant gene technology, cloning** and **gene therapy**. This has led to a sense of fear and distrust of technologies such as genetically modified foods. Related policies were developed to underpin any ongoing genomics research to advance knowledge and ensure genomics benefits the health of all humans (genome.gov/about-genomics/policy-issues). Overviews of key discoveries relating to genomics and key genetic advances are provided in Boxes 3.1 and 3.2, respectively.

Composition of DNA

Building Blocks

Cell nuclei contain large amounts of species-specific deoxyribonucleic acid (DNA). Another form of nucleic acid is **ribonucleic acid** (RNA). Nucleic acids are long **polymers** of molecules called **nucleotides** composed of several simple chemical compounds bound together in a regular pattern. These building blocks are **phosphoric acid,** a **pentose sugar** with five carbon atoms called **deoxyribose** and four **nitrogenous bases.** The bases are comprised of two **purines** (**adenine** and **guanine**) and two **pyrimidines** (**thymine** and **cytosine**) identified by the single letters A, G, T and C. In RNA, thymine is replaced by **uracil** (U). Box 3.3 details the DNA double-helix structure.

RNA is found in the cytoplasm, particularly concentrated in the **nucleolus,** whereas DNA is found mainly on the 46 chromosomes (arranged in 23 pairs in somatic cells). One chromosome of each pair originates from the

1865: The monk Gregor Mendel presented results of his experiments with garden peas. He had studied varieties of pea that differed in a single characteristic, such as tall and short plants or wrinkled and smooth seeds. He found an **inheritance pattern** where one of two characteristics—for example, tall plants—seemed to **dominate** the next generation (i.e., the **first filial (F1) generation**). These were called **dominant factors.** The opposite characteristic—short plants—disappeared, to reappear in the 'grandchildren' (the **second (F2) generation**). These were called **recessive factors.**

Mendel proposed that each pair of characteristics was controlled by a pair of factors, one of which was inherited from each parent plant. Pure-bred pea plants were **homologous** ('homo' means alike) and inherited two identical genes from their parents. The F1 generation produced all tall plants and resulted from the breeding of a tall plant with a short plant. However, they inherited two different genes from their parents and were **heterozygous** ('hetero' means different). The alternative versions of genes are called **allelomorphs,** usually shortened to **alleles.**

Mendel's Laws

Three main principles were developed:

i. The Law of Uniformity. When two homozygotes with different alleles are crossed, all the offspring of the F1 generation are identical and heterozygous. Characteristics do not blend and can reappear in subsequent generations.

ii. The Law of Segregation. Every individual possesses two genes for a particular characteristic; only one gene can be passed on in the ovum or sperm to the next generation.

iii. The Law of Independent Assortment. Members of different gene pairs segregate to offspring independently of one another. (This third law is not strictly true, because if two genes are situated closely together on the same **chromosome** (see later) they may be **linked** and inherited together).

1900: Rediscovery of Mendel's experiments and findings for genetic inheritance. Interest emerged when thread-like structures were seen in the nuclei of cells (i.e., chromosomes).

1909: W Johannsen, a Danish botanist, coined the word 'gene' to describe the Mendelian unit of heredity (Turnpenny & Ellard, 2017). New terms (genotype and phenotype) were introduced to differentiate between the genetic traits of an individual and outward appearance.

1952: **Deoxyribonucleic acid** (DNA) was identified as the universal genetic material.

1953: Structure of DNA double helix was first described by James D Watson and Francis H Crick. The power of **X-ray crystallography** revealed by Rosalind Franklin made their discovery possible (Streissguth, 2017).

1956: The exact number of 46 human chromosomes was identified.

The Human Genome Project

This **project** mapped all human genes to their chromosomes. The project, initiated in 1991 in the United States, investigated the mutation rates of DNA in response to exposure to radiation and chemicals. Completed in 2000, the project soon became international across numerous countries worldwide. The short-term hope was to enable better diagnosis and counselling for families with genetic disease (genome.gov/human-genome-project). In the longer term, the aim is to develop preventive strategies and treatments of genetic disorders (genome.gov/research-at-nhgri/Projects).

Detection of Abnormality

After the production of a karyotype, chromosomes can be identified by their size, banding patterns and the position of the centromere. Gross chromosomal defects can occur and where the gene can be identified, gene probes can be used to locate single gene defects. Commercial synthetic sections of DNA are available, which are attracted to the appropriate gene and can identify single base changes. Further advances are regularly achieved to identify or link genes. Recent genetic associations were made in relation to amyotrophic lateral sclerosis, the deteriorating disease suffered by the late Stephen Hawking. Others include *LGI2* in epilepsy and the gene *BOULE* responsible for sperm production, which is the first known gene to be *required* for sperm production in species ranging from insects to mammals.

DNA Technologies

Techniques include using enzymes called **restriction endonucleases** which cut DNA at a specific point, **polymerase chain reaction** and the **Southern blot technique.** DNA technology is in two main areas: **DNA cloning** (producing identical copies) and **DNA analysis.** Possible applications include medical cures, increased food production, crime detection and better energy production.

Chromosomes

Chromosomes take up different states depending on the stage of the **cell cycle** (Chapter 2). When the cell is not dividing, chromosomes are extended, and their **chromatin** is in the form of long, thin tangled threads known as **interphase** chromosomes. The highly condensed chromosomes in a dividing cell are called **mitotic** chromosomes (Alberts et al., 2019), which are much wider than the DNA double helix.

If the DNA of a single human cell was stretched out, it would be several metres long, yet the total length of the chromosomes placed end to end is less than 0.5 mm. DNA is packaged into chromosomes by coiling and folding (Turnpenny & Ellard, 2017). Besides the double helix, there is a secondary coiling around spherical molecules called **histones** to form **nucleosomes.** A tertiary coiling of nucleosomes forms the chromatin fibres which are then wound into a tight coil to make the chromosomes.

Circulating lymphocytes from peripheral blood are commonly used to study chromosomes, but skin or bone marrow cells can also be used. Fetal cells from the chorionic villi or amniotic fluid (**amniocytes**) can be sampled. The process of cell division is stopped during mitosis by adding **colchicines,** which prevents the formation of the spindle and arrests the

ovum and the other from the sperm. A cell containing two sets of chromosomes is described as **diploid.** Gametes are **haploid,** containing one of each pair of chromosomes. In 22 of the pairs, the chromosomes are identical; these pairs are called **autosomes.** The two chromosomes are termed **homologous.** The 23rd pair is the sex chromosomes: two X chromosomes in females and an X and a Y chromosome in males. Maternal and paternal chromosomes become closely apposed during meiosis and exchange segments of DNA between **homologues,** a phenomenon called **crossing over.**

cells in metaphase. Hypotonic saline solution is added, which destroys the cells and releases the chromosomes. These are photographed and then the chromosome images are cut out, laid out in a standard fashion and photographed again to produce a karyotype. Chromosomes are identified by their size, light and dark banding patterns and the position of the centromere.

At the time of DNA replication, the chromosomes consist of two identical strands called *sister chromatids* held

---

• BOX 3.3   The Double Helix

DNA holds the instructions for constructing, organizing and maintaining the body. It must be replicated accurately during mitosis (Chapter 2).

DNA molecules consist of a double helix structure made up of two complementary chains of nucleotides (Fig. 3.1). The double helix shape allows for DNA replication and protein synthesis to occur. The structure consists of two sugar–phosphate strands winding around each other, with base pairs stacked one above the other between these strands that point inwards to the centre of the double helix (Turnpenny & Ellard, 2017). The two chains are held together by hydrogen bonds between the base pairs. The hydrogen bonds are easily broken, a feature necessary for DNA replication. The sugar–phosphate molecules form the backbone of the chains (Fig. 3.1).

The structure Is stabilized by two other forms of bonds— hydrophobic and van der Waals interactions (Chapter 1)— between adjacent pairs. The twisted DNA unwinds and opens to allow a copy of the DNA to be made.

N.B. One of the two strands must be passed on to the next generation by means of ova and sperm.

---

together by a **centromere.** Centromeres consist of lengths of **repetitive DNA** and are responsible for the movement of the chromosomes that takes place in cell division. A chromosome is divided by its centromere into short and long arms. The short arm is referred to as 'p' and the long arm as 'q'. Chromosomes can be classified by the position of their centromeres. If located centrally the chromosome is **metacentric,** if intermediate it is **sub-metacentric** and if found at one end of the chromosome it is **acrocentric.** Acrocentric chromosomes may have stalks with satellites attached to them containing multiple copies of the genes for **ribosomal RNA.**

The tip of each chromosome arm is called the **telomere,** consisting of many repeats of a TTAGGG sequence which seals the ends of the chromosome to maintain its structural integrity. The length of these sequences is reduced each time the cell divides. This is part of normal cellular ageing; most cells can only undergo 50–60 divisions before becoming senescent.

Genes

The full complement of DNA is called the **genome.** Along the genome, about 60–70% of DNA is in the form of single or short repeats of single sequences called *low copy sequences,* whereas 30–40% consist of highly repetitive sequences appearing inactive. DNA is arranged in discrete segments called **genes,** and there may be 25,000–30,000 of these in the human genome. A rule of genetics says 'one gene, one protein'. However, genes often exist in families; for example,

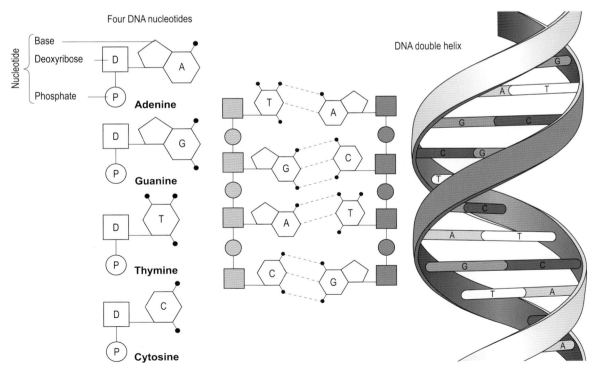

• Fig. 3.1 DNA double helix. (A) Sugar phosphate backbone and nucleotide pairing of the DNA double helix (P, phosphate; A, adenine; T, thymine; G guanine; C, cytosine). (B) Representation of the DNA double helix.

those coding for the various types of haemoglobin (Chapter 16) and those for antibodies (Chapter 29).

Genes code for **polypeptides,** which include enzymes, hormones, receptors and structural and regulatory proteins (Turnpenny & Ellard, 2017). The alternative alleles of any gene are present at a specific place, or locus, on each of a pair of chromosomes. If both parents contribute an identical allele for a locus, the new individual is **homozygous.** If the two alleles differ, the new individual is **heterozygous.**

Discrete single genes form about 25% of the DNA and are separated from each other by long runs of inactive, repetitive DNA sequences. It is not known why there is so much redundant DNA. The coding sequences of genes are called **exons** and the intervening non-coding sequences **introns.** Exons are usually interrupted by introns. Individual introns can be much larger than the exons, and some can contain a gene within a gene.

The Role of the Environment

Genes act in response to environmental changes (Chapter 15). These may be internal, such as a response to fluctuations in hormone level, or external, such as a response to a meal. The full range of genes inherited by an individual is called the **genotype.** The outward appearance of an individual (i.e., their physical, biochemical and physiological nature) is known as the **phenotype** and results from gene–environment interactions.

From DNA to RNA to Protein

Proteins are the working components of the cell. DNA stores the information. RNA (Fig. 3.2) carries out instructions encoded in DNA and synthesizes the proteins involved in cellular function (Jorde et al., 2019).

The Genetic Code

Twenty different amino acids are found in proteins. Because there are only four bases, more than one base must be necessary to specify a particular amino acid. Even two bases would not be enough, as 4^2 gives only 16 possibilities. However, 4^3 bases allow 64 possibilities of codons to occur with some redundancy. Each group of three nucleotides, called a **triplet codon** (Fig. 3.3), spells out each amino acid. The sequence of amino acids shapes a particular protein. There are also codons at the ends of genes that signify 'start' and 'stop'. The process of reading the DNA code which results in a functional protein product involves two processes: **transcription** and **translation** (see Box 3.4).

Mutations

Gene mutations are rare. A mutation or alteration in the arrangement or amount of genetic material in a cell arises either naturally or because of the effects of environmental challenges called *mutagens* such as radiation, chemical or physical stressors. Mutations can be minor changes in DNA such as **point mutations** (single base substitutions) or **macromutations** involving alterations such as **deletions** of large amounts of a chromosome.

Mutations often result in harmful or lethal defects. Point mutations cause amino acid substitutions resulting in faulty protein products. This may cause specific functional defects such as **cystic fibrosis** or **sickle cell disease.** Macromutations may cause syndromes as multiple changes in a particular chromosome leading to recognizable changes in the body as seen in Down syndrome (trisomy 21). **Nonsense mutations** involve the creation of a stop codon in an abnormal situation. The broken gene does not code for a protein

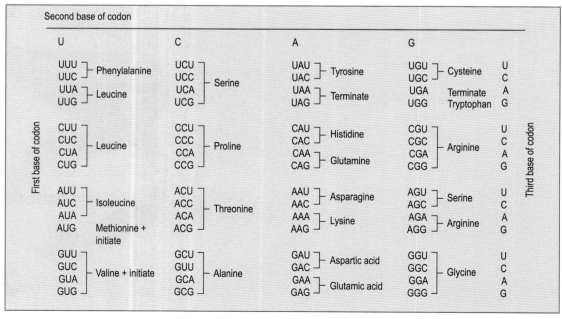

• **Fig. 3.2** Messenger RNA (mRNA) code words.

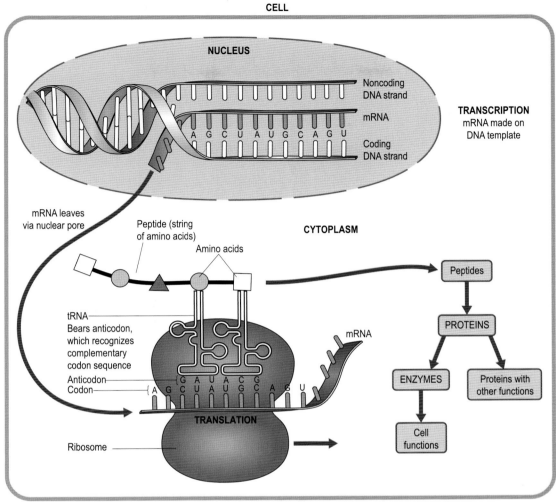

CELL

NUCLEUS

Noncoding DNA strand

mRNA

TRANSCRIPTION
mRNA made on DNA template

AGCUAUGCAGU

Coding DNA strand

mRNA leaves via nuclear pore

Peptide (string of amino acids)

Amino acids

CYTOPLASM

Peptides

tRNA
Bears anticodon, which recognizes complementary codon sequence

PROTEINS

Anticodon
Codon

GAUACG
AGCUAUGCAGU

TRANSLATION

mRNA

ENZYMES

Proteins with other functions

Ribosome

Cell functions

DNA makes RNA (transcription) makes protein (translation)

• **Fig. 3.3** The stages of protein synthesis translation.

• **BOX 3.4**   **Transcription and Translation**

Transcription

Three types of RNA are involved in the production of a protein:
1. Messenger RNA (mRNA) copies the genetic code of a stretch of DNA in the form of a sequence of bases that codes for a sequence of amino acids.
2. Transfer RNA (tRNA) carries the correct amino acids specified by the DNA to the ribosome and places them in the correct order.
3. Ribosomal RNA (rRNA) combines with proteins to make ribosomes, which have binding sites for the molecules needed to make a protein.

   In any gene, only one of the DNA strands acts as a template for a polypeptide, and it must be copied before it can be read (Fig. 3.3). This copying is called *transcription.* It must be accurate as mistakes may lead to an inactive

product. The information stored in the gene is transmitted from DNA to mRNA. Every base in the single-stranded mRNA is complementary to the DNA, but uracil replaces thymine. An enzyme called *RNA polymerase* tacks the bases onto the developing strand in the correct order.

Translation

After transcription, non-coding introns are excised, and the coding exons are spliced together to form mature mRNA. This is transported to the ribosomes in the cytoplasm for translation into a specific protein (Fig. 3.4). In the cytoplasm, a particular amino acid is bound to its tRNA for transporting to the ribosome, where it is linked up with others to form a polypeptide chain. The ribosome moves along the mRNA, linking up the amino acids to build the protein.

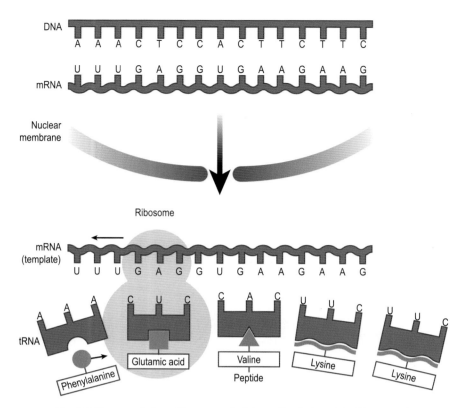

• **Fig. 3.4** Representation of how genetic information is translated into protein.

product. In **frameshift mutations** additions or deletions of a nucleotide alter the reading frame of the DNA to the left or the right so that triplet codons do not code for amino acids.

Regulation of Gene Expression

Every cell in the body (except gametes) has the full complement of genes. The cells making up organs have specialized functions, and only a small proportion of the genes will be active in a particular cell. Also, genes only make the amount of their protein product necessary for a particular body function. Genes may only function at specific phases of development of an organism and are activated and suppressed as needed (Turnpenny & Ellard, 2017).

Patterns of Inheritance

Dominant Genes

As previously mentioned, specific genes may be inherited as dominant, recessive or sex-linked. A dominant allele manifests its effects in heterozygotes as only one copy is needed to affect the phenotype. Except in cases of a new mutation, every child with that phenotype receives a copy of one allele from a similar parent. Most genes work normally, but if the gene codes for an abnormality where one parent is affected, a child will have a 1 in 2 chance of inheriting the gene and being affected.

The gene expression in the eye colour of the offspring is a common example. The rules of genetics dictate that eye colour often follows the traditional form of dominant and recessive interaction (Fig. 3.5). Examples of dominant or recessive genes influencing physical features and blood groups are presented in Table 3.1.

Recessive Genes

A recessive allele only affects the phenotype in homozygotes. People with one copy of the allele are carriers. If the gene codes for an abnormality, the children of two carriers will have a 1 in 4 chance of being affected or normal and a 1 in 2 chance of being a carrier (Fig. 3.6).

Sex-linked Genes

The X chromosome carries many genes involved in development and function. Males only have one X chromosome and are **hemizygous** for X chromosome genes. If there is an abnormal X chromosome gene, boys will be affected by an X-linked disorder. Females are usually heterozygous for such an abnormal X chromosome gene and will not be affected because of the opposing normal allele. However, homozygosity may rarely occur if an affected man and carrier woman have a daughter. These girls will be affected. In females, only one X chromosome is functional in each cell, and the other is randomly inactivated in the early embryo. This is called lyonization (Box 3.5).

Colour blindness in different forms is a common condition transmitted by sex-linked recessive genes. It affects more men than women and the most common form is red–green colour blindness (Fig. 3.7). The colours of brown, pale red,

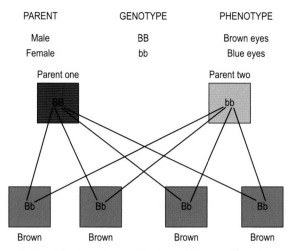

PARENT	GENOTYPE	PHENOTYPE
Male	BB	Brown eyes
Female	bb	Blue eyes

• **Fig. 3.5** Combination diagram illustrating the genetic outcomes of crossing a homozygous male with brown eyes.

TABLE 3.1	Examples of Autosomal Dominant and Recessive Traits	
Dominant Trait	**Recessive Trait**
Near or far sight	Normal vision
Curly hair	Straight hair
Dark brown hair	All other hair colours
Brown eye colour	Blue or grey eye colour
Normal skin pigment	Albinism
A or B antigen (A, B or AB blood group)	No A or B antigen (O blood group)
Rhesus antigen (Rh+ blood group)	No Rhesus antigen (Rh− blood group)

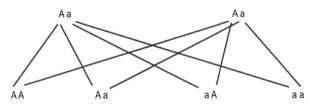

• **Fig. 3.6** In an autosomal-recessive disorder, the disease is only manifested if both parents are carriers of the abnormal gene (a); then there is a 1-in-4 chance that a child will have the disease.

green and orange all appear to be the same colour to that individual and can only be distinguished by their intensity.

Genomic Imprinting

It was discovered that genes on homologous chromosomes are not expressed equally. Different clinical features can arise depending on whether a gene was inherited from the mother or the father. This is genomic imprinting, which affects only a small proportion of the genome. Prader–Willi syndrome, characterized by short stature, obesity, small gonads and learning difficulty, occurs

In females, one of the X chromosomes is inactivated in each cell early in embryonic life. Inactivation occurs at around 15 days when the embryo consists of about 5000 cells. Their descendants retain the same activated X chromosome so that half the cells contain one activated X chromosome and half the other. This effect is called *lyonization* after its discoverer Dr Mary Lyon. Each female is a **mosaic** of half-paternal and half-maternal X chromosomes. Abnormal X chromosomes seem to be preferentially inactivated (Bainbridge, 2009; Turnpenny & Ellard, 2017).

In females or males with more than one X chromosome, any inactivated X chromosome can be seen during interphase as a dark mass of chromatin called *sex chromatin* or a **Barr body**. Looking for Barr bodies to determine sex is now an obsolete method due to the complexity of chromosomal abnormalities.

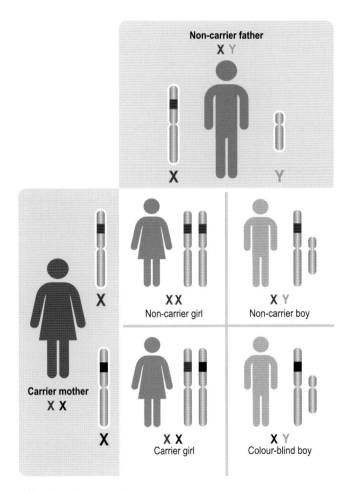

X : Normal gene on **X** chromosome

X : Abnormal colour blindness gene on **X** chromosome

Y : Normal **Y** chromosome (no gene present)

• **Fig. 3.7** Inheritance of sex-linked red–green colour blindness gene between generations.

in about 1 in 20,000 births. DNA analysis has shown it is nearly always the paternal homologue that is deleted. The remaining cases occur because of maternal disomy: two maternal and no paternal chromosome 15 (Turnpenny & Ellard, 2017).

Mitochondrial DNA

Each mitochondrion has its own circular double-stranded DNA called **mitochondrial DNA** (mtDNA) and is inherited only from the mother. The mitochondria in sperm are situated behind the head of the sperm in the neck, and as only the head enters the ovum, mitochondria are left outside with the tail. mtDNA codes for only 13 genes, some of which are important in cellular respiration. However, most mitochondrial proteins (about 1500) are coded for in the nuclear genome so that mitochondria rely on both genomes to carry out their functions (Lane, 2018). mtDNA has a higher rate of spontaneous mutation than nuclear DNA, and accumulation of mistakes may be responsible for some of the physical effects of ageing.

Mitochondrial inheritance may cause rare disorders affecting males and females but are transmitted only through their mothers. These disorders, which usually combine muscular and neurological features involving muscular weakness, are known as **mitochondrial myopathies.** Mitochondria are important in tissues with a high energy requirement, so it is not surprising that they are involved in abnormalities of the muscular and nervous systems.

Some Inherited Conditions

Most inherited disorders are a result of nuclear gene mutations, which are either dominant (Table 3.2), recessive (Table 3.3) or sex-linked (Table 3.4). Some may be due to a mutation in mtDNA (Table 3.5). Slight differences in a protein brought about by a mutation may cause devastating diseases such as cystic fibrosis or sickle cell disease. Some genes are **pleiotropic,** underpinning multiple functions; thus, an abnormality may affect multiple systems. In the recessive disorder phenylketonuria, low tyrosine levels lead to lack of pigment in hair, skin and eyes due to reduced melanin production.

Chromosomal Defects

About 50% of spontaneous abortions result from chromosomal defects occurring during oogenesis. Chromosomal defects may be present in up to 6% of all pregnancies. Numerical or structural changes may affect the autosomes or the sex chromosomes (see Box 3.6). People with chromosomal defects usually have characteristic phenotypes. One example relates to Down syndrome where the typical features may cause the children to look more like each other than to their relatives.

Structural Chromosomal Defects

Environmental factors may induce breaks in chromosomes, resulting in structural rearrangements called **macromutations.** Two of these—**inversion** and **translocation**—may be transmitted from parent to child.

- **Inversion** occurs if a segment of a chromosome breaks free and becomes reattached in reverse position. **Paracentric** inversion involves just one arm of the chromosome,

TABLE 3.2 Disorders of Systems caused by Dominant Genes

System	Disorder
Nervous	Huntington disease Neurofibromatosis
Bowel	Polyposis coli
Kidney	Polycystic disease
Eyes	Blindness
Ears	Deafness
Blood	Hypercholesterolaemia
Skeleton	Osteogenesis imperfecta Achondroplasia

TABLE 3.3 Some Recessively Inherited Conditions

System	Disorder
Metabolism	Cystic fibrosis Phenylketonuria
Nervous	Friedreich ataxia Tay–Sachs disease
Blood	Sickle cell anaemia Beta-thalassaemia
Ears	Congenital deafness
Eyes	Recessive blindness

TABLE 3.4 Some X-linked Disorders

System	Disorder
Locomotor	Duchenne muscular dystrophy
Blood	Haemophilia
Brain	Fragile X syndrome
Vision	Childhood blindness

TABLE 3.5 Some Mitochondrial Disorders

System	Disorder
Vision	Chronic progressive external ophthalmoplegia
Hearing	Aminoglycoside-induced deafness
Cardiovascular	Hypertrophic cardiomyopathy with myopathy

whereas **pericentric** inversion involves both arms and the centromere.

- **Translocation** is the transfer of a piece of one chromosome to another non-homologous chromosome. This may be a reciprocal translocation where two non-homologous chromosomes exchange pieces. If the translocation is balanced, the individual receives the normal complement of chromosomal material and there will be no abnormality. However, if the translocation results in extra chromosomal material, abnormality will occur. About 4% of people with Down syndrome receive their

---

• BOX 3.6   Numerical Chromosomal Defects

Many numerical defects arise during **failure of disjunction**. This is due to an error in cell division where the sister chromatids fail to separate at anaphase. This results in too few or too may chromosomes as detailed:

- **Polyploidy** means the presence of multiples of the haploid number of 23 chromosomes.
- **Triploidy** is the presence of 69 chromosomes. It may occur because the chromosomes of the second polar body fail to be ejected from the ovum or because of entry of two sperm into the ovum. It occurs in about 2% of fertilizations, and the zygote is lost early in development.
- **Monosomy** is when one of a chromosome pair is missing, leaving 45 chromosomes. This is only compatible with survival if the missing chromosome is an X. This results in a female with Turner syndrome.
- **Trisomy** is the presence of an extra chromosome. The usual cause is non-disjunction so that either the ovum or sperm carries 24 chromosomes instead of 23. At fertilization this results in 47 chromosomes. The most common condition is Down syndrome where there are three copies of chromosome 21 (Fig. 3.8). Non-disjunction occurs with increasing frequency as maternal age increases.
- **Mosaicism** results when the zygote develops into an individual with two genotypes or cell lines. The condition arises due to non-disjunction during early mitosis. The defects seen are less serious than those found in full monosomic or trisomic disorders.

third chromosome 21 translocated to another chromosome, often chromosome 14 or 15.

- **Deletion** is the loss of part of a chromosome. Loss of the termination of chromosome 5 causes Cri du chat syndrome where affected infants have a weak, cat-like cry, microcephaly, heart defects and mental impairment.
- **Duplication** is where a section of a chromosome is repeated, either within a chromosome, attached to another chromosome or as a separate fragment. This type of defect is less harmful as there is no loss of chromosomal material.
- **Isochromosome** is where the centromere divides horizontally instead of longitudinally; this occurs most often in the X chromosomes. Loss of the short arm of chromosome X is associated with features of **Turner syndrome.**

Advances in technology and scientific research have made a significant impact on the application of clinical practice. There is hope for diagnosis, prevention and treatment of conditions and situations. These also raise many ethical and moral issues. An overview of application to practice is presented in Box 3.7, with methods of gene therapy and stem therapies introduced in Boxes 3.8 and 3.9, respectively.

Conclusion

The moral and ethical issues accompanying gene technology are of major importance to the future of human health and medical treatment. It is essential for countries to develop safeguards ensuring that safety, privacy and confidentiality are not at risk. On a national and global scale, it is essential that any developments are made available to the maximum number of affected individuals. Biochemistry and its associated disciplines have real power to change the world. These developments need to be introduced in a regulated way while protecting the ethical and moral principles of the law and society.

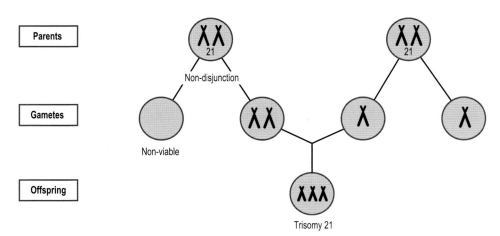

• Fig. 3.8 Non-disjunction of chromosome 21 leading to Down syndrome.

• BOX 3.7　Application to Practice

Therapeutic Advances in Technology

Hormones and enzymes can now be readily manufactured for medical applications. For example, human insulin has been used for years now in clinical practice. Other uses include pre-implantation genetic screening for disease and the sex of the embryo, fetal screening, screening of adults, gene replacement and stem cell therapies. Non-therapeutic uses, such as selecting attributes for a child or human cloning techniques, will continue to cause dilemmas.

Population Screening

The related ethical and moral debates continue and include the issues related to confidentiality and privacy of individuals accessing individual medical data. Population screening techniques are fraught with these issues from a personal, social, financial (insurance) and employment perspective.

Gene Therapy

This relates to the replacement of a deficient gene product or correction of an abnormal gene. When the gene enters the new cell, it may change the way the cell works or the chemicals that the cell secretes. Advances in molecular biology leading to the identification of many abnormal human genes and their products have led to possible treatments for some important diseases (Jorde et al., 2019).

These developments promise a new type of medicine. Regulatory bodies oversee the technical, therapeutic and safety aspects of gene therapy. Somatic cell therapy affecting only the individual tends to be more acceptable, whereas germ cell therapy is concerning as changes could be transmitted to future generations.

Over recent years, there have been successes such as therapy for X-linked severe combined immune deficiency (SCID), factor XI expression in haemophilia and some good effects in cancer and heart disease. These successes have involved only a few individuals (Jorde et al., 2019). Safety and cost may prevent gene therapy treatments from becoming widespread.

Important Considerations

Several technical aspects need to be overcome before gene therapy trials can take place:
1. The gene involved must have been cloned. This means not only the structural gene but also the sequences involved in its expression and regulation.
2. The specific targets—cell, tissue and organ—must be identified and accessible.
3. There must be an efficient vector system to carry the gene into the target cells.
4. There should be no harmful effects, such as malignancy, on the target cells.

• BOX 3.8　Methods of Gene Therapy

These can be divided into two groups: viral and non-viral.

Viral Agents

- **Retroviruses** are RNA viruses that can insert themselves into target cells, where their RNA is transformed into DNA and inserted into the cellular genome. They must be rendered inactive before use so that they cannot produce infection. The main problem with their use is that only very small stretches of DNA can be introduced.
- **Adenoviruses** are especially suitable for targeting the respiratory tract as they are more stable than retroviruses. They do not integrate into the genome, so there is no risk of mutagenesis. However, their effect is likely to be transient. As they contain **oncogenes** which are involved in the production of cancer, there is the danger of provoking malignancy.

- Other viruses such as the herpes virus, influenza virus and other RNA viruses could produce large quantities of the gene product but are likely to have the same problems already discussed. Viruses elicit an immune response which limits their repeated use.

Non-viral Agents

These tend to be safer methods but differ in their ability to produce sufficient gene product to be useful. They include:
- Direct injection of naked DNA
- Liposome-mediated transfer—DNA packaged in a lipid bilayer surrounding an aqueous vesicle
- Receptor-mediated endocytosis where specific receptors on the cell surface are targeted (genetherapynet.com/types-of-gene-therapy.html)

• BOX 3.9　Stem Cell Therapies

Stem cell therapy is the use of **stem cells** to treat or prevent a disease or condition. Bone marrow transplant is the most widely used **stem cell therapy**. Some **therapies** derived from umbilical cord blood are also in use.

After fertilization, the single cell and its early offspring are unspecified cells (**totipotent**) and can form any tissue in the body. The embryo-forming cells can become any tissue type. They are not capable of developing into the placenta and membranes. Stem cell therapy can be used for some genetic disorders, but risks of infection are high due to immunosuppression and

graft-versus-host disease. Stem cells derived from cord blood could overcome these problems. Sources include the embryonic inner cell mass, embryonic tissue retrieved after a termination of pregnancy, cord blood and some adult somatic cell lines (eurostemcell.org/cord-blood-stem-cells-current-uses-and-future-challenges).

Since the 1970s, skin stem cells have grown skin grafts for patients with severe and life-threatening burns on very large areas of the body. This solution is not perfect as the new skin has no hair follicles or sweat glands. The most widely used stem

• BOX 3.9   Stem Cell Therapies—cont'd

cell treatment is the transplantation of blood stem cells to treat diseases and conditions of the blood and immune system, or to restore the blood system after treatments for specific cancers. The number of patients treated with blood stem cells will continue to rise annually (≥48,000) in Europe and collaborating countries. Europe has approved a new stem cell-based treatment to repair damage to the cornea (the surface of the eye) after an injury like a chemical burn, called *Holoclar*.

Stem cell therapies can only be used once rendered safe and effective. All other therapies remain experimental until they have successfully passed thorough testing across all stages of clinical trials for a new therapy (sciencedaily.com/news/health_medicine/stem_cells/).

Recent progress shows that neurons suitable for transplantation can be generated from stem cells in culture and that the adult brain produces new neurons from its own stem cells in response to injury. These findings raise hope for the development of stem cell therapies in human neurodegenerative disorders.

Umbilical Cord Blood

Allogenic (tissues of two unalike individuals) stem cell transplantation has revolutionized the outcome for a wide range of malignant and non-malignant haematological conditions. Infusion of cord blood, which is very rich in highly proliferative stem cells, has been successfully used in children and young adults with some haematological and immunological disorders.

Embryonic Cells

In vitro fertilization and artificial growth of human embryos are needed to harvest cells from developing embryos. Research comes under vigilant monitoring and regulation in those countries where it is legal and supported. Removing cells from an aborted fetus raises clear ethical issues.

Adult Cells

Research into adult cells has indicated that some specialist **multipotent** cells may have the ability to produce other types of cells (Turnpenny & Ellard, 2017). Stem cells become dedicated to producing tissue with a specific function: for instance, blood stem cells are in the bone marrow and may also circulate in the bloodstream in small numbers. They continually replenish red cells, white cells and platelets. Some stem cells found in bone marrow have been able to produce liver cells. Caution is always required in this field.

In Utero Transplantation

Hereditary disorders revealed during prenatal scans could one day be cured before birth. This is one of the many reasons to move in utero gene therapy forward. Stem cell transplantation in utero may treat genetic disorders (DeWeerdt, 2018). The immature fetal immune system will tolerate novel cells, ending the need for a matched donor. Stem cells may be able to treat SCID, alpha- and beta-thalassaemia and sickle cell disease (Turnpenny & Ellard, 2017). In utero fetal gene therapy has been successful in mice with cystic fibrosis, so the possibility for treatment for the human fetus is real.

Somatic Cell Nuclear Transfer

Somatic cell nuclear transfer involves placing a somatic cell next to an ovum emptied of its nucleus. The two cells fuse together, and the resultant cell may be totipotent. If the newly created ovum was allowed to grow, cells from the inner cell mass would then give rise to pluripotent stem cell lines. The donor cell could be from the individual needing treatment, which would solve the problem of tissue rejection. The key ethical issue relates to the fact that the totipotent cell is a clone of the donor somatic cell.

Main Points

- Gregor Mendel proposed that each pair of characteristics in pea plants was controlled by a pair of factors, one inherited from each parent.
- The correct number of human chromosomes is 46. A cell containing two sets of chromosomes is referred to as *diploid*. One chromosome of each pair originates with the ovum and the other with the sperm.
- Gametes contain 23 chromosomes and are called *haploid*.
- In 22 pairs the chromosomes are identical, called *autosomes*. The 23rd pair are the sex chromosomes.
- The DNA molecule consists of a double helix made up of two complementary chains of nucleotides packaged into discrete chromosomes by coiling and folding.
- The genome is arranged in genes which carry the code for polypeptides.
- The genotype is the full complement of genes of an individual. The phenotype is their outward appearance.
- The process of reading the code of DNA involves transcription and translation.

- Genes may be dominant, recessive or sex-linked.
- Males have only one X chromosome and are hemizygous for X.
- In female cells, one X chromosome is deactivated at random, a process called *lyonization*.
- mtDNA is inherited only from our mothers. Mitochondrial inheritance may cause rare disorders that usually combine muscular and neurological features.
- Slight differences in a protein brought about by a genetic mutation may lead to devastating diseases such as sickle cell disease or cystic fibrosis.
- Fetal transplantation of pluripotent stem cells may treat genetic disorders because the fetal immune system will tolerate foreign cells.
- The Human Genome Project aims to achieve better diagnosis and counselling for families with genetic diseases and develop new preventive strategies and treatments for genetic disorders.

References

Alberts, B., Hopkin, K., Bray, D., Johnson, A.D., Lewis, J., Raff, M., Roberts, K., Walter, P., 2019. Essential Cell Biology, fifth ed. W.W. Norton & Company, New York.

Bainbridge, D., 2009. The X in Sex: How the X Chromosome Controls Our Lives, second ed. Harvard University Press, Cambridge.

DeWeerdt, S., 2018. Prenatal gene therapy offers the earliest possible cure. Nature 564, S6–S8.

Jorde, L.B., Carey, J.C., Bamshad, M.J., 2019. Medical Genetics, sixth ed. Elsevier, Philadelphia.

Lane, N., 2018. Power, Sex and Suicide: Mitochondria and the Meaning of Life, second ed. Oxford University Press, Oxford.

Streissguth, Y., 2017. Rosalind Franklin: DNA Discoverer (Women in Science). Essential Publishing, Essex.

Turnpenny, P.D., Ellard, S., 2017. Emery's Elements of Medical Genetics, fifteenth ed. Elsevier, London.

Websites

genome.gov/human-genome-project.

genome.gov/research-at-nhgri/Projects.

genetherapynet.com/types-of-gene-therapy.html.

eurostemcell.org/cord-blood-stem-cells-current-uses-and-future-challenges.

sciencedaily.com/news/health_medicine/stem_cells/.

Annotated recommended reading

Turnpenny, P.D., Ellard, S., 2017. Emery's Elements of Medical Genetics, fifteenth ed. Elsevier, London.

This book provides an excellent introduction to the complex subject of medical genetics. This subject continues to grow in importance with emerging advances evidenced by research-related activities. Interested readers will find clearly written text and good diagrams.

the-scientist.com.

This site provides current evidence-based information related to advances in life science and health.

cdc.gov/genomics.

This site provides current summaries of genomics and health impact information. Podcasts are available on genetic testing, disease and family health history.

genetherapynet.com/types-of-gene-therapy.html.

This information site about gene therapy provides current related activities and advances in this field.

4

The Female Reproductive System

LYNSAY MATTHEWS AND JEAN RANKIN

CHAPTER CONTENTS

This chapter details the anatomy of the female reproductive tract and the cyclical control of reproduction. It is crucial for students and midwives to have sound knowledge and understanding of the anatomy and physiology of the female reproductive organs and ovarian cycle. This fundamental knowledge is essential for their everyday practice and the care of women during pregnancy, childbirth and the puerperium.

Introduction

The female reproductive tract has the significant responsibility to carry, nurture and produce the offspring of sexual reproduction. In humans, this process involves the fusion of sex cells, known as **gametes.** Male and female gametes are known as **spermatozoa** and **oocytes** (or **ova**), respectively. Before the seventh week of gestation, there is no anatomical difference between male and female embryos. Two pairs of genital ducts are present: the **paramesonephric** or **Müllerian** (which develop into female genitalia) and the **mesonephric** or **Wolffian** ducts (which develop into male genitalia). If the embryo is XX, ovaries will form and the female ducts develop into female genitalia. If the embryo is XY, the presence of the *SRY* gene (sex-determining region Y) leads to formation of the testes and Sertoli cells (Johnson, 2018) (Chapter 5).

Anatomy of the Female Reproductive Tract

The soft tissues forming the organs of the female internal genitalia are situated in the pelvic cavity. Although the organs are separate structures, they form a continuous tract. The female reproductive tract is presented in Fig. 4.1. The organs include the vagina, uterus and cervix, uterine tubes and ovaries. The external genitalia are known as the *vulva.* Removal and/or injury to the external genitalia for non-medical reasons is known as **female genital mutilation (FGM)** (Box 4.1).

The Vulva

The vulva is formed by the labia majora, labia minora, clitoris, clitoral bulbs, mons veneris (mons pubis), vestibule and the greater vestibular glands (Bartholin glands) (Fig. 4.2).

The Labia Majora

The labia majora are two folds containing sebaceous and sweat glands embedded in adipose and connective tissue. They are covered with skin and form the lateral boundaries of the vulval cleft. The labia are homologues of the male scrotum. The labia unite anteriorly to form the **mons veneris** (mons pubis), an adipose pad over the symphysis pubis. The labia majora unite posteriorly to form the **posterior commissure.**

The Labia Minora

The labia minora are two delicate folds of skin containing some sebaceous glands. On the medial aspect, keratinized skin epithelium changes to squamous epithelium. Anteriorly, the labia minora are split into two parts. One passes over the clitoris to form its **prepuce** and the other passes beneath the clitoris to form a homologue of the frenulum in the male. Posteriorly, the two labia minora unite to form the **fourchette.**

The Clitoris

The clitoris is the homologue of the male penis. It is composed of erectile tissue and can enlarge and stiffen during sexual excitement. Only the **glans** and **prepuce** are normally visible, but the **corpus** can be palpated as a cord-like structure along the lower surface of the symphysis pubis.

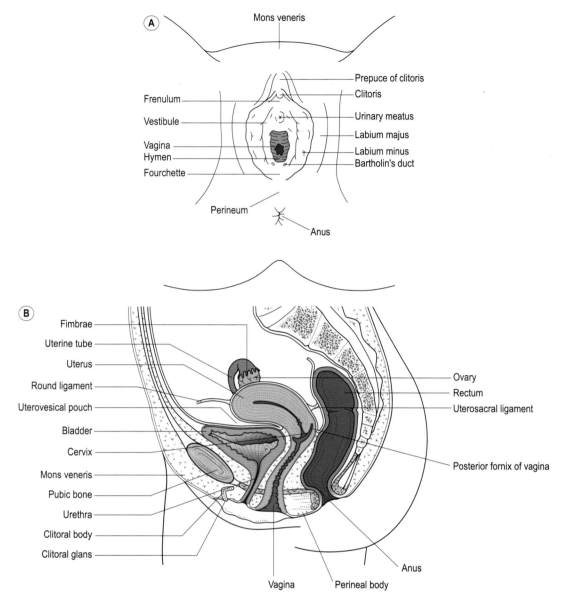

• **Fig. 4.1** The (A) female external genitalia and (B) female internal reproductive organs.

The Vestibule

The vestibule is the cleft between the labia minora into which the opening for both the urethra (urethral meatus) and vagina (vaginal orifice or introitus) are found.

Bartholin Glands

The **Bartholin glands** (the greater vestibular glands) are two pea-sized glands that are connected to the vestibule by ducts that are 2 cm long. These glands are homologues of **Cowper glands** in males. The ducts are lined with columnar epithelium which produce a mucoid secretion for lubrication during coitus.

Blood Supply

The vulva is highly vascular, receiving arterial supply from the internal pudendal arteries (branches of the internal iliac arteries) and the external pudendal arteries (branches of the femoral arteries). Venous drainage is usually by a plexus of veins which

drain into the internal iliac veins. The clitoris also has a plexus of veins which join the vaginal and vesical venous plexi.

Lymphatic Drainage

Lymphatic vessels form an interconnecting meshwork through the labia minora, prepuce, fourchette and vaginal introitus (orifice). These drain into the superficial and deep femoral nodes and the internal iliac nodes.

Nerve supply

Branches of the pudendal nerve and perineal nerve supply the vulval structures.

The Vagina

The vagina is a fibromuscular canal extending from the vulva to the uterus. The walls are normally in apposition.

The widest diameter of the vagina is anteroposterior in the lower one-third and transverse in the upper two-thirds. **This is important to remember when inserting vaginal speculae.** It runs upwards and backwards from the vestibule at

85% to the horizontal, which is parallel to the plane of the pelvic brim when the woman is standing erect.

The posterior wall ends blindly to form the vault of the vagina and is approximately 9 cm long. The anterior wall is shorter, 7 cm in length, due to the angle of the cervix. This cervical projection divides the vault of the vagina into four fornices, shallow anterior and lateral fornices and a more spacious posterior fornix. The walls of the vagina fall into transverse folds, or **rugae,** to allow for distension.

The entrance to the vagina is partially covered by the membranous **hymen** which has a few perforations to allow menstrual flow. This membrane varies in elasticity and is usually torn at the first coitus and more so at the first birth. Sometimes these perforations are absent (imperforate hymen) which can be a possible cause of failure to menstruate. Once ruptured, remnants are left called **carunculae myrtiformes.**

Layers of the Vagina

The vagina has three layers, including:
- An inner lining of stratified squamous non-keratinized epithelium. This is 10–30 cells deep and is continuous with the epithelium of the infravaginal cervix. The cells are divided into three layers, derived from the basement membrane and changing as they near the surface. These are the **parabasal cells, intermediate cells** and **superficial cells.**
- A middle layer of involuntary smooth muscle. The vagina varies in size, mainly caused by muscle tone and contraction in the pelvic floor muscles which are under voluntary control.
- An outer layer of vascular connective tissue containing elastic tissue, nerves and lymphatic and blood vessels.

The vaginal epithelium changes with the ovarian and menstrual cycles. There is further development and differentiation during pregnancy in response to circulating **oestrogens, progesterone** and **androgens.** The vaginal epithelium does not secrete mucus, but cervical secretions seep between the cells to moisten the vagina. Some cells contain glycogen which is metabolized by **Döderlein's bacillus,** producing lactic acid as a waste product. This results in a normal vaginal acid medium of pH 4.5, preventing pathogenic

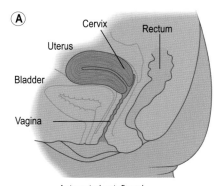

Anteverted anteflexed

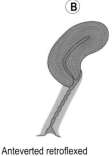

Anteverted retroflexed

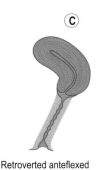

Retroverted anteflexed

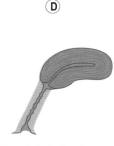

Retroverted retroflexed

● **Fig. 4.2** The anteverted and anteflexed position of the non-pregnant uterus. (A) normal position and (B–D) abnormal positions.

organisms from invading. The cells can also absorb drugs, particularly oestrogens.

Relations

- Anterior wall: urethra and base of bladder.
- Posterior wall: in close proximity to the anal canal, rectum and pouch of Douglas (a pouch of peritoneum).
- Lateral walls: pelvic connective tissue, **levatores ani** and the **bulbocavernousus muscle.**

Blood Supply

Arterial supply is from the vaginal and uterine arteries, which are both branches of the internal iliac artery. Venous drainage is by rich venous plexi in the muscular layer which drain to the internal iliac vein.

Nerve Supply

Nerve supply to voluntary vaginal muscle is via the pudendal nerve.

Vaginal Functions

- Escape of menstrual blood flow.
- Coitus with entry of the male penis.
- Birth of the fetus, placenta and membranes.

The Non-Pregnant Uterus

The uterus develops from fusion of the two embryonic Müllerian ducts (Johnson, 2018). It is a thick-walled, muscular, hollow, pear-shaped organ flattened in its anteroposterior diameter. Its lower third forms the cervix which projects into the vault of the vagina through its anterior wall. The uterus lies in the pelvic cavity in an **anteverted** (leans forward) and **anteflexed** (bent forward) position (Fig. 4.2). Its normal measurements are shown in Table 4.1.

Structure

The uterus (Fig. 4.3) consists of the body, which is 5 cm long, the narrow **isthmus** (0.5 cm long) and the cervix (2.5 cm long). The fundus is the area above and between the **uterine tubes** (Fallopian tubes), and the junction between each uterine tube and the uterus is called the **cornu** (plural cornua). A constriction at the upper end of the isthmus is called the **anatomical internal os,** and where the

TABLE 4.1	Measurements of the Non-pregnant Uterus	
Dimension	**Measurement**
Length, including cervix	7.5 cm
Breadth	5.0 cm
Depth	2.5 cm
Average thickness of walls	1.5 cm
Weight	60 g

endometrium meets the columnar cervical epithelium is called the **histological internal os.** The cavity has a triangular shape when viewed in coronal section and has a capacity of about 10 mL.

Although the cervix is continuous with and part of the uterus, it differs in its structure and function from the body of the uterus and will be described separately. The cervix is barrel-shaped and penetrated by the cervical canal. It is 2.5 cm long and separated from the body of the uterus by the isthmus. It is divided into two equal parts:

1. The **supravaginal cervix** lies above the vaginal vault and is surrounded by pelvic fascia, the **parametrium,** except posteriorly where it is in apposition with the **pouch of Douglas.**
2. The cone-shaped **infravaginal cervix** projects into the vagina and is covered by stratified squamous epithelium, continuous with the vaginal epithelium. It joins the columnar epithelium of the cervical canal at the external os, a site called the **squamocolumnar junction.** In some women the squamocolumnar junction may develop changes in what is known as the **transformation zone** that lead to cervical carcinoma (Tambouret & Wilbur, 2014). Early recognition of precancerous changes by cervical screening allows for life-saving surgical treatment.

Lining of the Uterus (Corpus)

The mucous lining, or **endometrium,** builds up from a layer of basal cells. It consists of **stroma** (connective tissue component of an organ) covered by a layer of ciliated cuboid cells. This layer dips down into the stroma to form mucus-secreting tubular cells opening into the uterine cavity (Fig. 4.4). The thickness varies depending on the phase of the menstrual cycle and is thinnest at the isthmus.

Lining of the Cervix

The spindle-shaped cervical canal connects the uterine cavity at the internal os with the vagina at the external os. The canal is lined by columnar mucus-secreting epithelium thrown into anterior and posterior folds from which circular folds radiate like branches from a tree trunk (the arbour vitae, or tree of life). The epithelium dips into the stroma in a complex system of crypts and tunnels separated by ridges of stroma consisting of 80% collagen, 10% muscle fibres and 10% blood vessels. Compound racemose glands secrete cervical mucus that varies in quality and quantity under the influence of the sex hormones.

Muscle Layer

The muscle layer, or **myometrium,** is made up of bundles of smooth muscle fibres. The outer longitudinal layer and the inner circular layer are not well developed in the non-pregnant uterus with most fibres running obliquely and interlacing surrounding blood vessels and lymphatic vessels. The proportion of muscle begins to diminish in the isthmus, being replaced by connective tissue until it reaches the 10% muscle content of the cervix.

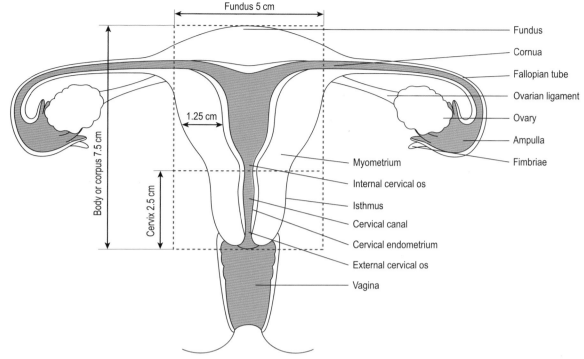

• **Fig. 4.3** The uterus, uterine tubes and ovaries.

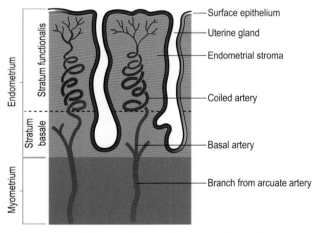

• **Fig. 4.4** The vascular supply to the endometrium.

Peritoneal Layer

The peritoneal layer is a double serosal layer known as the **perimetrium.** It covers the anterior and posterior surfaces but is absent from the narrow lateral surfaces. It is reflected off the uterus onto the superior surface of the bladder at the level of the anatomical internal os; **this is important for understanding the technique of lower segment caesarean section.**

Relations

- Anterior: uterovesical pouch and bladder.
- Posterior: pouch of Douglas and rectum.
- Lateral: broad ligaments, uterine tubes and ovaries.

- Superior: intestines.
- Inferior: vagina.

Supports

Four pairs of ligaments support the uterus: three pairs support its position in relation to the vagina (**cardinal**, also known as **transverse**, **pubocervical** and **uterosacral ligaments**) (Fig. 4.5) and one pair maintains uterine anteversion and anteflexion (the **round ligaments**) (Fig. 4.6) (Table 4.2). The **broad ligaments** are not true ligaments but thickened folds of peritoneum running from the uterus to the side walls of the pelvis.

Blood Supply

The blood supply to the uterus is complex and rich and is contributed to by both the **ovarian** and the **uterine** arteries (Fig. 4.7). The uterine artery, which is a branch of the internal iliac artery, enters at the level of the internal os and sends a small branch downwards to join the vaginal arteries in supplying the cervix and the vault of the vagina. The main branch of the uterine artery turns upwards and takes a tortuous path to anastomose (connect) with the ovarian artery which enters the broad ligament to supply the ovaries and uterine tubes. Anterior and posterior divisions anastomose with the opposite side of the uterus. Branches leaving these vessels at right angles supply blood to the myometrium; they enter the endometrium as the **basal arteries** (Fig. 4.4 and 4.8).

Venous Drainage

This is by the uterine and ovarian veins which then drain into the internal iliac arteries.

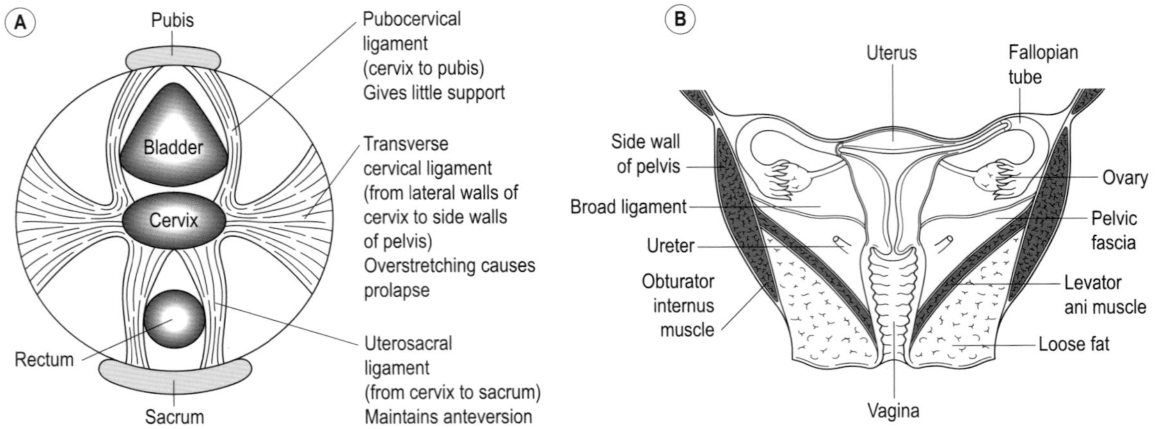

• **Fig. 4.5** The uterine ligaments. (A) Transverse and (B) coronal sections.

Lymphatic Drainage

Good lymphatic drainage of the uterus protects against uterine infection, especially after birth. There are three communicating networks of vessels and small nodes at the level of the endometrium, myometrium and subperitoneal layer of the uterus. The lymph is collected into major ducts and taken to lumbar and sacral nodes centrally and to inguinal, internal and external iliac nodes laterally.

Nerve Supply

The body of the uterus is supplied by autonomic nerves originating in the thoracic 11 and 12 and lumbar 1 vertebrae. Sensation from the body of the uterus is perceived as pain in response to stretch, infection and contraction. The cervix is innervated by the sacral plexus from sacral 2, 3 and 4 vertebral nerves. These pass through the **transcervical** or **Lee-Frankenhäuser nerve plexi.** Pain from the cervix is felt in response to rapid dilatation.

Functions of the Uterus

- To receive the fertilized ovum.
- To nurture and protect the developing embryo and fetus.
- To expel the fetus, placenta and membranes.

The Uterine Tubes (Fallopian Tubes)

The **uterine tubes** develop from the right and left embryonic Müllerian ducts. They are two small, muscular, hollow tubes 10 cm long. Each tube extends from a uterine cornu and travels to the side walls of the pelvis, turning downwards and backwards before reaching them. The tubes lie within the broad ligament and communicate with the uterus at their medial end and with the ovaries at their lateral end. There is a direct pathway between the vagina and the peritoneal cavity, thus a risk of entry of an ascending infection.

Structure

Each uterine tube is divided into four sections:
- The **interstitial part** is the narrowest part of the tube. Its lumen is only 1 mm in diameter and it runs within the uterine wall.
- The **isthmus** is a straight, narrow, thick section extending 2.5 cm laterally from the uterine wall.
- The **ampulla** is the longest and widest section. It extends 5 cm from the isthmus to the side walls of the pelvis. Its lumen is tortuous, relatively thin and distensible.
- The **infundibulum** or **fimbriated portion** is trumpet-shaped and ends in fimbriae or finger-like processes. It is the lateral 2.5 cm of the tube which turn downwards and backwards. Although the fimbriae have little or no contact with the ovary, they become very active during ovulation and sweep the ovarian surface.

The three layers of each uterine tube are:
1. An inner epithelial layer of cuboid cells arranged in **plicae** (folds), most pronounced in the ampulla. The complexity of the folds and the diameter of the lumen increase from the interstitial portion to the infundibular portion. Many cuboid cells are ciliated, whereas others are goblet cells and secrete mucus.
2. Involuntary muscle fibres in two layers, inner circular and outer longitudinal, make up the middle wall. These undergo peristaltic contractions during ovulation.
3. An outer covering of peritoneum on the superior, anterior and posterior surfaces but not on the inferior surface.

Relations

- Anterior, posterior and superior: the peritoneal cavity and intestines.
- Lateral: the side walls of the pelvis.
- Inferior: the broad ligaments and ovaries.
- Medial: the uterus.

Supports

The uterine tubes are held in position by their attachment to the uterus and broad ligaments.

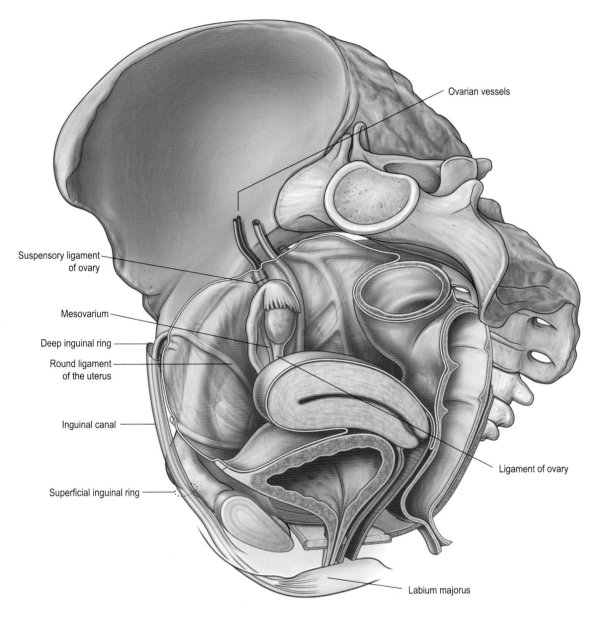

Ovarian vessels

Suspensory ligament
of ovary

Mesovarium

Deep inguinal ring

Round ligament
of the uterus

Inguinal canal

Superficial inguinal ring

Ligament of ovary

Labium majorus

• **Fig. 4.6** The uterus and broad ligament.

TABLE 4.2	**Ligaments Supporting the Uterus**	
Ligament	**Origin**	**Insertion**
Cardinal ligaments	Cervix	Side walls of pelvis
Pubocervical ligaments	Cervix	Under bladder to the pubic bones
Uterosacral ligaments	Cervix	Sacrum
Round ligaments	Cornua	Via inguinal canal to labia majora

Blood Supply, Lymphatic Drainage And Nerve Supply

These are shared with the ovaries and are described later.

Functions

- Mucus, cilia and peristaltic movements move the ovum towards the uterus.
- Fertilization normally takes place within the ampulla.
- The mucus secreted by the uterine tubes may provide nourishment for the ovum.

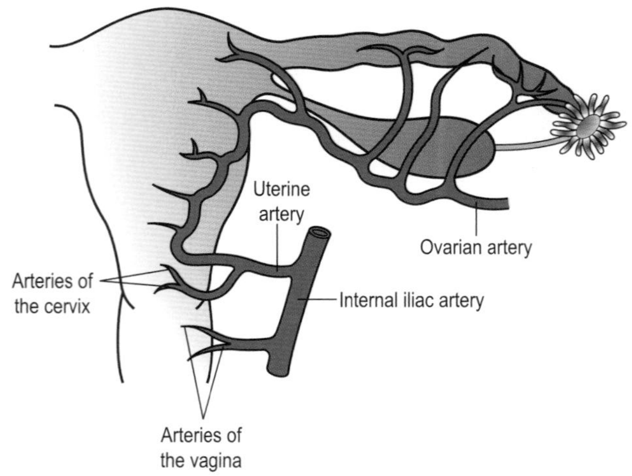

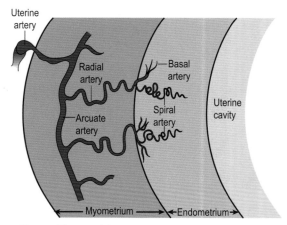

• **Fig. 4.7** The blood supply to the uterus and its appendages.

• **Fig. 4.8** The arterial supply to the uterine endometrium.

The Ovary

The two ovaries develop from the **embryonic gonadal ridges.** Undifferentiated primitive germ cells that began life on the wall of the yolk sac migrate into the gonadal ridges using amoebic movements at 6 weeks of embryological development. The female ovary is recognizable slightly later than the male testis, at about 10 weeks.

The mature ovaries consist of **interstitial tissue** and **follicles.** They are small almond-shaped glands measuring 3 cm × 2 cm × 1 cm and weighing just 6 g with a dull, pinkish-grey, uneven external appearance. They lie in a shallow peritoneal fossa adjacent to the lateral pelvic wall, outside the posterior layer of the broad ligaments and inside the peritoneum. The long axis of each ovary is in the vertical plane, but the position is influenced by movements of the uterus and broad ligament. If the uterus is retroverted, they may lie in the pouch of Douglas and cause pain during coitus. The uterine tubes arch over the ovaries. The ovaries produce progesterone and three types of oestrogen; the most potent is **oestradiol,** with **oestrone** second and **oestriol** third.

Macroscopic Structure

- The **medulla** is the inner part of the ovary which is directly attached to the broad ligament by the **mesovarium.** It consists of fibrous tissue containing blood vessels, lymphatics and nerves carried by the infundibulopelvic ligament.
- The **cortex** is the functional part of the ovary and consists of highly vascular stroma in which ovarian follicles are embedded.
- The **tunica albuginea** is a tough fibrous capsule forming the outer part of the cortex.
- The **germinal layer** consists of cuboid cells developed from modified peritoneum and is continuous with the broad ligament. It forms an outer covering for the ovary.

Microscopic Structure—The Follicles

Tiny sac-like structures called **ovarian follicles** at different stages of maturation are embedded in the ovarian cortex. These stages of maturation (Fig. 4.9) are brought about by neurohormonal changes. The **primordial follicle** contains an immature egg encased in a single layer of squamous-like follicle cells. These cells stay in a state of arrested development at the first **meiotic prophase** and will not complete their development until they are prepared for ovulation (Johnson, 2018).

Over 2 million primordial follicles are present in the fetal ovary before birth. No more are produced after birth. By the menarche only 200,000 remain. Only 300–400 will be shed at ovulation. It is not yet understood why these cells behave in this unusual way.

Development of the Mature Follicle

Each day a few primordial follicles begin to develop, but how these are selected is unknown (Johnson, 2018). A developing primordial follicle passes through three stages:
- First it becomes a **primary follicle** or **preantral follicle,** surrounded by two or more layers of cuboidal **granulosa cells.**
- It then becomes a **secondary follicle** or **antral follicle** (Graafian follicle).
- Finally it becomes a **preovulatory follicle.**

The granulosa and theca cells proliferate and differentiate, and the oocyte increases in size by a factor of 300. The granulosa cells divide to become several layers thick, and gap junctions develop, which allow easy transfer of molecules between cells. Secretion of fluid droplets leads to the formation of a single fluid-filled space called the **antrum** which separates the granulosa cells into distinct layers.

As the follicle continues to grow, the mature oocyte, surrounded by a dense mass of granulosa cells called the **cumulus oophorus,** becomes suspended in fluid called the **liquor folliculi.** It is attached to a stalk of granulosa cells which then breaks away and floats freely in the fluid. The follicle bulges out from the surface of the ovary. The theca cells differentiate into the **theca interna,** a highly vascularized glandular layer, and the **theca externa,** the dense, fibrous outer

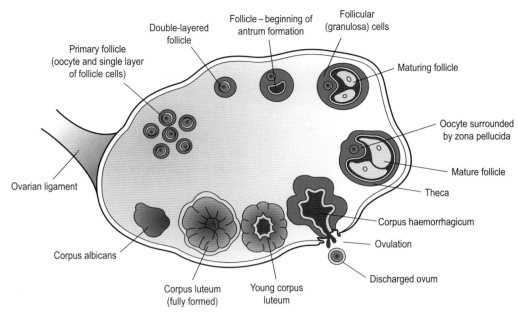

• **Fig. 4.9** Diagrammatic section of an ovary showing stages of follicular maturation.

capsule of the follicle. Glycoproteins secreted from the cell surface of the oocytes form a translucent layer called the **zona pellucida.**

Each month about 12 growing follicles emerge from the primordial follicles. One or occasionally more of the ripe follicles mature and rupture and the oocyte(s) escapes. After ovulation the ruptured follicle is transformed into a structure called the **corpus luteum** (yellow body) which, in the absence of a pregnancy, will degenerate in about 6 months into a **corpus albicans** (white body).

Relations

- Anterior: the broad ligaments.
- Posterior: the intestines.
- Lateral: the infundibulopelvic ligaments and the side walls of the pelvis.
- Superior: the uterine tubes.
- Medial: the uterus and ovarian ligament.

Supports

The ovary is held suspended in position:
- To the uterus by the ovarian ligament.
- To the posterior surface of the broad ligament by the mesovarium.
- To the side walls of the pelvis by the suspensory or infundibulopelvic ligament.

Blood Supply

The two long, slender ovarian arteries arise high up on the aorta. Each ovarian artery crosses over the pelvic brim laterally and enters the broad ligament where branches supply the uterine tube and the ovary. Each then anastomoses with its uterine artery to form the uterine blood supply. The right ovarian vein drains directly into the inferior vena cava, whereas the left ovarian vein first joins the left renal vein before draining into the inferior vena cava.

Lymphatic Drainage

Lymphatic drainage is into the lumbar glands.

Nerve Supply

The nerve supply of the ovary is well developed via the ovarian plexus. Sympathetic fibres and sensory nerves from the ovary run with the arteries to be relayed to the 10th thoracic segment of the spinal cord. The ovaries, like the testes, are extremely sensitive organs if handled or squeezed.

Functions of the Ovary

1. To produce ova.
2. To produce the female steroid hormones oestrogen and progesterone.

Cyclical Control of Reproduction

The organs of the female reproductive system prepare themselves for ovulation, fertilization and implantation via the interaction of two simultaneous hormonal cycles. These are the **ovarian cycle** (where the ovaries prepare an oocyte for ovulation) and the **menstrual cycle** where the uterus prepares for implantation of a fertilized ovum.

The cyclical changes that occur are an integrated process, but they can be discussed individually to achieve understanding. The following aspects will be considered:
1. The ovarian cycle.
2. The menstrual cycle.
3. Changes in other tissues.

The Ovarian Cycle

The ovarian cycle consists of two individual phases, known as the **follicular** phase and the **luteal** phase (outlined in Table 4.3). The average ovarian cycle lasts 28 days with ovulation on day 14. However, the cycle shows considerable variation in an individual woman and between women. It is usually the duration of the follicular phase leading up to ovulation that is variable. The cycle is responsive to stress, disease, allergies, physical activity and nutritional deficiencies.

The rhythm of the ovarian cycle and menstrual cycle is controlled by the **hypothalamus** and the **anterior pituitary gland** (Fig. 4.10). At least five groups of hormone-producing cells are found in the anterior lobe of the pituitary. Those concerned with reproduction include:

- Follicle-stimulating hormone (FSH).
- Luteinizing hormone (LH).
- Adrenocorticotrophic hormone.
- Prolactin.

Their function is regulated by neuronal substances from the hypothalamus (Moore, Persaud & Torchia, 2019). In particular, **gonadotrophin-releasing factor** (GnRH), released by the hypothalamus, is transferred to the anterior pituitary gland where it causes the release of the gonadotrophins FSH and LH.

The Ovary

Plasma levels of **oestrogen** and **progesterone** rise, reducing the production of GnRH in a negative-feedback mechanism. If pregnancy does not occur, the corpus luteum degenerates; FSH and LH therefore begin to rise on day 1 of the cycle and steadily increase towards the late follicular phase.

Ovulation is dependent upon a mid-cycle surge of LH and FSH. Although plasma levels of both hormones rise, the level of LH is higher and appears to be more important in causing ovulation. Ovulation occurs 24 hours after the surge. The capsule stretches and bursts, the follicle ruptures and the ovum is flushed into the abdominal cavity where it is picked up by the fimbriae of the uterine tubes. These waft the ovum into the **tubal ampulla** to await fertilization. Some women feel a pain at this time called **mittelschmerz.** The follicle now collapses to become the corpus luteum. If there is no pregnancy, the corpus luteum begins to regress after 14 days and production of oestrogen and progesterone declines rapidly. When plasma levels of these hormones become low enough, the anterior pituitary begins to produce FSH and LH and the cycle begins again.

Generally a single ovum is released in each cycle and the others that have begun developing regress to become **corpora atretica. Multiple pregnancy** can occur when more than one follicle develops simultaneously. The frequency of multiple ovulation increases with age and in Black women.

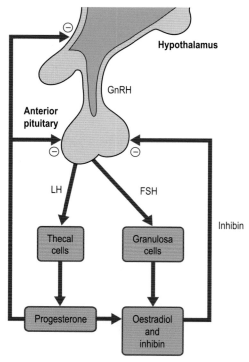

• **Fig. 4.10** Hormonal regulation of the menstrual cycle.

TABLE 4.3	**Phases of the Female Reproductive Cycle**	
Phase	**Timing**	**Characteristics**
Follicular phase	Ovarian cycle Day 1–14	The follicle in the ovary matures. This phase ends with ovulation.
Luteal phase	Ovarian cycle Day 15–28	This phase begins straight after ovulation and ends with menstruation.
Menstrual phase	Menstrual cycle Day 1–5	In the absence of pregnancy, the endometrium breaks down and results in menstruation.
Proliferative phase	Menstrual cycle Day 6–14	The lining of the uterus prepares for the next menstrual cycle by regrowth of the endometrial wall.
Secretory phase	Menstrual cycle Day 15–28	The corpus luteum secretes large amounts of progesterone, further preparing the endometrium for implantation.

Asian women are less likely than White women to have multiple ovulation.

Local Control of Growth and Development of the Oocytes

Local activities occur within the follicle for its growth and development. Some are carried out by theca cells, some by granulosa cells and some involve cooperation between both.

Oestrogen and Progesterone

During follicle development, LH stimulates the theca cells to produce **androstenedione** and **testosterone**. These are transported to the granulosa cells to be converted to oestrogen, which causes proliferation of granulosa and theca cells and further growth of the follicles. The follicle that develops most rapidly may produce larger amounts of oestrogen. This may inhibit the release of FSH by negative feedback to the pituitary gland, preventing further growth of the remaining follicles. Growth of the dominant follicle results in the oestradiol surge that immediately precedes ovulation. Within 12 hours, progesterone takes over as the dominant hormone produced by the theca and granulosa cells.

Other Hormones Involved Locally

Research related to in vitro fertilization has identified that steroid hormones (i.e., oestrogen and progesterone), and some peptide hormones, have a major influence on follicular development. It is worth mentioning two: **inhibin** and **growth hormone** (GH).

Inhibin may be one of the factors that determine the number of follicles released at ovulation. The rise in concentration of inhibin in follicular fluid may be in response to the surge in GnRH from the hypothalamus (Yding Andersen et al., 1993). Inhibin also affects sperm production (see Chapter 5). GH may increase the intraovarian production of **insulin-like growth factor 1** which amplifies the response of the granulosa cells to gonadotrophins (Adashi et al., 1985).

Triggering of Ovulation

The actions of FSH and oestrogen combine to induce the development of LH receptors on the granulosa cells. This coincides with the FSH and LH surge from the anterior pituitary gland. Ovulation occurs 24 hours later. Ovulation is facilitated by the local release of **prostaglandin E$_2$** (PGE$_2$) and the vasodilatory substances **histamine** and **bradykinin.** PGE$_2$ initiates breakdown of the follicular wall, whereas histamine and bradykinin cause local inflammation.

The Menstrual (Endometrial) Cycle

The menstrual cycle (sometimes referred to as the *uterine cycle*) is divided into three phases: **menstrual, proliferative** and **secretory** phases (Fig. 4.11). The menstrual and proliferative phases coincide with the follicular phase of the ovarian cycle and the secretory with the luteal phase (outlined in Table 4.3). The changing levels and interactions between

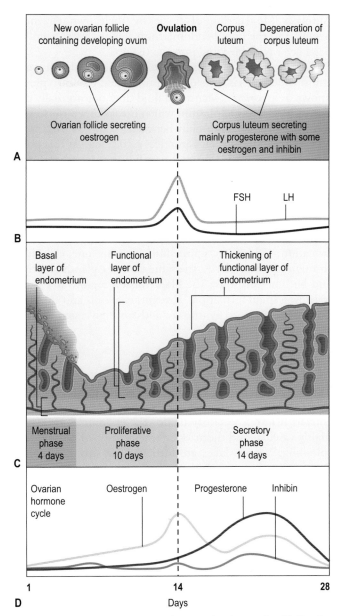

• **Fig. 4.11** Summary of one female reproductive cycle. (A) Ovarian cycle: maturation of follicle and development of corpus luteum. (B) Anterior pituitary cycle: luteinizing hormone (LH) and follicle-stimulating hormone (FSH) levels. (C) Uterine cycle: menstrual, proliferative and secretory phases. (D) Ovarian hormone cycle: oestrogen, progesterone and inhibin levels.

oestrogen and progesterone lead to alterations in endometrial tissue and selected tissues elsewhere. The endometrium is not totally dependent on ovarian hormones. It is itself an endocrine organ and secretes oestrogens, progesterone and prolactin.

Menstrual Phase—Days 1–5

As the corpus luteum degenerates, plasma progesterone, which has a shorter plasma half-life than oestrogen, falls more rapidly, changing the balance of the two hormones in favour of oestrogen. This causes the endometrium to become unstable. Fluid is lost from the tissues which shrink, compress the spiral arteries and cause endometrial anoxia.

Autolysis (destruction of tissue by their own enzymes) begins, and the upper endometrium sloughs away from the basal layer with bleeding into the tissues.

Oestrogen also increases the excitability of the myometrium which expels the sloughed tissue and blood (typically known as a 'period'). Menstrual fluid does not normally clot due to high levels of plasmin which breaks down fibrin as it forms. Blood loss is normally between 10 and 80 mL (mean of 35 mL) and an average iron loss of 0.5 mg. At this point the endometrium is thin and poorly vascularized and only the bases of the endometrial glands remain.

The Proliferative Phase—Days 6–14

Rising oestrogen levels cause rapid proliferation of stroma cells, and the endometrium thickens from 1 to 6 mm before ovulation. The outer epithelium remains one cell thick throughout the cycle. At the same time the glands lengthen and become tortuous. The blood vessels regrow and begin to show a spiral formation. The epithelial cells and the glandular cells begin to synthesize and store glycogen. At this point, ovulation occurs.

The Secretory Phase—Days 15–28

After ovulation the body prepares for a potential pregnancy. The corpus luteum secretes large amounts of progesterone which acts on the oestrogen-primed endometrium to convert it into a secretory tissue. The endometrium is now highly vascular and the arteries have developed pronounced spiralling. Venous lakes are formed. The stroma becomes even more oedematous, the cells themselves become larger and there is a further thickening of the endometrium to 6 mm. The endometrial glands secrete glycogen. The endometrial surface becomes folded and prepared for implantation, which occurs 7 days after ovulation. It is completed at 14 days after ovulation. In the absence of pregnancy, the next menstrual cycle would then begin.

Non-endometrial Sites of Hormone Action

The Myometrium

Excitability of the myometrium is dependent on the balance between progesterone and oestrogen. An increase in oestrogen brings about cyclical changes in the thickness of the myometrium and in muscle excitability. It stimulates spontaneous contractions. High levels of oestrogen also increase myometrial response to oxytocin. In contrast, progesterone reduces excitability.

The Cervix

The mucus secreted by the cervical glands during the follicular phase is watery and opaque, whereas that secreted after ovulation is thicker and clearer. Mucus secreted at the time of ovulation will crystallize in a fern-like pattern if left to dry on a glass slide.

The Vagina

During the follicular phase the cells of the vaginal epithelium are large and flat with an acidophilic cytoplasm. During the luteal phase they become polygonal and more basophilic. There is an increase in the glycogen content of the vagina, due partly to the secretory activity of the endometrium and partly to activity of the vaginal epithelial cells. Lactobacilli present in the vagina metabolize the glycogen to lactic acid, lowering the pH of the vagina from 6.5 during the follicular phase to pH of 4.5 in the luteal phase. This reduction in pH protects against infection.

The Uterine Tubes

During the follicular phase there is an increase in the number of ciliated cells. There is also an increase in the frequency and co-ordination of the peristaltic contractions of the muscle, reaching a maximum at the time of ovulation. Subsequently, the tubes become more inactive under the influence of progesterone.

Other Actions

Oestrogen causes:
- Development of the typical female shape.
- Growth of the breasts and nipples.
- Development of the adult reproductive organs.
- Control of FSH production by feedback mechanism.
- Maintenance of bone density.
- Reduction of capillary fragility.
- Increase in the ability of the cardiovascular system to withstand high blood pressures.
  Progesterone causes:
- Development of the secretory endometrium.
- Development of alveolar breast tissue before menstruation.
- Increase of the body temperature by 0.5°C after ovulation.
- Reduction of anxiety.
- Interaction with aldosterone receptors to cause retention of sodium and water.
  (Johnson, 2018)

Main Points

- There is no evidence of sexual difference between male and female embryos before the seventh week of gestation.
- The continuous tract of the female genitalia has a direct opening into the peritoneal cavity from the external environment. This is necessary for fertilization but increases the risk of pelvic infections.
- The vagina extends from the vulva to the uterus and is lined with stratified, squamous non-keratinized epithelium.

- The vagina has an acidic pH of 4.5 to prevent growth of pathogenic organisms.
- Endometrial thickness depends on the phase of the menstrual cycle.
- The cervix is divided into the supravaginal cervix and the infravaginal cervix.
- In some women the squamocolumnar junction may develop changes that lead to cervical carcinoma. Early

recognition by screening of precancerous changes allows for life-saving surgical treatment.

- The uterus receives the fertilized ovum, nurtures and protects the developing fetus and expels the fetus, placenta and membranes.
- The uterine tubes communicate with the uterus at their medial ends and the ovaries at their lateral ends.
- The ovaries consist of a medulla, cortex, tunica albuginea and germinal layer and produce ova and the female steroid hormones oestrogen and progesterone.
- The ovarian capsule stretches until it bursts, and the ovum is expelled into the abdominal cavity to be picked up by the fimbriae of the uterine tube.

- The average ovarian cycle lasts 28 days with ovulation on day 14. The control of the ovarian and menstrual cycles is via the hypothalamus and anterior pituitary gland.
- The menstrual and proliferative phases of the menstrual cycle coincide with the follicular phase of the ovarian cycle and the secretory phase with the luteal phase.
- Steroid hormones also affect the myometrium, cervix, vagina, uterine tubes and development of secondary sexual characteristics.
- The widest diameter of the vagina is anteroposterior in the lower one-third and transverse in the upper two-thirds, which is important to remember when inserting vaginal speculae.

References

Adashi, E.Y., Resnick, C.E., D'Ercole, A.J., Svoboda, M.E., Van Wyk, J.J., 1985. Insulin-like growth factors as intra-ovarian regulators of granulosa cell growth and function. Endocr. Rev. 6 (3), 400–420.

Johnson, M.H., 2018. Essential Reproduction, eighth ed. Wiley-Blackwell, Oxford.

Jones, L., Costello, B., Danks, E., Jolly, K., Cross-Sudworth, F., Latthe, P., et al., 2022. Views of female genital mutilation survivors, men and healthcare professionals on timing of deinfibulation surgery and NHS service provision: qualitative FGM Sister Study. Health Technol. Assess. 27 (3), 1–113.

Moore, K., Persaud, T.V.N., Torchia, M., 2019. The Developing Human, eleventh ed. Elsevier, London.

Okusanya, B.O., Oduwole, O., Nwachuku, N., Meremikwu, M.M., 2017. Deinfibulation for preventing or treating complications in women living with type III female genital mutilation: a systematic review and meta-analysis. Int. J. Gynaecol. Obstet. 136 (Suppl. 1), 13–20.

Tambouret, R.H., Wilbur, D.C., 2014. Glandular Lesions of the Uterine Cervix: Cytopathology with Histologic Correlates. Springer, New York.

United Nations Children's Fund (UNICEF), 2016. Female Genital Mutilation/Cutting: A Global Concern, 2016. Available at: https://www.unicef.org/reports/female-genital-mutilation-cutting.

World Health Organization, 2016. Female Genital Mutilation. Available at: http://who.int/mediacentre/factsheets/fs241/en/.

World Health Organization, 2023. Sexual and Reproductive Health: Types of Female Genital Mutilation. Available at: www.who.int/news-room/fact-sheets/detail/female-genital-mutilation.

Yding Andersen, C., Westergaard, L.G., Figenschau, Y., Bertheussen, K., Forsdahl, F., 1993. Endocrine composition of follicular fluid comparing human chorionic gonadotrophin to a gonadotrophin-releasing hormone agonist for ovulation induction. Hum. Reprod. 8 (6), 840–843.

Annotated recommended reading

Bainbridge, D., 2009. The X in Sex: How the X Chromosome Controls Our Lives, second ed. Harvard University Press, Cambridge.

This is a highly readable, entertaining account of all you need to know about the X chromosome.

Coad, J., Pedley, K., Dunstall, M., 2019. Anatomy and Physiology for Midwives, fourth ed. Elsevier, London.

This book provides a comprehensive and detailed overview of anatomy and physiology of the reproductive system relevant to clinical practice.

5

The Male Reproductive System

LYNSAY MATTHEWS

This chapter details the anatomy and physiology of the male reproductive system. This includes the hormonal control of male reproductive function and the physiology of sexual intercourse.

Introduction

Many aspects of fertility and infertility depend on the general health and sexual health of both partners (World Health Organization, 2023). Health and lifestyle factors of the male partner become important when planning and offering preconception care to prospective parents.

Anatomy of the Male Reproductive System

The male genitalia are mainly outside the body cavity, a situation necessary for both production and transfer of **spermatozoa** (the male germ cell). The organs are the scrotum, testis, rete and epididymis, ductus deferens, seminal vesicles, prostate gland, bulbourethral glands and penis with the urethra (Fig. 5.1).

The Scrotum and Testes

Embryonic Development

As discussed in the introduction to Chapter 4, *SRY* (sex-determining region Y gene) activity on the Y chromosome converts the indifferent gonad to a testis. In the absence of *SRY*, the gonad develops into an ovary. It is an efficient process; hence there are few true **hermaphrodites** (individuals who have both testicular and ovarian tissue). Once the gonad is established, the *SRY* gene is switched off. However, further differentiation is undertaken by the testicular **Sertoli cells** (see later), which secrete **Müllerian inhibiting hormone** and remain active until puberty, and the **Leydig cells** (see later) of the testis, which produce testosterone from 13–15 weeks of gestation (Johnson, 2018).

In the embryo, the testes develop high up on the lumbar region of the abdominal cavity. In the last few months of fetal life they descend through the abdominal cavity, over the pelvic brim and down the inguinal canal into the scrotal sac outside the body cavity. This descent occurs under the influence of testosterone and is completed by birth in 98% of boys.

The Mature Testis

At maturity, each testis measures 4 cm long and 3 cm in diameter and is surrounded by two coats: the outer **tunica vaginalis,** which is derived from peritoneum, and the **tunica albuginea,** the inner fibrous capsule. One testis sits in each pocket of the **scrotal sac.** The scrotum is a thin-walled sac covered with hairy, rugose skin, which is highly vascularized with a large surface area.

The temperature of the testes is maintained at 2–3°C below that of the body core to facilitate spermatogenesis (the production of mature spermatozoa). In a cold environment the **scrotal muscle** (dartos muscle) wrinkles the scrotal skin and reduces the size of the sac, and the **cremaster muscle** contracts and lifts the testes nearer to the body. In contrast, relaxation of these muscles allows the testes to be held away from the body to facilitate cooling.

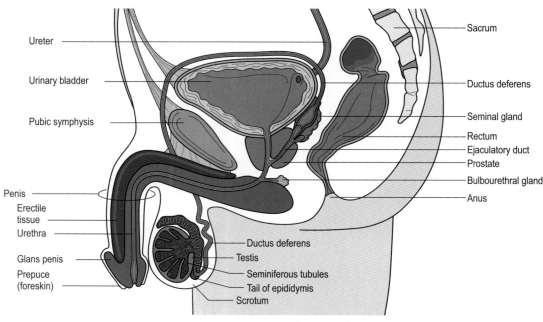

• **Fig 5.1** The male reproductive system.

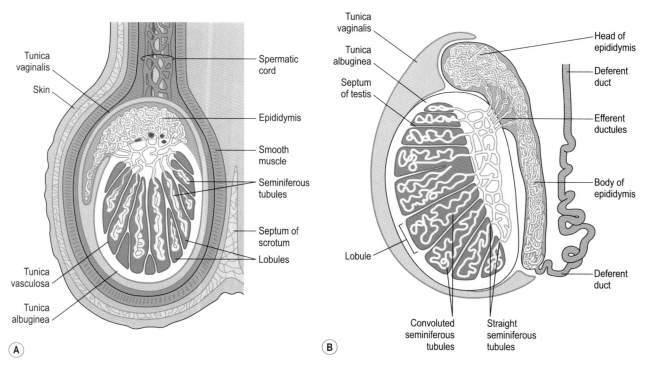

• **Fig. 5.2** The testis.

Structure

Each testis is divided into 200–300 wedge-shaped lobules by thin fibrous partitions that are extensions of the tunica albuginea (Fig. 5.2). Each lobule contains up to four **seminiferous tubules** which are highly coiled loops where the spermatozoa develop. They converge to form a straight tubule or **tubulus rectus.** This conveys the sperm into the **rete testis,** a tubular network on the posterior aspect of the testis. From here the sperm enter the **epididymis** which is in close apposition to the external surface of the testis. Macrophages that phagocytose dead sperm are found in the lumen of the epididymis. Interstitial tissue is packed around the **seminiferous tubules** and contains blood vessels and the **Leydig cells,** which secrete testosterone.

Blood Supply

The testes are supplied by the testicular arteries that arise from the abdominal aorta. The testicular veins form a network around the testicular artery called a **pampiniform**

plexus (tendril-like). This absorbs heat from the artery before the blood enters the testis.

Lymphatic Drainage
Lymphatic drainage is by the inguinal nodes.

Nerve Supply
There is both sympathetic and parasympathetic innervation by the autonomic system. There is also a rich sensory nerve supply, resulting in much pain and nausea if the testes are struck. The nerve fibres run with the blood vessels and lymphatics in the fibrous connective tissue sheath called the **spermatic cord.**

Function of the Testes
- To produce spermatozoa.
- To produce the hormones testosterone and inhibin.

Spermatogenesis (the Production of Spermatozoa)
Each testis consists of two separate compartments containing cells that produce sperm and those that produce hormones. There is a physical barrier, known as the **blood–testis barrier,** which limits free exchange of water-soluble materials. This barrier develops at puberty and is formed by multiple layers of gap and tight junctions surrounding each Sertoli cell (Johnson, 2018). Its functions are:
1. To prevent sperm from entering the systemic and lymphatic circulations where they could set up anti-sperm antibodies, leading to infertility.
2. To maintain distinct chemical environments on either side of the barrier to facilitate sperm development and health.

Sperm production occurs in the seminiferous tubules and has three phases:
1. Mitotic proliferation, which produces large numbers of cells. Seminiferous tubules contain two types of cells: germ cells and Sertoli cells. Primary germ cells are dormant from the fetal period of life and begin to increase in number at puberty. Germ cells originate from **spermatogonia.** Spermatogonia divide by mitosis continuously to ensure a constant supply of cells maturing towards sperm. After undergoing several mitotic divisions, they mature, become larger, and are known as **primary spermatocytes.** At this stage they are still **diploid** cells (i.e., they contain two complete sets of chromosomes, n = 46).
2. Meiotic division, which generates diversity and halves the chromosome number (haploid). Primary spermatocytes undergo the first meiotic division to form two secondary spermatocytes. They are now **haploid** cells (i.e., they contain one complete set of chromosomes, n = 23). Half of the secondary spermatocytes will receive the X chromosome and half the Y chromosome. Secondary meiosis results in four haploid cells called **spermatids.**
3. Cytodifferentiation, which packages the chromosomes for effective delivery.

Spermatids are found in close association with Sertoli cells. They provide nutrition and support to the sperm and are sometimes called **'nurse cells'.** Here the spermatids are transformed from basic cells into highly specialized sperm.

As a sperm matures, the chromatin of the nucleus condenses to become the head. One centriole develops into the tail, which is composed of a central filament of two microfibrils surrounded by a circle of nine fibrils. Mitochondria aggregate into the neck region, and the Golgi apparatus helps form the **acrosome cap.** This develops over the head of the sperm and contains enzymes called **hyaluronidases** and **proteases.**

The process takes about 70 days, and several hundred million sperm per day (about 400 per gram of testis per second) are produced continuously from puberty. As men age, the seminiferous tubules undergo involution, and extensive atrophy may be present by 70 years. The number of Sertoli cells remain the same, while germ cells reduce in number.

When sperm are fully formed, they are pushed along the duct system to the epididymis. The columnar epithelium of the epididymis is thought to secrete hormones, enzymes and nutrients to enable sperm maturation. Sperm can be stored in the epididymis for as long as 42 days.

The Duct System
The Epididymis
The **epididymis** is a comma-shaped, tightly coiled tube about 6 metres long. The head of the comma receives sperm from the efferent ductules of the testis. Here the sperm become more motile and fertile. However, they do not actively swim until ejaculated into the vagina. During ejaculation, the smooth muscle in the wall of the epididymis contracts strongly, expelling sperm from the tail portion into the ductus deferens.

The Vas (Ductus) Deferens
This muscular tube runs upwards from the epididymis, through the **inguinal canal** into the pelvic cavity. It can be felt where it passes over the pubic bone. Its terminus expands to form the ampulla and joins with the duct from the **seminal vesicle** to form the short **ejaculatory duct.** The two ejaculatory ducts pass into the **prostate gland** and empty into the **urethra.**

The wall of the **vas deferens** is composed of an outer layer of loose connective tissue and three layers of smooth muscle. The muscle undergoes rapid peristaltic contractions during ejaculation to pass the sperm forward. This movement is facilitated by the autonomic nerve supply. In the extra-abdominal portion, the ductus is accompanied by the **testicular artery,** the **pampiniform plexus** of veins, a nerve plexus, lymphatic vessels and the cremaster muscle. The whole complex is called the **spermatic cord.**

If no ejaculation occurs, sperm in the epididymis degenerate and phagocytic cells remove them. Vasectomy, or male sterilization, involves ligating and cutting the vas deferens. A man can still ejaculate (due to the presence of accessory gland fluids), but the operation prevents sperm from entering the ejaculate. Fertility may remain for 6–8 weeks because of viable sperm above the sectioned segment.

The Urethra

This is the terminal portion of the duct system and serves both urinary and reproductive systems. It is divided anatomically into three regions:

1. The prostatic urethra which exits from the bladder and is surrounded by the prostate gland.
2. The membranous urethra which passes through the urogenital diaphragm.
3. The spongy (penile) urethra which passes through the penis to exit at the external urethral meatus. The spongy urethra is about 15 cm long and is 75% of the total urethral length.

Accessory Glands

These include the paired seminal vesicles, the bulbourethral glands and the single prostate gland. They provide a transport medium, nutrients and the bulk of the ejaculate.

The Seminal Vesicles

The **seminal vesicles** lie behind the prostate gland and have the size and shape of fingers (i.e., 5–7 cm long). They have a capacity of 3 cm^3. They secrete an alkaline, sticky, yellowish fluid containing fructose, globulin, ascorbic acid and prostaglandins, accounting for 60% of the semen. Sperm and seminal fluid mix in the ejaculatory duct and enter the urethra together during ejaculation.

The Prostate Gland

The **prostate gland** is situated around the neck of the bladder and the first part of the urethra. It is about 3 cm in diameter in the normal adult and may involute or hypertrophy after middle age, resulting in urological problems. It produces a thin, acidic, milky fluid which contains enzymes, calcium and citrates. This fluid may act to stimulate motility in the sperm.

Semen

Semen is a milky-white, sticky fluid mixture of sperm and accessory gland secretions. It forms the transport medium and provides nutrients and chemicals to activate sperm. The **prostaglandins** in semen are thought to facilitate movement of sperm up the female reproductive tract by decreasing the viscosity of the cervical mucus and causing reverse peristalsis in the uterus. It is relatively alkaline with a pH of 7.2–7.6 which helps neutralize the acid medium of the vagina protecting the sperm and their motility.

Semen also contains a bacteriostatic chemical called **seminal plasmin** and clotting factors, including **fibrinogen,** which coagulate the semen shortly after it has been ejaculated. Once established in the vaginal vault, the **fibrinolysin** also contained in the semen causes it to liquefy so that the sperm can swim freely into the female duct system. The average ejaculate is about 3–6 mL and contains 60–200 million sperm.

The Bulbourethral (Cowper) Glands

These are tiny pea-sized glands below the prostate. They secrete thick, clear mucus that drains into the spongy urethra, acting as a lubricant before ejaculation.

The Penis

The **penis** normally hangs flaccidly from the perineum in front of the scrotum. It has an attached root and a free shaft that ends in an enlarged tip—the **glans penis.** Internally it has three long columns of erectile tissue (Fig. 5.3), consisting of two dorsal **corpora cavernosa** side by side and one **corpus spongiosum** containing the urethra. The erectile tissue is a spongy network of connective tissue and smooth muscle full of vascular spaces.

The root of the penis is broad and firmly fixed to the pubic rami by the proximal ends of the corpora cavernosa known as the **crus.** Each crus is surrounded by an **ischiocavernosus muscle.** The tip of the glans penis is perforated by the urethral meatus and is very well supplied by sensory nerve endings. It is the main male erogenous zone. In the resting state, the glans penis is covered by a folded cylinder of skin known as the **prepuce** or foreskin.

Hormonal Control of Male Reproductive Function

Male reproductive function is controlled by hormones from the hypothalamus, anterior pituitary lobe and testes. **Gonadotrophin-releasing hormone (GnRH)** from the hypothalamus influences the anterior pituitary to produce the same hormones as in the female: **follicle-stimulating hormone (FSH)** and **luteinizing hormone (LH).**

Actions of Luteinizing Hormone

LH acts on the interstitial tissue causing synthesis and release of testosterone. Plasma testosterone levels are directly related to plasma LH levels. Testosterone is an **anabolic androgenic steroid** molecule synthesized from cholesterol. Its functions are shown in Table 5.1.

Inhibin is a non-steroidal factor which may inhibit FSH secretion. It is possibly produced by the Sertoli cells and acts by a negative feedback loop.

Actions of Follicle-Stimulating Hormone

FSH binds to receptors (FSH-R) on Sertoli cells stimulated by the presence of androgens (Johnson, 2018). It seems to act on the later stages of sperm maturation and cannot initiate spermatogenesis in the absence of LH.

The Role of Prostaglandins in Reproduction

The group of chemical messengers known as the **prostaglandins** is active in multiple sites in the body and is involved

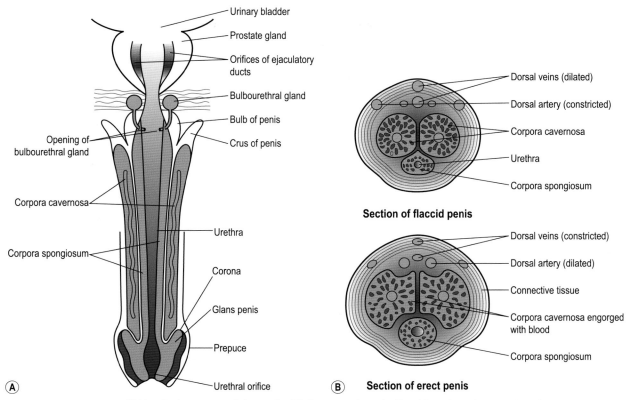

• **Fig. 5.3** (A) Detailed structure of the penis. (B) Cross-section of a flaccid penis and an erect penis.

TABLE 5.1   Functions of Testosterone

Action	Functions
Before birth	Masculinization of the reproductive tract and external genitalia Promotion of testicular descent
Sex-specific tissues	Growth and maturation at puberty Maintenance of reproductive tract throughout adult life Essential for spermatogenesis
Other reproductive effects	Increased libido and sex drive Control of gonadotrophic hormone secretion
Secondary sexual characteristics	Development of male distribution of body and facial hair Deepening of the voice due to thickening of the vocal cords and enlargement of the larynx
Other effects	Anabolic effect on protein production Growth of the long bones at puberty and fusion of epiphyses Increased secretion from sebaceous glands Possible role in aggressive behaviour

TABLE 5.2   Role of Prostaglandins in the Male and Female Reproductive Systems

- Promote sperm transport by causing smooth muscle contraction in male and female reproductive tracts.
- Increase uterine activity during menstruation.
- Play a role in ovulation by influencing follicular rupture.
- Mediate the renal vasodilation in pregnancy.
- Help prepare the cervix for labour by softening it.
- Probable mediation in the regulation of uterine contractions.

in many physiological processes (Table 5.2), including contraction and relaxation of smooth muscle, bronchodilation or bronchospasm, promotion of pain and inflammation and modulation of platelet aggregation. **Aspirin** is a prostaglandin inhibitor which is why it has so many pharmaceutical uses.

Prostaglandins are produced and act locally in the body. After they have acted, local enzymes rapidly inactivate them so that they do not gain access to the circulatory system. They are called prostaglandins because they were first isolated in semen and thought to be produced by the prostate gland.

The Physiology of Sexual Intercourse

In mammals, fertilization occurs internally; therefore sperm must be deposited inside the female body. In humans, there is significant psychological and social input to sexual behaviour, and arousal includes both cognitive and emotional factors. These are equally as important as the physiological aspects. Masters and Johnson (1966) described the classical response by both sexes as having four phases: **excitement,**

plateau, orgasm and **resolution.** This is known as the *'EPOR' model.*

The Male Response

In the male, two stages will be described: erection (which relates to the excitement phase) and ejaculation (which relates to the orgasm phase).

Erection

Erection is brought about by local stimulation of sensitive mechanoreceptors in the glans penis. When the man is sexually excited, increased parasympathetic and decreased sympathetic activity cause the arterioles in the erectile tissue of the corpora cavernosa and the corpus spongiosum to dilate and engorge with blood. Normally there is no parasympathetic control over blood vessels, and it is the variation in sympathetic stimulation that causes vasodilation and vasoconstriction. Erection is the major instance where both branches of the autonomic nervous system control blood vessels. Vasodilation is therefore accomplished more rapidly than usual.

Ejaculation

Sympathetic nerve impulses cause sequential contractions of smooth muscle in the prostate, epididymis, ductus deferens, ejaculatory duct and seminal vesicles. This causes **emission** where the genital ducts and accessory glands empty their contents into the posterior urethra. This is followed by the expulsion phase of **ejaculation** when the semen is expelled from the penis by a series of rapid muscle contractions. The filling of the urethra with semen triggers nerve impulses that activate skeletal muscles at the base of the penis to contract at 0.8-s intervals and forcibly expel the semen.

During ejaculation the sphincter at the base of the bladder is closed so that sperm do not enter the bladder and urine cannot be voided. **Orgasm** is a feeling of intense pleasure accompanied by involuntary rhythmic action of the pelvic muscles and generalized contraction of skeletal muscle throughout the body. This is followed by resolution with physical and psychological relaxation. Loss of erection follows due to venous drainage and vasoconstriction of the penile arterioles; this varies, depending on circumstances, from a few minutes to several hours. There is an absolute latent or refractory period during which subsequent erection cannot occur.

The Female Response

In the female, there is erection of the **clitoris** and erectile tissue in the **labia minora. Nipples** have erectile tissue and respond to sexual excitement. Lubrication from **Bartholin glands** facilitates entry of the penis. Orgasm may occur after movement of the penis in and out of the vagina. During the plateau phase, vasocongestion of the outer third of the vagina occurs which tightens the introitus around the penis. The uterus is raised upwards, lifting the cervix and enlarging the upper two-thirds of the vagina. This is called **ballooning** and increases the space for deposition of the ejaculate.

If orgasm occurs, the same pelvic muscle contractions as in the male occur, mostly in the engorged outer-third section of the vagina. This region is sometimes called the *orgasmic platform.* The uterus may contract, beginning at the fundus. During resolution, vasocongestion resolves and cardiac and respiratory changes return to normal (Johnson, 2018).

Cardiovascular and Respiratory Changes

In both sexes there are changes in the cardiovascular and respiratory systems. There is a marked increase in heart rate to between 100 and 170 bpm; systolic blood pressure may increase by 20–40 mmHg, respiration may double to 40/min and flushing of the chest, neck and face occurs.

Main Points

- The testes develop high in the abdominal cavity and descend into the scrotal sac in late fetal life.
- Testicular temperature is maintained at 2–3°C below the body core, thereby facilitating spermatogenesis.
- The male genital and urinary systems share a common outlet through the urethra.
- The testes produce spermatozoa and the hormones testosterone and inhibin.
- Seminiferous tubules contain two types of cells: germ cells and Sertoli cells.
- Primary spermatocytes (diploids) undergo the first meiotic division to form two secondary spermatocytes (haploids), of which half receive an X chromosome and half a Y chromosome.
- As men age, the seminal tubules undergo involution, with possible extensive atrophy by age 70 years.
- Fully formed sperm are pushed along the duct system to the epididymis where they mature and become motile. Sperm can be stored in the epididymis for 42 days.
- Interstitial tissue packed around the seminiferous tubules contains Leydig cells which secrete testosterone.
- The accessory glands of the male reproductive system provide a transport medium and nutrients. The average ejaculate is about 3–6 mL and contains 60–200 million sperm.
- The penis has three long columns of erectile tissue: two dorsal corpora cavernosa and one corpus spongiosum containing the urethra.
- Control of male reproduction is by the hypothalamus, anterior pituitary gland and testes. GnRH influences the anterior pituitary gland to produce FSH and LH. LH produces testosterone. Inhibin may inhibit FSH secretion and prevent sperm manufacture by a negative-feedback loop.

References

Johnson, M.H., 2018. Essential Reproduction, eighth ed. Wiley-Blackwell, Oxford.

Masters, W., Johnson, V., 1966. Human Sexual Response. J&A Churchill, London.

World Health Organization, 2023. Infertility. Available at who.int/news-room/fact-sheets/detail/infertility.

Annotated recommended reading

Johnson, M.H., 2018. Essential Reproduction, eighth ed. Wiley-Blackwell, Oxford.

All the major areas of reproduction are covered in this book. In particular, the section on sexual differentiation and regulation of gonadal function is recommended.

6

Fertility Control

LYNSAY MATTHEWS AND JEAN RANKIN

CHAPTER CONTENTS

This chapter focuses on aspects related to fertility control, including the range and effectiveness of methods of contraception. This chapter will help students and midwives recognize the different needs of women in relation to reproduction, sexual health and family planning.

Introduction

Fertility control is of prime concern for women from puberty to menopause. Young sexually active women may well become pregnant on their first sexual encounter and should take precautions against pregnancy. Fertility is the capacity to conceive normally; infertility is when conception has not occurred after a year of unprotected sex in the reproductive period of life (World Health Organization [WHO], 2023a). **Fecundity** is when the fertility capacity of people produces offspring leading to birth rate or natality rate. The human species is not as fertile as some mammalian species. The fecundity rate alters according to age in the human childbearing-aged population. The fecundity rate is 25% between 20 and 30 years of age, decreasing to below 10% above the age of 35. The median age at last birth is 40–41 years in most studied populations experiencing natural fertility (Vander Borght & Wyns, 2018).

There is a 1-in-5 chance of conceiving at the most fertile time. At birth, the female ovary contains immature ova which remain in limbo until puberty. Under hormonal influence, one ovum matures at each ovarian cycle. Men produce an almost infinite supply of spermatozoa continuously.

Contraception has been an issue since the link was made between sexual behaviour and pregnancy. In modern times, contraception has become legal in most countries. The United Nations (2019) estimated that 1.9 billion women worldwide were of reproductive age (15–49 years). Box 6.1 summarizes the trends in contraceptive use worldwide. When considering religious, moral and cultural issues, it is unlikely that one method will ever become universal.

Ideally, the method of contraception used should be 100% effective, painless, easy to use independently of the user's memory, cheap, accessible and without medical control. It needs to be safe, with life-threatening problems from pregnancy always measured against the safety of any contraception used. All maternity providers need to have a comprehensive understanding of family planning and spacing, as well as the myriad of methods employed to control fertility and reduce unwanted pregnancies.

Contraception and Population Growth

The world's population has grown from 2.5 billion in 1950 to 8 billion in 2022. Worldwide, approximately 2 billion women are in reproductive years with an estimated 922 million women (or partners) using contraceptive methods (see Table 6.1). Fertility rates are highest in the poorest countries and among the poorest people in these countries (O'Neill, 2022). Reproduction and contraception constitute a significant health issue for both women and men, with much of the world's population being young and still to have their families. It is estimated that 60% of the world's population will live in urban communities by the year 2030. This will mean environmental change, population change and planning for sustainable resources. Table 6.2 presents the worldwide prevalence of usage of contraception methods.

The Effectiveness of Contraception

Contraceptive prevalence worldwide is variable. Numerous studies have shown that unplanned pregnancies are pivotal in poverty rates amongst women (Bernstein & Jones, 2019). Worldwide, the contraceptive effect of breastfeeding

The prevalence of methods has changed slowly at global and regional levels:

- Use of the pill, intrauterine devices (IUDs), calendar (rhythm) methods and withdrawal has remained relatively stable over the past 25 years.
- Female sterilization has declined from 13.7% to 11.5% (between 1994 and 2019).
- Male sterilization has declined from 3.0% to 0.8% (between 1994 and 2019).
- Male condom use has more than doubled from 4.5% to 10.0% (between 1994 and 2019) with the largest increase in Eastern and South-Eastern Asia (5.0% to 17.0%). There are cultural differences, with Japan having 34.9% users of male condoms.
- Rapid increase in use of implants, injectables and male condoms in sub-Saharan African countries, Latin America and the Caribbean.
- Calendar (rhythm) methods and withdrawal remain the two most commonly used traditional methods, but their prevalence has been declining since 1994 with the sharpest declines in Europe and North America.
- The largest recorded increases were in numbers of women relying on male condoms (from 64 million to 189 million) or on injectables (from 17 million to 74 million).

(United Nations, 2019)

TABLE 6.1   **Family Planning Needs for Women Worldwide (15–49 Years)**

Need/Methods	Estimated Number	%
Modern methods	842 million	44%
Traditional methods	80 million	4%
Unmet needs	790 million	42%
No need	190 million	10%

(United Nations, 2019)

TABLE 6.2   **Usage of Contraceptive Methods Worldwide (Estimated Number of Women of Reproductive Age (15–49 Years))**

Method	Prevalence	Percentage (%)
Female sterilization	210 million	24%
Male condom	189 million	21%
Pill	150 million	16%
Intrauterine device	150 million	17%
Injectables	74 million	8%
Withdrawal (coitus interruptus)	47 million	5%
Calendar method (rhythm)	29 million	3%
Male sterilization	16 million	2%
Implants	23 million	2%
Other	15 million	2%

(United Nations, 2019)

probably has as much impact as all forms of contraception. It is expected that contraceptive use will increase as education increases in under-developed countries. The link between the social determinants of health and contraceptive use is obvious when comparing regional differences (Bernstein & Jones, 2019). For example, religious and other cultural factors are important in couples' decisions about family size and contraception.

Calculating Effectiveness

A mathematical concept used to assess the effectiveness of contraceptive methods is the **failure rate per hundred woman-years (HWY)**, or the number of pregnancies if 100 women were to use the method for 1 year (Table 6.3). It is also known as the **Pearl Index** (Guillebaud, 2019). This would be truly representative of a method's effectiveness, but it is complicated by factors such as changes in fertility with age, motivation to use the method correctly every time and the small number of women who may be infertile. It is difficult to differentiate between failure of the method and failure of the user to comply with instructions (Guillebaud, 2019). Failure often occurs in the early months after commencement of any method which becomes more reliable as skills in use develop.

Physiological Application of Contraception

The reproduction stages of male and female gametes (Fig. 6.1) identify sites for the development of effective methods of contraception (Fig. 6.2).

Contraceptive methods are usually categorized into hormonal, intrauterine contraceptive device (IUCD) (Fig.6.3), barrier (including surgical intervention) and natural methods. Table 6.4 summarises the advantages, disadvantages and contraindications of the contraceptive methods.

Hormonal-based Contraceptive Approaches

All ova available for reproduction are already present in the woman's ovaries at birth (Coad, Pedley & Dunstall, 2019). Therefore, it is not a matter of preventing ovum production, but of preventing their maturation and ovulation by suppressing follicle-stimulating hormone (FSH) and luteinizing hormone (LH) at the pituitary level. This, in turn, will prevent the feedback mechanisms between the hypothalamus and the pituitary gland. This is the underlying principle of hormonal-based contraceptive methods.

TABLE 6.3	Methods and their Failure Rates Per Hundred Woman-Years (HWY)	
Method		**Failure Rate Per HWY**
Male sterilization		0–0.15
Female sterilization		0–0.5
Injectable progestogen		0–1
Hormone implant or rod		0.1
Combined oestrogen with progestogen pill		0.1–7
Progestogen-only pill		0.3–4
Progestin intrauterine device (IUD)		0.3–0.7
Combined injectable contraceptive (CIC)		0.5–3
Copper IUD		0.6–0.8
Symptothermal method (temperature + cervical mucus)		1–4
Female barrier methods		2–12
Male condom		2–13
Female condom		5–21
Calendar method (rhythm)		15–24
Withdrawal (coitus interruptus)		20–25
Chemical contraceptives (spermicides) (used alone)		28
No contraception		85

Women: Combined Hormonal Contraception

Combined hormonal contraception (CHC) contains oestrogen and progestogens delivered as a pill (COC), transdermal patch (CTP) or vaginal ring (CVR) (Faculty of Sexual and Reproductive Health [FSRH], 2020a). The word 'combined' is used because the preparations include oestrogens and progestogens. The synthetic oestrogen is **ethinyloestradiol.** The synthetic progestogens used are various and include **norethisterone, levonorgestrel** and **gestodene**. The oestrogen component inhibits FSH release and stops the maturation of the follicle, whereas the progestogen inhibits the release of LH, preventing ovulation.

Combined Oral Contraception

Combined oral contraception (COC) has been used by women worldwide for almost 60 years, with significant changes in dosage and preparation over time. Some of the side effects occur because the altered physiology of taking the combined pill mimics that of pregnancy. For example, any cardiovascular-related risks occur because of increased clotting factors, platelet aggregation and increased serum lipids. Other risk factors include a family history of thrombosis or an anticlotting disorder, obesity and cigarette smoking which greatly increase the risk of thromboembolism in pill users.

Other Combined Methods: Combined Transdermal Patch and Combined Vaginal Ring

- The combined transdermal patch (CTP) is applied to the skin and changed every 7 days. There is a patch-free week after 3 weeks, when a withdrawal bleed will occur.
- The combined vaginal ring (CVR) is inserted into the vagina for 3 weeks, removed for 7 days (ring-free week) and then a new ring is inserted.

Both of these methods are relatively new. Although evidence is emerging, further research is needed over time to demonstrate their effects on health-related outcomes.

Emergency Contraception

Sperm are viable in the female genital tract for about 5 days. If ovulation occurs within those 5 days, fertilization could take place and a woman is at risk of pregnancy. A judicial review in 2002 concluded that pregnancy begins at implantation. It is currently accepted that any intervention given for emergency contraception (EC) must act either to prevent fertilization or to prevent implantation, rather than by disrupting established implantation. The shortest time from ovulation to implantation is 6 days (although usually longer – over 80% of pregnancies implant 8–10 days after ovulation). Women may have cultural or religious reasons for avoiding a method of EC that could have its effect after fertilization. In the UK, three methods of EC are currently available: the copper IUD (Cu-IUD), oral ulipristal acetate and oral levonorgestrel (FSRH, 2020b).

Oral preparations prevent or delay the release of a woman's egg from the ovary (ovulation) and possibly the attachment of the woman's egg to the wall of the uterus. The Cu-IUD works by having a toxic effect on sperm and ova by adversely affecting the motility and viability of sperm and the viability and transport of ova. Family planning services provide up-to-date information on EC for users (including women breastfeeding) and health practitioners (www.fpa.org.uk; www.familyplanning.org.nz).

Barrier Methods of Contraception

The Female Diaphragm

The female diaphragm (Fig. 6.4) is made of polyurethane and covers the cervix when inserted into the vagina. It must be fitted to the individual, and any weight loss or gain of more than 7 lb (3 kg) necessitates refitting. Cervical and vault caps which adhere to the cervix by suction are less commonly used (Fig. 6.4). Diaphragms must be used with a spermicidal preparation and should be left in situ for 6 h for the sperm to be killed (BNF & NICE, 2019) (Fig. 6.5).

The Male Condom

These tubular devices have been made from various materials. Currently condoms are made from polyurethane and latex. They must be placed on the erect penis before sexual contact, as there may be sperm in the fluid released from the tip of the penis after arousal. They are already lubricated. The additional use of oil-based lubricants can damage latex condoms, rendering them ineffective. After coitus, the penis

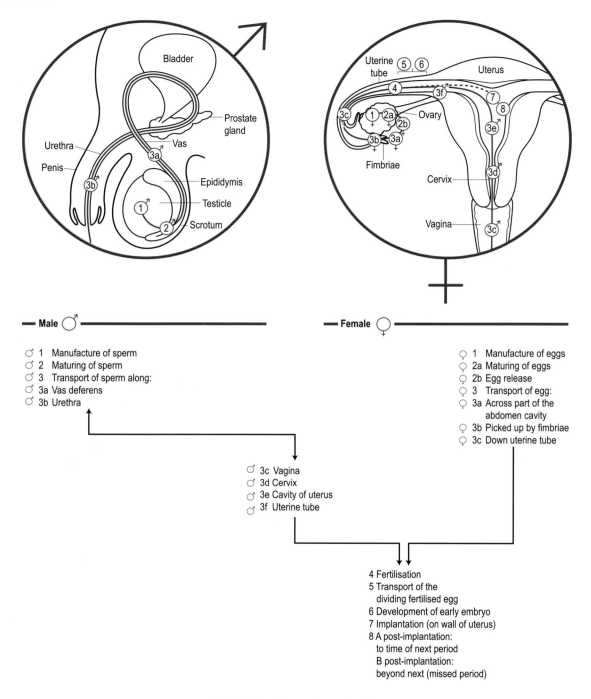

• **Fig. 6.1** The stages of reproduction.

must be removed from the vagina before the erection is lost with no further genital contact (Fig. 6.6).

The Female Condom

These are made of polyurethane, which is tougher and finer than rubber. The device lines the vagina with an inner rim that fits into the vaginal fornices and an outer rim around the vulva. They are lubricated to aid penile insertion.

Spermicidal Preparations

Spermicidal contraceptives are useful additional safeguards and are efficient at killing spermatozoa. As many millions of sperm may be released per ejaculation, these preparations should not be used alone, as they do not give adequate protection unless fertility is already significantly diminished. Chemical preparations include foaming tablets, aerosols, films, creams, pessaries and jellies. Spermicides may reduce the incidence of sexually transmitted organisms.

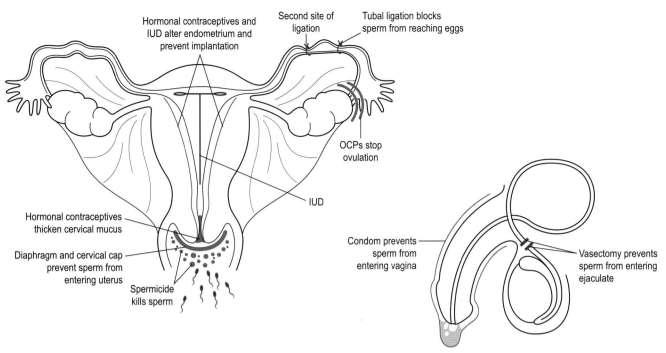

• **Fig. 6.2** Mechanisms by which contraceptives work.

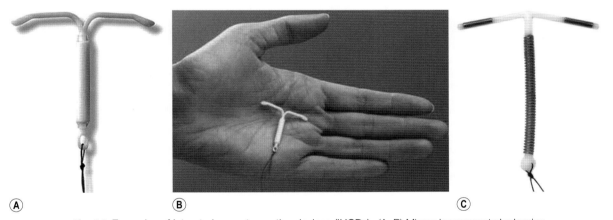

• **Fig. 6.3** Examples of intrauterine contraceptive devices (IUCDs). (A, B) Mirena levonorgestrel-releasing IUCD; (C) TTC 380 copper-loaded IUCD.

Sterilization

Fertilization occurs in the ampulla of the uterine tube; the zygote then travels down the tube to the uterus. Female sterilization aims to seal a section of the uterine tube to prevent spermatozoa reaching the ovum (Fig. 6.7). Spermatozoa travel up the vas deferens towards the urethra to be ejaculated into the vagina. Male sterilization or vasectomy aims to remove a section of the vas deferens to prevent the spermatozoa entering the ejaculatory fluid (Fig. 6.8). Other techniques include flushing the vas deferens with fluid and blocking the cut ends with body tissue (Cook et al., 2014). Clips are applied to increase the chance of reversal, but this procedure must be considered permanent as reversal involves microsurgery and may not be successful. After vasectomy, it may take up to 20 ejaculations to clear spermatozoa from the ducts, and ejaculate should be tested until two clear specimens are obtained.

TABLE 6.4	**Contraceptive Methods**		
Type	**Advantages**	**Disadvantages**	**Contraindications**
Hormonal Contraception			
Combined hormonal contraception (CHC) Combined oral contraception (COC) Combined transdermal patch (CTP) Combined vaginal ring (CVR)	Convenient and 99% effective (when used as prescribed) Reduced risk of endometrial, ovarian and colorectal cancer Predictable bleeding patterns, reduction in menstrual bleeding and pain, and management of **polycystic ovary syndrome (PCOS), endometriosis, premenstrual syndrome (PMS) and premenstrual dysphoric disorder (PMDD)**	Must be taken as prescribed. Does not prevent sexually transmitted infections (STIs) May experience irregular bleeding for the first two cycles Associated health risks: • Increased risk of venous thromboembolism (dependent on combination of hormones) • Very small increased risk of myocardial infarction (MI) and ischaemic stroke that appears to be greater with higher doses of oestrogen in COC • Small increased risk of breast cancer which reduces with time after stopping CHC • Small increased risk of cervical cancer when CHC is used for more than 5 years with risk reducing to zero after 10 years	High body mass index (BMI) ≥30 Women with history of heart attack, stroke or deep venous thrombosis (DVT) and/or family history of DVT Hypertension with no related cardiovascular risk Age >40 years, a non-smoker aged >35 years, or a smoker aged >35 smoking 15 cigarettes per day Immobilized (increased risk of DVTs), experiences leg pain Migraines and prolonged headaches CHC should be discontinued with: • Abdominal pain, breathlessness, blood-stained sputum, loss or partial sight loss or paraesthesia • Allergic reaction presents as jaundice • Preparing for major operative surgery (Guillebaud, 2019)
Progesterone-only pill (POP) also known as mini pill	Convenient and 99% effective (when used as prescribed) Can be used for all medically eligible individuals between menarche and 55 years of age Limited evidence suggests no increased risk of: • Thromboembolism • Myocardial Infarction • Breast cancer Provides protection against some bacterial pathogens due to thickened cervical mucus, thus reducing the risk of pelvic inflammatory disease Good option if women are sensitive to oestrogens found in other forms of hormonal-based contraceptives POP prescribed at any age and is an alternative to COC if the woman is currently a smoker and/or <35 years	Must be taken as prescribed Unpredictable bleeding patterns Does not protect against STIs	History of: • Severe renal insufficiency or acute renal failure • Hyperkalaemia or untreated hypoaldosteronism (e.g., Addison's disease)

TABLE 6.4   Contraceptive Methods—cont'd

Type	Advantages	Disadvantages	Contraindications
Long-acting reversible contraception (LARC) Progestogen-only injectable contraceptives	Progestogens increase the stability of red blood cells and may benefit women with sickle cell disease Option for women who cannot take oral preparations where absorption is poor or if the large intestine has been removed Beneficial for young girls who may forget the pill	Common adverse effects reported in 5% of users (Perry, 2014): • Backache • Depression • Acne • Hot flushes • Breast pain • Alopecia • Nausea • Bloating, weight gain May have heavy, irregular bleeding which settles after a few months Delayed return of fertility Injections need to be repeated every 12 weeks (8 weeks for Noristerat) Long-term use results in lower-than-average bone mineral density–stabilizes after 3 years of use (Zhang et al., 2013) Risk of repeated pregnancies may outweigh the side effects of the progestogen injection	Family history of osteoporosis Smoking Taking steroids Excessive alcohol intake Eating disorders Coeliac disease If breast cancer diagnosed within 5 years
Progestogen-only subdermal implants	Depending on the implant, the contraceptive effect lasts 3–5 years. Other advantages are: • May stop periods • Convenient, no pills to remember and no interruption to sexual intercourse • Can be removed anytime • No contraindications with breastfeeding	May cause irregular bleeding, partly due to its effect on the endometrium Side effects of progesterone implants are similar to the other progesterone forms of contraception previously discussed	
Progestogen-only intrauterine systems (Mirena IUCD)	Widely used and highly effective (up to 99%)	**Menstrual disorders** – some women have an increased duration of blood loss. This is not a straightforward lengthening of the menstrual phase of the cycle. Light loss 2–3 days before true bleeding and with a similar tailing off with light bleeding afterwards. The only IUCD without this effect is the progesterone-containing type **Fetal abnormalities** – no abnormalities recorded with an IUCD in situ Miscarriage is more common, occurring in about 50% of pregnancies, and ectopic pregnancy may occur In continuing pregnancies, premature onset of labour may occur if the IUCD remains in situ	

Continued

TABLE 6.4 **Contraceptive Methods—cont'd**

Type	Advantages	Disadvantages	Contraindications
Copper intrauterine devices (non-hormonal)	Widely used and 98% effective Highly effective emergency contraceptive (EC) method	**Infection** – risk with IUCDs is very low (Hubacher, 2014) Women with healthy tracts are at no greater risk of ectopic or subsequent infertility Risk of pelvic inflammatory disease is greatest with an STI **Fetal abnormalities** – as previously reported for other IUCDs	Providers of emergency contraceptives should be aware that breastfeeding women have a higher relative risk of uterine perforation during insertion of intrauterine contraception than non-breastfeeding women. However, the absolute risk of perforation is low
Emergency contraception (EC) also known as the morning-after pill	Effective	Side effects reported include nausea, vomiting, dizziness and headache	Breastfeeding women will need specific up to date advice The use of Levonelle 1500 is not advised if the woman has any of the following: • Disease of small bowel (such as Crohn's disease) that inhibits the absorption of the drug • Severe liver problems • History of ectopic pregnancy (where the baby develops somewhere outside the uterus) • History of salpingitis (inflammation of the Fallopian tubes)
Barrier Methods (Including Surgical Interventions)				
Female diaphragm	Efficient alternative to hormonal contraception Possible protection against some STIs Provides women with control over fertility	Allergy to rubber material or spermicide Possible to experience discomfort (e.g., uterine prolapse). Difficult to maintain in situ Recurrent cystitis Use may be distasteful to some women	History of allergic reactions. Women who may forget to insert before coitus
Male condom	Cheap, easily purchased and successful. Provides barriers to various organisms and help in the prevention of the spread of STIs	Relies on the integrity of the condom and the experience of the user	
Female condom	Women have the control over their contraception	Further development and research evidence for effectiveness is required	
Spermicides	Convenient and easy to use Some protection against STI	Should be used in combination with other methods	Allergies
Sterilisation	Female and male sterilization are effective	Short-term risk includes infection or haematoma No long-term health problems	
Natural Methods				
Withdrawal	Easy to use	No need for medical supervision	
Calendar (rhythm) method	Effective if the woman is motivated and committed	One key limitation – cycles need to be between 23 and 25 days	Unstable length of cycle

TABLE 6.5	The Timing of Contraceptive Methods
Method of Contraception	**Timing of Use Postnatally**
Lactational amenorrhoea method (*effective* when baby is exclusively breastfeeding)	Immediate (First 6 months only)
Natural methods	As soon as required
Barrier methods (condom, femidom)	As soon as required
Implant	3 weeks (21 days)
Progesterone-only pill (POP) – mini pill	3 weeks (21 days)
Emergency contraception – progesterone only (e.g., Levonelle [levenorgestrel]; ellaOne [Ulipristal]; and copper IUCD	3 weeks (21 days) (Levonelle – suitable for women irrespective of feeding method; ellaOne is more suitable for non-breastfeeding women) oral ulipristal acetate (UPA) 30 mg (single dose) and oral levonorgestrel (LNG) 1.5 mg (single dose)
Emergency IUCD	4 weeks (28 days) Can be inserted 5 days (120 hours) after unprotected sex or within 5 days of the earliest time an ovum could have been released
Injection	3 weeks (21 days, **if not** breastfeeding)
Injection	6 weeks (42 days) **if** breastfeeding
Intrauterine contraceptive devices (IUCDs)	*Can be fitted 48 hours after birth – **additional contraception is required** for protection.* From 4 weeks (28 days)
Diaphragms and caps	6 weeks
Female sterilization	Not advisable shortly following birth
Vasectomy	Not advisable following birth

Adapted from FSRH, 2020b; Steen, Jackson & Brown, 2020.

Natural Methods

Preventing Ejaculation into the Vagina

Various contraceptive techniques of preventing ejaculation into the vagina are practiced, despite their relatively high failure rate. These methods, which are easy to use and do not need medical supervision, include:

- Withdrawing the penis from the vagina at climax, termed *coitus interruptus.*
- Avoiding ejaculation, or coitus reservatus.

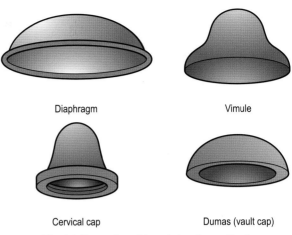

Diaphragm　　　　　Vimule

Cervical cap　　　　Dumas (vault cap)

• **Fig. 6.4** Examples of female barrier methods.

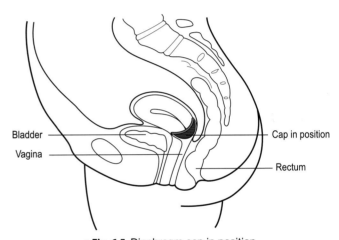

Bladder　　　　　　　　　　Cap in position

Vagina　　　　　　　　　　　Rectum

• **Fig. 6.5** Diaphragm cap in position.

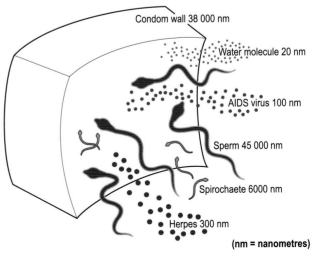

Condom wall 38 000 nm

Water molecule 20 nm

AIDS virus 100 nm

Sperm 45 000 nm

Spirochaete 6000 nm

Herpes 300 nm

(nm = nanometres)

• **Fig. 6.6** The condom barrier.

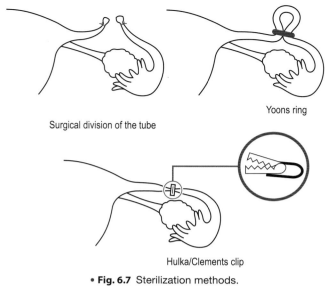

Surgical division of the tube

Yoons ring

Hulka/Clements clip

• **Fig. 6.7** Sterilization methods.

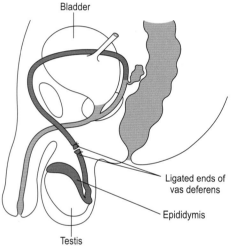

Bladder

Ligated ends of vas deferens

Epididymis

Testis

• **Fig. 6.8** Ligation of the vas deferens.

- Coitus intracrura where the penis is placed between the thighs of the woman.
- Coitus saxonicus, where hard pressure to the male perineum just before ejaculation results in retrograde ejaculation into the bladder. This is an unusual and difficult but effective technique.
- Anal intercourse may be used.

Timing, Temperature and Cervical Mucus

Each ovulatory cycle has a brief window when the ovum is available for fertilization. It is assumed that pregnancy will not occur if intercourse is avoided at that time. The calendar or timing method has been used successfully in women with a regular menstrual cycle.

Methods of pinpointing ovulation have been developed when this may occur irregularly. These rely on two changes brought about by the secretion of progesterone (i.e., the change in cervical mucus and the rise in core temperature) (Fig. 6.9). The symptothermal method combines these two indicators of fertility: (i) measurement of basal body temperature with a thermometer every morning upon awakening (at approximately the same time every day) and (ii) evaluation of cervical mucus and its texture, consistency, and colour every day. Basal body temperature is now considered to be unreliable as a predictor of ovulation and its use is discouraged (NICE, 2017; Su et al., 2017). During the fertile period of the menstrual cycle, the cervical mucus is reported to be clear and stringy. It can be stretched between two fingers to a length of at least 6 cm due to an increase in oestrogen at the end of the follicular phase before ovulation. This watery consistency is meant to facilitate sperm mobilization for the process of fertilization. Change in cervical mucus can be detected approximately 4–7 days before ovulation.

Lactational Amenorrhoea Method

The lactational amenorrhoea method is a temporary method of contraception for new mothers whose monthly bleeding has not returned. During this period, eggs are not released and so pregnancy cannot occur. Exclusively breastfeeding mothers can use this as a natural method of contraception in the first 6 months.

Abortion

For some women, abortion may be the only answer to an unwanted or dangerous pregnancy, with the most vulnerable women being adolescents and women aged 45 and over. In the UK, this procedure to terminate the pregnancy is legally guided by The Abortion Act (1967, C.87).

Infections Affecting Reproductive Health

It is important to differentiate between infection and normal flora in diagnosing vaginal infection (Farthing, 2018). However, infections may impact on fertility and reproductive health by ascending through the reproductive tract. Sexually transmitted infections (STIs) can cause serious complications and long-term health problems for women, such as pelvic inflammatory disease, ectopic pregnancy and miscarriage (Greenhouse, 2018). Untreated gonorrhoea and chlamydia can cause infertility in both men and women (WHO, 2023b). Some examples of vaginal infections are summarized in Table 6.6.

Future Focus

Following birth, women and partners need to focus on appropriate contraceptive methods in relation to planning the timing of any future pregnancies. To date, there remains insufficient evidence to suggest that postpartum contraception education is effective (Lopez et al., 2015). There is no perfect contraceptive method. Many unplanned pregnancies remain, particularly in very young women. Women and their partners in childbearing years need to acquire information and education about contraceptive and family spacing education to help reduce unplanned and unwanted pregnancies. Ongoing research is important to investigate ever simpler and acceptable contraception methods while supporting women and their partners to find and correctly use their chosen methods from what is available and appropriate to their unique needs.

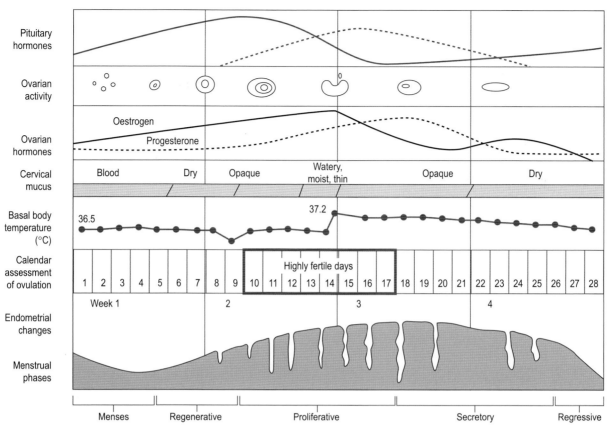

• **Fig. 6.9** Physiological changes in the menstrual cycle in conjunction with physiological methods of 8 + 78 birth control.

TABLE 6.6	Vaginal Infections
Infection	**Characteristics**
Vaginal candidiasis	This fungal infection is caused by *Candida* and is commonly referred to as 'thrush'. The most common species is *Candida albicans*. Thrush causes vaginal irritation and vaginitis and is readily treated. However, *Candida* can be transmitted to a sexual partner. Some 10% of women will develop recurrent infections. Predisposing factors include oral contraceptives, diabetes and pregnancy.
Bacterial vaginosis	This infection is mainly associated with the organism *Gardnerella vaginalis*. Some 50% of infected women are asymptomatic and the vagina is not usually (the term 'vaginosis' is used rather than vaginitis). The discharge has a characteristic fishy amine smell. Bacterial vaginosis may be associated with pelvic inflammatory disease and postoperative pelvic infection.
Trichomoniasis	Trichomoniasis is an STI caused by the parasite *Trichomonas vaginalis* (flagellated organism). The infection can damage the vaginal epithelium, increasing a woman's susceptibility to infection by HIV. A woman with this STI needs to be referred to a genitourinary medicine clinic for contact tracing. It can cause dyspareunia.
Chlamydia	Chlamydia is the most common bacterial STI, often with no signs or symptoms of infection. This STI usually clears spontaneously within 1 or 2 years. Usually, the infection does not cause any significant harm. However, individuals are frequently co-infected with gonorrhoea which does have significant harm.
Gonorrhoea and Syphilis	Gonorrhoea is an STI caused by bacteria – *Neisseria gonorrhoeae* or *N. gonococcus*. It is routinely screened for in pregnancy as the infection can also be passed to the baby. Without treatment, gonorrhoea can cause permanent blindness in a newborn baby. Syphilis is uncommon among women in the UK. It does cause severe complications to individuals.
Non-specific infections	The presence of foreign bodies; for example, ring pessary, continual use of tampons and/or the presence of an intrauterine contraceptive device.

Main Points

- The calculation of the failure rate per HWY is used to assess the effectiveness of contraceptive methods.
- CHC contains oestrogen and a progestogen delivered as a pill (COC), transdermal patch (CTP) or vaginal ring (CVR).
- COC prevents the maturation of ova and ovulation. Risks include its oestrogen content, cigarette smoking, obesity, a sedentary way of life and a family history of thrombosis.
- Progestogen adds to the contraceptive effect by thickening cervical mucus, making the endometrium unsuitable for implantation and reducing uterine tube motility.
- Women with malabsorption disorders should not be prescribed oral COC.
- Research currently focuses on stopping spermatogenesis by reducing feedback mechanisms and the production of GnRH.
- Milk production is not diminished when women take a progesterone-only pill.
- Barrier contraception methods include the diaphragm, the male condom, the female condom and spermicidal preparations. Some methods may prevent the spread of STIs.
- Natural methods include preventing ejaculation taking place in the vagina, timing and cervical mucus testing and control of coital frequency.
- Modern methods of postcoital contraception interrupt implantation or even ovulation depending on the time in the menstrual cycle (e.g., IUCD insertion and emergency contraceptive pill).
- The three methods of emergency contraception in the UK are the Cu-IUD, oral ulipristal acetate and oral levonorgestrel.

References

Abortion Act 1967, c. 87. Available at: https://www.legislation.gov.uk/ukpga/1967/87/contents.

Bernstein, A., Jones, K.M., 2019. The Economic Effects of Contraceptive Access: A Review of the Evidence. Institute for Women's Policy Research, Washington, DC.

BNF & NICE, 2019. Contraceptives. Available at: https://bnf.nice.org.uk/treatment-summaries/contraceptives-hormonal/.

Coad, J., Pedley, K., Dunstall, M., 2019. Anatomy and Physiology for Midwives, fourth ed. Elsevier, London.

Cook, L.A., Van Vliet, H.A.A.M., Lopez, L.M., Pun, A., Gallo, M.F., 2014. Vasectomy occlusion techniques for male sterilization. Cochrane Database Syst. Rev. 2014 (3),CD003991.

Faculty of Sexual and Reproductive Health (FSRH), 2020a. FSRH clinical guideline: combined hormonal contraception. Amended 2020. Available at: https://www.fsrh.org/documents/combined-hormonal-contraception/.

Faculty of Sexual and Reproductive Health (FSRH), 2020b. FSRH Clinical Guideline: Progestogen-Only Pills (August 2022, Amended November 2022). Available at: https://www.fsrh.org/documents/cec-guideline-pop.

Farthing, A., 2018. Clinical anatomy of the pelvis and reproductive tract. In: Edmonds, D.K., Lees, C., Bourne, T.H. (Eds.), Dewhurst's Textbook of Obstetrics and Gynaecology, ninth ed. Wiley, Oxford.

Greenhouse, P., 2018. Sexually transmitted infection. In: Edmonds, D.K., Lees, C., Bourne, T.H. (Eds.), Dewhurst's Textbook of Obstetrics and Gynaecology, ninth ed. Wiley, Oxford.

Guillebaud, J., 2019. Contraception Today, ninth ed. CRC Press, Informa Healthcare, New York.

Hubacher, D., 2014. Intrauterine devices & infection: review of the literature. Indian J. Med. Res. 140 (1), S53–S57.

Lopez, L.M., Grey, T.W., Hiller, J.E., Chen, M., 2015. Education for contraceptive use by women after childbirth. Cochrane Database Syst. Rev. 2015 (7),CD001863.

National Institute for Health and Care Excellence (NICE), 2017. Fertility: Assessment and Treatment. Available at: https://www.nice.org.uk/guidance/cg156.

New Zealand Family Planning, 2022. Available at: www.familyplanning.org.nz/.

O'Neill, S.A., 2022. Fertility Rate of the World and Continents 1950-2020. Available at: https://www.statista.com/statistics/1034075/fertility-rate-world-continents-1950-2020/.

Perry, M., 2014. Depo-Provera: a review of contraceptive efficacy. Pract. Nurs. 25 (2), 77–80.

Steen, M., Jackson, K., Brown, A., 2020. Physiology and care during the puerperium. In: Marshall, J.E., Raynor, M. (Eds.), Myles' Textbook for Midwives, seventeenth ed. Elsevier, London.

Su, H.W., Yi, Y.C., Wei, T.Y., Chang, T.C., Cheng, C.M., 2017. Detection of ovulation, a review of currently available methods. Bioeng. Transl. Med. 2 (3), 238–246.

United Nations, 2019. Contraceptive Use by Method 2019: Data Booklet (ST/ESA/SER.A/435). Available at: www.un.org/development/desa/pd/content/contraceptive-use-method-2019.

Vander Borght, M., Wyns, C., 2018. Fertility and infertility: definition and epidemiology. Clin. Biochem. 62, 2–10.

World Health Organization (WHO), 2023a. Infertility. Available at: https://www.who.int/news-room/fact-sheets/detail/infertility.

World Health Organization (WHO), 2023b. Sexually Transmitted Infections. Available at: www.who.int/news-room/fact-sheets/detail/sexually-transmitted-infections-(stis).

Zhang, M.H., Zhang, W., Zhang, A.D., Yang, Y., Gai, L., 2013. Effect of depot medroxyprogesterone acetate on bone mineral density in adolescent women. Chinese Med. J. 126 (21), 4043–4047.

Annotated recommended reading

National Institute for Health and Care Excellence (NICE), 2016. Contraception: Quality Standard [QS129]. Available at: www.nice.org.uk/guidance/qs129.

National Institute for Health and Care Excellence (NICE), 2017. Sexually Transmitted Infections: Condom Distribution Schemes: NICE Guideline [NG68]. Available at: www.nice.org.uk/guidance/ng68.

National Institute for Health and Care Excellence (NICE), 2019. Long-acting Reversible Contraception: Clinical Guideline [CG30]. Available at: www.nice.org.uk/guidance/cg30.

These NICE websites provide evidence-based guidance and standards on fertility-related issues.

Faculty of Sexual and Reproductive Health. Available at: https://www.fsrh.org//.

FSRH is a faculty of the Royal College of Obstetricians and Gynaecologists. This is an excellent site offering a wide range of sexual and reproductive health resources for health professionals including up-to-date evidence-based publications, standards and learning resources.

Useful websites

The following sites are useful for anyone: students, midwives, family planning and other public health providers and their clients. They provide up-to-date, evidence-based information and advice covering a range of fertility and contraceptive aspects. Family planning websites are usually available in a wide range of countries. Interested readers may prefer to locate the nearest country's website for appropriate guidance.

Family Planning Association (UK) – www.fpa.org.uk.

FP 2030 – https://fp2030.org/.

New Zealand Family Planning – www.familyplanning.org.nz/.

FertilityUK – www.fertilityuk.org/.

Faculty of Sexual and Reproductive Health (UK) – https://www.fsrh.org/.

NICE British National Formulary – https://bnf.nice.org.uk/.

7

Infertility

LYNSAY MATTHEWS AND JEAN RANKIN

CHAPTER CONTENTS

Increasingly, midwives will encounter families who have required assistance in conceiving. Therefore, students and midwives need to have up-to-date knowledge and understanding about infertility including the possible causes, investigations and the available treatment. It is essential that they are also aware of the physical and psychological effects that infertility has on the family and parenting.

Introduction

In 1978 the first baby was born following in vitro fertilization (IVF; i.e., 'test tube'). This resulted in couples actively seeking advice and help to conceive using assisted reproductive technologies (ART) (Gurevich, 2022). Reproductive medicine has since pioneered the use of donated sperm through intrauterine insemination (IUI). This was initially offered to heterosexual couples with male factor infertility. Fertility treatment now facilitates more families to become

parents including single women with no partner, same-sex relationships (Wrande et al., 2022) and older age groups (Human Fertilisation & Embryology Authority [HFEA], 2020). Since 1991, approximately 390,000 babies have been born in the UK following 1.3 million IVF cycles and over 260,000 donor insemination (DI) cycles (HFEA, 2021a).

Defining Infertility

Infertility is a disease of the male or female reproductive system defined by the failure to achieve a pregnancy after 12 months or more of regular unprotected sexual intercourse (World Health Organization [WHO], 2018; Zegers-Hochschild, 2017). Primary infertility refers to the inability to have a pregnancy whilst secondary infertility occurs when there is the inability to have another pregnancy following a previous successful pregnancy (WHO, 2020). The global burden of infertility has increased between 1990 and 2017 (Sun et al., 2019). Although infertility may affect millions of people of reproductive age, prevalence rates are difficult to determine due to the presence of both male and female factors (WHO, 2023a). Estimates have suggested that between 48 million couples and 186 million individuals live with infertility worldwide (WHO, 2023a). Infertility affects as many as one in seven couples in developed countries and one in four couples in developing countries (Mascarenhas et al., 2012). The WHO (2020) ranked infertility as the highest serious global disability among populations under the age of 60 years.

Infertility has a major impact on individuals, their families and communities (WHO, 2023b). For couples who have difficulty conceiving, the desire to have a baby may be all-consuming. This is a life crisis with psychological, emotional and sociocultural consequences on individuals and couples (Anokye et al., 2017; Lordăchescu et al., 2021) (Box 7.1). For women, the socially valued status of motherhood is threatened (Taebi et al., 2021), and for men their masculinity (Dolan et al., 2017). Although infertility affects both sexes equally, it is women who are most frequently blamed (Hasanpoor-Azghady et al., 2019; Taebi et al., 2021). These factors potentially cause disharmony in relationships with each other and within families. To seek help, the couple must recognize that a problem exists, and a third party comes into their intimate lives. Infertility clinics,

• BOX 7.1   **Psychological and Social Issues**

Individuals and couples with infertility problems experience a range of psychological, emotional and social issues (Anokye et al., 2017; Lordăchescu et al., 2021; Vioreanu, 2021). Psychological effects experienced can be profound and relate to depression, anxiety, low self-esteem, frustrations and despondency. Worldwide, the inability to conceive children can be a stressful situation for individuals and couples. Whilst women clearly experience stress (de Berardis et al., 2014), it remains unclear if infertility is caused by the stress (Rooney & Domar, 2018).

In the first instance, it is women who are more prone to feelings of shame, feelings of low self-esteem, guilt and acute distress (Taebi et al., 2021). With prolonged infertility problems, partners can also suffer from these effects (Dolan et al., 2017). Women using assisted reproduction may experience pregnancy loss or consecutive pregnancy losses. This loss can trigger prolonged grief and mourning (Bashiri, Halper & Orvieto, 2018; de Castro et al., (2021)). Evidence suggests that abortion, fetal death or even reproductive treatment failure represent a source of suffering that could have a devastating effect on the psychological wellbeing of infertile couples (de Castro et al., (2021); Doyle & Carballedo, 2014; Hasanpoor-Azghdy, Simbar & Vedadhir, 2014) and could lead to prolonged grief responses among women and their partners (Gameiro & Finnigan, 2017).

During the unprecedented COVID-19 pandemic, the suspension of fertility treatment had a negative impact on women's mental health and quality of life (Gordon & Balsom, 2020).

Infertility can have life-changing negative social effects on couples including exclusion, verbal and physical abuse, divorce and stigma (Anokye et al., 2017; Dolan et al., 2017; Taebi et al., 2021). In some cultures, childless women suffer discrimination and ostracism (Almas & Sabahat, 2022; Sembuya, 2010; Tedros, 2019). In addition to these psychological and social factors, murder and suicide are linked to infertility (Shani et al., 2016).

Psychosocial support and counselling before, during and after artificial reproductive technologies is crucial for couples experiencing infertility problems (NICE, 2017a; Patel, Sharma and Kumar, 2018; Vioreanu, 2021).

counselling and fertility support groups play a valuable role in helping couples cope with the range of psychological, emotional and social issues experienced (Patel, Sharma & Kumar, 2018).

The Causes of Male and Female Infertility

Fig. 7.1 outlines the main causes of infertility. Relevant investigations are needed to ensure:

1. Adequate numbers of sperm are deposited around the cervix (postcoital test).
2. The endometrium is in an appropriate state to receive the fertilized ovum (endometrial biopsy).
3. The fallopian tubes are patent (laparoscopy, salpingography).
4. Ovulation occurs (endometrial biopsy, hormonal assays).
5. The woman is psychologically prepared for pregnancy.

Table 7.1 indicates the frequency of infertility causes in UK couples.

Investigations for Infertility

Risk factors threatening optimal fertility include increasing age for females, excessive or very low body fat, lifestyle/environmental factors and medical and reproductive history for couples. Reproductive history needs to include coitus and sexually transmitted infections (STIs) and diseases (STDs). Not all STIs result in disease. An initial high-quality assessment of general health (men and women) needs to be performed, typically including investigations such as screening for *Chlamydia trachomatis*. Assessment of lifestyle behaviours is required to ascertain modifiable factors such as weight loss or weight gain, alcohol intake, smoking, folic acid intake, prescribed and recreational drug use. Changes to these behaviours have the potential to improve natural conception rates and enhance the effectiveness of fertility treatments (National Institute for Health and Care Excellence [NICE], 2017a).

Male Infertility

The exact rate of male infertility is difficult to determine worldwide (Barratt et al., 2017). It is found in half of involuntarily childless couples and can be related to idiopathic genetic defects or environmental effects (Leslie et al., 2022). To date, there remain no definitive causative links to the decline in sperm counts. A diagnostic assessment will include physical examination, medical and reproductive history and semen analysis.

The recent SARS-CoV-19 virus (if the condition was severe) caused reduced fertility and even infertility in some recovered males. Although further investigations are required, the virus appears to affect the testis by direct cellular infection and with side effects from the various antiviral and immunological therapies used (Ardestani Zadeh & Arab, 2021).

Semen Analysis and Sperm Deposition

Specimens of semen are collected into a clean, dry glass jar. The specimen should preferably be produced by masturbation after 2 days of abstinence from coitus, kept at room temperature and taken to the laboratory within 1 hour of collection. Ideally, as a fertility test, an average of three specimens at 2- to 3-week intervals provides a calculation of semen value.

The WHO (2021) normal values for semen in the sample are as follows:

- Volume – 1.5 mL or more.
- Sperm concentration – 15 million/mL or more.
- Total sperm number – 39 million spermatozoa per ejaculate or more.
- Total sperm motility (i.e., ability to swim) – 40% or more motile or 32% or more with progressive motility.
- Vitality – 58% or more live spermatozoa.
- Morphology (size and shape) – normal form 4.0% or more.
- pH level – 7.2 or higher.

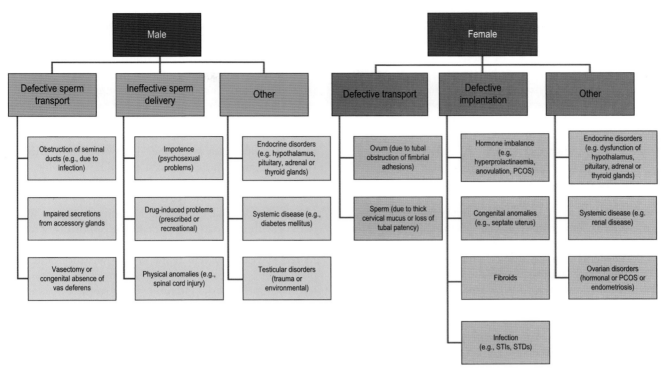

• **Figure 7.1** Main causes of infertility in males and females.

TABLE 7.1	The Main Causes of Infertility in UK Couples	
Cause		**Approx. Percentage Frequency**
Uterine or peritoneal disorders		10
Tubal damage		20
Ovulatory problems		25
Male factors (e.g., sperm defects)		30
Unexplained (no identified male or female cause)		25

Infertility affects an estimated 1 in 7 couples.
In 40% of cases, disorders are found in both the man and the woman.
Uterine or endometrial factors, gamete or embryo defects, and pelvic conditions play a role.

Percentages indicate approximate prevalence.
NICE, 2017a

Defective Spermatogenesis

The aetiology of sperm production is related to gene mutations, stress from the environment and chromosomal abnormalities, all affecting spermatogenesis (Leslie et al., 2022). An elevated body mass index (BMI) in males is associated with infertility, although numerous studies have shown that most mechanisms leading to reduced fertility are reversible (Katib, 2015). Recent findings reported that central obesity had a potential role to play in progressive motility and total sperm count, but the role did not extend to affecting normal morphology and concentration (Keszthelyi et al., 2020). Hypotestosteronaemia found in men with obesity is the prime hormonal defect leading to impaired spermatogenesis (Katib, 2015).

Absence of sperm (azoospermia) is uncommon and may be due to defective spermatogenesis or blockage. Whilst 15% of male infertility can be identified as due to genetic factors, the aetiology is still unknown in approximately 50%, termed *idiopathic infertility*. Biopsy of the testes and epididymis will show whether sperm are being produced and, if present, obtained for fertility treatments such as IUI or intracytoplasmic sperm injection (ICSI).

The debate continues relating to varicoceles (enlargement of veins in the scrotum) and if they cause raised testicular temperature and affect spermatogenesis. Improvements in semen quality following varicocelectomy do not always result in spontaneous pregnancy and some men with varicoceles are able to father children, even without intervention (Jensen et al., 2017). Varicoceles should not be routinely treated as evidence to date has not yet demonstrated improved fertility (NICE, 2017a). Men should be aware there is an association between reduced semen quality and smoking, elevated BMI (≥ 30 kg/m^2), alcohol consumption greater than 3–4 units per day, elevated scrotal temperature and exposure to hazards (NICE, 2017a).

Where significant levels of sperm antibodies are found to be coating the sperm, there is some speculation that it reduces their ability to progress normally through the female reproductive system. In these circumstances, it is always necessary to perform ICSI (Barberán et al., 2020). Antibodies are mainly found where the man has experienced trauma to the testes, testicular surgery or vasectomy reversal (Lotti et al., 2018). The significance of antisperm antibodies remains unclear and the effectiveness of systemic corticosteroids is uncertain (NICE, 2017a).

Erectile and Ejaculatory Failure

Disorders related to erectile and ejaculatory failure are causes of infertility (Capogrosso et al., 2021). In males of infertile couples, the prevalence of erectile dysfunction increases as a function of semen quality impairment severity (Lotti et al., 2016). For men diagnosed with failure in ejaculation, artificial insemination by the husband/partner's semen via IUI or ISCI may be useful, with or without ovarian stimulation (Barberán et al., 2020).

Female Infertility

Specific investigations would include:
- Endocrinology screening.
- Confirmation of rubella immunity.
- Cervical cytology.
- Screening for infections such as *C. trachomatis.*
- Ultrasound to assess the uterus and uterine tubes.
- Hysterosalpingography to assess tubal patency.
- Laparoscopy—observation of pelvic organs (Mahran et al., 2017).

Further investigations will be required relating to specific comorbidities (NICE, 2017a).

Ovulation

Women who experience regular monthly menstrual cycles are likely to be ovulating and can have their cycle confirmed by hormonal studies. Serum progesterone in the mid-luteal phase of their cycle (day 21 of a 28-day cycle) will confirm ovulation. Women with prolonged irregular cycles should have their serum progesterone levels checked weekly, starting later in the cycle and continuing until the next menstrual cycle begins. Women with irregular cycles should have serum levels of follicle-stimulating hormone and luteinizing hormone (gonadotrophins) measured (NICE, 2017a).

Monitoring cervical mucus and identifying the change to copious, clear and stretchy mucus at the time of ovulation can assist in ensuring intercourse occurs at an opportune time. The use of basal body temperature as ovulation prediction is unreliable and now discouraged (NICE, 2017a; Su et al., 2017).

Ovarian stimulation produces multiple mature ova for harvesting which may then be used for IVF or stored for future use as ova. For women diagnosed with explained infertility, ovulation stimulation, such as clomiphene citrate, can be used in conjunction with IUI (NICE, 2017a). There is the associated risk of a multiple pregnancy occurring (Evans et al., 2020). Artificial stimulation of the ovary carries the risk of hyperstimulation syndrome, a potentially fatal condition. Therefore, women must be informed of early signs and symptoms of the syndrome and carefully observed.

Women are born with a finite number of oocytes; hence, fecundity decreases with age. Delayed childbearing has resulted in an increase in access to ART worldwide. However, the success of treatment dramatically reduces between the ages of 35 (41% success after one cycle) and 42 years (4%) (MacDougall, Beyene & Nachtigall, 2013). Women with or without a partner may take the opportunity to cryopreserve their eggs to preserve their fertility (HFEA, 2022). In recent years, ovarian tissue cryopreservation and transplantation is becoming a successful method of preserving fertility in prepubertal girls and young women with primarily cancer diseases and undergoing gonadotoxic therapy. This offers them the chance of them becoming biological mothers in the future (Kristensen & Andersen, 2018).

Polycystic Ovary Syndrome

Polycystic ovary syndrome (PCOS) is the most common hormonal disorder in women and accounts for approximately 80% of women with anovulatory infertility (Balen et al., 2016). PCOS can be confirmed by the presence of hyperandrogenism, anovulation with menstrual irregularities and polycystic ovaries (Trikudanathan, 2015). Obesity and insulin resistance are features of the syndrome. These hormone imbalances affect the ovary, thickening the thecal layer, ceasing ovulation and creating the menstrual abnormalities. Not all women with PCOS have every symptom, and when presenting with infertility the relevant problem must be treated to enable pregnancy to occur.

Tubal Patency

Fertilization takes place in the fallopian tube, and the zygote moves through the tube and enters the uterus where it will implant and develop. Patency of the tubes is essential for the sperm to move toward the egg and for the zygote to move into the uterine cavity. However, infection can ascend through the cervix and uterus to affect the uterine tubes (salpingitis), the ovaries and the pelvic peritoneum, causing pelvic inflammatory disease (PID). Adhesions may distort the tubes, or the endothelial folds lining the tubes may be functionally damaged and blocked with reduced or absent ciliated cells or peristaltic movements.

The most common organisms implicated in PID are those causing chlamydial infection and gonorrhoea (Tsevat et al., 2017). Women presenting with infertility and diagnosed with PID may have no recollection of an infection. Current and past infections can be treated, if necessary, in both partners. The incidence of bacterial vaginosis tends to be higher in women suffering from tubal infertility. To investigate and diagnose tubal patency, hysterosalpingography can be performed by injecting a radio-opaque contrast medium through the cervix and monitoring its passage through the uterus and uterine tubes using X-rays. A laparoscopy can also examine tubal function and general pelvic structures.

Endometriosis

Endometriosis is a disease characterised by the presence of tissue similar to the lining of the uterus growing outside the uterus, causing pain and/or infertility (WHO, 2023c). The life-impacting pain caused by this complex chronic condition is due to the external endometrial tissue becoming reactive to the hormonal changes during the menstrual cycle. This chronic debilitating disease may impair fertility either by itself or in conjunction with other fertility-reducing factors (NICE, 2017b). The effects of endometriosis will probably impact on the pelvic cavity, ovaries, fallopian tubes or uterus (WHO, 2023c). This may range from anatomical distortions due to chronic inflammatory response, adhesions and fibrosis to endocrine abnormalities and immunological disturbances (Králíčková & Vetvicka, 2015).

Treatment of endometriosis-associated infertility requires some form of restorative surgery to remove endometrial deposits, as well as pituitary suppressive agents such as analogues of gonadotrophin-releasing hormone to suppress the endometrial deposits or assisted reproduction (Fadhlaoui, Bouquet de la Jolinière & Feki, 2014; Tanbo & Fedorcsak, 2017). Women with endometriosis do not respond well to ovarian hyperstimulation.

Reproductive Technologies

Once a diagnosis is confirmed, treatment falls into three categories (NICE, 2017a):
i. Medical treatment to restore fertility (e.g., the use of drugs for ovulation induction).
ii. Surgical treatment to restore fertility (e.g., laparoscopy for ablation of endometriosis).
iii. ART (i.e., any treatment dealing with means of conception other than vaginal intercourse).

ART frequently involve the handling of gametes or embryos and require the ability of the embryologist to manipulate ova and sperm outside the body. Developmental fertility research for the purpose of reproduction is sensitive and fraught with ethical concerns. In recent years, there has been significant progress made in genome editing of stem cells to adapt into fertility treatment (Wang et al., 2019). Without the concerns of ethical problems, ongoing research into the field of artificial gametes and embryos will have a profound and lasting effect for reproduction. Artificial embryos will become a powerful research platform for early embryo development, especially human embryonic development (Zhang et al., 2020).

Table 7.2 outlines the abbreviations and processes used in assisted conception.

Sperm, Ova and Embryo Donation

For some couples, using donated ova and/or sperm or embryos is essential in the treatment of infertility. Donors are carefully selected for health and family history of diseases and should be under the age of 35. Careful matching between the donor and recipient couples is facilitated between fertility clinic counsellors. Whilst gamete donation

TABLE 7.2	Terminologies for Assisted Conception Techniques
Term	**Explanation**
AHR	Assisted human reproduction
AIH	Artificial insemination by husband/partner treats problems with sperm delivery, antisperm antibodies and where semen has been stored before chemotherapy or radiotherapy. AIH is also known as homologous insemination.
AID	Artificial insemination by donor to prevent risk of transmission of a hereditary disease or Rhesus factor incompatibility, where sperm are totally abnormal on semen analysis
ART	Assisted reproductive technology
DI	Donor insemination
ET	Embryo transfer
IUI	Intrauterine insemination (also known as artificial insemination). This treatment involves the injection of better-quality sperm directly into the uterus.
IVF	In vitro fertilization: conception takes place outside the body
IVM	Use of immature ova, before conception in vitro
GIFT	Gamete intrafallopian transfer: sperm and ova are inserted into the uterine tube for conception to take place in a natural way
ZIFT	Zygote intrafallopian transfer: fertilized ovum replaced into the uterine tube after conception in vitro
ICSI	Intracytoplasmic sperm injection: sperm is manipulated via a pipette into the ova and then implanted into the uterus
MESA	Microsurgical epididymal sperm aspiration: the extraction of sperm from the epididymis
TESA	The aspiration of sperm from the testes
PGD	Preimplantation genetic diagnosis
PICSI	Physiological intracytoplasmic sperm injection (PICSI) selects sperm to use in ICSI treatment. PICSI identifies sperm that can bind to HA and select for use in treatment. No evidence to date.

may increase the opportunity of success, it brings emotional challenges from the loss of biological connection (Shepherd et al., 2018). Before accessing donor oocyte/sperm, it is essential that counselling is provided to ensure that the associated risks are well outlined.

In some countries, gamete and embryo donation follow specific guidelines, like the HFEA in the UK. In New Zealand, the Ethics Committee on Assisted Reproductive Technology (ECART) reviews, determines and monitors all embryo and egg donations and human reproductive research (ECART, 2021). Both countries maintain a register of donors so that any child born after gamete sperm or ovum donation has access to details about their biological parentage.

Principles of IVF

IVF is a common treatment for people who are unable to conceive naturally. IVF assists in conception by using laboratory techniques to assist sperm and egg to unite and produce an embryo which is then inserted into the uterus. The HFEA (2018) explains the sequence of phases in the technique of IVF:

- Superovulation.
- Egg recovery; sperm recovery.
- Fertilization.
- Preparation for pregnancy.
- Embryo transfer.

Superovulation involves using drugs to stimulate development of multiple ova. The investigations necessary to ensure that the phase of egg recovery results in mature ova involve frequent blood tests for oestradiol levels and ultrasound scans for follicle tracking. Egg recovery occurs usually under the guidance of ultrasound, with the egg being aspirated out of the follicle via a needle inserted through the vagina into the ovaries. The partner's or donor's sperm is added to the collected ova. Fertilization occurs with the partner or donor sperm in an incubator over approximately 14 hours. The embryos that begin to develop are assessed for quality. Cleavage-stage embryos are those that are grown for 2–3 days before transfer. Blastocysts are those that are grown in a laboratory incubator for 5–6 days before they are transferred into the uterus. Not all embryos will develop to blastocyst stage; overall a higher proportion of younger women will have blastocyst-stage embryos transferred. Many fertility clinics limit the number of embryos implanted into the uterus to one embryo to reduce the incidence of multiple pregnancy and ensure a positive outcome for ART. Remaining embryos are cryopreserved for future use. The woman receives hormones to prepare the endometrial lining for pregnancy, and the transfer is simple using a catheter inserted through the vagina and into the uterus.

Intracytoplasmic Sperm Injection

In the treatment of male infertility, ICSI has been revolutionary in making it possible for the baby's father to be the genetic parent (Barberán et al., 2020). Sperm are put into a solution that slows down motility to make them easier to work with. A microneedle is used to inject a single spermatozoon directly into the oocyte cytoplasm from the previously obtained oocyte as detailed earlier. The technique continues exactly as for IVF and embryo transfer. Although ICSI improves fertilization rates compared with IVF, the overall achievement rate of a pregnancy is no different (NICE, 2017a).

Surrogacy

When infertility treatment with IVF or ICSI fails (with or without donor oocyte/sperm), the only alternatives would be surrogacy or adoption. Surrogacy may be traditional whereby the surrogate's own ova are used with no requirement for fertility clinic services. Arrangements for surrogacy may be gestational, whereby at a fertility clinic the recipient parents' embryo is placed into the surrogate's uterus for her to gestate (HFEA, 2016). Many unanswered questions remain about the role of surrogacy where it is more readily acceptable in some countries than others. In some countries, surrogates may receive payment (e.g., United States), whereas in others payment is illegal (e.g., UK and New Zealand). Surrogacy has implications for the family's values and beliefs regarding informing the child of its origins and his/her surrogate mother.

Statistics and Conclusions

Clinical advances in the field of ART have revolutionized the treatment of infertility and improved the success rates of IVF. Based on records from 2019 (HFEA, 2021b), success rates vary across age and ethnic groups. Birth rates for women under 35 years were 32% per embryo transferred, compared to below 5% for women aged ≥43 years when using their own eggs. A considerable increase in the chance of a live birth to 30% is noted for all age groups when using donor eggs. The multiple birth rate reduced to the lowest of 6%. Box 7.2 summarizes the related differences when considering women from various ethnic backgrounds (HFEA, 2021b). The reasons are uncertain but may include socioeconomic-related pre-existing health conditions such as obesity.

Treatment using ART comes with considerable physical implications and financial costs. The psychological effects of undergoing fertility treatments have been likened to being on an emotional 'roller coaster'. For those in developing countries, there remains inequity of access.

To provide care for the increasing number of women who have conceived in this manner, maternity care providers require a clear understanding of infertility and ART procedures. Recognizing the underlying maternal factors as causative factors in complicated pregnancies, rather than ART alone, is important (Talaulikar & Arulkumaran, 2013). An increased risk of structural and chromosomal fetal anomalies requires serum and ultrasound

- IVF birth rates lowest for women from Black ethnicities.
- From 2014–2018, birth rates were lower among Black African and South Asian women in contrast to higher birth rates for White and mixed ethnicities.
- Black women aged 30–34 years had an average birth rate per embryo transferred of 23%, compared to average birth rates of 30% for mixed and White ethnicities.
- Endometrial receptivity may vary by ethnicity, and fibroids are three times more common in the Black population and are associated with reduced IVF success.
- Higher rates of tubal factor infertility were recorded among Black women (31%) compared to all women (18%).
- Asian women had the highest rates of ovulatory disorder at 25%, compared to the average of 20%.
- Black women are at a five times greater risk than White women of dying during pregnancy.
- Black women had the highest rate of multiple embryo transfer (46% of cycles), while White women had the lowest (38%) from 2014–2018.
- In 2018, IVF treatment was predominantly used by White women (78%), followed by Asian (14%), Black (3%), other (3%) and mixed-ethnicity (2%) women.
- For DI, the proportions of women by ethnicity in 2018 were: White (92%), followed by Asian (3%), Black (2%), mixed (2%) and other (1%).

HFEA, 2021b

Health professionals involved with women in reproductive years need the knowledge and information to appropriately provide accurate advice and evidence-based guidance to women and couples experiencing difficulties in conceiving.

Knowledge required:
- Main causes of infertility for women and for men.
- Investigations a women/couple might undergo to determine whether they are fertile.
- Different procedures (e.g., ICSI) involved and when they might be used.
- What IVF involves for the woman and couple.
- The differences between traditional and gestational surrogacy.

Information and advice relating to:
- Lifestyle factors that may reduce fertility for the woman or man.
- The range of information available for women/couples who are having difficulties conceiving.
- Ethical and social issues possibly experienced.
- Support groups, available professional support and potential psychological therapies.
- The use of surrogates from other countries.
- The implications of sperm, ova or embryo donation for the recipient woman and her partner and the future child.

monitoring, including fetal growth if restriction is suspected. Despite these known risks and the psychological impact of infertility and ART, people will continue to access ART to become parents. Across the infertility–pregnancy continuum, health professionals should be aware of the emotional distress and physical morbidity experienced by women and their partners in their quest to become parents. Their care needs to be informed, non-judgmental and tailored to each woman and her family. Clinical Application 7.1 discusses the knowledge and information required by health professionals.

Main Points

- The WHO defines infertility as a failure to achieve a clinical pregnancy after 12 months or more of regular unprotected sexual intercourse.
- Estimates indicate that between 48 million couples and 186 million individuals live with infertility worldwide.
- Infertility may result in psychological, emotional and sociocultural consequences for individuals and couples.
- The general lifestyles of both partners should be investigated.
- Male infertility can be related to idiopathic genetic defects or environmental effects with a decline in sperm counts.
- Males should be informed of the association between reduced semen quality and smoking, elevated BMI (≥ 30 kg/m^2), alcohol consumption greater than 3–4 units per day, elevated scrotal temperature and exposure to hazards.

- Women have a finite number of oocytes resulting in fecundity decreasing with age.
- Ultrasound scanning can detect a ripening Graafian follicle and a thickening endometrium.
- Women with irregular cycles should have serum levels of follicle-stimulating hormone and luteinizing hormone (gonadotrophins) measured.
- The use of basal body temperature as ovulation prediction is unreliable and now discouraged.
- PCOS, the most common hormonal disorder in women, can be confirmed by the presence of hyperandrogenism, anovulation with menstrual irregularities, and polycystic ovaries.
- Ascending infection is a common cause of tubal patency loss, which, with pelvic adhesions, distorts the uterine tubes.
- IVF treatment consists of a series of steps: superovulation, egg recovery, fertilization and embryo transfer.

References

Almas & Sabahat, 2022. Practice of FGM/FGC as customary/cultural ritual in a particular community in Pakistan. Multicult. Educ. 8 (3), 320–331.

Anokye, R.A., Acheampong, E., Mprah, W.K., Ope, J.O., Barivure, T.N., 2017. Psychosocial effects of infertility among couples attending St. Michael's Hospital, Jachie-Pramso in the Ashanti Region of Ghana. BMC Res. Notes 10, 690.

Ardestani Zadeh, A., Arab, D., 2021. COVID-19 and male reproductive system: pathogenic features and possible mechanisms. J. Mol. Histol. 52 (5), 869–878.

Balen, A.H., Morley, L.C., Misso, M., Franks, S., Legro, R.S., Wijeyaratne, C.N., et al., 2016. The management of anovulatory infertility in women with polycystic ovary syndrome: an analysis of the evidence to support the development of global WHO guidance. Hum. Reprod. Update 22 (6), 687–708.

Barberán, A.C., Boel, A., Meerschaut, F.V., Stoop, D., Heindryckx, B., 2020. Diagnosis and treatment of male infertility-related fertilization failure. J. Clin. Med. 9 (12), 3899.

Barratt, C.L.R., Björndahl, L., De Jonge, C.J., Lamb, D.J., Osorio Martini, F., McLachlan, R., et al., 2017. The diagnosis of male infertility: an analysis of the evidence to support the development of global WHO guidance-challenges and future research opportunities. Hum. Reprod. Update 23 (6), 660–680.

Bashiri, A., Halper, K.I., Orvieto, R., 2018. Recurrent implantation failure-update overview on etiology, diagnosis, treatment and future directions. Reprod. Biol. Endocrinol. 16, 121.

Capogrosso, P., Jensen, C.F.S., Rastrelli, G., Torremade, J., Russo, G.I., Raheem, A.A., et al., 2021. Male sexual dysfunctions in the infertile couple–recommendations from the European Society of Sexual Medicine (ESSM). Sex. Med. 9 (3), 100377.

de Berardis, D., Mazza, M., Marini, S., Del Nibletto, L., 2014. Psychopathology, emotional aspects and psychological counselling in infertility: a review. La Clinica Terapeutica 165 (3), 163–169.

de Castro, M.H.M., Mendonça, C.R., Noll, M., de Abreu Tacon, F.S., do Amaral, W.N., 2021. Psychosocial aspects of gestational grief in women undergoing infertility treatment: a systematic review of qualitative and quantitative evidence. Int. J. Environ. Res. Publ. Health 18 (24), 13143.

Dolan, A., Lomas, T., Ghobara, T., Hartshorne, G., 2017. 'It's like taking a bit of masculinity away from you': towards a theoretical understanding of men's experiences of infertility. Sociol. Health Illness 39 (6), 878–892.

Doyle, M., Carballedo, A., 2014. Infertility and mental health. Adv. Psychiatr. Treat. 20 (5), 297–303.

Ethics Committee on Assisted Reproductive Technology (ECART), 2021. Available at: https://ecart.health.govt.nz/.

Evans, B.M., Stentz, N.C., Richter, K.S., Schexnayder, B., Connell, M., Healy, M.W., et al., 2020. Mature follicle count and multiple gestation risk based on patient age in intrauterine insemination cycles with ovarian stimulation. Obstet. Gynecol. 135 (5), 1005–1014.

Fadhlaoui, A., Bouquet de la Jolinière, J., Feki, A., 2014. Endometriosis and infertility: how and when to treat? Front. Surg. 1, 24.

Gameiro, S., Finnigan, A., 2017. Long-term adjustment to unmet parenthood goals following ART: a systematic review and meta-analysis. Hum. Reprod. Update 23 (3), 322–337.

Gordon, J.L., Balsom, A.A., 2020. The psychological impact of fertility treatment suspensions during the COVID-19 pandemic. PLoS One 15 (9), e0239253.

Gurevich, R., 2022. Fertility Treatment. Available at: https://www.verywellfamily.com/fertility-treatment-overview-4581820.

Hasanpoor-Azghdy, A.B., Simbar, M., Vedadhir, A., 2014. The emotional-psychological consequences of infertility among infertile women seeking treatment: results of a qualitative study. Iran. J. Reproductive Med. 12 (2), 131–138.

Human Fertilisation & Embryology Authority (HFEA), 2016. Surrogacy. Available at: https://www.hfea.gov.uk/treatments/explore-all-treatments/surrogacy/.

Human Fertilisation & Embryology Authority (HFEA), 2018. In Vitro Fertilisation (IVF). Available at: https://www.hfea.gov.uk/treatments/explore-all-treatments/in-vitro-fertilisation-ivf/.

Human Fertilisation & Embryology Authority (HFEA), 2020. Family Formations in Fertility Treatment 2018: UK IVF and DI Statistics for Heterosexual, Female Same-Sex and Single Patients. Available at: https://www.hfea.gov.uk/media/3234/family-formations-in-fertility-treatment-2018.pdf.

Human Fertilisation & Embryology Authority (HFEA), 2021a. Fertility Treatment in 2019: Trends and Figures. Available at: https://www.hfea.gov.uk/about-us/publications/research-and-data/fertility-treatment-2019-trends-and-figures.

Human Fertilisation & Embryology Authority (HFEA), 2021b. Ethnic Diversity in Fertility Treatment 2018: UK Ethnicity Statistics for IVF and DI Fertility Treatment. Available at: https://www.hfea.gov.uk/about-us/publications/research-and-data/ethnic-diversity-in-fertility-treatment-2018/.

Human Fertilisation & Embryology Authority (HFEA), 2022. Fertility Treatment. Available at: https://www.hfea.gov.uk/treatments/fertility-preservation/egg-freezing/.

Iordăchescu, D.A., Paica, C.I., Boca, A.E., Gică, C., Panaitescu, A.M., Peltecu, G., et al., 2021. Anxiety, difficulties, and coping of infertile women. Healthcare 9, 466.

Jensen, C.F.S., Østergren, P., Dupree, J.M., Ohl, D.A., Sønksen, J., Fode, M., 2017. Varicocele and male infertility. Nat. Rev. Urol. 14 (9), 523–533.

Katib, A., 2015. Mechanisms linking obesity to male infertility. Cent. European J. Urol. 68 (1), 79–85.

Keszthelyi, M., Gyarmathy, V.A., Kaposi, A., Kopa, Z., 2020. The potential role of central obesity in male infertility: body mass index versus waist to hip ratio as they relate to selected semen parameters. BMC Publ. Health 20, 307.

Kirstensen, S.T., Andersen, C.Y., 2018. Cryopreservation of ovarian tissue: opportunities beyond fertility preservation and a positive view into the future. Front. Endocrinol. 9, 347.

Králíčková, M., Vetvicka, V., 2015. Immunological aspects of endometriosis: a review. Ann. Transl. Med. 3 (11), 153.

Leslie, S.W., Siref, L.E., Soon-Sutton, T.L., Khan, M.A.B., 2022. Male infertility. In: In StatPearls [Internet]. StatPearls Publishing, Treasure Island.

Lotti, F., Corona, G., Castellini, G., Maseroli, E., Fino, M.G., Cozzolino, M., Maggi, M., 2016. Semen quality impairment is associated with sexual dysfunction according to its severity. Hum. Reprod. 31 (12), 2668–2680.

Lotti, F., Baldi, E., Corona, G., Lombardo, F., Maseroli, E., Degl'Innocenti, S., et al., 2018. Epididymal more than testicular abnormalities are associated with the occurrence of antisperm antibodies as evaluated by the MAR test. Hum. Reprod. 33 (8), 1417–1429.

MacDougall, K., Beyene, Y., Nachtigall, R., 2013. Age shock: misperceptions of the impact of age on fertility before and after IVF in women who conceived after age 40. Hum. Reprod. 28 (2), 350–356.

Mahran, A., Abdelraheim, A.R., Eissa, A., Gadelrab, M., 2017. Does laparoscopy still has a role in modern fertility practice? I Int. J. Reprod. Biomed. 15 (12), 787–794.

Mascarenhas, M., Flaxman, S., Boerma, T., Vanderpoel, S., Stevens, G.A., 2012. National, regional, and global trends in infertility prevalence since 1990: a systematic analysis of 277 health surveys. PLoS Med. 9 (12), e1001356.

National Institute for Health and Care Excellence (NICE), 2017a. Fertility: Assessment and Treatment. Available at: https://www.nice.org.uk/guidance/cg156.

National Institute for Health and Care Excellence (NICE), 2017b. Endometriosis: Diagnosis and Management. Available at: www.nice.org.uk/guidance/ng73.

Patel, A., Sharma, P.S.V.N., Kumar, P., 2018. Role of mental health practitioner in infertility clinics: a review on past, present and future directions. J. Hum. Reprod. Sci. 11 (3), 219–228.

Rooney, K.L., Domar, A.D., 2018. The relationship between stress and infertility. Dialogues Clin. Neurosci. 20 (1), 41–47.

Sembuya, R., 2010. Mother or nothing: the agony of infertility. Bull. World Health Organ. 88, 881–882.

Shani, C., Yelena, S., Reut, B.K., Adrian, S., Sami, H., 2016. Suicidal risk among infertile women undergoing in-vitro fertilization: incidence and risk factors. Psychiatr. Res. 240, 53–59.

Shepherd, L., Kardzhieva, D., Bussey, L., Lovell, B., 2018. The role of emotions in predicting sperm and egg donation. J. Appl. Soc. Psychol. 48 (4), 217–226.

Su, H.W., Yi, Y.C., Wei, T.Y., Chang, T.C., Cheng, C.M., 2017. Detection of ovulation, a review of currently available methods. Bioeng. Transl. Med. 2 (3), 238–246.

Sun, H., Gong, T.T., Jiang, Y.T., Zhang, S., Zhao, Y.H., Wu, Q.J., 2019. Global, regional, and national prevalence and disability-adjusted life-years for infertility in 195 countries and territories, 1990–2017: results from a global burden of disease study. Aging 11 (23), 10952–10991.

Taebi, M., Kariman, N., Montazwei, A., et al., 2021. Infertility stigma: a qualitative study on feelings and experiences of infertile women. Int. J. Fertil. Steril. 15 (3), 189–196.

Talaulikar, V., Arulkumaran, S., 2013. Maternal, perinatal and long-term outcomes after assisted reproductive techniques (ART): implications for clinical practice. Eur. J. Obstet. Gynecol. Reprod. Biol. 170 (1), 13–19.

Tanbo, T., Fedorcsak, P., 2017. Endometriosis-associated infertility: aspects of pathophysiological mechanisms and treatment options. Acta Obstet. Gynecol. Scand. 96 (6), 659–667.

Tedros, A.G., 2019. Together for a Healthier World. Available at: https://www.who.int/director-general.

Trikudanathan, S., 2015. Polycystic ovarian syndrome. Med. Clin. 99 (1), 221–235.

Tsevat, M.D.G., Wiesenfeld, H.C., Parks, C., et al., 2017. Sexually transmitted diseases and infertility. Am. J. Obstet. Gynecol. 216 (1), 1–9.

Vioreanu, A., 2021. The psychological impact of infertility. Directions for the development of interventions. Ment. Health: Global Challenges Journal 4 (1).

Wang, J., Liu, C., Fujino, M., et al., 2019. Stem cells as a resource for treatment of infertility-related diseases. Curr. Mol. Med. 19 (8), 519–546.

World Health Organization (WHO), 2018. International Classification of Diseases. 11th revision. WHO Press, Geneva.

World Health Organization (WHO), 2020. Multiple Definitions of Infertility. Available at: https://www.who.int/news/item/04-02-2020-multiple-definitions-of-infertility.

World Health Organization (WHO), 2021. WHO Laboratory Manual for the Examination and Processing of Human Semen, sixth ed. WHO Press, Geneva.

World Health Organization (WHO), 2023a. Infertility Prevalence Estimates, 1990-2021. Available at: https://www.who.int/publications/i/item/978920068315.

World Health Organization (WHO), 2023b. Infertility. Available at: https://www.who.int/news-room/fact-sheets/detail/infertility.

World Health Organization (WHO), 2023c. Endometriosis. Available at: https://www.who.int/news-room/fact-sheets/detail/endometriosis.

Wrande, T., Kristjansdottir, B.H., Tsiartas, P., et al., 2022. Live birth, cumulative live birth and perinatal outcome following assisted reproductive treatments using donor sperm in single women vs. women in lesbian couples: a prospective controlled cohort study. J. Assist. Reprod. Genet. 39 (3), 629–637.

Zegers-Hochschild, F., Adamson, G.D., Dyer, S., et al., 2017. The international glossary on infertility and fertility care, 2017. Fertil. Steril. 108 (3), 393–406.

Zhang, P., Fan, Y., Tan, T., et al., 2020. Generation of artificial gamete and embryo from stem cells in reproductive medicine. Front. Bioeng. Biotechnol. 8, 781.

Annotated recommended reading

National Institute for Health and Care Excellence (NICE), 2017a. Fertility: Assessment and Treatment. Available at: https://www.nice.org.uk/guidance/cg156.

This easy-to-read evidence-based guideline was updated in 2017 and details the treatment of infertility from the context of the United Kingdom. Information on lifestyle risk factors with appropriate guidance is provided for health professionals to support individuals and couples who are experiencing fertility difficulties.

Patel, A., Sharma, P.S.V.N., Kumar, P., 2018. Role of mental health practitioner in infertility clinics: a review on past, present and future directions. J. Hum. Reprod. Sci. 11 (3), 219–228.

This paper provides an excellent review of the psychological, emotional and social factors impacting on infertile couples. It highlights the appropriateness of structured psychological interventions and the application of psychotherapy.

8

Preconception Matters

HORI SOLTANI AND FRANKIE FAIR

CHAPTER CONTENTS

This chapter focuses on preconception care and key factors relating to lifestyle and the environment that can impact on reproductive health and pregnancy outcomes. These factors include nutrition, smoking, alcohol, radiation, toxic waste, pre-existing diseases and drug ingestion and their interaction with the physiology of conception.

Introduction

Preconception care is a preventative approach through which biomedical, behavioural, social, environmental and psychosocial risk factors are identified before pregnancy or very early in pregnancy to optimize maternal and neonatal health outcomes. Preconception interventions are targeted at women, their partners and families to ensure a comprehensive approach.

It is estimated that between 7–10% of birth defects result from environmental agents such as infections and drugs. A further 20–25% of birth defects are believed to have multifactorial inheritance with a complex interaction between genetic and environmental factors (Moore et al.,

2019). The World Health Organization (WHO, 2023) estimated that 94% of severe birth defects occur in low- and middle-income countries where women frequently have poorer nutrition, less access to healthcare and screening and increased exposure to pollutants and infection.

The Healthy Gamete

There is no clear demarcation between the health of the gametes immediately before conception and the developing embryo, with both stages vulnerable to disruption. In the female fetus, the primary oocytes have already undergone their first reduction division early in the first trimester of fetal life. It is generally believed that females generate no new ova after the fifth month of fetal life. However, mechanisms for potential generation of new ova have recently been identified within adult mammals (Porras-Gómez & Moreno-Mendoza, 2017). In this arrested stage of development, oocytes are relatively resistant to mutagenic damage, although may still be vulnerable to chemotherapy, radiation and some environmental toxins. The continuously produced sperm are at high risk of environmental insult, with 75–80% of de novo human mutations believed to derive from the paternal gametes (Aitken, 2022).

After fertilization, until the zygote undergoes cleavage, so few cells are present that either the fetus will be affected by mutations and aborted spontaneously or it will not be affected and will continue to develop. The former may account for a considerable proportion of unexplained pregnancy losses within the first 6 weeks.

Prepregnancy Care Provision

The preconception period is traditionally seen as the 3 months prior to conception, with this also being the average time for fertile couples to conceive (Stephenson et al., 2018). The days to weeks prior to conception are important from a biological perspective when sensitivity to micronutrient deficits, smoking, drugs and alcohol are highest. However, a longer time period of months to years is necessary from a public health perspective to address risk factors such as diet and obesity (Stephenson et al., 2018).

Poor parental lifestyle during gamete maturation, fertilization and early embryonic development can cause epigenetic alterations. For example, DNA methylation (which controls gene expression) can be altered, which can have a long-term impact on offspring cardiovascular, immune, neural and metabolic health (Fleming et al., 2018). Therefore, the periconceptional period is of crucial importance for reducing maternal and neonatal mortality and enhancing lifelong offspring development.

One difficulty inherent in the concept of preconceptual care for health professionals is that many babies are conceived accidently, with an estimated 44% of pregnancies, leading to 23% of all births worldwide being unplanned (Bearak et al., 2018). For most of those who plan their conception, by the time their pregnancy is confirmed, they have already gone through the most vulnerable stage of embryogenesis. Embryogenesis is completed by the eighth week of pregnancy when many women have not yet attended their first antenatal visit. Additional barriers to preconception care include lack of provider knowledge, lack of parental knowledge of the need for preconception care and system-level issues such as lack of time and guidance (Goossens et al., 2018). However, there is evidence from randomized trials as well as retrospective, prospective and case control studies to indicate that preconception counselling improves pregnancy outcomes. A scoping review has found that women receiving prepregnancy care had improved pregnancy health behaviours including increased smoking cessation, healthy weight status and folic acid use and decreased alcohol use (Toivonen et al., 2017). There are debates concerning appropriate location, timing and format of preconception care provision. It has been suggested that young girls or women of childbearing age should be opportunistically educated at school or in primary care settings, with special programmes established to target the groups most in need. Examples include low socioeconomic status, smokers, women with obesity or those at high risk of complications due to underlying health conditions (diabetes or epilepsy). The aims of prepregnancy care are presented in Box 8.1.

Chronic Health Conditions

The benefits of preconception care are most evident in those with pre-existing or chronic diseases. Any pre-existing condition or disease requires specialist consultation before or very early in pregnancy. However, several common conditions are discussed below for information:

> **• BOX 8.1   Aims of Prepregnancy Care**
>
> - Assess potential risks to mother or infant by reviewing personal and family history, lifestyle risks and environmental exposure to teratogens, as well as undertaking a physical examination.
> - Counsel and educate with the aim to change risk behaviours (e.g., smoking, alcohol use, nutrition).
> - Manage chronic conditions and prevent adverse outcomes (e.g., pre-existing diabetes and addressing other conditions through vaccination, folic acid supplementation) (Atrash & Jack, 2020).

- **Diabetes**—Preconception care accompanied with good glycaemic control lowers the risk of fetal abnormalities, preterm birth and perinatal death in diabetic pregnancies (Wahabi et al., 2020).
- **Epilepsy**—Antiepileptic medications may be teratogenic; therefore adjusting the required dose may help in reducing potential risks.
- **Cardiac diseases**—Collaboration with cardiologists is crucial.
- **Oral anticoagulants**—Changing to injectable medication may reduce the risk of teratogenicity.
- **Hypothyroidism**—The thyroid gland is important in human metabolism; thus timely intervention to adjust thyroid levels could reduce the risk of abnormal fetal neurological development.
- **Phenylketonuria**—A diet reduced in phenylalanine before and during pregnancy can prevent damage to fetal brain development for women with this condition.
- **Mental health**—Minor and major forms of mental health should be screened and supportive care offered.
- **Acne**—Treatment with isotretinoin should be stopped because of the risk of teratogenicity.

General Health Care

The medical, obstetrical, social and family history of both the man and the woman should be taken, with known personal or familial health problems discussed. A gynaecological examination should be carried out to check for sexually transmitted diseases, as well as screening of blood and urine. Any infections should be treated, dietary problems discussed and possible work and lifestyle hazards considered.

As a general risk assessment, the main relevant issues screened for by making simple enquiries are summarized elsewhere (Atrash & Jack, 2020). Specific aspects are discussed below.

Socio-demographic History

The impact of maternal age on pregnancy outcome at both ends of the reproductive age is important. Teenagers are more likely to be anaemic (Pavord et al., 2019) and at risk of having growth-restricted infants, preterm labour and higher infant mortality, although they have a lower risk of gestational diabetes, caesarean section and instrumental birth (Marvin-Dowle & Soltani, 2020). Most teenage pregnancies are unplanned; therefore they rarely present for preconception care. Early pregnancy counselling could still be helpful. Pregnancies in later life (after 35 years) are substantially more at risk of obstetric complications (e.g., chromosomal abnormalities, gestational hypertension, gestational diabetes [GDM], preterm birth, low birthweight [LBW], perinatal mortality) (Avançada et al., 2019).

Socially disadvantaged women, asylum seekers and women at risk of mental health problems require integrated care from an early stage of pregnancy or ideally before pregnancy. However, providing preconception care can be more challenging for such women due to reduced access to routine care and a non-compliant behavioural pattern.

Providing creative outreach services and/or opportunistic care targeting such vulnerable groups can reduce maternal and neonatal health inequalities.

Nutrition and Weight

Establishing a balanced diet and a healthy lifestyle before pregnancy increases the likelihood of a successful pregnancy. Prepregnancy weight is positively related to infant birthweight. Body mass index (BMI, weight/height^2) is used to ascertain the optimum weight for an individual.

The WHO (2010) provides BMI ranges as a guide for nutritional status (see Table 8.1). Achieving a BMI within the normal weight range prior to pregnancy is recommended as nutritional deficiencies are seen at both ends of the scale.

Poor Nutrition

Retrospective studies during famine provide information about effects of food restriction on the human fetus. The Dutch famine of 1944–1945 showed more early pregnancy perinatal mortality in undernourished women and reduced fertility with sudden falls in energy intake (Barker, 1992). Acute energy deprivation may be different from chronic nutritional deprivation where maternal metabolism adjusts to optimize nutrient availability for the growing fetus. Additionally, the environmental stresses also present within such retrospective studies limit their applicability and generalizability. An estimated 2 billion people worldwide are deficient in micronutrients, with women being especially vulnerable due to menstruation and the additional nutritional demands of pregnancy (Darnton-Hill, 2018). Micronutrient deficiencies during pregnancy vary depending on season, deprivation and country socioeconomic status, but commonly include iron, zinc, vitamin B complex and vitamins D, E and A (Gernand et al., 2016). Teenagers are also especially vulnerable to poor nutrition and micronutrient intake, with 99% of women aged 18–25 years in the UK and 92% in Australia not consuming five portions of fruit and vegetables a day and 38% having diets deficient in iron in the UK (Stephenson et al., 2018). Teenagers are also more likely to eat more snacks, processed food and fizzy drinks (Marvin-Dowle et al., 2018). Being undernourished prior to conception is associated with fetal abnormality (Mezzasalma et al., 2021), preterm birth and LBW (Caut et al., 2022).

TABLE 8.1 BMI Ranges

BMI (kg/m^2)	Status
• Less than 18.5	Underweight
• 18.5–24.9	Normal weight
• 25.0–29.9	Pre-obesity
• 30.0–34.9	Obesity (class I)
• 35.0–39.9	Obesity (class II)
• Above 40.0	Obesity (class III)

(WHO, 2010)

Obesity

Obesity is a growing problem in many countries, particularly in industrialized societies such as the UK (Baker, 2021). Obesity is associated with increased risk of complications such as GDM, pre-eclampsia, thrombophlebitis, maternal infection, caesarean delivery and macrosomia (D'Souza et al., 2019; Santos et al., 2019; Wang et al., 2021). Women with obesity are prone to further development of obesity after pregnancy, particularly the central type of obesity (Soltani & Fraser, 2000). Additionally, women with obesity diagnosed with GDM are at increased risk of type II diabetes development in later life (Li et al., 2020).

Dieting is not advised during pregnancy (NICE, 2010) and lifestyle interventions during pregnancy for women with overweight or obesity can reduce weight gain but have limited impact on maternal or child health outcomes (Fair & Soltani, 2021). Prepregnancy weight is believed to have the largest influence on pregnancy outcomes; therefore adjusting maternal diet and weight before conception is essential (Marshall et al., 2022). A dual approach is required that targets women who are planning pregnancy, as well as improving population health in general (Barker et al., 2018). Lifestyle intervention research prior to conception is mainly performed among women with overweight or obesity seeking assisted reproduction. Findings suggest greater weight loss in intervention groups, but no reduction in adverse pregnancy outcomes such as preterm birth, pre-eclampsia or GDM (Lan et al., 2017). However, a recent review has suggested that higher levels of physical activity prior to pregnancy decrease the odds of GDM and pre-eclampsia (Daly et al., 2022). In one study, 65% of women with obesity were willing to defer the removal of contraceptive devices by 6 months to follow a weight-loss plan (Brackenridge et al., 2018).

Specific Nutrient Requirements

Suboptimal dietary deficiencies are common, especially in areas of high unemployment and poverty or people with dietary restrictions (vegans or vegetarians).

There is mounting evidence implicating specific dietary deficiencies affecting the process of organogenesis in the embryo, especially related to folic acid and zinc. Although the mechanism is unclear, studies show that supplementation with folate/folic acid around conception can prevent neural tube defects (NTD) in the fetus (Daly et al., 2022). Women are encouraged to eat folate-rich foods (e.g., green beans, peas and dark green leafy vegetables) and avoid overcooking them. Adequate consumption of folate is difficult to achieve through diet alone; therefore women planning a pregnancy are advised to take a daily supplement of 0.4 mg folic acid when trying to conceive until the 12th week of pregnancy (NICE, 2014). Furthermore, in many countries, fortification of foods such as breakfast cereals and flour is undertaken to reduce NTD. Other benefits of folic acid supplementation include decreased pre-eclampsia, LBW, infants small for gestational age (SGA), stillbirth and autism (Bulloch et al., 2018; Chen et al., 2021; Jonker et al., 2019).

Low zinc levels in both maternal blood samples and cord blood are associated with lower birthweight (Atazadegan et al., 2022). There is also some evidence that in utero exposure to high zinc levels reduces the risk of cleft palate (Ni et al., 2019). However, there is insufficient evidence to suggest that zinc supplementation during pregnancy can improve maternal or neonatal outcomes (Carducci et al., 2021). Consumption of foods rich in zinc such as oyster, meat, seeds, nuts and legumes should be encouraged.

Additionally, women should be made aware of the need for vitamin D supplementation once pregnant, especially if they belong to a group at higher risk of deficiency such as those with low exposure to the sun, with darker skin or teenagers (NICE, 2017).

Excessive intake of fat-soluble vitamins is harmful. Evidence suggests a potential risk of teratogenicity with doses of vitamin A above 10,000 IU per day, with increased risk of miscarriage and anomalies of the urinary tract reported (Bastos Maia et al., 2019). Although its role in causing human abnormalities is not fully confirmed, women in the UK who might become pregnant are usually advised to avoid vitamin A supplements and sources rich in vitamin A (e.g., liver) (British Dietetic Association, 2021).

Paternal Nutrition

The importance of nutrition in male fertility is also increasingly being investigated and recognized. Paternal obesity is linked to increased infertility by impacting sperm quantity and quality, such as reduced motility and increased abnormalities (Fleming et al., 2018). Consuming a diet containing lots of processed meats and fatty or sweet products has been associated with fewer morphologically normal sperm, reduced sperm motility and a decreased sperm count, especially for saturated fats (Fleming et al., 2018; Nassan et al., 2018). In contrast, consuming a diet rich in fish, omega-3 polyunsaturated fats, antioxidants, fruits and vegetables is related to a higher percentage of morphologically normal sperm and a higher mobile sperm count (Nassan et al., 2018). Nutrition can also influence seminal fluid composition which can further impact offspring development (Fleming et al., 2018).

Milk Products

Lower proportions of sperm with normal morphology and reduced sperm motility have been associated with increased consumption of dairy foods, particularly full-fat dairy products such as cheese (Salas-Huetos et al., 2017). Oestrogen, which is naturally present in dairy products, may partially contribute to these changes. However, low-fat dairy products are also known to increase circulating insulin and insulin-like growth factor 1, which may account for the higher sperm concentrations and motility noted with low-fat dairy products (Salas-Huetos et al., 2017). Additionally, other pollutants in milk such as pesticides may be the cause of sperm abnormalities (Afeiche et al., 2013).

Drugs

Drugs may be teratogenic, reduce absorption of nutrients or interfere with normal growth and development. The placenta is not a complete barrier against all chemicals.

Many people are exposed to drugs used to treat medical conditions. These may be essential for treatment and difficult to withdraw or reduce. Sometimes they can be substituted by less toxic drugs or stopped altogether during pregnancy. Women of childbearing age should only take medicines under medical supervision, and medical practitioners should be alert to the teratogenic side effects of drugs or their interactions.

Women are advised to allow 3 months after discontinuing hormonal contraceptives before trying to conceive. This allows the body time to readjust its hormonal system, resume physiological menstrual cycles and regulate the level of minerals and vitamins which may be affected by hormonal contraceptives. Mineral and vitamin levels may also be affected by intrauterine devices, especially if they contain copper which can interfere with zinc absorption and cause zinc deficiency.

Drugs may be taken for recreational reasons because of their mood-altering abilities. Such substances include alcohol, tobacco and caffeine, as well as addictive drugs such as cocaine (and its derivative crack), marijuana and heroin. It is difficult to ascertain whether they are being taken and to help people stop taking them. With appropriate referral systems, preconception counselling would be most effective for women who habitually use drugs, as drug misuse is associated with malnutrition, alcohol misuse, smoking and a higher risk of sexually transmitted diseases.

Smoking

The dangers of smoking for general health and during pregnancy are well documented. Many harmful chemicals such as polycyclic aromatic hydrocarbons, carbon monoxide, cyanide, lead and cadmium are inhaled in cigarette smoke. The effects of smoking on reproduction are increased infertility, increased risk of an early natural menopause (Zhu et al., 2018), reduced number and motility of sperm and increased number of abnormal sperm (Montagnoli et al., 2021). Smoking during pregnancy has been associated with reduced fetal growth (especially in women smoking 15 or more cigarettes a day) (Di et al., 2022), increased risk of sudden infant death syndrome (Anderson et al., 2019), 45% increased odds of stillbirth, and increased spontaneous abortions, fetal malformations, preterm labour and reduced length of gestation (Avşar et al., 2021). Long-term smoking during pregnancy has been linked to increased risk of obesity, attention deficit hyperactivity disorder, school-aged learning difficulties (Avşar et al, 2021) such as an increased risk of poor spelling, writing and numerical ability at 14 years of age (Ayano et al., 2021) and reduced immunocompetence (Avşar et al, 2021).

While no trials show that a reduction in smoking prior to pregnancy can improve outcomes, observational studies have shown improved pregnancy outcomes from reducing smoking prior to pregnancy, with no difference in LBW between women who stopped smoking prior to conception and those who had never smoked (Xaverius et al., 2019). Current evidence suggests that e-cigarettes are associated with similar adverse neonatal outcomes during pregnancy to traditional cigarettes (Kim & Oancea, 2020); therefore, stopping all forms of smoking prior to pregnancy is recommended. Given gaps in pregnancy planning, interventions such as smoke-free legislation are essential to not only improve whole population health, but also to benefit women with unplanned pregnancies (Stephenson et al., 2018).

Alcohol Consumption

Alcohol can impact male fertility as it is a direct testicular toxin. This leads to reduced semen quality, and animal studies also suggest atrophy of seminiferous tubules and changes to the number and morphology of Leydig cells (Finelli et al., 2022).

Alcohol consumption during pregnancy is also hazardous to the growing baby. There is growing recognition of fetal alcohol spectrum disorder, with a prevalence globally estimated to be 0.77%, but the prevalence in Europe and North America is estimated to be 2–5% and as high as 11% in South Africa (Lange et al., 2017). When alcohol is consumed by mothers, it reaches the fetus quickly, and there is no known safe level. The embryo is vulnerable to the damaging effects of alcohol at all stages of development, with the impact of alcohol on the fetus dependent on timing of consumption. Adverse effects include increased risk of miscarriage, physical defects, LBW, preterm birth, and behavioural problems such as hyperactivity and reduced attention span. Drinking alcohol also affects the mother's health by reducing absorption of vitamins and minerals. It is therefore recommended that women abstain from drinking when deciding to conceive and throughout the pregnancy (NICE, 2021).

Infection

Successful preconception care should investigate and treat any maternal infection and give appropriate advice to prevent infection, as it can adversely affect the pregnancy outcome. Urinary or genital infections may lead to preterm labour or miscarriage, and systemic infections may cause reproductive problems such as infertility and congenital defects.

Vaccination to confer immunity to **rubella** may be available, or when no vaccine is available, advice is given on how to minimize the risk of infection during pregnancy. Rubella acquired in the first trimester of pregnancy is associated with miscarriage or stillbirth. For surviving babies, 90% will have been congenitally infected with lifelong consequences from the associated congenital malformations (Singh, 2020). Routine rubella screening is offered to women in most Western countries; however rubella vaccination is contraindicated during pregnancy. Antenatal screening for rubella therefore only identifies the need for postpartum immunization to protect future pregnancies. Due to some controversial evidence regarding the measles, mumps and rubella (MMR) vaccination, there has been a decline in the number of children vaccinated against these diseases. There are also some women who give birth from abroad where vaccination against MMR is not widely offered. Preconception screening for at-risk women can play a protective role for their future pregnancies. After immunization, pregnancy should be avoided for at least a month.

The **Zika** virus came to international attention when it was linked to multiple cases of microcephaly diagnosed in neonates in Brazil. Although mainly caught from a mosquito bite, it can also be passed on through sexual intercourse. The virus is asymptomatic for many adults. Therefore, both men and women are advised to avoid conception for three months after visiting areas at risk of exposure to the Zika virus.

Numerous vaccines are also recommended once a woman becomes pregnant. These include **influenza**, which has been shown to reduce preterm birth and LBW (Giles et al., 2018) as well as influenza-related hospitalizations in the first 6 months of life for the infant (Jarvis et al., 2020). Similarly, women receiving the **whooping cough** vaccine from 18–20 weeks of pregnancy pass protective maternal antibodies across the placenta. This vaccine is highly effective at reducing whooping cough cases and subsequent hospitalization in infants under 3 months of age (Kandeil et al., 2020). The recent global **SARS-CoV-2** (COVID-19) pandemic has highlighted the vulnerability of pregnant women. Although evidence is still limited, it suggests that pregnant women infected with SARS-CoV-2 are at increased risk of pre-eclampsia, preterm birth, LBW and maternal mortality (Marchand et al., 2022), particularly for those with comorbidities such as obesity. Pregnant women are therefore recommended to be up to date with their COVID-19 vaccinations. In all cases, it is important that informed choice is facilitated, particularly where the balance of benefit and harm may be debatable at an individual level.

Toxoplasmosis caused by the parasite *Toxoplasma gondii*, which is found in soil and vegetation, multiplies at refrigerator temperatures (4–6°C or above), and *Listeria monocytogenes* can cause miscarriage, perinatal mortality or fetal abnormalities. Women planning a pregnancy or already pregnant should be advised on handling cat litter trays and to cook meat thoroughly to avoid toxoplasmosis. Additionally, all cat owners should not throw the contents of their cat litter tray down their toilet as the *T. gondii* parasite is not eliminated by current sewage treatments, and so can contaminate drinking water supplies.

To avoid **listeriosis,** women should be informed of hygienic food handling and to avoid eating soft, ripened cheeses such as Brie and blue-vein types. Cooked chilled meals and ready-to-eat poultry should be reheated until piping hot before consumption.

At the preconception clinic, women could be screened for other sexually transmitted or blood-borne infections such as chlamydia, syphilis, HIV and hepatitis B. Most bacteria are too large to cross the placenta, but viruses and the spirochaete of syphilis-causing *Treponema pallidum* can penetrate the placental membrane to infect the fetus.

Haemoglobinopathies

Genetic disorders affecting the shape and structure of haemoglobin in red blood cells can lead to a reduced oxygen-carrying capacity. Sickle cell disease is the most common haemoglobinopathy in the UK, with thalassaemia being less common. There is more prevalence of these disorders found in individuals in particular ethnic groups and others originating from specific countries (see Chapter 33). Sickle cell disease and thalassaemia are controlled by recessive genes; thus healthy people can be haemoglobinopathy carriers, with a 25% chance of each pregnancy being affected if both parents are carriers. Ideally, targeted screening should be offered to high-risk individuals before conception to provide an opportunity to discuss options, including diagnostic genetic testing, with counselling and support in making informed choices.

Hair Mineral Analysis

Hair analysis, which involves taking a sample of scalp hair and measuring mineral content, is regarded as fringe research but it can be useful. Some toxins are eliminated from blood and stored in body tissues, with hair showing traces of whatever has passed into the follicle in the previous 6–8 weeks. The following minerals can be tested through hair analysis (Mikulewicz et al., 2013):

- Essential minerals: calcium, magnesium, potassium, iron, chromium, cobalt, copper, manganese, nickel, selenium and zinc.
- Toxic minerals: aluminium, cadmium, mercury and lead. The last two are discussed later.

However, caution over interpretation of hair analysis during pregnancy may be required as zinc levels decrease and magnesium levels increase with maternal age and magnesium levels decrease with gestational age (Kocyłowski et al., 2018).

Environmental Issues

Toxins

Toxins can be natural or manufactured and are explained next.

Natural Toxins

Many natural toxins were developed by plants as a defence against being eaten and are well tolerated by humans. Examples include the tannins and alkaloids found in acorns or the cyanide in apples and apricots, where although the flesh is nutritious, the seeds in quantity are poisonous.

Defence Systems

Animals, including humans, have developed defence systems against plant toxins. The first line of defence is avoidance mediated by sight, smell and taste. The next line of defence is to expel toxins by vomiting and diarrhoea. One hypothesis is that the food aversion, nausea and vomiting experienced by about 80% of women in early pregnancy are protective against possible ingested toxins (American College of Obstetricians and Gynecologists' Committee, 2018). Other defence mechanisms include stomach acids and enzymes which neutralize some toxins and cells in the epithelial lining of the stomach which secrete a thin layer of protective mucus to prevent toxin absorption. Additionally, the liver has a wide range of enzymes that can render some toxins harmless.

Manufactured Toxins

The development of the chemical industry has resulted in contamination of the environment by vast quantities of synthetic pollutants such as organochlorine pesticides, polychlorinated biphenyls and polybrominated diphenyl ethers (PBDEs), all of which have long half-lives and accumulate in fatty tissues (Björvang et al., 2020). Pesticides (e.g., DDT) may disrupt reproductive development by interfering with the thyroid, oestrogen, androgen and neuroendocrine systems (Kabir et al., 2015). Worldwide use of pesticides is increasing, and it is believed that approximately 350,000 synthetic chemicals are now in use, some of which, although banned in Western countries (e.g., DDT), are still used in developing countries. Many of these chemicals are not easily biodegraded, and so the problem is likely to be with us for years to come. Some studies have suggested that parental exposure to pesticides or chemical pollutants such as perfluorooctanoic acids (PFOAs, found in oil and grease repellents) at high doses before or during pregnancy may be associated with SGA, stillbirth and congenital malformations. However the most recent systematic review suggested there is inadequate and inconsistent current evidence regarding this (Kirk et al., 2018). Exposure to phthalates used in plastics, paints and adhesives in males during adulthood has been linked to decreased sperm concentration and motility and increased time to pregnancy (Radke et al., 2018). The observed adverse associations alert us to the importance of regulatory legislation to control chemical waste and human exposure to them.

Human Infertility

Recent literature reviews have suggested a fall in sperm count of about 52.4% globally between 1973 and 2011 (Levine et al., 2017) and of about 32.5% within European men over the last 50 years (Sengupta et al., 2018), highlighting a decline in male fertility. Potential causes include lifestyle factors such as smoking, alcohol consumption and changes to diet composition, all of which can impact spermatogenesis. Additionally, increasing agricultural and industrial activity over recent decades has led to numerous environmental pollutants which have also been suggested to reduce male fertility (Sengupta et al., 2018). Continued investigation is however still needed into the impact of lifestyle, nutrition, body characteristics (e.g., BMI) and endocrine disruptors on male fertility.

River Pollution

Research has found that rivers are polluted with many endocrine-disruptive chemicals. These can occur naturally (e.g., hormones such as oestrogen, progesterone and testosterone) or they can be synthetically produced such as polycyclic aromatic hydrocarbons, ethinyl oestradiol (one of the two active ingredients of the contraceptive pill) or in other chemicals such as bisphenol A and phthalates found in plastics, organochlorine pesticides, and nonylphenols in detergents and domestic cleaners (Kasonga et al., 2021; Tang et al., 2020). Male embryos exposed to endocrine-disrupting chemicals from wastewater in utero have been linked to male reproductive disorders such as subfertility, undescended testes and testicular cancer (Kasonga et al., 2021). Additionally, there are numerous reports of the impact of these chemicals on wildlife including the feminization of fish with high percentages of intersex fish noted including the presence of oocytes in male testes, as well as thinning of birds' eggshells and population decline (Kasonga et al., 2021).

Unto the Third Generation

Environmental factors are probably as important in gametogenesis as in fetal development. The effect must, however, be considered over three generations as the ova of today's childbearing woman were developed while they were still in utero, as were the numbers of Sertoli cells in today's childbearing men.

Heavy Metals

Lead

Lead has been known to be toxic to the fetus for over 100 years. Lead is stored in the bones and may enter the fetus alongside the calcium mobilized from bone to supply fetal skeletal needs or through breastmilk during lactation. Lead exposure in early life affects mental development. In recognition of these detrimental effects, legislation protects pregnant women by stating that employers must remove them from working environments where significant exposure to lead would occur (Health and Safety Executive (UK) 2012).

Mercury

Organic mercury was shown to be exceedingly toxic when methylmercury was discharged into the Minamata Bay area of Japan in the 1950s. The mercury entered the food chain through fish, resulting in an increase in children born with cerebral palsy and other neurological abnormalities (Sakamoto et al., 2018). Mercury is still released into the atmosphere through coal-fired plants, waste incineration, mining and other industrial processes. This mercury enters the waterways through run-off or the settling of airborne particles, resulting in the presence of mercury in many fish. As smaller fish are eaten by bigger fish, mercury biomagnifies up the food chain, with the highest amounts of mercury seen in predatory fish such as tuna and shark. Women trying to conceive or who are pregnant are advised to minimize their consumption of tuna to reduce the possible impact of mercury on the developing fetal nervous system (British Dietetic Association, 2021).

Radiation

Radiation can be divided into ionizing radiation, such as that emitted by X-rays, nuclear medicine and atomic weapons testing, and non-ionizing radiation, emitted as ultraviolet and infrared rays and by microwaves, radar and radiofrequency waves. Visual display units are widely used in both the home and the workplace and release low levels of electromagnetic radiation.

Ionizing Radiation

Ionizing radiation damages DNA by transferring its energy into living cells. Atoms lose electrons and develop an electric charge. These charged particles penetrate the body and damage molecules, producing free radicals and oxidizing agents which break and damage DNA. An intense dose can kill cells and is used for this purpose in radiotherapy for cancer.

Diagnostic X-rays

There is no evidence that birth defects are caused by diagnostic levels of radiation. However, due to its potential harmful effects, limited maternal exposure to X-rays throughout the gestational period is advised unless it is an emergency. While shielding of the gonads of both men and women during diagnostic X-rays to prevent possible gamete damage has been practised for many years, with modern advances in equipment and optimisation, the benefits provided by this are now considered negligible (Jeukens et al., 2020).

Environmental Radiation

Humans are exposed to low-level natural background radiation, stemming mainly from natural γ-radiation from uranium in the ground and radon, its decay product. High doses of radon are associated with some birth defects, some cancers and chronic obstructive pulmonary disease, and are potentially linked with neurodegenerative diseases (Nayak et al., 2022).

The after-effects on health due to atomic bombs and nuclear accidents are presented in Box 8.2.

Non-ionizing Radiation

In relation to non-ionizing radiation (electromagnetic fields), the four types of electromagnetic fields are summarized in Table 8.2.

Research suggests a potential link between the incidence of childhood leukaemia diagnosed before the age of 5 years and exposure to electromagnetic fields produced by high-voltage power lines and transformer stations (Amoon et al., 2018). Some studies have revealed clusters of effects, including increased miscarriages and congenital defects; however, the multiple confounders within observational studies means correlation does not necessarily imply causation

• BOX 8.2 Atomic Bombs and Nuclear Accidents

Radiation is most damaging on the DNA of rapidly dividing cells such as spermatozoa, the ovum in late menstrual cycle and the early embryo. In 1945, after the dropping of atomic bombs at Hiroshima and Nagasaki in Japan by Americans, fetuses were found to be very sensitive to radiation, as many babies born to survivors were dead or deformed. The proposed critical exposure time for neurobehavioural abnormalities is between 8 and 15 weeks of gestation, as the fetal central nervous system develops rapidly at this stage (Kamiya et al., 2015). Instances of leukaemia, lung cancer, breast cancer and thyroid cancer have increased amongst atomic bomb survivors, with those exposed in utero having a similar risk of cancer to those exposed during childhood (Kamiya et al., 2015). Over the last 50 years, the increased risk of thyroid cancers, but not non-cancer thyroid dysfunction, has persisted in Japanese atomic bomb survivors, with the risk being highest among those who were youngest when exposed to the radiation (Imaizumi et al., 2017).

Chernobyl and Fukushima

The Chernobyl nuclear reactor accident (1986) was 'the worst nuclear accident in history'. Hot air carried fission products, far more reactive than uranium and plutonium, into the atmosphere. The Fukushima accident occurred in 2011 after a tsunami damaged the nuclear power plant. Both Chernobyl and Fukushima nuclear reactor disasters have been rated at the highest possible level on the international nuclear events scale.

Radiation exposure after a nuclear disaster is different from after a bomb, as it is protracted rather than an acute single event (Hatch et al., 2019). However, long-term follow-up from the area surrounding Chernobyl has suggested similar increases in thyroid cancer among those in utero at the time of the disaster, as well as among children and adolescents (Hatch et al., 2019). This is believed in part to be due to consumption of dairy products heavily contaminated with radioactive iodine (Drozdovitch, 2021). Workers present at the Chernobyl accident or who attempted to contain the explosion were shown to have a high incidence of malformed sperm and decreased sperm motility (De Felice, 2018). Higher rates of birth defects (e.g., spina bifida and cleft palate) were seen across numerous European countries after the Chernobyl reactor meltdown (Mangano & Sherman, 2015). More recently, a significant increase in five birth defects (anencephaly, cleft lip and palate, Down syndrome, gastroschisis and spina bifida) has been detected in the Western states of the United States compared with the rest of the United States after the Fukushima nuclear disaster (Mangano & Sherman, 2015).

TABLE 8.2	Types of Electromagnetic Fields
1.	Extremely low-frequency electromagnetic fields (<300 Hz): generated by some domestic electrical appliances (even when switched off but connected to a power source), power lines and military equipment.
2.	Intermediate-frequency electromagnetic fields (300 Hz–10 MHz): generated around high-voltage power lines and domestic electrical equipment such as computer displays.
3.	High-frequency electromagnetic fields (10 MHz–3000 GHz): generated by laptops, Wi-fi, televisions, microwave ovens and mobile phones.
4.	Static electromagnetic fields have zero frequency and are produced by MRI machines and in geomagnetism.

Jangid et al., 2022

(Jangid et al., 2022). There is some evidence of the detrimental effect of electromagnetic fields on male fertility, with sperm mobility and sperm count decreased with increased exposure to mobile phone radiation (Sciorio et al., 2022). While microwave ovens are generally deemed safe, they should not be used if broken or defective and pregnant women are advised to avoid standing directly in front of them when switched on.

Chemical Weapons

Chemical weapons, such as those used in conflicts by Iraq against Iran and its own Kurdish people, can have devastating consequences on reproduction, with decreased sperm count and increased infertility, miscarriage and congenital anomalies.

Main Points

- Pregnancy outcome is improved markedly when couples are screened and given preconception advice to optimize health before pregnancy.
- Long-term health problems should be stabilized, infections treated and lifestyle issues addressed.
- Sperm are at risk of environmental insult. Ova in a state of arrested development are relatively resistant to mutagenic damage until just before ovulation. The zygote is resistant to genetic injury during cleavage, but after 16 days intense organogenesis begins and sensitivity is high.
- Systemic infections may cause reproductive problems (e.g., infertility and congenital defects). Specific infectious diseases can be prevented by vaccination and advice on how to avoid or reduce contact with infected individuals/groups.
- Drugs and alcohol may damage sperm and ova or adversely affect nutrient absorption so that essential nutrients are absent at crucial times during embryonic development.
- The development of the chemical industry has resulted in vast quantities of synthetic chemicals being released into the environment, which may disrupt human reproduction. Lead and mercury are exceedingly toxic to the developing nervous system.
- Environmental factors are important in gametogenesis and fetal development and may cause an impact over three generations. The ova of today's childbearing women

were developed while they were still in utero, as were the number of Sertoli cells in today's prospective fathers.
- Ionizing radiation damages DNA. Leukaemia, lung cancer and thyroid cancer are increased among atomic bomb survivors and among those exposed in utero.

- The health effects of electromagnetic fields on reproductive health are still unclear.
- Other agents affecting reproductive health are chemical weapons due to the detrimental effects on the developing fetus.

References

Afeiche, M., Williams, P.L., Mendiola, J., Gaskins, A.J., Jørgensen, N., Swan, S.H., et al., 2013. Dairy food intake in relation to semen quality and reproductive hormone levels among physically active young men. Hum. Reprod. 28 (8), 2265–2275.

Aitken, R.J., 2022. Role of sperm DNA damage in creating de-novo mutations in human offspring: the 'post-meiotic oocyte collusion' hypothesis. Reprod. Biomed. Online 45 (1), 109–124.

American College of Obstetricians and Gynecologists' Committee, 2018. ACOG practice bulletin 189: nausea and vomiting of pregnancy. Obstet. Gynecol. 131 (1), e15–e30.

Amoon, A.T., Crespi, C.M., Ahlbom, A., Bhatnagar, M., Bray, I., Bunch, K.J., et al., 2018. Proximity to overhead power lines and childhood leukaemia: an international pooled analysis. Br. J. Cancer 119 (3), 364–373.

Anderson, T.M., Lavista Ferres, J.M., Ren, S.Y., Moon, R.Y., Goldstein, R.D., Ramirez, J.M., et al., 2019. Maternal smoking before and during pregnancy and the risk of sudden unexpected infant death. Pediatrics 143 (4), e20183325.

Atazadegan, M.A., Heidari-Beni, M., Riahi, R., Kelishadi, R., 2022. Association of selenium, zinc and copper concentrations during pregnancy with birth weight: a systematic review and meta-analysis. J. Trace Elem. Med. Biol. 69, 126903.

Atrash, H., Jack, B., 2020. Preconception care to improve pregnancy outcomes: the science. J. Hum. Growth Dev. 30 (3), 355–362.

Avançada, I.M., da Gravidez, D.A., Meta-Análise, U., 2019. Advanced maternal age: adverse pregnancy outcomes of pregnancy, a meta-analysis. Acta Med. Port. 32 (3), 219–226.

Avşar, T.S., McLeod, H., Jackson, L., 2021. Health outcomes of smoking during pregnancy and the postpartum period: an umbrella review. BMC Pregnancy Childbirth 21 (1), 254.

Ayano, G., Betts, K., Dachew, B.A., Alati, R., 2021. Maternal smoking during pregnancy and poor academic performance in adolescent offspring: a registry data-based cohort study. Addict. Behav. 123, 107072.

Baker, C., 2021. Research Briefing. Obesity Statistics. House of Commons Library Briefing Paper, p. 3336.

Barker, D.J.P., 1992. Fetal and Infant Origins of Adult Disease. BMJ Books, London.

Barker, M., Dombrowski, S.U., Colbourn, T., Fall, C.H.D., Kriznik, N.M., Lawrence, W.T., et al., 2018. Intervention strategies to improve nutrition and health behaviours before conception. Lancet 391 (10132), 1853–1864.

Bastos Maia, S., Rolland Souza, A.S., Costa Caminha, M.F., Lins da Silva, S., Callou Cruz, R.S.B.L., Carvalho Dos Santos, C., et al., 2019. Vitamin A and pregnancy: a narrative review. Nutrients 11 (3), 681.

Bearak, J., Popinchalk, A., Alkema, L., Sedgh, G., 2018. Global, regional, and subregional trends in unintended pregnancy and its outcomes from 1990 to 2014: estimates from a Bayesian hierarchical model. Lancet Global Health 6 (4), e380–e389.

Björvang, R.D., Gennings, C., Lin, P.I., Hussein, G., Kiviranta, H., Rantakokko, P., et al., 2020. Persistent organic pollutants, prepregnancy use of combined oral contraceptives, age, and time-to-pregnancy in the SELMA cohort. Environ. Health 19 (1), 67.

Brackenridge, L., Finer, N., Batterham, R.L., Pedram, K., Ding, T., Stephenson, J., et al., 2018. Pre-pregnancy weight loss in obese women requesting removal of their intra uterine contraceptive device in order to conceive: a pilot study of full meal replacement. Clin. Obes. 8 (4), 244–249.

British Dietetic Association, 2021. Pregnancy and Diet: Food Fact Sheet. Available from: https://www.bda.uk.com/resource/pregnancy-diet.html.

Bulloch, R.E., Lovell, A.L., Jordan, V.M.B., McCowan, L.M.E., Thompson, J.M.D., Wall, C.R., 2018. Maternal folic acid supplementation for the prevention of preeclampsia: a systematic review and meta-analysis. Paediatr. Perinat. Epidemiol. 32 (4), 346–357.

Carducci, B., Keats, E.C., Bhutta, Z.A., 2021. Zinc supplementation for improving pregnancy and infant outcome. Cochrane Database Syst. Rev. 3 (3), CD000230.

Caut, C., Schoenaker, D., McIntyre, E., Vilcins, D., Gavine, A., Steel, A., 2022. Relationships between women's and men's modifiable preconception risks and health behaviors and maternal and offspring health outcomes: an umbrella review. Semin. Reprod. Med. 40 (03/04), 170–183.

Chen, H., Qin, L., Gao, R., Jin, X., Cheng, K., Zhang, S., et al., 2021. Neurodevelopmental effects of maternal folic acid supplementation: a systematic review and meta-analysis. Crit. Rev. Food Sci. Nutr. 1–17.

Daly, M., Kipping, R.R., Tinner, L.E., Sanders, J., White, J.W., 2022. Preconception exposures and adverse pregnancy, birth and postpartum outcomes: umbrella review of systematic reviews. Paediatr. Perinat. Epidemiol. 36 (2), 288–299.

Darnton-Hill, I., 2018. Prevalence, causes and consequences of micronutrient deficiencies. 'The gap between need and action', Chapter 2. In: Mannar, M.G.V., Hurrell, R.F. (Eds.), Food Fortification in a Globalized World. Academic Press, Cambridge, Massachusetts.

De Felice, F., Marchetti, C., Marampon, F., Cascialli, G., Muzii, L., Tombolini, V., 2018. Radiation effects on male fertility. Andrology 7 (1), 2–7.

Drozdovitch, V., 2021. Radiation exposure to the thyroid after the Chernobyl accident. Front. Endocrinol. 11, 569041.

D'Souza, R., Horyn, I., Pavalagantharajah, S., Zaffar, N., Jacob, C.E., 2019. Maternal body mass index and pregnancy outcomes: a systematic review and metaanalysis. Am. J. Obstet. Gynecol. MFM 1 (4), 100041.

Fair, F., Soltani, H., 2021. A meta-review of systematic reviews of lifestyle interventions for reducing gestational weight gain in women who are overweight or obese. Obes. Rev. 22 (5), e13199.

Finelli, R., Mottola, F., Agarwal, A., 2022. Impact of alcohol consumption on male fertility potential: a narrative review. Int. J. Environ. Res. Publ. Health 19 (10), 328.

Fleming, T.P., Watkins, A.J., Velazquez, M.A., Mathers, J.C., Prentice, A.M., Stephenson, J., et al., 2018. Origins of lifetime health around the time of conception: causes and consequences. Lancet 391 (10132), 1842–1852.

Gernand, A.D., Schulze, K.J., Stewart, C.P., West Jr., K.P., Christian, P., 2016. Micronutrient deficiencies in pregnancy worldwide: health effects and prevention. Nat. Rev. Endocrinol. 12 (5), 274–289.

Giles, M.L., Krishnaswamy, S., Macartney, K., Cheng, A., 2018. The safety of inactivated influenza vaccines in pregnancy for birth outcomes: a systematic review. Hum. Vaccines Immunother. 15 (3), 687–699.

Goossens, J., De Roose, M., Van Hecke, A., Goemaes, R., Verhaeghe, S., Beeckman, D., 2018. Barriers and facilitators to the provision of preconception care by healthcare providers: a systematic review. Int. J. Nurs. Stud. 87, 113–130.

Hatch, M., Brenner, A.V., Cahoon, E.K., Drozdovitch, V., Little, M.P., Bogdanova, T., et al., 2019. Thyroid cancer and benign nodules after exposure in utero to fallout from Chernobyl. J. Clin. Endocrinol. Metab. 104 (1), 41–48.

Health and Safety Executive (UK), 2012. Lead and You. Working Safely with Lead. HSE, London.

Imaizumi, M., Ohishi, W., Nakashima, E., Sera, N., Neriishi, K., Yamada, M., et al., 2017. Thyroid dysfunction and autoimmune thyroid diseases among atomic bomb survivors exposed in childhood. J. Clin. Endocrinol. Metab. 102 (7), 2516–2524.

Jangid, P., Rai, U., Sharma, R.S., Singh, R., 2022. The role of non-ionizing electromagnetic radiation on female fertility: a review. Int. J. Environ. Res. Publ. Health 33 (4), 358–373.

Jarvis, J.R., Dorey, R.B., Warricker, F.D.M., Alwan, N.A., Jones, C.E., 2020. The effectiveness of influenza vaccination in pregnancy in relation to child health outcomes: systematic review and meta-analysis. Vaccine 38 (7), 1601–1613.

Jeukens, C.R.L.P.N., Kütterer, G., Kicken, P.J., Frantzen, M.J., van Engelshoven, J.M.A., Wildberger, J.E., et al., 2020. Gonad shielding in pelvic radiography: modern optimised X-ray systems might allow its discontinuation. Insights Imag. 11 (1), 15.

Jonker, H., Capelle, N., Lanes, A., Wen, S.W., Walker, M., Corsi, D.J., 2019. Maternal folic acid supplementation and infant birthweight in low- and middle-income countries: a systematic review. Matern. Child Nutr. 16 (1), e12895.

Kabir, E.R., Rahman, M.S., Rahman, I., 2015. A review on endocrine disruptors and their possible impacts on human health. Environ. Toxicol. Pharmacol. 40 (1), 241–258.

Kamiya, K., Ozasa, K., Akiba, S., Niwa, O., Kodama, K., Takamura, N., et al., 2015. From Hiroshima and Nagasaki to Fukushima 1. Long term effects of radiation exposure on health. Lancet 386 (9992), 469–478.

Kandeil, W., van den Ende, C., Bunge, E.M., Jenkins, V.A., Ceregido, M.A., Guignard, A., 2020. A systematic review of the burden of pertussis disease in infants and the effectiveness of maternal immunization against pertussis. Expert Rev. Vaccine 19 (7), 621–638.

Kasonga, T.K., Coetzee, M.A.A., Kamika, I., Ngole-Jeme, V.M., Benteke Momba, M.N., 2021. Endocrine-disruptive chemicals as contaminants of emerging concern in wastewater and surface water: a review. J. Environ. Manag. 277, 111485.

Kim, S., Oancea, S.C., 2020. Electronic cigarettes may not be a "safer alternative" of conventional cigarettes during pregnancy: evidence from the nationally representative PRAMS data. BMC Pregnancy Childbirth 20 (1), 557.

Kirk, M., Smurthwaite, K., Bräunig, J., Trevenar, S., D'Este, C., Lucas, R., et al., 2018. The PFAS Health Study: Systematic Literature Review. The Australian National University, Canberra.

Kocyłowski, R., Lewicka, I., Grzesiak, M., Gaj, Z., Sobańska, A., Pozna-niak, J., et al., 2018. Assessment of dietary intake and mineral status in pregnant women. Arch. Gynecol. Obstet. 297 (6), 1433–1440.

Lan, L., Harrison, C.L., Misso, M., Hill, B., Teede, H.J., Mol, B.W., et al., 2017. Systematic review and meta-analysis of the impact of preconception lifestyle interventions on fertility, obstetric, fetal, anthropometric and metabolic outcomes in men and women. Hum. Reprod. 32 (9), 1925–1940.

Lange, S., Probst, C., Gmel, G., 2017. Global prevalence of fetal alcohol spectrum disorder among children and youth. A systematic review and meta-analysis. JAMA Pediatr. 171 (10), 948–956.

Levine, H., Jørgensen, N., Martino-Andrade, A., Mendiola, J., Weksler-Derri, D., Mindlis, I., et al., 2017. Temporal trends in sperm count: a systematic review and meta-regression analysis. Hum. Reprod. Update 23 (6), 646–659.

Li, Z., Cheng, Y., Wang, D., Chen, H., Chen, H., Ming, W.K., et al., 2020. Incidence rate of type 2 diabetes mellitus after gestational diabetes mellitus: a systematic review and meta-analysis of 170,139 women. J. Diabetes Res. 2020, 3076463.

Mangano, J., Sherman, J.D., 2015. Changes in congenital anomaly incidence in west coast and pacific states (USA) after arrival of Fukushima fallout. Open J. Pediatr. 5 (1), 76–89.

Marchand, G., Patil, A.S., Masoud, A.T., Ware, K., King, A., Ruther, S., et al., 2022. Systematic review and meta-analysis of COVID-19 maternal and neonatal clinical features and pregnancy outcomes up to June 3, 2021. AJOG Global Rep. 2 (1), 100049.

Marshall, N.E., Abrams, B., Barbour, L.A., Catalano, P., Christian, P., Friedman, J.E., et al., 2022. The importance of nutrition in pregnancy and lactation: lifelong consequences. Am. J. Obstet. Gynecol. 226 (5), 607–632.

Marvin-Dowle, K., Soltani, H., 2020. A comparison of neonatal outcomes between adolescent and adult mothers in developed countries: a systematic review and meta-analysis. Eur. J. Obstet. Gynecol. Reprod. Biol. X 6, 100109.

Marvin-Dowle, K., Kilner, K., Burley, V., Soltani, H., 2018. Differences in dietary pattern by maternal age in the Born in Bradford cohort: a comparative analysis. PLoS One 13 (12), e0208879.

Mezzasalma, L., Santoro, M., Coi, A., Pierini, A., 2021. Association between maternal body mass index and congenital anomalies: a case control study in Tuscany (Italy). 114 (3–4), 116–123.

Mikulewicz, M., Chojnacka, K., Gedrange, T., Górecki, H., 2013. Reference values of elements in human hair: a systematic review. Environ. Toxicol. Pharmacol. 36 (3), 1077–1086.

Montagnoli, C., Ruggeri, S., Cinelli, G., Tozzi, A.E., Bovo, C., Bortolus, R., et al., 2021. Anything new about paternal contribution to reproductive outcomes? A review of the evidence. The World Journal of Men's Health 39 (4), 626–644.

Moore, K.L., Persaud, T.V.N., Torchia, M.G., 2019. Before We Are Born: Essentials of Embryology and Birth Defects, tenth ed. Elsevier, Philadelphia.

Nassan, F.L., Chavarro, J.E., Tanrikut, C., 2018. Diet and men's fertility: does diet affect sperm quality? Fertil. Steril. 110 (4), 570–577.

Nayak, T., Basak, S., Deb, A., Dhal, P.K., 2022. A systematic review on groundwater radon distribution with human health consequences and probable mitigation strategy. J. Environ. Radioact. 247, 106852.

Ni, W., Yang, W., Yu, J., Li, Z., Jin, L., Liu, J., et al., 2019. Association between selected essential trace element concentrations in umbilical cord and risk for cleft lip with or without cleft palate: a case-control study. Sci. Total Environ. 661, 196–202.

NICE (National Institute for Health and Care Excellence), 2010. Weight Management before, during and after Pregnancy. NICE PHG27. NICE, London.

NICE (National Institute for Health and Care Excellence), 2014. Maternal and Child Nutrition. NICE PH11. NICE, London.

NICE (National Institute for Health and Care Excellence), 2017. Vitamin D: Supplement Use in Specific Population Groups. NICE PH56. NICE, London.

NICE (National Institute for Health and Care Excellence), 2021. Antenatal Care. NICE Guideline NG201, NICE, London.

Pavord, S., Daru, J., Prasannan, N., Robinson, S., Stanworth, S., Girling, J., BSH Committee, 2019. UK guidelines on the management of iron deficiency in pregnancy. Br. J. Haematol. 188 (6), 819–830.

Porras-Gómez, T.J., Moreno-Mendoza, N., 2017. Neo-oogenesis in mammals. Zygote 25 (4), 404–422.

Radke, E.G., Braun, J.M., Meeker, J.D., Cooper, G.S., 2018. Phthalate exposure and male reproductive outcomes: a systematic review of the human epidemiological evidence. Environ. Int. 121 (1), 764–793.

Sakamoto, M., Tatsuta, N., Izumo, K., Phan, P.T., Vu, L.D., Yamamoto, M., et al., 2018. Health impacts and biomarkers or prenatal exposure to methylmercury: lessons from Minamata, Japan. Toxics 6 (3), 45.

Salas-Huetos, A., Bulló, M., Salas-Salvadó, J., 2017. Dietary patterns, foods and nutrients in male fertility parameters and fecundability: a systematic review of observational studies. Hum. Reprod. Update 23 (4), 371–389.

Santos, S., Voerman, E., Amiano, P., Barros, H., Beilin, L.J., Bergström, A., et al., 2019. Impact of maternal body mass index and gestational weight gain on pregnancy complications: an individual participant data meta-analysis of European, North American and Australian cohorts. BJOG An Int. J. Obstet. Gynaecol. 126 (8), 984–995.

Sciorio, R., Tramontano, L., Esteves, S.C., 2022. Effects of mobile phone radiofrequency radiation on sperm quality. Zygote 30 (2), 159–168.

Sengupta, P., Borges Jr., E., Dutta, S., Krajewska-Kulak, E., 2018. Decline in sperm count in European men during the last 50 years. Hum. Exp. Toxicol. 37 (3), 247–255.

Singh, C., 2020. Rubella in pregnancy. J. Fetal Med. 7 (8302), 37–41.

Soltani, H., Fraser, R.B., 2000. A longitudinal study of maternal anthropometric changes in normal weight, overweight and obese women during pregnancy and postpartum. Br. J. Nutr. 84 (1), 95–101.

Stephenson, J., Heslehurst, N., Hall, J., Schoenaker, D.A.J.M., Hutchinson, J., Cade, J.E., et al., 2018. Before the beginning: nutrition and lifestyle in the preconception period and its importance for future health. Lancet 391 (10132), 1830–1841.

Tang, Z.R., Xu, X.L., Deng, S.L., Lian, Z.X., Yu, K., 2020. Oestrogenic endocrine disruptors in the placenta and the fetus. Int. J. Mol. Sci. 21 (4), 1519.

Toivonen, K.I., Oinonen, K.A., Duchene, K.M., 2017. Preconception health behaviours: a scoping review. Prev. Med. 96, 1–15.

Wahabi, H.A., Fayed, A., Esmaeil, S., Elmorshedy, H., Titi, M.A., Amer, Y.S., et al., 2020. Systematic review and meta-analysis of the effectiveness of pre-pregnancy care for women with diabetes for improving maternal and perinatal outcomes. PLoS One 15 (8), e0237571.

Wang, A.M., Lee, A.J., Clark, S.M., 2021. The effects of overweight and obesity on pregnancy-related morbidity. Clin. Exp. Obstet. Gynecol. 48 (5), 999–1009.

WHO (World Health Organization), 2023. Birth defects. Available from: https://www.who.int/news-room/fact-sheets/detail/birth-defects.

WHO (World Health Organization), 2010. A healthy lifestyle – WHO recommendations. Available from: https://www.who.int/Europe/news-room/fact-sheets/item/a-healthy-lifestyle---WHO-recommendations.

Xaverius, P.K., O'Reilly, Z., Li, A., Flick, L.H., Arnold, L.D., 2019. Smoking cessation and pregnancy: timing of cessation reduces or eliminates the effect on low birth weight. Matern. Child Health J. 23 (10), 1434–1441.

Zhu, D., Chung, H.F., Pandeya, N., Dobson, A.J., Cade, J.E., Greenwood, D.C., et al., 2018. Relationships between intensity, duration, cumulative dose, and timing of smoking with age at menopause: a pooled analysis of individual data from 17 observational studies. PLoS Med. 15 (11), e1002704.

Annotated recommended reading

Moore, K.L., Persaud, T.V.N., Torchia, M.G., 2019. Before We Are Born: Essentials of Embryology and Birth Defects, tenth ed. Elsevier, Philadelphia.

This embryology textbook has a very good chapter on human birth defects, including sections on genetical and environmental factors and multifactorial inheritance.

Goossens, J., De Roose, M., Van Hecke, A., Goemaes, R., Verhaeghe, S., Beeckman, D., 2018. Barriers and facilitators to the provision of preconception care by healthcare providers: a systematic review. Int. J. Nurs. Stud. 87, 113–130.

This article provides an excellent overview of the barriers faced by healthcare providers around the provision of preconception care.

Fleming, T.P., Watkins, A.J., Velazquez, M.A., Mathers, J.C., Prentice, A.M., Stephenson, J., et al., 2018. Origins of lifetime health around the time of conception: causes and consequences. Lancet 391 (10132), 1842–1852.

This article provides the biological mechanisms by which the periconceptional period impacts on offspring lifetime health.

Website

https://www.nice.org.uk.

This site provides the reader with a range of the most up-to-date high-quality evidence-based guidelines, evidence and best practice resources.

Pregnancy—The Fetus

This section is concerned with the development and growth of the fetus, placenta and membranes. The topic is presented in some detail as the developments in treatment of infertility and in the detection and management of fetal abnormalities are expanding rapidly. The care of the childbearing woman includes complex screening tests for fetal well-being. Therefore it is essential for the midwife to have relevant knowledge and experience to appropriately support women and their families. Chapter 9 discusses general points about embryological development, with Chapters 10 and 11 detailing the development of individual systems. Chapter 12 describes the development and function of the placenta and membranes and the nature of amniotic fluid. Chapter 13 explores fetal growth and development, and Chapter 14 discusses some common fetal problems. Finally, the important topic of the causes, diagnosis and management of common congenital anomalies is discussed in Chapter 15.

9

General Embryology

SONYA MACVICAR

CHAPTER CONTENTS

This is the first of three chapters detailing the development of the embryo and fetus. This chapter outlines the general principles of embryology and introduces gametogenesis, fertilization and related terminology. An overview of the initial programming of the embryo includes early cell division–cleavage, differentiation and morphogenesis. Thereafter, development of the embryo, blastocyst and implantation are covered with development and differentiation of the germ layers and organogenesis.

Introduction

Embryology is the term used to describe the developmental processes that take the human from one fertilized egg to a fetus ready to be born.

Embryology

Due to ethical considerations, discoveries about the development of the human embryo are gained by research into the development of other species (The Human Fertilisation and Embryology Act, 2008). There are surprising similarities in the basic processes of development between species, including cell division and differentiation, pattern formation, change in form and growth (Wolpert, Tickel & Arias, 2019).

The study of embryology enables us to understand the causes of congenital abnormalities. These are present in about 6% of live births, of which half are detected at birth and half during the first year of life. At least half of all conceptuses are malformed, and these are usually aborted spontaneously (Moore, Persaud & Torchia, 2018).

Gametogenesis

Gametogenesis (gamete formation) is the formation of the sperm and ova (Moore, Persaud & Torchia, 2018). The primary spermatocytes and primary oocytes are diploid cells, having 46 chromosomes. **Meiosis** results in reduction of chromosomes to the **haploid** 23 found in the mature sperm and ovum (Fig. 9.1). Independent assortment of maternal and paternal chromosomes occurs amongst the gametes (Chapter 3). This recombination of genetic material ensures that each gamete is a mixture of maternal and paternal genes. After fertilization of an ovum by a sperm, the resulting zygote gains its full complement of 46 chromosomes.

Oogenesis

Primary **oocytes** are present in a female ovary before birth. **Oogenesis** (the process of transforming oocytes into ova) begins before the person's birth but is not completed until after puberty (Moore, Persaud & Torchia, 2018). By the time a girl is born, her **primary oocytes** have undergone the prophase of meiosis. Just before ovulation, a surge of follicle-stimulating hormone (FSH) and luteinizing hormone (LH) results in maturation of the ovum (Fig. 9.2) and completion of the first meiotic division (Fig. 9.3).

The process results in the formation of a **secondary oocyte** and a non-functional cell called the first **polar body.** The secondary oocyte receives 23 chromosomes, including an X

Normal gametogenesis

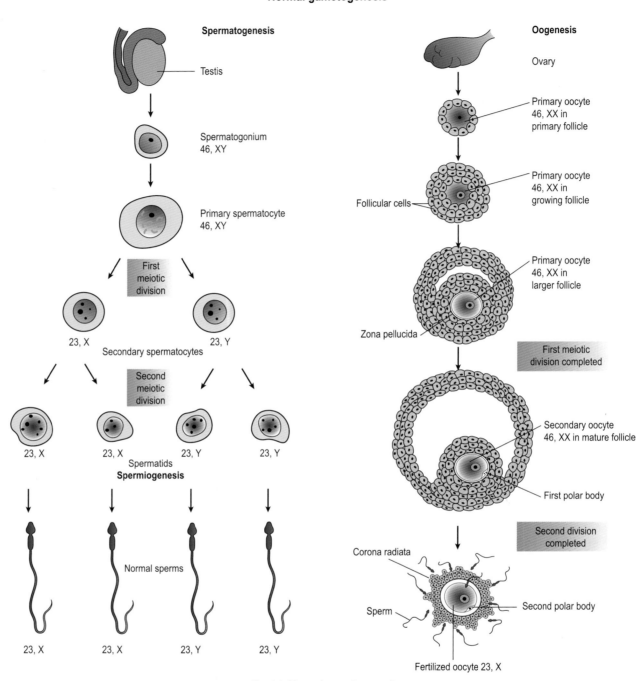

• **Fig. 9.1** Normal gametogenesis.

chromosome, and the first polar body receives the other 23 chromosomes. At ovulation, the secondary oocyte begins the second meiotic division but becomes arrested in metaphase. This division only completes if penetrated by a sperm. The result is one mature ovum with a second polar body. These polar bodies degenerate (Schoenwolf et al., 2021).

Spermatogenesis

Spermatogenesis is the process by which **spermatogonia** develop into mature sperm cells (Moore, Persaud &

Torchia, 2018). Spermatozoa are produced in the seminiferous tubules of the testes (Chapter 5). **Primary spermatocytes** begin to increase in number from puberty. In a functioning testis, germ cells are present at various stages of development, all originating from spermatogonia which divide continuously by mitosis to ensure a constant supply of cells. Spermatogonia divide and grow to become primary spermatocytes: diploid cells with 46 chromosomes.

These undergo the first meiotic division to form two **secondary spermatocytes** with only 23 chromosomes. Half receive an X chromosome and half a Y chromosome. Secondary meiosis

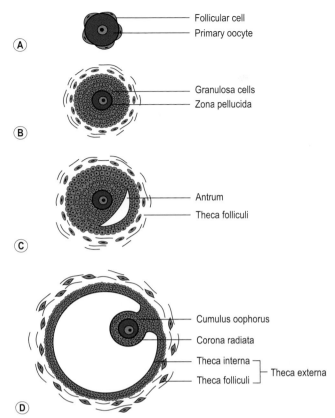

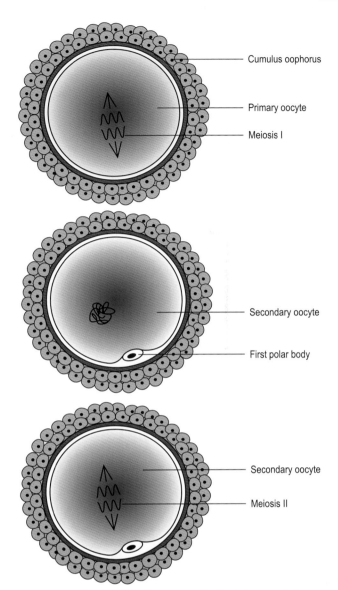

• **Fig. 9.2** The stages of development in the follicle. (A) Primordial follicle, (B) primary follicle, (C) secondary follicle, (D) Graafian follicle.

results in four haploid **spermatids** which are transformed into mature **spermatozoa.** As a sperm matures, an **acrosome cap** develops, containing the enzymes *hyaluronidases* and proteases. The mature sperm can be seen in (Fig. 9.4).

Gamete Size

The oocyte is a massive cell compared with the sperm cell. It is immotile in contrast to the highly motile sperm (Moore, Persaud & Torchia, 2018). Usually only one oocyte is released at ovulation which contains all the material necessary for early embryonic growth and development. In sharp contrast, the mature sperm has lost most of its cytoplasm, is very small and millions are released at ejaculation. About 1000 sperm will reach the oocyte, and these will all be needed to allow just one to enter and form a diploid zygote—the first cell of a unique human being.

Fertilization

Several processes take place to facilitate fertilization. These include capacitation, the acrosome reaction and blocks to polyspermy (i.e., the entry of multiple sperm) (Table 9.1).

Results of Fertilization

• The number of chromosomes is restored to the diploid (23 pairs, 46 chromosomes).

• **Fig. 9.3** Events within the zona pellucida before ovulation.

• The new individual inherits a unique set of genes from both its parents.
• Sex determination occurs.
• Initiation of cleavage stimulates the zygote to begin mitotic cell division.

The Embryo

Terminology

The term **'conceptus'** refers to the products of fertilization and comprises the embryo and its supporting tissues (adnexa). The **preimplantation period** is the time between fertilization and implantation and lasts about 6 days. The conceptus is called an *embryo* from implantation until the end of the eighth week after fertilization, when it becomes known as a **fetus.** The size of the embryo is expressed as the **crown–rump length** (from the crown of the head to the terminal part of the caudal end), in contrast to the length of the fetus which is measured from crown to heel.

TABLE 9.1	Processes which Facilitate Fertilization
Process	**Key Points**
Capacitation	• The process of maturation enabling a freshly ejaculated sperm to fertilize an ovum. • Glycoproteins are removed from the surface of the acrosome cap.
The acrosome reaction	• The acrosome develops perforations in its cap, and the contents of the acrosomal vesicle are released. This is known as the **acrosome reaction.** • Lytic (digestive) enzymes are released around the oocyte and digest the first physical barrier. They disperse the corona radiata follicular cells, allowing the head of one sperm to contact the zona pellucida. • Other enzymes, such as acrosin, are released which produce an opening in the zona pellucida (Wolpert, Tickel & Arias, 2019). • The sperm cell membrane and the sperm nucleus pass into the ovum (Fig. 9.4).
Blocks to polyspermy	• These blocks ensure that the fertilized ovum only contains 46 chromosomes (Fig. 9.5). • **Fast block**—The electrical resting potential of the oocyte plasma membrane changes from negative to positive, preventing other sperm from entering. This is a brief reaction, and the resting potential soon returns to a negative charge. • **Slow block** (cortical reaction)—The brief depolarization causes (i) the ovum to swell and detach any remaining sperm in contact with it and (ii) activate the secondary oocytes to complete the secondary meiotic division and expel the second polar body. The ovum is now mature. Its nucleus is now called the **female pronucleus.** Once the head of the sperm enters the cytoplasm of the ovum, its head enlarges to form the **male pronucleus.** The male and female pronuclei fuse, and paternal and maternal chromosomes intermingle.

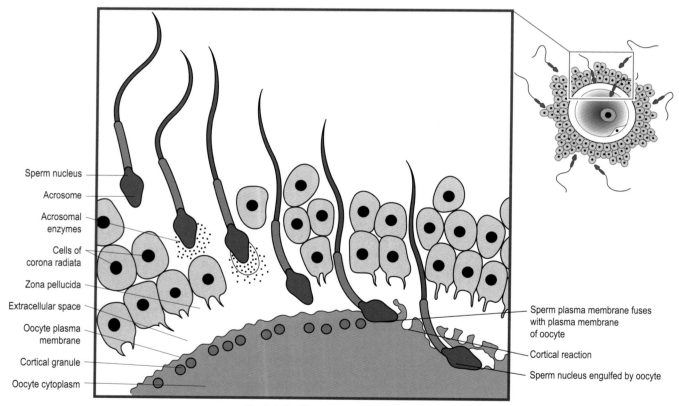

Labels (left): Sperm nucleus; Acrosome; Acrosomal enzymes; Cells of corona radiata; Zona pellucida; Extracellular space; Oocyte plasma membrane; Cortical granule; Oocyte cytoplasm

Labels (right): Sperm plasma membrane fuses with plasma membrane of oocyte; Cortical reaction; Sperm nucleus engulfed by oocyte

• **Fig. 9.4** Fertilization and cortical reaction.

Programming the Embryo

The information to make an embryo is in the DNA of the zygote. Although the sperm and ovum contribute 23 chromosomes each, it is the ovum that contributes the organelles and mitochondrial DNA. Regulatory genes control development by influencing where and when proteins are made. Developmental processes include (Wolpert, Tickel & Arias, 2019):

• Pattern formation.
• Differentiation.
• Morphogenesis.
• Development of the germ layers.
• Growth.

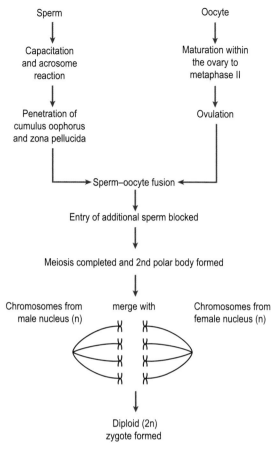

• **Fig. 9.5** Events leading up to fertilization.

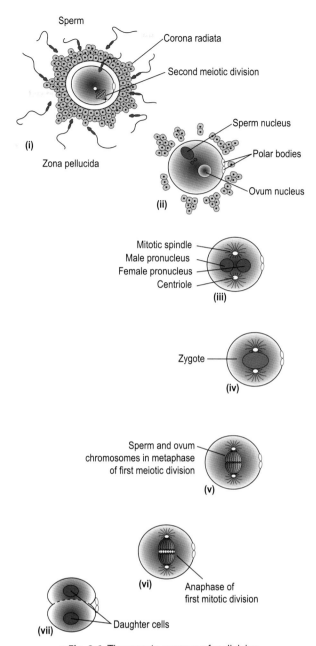

• **Fig. 9.6** The zygote prepares for division.

Pattern Formation

Cells in the embryo 'know' where and when to change shape and position, and cell movements are part of the embryo's developmental programme.

Cellular processes include:
- Somatic cell division where daughter cells receive identical genetic information.
- Cell differentiation to make up different embryological tissues.
- Induction where cells interact and one type of cell influences another.
- Migration of cells.
- Programmed cell death (apoptosis) to remove redundant cells.

Early Cell Division–Cleavage

Early in pregnancy, growth and development are very similar in human embryos but the exact days when embryonic features develop can vary. Days of development are counted from the moment of fertilization. Within 24 hours, the large zygote undergoes mitosis and splits into smaller cells (Fig. 9.6). This is called **cleavage,** and the daughter cells

are called **blastomeres.** There is synthesis of new DNA but no increase in the amount of cytoplasm, so the size of the blastomeres diminishes with each cleavage (Moore, Persaud & Torchia, 2018). The zygote continues its journey down the uterine tube, and by the fourth day there are between 16 and 20 cells. The embryo is now called a **morula** (Fig. 9.7).

Differentiation

Humans have about 350 different cell types and the embryo builds up different tissue types by combining proteins. There are two important classes of proteins:

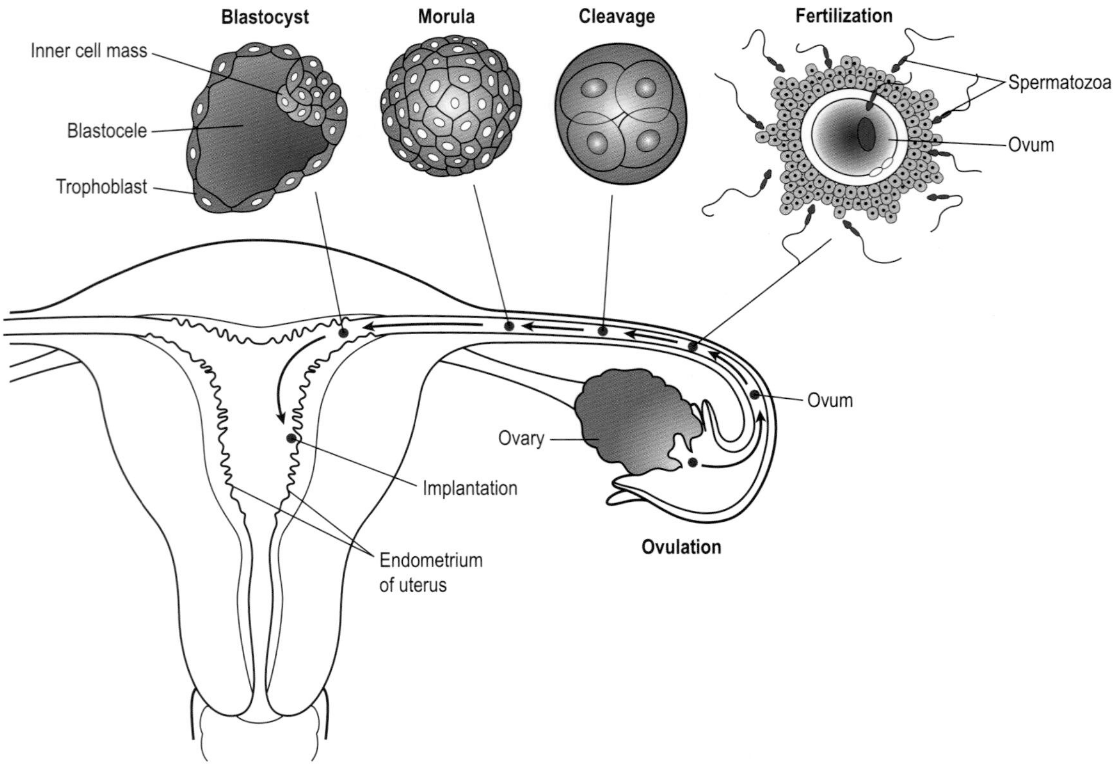

• **Fig. 9.7** Fertilization and early embryonic development.

1. Transmembrane proteins needed for cell adhesion and cell signalling.
2. Gene regulatory proteins.

Development is led by cell–cell interactions and by differential gene expression.

A handful of genetically controlled cell–cell signals are used to cause cells to differentiate to form a complex multicellular individual. All these signals are genetically controlled:

- Sister cells may differ because of asymmetrical cell division.
- Sister cells may compete, inhibiting the development of those next to them (lateral inhibition).
- A group of similar cells may be exposed to different signals, called **morphogens,** from outside the group.

Morphogenesis

Regulatory Genes

Cells in different parts of the embryo change shape and function to carry out their developing roles. Genes in the cell nuclei interact with environmental factors to bring about the huge variety of cell types. Eggs and embryos show **polarity,** which means one end is distinguishable from the other even before organized development has begun.

All vertebrates have a similar basic **body plan** with a segmented vertebral column and the brain at the anterior end. These structures mark the **anteroposterior axis,** the axis running from head to tail. The vertebrate body also has a distinct **dorsoventral axis** (back to belly) with the mouth on the ventral side.

Finally, although vertebrates are bilaterally symmetrical for many structures such as eyes, ears and limbs, the right-to-left symmetry is broken to allow differentiation of the internal organs such as the heart, spleen and liver. This left-to-right specification is different from the other two axes and only develops after they have been set.

Something in the embryonic environment turns on **developmental genes** which control how cells divide, multiply and move around the embryo. Regulatory genes control patterning in the embryo by a cascade of these gene products. The most important discovery was of the **homeobox,** a discrete portion of DNA with a specific order of genes present in most animals (Moore, Persaud & Torchia, 2018).

The Homeobox

Genes control **segmentation** in the developing embryo so that the correct positioning of organs occurs. These genes are referred to as **HOM genes** in invertebrates and **Hox genes** in vertebrates, including humans (Carlson, 2019). Different homeobox genes are switched on in the order they are positioned in the Hox complex to produce different protein products (Wolpert, Tickel & Arias, 2019; Alberts et al., 2022). These subdivide the embryo into discrete **homeodomains** before differentiation into specific tissue types, organs and systems. Homeobox genes may be switched on sequentially by **chemical gradients.**

Morphogens

Cytoplasm, located at the ends of the zygote, produces substances that govern the pattern of tissue development. These are called **morphogens** and they spread from a localized source to form a concentration gradient across a developing tissue, activating other genes when they reach specific concentrations.

Induction

In 1935, Hans Spemann won the only Nobel Prize awarded for embryology for discovering what organizes the embryo's development (Shampo & Kyle, 1999). He demonstrated that a nervous system will only develop if future muscle and adjacent cells move from the outside of the embryo to a situation underneath the outer layer. This cellular movement and the migrated cells produce a signal that causes the overlying sheet of cells to induce the development of the nervous system. The influencing tissues are called **inductors** or organizers. The inductor needs to be near but not necessarily in contact with the tissue to be induced. It is generally accepted that some signal passes from inductor to induced tissue. There needs to be a sufficiently large community of cells for induction to occur. This is referred to as the **community effect.**

Cell Communication

Cells communicate with each other in different ways. In some tissues the inductor may be a **diffusible molecule** passing directly from one tissue to another. In other tissues the message is mediated by an **extracellular matrix** (ECM) secreted by the inductor, which contacts with the reacting tissue. Some tissues react to **direct physical contact** between the inducing and reacting tissues (Moore, Persaud & Torchia, 2018), and cells receive cues from their neighbouring cells about where they should be and how they should behave. **Tissue-specific proteins** create cell recognition and accumulation. The originators of a group of cells may specify where it travels to and the tissue it forms.

Programmed Cell Death

Programmed cell death, or **apoptosis**, plays a major part in the final pattern of cells, especially in the formation of body cavities. It is controlled by mitochondrial gene products (Lane, 2018). Cells in some tissues are overproduced, and those that are not needed commit suicide (Alberts et al., 2022). Cell death is a normal feature of the development of the nervous system, limbs, skeleton and heart, as the following examples explain:

- In limb formation, cell death helps achieve the final shape, such as the disappearance of webbing between the fingers.
- In the developing brain and nervous system, over 50% too many axons arrive at target cells. The first to arrive make the best connections and send signals back in the form of nerve growth factor which sustains neurons. There is no room for new arrivals which cannot obtain nourishment and die.
- Too many cells are made in the development of tubes such as blood vessels, and the tube is hollowed out by cell death.

Development of the Embryo

The Blastocyst

The group of cells continues cleaving for the first 4 days. The first three cleavages are synchronous but later cleavages are asymmetrical. There is also polarization, with internal cells differing from external cells. The inner cells divide less frequently and remain large and round, whereas the outer cells in contact with the zona pellucida become flattened. At this point the cells lose their **totipotency** and begin to differentiate. They are destined to become specific parts of the embryo.

On the fifth day, the zona pellucida is digested by uterine secretions and the embryo 'hatches'. Fluid accumulates in the space between the peripheral and central cells of the morula, and it becomes the hollow **blastocyst.** The inner cell mass of the blastocyst is the **embryoblast** and will become the embryo. The flattened outer cells are called the **trophoblast** and will form the placenta (Fig. 9.8).

Implantation

On the sixth day, the embryoblast begins to implant into the endometrium, most commonly on the posterior wall of the uterus. Where the trophoblastic cells contact the endometrium, they undergo rapid DNA synthesis and become cuboid in shape to form the cytotrophoblast. The daughter cells shed their plasma membranes to form a mass of protoplasm with nuclei and organelles called a **syncytium.** The mass of tissue is called the **syncytiotrophoblast** (Fig. 9.8), which has the dual role to produce enzymes that attack the endometrium and hormones that allow the pregnancy to continue.

The Effects of Enzymatic Erosion

As the enzymes erode the endometrium, the uterine glands release their content to nourish the embryo and the blastocyst begins to enlarge. Nutrition is also provided by the stroma cells which undergo changes known as the **decidual reaction** and become swollen with glycogen and lipid. The change commences at the implantation site and spreads within a few days throughout the whole endometrium except for the lining of the cervix. The endometrium is now known as the **decidua.**

At the implantation site, new blood capillaries fed by branches of the spiral arteries and drained by the endometrial veins develop and dilate (Fig. 9.9). The conceptus is completely embedded in the compact layer of the endometrium by the 12th day and is covered by the overlying uterine epithelium. Erosion of these sinuses results in maternal blood entering the syncytiotrophoblast to collect in a labyrinth of little pockets called **lacunae. Human chorionic gonadotrophin** (hCG) is secreted into the lacunae by the trophoblast, enters the maternal circulation and maintains the corpus luteum. This ensures the continued production of oestrogen and progesterone for maintenance of the pregnancy until produced by the placenta at 12 weeks.

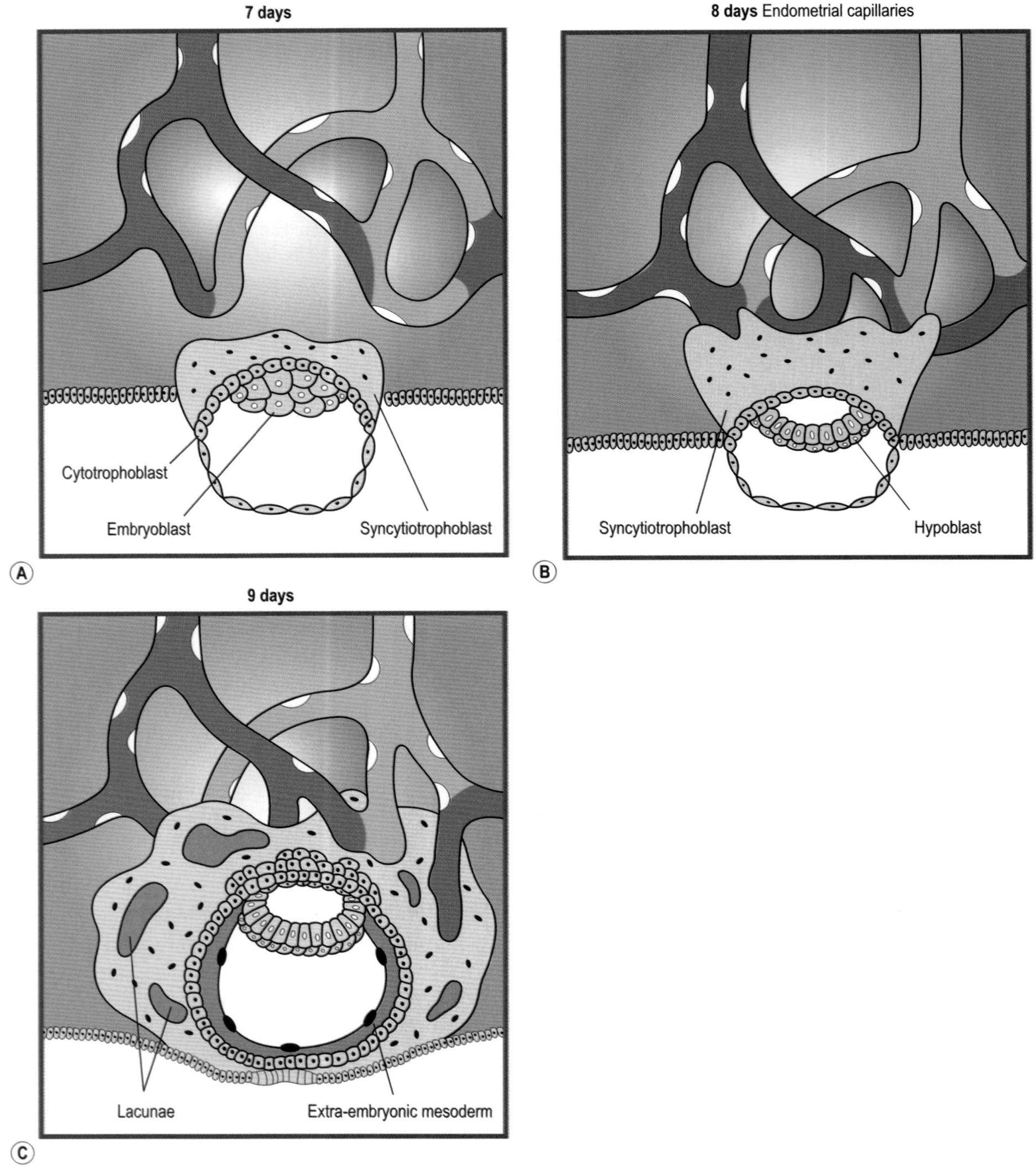

7 days

(A)

8 days Endometrial capillaries

(B)

9 days

(C)

• **Fig. 9.8** The implanting conceptus on days 7 (A), 8 (B) and 9 (C) after fertilization. The developing conceptus rapidly contacts with endometrial capillary loops (uterine glands are not represented).

Development of the Germ Layers

The Bilaminar Embryonic Disc

By the second week of development the cells are well organized, and the inner cell mass forms a flattened disc consisting of two layers known as the **bilaminar embryonic disc.** The inner layer or epiblast is composed of tall columnar epithelium, and the outer layer or **hypoblast** is composed of low cuboidal epithelium.

The margins of the epiblast create a thin epithelial layer, the **amnion,** and the epiblast and amnion form the amniotic sac. The sac grows more rapidly than the embryo and comes to surround the embryo. The cell margins of the hypoblast also divide rapidly to form branched cells that line the cavity of the blastocyst. This lining is called the **extraembryonic mesoderm.**

This cavity splits the mesoderm into a **visceral layer,** which is included in the **umbilical vesicle** formerly known

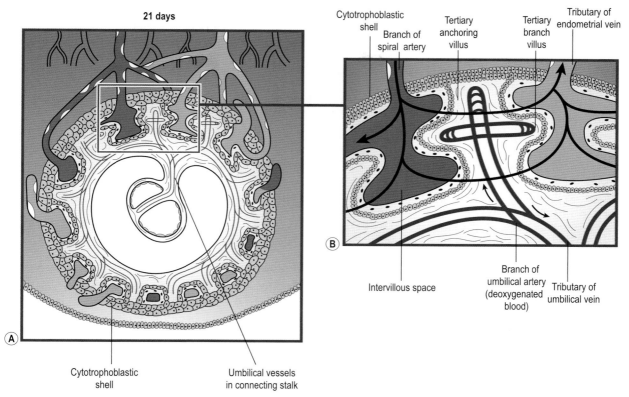

• **Fig. 9.9** Chorionic vesicle, day 21. (B) Enlargement of upper part of (A) showing the circulation of embryonic and maternal blood.

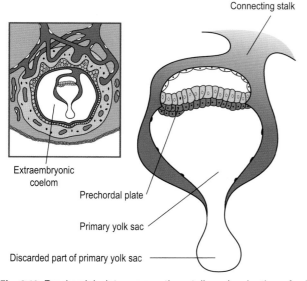

• **Fig. 9.10** Prechordal plate, connecting stalk and reduction of primary yolk sac.

as the **yolk sac** (Fig. 9.10) but renamed as it contains no yolk (Moore, Persaud & Torchia, 2018), and a **parietal layer,** which contributes to the **chorion** together with the trophoblast. The visceral and parietal extraembryonic mesoderm are linked by a **connecting stalk** that develops into the **umbilical cord.** Towards the end of the second week the flattened disc becomes ovoid. The cranial (head end) part

of the hypoblast thickens to form the prechordal plate, the future site of the mouth and an important organizer of the head region (Moore, Persaud & Torchia, 2018).

The Trilaminar Embryo

During **embryogenesis,** cells migrate through the embryo, differentiating into specific cell types to form organs and systems. The formation of the **primitive streak, gastrulation** and formation of the notochord are important in creating the body plan (Moore, Persaud & Torchia, 2018). They will be described separately although they occur simultaneously and are interlinked in the embryo.

The Primitive Streak

At the beginning of the third week, a thick linear band of embryonic epiblast appears caudally, in the dorsal aspect of the embryonic disc. It is the site of enormous cell activity when the first wave of migration forms the middle layer of the embryo, and the basic body plan is laid down with cranial and caudal ends. The primitive streak elongates by adding cells to its caudal end, and the cranial end enlarges to form a **primitive node.**

The primitive streak continues to form mesodermal cells until the end of the fourth week. Embryonic mesodermal cells migrate in three directions: laterally to the margins of the embryonic disc, cranially alongside the notochord and caudally around the cloacal membrane. If cell formation and migration persist beyond the fourth week, it can give rise to a multi-tissued tumour called a **sacral teratoma.**

Gastrulation

Gastrulation is a process of invagination by which the inner cell mass becomes the trilaminar embryo. It begins in the first week with the formation of the hypoblast, continues during the second week with the formation of the epiblast and is completed during the third week. It ends when the three primary germ layers of **ectoderm, mesoderm** and **endoderm** are in situ and the embryo is a trilaminar disc. A human is just a complex elaboration of these three layers.

Epiblastic cells dip through the primitive streak and spread laterally beneath it, with movement occurring simultaneously over many parts of the embryo. Sheets of cells stream past each other, contracting and expanding. Some cells displace the underlying hypoblast to form the embryonic endoderm, whilst the rest form the embryonic mesoderm or mesenchyme. Epiblastic cells that remain on the surface form embryonic ectoderm. The endoderm migrates inside the wall of the umbilical vesicle, and a finger of the umbilical vesicle becomes pinched off and extends into the connecting stalk to form the allantois.

Development of Body Cavities

Late in the second week fluid-filled spaces appear in the cranial half of the embryonic mesoderm. These coalesce during the third week to form the U-shaped **embryonic coelom.** The bend of the U at the cranial end forms the **pericardial coelom.** This is divided by the **septum transversum** from the caudal two arms of the U, which form the **pericardioperitoneal or pleural canals** leading to two branches of the **peritoneal coelom.** This results in the development of three body cavities: a pericardial cavity around the heart, two smaller **pleural canals** and a large **peritoneal cavity.** The first two are divided from the peritoneal cavity by the **diaphragm.**

Formation of the Notochord

The notochordal process grows out cranially from beneath the ectoderm until it reaches the prechordal plate. Where the prechordal plate is firmly attached to the ectoderm and remains bilaminar, it forms the **oropharyngeal membrane** or future site of the mouth. Caudal to the primitive streak is a circular area which also remains bilaminar, called the **cloacal membrane** or future site of the anus and urogenital orifices. The notochord develops from the notochordal process. Mesodermal cells gather around it to form the **vertebral column,** and it is almost completely formed by the end of the third week. It disappears once it is surrounded by the vertebral bodies.

Organogenesis

From 3 weeks, the embryo enters the vulnerable stage of organogenesis, which is complete by 8 weeks (Fig. 9.11).

Organs are made up of cell types that originate from different sources and obey different instructions. From about days 20–30, the dorsal surface of the embryo looks segmented with the appearance of **paired somites** (distinct blocks of embryonic tissue on either side of the notochord) (Wolpert, Tickel & Arias, 2019). Somite formation begins at the anterior end of the embryo and proceeds posteriorly with each pair of somites being formed simultaneously. The vertebral column develops from the somites and segmentally innervates muscles of the trunk. Somites are still visible at 6 weeks but have differentiated by 8 weeks.

Differentiation of the Germ Layers

Fig. 9.12 summarizes the tissues and organs developing from the three layers.

Ectoderm

- Tissues derived from neuroectoderm include the central and peripheral nervous systems, the retina of the eye and the posterior lobe of the pituitary gland.
- Tissues derived from surface ectoderm include the outer layer of the skin (the epidermis) with its hair follicles and cutaneous glands, including the breasts, the lens of the eye, the special sense cells of the inner ear, the anterior lobe of the pituitary gland and the enamel of the teeth.

Neurulation

Neurulation is development of the brain and nervous system. The notochord induces its overlying ectoderm to thicken and form a neural plate. These cells are called the **neuroectoderm** and differ from the remaining surface ectoderm. A flat sheet of cells on the upper surface of the embryo folds up into a tube which will develop into the brain and spinal cord. On about day 18, the neural plate develops a midline neural groove with lateral neural folds. From 4 weeks, the folds come together to form the neural tube.

Fusion of the folds begins at the level of the fourth pair of somites and proceeds simultaneously in cranial and caudal directions. Cells near to the crests of the neural folds escape from the neural tube during closure and come to lie on either side to form the neural crest. The two open ends of the neural tube are termed **neuropores.** The cranial neuropore closes at about day 25 and the caudal neuropore at about day 27. The neural tube becomes the brain and spinal cord. The neural canal within the tube becomes the **ventricular system** of the brain and the central canal of the spinal cord. This early closure of the neural tube has implications for the causation and prevention of open neural tube defects.

Mesoderm

Nearest the midline axis of the embryo is the **paraxial mesoderm** which segments to form the somites. Next

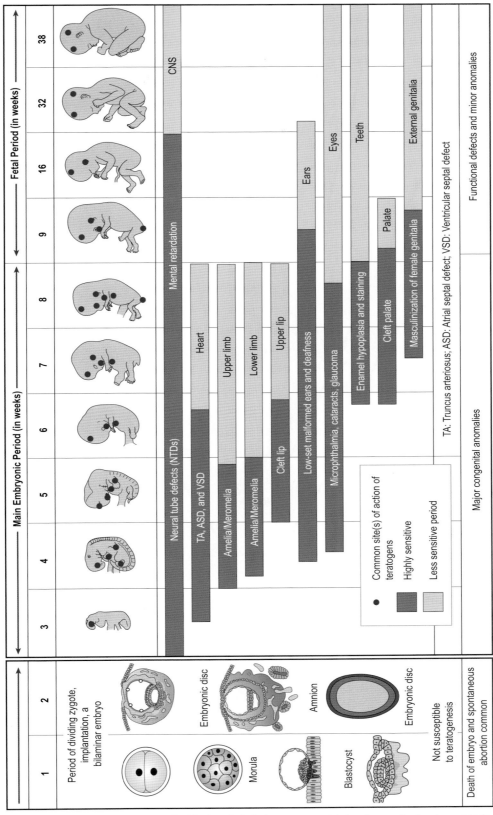

• **Fig. 9.11** Schematic illustration of critical periods in human prenatal development, showing periods of sensitivity to teratogens.

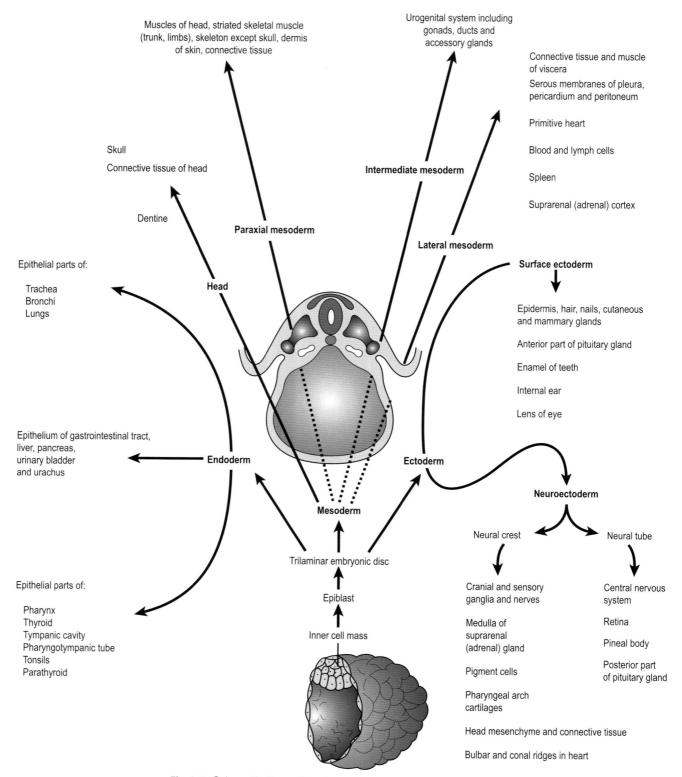

Muscles of head, striated skeletal muscle (trunk, limbs), skeleton except skull, dermis of skin, connective tissue

Urogenital system including gonads, ducts and accessory glands

Connective tissue and muscle of viscera

Serous membranes of pleura, pericardium and peritoneum

Primitive heart

Blood and lymph cells

Spleen

Suprarenal (adrenal) cortex

Intermediate mesoderm

Skull

Connective tissue of head

Dentine

Paraxial mesoderm

Lateral mesoderm

Head

Surface ectoderm

Epithelial parts of:

Trachea
Bronchi
Lungs

Epidermis, hair, nails, cutaneous and mammary glands

Anterior part of pituitary gland

Enamel of teeth

Internal ear

Lens of eye

Epithelium of gastrointestinal tract, liver, pancreas, urinary bladder and urachus

Endoderm

Ectoderm

Neuroectoderm

Mesoderm

Neural crest

Neural tube

Trilaminar embryonic disc

Epiblast

Inner cell mass

Cranial and sensory ganglia and nerves

Medulla of suprarenal (adrenal) gland

Pigment cells

Pharyngeal arch cartilages

Head mesenchyme and connective tissue

Bulbar and conal ridges in heart

Central nervous system

Retina

Pineal body

Posterior part of pituitary gland

Epithelial parts of:

Pharynx
Thyroid
Tympanic cavity
Pharyngotympanic tube
Tonsils
Parathyroid

• **Fig. 9.12** Schematic illustration of the derivatives of the three germ layers.

to the somites, but not undergoing segmentation, is the **intermediate mesoderm** and outside that is the **lateral plate.** The lateral plate is divided into **somatic mesoderm** lying just beneath the body wall and **splanchnic mesoderm** lying next to the endoderm of the umbilical vesicle.

Tissues derived from mesoderm are:
- From the paraxial mesoderm cranial to the somites: part of the skull and the muscles of the face and jaws.
- From the somites: the vertebral column and the skeletal musculature of the trunk and connective tissue or dermis of the skin.

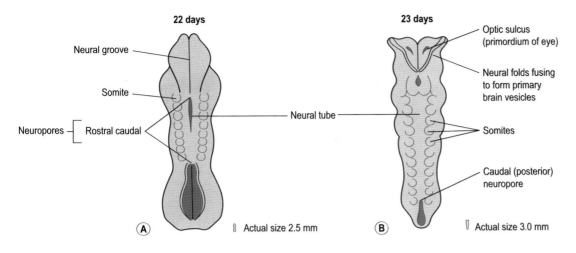

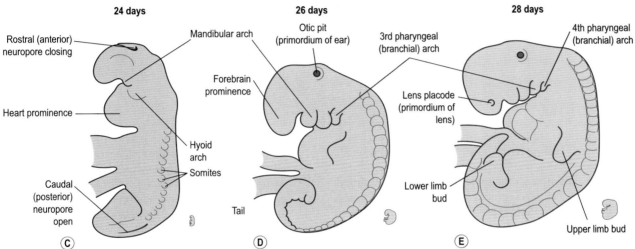

• **Fig. 9.13** (A, B) Dorsal views of embryos early in the 4th week showing 8 and 12 somites, respectively. (C–E) Lateral views of older embryos showing 16, 27 and 33 somites, respectively. The rostral neuropore is normally closed by days 25–26 and the caudal neuropore by the end of 4 weeks.

- From the intermediate mesoderm: the kidneys and ureters, the gonads, the ductus deferens and the uterus and uterine tubes.
- From the somatic mesoderm: the limb skeleton and muscles, the sternum and anterior part of the ribs.
- From the splanchnic mesoderm: the cardiovascular system and blood, the spleen and smooth muscle of the gastrointestinal tract.

Endoderm

Tissues derived from endoderm include the epithelial linings of the alimentary tract and its glands, the liver, the pancreas, the epithelial lining of the lower respiratory tract and of the bladder and urethra.

Folding of the Embryo

Folding of the embryo changes its shape and the relationships of the organs (Fig. 9.13). Neurulation is a good example. A flat sheet of cells on the upper surface of the embryo folds up into a tube which develops into the brain and spinal cord. Events in the longitudinal and transverse planes are described separately.

Longitudinal Folding

Longitudinal folding brings about flexion and development of the head and tail folds (Fig. 9.14) and an hour-glass constriction and partial extrusion of the umbilical vesicle. The portion of the umbilical vesicle retained in the embryo becomes the gut, whereas that extruded becomes the **vitelline duct** (which remains attached to the gut at the **vitellointestinal communication** and eventually disappears). When flexion is complete the brain overhangs the developing heart, and the heart is ventral to the foregut. The midgut faces into the vitelline duct, and the hindgut extends from the vitellointestinal communication to the cloacal membrane.

Transverse Folding

The lateral margins of the embryonic disc form the lateral body folds which turn the embryo from a disc into a cylinder. The peritoneal coelom on each side initially open into the extraembryonic coelom. Transverse folding directs these two openings ventrally and, with the constriction of the umbilical vesicle, the two openings communicate across the midline to form the peritoneal cavity.

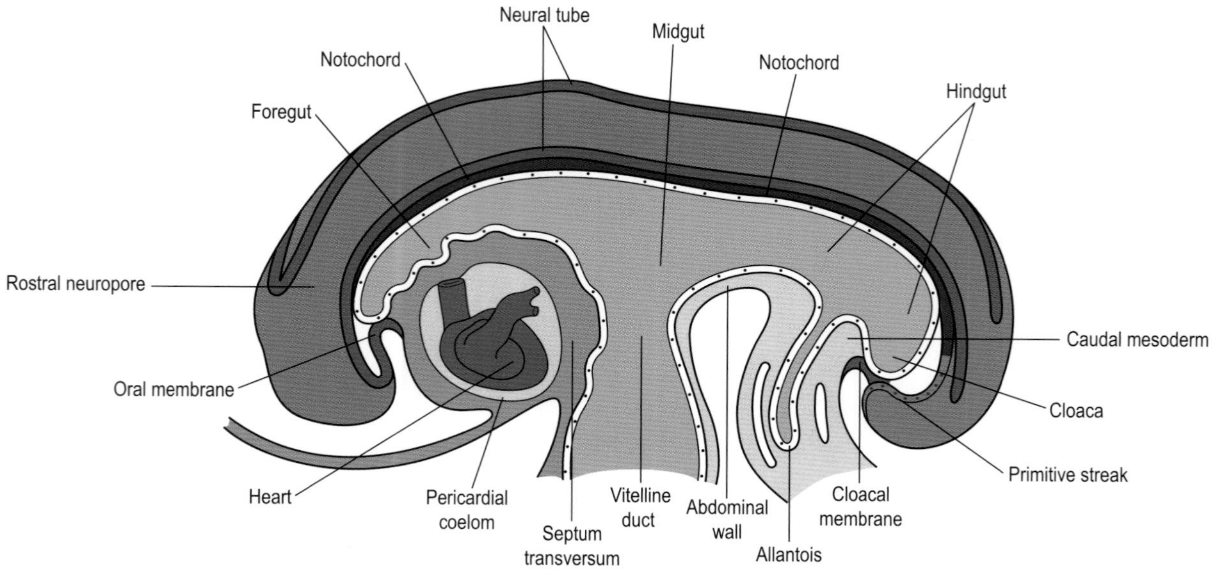

• **Fig. 9.14** Longitudinal section of embryo, day 25.

Main Points

- Gametogenesis allows the independent assortment of maternal and paternal chromosomes amongst the gametes.
- The oocyte contains all the material necessary for embryonic growth and development. When one sperm enters an oocyte, the first diploid cell of a new human is formed.
- The acrosome reaction occurs when a capacitated sperm meets the corona radiata of the oocyte. Lytic enzymes disperse the follicular cells of the corona radiata, allowing the head of the sperm to enter.
- During embryogenesis, cells change shape and position to form body systems. Cellular processes include cell division, cell differentiation, cell migration and apoptosis.
- Mitotic cleavage splits the large zygote into smaller cells called *blastomeres*. By day 4 after fertilization there are 16–20 cells, and the conceptus is called a *morula*.
- Regulation of embryonic development is by a cascade of gene products. Homeobox genes produce proteins which control segmentation so that the correct positioning of organs occurs.
- During early development some embryonic tissues influence the development of adjacent tissues. These influencing tissues are called *inductors* or *organizers*.
- Cleavage continues with polarization, with internal cells differing from external cells. Inner cells divide less frequently, remaining large and round, whereas the outer cells, in contact with the zona pellucida, become flattened.
- On day 5, the zygote hatches as the zona pellucida is digested by uterine secretions. Fluid accumulates, and the morula becomes a blastocyst, the inner embryoblast becomes the embryo, and the flattened outer trophoblast the placenta.

- On day 6, the embryo begins to implant into the endometrium and trophoblast cells touching the endometrium become cuboid, forming the cytotrophoblast.
- Daughter cells form the syncytiotrophoblast, producing enzymes that erode the endometrium. Hormones such as hCG are released to maintain the corpus luteum and until the placenta can produce sufficient oestrogen and progesterone.
- During embryogenesis, cells migrate throughout the embryo to differentiate into specific tissues forming organs. Formation of the primitive streak, gastrulation and formation of the notochord create the body plan.
- The dorsal embryonic surface develops paired somites at days 20–30, from which arise the vertebral column and segmentally innervated trunk muscles.
- The embryonic ectoderm gives rise to the epidermis, central and peripheral nervous systems, the eye and the inner ear.
- Embryonic endoderm gives rise to the epithelial lining of the gastrointestinal and respiratory tracts, parenchyma of the tonsils, thyroid and parathyroid glands, thymus, liver and pancreas.
- The embryonic mesoderm gives rise to all skeletal muscles and blood cells; all visceral smooth muscle coats; all linings of blood vessels and body cavities; the reproductive and excretory systems; and most of the cardiovascular system.
- During neurulation, a flat sheet of cells on the upper surface of the embryo folds into a tube which develops into the brain and spinal cord.
- Longitudinal and transverse folding of cell sheets forms the basis of the early development of organs.

References

Alberts, B., Heald, R., Johnson, A., Morgan, D., Raff, M., Roberts, K., et al. 2022. Molecular Biology of the Cell, seventh ed. Norton & Company, New York.

Carlson, B.M., 2019. Human Embryology and Developmental Biology, sixth ed. Elsevier, New York.

Human Fertilisation and Embryology Act 2008. Available at: https://www.legislation.gov.uk/ukpga/2008/22.

Lane, N., 2018. Power, Sex and Suicide: Mitochondria and the Meaning of Life. Oxford University Press, Oxford.

Moore, K.L., Persaud, T.V.N., Torchia, M.G., 2018. The Developing Human, eleventh ed. Elsevier, London.

Schoenwolf, G.C., Bleyl, S.B., Brauer, R., Francis-West, P.H., 2021. Larsen's Human Embryology, sixth ed. Elsevier, New York.

Shampo, M.A., Kyle, R.A., 1999. Hans Spemann – contributions to embryology. Mayo Clin. Proc. 74, 474.

Wolpert, L., Tickel, C., Arias, A., 2019. Principles of Development, sixth ed. Oxford University Press, Oxford.

Annotated recommended reading

Moore, K.L., Persaud, T.V.N., Torchia, M.G., 2018. The Developing Human: Clinically Oriented Embryology, eleventh ed. E-Book Elsevier, New York.

This e-textbook clearly describes embryo development week by week and provides a detailed resource for understanding the origin of congenital defects. The illustrations are very good, with animations. This e-textbook is recommended for both students and practitioners to peruse.

Schoenwolf, G.C., Bleyl, S.B., Brauer, R., Francis-West, P.H., 2021. Larsen's Human Embryology, sixth ed. Elsevier, New York.

This e-textbook offers a straightforward approach to a highly complex subject. The comprehensive content examines both molecular biological and clinical aspects of embryology with applications linked to an advancing knowledge base.

10

Embryological Systems 1—Trunk, Head and Limbs

LYNSAY MATTHEWS

This chapter introduces the timing and process in the development of the normal body systems. Development of the structures and soft tissues related to the trunk, skull, brain, spinal cord, head and neck, the face, ears and eyes and limbs are outlined. Students and midwives are not expected to be experts in embryology but they do need to have basic knowledge and understanding.

Introduction

The normal development of the organs and structures of the selected body systems are outlined using straightforward explanations. This approach provides a knowledge base for the basic understanding of the development of congenital abnormalities.

The Trunk

Skeletal Features

The Vertebral Column

There are three phases in the development of the vertebral column (Fig. 10.1): **precartilaginous, cartilaginous** and **bony** (Moore, Persaud & Torchia, 2018).

Precartilaginous Phase

Precursors of vertebrae are called **sclerotomes.** They are derived from **somites.** Mesenchymal cells surround the **notochord** forming the segmented **mesenchymal vertebral column.** The cranial end of each mesenchymal vertebra is thinner than the caudal ends. The cells at the interface between the two form an **intervertebral disc,** and the remainder of the condensed structure merges with the caudal vertebrae to form the **centrum.** This is an intersegmental structure formed from parts of two sclerotomes. From the upper part of the centrum, a pair of **neural arches** grow and surround the neural tube, giving rise to pairs of costal and transverse processes.

Cartilaginous Phase

Chondrification centres appear in the centrum and neural arch late in week 5. In the 12 thoracic vertebrae, the cartilaginous coastal processes which will develop into the ribs become detached from their parent neural arches by the formation of synovial joints. Synovial joints also appear between the costal and transverse processes. The remaining costal processes are incorporated into the vertebrae.

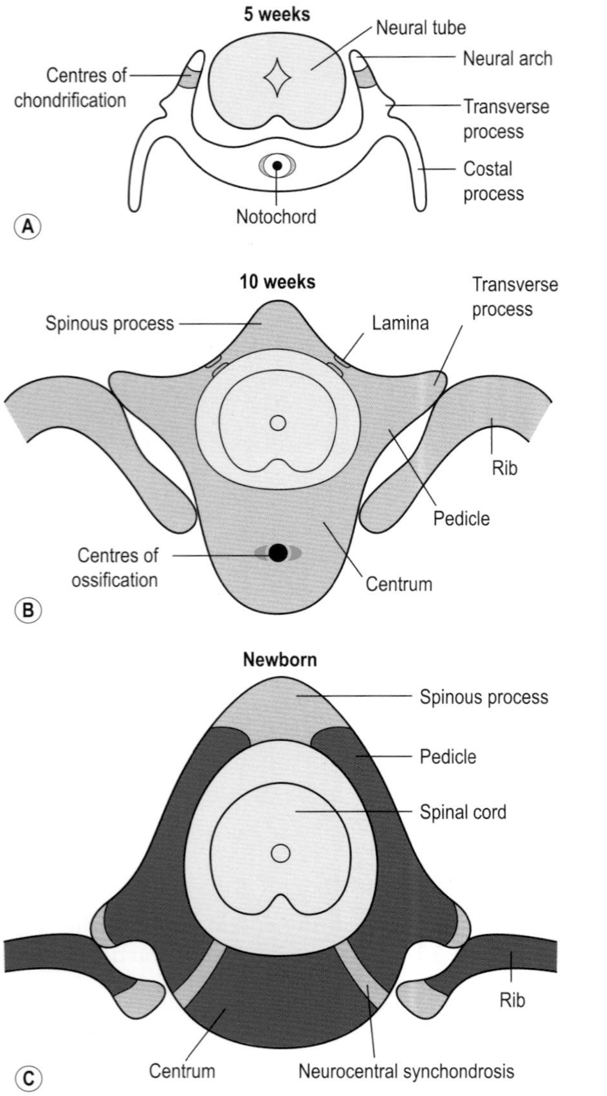

• **Fig. 10.1** (A) Blastemal vertebra with centre of chondrification *(shaded dark)*, (B) cartilaginous vertebra with centres of ossification *(shaded dark)*, (C) bony vertebra.

Bony Phase

During week 8, **ossification centres** appear in the centrum, in neural arches and in the ribs. Ossification of the skeleton is not completed until the 25th year.

Ribs and Sternum

As the lateral body folds in week 4, the somatic mesoderm is penetrated by the thoracic costal processes. These induce the mesoderm to add to their tips, completing the formation of the prechondrial ribs. Two sternal bars develop in the ventral part of the somatic mesoderm. These meet in the midline and unite to form a prechondrial sternum. The **xiphisternum** often remains bifid. The ventral ends of the seven cranial costal processes fuse with the sternum (Moore, Persaud & Torchia, 2018).

Soft Tissues

During week 4, the somites subdivide into three kinds of mesodermal primordia: myotomes, dermatomes and sclerotomes (Schoenwolf et al., 2021).

Myotomes

Myotomes give rise to all muscles linking the vertebrae and skull together, and to the muscles of the abdominal and thoracic walls. Spinal nerves divide into **dorsal** and **ventral** rami. Dorsal rami supply the muscles with motor fibres, and ventral rami supply the muscles and their overlying dermatome with sensory fibres. Limb muscles are not formed from myotomes.

Dermatomes

Dermatomes merge to form the **dermis** layer of the skin. Each dermatome is accompanied by sensory nerve fibres derived from the level of the spinal cord where the dermatome originates. That is why neurologists divide the body surface into regions called **dermatomes.**

The Skin and Mammary Glands

Although the dermis develops from the dermatomes, the **epidermis** and its appendages are derived from surface ectoderm which begins as a single cuboidal layer but becomes two-layered in month 2. The superficial layer is shed, leaving the underlying germinal layer to form the structures of the skin. In month 3, the epidermis becomes stratified and its basal layer sends pegs down into the dermis to form the root sheath of the hair follicles. **Lanugo,** which is very soft fine hair, grows all over the body. Lanugo is shed shortly before birth and replaced by true or **vellus hair** derived from a second set of hair follicles.

During month 5, the sebaceous glands bud into the dermis from the root sheath and the sweat glands grow down from the epidermis. Secretions from sebaceous glands become vernix caseosa when mixed with peridermal cells. Mammary glands appear in week 6 as paired strips of longitudinal ectodermal thickening on the ventral surface of the embryo called the *mammary ridge.* In humans, only one pair of breasts forms from the thoracic part of the ridge. The rest of the ridge disappears.

The Skull

The skull forms from mesenchyme around the developing brain. It consists of the neurocranium which encloses the brain and the viscerocranium making up the bones of the face. The base of the skull, or **chondrocranium,** develops out of cartilage, whereas the **vault bones** (Chapter 24) develop from membrane (Moore, Persaud & Torchia, 2018). Intramembranous ossification begins from the fourth month, with separate ossification centres giving rise to the parietal bones, frontal bones, occipital bone and the squamous part of the temporal bones.

The Viscerocranium

All facial bones ossify in membrane, starting with the mandible early in week 6. Detailed development of the face is given later.

The Teeth

Tooth buds form from thickened ectoderm called the **dental lamina**: 10 in the upper jaw and 10 in the lower jaw. These are responsible for the deciduous (milk) teeth. Later, the dental lamina forms the buds of the permanent dentition. Permanent molars do not have precursors in the deciduous dentition but develop from a backwards extension of the dental lamina. The crowns of the teeth begin when cells called **odontoblasts** form predentine, which later calcifies to become dentine. Calcification signals cells called **ameloblasts** to lay down enamel on the surface of the dentine. Central cells constitute the pulp of the tooth, which is richly supplied with blood and sensory nerve endings as many of us can testify!

The outer and inner enamel epithelia fuse to form the **epithelial root sheath.** Predentine and dentine are induced to form the root of the tooth. Mesoderm of the dental sac produces a specialized form of bone called *cement* and the **periodontal ligament** which anchors the cement to the wall of the tooth socket. Eruption of the deciduous teeth occurs between 6 months and 2 years after birth.

The Brain

Chapter 26 describes the complex adult brain and central nervous system. The neural tube cranial to the fourth pair of somites develops into the brain (Moore, Persaud & Torchia, 2018). The human nervous system begins to form 19 days after fertilization and is the earliest system to differentiate. Primary brain vesicles are:
- Forebrain—prosencephalon.
- Midbrain—mesencephalon.
- Hindbrain—rhombencephalon.

From 4 weeks the major regions of the brain are distinct, and neurons begin to differentiate from the epithelium of the neural tube. The thalamus and **hypothalamus** are differentiated by week 5. By the end of week 8, the head is equal to half the length of the embryo and controls first movement of the limbs.

The Changing Shape of the Brain

The brainstem buckles and a cervical flexure appears at the junction of the brainstem and spinal cord. A midline flexure moves the mesencephalon to the summit of the brain. The rhombencephalon folds on itself, causing the walls of the neural tube to expand into the fourth ventricle. The dorsal region of the prosencephalon expands on either side to form the cerebral hemispheres or **telencephalon.** Within the cerebral hemispheres, the neural tube dilates to form the **lateral ventricles.**

The remainder of the prosencephalon straddles the midline and is known as the **diencephalon.** The third ventricle, a cavity within the diencephalon, communicates with the fourth ventricle through the **aqueduct of Sylvius.** An outgrowth from the diencephalon becomes the two retinas and optic nerves. The cranial end of the rhombencephalon gives rise to the **pons** and the **cerebellum,** whereas the caudal end becomes the **medulla oblongata.**

The Forebrain

Neurons migrate from the ventricular zone of the telencephalon to the surface to form the cerebral cortex. The frontal, parietal, occipital and temporal lobes are present by 12–14 weeks. Two **commissures** of nerve fibres link the two cerebral hemispheres. The anterior commissure links the olfactory regions, and the larger corpus callosum links areas of the cerebral cortex.

Other Brain Structures

The diencephalon gives rise to the **pineal gland,** the paired thalami and the hypothalamus. The **basal ganglia** develop immediately below the thalamus and help control body movement.

Blood Supply to the Brain

Arterial blood supply develops from cranial segments of the **dorsal aortae,** comprising two internal carotid arteries and two **vertebral arteries.** Internal carotid arteries branch to form the **anterior, middle** and **posterior cerebral arteries.** Each vertebral artery gives off a branch to supply the cerebellum and medulla oblongata before uniting with its partner to form the **basilar artery.** This gives off two pairs of arteries to the cerebellum and upper brainstem before dividing into two terminal branches that link up with the ends of the internal carotid arteries to form the intercommunicating **circle of Willis.** Venous drainage is discussed in Chapter 24.

The Spinal Cord

Following closure of the neural tube and formation of the somites, the neural crest cells form clusters corresponding to the somites. Corresponding levels of the neural tube develop from the primitive streak during a process of secondary neurulation. At first the neural tube is solid but becomes canalized by caudal extension of the neural canal.

Zones of the Spinal Cord

During the fifth week, three zones can be distinguished in the side walls of the neural tube. From inner to outer, these are the **ventricular, intermediate** and **marginal zones.**
- The ventricular zone is where neuroepithelial cells divide. After several cell divisions daughter cells move out of the ventricular zone; the first ones become neurons and the last become the connective tissue cells called **neuroglia.**

- The intermediate zone is the forerunner of the grey matter of the spinal cord. Cells called **neuroblasts** from the ventricular zone differentiate into neurons. **Glioblasts** enter the intermediate zone and become **astrocytes,** the structural support of the central nervous system (CNS), and oligodendrocytes form the **myelin sheaths.** Phagocytic microglial cells develop from blood monocytes and migrate from the capillary bed to the CNS during month 3.
- The marginal zone is the forerunner of the white matter of the spinal cord. Small neurons invade the marginal zone and emit axons alongside the grey matter to form pathways that link different levels of the spinal cord.

During week 6, an accumulation of neuroblasts in the dorsolateral plate gives rise to the sensory **dorsal horn** of grey matter. The dorsal horn communicates with neural crest cells outside the neural tube to form **dorsal root ganglia.** Large accumulations of cells in the ventrolateral plate form the motor **ventral horn** of grey matter. Axons emerging from the ventral horn form the **ventral nerve roots,** joining with peripheral processes to form mixed spinal nerves.

During weeks 7–10, the spinal cord is formed. The neural canal shrinks to become the central canal of the spinal cord. Cells left behind in the ventricular zone develop cilia and become the lining cells of the central canal called **ependymal cells.** The discrete ascending and descending columns of the spinal cord white matter are finalized.

Cells from the Neural Crest

Neural crest cells are **pluripotent** and give rise to the following cell types, many of which are involved in the regulation of body systems:
- Dorsal root ganglia cells.
- Autonomic ganglion cells.
- Chromaffin cells of the adrenal medulla.
- Schwann cells that produce myelin sheaths.
- Pia mater and arachnoid mater (cerebral membranes).
- Skin melanocytes.
- Connective tissue in the wall of the heart and great vessels.
- Parafollicular cells of the thyroid gland.
- Glomus cells of the carotid and aortic bodies.
- Much of the craniofacial skeleton.
- Odontoblasts of developing teeth.

Structures of the Head and Neck

Pharyngeal Apparatus

The pharyngeal apparatus (refer to Moore, Persaud & Torchia (2018) for more detail) consists of:
- Pharyngeal arches.
- Pharyngeal pouches.
- Pharyngeal grooves.
- Pharyngeal membranes.

Pharyngeal Arches

Head and neck mesoderm originates from two sources: the paraxial mesoderm and the neural crest. The pharyngeal arches (formerly branchial) begin to develop early in week 4. During week 5, a side view of the embryo shows five pairs of arches numbered I, II, III, IV and VI in craniocaudal sequence. In mammals, a pair numbered V may be transient or never develop (Schoenwolf et al., 2021).

These arches are remnants of the gill (branchial) arches found in fishes. In mammals, there are no gill arches and the pharyngeal arches are linked by mesoderm (Fig. 10.2). On the surface ectoderm there are thickenings called *placodes*; three of these are the nasal placode, lens placode and otic placode, whilst another four contribute sensory ganglion cells to the cranial nerves. Most malformations of the head and neck happen during transformation of pharyngeal arch structures to their final form.

The Structure of the Pharyngeal Arches

Every arch contains the following structures:
1. Migrated neural cells surrounding a central core of mesenchyme cells.
2. Unsegmented mesoderm which forms muscle and bone.
3. A branch of the dorsal aorta on the same side as the pharyngeal arch.
4. A nerve, carrying motor fibres called *branchial efferents,* supports the striated muscles.
5. An external covering of ectoderm.
6. An internal covering of endoderm.

Pharyngeal Pouches and Grooves

Pockets called *pharyngeal pouches* develop from endoderm between the pharyngeal arches. There are four well-defined pairs and a rudimentary fifth pair. The primitive pharynx develops from the foregut and widens cranially. It is lined by endoderm covering the internal surfaces of the pharyngeal arches. Externally the pharyngeal arches are separated by pockets of ectoderm called *pharyngeal grooves.*

Derivatives of the Pharyngeal Arches
First Pharyngeal Arch

The first pair, or **mandibular arches,** are involved in the development of the face. The cartilage of this arch forms **Meckel cartilage** which serves as a template for the mandible. During week 6, the mandible develops around the ventral portion of the cartilage by ossification of surrounding membrane, and the cartilage mostly disappears. The dorsal end of Meckel cartilage is incorporated into the middle ear to form the **malleus** and **incus.** The **mandibular prominence** and the **maxillary prominence** develop from the dorsal part of each mandibular arch.

Second Pharyngeal Arch

The second pair, or **hyoid arches,** have a much smaller skeletal component than the first pair. Their dorsal ends form the **stapes** of the middle ear and the **styloid process** of the

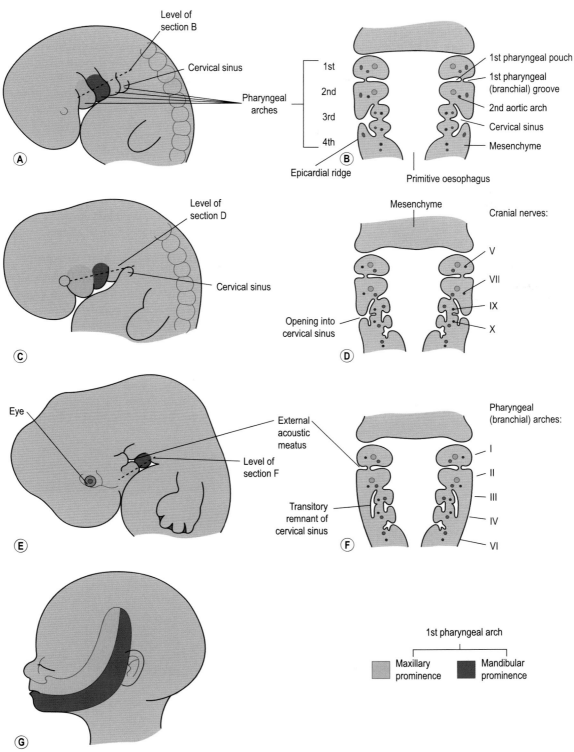

• **Fig. 10.2** (A) Lateral view of the head, neck and thoracic regions of an embryo (about 32 days), showing pharyngeal arches and the cervical sinus. (B) Diagrammatic section through the embryo at the level shown in (A) illustrating growth of a second arch over the third and fourth arches. (C) An embryo of about 33 days. (D) Section of embryo shown in (C), illustrating early closure of the cervical sinus. (E) An embryo of about 41 days. (F) Section of an embryo at the level shown in (E), showing transitory cystic remnant of the cervical sinus. (G) Drawing of a 20-week fetus illustrating the area of the face derived from the first pair of pharyngeal arches.

temporal bone. The ventral ends form part of the hyoid bone. Most of the mesoderm migrates to form the muscles of facial expression. The sensory facial nerve supplies the muscles formed from the hyoid arches.

Third Pharyngeal Arch

The third pair forms the posterior part of the tongue and the lower half of the hyoid bone. The **stylopharyngeus muscle** running from the styloid process to the pharynx is the only muscle formed from this arch. It is innervated by the **glossopharyngeal nerve,** which also carries the sensory fibres for taste in the posterior part of the tongue. The artery of this arch persists as part of the carotid artery.

Fourth and Sixth Pharyngeal Arches

These form the cartilage, ligaments and muscles of the larynx. Nerve supply to the muscles is via the vagus nerve through laryngeal and pharyngeal branches. The left artery of the fourth arch contributes to the aorta, whereas the right one forms most of the right subclavian artery.

Derivatives of the Pharyngeal Pouches

The derivatives of the pharyngeal pouches are:
- First pouch: the Eustachian tube and the middle ear cavity.
- Second pouch: the tonsils.
- Third pouch: the thymus gland and inferior parathyroid gland.
- Fourth/fifth pouches: superior parathyroid gland, parafollicular and C cells of the thyroid gland.

The thyroid gland is the first endocrine gland to develop, arising during week 4 from a thickening of endoderm on the floor of the **pharynx.** Two lobes are formed, joined by an isthmus. By 7 weeks, the thyroid gland reaches its final destination in the neck.

The tongue develops from five tongue buds on the floor of the pharynx at the end of week 4. Two distal tongue buds develop on each side of the median tongue bud and overgrow it to form the anterior or oral two-thirds of the tongue. The posterior part of the tongue develops from mesoderm in the third and fourth pharyngeal arches.

Derivatives of the Pharyngeal Grooves

The first pharyngeal groove is the only one that contributes to final structures. It forms the **external canal of the ear.** Others form a deep ectodermal depression called the *cervical sinus* during week 5. The **cervical sinus** is obliterated by week 7, giving the neck a smooth contour.

The Face

The development of the face is complex, and it is not possible to cover every detail (Fig. 10.3). The primitive mouth

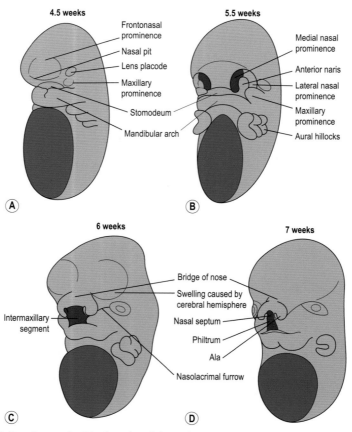

• **Fig. 10.3** Development of the face (medial nasal processes and intermaxillary segment are shaded dark).

begins as a slight depression of the surface ectoderm called the **stomodeum.** It is separated from the foregut by the **oropharyngeal membrane** which ruptures about day 24 to bring the digestive tract into contact with the amniotic cavity. Early in week 4, five prominences emerge around the stomodeum: the **frontonasal** prominence, two pairs of mandibular and two pairs of **maxillary prominences.** These merge with each other and are covered by surface ectoderm.

The mandibular prominence forms the lower jaw or mandible, and the maxillary prominence gives rise to the upper jaw or **maxilla,** the **zygomatic bone** and the squamous portion of the temporal bone, as well as the outer parts of the upper lip. Mandibular arch mesoderm forms the muscles of mastication which are inserted into the mandible. These muscles are innervated by the mandibular branch of the trigeminal nerve. The skin of the face and mucous membranes are formed from mandibular arch ectoderm. They receive a somatic sensory nerve supply from three branches of the **trigeminal nerve**: ophthalmic, maxillary and mandibular.

By the end of week 4, bilateral thickenings of the ectoderm called **nasal placodes** appear. The formation of the nose, palate and upper lip begins early in week 5 when the two nasal placodes recede into **nasal pits** whose openings become the nostrils. A week later the frontonasal prominence extends onto both sides of the nasal pits to form the medial and lateral nasal prominences. The two medial nasal prominences merge across the midline to form the **intermaxillary segment.** During week 7, this produces three midline structures: the lower border of the nasal septum, the **philtrum** of the upper lip and the **primary palate.** If these structures fail to develop, cleft lip and palate result.

The Ears

The Outer and Middle Ear

The **pinna** (auricle) of the ear develops from six **aural hillocks,** three on the first pharyngeal arch and three on the second. It begins in the upper part of the neck and is displaced cranially during development of the mandible. The first pharyngeal cleft gives rise to the **external acoustic meatus** (outer ear canal). The middle ear cavity extends outwards from the first pharyngeal pouch during week 5. Where it contacts the outer ear canal, a thin layer of mesoderm forms the **tympanic membrane** (ear drum). Ear ossicles develop from the dorsal ends of the first and second pharyngeal arches.

The Inner Ear

At the end of week 3, an **otic placode** develops on either side of the head. These sink below the surface to form **otic vesicles** which develop into the **vestibular** and **cochlear sacs.** Three plate-like extensions of the vestibular sac become the **semicircular canals**, and the remainder of the sac becomes the **utricle.** From the cochlear sac the **cochlea** with the **organ of Corti** arises and the rest becomes the **saccule.** A shell of chondrified mesoderm surrounds the

membranous labyrinth and ossifies into the bony labyrinth. The **vestibulocochlear nerve** originates from neural crest cells. The inner ear, tympanic cavity and ossicles are almost fully sized at birth, but the outer ear is short and easily damaged by insertion of objects into the canal.

The Eyes

In week 4, two important events occur in the development of the eye:
1. The **optic vesicles** develop as an outgrowth of the diencephalon, remaining attached to it by the **optic stalk.**
2. Under the inducing influence of the optic vesicles the lenses develop as an in-growth of surface ectoderm—the **lens placode.**

As the lens vesicle sinks inwards, the optic vesicle becomes a double-walled optic cup by invagination. This creates the **optic fissure** on the under-surface of the optic cup and stalk. Before the lips of the optic fissure come together during week 6, it is infiltrated by mesenchyme (Fig. 10.4). Within the cup the mesenchyme produces a gelatinous secretion that fills the **vitreous component** of the eye. During weeks 5 and 6, a shell of mesenchyme covers the outer surface of the optic cup and differentiates into the vascular **choroid coat** of the eyeball and the outer fibrous coat consisting of the **sclera** and **cornea.** The six extraocular muscles develop from mesoderm. Cells in the posterior wall of the **lens vesicle** elongate and lay down **primary lens fibres. Secondary lens fibres** are laid down later by cells migrating into the interior from the margins of the lens.

The Optic Cup

The outer epithelium of the optic cup accumulates **melanin pigment** and becomes the pigmented layer of the **retina.** Around the rim of the cup the outer and inner layers form the **ciliary body** and the **iris.** Ciliary muscles develop from ectomesenchymal cells in the ciliary body, and the sphincter and dilator pupil muscles develop from the posterior epithelium of the iris. The inner epithelium of the optic cup becomes the nervous layer of the retina. Axons of these neurons converge on the optic stalk to form the **optic nerve** which is an extension of the CNS white matter.

Ciliary processes secrete **aqueous humour** between the cornea and the lens. The anterior chamber is between the iris and cornea. The posterior chamber is between the iris and lens. Aqueous humour moves from posterior to anterior chamber through the pupil and then into a small vein encircling the eye at the anterior margin of the choroid coat called the **canal of Schlemm.** The eye is complete by 20 weeks (Fig. 10.5).

The Eyelids and Lacrimal Apparatus

Eyelids develop from mesodermal folds lined by surface ectoderm that grow to meet each other during the second week. From months 3–6, the eyelids are fused, allowing

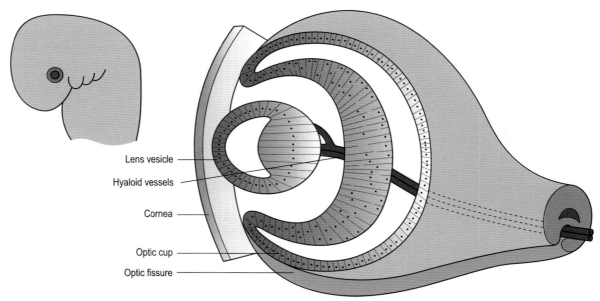

• **Fig. 10.4** The eye at 6 weeks, showing the optic fissure.

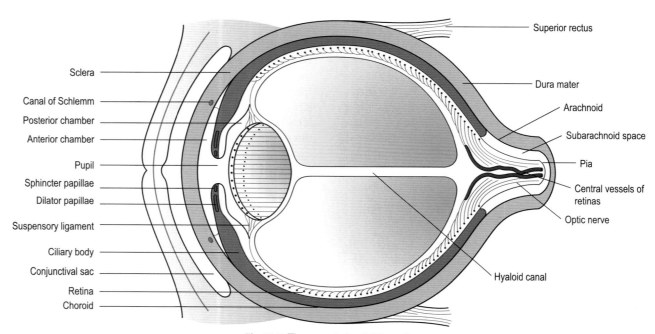

• **Fig. 10.5** The eye at about 20 weeks.

clinicians to estimate the gestational age of a very premature baby. The **lacrimal glands** develop from the outer part of the conjunctival sac and are exocrine glands. It is said that newborns do not produce tears, but there is a continuous lacrimal secretion to protect the cornea.

The Limbs

Development of the Limbs

Limbs form from somatic mesoderm of the lateral body wall in the typical **craniocaudal developmental pattern** (Moore, Persaud & Torchia, 2018) (Fig. 10.6).

Minute upper limb buds appear in the middle of week 4 at the level of the cervical somites. The lower limb buds appear 2 days later at the level of the lower lumbar somites.

Development of the limbs is regulated by **Hox genes** (Wolpert, Tickle & Arias, 2019). Proliferation of somatic mesodermal cells is induced in each limb by the **apical ectodermal ridge** (AER), a thickening of surface ectoderm over the limb bud (Schoenwolf et al., 2021). This covers the whole surface at first but is later confined to the growing tip of the limb. The limb bud is covered with loose mesenchyme. Cell division in the mesenchyme is restricted to a progress zone immediately below the AER. Daughter cells separate out from this zone to add to the limb's length.

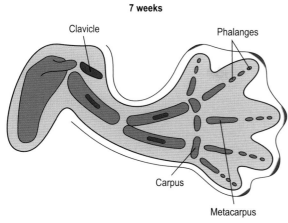

7 weeks

Clavicle

Phalanges

Carpus

Metacarpus

• **Fig. 10.6** Upper limb skeleton at 7 weeks. Centres of ossification (*dark blue*) have appeared in the clavicle and in three major long bones.

The skeleton is the first part of the limb to demonstrate differentiation and is seen as a condensation of mesenchymal cells in the proximal part of the limb bud. Joint formation occurs by the transverse splitting of precartilaginous rods rather than the coming together of separate limb elements. A gene product, known as Indian hedgehog, is known to act on the developing cartilage (Carlson, 2019).

Formation of the Hands and Feet

During week 5, the hands and feet develop as flat limb plates. The AER breaks up into five ridges that mark the positions of the future digits. Each of these lays down a rod of mesoderm called **digital rays.** Webs of loose mesenchyme connect the rays, but apoptosis (programmed cell death) creates **interdigital clefts.**

Development and Rotation of the Limbs

The limb skeleton passes through the precartilaginous, cartilaginous and ossification stages except for the clavicle which develops from membrane. During week 5, condensations of the limb mesenchyme form a rough skeletal plan. By the end of week 6, the skeleton is fully cartilaginous. Ossification centres are present in the limb long bones by week 12. Ossification of the ankle bones begins late in fetal life, but the wrist bones remain cartilaginous until after birth. At first, the limbs grow out laterally from the trunk but during week 8 the limbs rotate to their normal position. Elbow and knee creases appear.

Muscles and Nerves of the Limbs

Skeletal muscle of limbs develops from cells that migrate from the nearest somites, whereas tendons develop from somatic mesoderm already present in the limb buds. Spinal nerves called *ventral rami* invade the limbs before rotation with mixed nerves carrying both motor and sensory fibres. The 31 pairs of spinal nerves are named by the first letter of the name and number of each vertebra from top downwards:

• Cervical: C1–8.
• Thoracic: T1–12.
• Lumbar: L1–5.
• Sacral: S1–5.

There is also one coccygeal nerve. Upper limbs receive nerves from vertebrae C5 to T1, whereas the lower limbs receive nerves from vertebrae L2 to S2.

Blood Supply to the Limbs

Limb buds are invaded early by branches of the **intersegmental** blood vessels. A single axial artery is later replaced by new blood vessels. In the upper limb these are **axillary, brachial** and **interosseous** arteries, with the brachial artery branching into the **radial** and **ulnar** arteries supplying the forearm and hand. In the lower limb, the **popliteal** and **peroneal** arteries replace the axial artery, with the **femoral** artery developing to join the popliteal artery. The femoral artery branches into the anterior and posterior tibial arteries to supply the lower leg and foot.

Main Points

• The human nervous system is the first system to differentiate. By day 19, three primary brain vesicles are present: the prosencephalon, mesencephalon and rhombencephalon. Frontal, parietal, occipital and temporal lobes are present by 14 weeks.
• During week 3, lanugo, very soft fine hair, grows all over the body.
• Between weeks 3 and 6, development of the eye takes place. Eyelids develop during month 2 but are fused between months 3 and 6.
• The primitive mouth begins as a slight depression of surface ectoderm called *stomodeum.* It is separated from the foregut by the oropharyngeal membrane and ruptures at about day 24, bringing the digestive tract into contact with the amniotic cavity.
• The thyroid gland is the first endocrine gland to develop, arising during week 4 from a thickening of endoderm on the floor of the pharynx.
• Upper limb buds appear in the middle of week 4 at the level of lower cervical somites, and lower limb buds appear 2 days later at the level of the lower lumbar somites. Development of the limbs is regulated by Hox genes.
• Three phases—the precartilaginous, cartilaginous and bony phases—lead to development of vertebrae. Chondrification centres appear in the centrum and neural arch late in week 5. Ossification centres appear in the centrum, neural arches and in the ribs by week 8.
• During week 5, hands and feet develop as flat limb plates. Five epidermal apical ridges mark positions of future digits. At first, limbs grow out laterally from the trunk but rotate into normal position in week 8.
• Mammary glands appear in week 6 as paired longitudinal strips of ectodermal thickening on the ventral surface of the embryo.

- At first the neural tube is solid, but it becomes canalized by caudal extension of the neural canal. During weeks 7–10, the spinal cord is finalized.
- Myotomes give rise to the muscles of the head and trunk. Dermatomes merge to form the dermis of the skin. Each dermatome is accompanied by sensory nerve fibres derived from the level of the spinal cord where the dermatome originates.
- The skull is divided into the neurocranium enclosing the brain, and the viscerocranium making up the bones of the face. Ossification gives rise to the parietal bones, frontal bones, occipital bone and squamous portion of the temporal bone of the vault.
- Twenty tooth buds form from thickened ectoderm called *dental lamina*. These form the basis of the deciduous teeth. Later dental lamina forms the buds of the permanent dentition.
- Two commissures of nerve fibres link the right and left cerebral hemispheres: the anterior commissure connects the olfactory regions, and the corpus callosum links matched areas of the cerebral cortex.

References

Carlson, B.M., 2019. Human Embryology and Developmental Biology, sixth ed. Elsevier Saunders, Philadelphia.

Moore, K.L., Persaud, T.V.N., Torchia, M.G., 2018. The Developing Human: Clinically Oriented Embryology, eleventh ed. Elsevier, Philadelphia.

Schoenwolf, G.C., Bleyl, S.B., Brauer, R., Francis-West, P.H., 2021. Larsen's Human Embryology, sixth ed. Elsevier, New York.

Wolpert, L., Tickle, A., Arias, A.M. (Eds.), 2019. Principles of Development, sixth ed. Oxford University Press, Oxford.

Annotated recommended reading

Carlson, B.M., 2019. Human Embryology and Developmental Biology, sixth ed. Elsevier Saunders, Philadelphia.

This book provides much more detail for the reader interested in finding out further information on fetal development.

Moore, K.L., Persaud, T.V.N., Torchia, M.G., 2018. The Developing Human: Clinically Oriented Embryology, eleventh ed. Elsevier, Philadelphia.

This textbook clearly describes embryo development week by week and provides an excellent source for understanding the origin of congenital defects. The illustrations on specific aspects of fetal development are excellent.

Schoenwolf, G.C., Bleyl, S.B., Brauer, R., Francis-West, P.H., 2021. Larsen's Human Embryology, sixth ed. Elsevier, New York.

This e-textbook offers a straightforward approach to a highly complex subject. The comprehensive content examines both molecular biological and clinical aspects of embryology with applications linked to an advancing knowledge base.

11

Embryological Systems 2—Internal Organs

LYNSAY MATTHEWS AND JEAN RANKIN

CHAPTER CONTENTS

This chapter introduces the timing and processes involved in the development of the internal organs and structures of the body systems. Development (with related structures) of the cardiovascular system, lower respiratory tract and diaphragm, the alimentary, urinary and genital tracts and the reproductive system are outlined. Indicators to estimate embryonic age are introduced.

Introduction

The normal development of the internal organs is essential to keep an individual alive and perpetuate the species.

The Cardiovascular System

The cardiovascular system develops early in the embryo from the end of week 2 before the system becomes too large to receive nourishment by diffusion. From the end of week 3, the embryo must obtain nutrients from the maternal circulation. The cardiovascular system can pump blood around embryonic vessels early in week 4.

Vasculogenesis and Angiogenesis

The formation of the embryonic vascular system during week 3 involves **vasculogenesis** which is the formation of vascular channels from cells called *angioblasts* (Fig. 11.1). **Angiogenesis** is the formation of new vessels by budding and branching from pre-existing vessels.

To summarize blood vessel formation from ~17 days:

- Mesenchymal cells in the extraembryonic mesoderm lining the **umbilical vesicle** differentiate into central **angioblasts.** These join to form **blood islands** which are associated with the umbilical vesicle (yolk sac).
- Small cavities appear within the blood islands.
- Peripheral angioblasts flatten to form endothelial cells. These arrange themselves around cavities in the blood island to form endothelium.
- The endothelial-lined cavities fuse to form networks of endothelial channels (vasculogenesis).
- Vessels sprout into adjacent areas by endothelial budding and fuse with other vessels.

Blood cells develop from **multipotent stem cells** in the mesoderm of the **umbilical vesicle** and **allantois** at the end of week 3 and then in specialized sites along the aorta (Wolpert, Tickle & Arias, 2019). Later blood cells develop in the liver, spleen, bone marrow and lymph nodes (Moore, Persaud & Torchia, 2018).

All red cells contain the pigment **haemoglobin,** but in cells made in the umbilical vesicle and liver the haemoglobin is fetal haemoglobin. This fetal haemoglobin takes up and releases oxygen and carbon dioxide more readily than

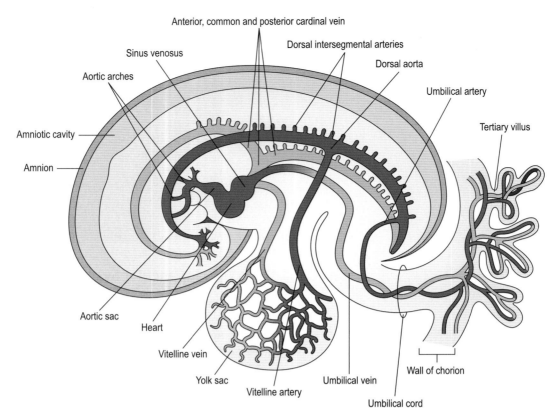

• **Fig. 11.1** Diagram of the primitive cardiovascular system in an embryo of ~20 days, viewed from the left side. Observe the transitory stage of paired symmetric vessels. Each heart tube continues dorsally into a dorsal aorta that passes caudally. Branches of the aortae are umbilical arteries, establishing connections in the chorion; vitelline arteries to the yolk sac; and dorsal intersegmental arteries to the body of the embryo. Vessels on the yolk sac form a vascular plexus that is connected to the heart tubes by vitelline veins. The anterior cardinal veins return blood from the head region. The umbilical vein carries oxygenated blood and nutrients from the chorion to the embryo. The arteries carry poorly oxygenated blood and waste products to the chorionic villi for transfer to the maternal blood.

does adult haemoglobin. Red cells produced by bone marrow are mature and contain adult haemoglobin.

The Primordial Cardiovascular System

Heart and great vessels develop from mesenchymal cells in the **cardiogenic area,** and by 22 days the heart begins to beat.

Three parts of the embryonic arterial system develop:
1. A pair of **umbilical arteries** carries blood to the placenta.
2. **Vitelline arteries** arise from the **dorsal aortas** linking up with the newly developed capillary bed. These eventually become the **mesenteric arteries** supplying the gut.
3. **Intersegmental arteries** supply blood to somites and the neural tube.

As pharyngeal arches form during weeks 4 and 5, they are supplied by paired **aortic arches** arising from the aortic sac and terminating in the dorsal aortas running the length of the embryo. The paired dorsal aortas soon fuse to form a single dorsal aorta.

About 30 branches of the dorsal aorta, called **dorsal intersegmental arteries,** carry blood to somites and their derivatives. Those in the neck join to form a **vertebral artery** on either side of the neck. In the thorax these become the

intercostal arteries. Most of the abdominal branches become **lumbar arteries,** but the fifth pair of lumbar intersegmental arteries remains as the **common iliac arteries.** The sacral intersegmental arteries become **lateral sacral arteries.**

Three pairs of veins drain into the tubular heart of the 4-week embryo:
1. **Umbilical veins** form in the body stalk. Only the left vein persists to carry oxygenated blood to the embryo.
2. The **vitelline veins** carry blood from the umbilical vesicle to the heart tube.
3. **Common cardinal veins** return poorly oxygenated blood from the embryo.

Development of the Heart

The **primordium** (primitive form) of the heart is visible at 18 days and begins to beat at 22 days. Before the head fold develops, cardiogenic mesoderm occupies the floor of the pericardial coelom and gives rise to a pair of **endothelial heart tubes.** These unite to form a single heart tube, and a **primordial myocardium** develops. A **pericardial sac** forms around the heart tube. The tubular heart elongates and forms a series of alternating dilatations and constrictions:

- Truncus arteriosus.
- Bulbus cordis.
- Ventricle.
- Atrium.
- Sinus venosus.

Because the bulbus cordis and the ventricle grow faster than the other regions, the heart tube buckles to form a twisted U shape called the **bulboventricular loop.** The **atrioventricular canal** divides the primordial atrium and ventricle. The truncus arteriosus is continuous with the aortic sac from which the aortic arches arise. The sinus venosus receives the umbilical, vitelline and common cardinal veins mentioned earlier.

Blood Flow Through the Early Heart

Blood flows via veins from the umbilical vesicle, embryo and chorionic villi to the venous sinuses and into the primitive atrium. The blood then passes through the atrioventricular canal into the primordial ventricle. The ventricle contracts, and blood is pumped through the bulbus cordis and truncus arteriosus into the aortic arches. It then passes into the dorsal aortas to return to the umbilical vesicle and early placenta.

Partitioning of the Heart

Partitioning of the heart begins in the middle of week 4. The primitive atrium is partitioned into two by the growth and fusion of two septa: the **septum primum** from the dorsocranial wall and the **septum secundum** from the ventrocranial wall. An opening with a flap-like valve formed by the septum secundum is left between the atria to accommodate a left-to-right shunt of blood across the atria. This is the **foramen ovale** which closes at birth (Moore, Persaud & Torchia, 2019).

Division of the primitive ventricle begins at the end of week 4 with the development of a ridge of tissue called the **interventricular septum.** An **interventricular foramen** closes at the end of week 7, and the pulmonary arterial trunk taking blood to the lungs then communicates with the right ventricle and aorta carrying blood to the body with the left ventricle. Formation of two atria and two ventricles completes the fetal circulation.

Valves and their supporting **papillary muscles** and **chordae tendineae** and the tissue forming the **conducting system** of the heart begin developing at about 5 weeks and are in place by the end of **organogenesis.** The development of the heart and great vessels is complex, leading to the possibility of many different types of malformation.

The Lower Respiratory Tract

Development of the Laryngotracheal Tube

A median **laryngotracheal groove** appears on the floor of the primitive pharynx in the middle of week 4. This is converted by the development of a septum to the **laryngotracheal tube** with an opening into the pharynx. The epithelial lining of the cranial end of this tube, the laryngeal cartilages

and the vocal cords develop from the fourth and sixth pharyngeal arches (Carlson, 2019). The cranial epithelium becomes the epithelial lining of **larynx** and **trachea,** and the caudal part lines the **bronchial tree. Tracheo-oesophageal folds** grow towards each other to form a septum that divides the cranial part of the foregut into the laryngotracheal tube and oesophagus (Fig. 11.2).

Development of the Lungs

Lung buds develop as a bulge in the caudal part of the laryngotracheal tube during week 4. It splits to form two bronchial buds giving rise to **primary bronchi.** Bronchial buds invaginate the **pericardioperitoneal canals** which become pleural cavities. Epithelium covering the outside of bronchial buds becomes the **visceral pleura,** and the epithelium lining pericardioperitoneal canals becomes the **parietal pleura.** Connections between the two pleural cavities and the pericardial cavity containing the heart become closed off. Two primary bronchi divide into secondary and lobar bronchi and then into segmental bronchi lined with cuboid epithelium to serve three lobes in the right lung and two in the left lung. During month 7, respiratory **bronchioles** become more abundant and terminate in **alveolar ducts** and **sacs.**

From weeks 5–17 the developing lungs are in the **pseudoglandular period,** resembling an exocrine gland, and respiration is not possible. In the **canalicular period,** from weeks 16–25, air passages become patent and blood capillaries surround the future alveoli. From 24 weeks until birth, alveoli develop in the **terminal sac period,** and respiration and survival become possible. Budding of alveolar ducts and sacs continues for the first 8 years of life. This is the **alveolar period** (Carlson, 2019; Moore, Persaud & Torchia, 2018).

At first terminal sacs are lined by **type 1 alveolar cells** which take part in gas exchange. By 24 weeks, **type 2 alveolar cells** are found which secrete **surfactant.** This lowers surface tension between the alveolar epithelium and inspired air. Babies born before 34 weeks may develop **respiratory distress syndrome** because of insufficient surfactant production.

The Diaphragm

The diaphragm is complex with five elements contributing to its formation:
- The third to fifth somites contribute cells that form the muscles of the diaphragm.
- Ventral extension of the pleural sacs forms diaphragmatic connective tissue.
- The oesophageal mesentery supplies connective tissue around the oesophagus and inferior vena cava.
- The septum transversum gives rise to the fibrous tissue of the central tendon.
- Pleuroperitoneal membranes contribute connective tissue surrounding the central tendon.

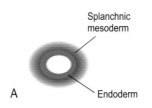

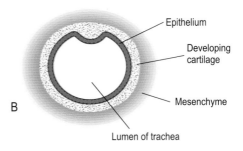

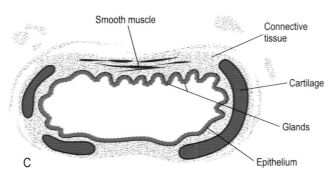

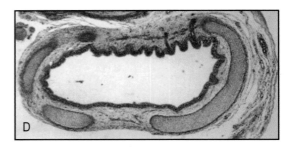

• **Fig. 11.2** Transverse sections through the laryngotracheal tube illustrating progressive stages in the development of the trachea. (A) 4 weeks. (B) 10 weeks. (C) 12 weeks (drawing of micrograph in D). Note that the endoderm of the tube gives rise to the epithelium and glands of the trachea, and that the mesenchyme surrounding the tube forms the connective tissue, muscle and cartilage. (D) Photomicrograph of a transverse section of the developing trachea at 12 weeks.

The Alimentary Tract

The primitive gut begins to form during week 4 when the dorsal part of the umbilical vesicle becomes incorporated into the embryo. The endoderm of this primitive gut gives rise to most of the epithelial lining and glands of the digestive system. By the middle of week 4, the alimentary tract consists of **foregut, midgut** and **hindgut,** each with different arterial blood supply (Carlson, 2019; Schoenwolf et al., 2021). Epithelial linings of the cranial and caudal ends of the gut, the **stomodeum** and the **anal pit** are derived from ectoderm. Muscular and fibrous parts of the digestive tract form from splanchnic mesoderm.

The Foregut

By week 5, the foregut is visibly divided into the oesophagus, stomach and proximal duodenum (Fig. 11.3).

The Oesophagus

Although the **oesophagus** is part of the alimentary tract, it is in close proximity to the respiratory tract and is a thoracic structure. As the thoracic cavity lengthens and heart and lungs descend into it, the oesophagus also lengthens. Upper and lower parts of the oesophagus differ in origin. Pharyngeal arch mesoderm contributes striated muscle to its upper part, and this is supplied by the recurrent laryngeal branches of the vagus nerve. Splanchnic mesoderm contributes smooth muscle to its lower part, and nerve supply is autonomic from the neural crest.

The Stomach

The stomach begins as a spindle-shaped dilatation of the caudal end of the foregut. It is attached to the dorsal wall of the abdominal cavity by dorsal mesentery. During weeks 5 and 6, the dorsal border elongates to form the convex **greater curvature** of the stomach whilst the ventral border forms the concave **lesser curvature.** The stomach now rotates clockwise on its axis through 90 degrees, taking the **dorsal mesentery** to the left. This rotation ensures that the liver becomes a right-sided organ and the spleen a left-sided organ (Schoenwolf et al., 2021).

The Duodenum

The **duodenum** develops from the caudal part of the foregut and cranial end of the midgut. The junction of the two parts is just distal to the common bile duct.

The Liver, Gall Bladder, Pancreas and Spleen

About day 24 the endoderm thickens directly caudal to the **septum transversum** to form the **hepatic diverticulum,** or liver bud, which grows out of the duodenum. The liver bud gives off the **gall bladder** and **biliary duct system.** The hepatic diverticulum divides into left and right hepatic buds, which develop into lobes of the liver. The stalk of the gall bladder becomes the **cystic duct,** and stalks of the hepatic buds become **hepatic ducts.** The **bile duct** is formed by the union of the conjoined hepatic ducts with cystic ducts. Hepatic buds produce a network of **hepatocytes** arranged in branching and anastomosing plates.

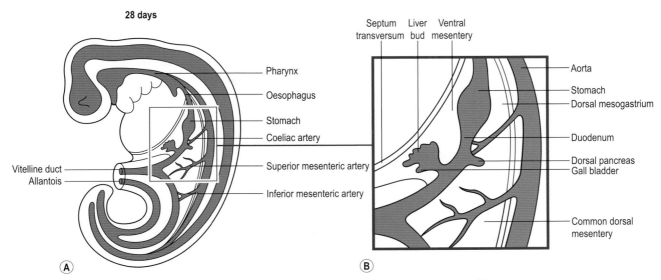

28 days

Pharynx
Oesophagus
Stomach
Coeliac artery
Superior mesenteric artery
Inferior mesenteric artery

Vitelline duct
Allantois

Septum transversum
Liver bud
Ventral mesentery

Aorta
Stomach
Dorsal mesogastrium
Duodenum
Dorsal pancreas
Gall bladder
Common dorsal mesentery

(A)　(B)

• **Fig. 11.3** (A) Digestive system at 4 weeks. (B) Enlargement from (A).

The **pancreas** develops as two separate structures. The smaller ventral pancreas arises from the hepatic diverticulum, which becomes the bile duct, to form the uncinate process of pancreas. The larger dorsal pancreas arises from the duodenum to form the head, body and tail. The main **pancreatic duct** enters the duodenum with bile duct.

The **spleen** develops from mesenchymal cells between layers of the dorsal mesentery. It appears around week 5 on the left side of the abdomen. The spleen is seeded by **haematopoietic cells** from the wall of the umbilical vesicle and manufactures both fetal red and white blood cells in the middle trimester of pregnancy.

Development of the Veins of the Liver

Vitelline veins infiltrate between the hepatocytes to form the **liver sinusoids.** The **portal vein,** draining the entire gut below the diaphragm, also develops from segments of the two vitelline veins. During week 5, the right umbilical vein disappears while the left one enlarges to receive returning placental blood. During weeks 6–8, a large vascular shunt called the **ductus venosus** diverts oxygenated blood from the left umbilical vein to the right hepatic vein, ensuring that the highly metabolic liver receives sufficient oxygen and nutrients (Moore, Persaud & Torchia, 2019).

The Midgut

Derivatives of the midgut are the **small intestine, the caecum** and **vermiform appendix, ascending colon** and the right half of the **transverse colon.** During week 6, the midgut lengthens and, because of the rapid growth of liver and kidneys, there is insufficient room in the abdominal cavity. As the intestine elongates, it moves outside of the embryonic abdomen herniating into the base of the umbilical cord. This is termed the *physiological umbilical herniation of the midgut* (Moore, Persaud & Torchia, 2018).

As it enters the umbilical cord, the midgut twists 90 degrees counter-clockwise (to face the embryo). By 10–11 weeks, the peritoneal coelom has increased sufficiently in size to allow the intestines to slide back into the abdominal cavity. The small intestine returns first, and the colon follows to frame it. The caecum and appendix enter last to lie on the right side below the liver.

The Hindgut: the Rectum and Anal Canal

The hindgut extends from the midgut to the **cloacal membrane.** The **cloaca** will form the bladder and urethra by week 7 with development of the **urorectal septum,** formed by migration of cells from the **urogenital tubercle.** It forms the **urogenital sinus** ventrally and the **rectum** and upper **anal canal** dorsally. The upper half of the anal canal is lined by columnar epithelium continuous with the rectum, whereas the lower half develops from the anal pit and is lined with stratified epithelium continuous with the epidermis of surrounding skin.

The urorectal septum fuses with the cloacal membrane by the end of week 6 to form the **dorsal anal membrane** and the larger **urogenital membrane.** The anal membrane ruptures at the end of week 7 to form the anal orifice. Absent anus (imperforate anus) occurs in 1 in 5000 births. The mesoderm of the urogenital septum persists as the **perineal body.**

The Urinary and Genital Tracts

The urinary and genital systems are closely related and develop from intermediate mesoderm, with the urinary system developing before the genital system. During embryonic folding, the intermediate mesoderm is carried ventrally and loses contact with the somites. A longitudinal ridge of mesoderm on either side of the primitive aorta is called the **urogenital ridge.** Part of this ridge, the **nephrogenic cord,** gives rise to the urinary system, and the **gonadal** or **genital ridge** gives rise to the genital system.

The Kidneys and Ureters

Three pairs of kidneys appear in succession during development:

- The **pronephros** appears in week 4 (non-functional in mammals and disappears).
- The **mesonephros** exists between weeks 4 and 8 (disappears in mammals).
- Finally, the **metanephros** or mammalian kidney appears.

Development of the Collecting System

The metanephros develops from the **metanephric diverticulum,** a dorsal bud from the mesonephric (Wolffian) ducts and a mass of metanephric mesoderm. The stalk of each **metanephric diverticulum** becomes the **ureter.** As this ureter advances towards the kidney, it acquires a lumen by apoptosis and its tip hollows out to become the **renal pelvis.** The ureteric bud keeps dividing to form generations of **collecting tubules** (Fig. 11.4). The first four generations

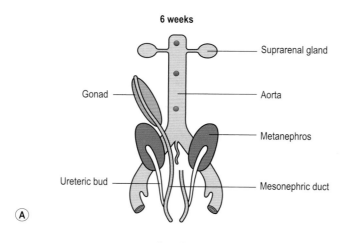

6 weeks

Suprarenal gland

Gonad

Aorta

Metanephros

Ureteric bud

Mesonephric duct

(A)

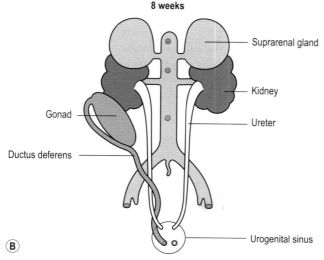

8 weeks

Suprarenal gland

Gonad

Kidney

Ductus deferens

Ureter

Urogenital sinus

(B)

• **Fig. 11.4** Renal ascent. (A) At 6 weeks, (B) at 8 weeks.

enlarge to become **major calyces** and the next four become **minor calyces** of the kidney. The remaining generations form the collecting tubules.

Cells of the intermediate mesoderm surrounding the kidney form a **metanephric cap** over the renal pelvis. A cluster of metanephric cells gathers at the tip of each collecting tubule to form a **nephron.** The kidneys ascend into the abdomen to contact with **adrenal glands** by week 8. The fetal kidney produces small amounts of urine from 9 weeks and is more functional from 15 weeks with excretion of urine into the amniotic cavity. Renal arteries develop to supply blood.

The Bladder and Urethra

Between the umbilicus and the cloacal membrane, caudal mesoderm forms a midline swelling called the **genital tubercle.** Migration of cells form the **urogenital sinus** which gives rise to the bladder and urethra. The urogenital sinus has three parts:

1. A **vesical part** expands to form the bladder and receive the two ureters.
2. A narrow **pelvic part** forms the lining epithelium of prostatic and membranous parts of the **urethra.** In females, the pelvic part lines the short urethra.
3. A **phallic part** extends ventrally beneath the **penis.** At first the urethra opens on the underside of the penis behind the developing **glans.** During month 4, a glandular urethra opens at the tip of the glans. The **prepuce** is an outgrowth of skin from the glans.

As the bladder enlarges, the caudal parts of the mesonephric ducts are incorporated into its dorsal wall so that the ureters open into the urinary bladder.

The Suprarenal Glands

The cortex and medulla of the **suprarenal glands** are formed from separate tissues. The cortex develops from mesoderm, and the medulla develops from neural crest cells. The medullary **chromaffin cells** are modified sympathetic ganglion cells whose chief secretion is adrenaline (epinephrine).

The Reproductive System

Gonads can be identified about week 5 and develop from three sources. The gonadal ridges on the medial side of the mesonephros include cells from two sources: the **coelomic epithelium** and underlying **intermediate mesoderm.** The epithelium releases a chemical that attracts a third source of cells, **primordial germ cells,** which become ova or sperm. About 100 are present on the caudal surface of the umbilical vesicle during week 4. These migrate into the interior of the gonadal ridge and are enclosed in columns of epithelial cells called **sex cords.** Initially the indifferent gonads are the same in male and female but soon differentiate into recognizable male and female structures from week 7 (Fig. 11.5).

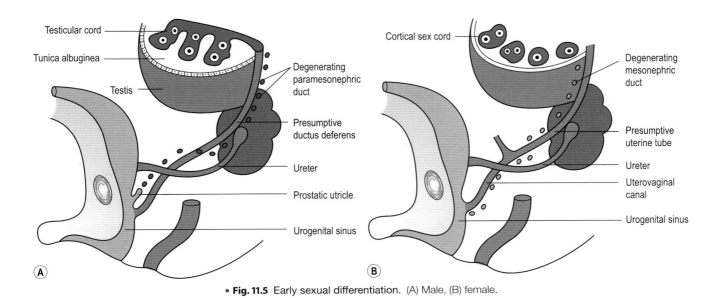

• **Fig. 11.5** Early sexual differentiation. (A) Male, (B) female.

Testes and the Male Genital Tract

In the presence of the *SRY* (sex-determining region Y) gene around day 50, intermediate mesoderm forms the **tunica albuginea.** Sex cords become **testicular cords,** and the primordial germ cells become **prospermatogonia.** Testicular cords are gathered into lobules separated by testicular septa derived from the tunica albuginea. The inner ends of the cords are linked together in a network called the **rete testis.** Two sets of endocrine cells form in the lobules:

1. Sertoli cells are the most numerous and produce a **Müllerian duct inhibitory factor** which causes regression of the paramesonephric ducts during week 9.
2. Leydig cells secrete **testosterone** which ensures the survival and growth of the **Wolffian ducts** and the formation of the epididymis, ductus deferens and ejaculatory duct.

The testes descend gradually from their original site in the lumbar region into the scrotal sac, usually by term. They are accompanied by a pocket of peritoneum called the **processus vaginalis** which becomes the **tunica vaginalis** on completion of descent. Testes are accompanied by the ductus deferens, testicular blood vessels, nerves and lymphatics constituting the spermatic cords. In females, the Wolffian ducts disappear by programmed cell death without any ovarian influence. Remnants found in the broad ligament may form **parovarian cysts.**

Ovaries and the Female Genital Tract

In the absence of *SRY*, no tunica albuginea forms. Sex cords accumulate in the outer cortex of the gonadal ridge. This becomes filled with **primordial follicles** consisting of an oocyte derived from primordial germ cells, an inner shell of follicular cells and an outer shell—the theca. The number of primordial follicles reaches a maximum of 6–7 million in week 15. Programmed cell death reduces this number drastically so that 2 years after birth only 1 million remain and at puberty only 300,000. The ovary descends from the abdominal lumbar region into the pelvis after week 12.

Upper and middle sections of the Müllerian tubes form the epithelial lining of the uterine tubes, and the lower segments fuse into one during week 9. This becomes the **uterovaginal canal** which eventually forms the epithelial lining of the uterus. Muscle walls of the uterine tubes and uterus are formed from splanchnic mesoderm.

The Vagina

If the Müllerian system develops, a small tubercle called the *Müllerian eminence* gives rise to the **vaginal plate.** This lengthens along the dorsal wall of the urogenital sinus. The lumen of the vagina is formed by canalization from below upwards and extends around the cervix to form the fornices. The hymen is left as a partition between the vagina and the vestibule.

The External Genitalia

Early in month 3, it is not possible to see a sexual difference. Externally the phallic urethra is an open groove flanked by paired inner urogenital folds and outer genital swellings derived from mesenchyme.

- In males, the matching pairs come together under the influence of testosterone. Urogenital folds unite below the urethral groove to complete the spongy urethra, and the genital swellings form the two halves of the scrotum. A line of union at the junction of the two halves of the scrotum is called the *scrotal raphe,* and the line of union of the urogenital folds is marked by the urethral raphe.
- In females, the matching pairs stay apart, and there is growth in situ of the urogenital folds and genital swellings. The phallus forms the clitoris with a small glans at

its tip. The urethral groove and the phallic part of the urogenital sinus remain open as the vestibule and the urogenital folds become the labia minora and the genital swellings become the labia majora.

Estimation of Embryonic Age

By 8 weeks the embryo is recognizably human, although the head is rounder and large in proportion to the body. The remainder of pregnancy is concerned mainly with growth and maturation. The usual calculation of embryonic age is made by ascertaining the date of the first day of the last menstrual period (LMP). External features and measurements are useful, and careful ultrasound scanning can confirm the age of a viable embryo in utero. At 4 weeks after fertilization (6 weeks from the first day of the LMP), the embryo and its sac measure 5 mm in length. One week later, discrete embryonic features can be visualized and crown–rump measurements can be made.

Main Points

- Three pairs of veins drain into the tubular heart (4-week embryo). Umbilical veins form in the body stalk, but only the left one persists to carry oxygenated blood to the embryo. Vitelline veins carry blood from the umbilical vesicle to the heart tube. Common cardinal veins return poorly oxygenated blood from the embryo.
- Lung buds split to form two bronchial buds dividing into secondary bronchi serving the three lobes of the right lung and the two lobes of the left lung.
- During month 7, respiratory bronchioles terminate in alveolar ducts and sacs lined by type 1 alveolar cells.
- At the end of month 6 (24 weeks), type 2 alveolar cells secreting surfactant appear.
- By week 4, the alimentary tract consists of foregut, midgut and hindgut.
- During weeks 5 and 6, the dorsal border elongates to form the greater curvature of stomach and the ventral border forms the lesser curvature.
- On day 24, the liver bud grows out from the duodenum and gives off the gall bladder and biliary duct system. Bile duct is formed from the union of hepatic and cystic ducts.
- The spleen appears around week 5.
- The cloaca forms the bladder and urethra with development of the urorectal septum.
- The anal membrane ruptures by week 7 to form the anal orifice.

- The urogenital ridge gives rise to the nephrogenic cord, the primordium of the urinary system. The genital ridge gives rise to the genital system. Three pairs of kidneys appear in succession during development. The last is the metanephros, or permanent mammalian kidney.
- Epithelium cells from the gonadal ridge release a chemical attracting primordial germ cells, which will form ova or sperm.
- Gonads are identical in males and females up to week 7.
- Two pairs of genital ducts are present: the Wolffian ducts are forerunners of the male genital tract, and the Müllerian ducts are forerunners of the female genital tract. In the absence of the trigger *SRY* gene, all fetuses become female. *SRY* triggers formation of the testes.
- Early in month 3, the phallic urethra is an open urethral groove flanked by paired urogenital folds and outer genital swellings.
- In males, testosterone influences the matching pairs to come together to complete the spongy urethra, and the genital swellings form two halves of the scrotum.
- In females, the urethral groove and the phallic part of the genital sinus remain open. The urogenital folds become the labia minora whilst the genital swellings become the labia majora. The phallus forms the clitoris with a small glans at its tip.
- By 8 weeks, the embryo is recognizably human.

References

Carlson, B.M., 2019. Human Embryology and Developmental Biology, sixth ed. Elsevier Saunders, Philadelphia.

Moore, K.L., Persaud, T.V.N., Torchia, M.G., 2018. The Developing Human: Clinically Oriented Embryology. Elsevier Health Sciences, New York.

Moore, K.L., Persaud, T.V.N., Torchia, M.G., 2019. Before We are Born. Essentials of Embryology and Birth Defects, tenth ed. Elsevier, Philadelphia.

Schoenwolf, G.C., Bleyl, S.B., Brauer, R., Francis-West, P.H., 2021. Larsen's Human Embryology, sixth ed. Elsevier, New York.

Wolpert, L., Tickle, A., Arias, A.M. (Eds.), 2019. Principles of Development, sixth ed. Oxford University Press, Oxford.

Annotated recommended reading

Moore, K.L., Persaud, T.V.N., Torchia, M.G., 2019. Before We are Born. Essentials of Embryology and Birth Defects, tenth ed. Elsevier, Philadelphia.

This book covers the essentials of normal and abnormal human development including embryogenesis, causes of birth defects and the role of genes in human development. It includes numerous illustrations.

Schoenwolf, G.C., Bleyl, S.B., Brauer, R., Francis-West, P.H., 2021. Larsen's Human Embryology, sixth ed. Elsevier, New York.

This e-textbook offers a straightforward approach to a highly complex subject. The comprehensive content examines both molecular biological and clinical aspects of embryology with applications linked to an advancing knowledge base.

12

The Placenta, Membranes and Amniotic Fluid

SHONA MONTGOMERY AND JEAN RANKIN

CHAPTER CONTENTS

This chapter details the placenta, membranes and amniotic fluid. This includes implantation, development and a description of the mature placenta. The functions are explained and anatomical variations described. Students and midwives need to have knowledge and understanding of this organ to recognize potential problems and initiate appropriate interventions that may save babies lives.

Introduction

The placenta is arguably the most important organ of the body, but paradoxically the most poorly understood (Burton & Fowden, 2015). The placenta is vital for normal in utero development in mammals. It is the largest fetal organ and the first organ to develop (Turco & Moffett, 2019). During its transient existence, the principal function of the placenta is to supply the fetus, and in particular, the fetal brain, with oxygen and nutrients (Burton & Fowden, 2015). The development of the mature placental structure is adapted for this purpose by having a large surface area for exchange and a thin interhaemal membrane separating the maternal and fetal circulations. The process in development involves adopting strategies that are essential to facilitating transfer, including remodelling of the maternal uterine arteries that supply the placenta to ensure optimal perfusion (Tal & Taylor, 2021). Establishing the maternal circulation to a haemochorial placenta where the maternal–fetal interface is represented by maternal blood bathing the trophoblast surface is a major haemodynamic challenge (Burton & Fowden, 2015; Tal & Taylor, 2021).

Implantation and Early Placental Development

In preparation for implantation, the **trophoblasts** produce human chorionic gonadotrophin (hCG), and the action of this hormone promotes vascularity of the endometrium. This lining of the uterus undergoes a series of structural changes to become prepared and receptive to the implanting embryo. This process is referred to as decidualization and the uterine lining (endometrium) is named the **decidua** during pregnancy. Box 12.1 summarizes key information related to the structural changes necessary to support development of the placenta.

Implantation starts the process and occurs where there is a synchronicity between a receptive endometrium and the blastocyst (Aplin & Ruane, 2017). This process is mediated by a coordinated sequence of interactions between embryonic and maternal cells (Blackburn, 2018). Implantation into the decidua (endometrium) involves apposition, adhesion and invasion (Aplin & Ruane, 2017; Okada, Tsuzuki & Marata, 2018; Tal & Taylor, 2021). The placenta is derived from embryonic trophoblast cells and a few inner-cell mass

- Decidualization refers the functional and morphological changes that occur in the endometrium to form the decidual lining into which the blastocyst implants.
- Increasing hormone levels of progesterone result in enlargement of the connective tissue of the endometrium, vascular changes and the cells differentiating into decidual cells (Tal & Taylor 2021).
- **Decidual reaction** refers to the cellular and vascular changes taking place in the endometrium in preparation for implantation.
- Endometrium is referred to as decidua during pregnancy (this lining is shed following pregnancy).
- **Trophoblasts** have a potent invasive capacity (Haram et al 2020). This is moderated by the decidua which secretes cytokinenes and protease inhibitors to modulate this trophoblastic invasion.
- The *Layer of Nitabusch* is a collagenous layer lying between the endometrium and myometrium which assists in preventing invasion of cells outwith the decidua.
- The human placenta is haemomonochorial as maternal blood makes direct contact rather than via blood vessels (haemo), while on the fetal side there is a single intact layer of trophoblast (monochorial) between maternal blood and the fetal vascular compartment (Huppertz & Kingdom 2018).

TABLE 12.1 **Placental Development: Key Timelines**

Blastocyst Stage	Differentiation of the Trophoblast Lineage
Day 7–8 post-conception	Pre-lacunar stage of placental development
Day 8–9 post-conception	Lacunar stage of placental development
Day 12 post-conception	Implantation completed, embryo completely surrounded by placenta
Day 14 post-conception	Differentiation of extravillous trophoblast
Day 20 post-conception	Development of placental vessels and blood cells independent of vessel development in the embryo proper
Week 12	Onset of maternal flow within the intervillous space, development of the chorion laeve
First trimester	Histiotrophic nutrition (*nourishment through uterine glands*)
Second and third trimester	Haemotrophic nutrition (*nourishment through maternal blood flow*)

Huppertz & Kingdom, 2018.

mesodermal cells. The trophoblastic cells overlying the inner cell mass are known as the polar trophoblast; it is these cells that begin the process of adhesion and implantation (Coad, Pedley & Dunstall, 2019).

Implantation is outlined in the following sequence (Blackburn, 2018):
1. Loss of the pellucida (5 days after fertilization, hatching of the blastocyst occurs followed by rapid proliferation of the trophectoderm to form the trophoblast cell mass).
2. The blastocyst aligns and adheres to the endometrial luminal surface between the opening of uterine glands (which stimulates the decidual reaction).
3. The epithelium of the endometrial surface erodes with the blastocyst burrowing beneath the surface as uterine stromal cells encapsulate it.
4. Placental trophoblasts migrate into the endometrium with disruption of capillary beds.
5. Maternal capillary beds remodel to form blood-filled trophoblastic lacunae.

With hatching, the blastocyst acquires the ability to attach to the uterus. Implantation and placentation both require substances and many signalling pathways with ongoing communication (cross talk) between the developing blastocyst and maternal endometrium. The process of implantation is unstable and extremely aggressive. This involves chemical mediators, prostaglandins and proteolytic enzymes released by both the decidua and the trophoblasts and the invasion of maternal connective tissue (Bailey, 2020). Table 12.1 summarizes the key timeline for placental development. The pre-lacunar and lacunar stages occurring during implantation and early development are detailed in Box 12.2.

Development of the Chorionic Villi and Vascular Network

By the end of the second week, trophoblastic cells have formed finger-like projections called **primary chorionic villi** all around the embryo. Early in the third week, a core of loose connective tissue developed from embryonic mesenchyme invades each primary chorionic villus to form the **secondary chorionic villi.** Some of the mesenchymal cells in the core differentiate into fetal blood capillaries, forming mature **tertiary chorionic villi**.

By 15–20 days, there is an established and functioning **arteriocapillary venous network** connected to the embryonic heart vessels. By the end of the third week, fetal blood circulates through the chorionic villi and exchange of substances between maternal and fetal circulations begins (Figs 12.1 and 12.2).

In normal pregnancy, decidual and myometrial arteries change to convert them to **uteroplacental arteries.** Two types of **migratory cytotrophoblast** (MC) cause this:
1. Endovascular MCs invade numerous spiral arterioles on the decidua and myometrium and replace arterial endothelium, destroying muscle and elastic tissues in the tunica media. Tissues are replaced by maternal fibrinoids.

• BOX 12.2   Early Development of the Placenta

Pre-lacunar Stage

The human placenta develops from the trophectoderm, the outer layer of the pre-implantation embryo, which forms at ~5 days post-fertilization. At this stage, the pre-implantation embryo (termed **blastocyst**) is segregated into two lineages: the **inner cell mass** (ICM) and the trophectoderm. The blastocyst contacts the endometrium (apposition) and then the process of placentation commences. Nearby maternal blood vessels ensure there is optimum flow of blood to the placenta (Bailey, 2020).

Initial trophoblastic cells, collectively called the cytotrophoblast, give rise to the syncytiotrophoblast (trophoblast without cells) that have undergone nuclear division without forming daughter cells. The cells quickly invade the uterine lining and allow the embryo to embed. This involves a plug of blood clot and cellular debris closing over the point of entry. Following attachment to the uterine surface epithelium, the trophectoderm fuses to form a primary syncytium. The cytotrophoblasts form a double layer and cells further differentiate into various types of syncytiotrophoblasts. The trophoblastic cell columns anchor the placenta (*see formation of the cytotrophoblastic shell*).

Lacunar Stage (Day 8–9 Post-conception)

By the first missed menstrual period, the blastocyst is completely embedded (~8–10 days), and the decidual reaction spreads outwards from the embedding site. The uterine glands secrete nutrients (e.g., glycogen) to maintain the developing embryo until the intraplacental blood flow is fully developed and established by weeks 10–12 (Huppertz & Kingdom, 2018).

Following implantation, the primary syncytium rapidly invades through the surface epithelium into the underlying decidual glands. Maternal endometrial capillaries surrounding the embryo swell to form **sinusoids** eroded by the increasing number of invasive syncytiotrophoblasts. Small fluid-filled spaces called **lacunae** appear in the syncytiotrophoblast and become filled with a mixture of blood from the sinusoids and secretions from the eroded **endometrial** glands (Moore, Persaud & Torchia, 2018). The lacunae fuse to form the **intervillous spaces** of the placenta through which maternal blood begins to flow. This is the villous stage of development (see *Development of the chorionic villi and vascular network*).

The development of the lacunar system subdivides the placenta into three regions of the decidua based on their relation to the implantation site:
1. The **decidua basalis** lies beneath the conceptus, forming the *maternal component* of the placenta.
2. The **decidua capsularis** overlies *the developing embryo* (conceptus).
3. The **decidua vera** or parietalis lines the remainder of the uterine cavity.

Mesodermal tissue from the developing embryo migrates through the primitive streak and joins trophoblast extensions to form the connecting stalk. This mesoderm gives rise to the umbilical blood vessels, ultimately becoming the umbilical cord. The embryo, its umbilical vesicle and the early amniotic sac are suspended in the **chorionic sac**. This chorionic sac consists of a layer of mesoderm nearest the embryo, the cytotrophoblast and the syncytiotrophoblast nearest the endometrium. The amniotic sac is nearest to the uterine wall and is divided from the chorion by a fluid-filled cavity called the **extraembryonic coelom**.

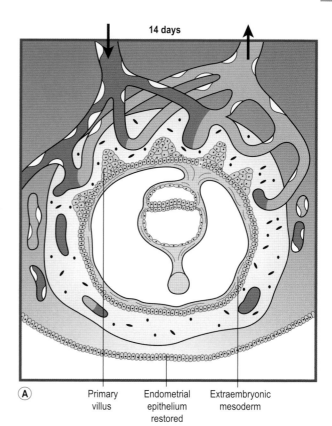

(A)   Primary villus   Endometrial epithelium restored   Extraembryonic mesoderm

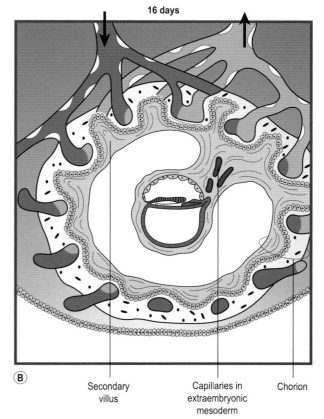

(B)   Secondary villus   Capillaries in extraembryonic mesoderm   Chorion

• **Fig. 12.1** Formation of the chorionic vesicle. (A) Primary chorionic villi are small, nonvascular, and contain only the trophoblast. (B) Secondary chorionic villi have a core of loose connective tissue growing into the primary chorionic villi. The villi increase in size and branch, while the mesoderm grows into them. At this point the villi contain trophoblast and mesoderm.

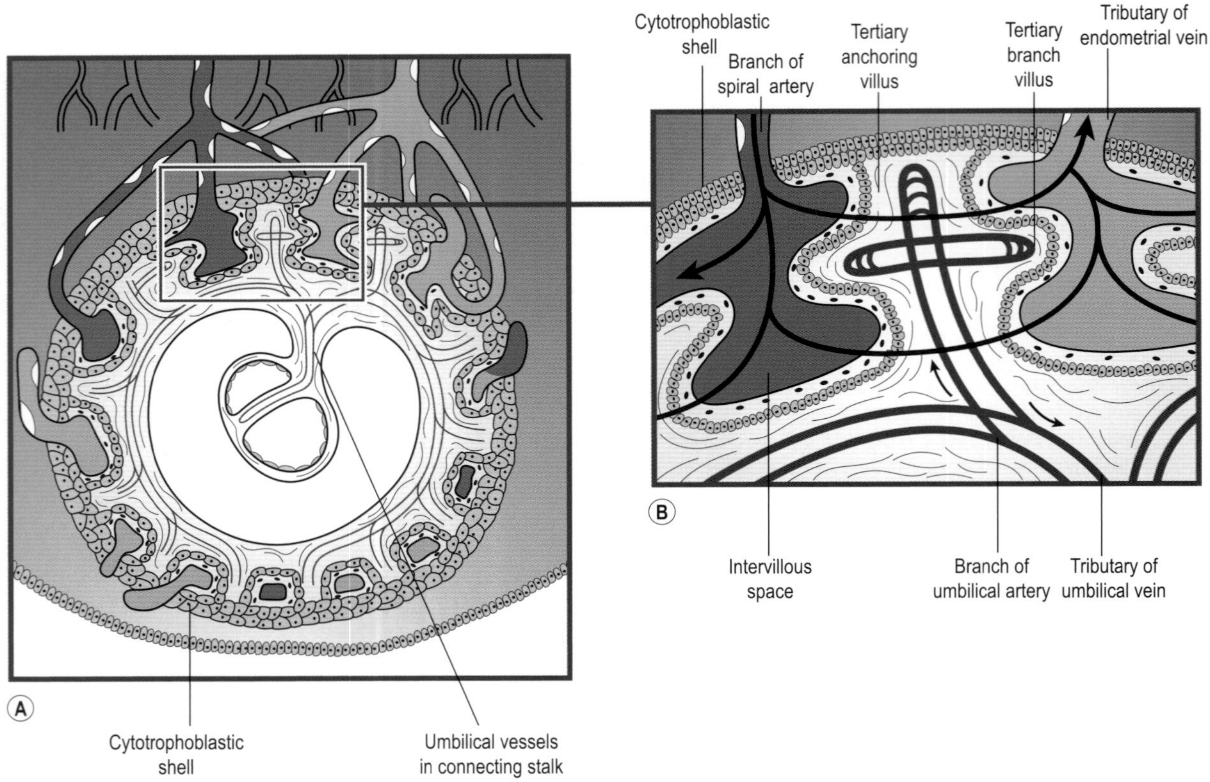

• **Fig. 12.2** (A) Chorionic vesicle at 21 days. (B) Enlargement of the upper part of (A) showing the circulation of embryonic and maternal blood.

The migration takes place in two waves: at 6–10 weeks and 14–16 weeks.

2. Interstitial (stromal) MCs destroy the ends of decidual blood vessels, promoting blood flow into the lacunae. The maternal arteries are functionally denervated so that they are completely dilated and unresponsive to a pressor substance or autonomic neural control. Local prostacyclin maintains vasodilation of the uterine radial arteries.

Until the eighth week, the entire surface of the chorionic sac is covered by villi. As the sac grows, the chorionic villi associated with the decidua capsularis become compressed. This reduces their blood supply, and these chorionic villi degenerate to become the **chorion laeve** (smooth) and then the **chorionic membrane.** The chorionic villi of the decidua basalis branch to form the **chorion frondosum,** or fetal part of the placenta.

Formation of the Cytotrophoblastic Shell

The cytotrophoblastic cells proliferate and extend through the syncytiotrophoblast to form a **cytotrophoblastic shell.** This is the external layer of the cytotrophoblasts found on the maternal surface of the placenta. The shell attaches the chorionic sac to the maternal endometrium by specialized chorionic villi called **stem** or **anchoring villi.** Villi branch and grow from the sides of the stem: it is here where the main exchange of materials between maternal and fetal circulations occurs.

Until about 20 weeks, the placental membrane (Fig. 12.3) consists of four layers separating the two circulations: syncytiotrophoblast, cytotrophoblast, connective tissue of the mesenchyme core and the endothelium of the fetal capillary (Moore, Persaud & Torchia, 2018). As the conceptus grows, the decidua capsularis bulges into the uterine cavity and eventually fuses with the decidua vera. By 22 weeks, the decidua capsularis has degenerated and disappeared (Fig. 12.4). Maternal and fetal circulations do not mingle unless there is damage to the villi. As pregnancy advances, this placental membrane becomes thinner and fetal capillaries lie very close to the syncytiotrophoblast.

Later Placental Development

By 16 weeks, the placenta reaches full thickness; no new lobes or stem villi will develop thereafter. Circumferential growth continues with the branching of villi. The size and number of maternal capillaries continue to increase, as does the surface area for gas exchange. The vascular network is established with a clearly defined and functioning fetalmaternal unit (see *placental circulation*). Cellular proliferation stops at 35 weeks, but cellular hypertrophy continues until term and there is scope for the fetus to signal to the placenta if the fetal needs are not being met.

At each stage of placental development, genetic variants, exposure to infection, poor vascular function, oxidative stress or failure of normal development can all lead to abnormal formation. Many complications of pregnancy have their origins in abnormal development of the placenta in the first trimester. These include pre-eclampsia, fetal growth restriction (FGR), unexplained stillbirth, placental abruption and preterm labour. These conditions are responsible for a high proportion of maternal and neonatal morbidity and mortality

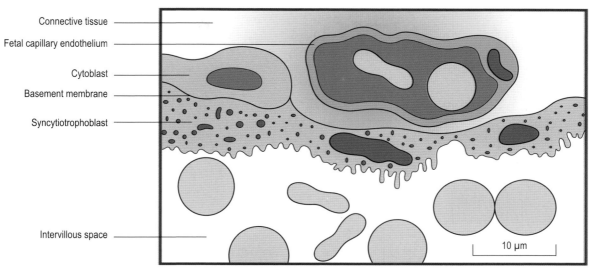

Connective tissue

Fetal capillary endothelium

Cytoblast

Basement membrane

Syncytiotrophoblast

Intervillous space

10 μm

• **Fig. 12.3** Structure of the placental membrane. All erythrocytes are coloured grey.

seen in all populations, but particularly in sub-Saharan Africa (Graham et al., 2016; Turco & Moffett, 2019).

The Mature Placenta

Appearance

The placenta is a flattened discoid organ about 22 cm in diameter and 2.5 cm thick at the centre (Huppertz & Kingdom, 2018). The placenta thickness thins out towards its circumference where it is continuous with the chorion. The weight of the placenta at term is approximately 470 g (450–500g) which makes it directly proportional to the weight of the baby (Huppertz & Kingdom, 2018). The ratio of fetal size to that of the placenta is 7:1; however maternal complications and placental pathological issues may affect placental weight (Rampersad, Cervar-Zivkovic & Nelson, 2011).

There are two distinct surfaces (Fig. 12.5): the **maternal surface** attached to the decidua and the **fetal surface** covered with amnion into which the umbilical cord inserts.

On inspection following birth, the maternal surface of the placenta is a dark red colour because it contains maternal blood. The surface is formed of about 20 **cotyledons** (lobes) separated by **sulci** (grooves). The decidua dips down into these sulci to form septa. The lobes are made up of **lobules,** each containing a tertiary villus and branches.

The fetal surface of the placenta is a shiny greyish white colour because it is covered by amniotic membrane (the inner most layer). From the insertion of the umbilical cord, branches of the single umbilical vein and two umbilical arteries spread out and dip down into the tissue. The amnion can be peeled off the surface, leaving the chorionic plate, which is the portion continuous with the chorion.

The Membranes

The placental membranes are known as the **amnion** and **chorion,** which grow until about 28 weeks and then increase their size by stretching. They resist rupture as the fetus grows,

mainly due to the strength of the amnion. Spontaneous rupture of the membranes during labour is probably brought about by increased intrauterine pressure; as the uterus contracts the intrauterine space is reduced and the amniotic fluid cannot be compressed. The amnion and chorion are not fused and contain up to 200 mL of amniotic fluid between them.

The outer chorion adheres closely to the decidua, but the amnion moves over it aided by mucus. This may lead to rupture of the amnion with the formation of amniotic bands which may constrict or amputate fetal limbs (Blackburn, 2018). The chorion is a thick, opaque, friable membrane that varies at term from 0.02–0.2 mm thick. It consists of four layers of tissue (Fig. 12.6), which atrophy as pregnancy advances. The cells of the chorion laeve are metabolically active, producing enzymes that can reduce the level of locally produced progesterone and a protein that can bind progesterone. The chorion also produces prostaglandins, oxytocin and platelet-activating factor, which are stimulators of myometrial activity.

The inner amnion is tough, smooth and translucent and lines the chorion and the surface of the placenta, continuing over the outer surface of the umbilical cord. At term, it is about 0.02–0.5 mm thick and consists of five layers (Fig. 12.6). It is lined with non-ciliated epithelial cells which may help in the formation and regulation of amniotic fluid. The amnion also produces prostaglandins, particularly PGE_2, which may help initiate the onset of labour. A rising ratio between oestradiol and progesterone may regulate the activity of prostaglandin. This may play an important part in the onset of labour by increasing the number of myometrial oxytocin receptors (Johnson, 2018).

The Umbilical Cord

The umbilical cord, or **funis,** is usually attached to the centre of the placental fetal surface. It is 1–2 cm in diameter and varies in length from 30–90 cm with an average of 50 cm. There are normally two **umbilical arteries** and one **umbilical vein** surrounded by a mucoid connective tissue called

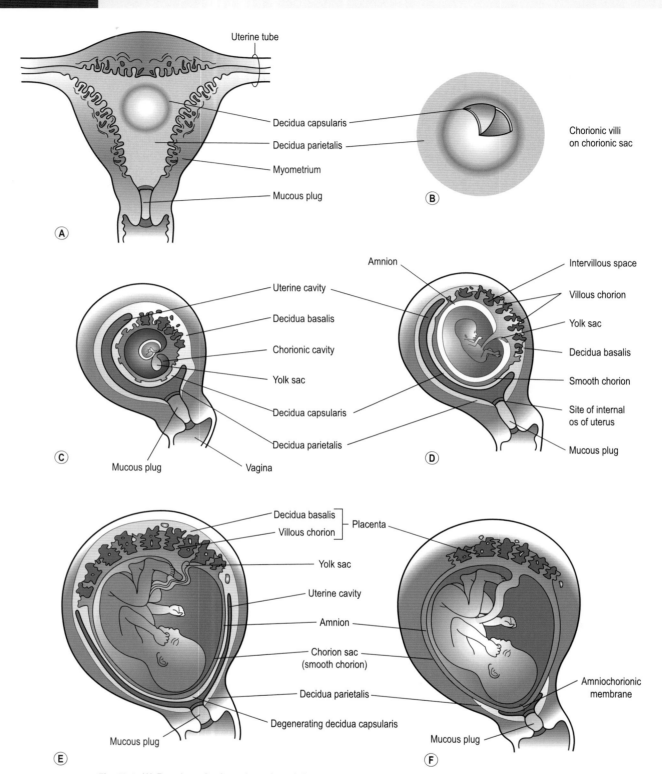

• **Fig. 12.4** (A) Drawing of a frontal section of the uterus showing the elevation of the decidua capsularis caused by the expanding chorionic sac of an implanted 4-week embryo. (B) Enlarged drawing of the implantation site shown in (A); the chorionic villi have been exposed by cutting an opening in the decidua capsularis. (C–F) Drawings of sagittal sections of the decidua. In (F), the amnion and chorion are fused with each other and the decidua parietalis, thus obliterating the uterine cavity. Note that the chorionic villi persist only where the chorion is associated with the decidua basalis; here they have formed the villous chorion.

Wharton jelly. The umbilical vein is longer than the arteries that spiral around it. The vessels are longer than the cord, and non-significant loops of vessel called **false knots** may be seen. Rarely a **true knot** may be present which can possibly cause the blood vessels to become occluded. This rare occurrence will cause fetal distress, especially during labour.

The Umbilical Vesicle (Yolk Sac) and Allantois

By 9 weeks, the umbilical vesicle has shrunk to a pear-shaped remnant about 5 mm in diameter. Once its functions in producing blood cells during weeks 3–5 are completed, it becomes detached from the gut and remains present in the umbilical cord (Coad, Pedley & Dunstall, 2019). The **allantois** is an important structure for the exchange of gases and removal of urinary waste. This structure degenerates, forming the **urachus** (median umbilical ligament) that connects the umbilicus to the urinary bladder.

The Placental Circulation

The placental villi form a large surface area for substance exchange between maternal and fetal circulations. The

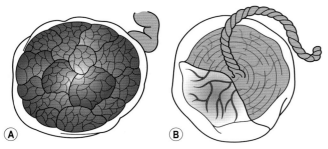

• **Fig. 12.5** The placenta. (A) The maternal surface, showing cotyledons. (B) The fetal surface.

increased maternal blood flow experienced during pregnancy is mediated by the low-resistance uteroplacental circuit (Blackburn, 2018). Table 12.2 summarizes the placental circulation. The fetal circulation is described in detail in Chapter 48.

Anatomical Variations of the Placenta

Placentas may be abnormally shaped. It is essential to examine the placenta and seek medical aid if the placenta appears incomplete or abnormal in shape. A range of abnormal placentae is presented in Table 12.3.

Functions of the Placenta

During its transient existence, the placenta performs actions which will later be taken on by diverse separate organs of the baby. These organs include the lungs, liver, gut, kidneys and endocrine glands. The key placental function is the **transport of nutrients** to the fetus and **waste products** away from the fetus. It has an **immunological role** in preventing fetal rejection and provides **protection** for the fetus against environmental hazards. It also acts as an **endocrine organ.** Several hormones, including hCG, human placental lactogen (hPL), placental prolactin, relaxin, progesterone and oestrogens, are synthesized by the syncytial trophoblast and released into the maternal circulatory system (Blackburn, 2018).

The mnemonic SERPENT acts as a memory aid for students to prompt recall of the functions (see Box 12.3).

Storage

The placenta metabolizes glucose, stores it in the form of glycogen and reconverts it to glucose as required. The placenta can also store fat-soluble vitamins and iron.

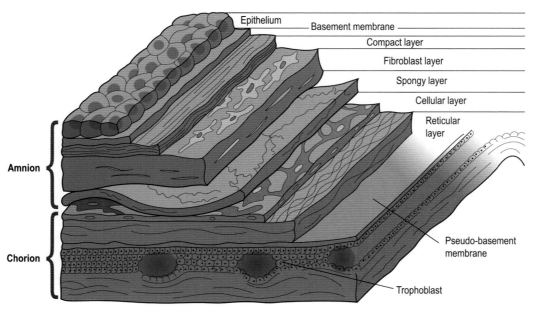

• **Fig. 12.6** Layers of the human amnion and chorion.

TABLE 12.2 The Placental Circulation

Maternal placental circulation	In placental development, the villi bathe in the lacunae or lakes of blood formed by the syncytiotrophoblasts eroding maternal blood vessels. Maternal blood, from the spiral endometrial arteries, pulses between the intervillous spaces. This occurs temporarily outside of maternal circulation.
	Maternal blood enters the intervillous space in spurts via 80–100 endometrial spiral arteries. Blood flows slowly over the surface of the villi and substances are exchanged in both directions. The maternal blood reaches the floor of the intervillous space where it drains into the endometrial veins (Figs. 12.7–12.9). Any interference with the uteroplacental circulation will result in fetal hypoxia and may restrict fetal growth or cause death.
	Blood enters at a higher pressure than the blood already present in the intervillous spaces. Blood spurts in the direction of the chorionic plate. The pressure dissipates and the blood flows slowly over the branch villi. An estimated 150 mL of blood flows into the intervillous space 3–4 times per minute (Bailey, 2020; Moore, Persaud & Torchia, 2018). As the blood circulates, this enables some of the villi to absorb nutrients and oxygen and to excrete waste products. These are known as the nutritive villi. The blood returns to the maternal circulation via endometrial veins. The anchoring villi are more deeply attached to the decidua.
	Reductions in uteroplacental blood flow can result in fetal hypoxia and intrauterine growth restriction. If severe, it can lead to fetal death.
Fetal placental circulation	Fetal blood vessels:
	Two umbilical arteries – transport poorly oxygenated blood to the placenta from the fetus.
	One umbilical vein – transports highly oxygenated blood to the fetus.
	Deoxygenated blood leaves the fetus and passes into the two umbilical arteries, which carry it to the placenta. Within the chorionic villi, the fetal blood is brought very close to maternal blood from which it picks up oxygen. The oxygenated blood enters the umbilical vein which returns it to the fetus.
	The umbilical cord attaches to the placenta, the umbilical arteries subdivide into chorionic arteries that branch outwards and downwards to the chorionic plate and ultimately into the network of chorionic villi.
	There is a large surface area here for gaseous and metabolic exchange of substances through the extensive arteriocapillary venous system. The highly oxygenated fetal blood in the fetal capillaries passes into the thin-walled veins. At the site of attachment of the umbilical cord to the placenta, the veins converge into one umbilical vein transporting highly oxygenated blood (Fig. 12.8).

TABLE 12.3 Abnormal Placentae

Succenturiate lobe	A separate placental lobe is linked by blood vessels to the main placenta. Failure to deliver this succenturiate lobe may lead to infection and haemorrhage. Each placenta must be examined for a hole in the membranes with blood vessels leading away from it (Fig. 12.10).
Circumvallate placenta	An opaque thickened ridge is seen on the fetal surface of the placenta which forms because of doubling back of the membranes (Fig. 12.11). The membranes may leave the placenta nearer to the centre than normal. It is associated with an increased risk of growth retardation.
Bipartite and tripartite placenta	A placenta may be divided into two or three fairly equal lobes (Fig. 12.12).
Velamentous	The umbilical cord insertion is into the membranes outside the placental boundary (Fig. 12.13). Rarely the umbilical vessels cross the internal os, a condition known as *vasa praevia*. A massive haemorrhage may occur if these vessels rupture during labour. This can result in an adverse fetal outcome.
Battledore placenta	The umbilical cord is inserted into the edge of the placenta. This position renders the cord at risk of prematurely tearing from the placenta during the third stage of labour.
Infarcts and calcification	**Infarcts** on the maternal surface of the placenta are patches caused by localized death of placental tissue resulting from an interruption of blood supply. When newly formed, they are red but degenerate into white fibrous patches. These are found on many placentas but they are more commonly associated with pregnancy hypertension.
	Calcifications appear as small, gritty greyish-white patches on the surface of the placenta, especially if the pregnancy is post-term. These are deposits of lime salts and are of no significance.
	Chapter 31 discusses the major placental pathologies of abruptio placentae and placenta praevia.

Endocrine

The many endocrine functions of the placenta are varied and complex and require both maternal and fetal input.

• BOX 12.3 Summary: Functions of the Placenta

(SERPENT)
Storage
Endocrine
Respiratory
Protection
Excretory
Nutrition
Transfer

Bailey (2020).

Although the maternal part of the placenta and the decidua secrete the hormones **prolactin, relaxin** and **prostaglandins,** decidual production of these hormones probably influences pregnancy most. **Pregnancy-associated placental protein A** (PAPP-A) is produced by the decidua and the placental trophoblasts. These decidual hormones target the fetoplacental unit and bind to the fetal membranes and trophoblasts.

The fetoplacental hormones alter maternal metabolic processes to benefit the fetus. They can be divided into two groups: **steroid hormones** and **protein hormones.** Steroid hormones such as oestriol require both maternal and fetal precursors, so monitoring maternal oestriol levels during pregnancy is a useful indicator of fetal well-being (Coad, Pedley & Dunstall, 2019). Steroid hormones are found in higher concentrations in fetal blood than in maternal blood.

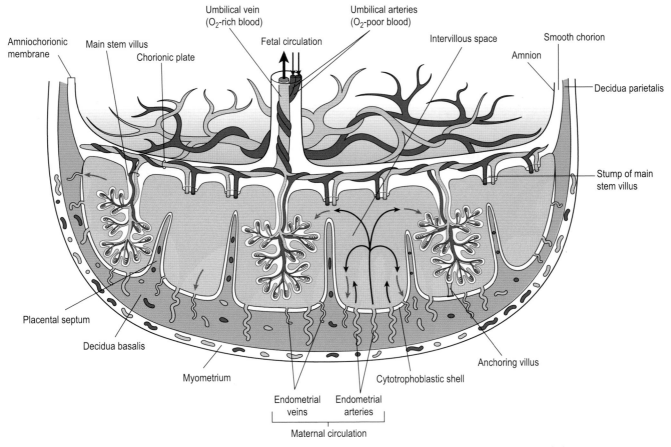

• Fig. 12.7 Schematic drawing of a transverse section through a full-term placenta, showing the relation of the villous chorion (fetal part of the placenta) to the decidua basalis (maternal part of the placenta, the fetal circulation and the maternal placental circulation). Maternal blood flows into the intervillous spaces in funnel-shaped spurts from the spiral arteries, and exchanges of material between the mother and the embryo/fetus occur. The inflowing arterial blood pushes venous blood out of the intervillous space into the endometrial veins, which are scattered over the entire surface of the decidua basalis. Note that the umbilical arteries carry poorly oxygenated fetal blood (shown in dark grey) to the placenta and that the umbilical vein carries oxygenated blood (shown in light grey) to the fetus. Note also that the cotyledons are separated from each other by placental septa, projections of the decidua basalis. Each cotyledon consists of two or more main stem villi and their many branches. In this drawing, only one stem villus is shown in each cotyledon, but the stumps of those that have been removed are indicated.

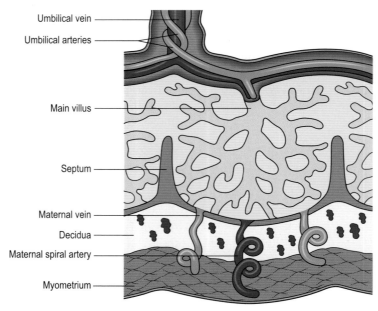

Umbilical vein

Umbilical arteries

Main villus

Septum

Maternal vein

Decidua

Maternal spiral artery

Myometrium

• **Fig. 12.8** Blood flow around chorionic villi.

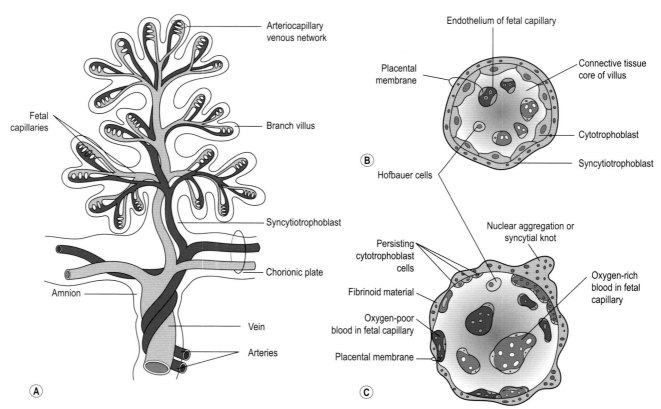

Arteriocapillary venous network

Fetal capillaries

Branch villus

Syncytiotrophoblast

Chorionic plate

Amnion

Vein

Arteries

Ⓐ

Endothelium of fetal capillary

Placental membrane

Connective tissue core of villus

Cytotrophoblast

Syncytiotrophoblast

Ⓑ

Hofbauer cells

Nuclear aggregation or syncytial knot

Persisting cytotrophoblast cells

Fibrinoid material

Oxygen-rich blood in fetal capillary

Oxygen-poor blood in fetal capillary

Placental membrane

Ⓒ

• **Fig. 12.9** (A) Drawing of a stem chorionic villus showing its arteriocapillary venous system. The arteries carry poorly oxygenated fetal blood and waste products from the fetus, whereas the vein carries oxygenated blood and nutrients to the fetus. (B, C) Drawings of sections through a branch villus at 10 weeks and full-term, respectively. The placental membrane, composed of extra fetal tissues, separates the maternal blood in the intervillous space from the fetal blood in the capillaries in the villi. Note that the placental membrane becomes very thin at full term. Hofbauer cells are thought to be phagocytic.

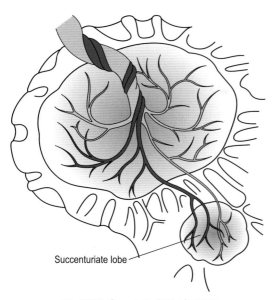

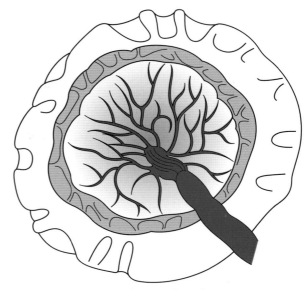

• **Fig. 12.10** Succenturiate placenta.

• **Fig. 12.11** Circumvallate placenta.

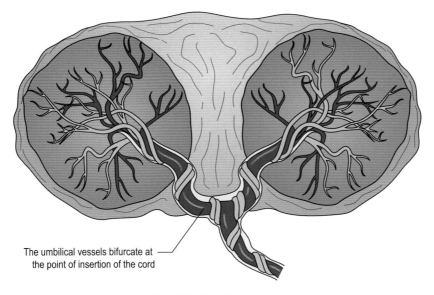

The umbilical vessels bifurcate at the point of insertion of the cord

• **Fig. 12.12** Bipartite placenta.

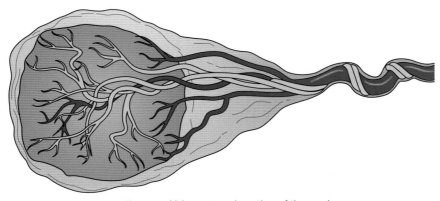

• **Fig. 12.13** Velamentous insertion of the cord.

The placenta produces specific protein hormones in substantial amounts, as well as small quantities of every protein in the adult body. The manufacture of protein hormones does not appear to need fetal input but may be linked to the amount of active trophoblastic tissue. They are found only in maternal blood and are implicated in changing maternal physiology. There does not appear to be a feedback mechanism for controlling their production. The syncytiotrophoblast produces its own **luteinizing hormone–releasing hormone** which controls hCG production in the same cell.

The Protein Hormones

The main placental protein hormones are:

- hCG.
- hPL.
- Schwangerschaftsprotein 1 (SP$_1$).
- PAPP-A.
- Pregnancy-associated protein B (PAPP-B).
- Placental protein 5 (PP5).

These hormones are analogous to some anterior pituitary hormones (see Box 12.4). For example, hCG has a similar structure to luteinizing hormone, and hPL is similar to prolactin and growth hormone.

The Steroid Hormones: Oestrogens

Three oestrogens are important: **oestrone, oestradiol** and **oestriol.** In the non-pregnant woman, oestriol is derived from oestradiol and oestrone, whereas in pregnancy it is synthesized by the fetoplacental unit. The fetal liver and suprarenal glands are important in oestriol production, which is a direct measure of fetal well-being. **Pregnenolone sulphate,** the precursor of all fetoplacental steroids, is converted to oestrogens by placental enzymes.

Oestrogen Levels in Normal Pregnancy

Most tissues and organs are affected by oestrogens in pregnancy. Oestrogens are growth stimulators and cause hypertrophy and hyperplasia of uterine muscle, as well as growth and development of the breasts. In a normal pregnancy, maternal serum levels of all three hormones rise but the curve for oestriol is the most useful, showing a steep rise from 34–36 weeks. This late surge may not occur if pregnancy pathology affects the fetus. The curve may flatten out or even fall away. Serial assays of oestriol are no longer thought to be useful in assessing fetal well-being.

The Steroid Hormone: Progesterone

Progesterone is produced by the syncytiotrophoblast. Some are sent to the maternal circulation and some to the fetus. Production is via cholesterol through pregnenolone to progesterone. Progesterone is broken down into the inactive substance pregnanediol and excreted in maternal urine.

The Function of Progesterone in Pregnancy

Ovarian progesterone plays a part in the transport and implantation of the ovum. Progesterone is involved in endometrial development in the second part of the menstrual

---

• BOX 12.4 Placental Protein Hormones

Human Chorionic Gonadotrophin

Human chorionic gonadotrophin (hCG) is a glycoprotein consisting of two subunits, a small α (alpha) subunit and a larger β (beta) subunit, joined by a disulphide bond. The β subunit is probably the biologically active one. In early pregnancy, there is a rapid increase in hCG production, with the urinary rate doubling every 36–48 hours. The curve flattens out at 9 weeks then declines. The lower level is maintained until just before term when there is another rise. Plasma concentration rises from 7–100 IU/mL (international units/mL). Pregnancy test kits contain antibodies which bind to the β subunit and can be detected in maternal blood 9 days after fertilization.

hCG influences the ovary to produce extra oestrogen and progesterone which maintains pregnancy. The amount of hCG also appears to influence the level of placental progesterone production. There is no association between insufficient hCG production and spontaneous abortion. A placental abnormality called hydatidiform mole produces large amounts of hCG (Chapter 31).

Human Placental Lactogen

Human placental lactogen (hPL) is produced by the syncytiotrophoblast and consists of 190 amino acids, of which 163 are found in human growth hormone. It is the only placental protein that does not contain carbohydrate. Maternal blood levels of hPL rise from 0.3 µg at 10 weeks to 5.4 µg at 36 weeks. There is then a fall until delivery, which may correspond to a fall in functioning placental tissue. Maternal plasma hPL has been used to check placental function.

In pregnancy, hPL probably acts as a growth promoter affecting carbohydrate metabolism. It causes the mobilization of free fatty acids and antagonizes the action of insulin. Pregnant women must manufacture more insulin, and where the insulin reserve is poor, carbohydrate metabolism may be compromised, especially in diabetic women, (i.e., hPL is diabetogenic).

Schwangerschaftsprotein 1 (SP$_1$)

SP$_1$ is a glycoprotein present in large amounts. It can be detected in early pregnancy and is easily measured in late pregnancy. This hormone may affect immunosuppression, preventing fetoplacental rejection.

Pregnancy-associated Proteins A and B

A series of pregnancy-associated proteins were discovered in the early 1970s. Of these, PAPP-A and PAPP-B are produced by the trophoblast. PAPP-A is a large zinc-binding glycoprotein detectable in maternal plasma early in pregnancy with a rising concentration as pregnancy progresses right up to the onset of labour. Low levels may be associated with poor fetal growth and may be involved in preventing rejection of the fetoplacental unit by the cellular lymphocyte component of the maternal immune system. PAPP-B is the largest placental glycoprotein and rises throughout pregnancy, with the steepest part of its concentration curve after 30 weeks. It can be used to assess placental well-being in diseases such as pre-eclampsia and diabetes mellitus.

Placental Protein 5

PP5 is a small glycoprotein with different properties from the others. It is found in the stroma of the chorionic villi, as well as in the syncytiotrophoblast. It may inhibit the proteolytic activity of trypsin and may inhibit protease activity in the placenta.

cycle, and the decidual reaction is caused by progesterone secretion for 48 hours followed by superimposed oestrogen. Progesterone has a sedative effect on uterine muscle contractibility. With relaxin, it may alter membrane potential in myometrial cells to reduce contractile impulses. Progesterone relaxes all smooth muscles during pregnancy, leading to many minor disorders of pregnancy. It competes with aldosterone for binding sites in the kidney, leading to urinary sodium loss. Aldosterone secretion is increased to counteract this. There is little evidence that in women a fall in progesterone initiates the onset of labour, and the oestrogen:progesterone ratio does not appear to change significantly in humans (Johnson, 2018).

Progesterone Levels in Normal and Abnormal Pregnancy

It used to be thought that progesterone levels were indicative of fetal well-being and that low levels caused spontaneous abortion, but progesterone treatment was unsuccessful, and low levels follow rather than cause fetal compromise. There is no agreement on normal levels, as they fluctuate throughout pregnancy, but the average is from 275 nmol/mL at 32 weeks to 450 nmol/mL at term (Johnson, 2018). Progesterone is stored in body fat and may act as a buffer against transient low production.

Respiration

The major respiratory gases, oxygen and carbon dioxide, are moved between mother and fetus by simple transfer down a partial pressure concentration gradient. This becomes complex by maternal and fetal differences in haemoglobin concentration and type. Respiratory exchange may be compromised if there is interruption to blood flow by maternal or fetal disease.

Fetal Oxygen Supply

Most oxygen (O_2) in maternal and fetal blood is bound to haemoglobin in the form of **oxyhaemoglobin** (HbO_2). Maternal blood arrives in the intervillous spaces of the placenta saturated with O_2 at a partial pressure (Po_2) of about 50 mmHg. Fetal blood arrives in the placenta with a low O_2 content and a low Po_2 of 20 mmHg, rising to only 30 mmHg after oxygenation. Therefore, O_2 diffuses readily down the partial pressure gradient from mother to fetus. The diffusion gradient is enhanced in three ways (Hall & Hall, 2020):

1. By an increased affinity for O_2 of fetal haemoglobin (HbF), which combines more readily with O_2 than does adult haemoglobin (HbA).
2. The haemoglobin concentration in fetal blood is about 50% more than in the mother's blood.
3. The Bohr effect means that haemoglobin can carry more O_2 at a low Pco_2 than at a high Pco_2 (see excretion of CO_2 later).

Fetal systemic Po_2 is much lower than that of an adult, and parts of the fetal vascular tree are extremely sensitive to O_2. Because of this, after the onset of respiration at birth, a rise in Po_2 leads to closure of the ductus arteriosus and constriction of the umbilical vessels.

Carbon Dioxide

Most fetal metabolic processes are aerobic and depend on a constant oxygen supply. The fetus produces carbon dioxide (CO_2) for excretion. The much higher lipid solubility of CO_2 over O_2 results in a much more rapid transfer of the gas over cell membranes.

Protection

The placental membrane is a barrier against most bacteria, which are too large to penetrate it, but the organisms causing syphilis and tuberculosis can cross the barrier, resulting in **transplacental infection.** Most infections that cause fetal abnormality, however, are viral such as rubella, first recognized in 1941. Drugs with a small molecular structure may cross to the fetus, and some cause fetal abnormalities. Other drugs such as antibiotics may be beneficial in treating intrauterine infections such as fetal syphilis. Towards the end of pregnancy there is a transfer by pinocytosis of immunoglobulin G (IgG), conferring passive immunity for the first 3 months of extrauterine life.

Immunological Role

The trophoblast appears to have immunological properties that make it inert so that maternal antibodies do not reject the fetus as foreign tissue (see Chapter 29).

Excretion

Besides carbon dioxide, the placenta also passes other metabolic by-products such as urea, uric acid and bilirubin to the maternal circulation for excretion.

Nutrition

The fetus needs **amino acids** for cell building, **glucose** for energy, **calcium** and **phosphorus** for bones and teeth and iron and other minerals for the formation of blood. Simple forms of nutrients such as amino acids, glucose and fatty acids pass from maternal to fetal blood through the walls of the villi. The placenta selects substances and will deplete maternal supplies if necessary. Water, electrolytes and water-soluble vitamins diffuse across the cell membranes from mother to fetus.

Transfer of Substances

The fetus is completely dependent on the mother for respiration, nutrition, excretion and protection, and the placenta acts as the fetal lungs, alimentary tract, kidneys and endocrine system. The placenta grows throughout pregnancy and as the fetus grows rapidly in the second half of pregnancy, the placenta keeps pace with fetal needs by the increased maternal and fetal blood flow.

New villi are formed until term when their surface area exposed to maternal circulation is about 11 m². By late pregnancy, there is thinning of the syncytium in small areas known as **vasculosyncytial membranes.** There are fewer microvilli, and the syncytium is closely applied to the capillary basement membrane. Many **intracellular vesicles** enable the transfer of macromolecules such as immunoglobulins.

Mechanisms of Transfer

Substances such as gases, nutrients, waste materials and drugs are transported across the placental membrane (to and from the fetus) by the usual cellular membrane systems. These include:

- Simple diffusion of lipid-soluble substances.
- Water pores transfer water-soluble substances as a result of osmotic and potentially hydrostatic forces.
- Facilitated diffusion of substances such as glucose by carrier proteins.
- Active transport mechanisms against a concentration gradient of ions such as calcium and phosphate, of amino acids and of some vitamins.
- Endocytosis (pinocytosis) of macromolecules.

Transport across the placenta increases as pregnancy progresses and the placenta develops and increases in size. The rate of transfer is influenced by increased maternal and fetal blood flow, increased fetal demands and other factors such as maternal nutritional status, exercise and disease. Hypertensive disorders and pre-eclampsia decrease nutrient transfer and alcoholism impairs placental uptake of glucose and amino acids.

Carbohydrate Transfer

Glucose is a principal substrate for energy production, which the fetoplacental unit utilizes for the synthesis of macromolecules not obtained from the mother. The main form of glucose transport is facilitated diffusion via a carrier protein. Some glycogen is stored in the placenta and may help supply its own needs. The healthy placenta has a capacity for glucose transfer that far exceeds fetal needs. The transfer is affected by maternal blood glucose levels and by insulin.

Amino Acid Transfer

Fetal proteins are synthesized from amino acids obtained via carrier systems from the maternal circulation. The fetus accumulates amino acids against a concentration gradient, and the placenta contains more amino acids than either maternal or fetal circulations (Broughton Pipkin, 2018).

Lipid Transfer

The fetus synthesizes fatty acids from carbohydrate and short-chain organic acids, compensating for their absence in the diet of strict vegetarians. The fetus also probably obtains and stores fatty acids from the mother by passive transfer. Cholesterol also crosses the placenta.

Vitamin Transfer

Because **vitamins** cannot be synthesized in the body, the fetus is dependent on its mother for their supply. The lipid-soluble vitamins A, D and E pass from maternal to fetal blood down a concentration gradient. Water-soluble vitamins (e.g., vitamin C) appear to be transferred to the fetus against a gradient and cannot be passed back to the maternal circulation.

Trace Element Transfer

Small amounts of crucial trace elements, including iron, zinc and copper, are transferred to the fetus.

Water and Electrolyte Transfer

Water balance is achieved by a diffusional gradient brought about by hydrostatic pressure and colloid osmotic pressure (see Chapter 17). Solutes such as sodium, potassium, calcium and phosphate (PO_4) are also freely transferred between maternal and fetal fluid circulations. The maternal and fetal fluid compartments are finely balanced, and this can be disturbed by administration of hypotonic intravenous solutions such as 5% dextrose to the mother, especially if it contains the **antidiuretic oxytocin.** Transfer of water to the fetus results in fetal **hyponatraemia.**

Amniotic Fluid

During early embryonic development, the amnionic cavity increases in size and finally surrounds and encases the complete embryo. Fluid accumulation within the amnionic cavity leads to complete separation of the embryo from surrounding extraembryonic tissues, leaving only the developing umbilical cord as the connection between placenta and embryo (Huppertz & Kingdom, 2018). Amniotic fluid surrounds the fetus to provide a protected, low-resistance environmental space suitable for fetal movements, growth and development (Blackburn, 2018; Qazi et al., 2017).

Amniotic fluid (liquor amnii) is an alkaline, clear, pale straw-coloured fluid consisting of about 99% water and 1% organic and inorganic substances in solution. It is contained within the amniotic sac. It is derived mainly from the maternal circulation across the amniotic and chorionic membranes and is exuded from the fetal surface. It contains growth-promoting and bacteriostatic properties. Amniotic fluid has an important role to play in the protection of the fetus.

Sources and Production of Amniotic Fluid

- Before keratinization of the fetal skin there is free exchange of fluid and solutes between the fetus and the amniotic cavity.
- Amniotic fluid may be secreted by the amniotic membrane cells. Between 4 and 8 weeks of gestation, amniotic fluid increases to about 20 mL.
- From the 11th week, the fetus excretes urine into the amniotic fluid, and the volume increases to 350 mL at 20 weeks, 700–1000 mL by 37 weeks and then declines slightly until term.
- Fluid is also secreted by the fetal respiratory and gastrointestinal tracts.

- Diffusion from maternal interstitial fluid across the amniochorionic membrane from the decidua is probably the main source (Moore, Persaud & Torchia, 2018).

Circulation of Amniotic Fluid

Amniotic fluid is in a constant state of circulation (Moore, Persaud & Torchia, 2018). The net volume turnover of amniotic fluid is approximately 1000 mL/day with the turnover rate independent of volume (Blackburn, 2018). The fetal gastrointestinal tract is a major pathway for its removal. It is swallowed by the fetus and absorbed into its bloodstream; large amounts diffuse across the placenta into the maternal circulation, and some is excreted by the fetus into the amniotic sac. In the second half of pregnancy, the chief sources of amniotic fluid are the fetal kidneys, which contribute 700 mL/day, and the fetal lungs, which contribute 350 mL/day (Fig. 12.14).

Content of Amniotic Fluid

During the first half of pregnancy, the fetal skin is not a barrier to fluid and is a site for water and solute transfer. The composition of amniotic fluid in early pregnancy is similar to fetal tissue fluid. After keratinization of the fetal skin at 17 weeks, the continuity between amniotic fluid and fetal extracellular fluid is lost and the pattern of content and flow changes.

In the latter half of pregnancy, osmolality decreases to about 90% of maternal plasma, and the composition of amniotic fluid resembles that of dilute urine (Blackburn, 2018).

Mature amniotic fluid contains electrolytes, proteins and protein derivatives such as urea and creatinine, carbohydrates, lipids, hormones, enzymes, desquamated fetal cells, vernix and lanugo. Sodium and chloride content decreases and urea, uric acid and creatinine increase as the fetal kidney matures. Increasing amounts of phospholipids from the lungs appear as the fetal lungs mature.

Regulation of Amniotic Fluid Quantity

Decidual prolactin and **prostaglandins** (PGE_2) from the amnion may regulate amniotic fluid volume. The concentration of prolactin in amniotic fluid is up to 10 times that of maternal circulation, increasing sharply in the second trimester and declining to a lower plateau after 34 weeks. Prolactin may regulate amniotic fluid volume by controlling electrolyte exchange across the chorioamniotic membrane. PGE_2 may regulate amniotic fluid by removing it into the maternal circulation to counterbalance the large volume of fetal urine produced in the second half of pregnancy.

Functions of Amniotic Fluid

Amniotic fluid is critical to the normal development of the fetus. Amniotic fluid (Moore, Persaud & Torchia, 2018):
- Supports free movement of the fetus, aiding musculoskeletal development.
- Permits symmetric external growth of the embryo and fetus.
- Has bacteriostatic properties which act as a barrier to infection.
- Permits normal fetal lung development.
- Prevents adherence of the amnion to the embryo and fetus.
- Cushions the embryo and fetus against injuries.
- Helps control the embryo's body temperature by maintaining a constant environmental temperature.
- Assists in maintaining homeostasis of fluid and electrolytes.

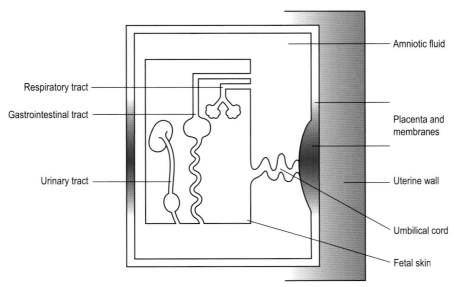

• **Fig. 12.14** Pathways of amniotic fluid production and exchange.

Clinical Implications: Abnormalities of Quantity

Abnormalities of the fetus are related to abnormalities of amniotic fluid quantity (Moore, Persaud & Torchia, 2018). In fetal conditions such as renal agenesis or urethral obstruction with obstruction to urine flow, amniotic fluid volume is very low (oligohydramnios). If the fetus cannot swallow, as in oesophageal atresia or anencephaly, there is more than 2000 mL of amniotic fluid (polyhydramnios).

Polyhydramnios

One of the most common anomalies found on ultrasound examination is polyhydramnios (Blackburn, 2018). It affects up to 1.5% of all pregnancies. Polyhydramnios may be chronic or acute:

- Chronic polyhydramnios is more common and is gradual in onset from about the 30th week of pregnancy.
- Acute polyhydramnios is rare, occurring at about the 20th week of pregnancy and is associated with monozygotic twins and occasionally with severe fetal abnormality.

Fetal causes are associated in 20% of cases and maternal causes are associated in 20% (Box 12.5). In 60% of cases, there is no known cause. Clinical management is presented in Box 12.6.

Oligohydramnios

Oligohydramnios occurs when the amount of amniotic fluid is less than 500 mL at term. It may be much less than this and affects up to 5% of pregnancies. This complication is serious and is associated with poor perinatal outcomes (Qazi et al., 2017). Oligohydramnios may be associated with fetal renal impairment, severe fetal growth retardation and usually with maternal disease such as hypertension or chronic renal disease (Blackburn, 2018). Management depends on the length of gestation, the maturity of the fetus, fetal and maternal health and the relative risks of conservative management or delivery. The means of delivery are aimed at achieving maximum safety for mother and fetus. Maternal fluid and hydration status can significantly increase the volume of amniotic fluid (Blackburn, 2018; Gizzo et al., 2015; National Institute for Health and Care Excellence [NICE], 2006).

The causes of oligohydramnios are listed in Box 12.7, and clinical management is detailed in Box 12.8.

Diagnostic Uses of Amniotic Fluid

Biophysical Profile

A biophysical profile (BPP) is a non-invasive test of fetal well-being using ultrasound imaging. It is not clear whether there is any benefit to this testing. Further research is suggested. Four variables are measured (Lalor et al., 2008):

- Fetal tone.
- Somatic movements.
- Breathing movements.
- Amniotic fluid volume.

• BOX 12.5 The Causes of Polyhydramnios

Fetal Causes

- Multiple pregnancy.
- Central nervous system anomalies: anencephaly, hydrocephaly, spina bifida.
- Gastrointestinal anomalies: oesophageal atresia, small bowel atresia, diaphragmatic hernia.
- Cardiac anomalies.
- Haematological anomalies: α-thalassaemia, fetalmaternal haemorrhage.
- Skeletal malformations: achondroplasia, osteogenesis imperfecta.
- Chromosome/genetic abnormalities.
- Intrauterine infections: rubella, syphilis, toxoplasmosis.

Maternal Causes

- Diabetes mellitus.
- Rhesus isoimmunization.

Placental Causes

- Placental chorioangioma.
- Circumvallate placenta syndrome.

• BOX 12.6 Polyhydramnios: Clinical Management and Considerations

Polyhydramnios can be suspected if:

- The uterus is large for gestational age.
- There is easy ballottement of the fetus.
- Fetal parts are difficult to find.
- The fetal heart is muffled.
  Maternal symptoms include breathlessness, vulval varicosities, oedema and gastric problems.
  Diagnostic tests include:
- Ultrasound examination to detect fetal and placental abnormalities and to confirm gestational age.
- Studies of **fetal karyotype** to rule out chromosomal or genetic abnormalities.
- Fetal swallowing studies.
- Screening for intrauterine infection.
- Maternal antibody screening and diabetic screening.
  Maternal comfort will be improved by resting upright in bed to aid breathing. Antacids may be required to relieve heartburn and nausea. Amniotic fluid may be removed to conserve pregnancy.

Complications

Associated with an increase in maternal and fetal mortality.
Maternal complications: pregnancy-induced hypertension and respiratory discomfort.
Fetal mortality is associated with conditions incompatible with life and morbidity with minor abnormalities and preterm birth.
Obstetric complications include unstable lie, malpresentation, cord presentation and prolapse, preterm labour, premature rupture of membranes, placental abruption and postpartum haemorrhage.

Maternal causes: uteroplacental inefficiency, hypertension, diabetes, pre-eclampsia, hypovolaemia and elevated second-trimester α-fetoprotein (Qazi et al., 2017).
Post-term pregnancy (more than 42 weeks).
Intrauterine growth retardation.
Premature rupture of membranes (PROM).
Fetal renal anomalies: renal agenesis (Potter syndrome), urethral obstruction, prune belly syndrome, multicystic and dysplastic kidneys.
Fetal non-renal anomalies: triploidy, thyroid gland agenesis, skeletal dysplasia, congenital heart block, twin–twin transfusion syndrome.
Chronic abruptio placentae.

Fetal heart rate monitoring can be added as a modification.

Amniocentesis

Cellular and biochemical components of amniotic fluid change with gestational age and provide useful indicators of fetal well-being and maturity (Blackburn, 2018). Although the procedure is considered safe, there are possible complications of abortion, infection, haematoma, leakage of amniotic fluid or preterm labour. Amniotic fluid analysis can be used as follows:

- Cells can be used for genetic and chromosomal studies.
- α-Fetoprotein can assess the likelihood of neural tube defects or as part of a triple test for Down syndrome.
- Creatinine levels increase as the fetus matures.
- Bilirubin estimates can monitor red blood cell haemolysis in Rhesus factor incompatibility.
- The ratio of the phospholipids lecithin and sphingomyelin can be used to assess lung maturity.
- Enzyme studies of cultured cells can help diagnose many inborn errors of metabolism.

Diagnosis

The condition may be suspected on abdominal examination if the following findings are present:
- The uterus appears smaller than expected for gestational age.
- The mother has noticed a reduction in fetal movements.
- The uterus feels compact, and fetal parts are easily felt.
   Ultrasound examination confirms the absence of normal amniotic fluid pockets.

Amnioinfusion is the infusion of an isotonic fluid into the abdominal cavity such as normal saline or Ringer's lactate solution to correct oligohydramnios. The procedure can be performed for prophylactic, diagnostic or therapeutic reasons. Two techniques (transabdominal or transvaginal) can be used for this procedure and the procedure is deemed a safe and effective option for the prevention of fetal distress in pregnancies with oligohydramnios (Qazi et al., 2017). This procedure can be repeated (serial amnioinfusion) if necessary. It is performed in the antenatal period or in labour to:
- Replace fluid in conservative treatment of PROM.
- Prevent the development of fetal lung hypoplasia.
- Decrease cord compression and reduce fetal distress during labour.
- Dilute meconium.
   This procedure should only be carried out by specialists in invasive neonatal medicine. Parents need to be made aware of the risks and benefit.

Complications

Prognosis is poor mainly due to PROM and fetal abnormalities. Pulmonary hypoplasia affects 60% of fetuses deprived of amniotic fluid for several weeks. It is generally lethal with small, immature lungs, poor surfactant levels and pulmonary hypertension. Oligohydramnios is often associated with amnion nodosum. Yellow-grey nodules consisting of desquamated fetal epidermal cells, lanugo and vernix are found in and on the amnion and on the fetal surface of the placenta, probably because of its close application to the fetus.

Main Points

- The placenta is derived from extraembryonic trophoblast with a few inner-cell mass mesodermal cells.
- The cytotrophoblast gives rise to the syncytiotrophoblast, which invades the endometrium to allow embedding. Lacunae fuse to form intervillous spaces.
- The chorionic villi of the decidua capsularis degenerate and form the chorion laeve, which becomes the chorionic membrane. The villi of the decidua basalis branch to form the fetal part of the placenta. The outer chorion and the inner amnion form the fetal sac.
- The placenta produces protein hormones and steroid hormones.
- Fetal growth depends on placental transfer of nutrients and oxygen. Oxygen and carbon dioxide cross the syncytiotrophoblast and the fetal capillary epithelium down a partial pressure concentration gradient. Nutrients, trace elements and vitamins pass from maternal to fetal blood through the walls of the villi.
- The placenta excretes urea, uric acid and bilirubin into the maternal circulation.
- Water and solute balance is achieved by diffusional gradients, and these substances are freely transferred between maternal and fetal circulations.
- Mature amniotic fluid contains electrolytes, proteins, urea and creatinine, carbohydrates, lipids, hormones, enzymes, desquamated fetal skin cells, vernix and lanugo.
- Sodium and chloride content decrease and urea, uric acid and creatinine increase as the fetal kidneys mature.
- Amniotic fluid is constantly being replaced, and the fetal gastrointestinal tract is a major pathway for its removal. Prolactin and prostaglandins may regulate amniotic fluid volume.

- Amniotic fluid provides space for fetal growth and movement and protects the fetus from injury and infection. A constant temperature is maintained.
- The BPP could be an accurate predictor of fetal danger, but so far does not show effects on pregnancy outcome.

- Cellular or biochemical components of amniotic fluid provide useful indicators of fetal well-being and maturity.
- Risks associated with amniocentesis include abortion, infection, haematoma, haemorrhage, leakage of amniotic fluid and preterm labour.

References

Aplin, J.D., Ruane, P.T., 2017. Embryo–epithelium interactions during implantation at a glance. J. Cell Sci. 130 (1), 15–22.

Bailey, J., 2020. Hormone cycles: fertilization and early development. In: Marshall, J.E., Raynor, M.D. (Eds.), Myles Textbook for Midwives, seventeenth ed. Elsevier, London.

Blackburn, S.T., 2018. Maternal, Fetal and Neonatal Physiology: A Clinical Perspective, fourth ed. Elsevier Saunders, Missouri.

Broughton Pipkin, F.B., 2018. Maternal physiology. In: Edmonds, D.K., Lees, C., Bourne, T. (Eds.), Dewhurst's Textbook of Obstetrics and Gynaecology, ninth ed. Wiley-Blackwell, Oxford.

Burton, G.J., Fowden, A.F., 2015. The placenta: a multifaceted, transient organ. Philos. Trans. R. Soc. Lond. B Biol. Sci. 370 (1663), 20140066.

Coad, J., Pedley, M., Dunstall, K., 2019. Anatomy and Physiology for Midwives, fourth ed. Elsevier, Edinburgh.

Gizzo, S., Noventa, M., Vitagliano, A., Dall'Asta, A., D'Antona, D., Aldrich, C.J., et al. 2015. An update on maternal hydration strategies for amniotic fluid improvement in isolated oligohydramnios and normohydramnios: evidence from a systematic review of literature and meta-analysis. PLoS One 10 (12), e01144334.

Graham, W., Woodd, S., Byass, P., Filippi, V., Gon, G., Virgo, S., Chou, D., Hounton, S., Lozano, R., Pattinson, R., Singh, S., 2016. Diversity and divergence: the dynamic burden of poor mental health. Lancet 388 (10056), 2164–2175.

Hall, J.E., Hall, M.E., 2020. Guyton and Hall Textbook of Medical Physiology, fourth ed. Elsevier Saunders, Philadelphia.

Haram, K., Mortensen, J.H., Myking, O., Roald, B., Magann, E.F., Morrison, J.C., 2020. Early development of the human placenta and pregnancy complications. J. Matern. Fetal Neonatal Med. 33 (20), 3538–3545.

Huppertz, B., Kingdom, J.C.P., 2018. The placenta and fetal membranes. In: Edmonds, D.K., Lees, C., Bourne, T. (Eds.), Dewhurst's Textbook of Obstetrics and Gynaecology, ninth ed. Wiley-Blackwell, Oxford.

Johnson, M.H., 2018. Essential Reproduction, eighth ed. Wiley-Blackwell, Oxford.

Lalor, J.G., Fawole, B., Alfirevic, Z., Devane, D., 2008. Biophysical profile for fetal assessment in high risk pregnancies. Cochrane Database Syst. Rev. 2008 (1), CD000038.

Moore, K., Persaud, T.V.N., Torchia, M., 2018. The Developing Human, eleventh ed. Elsevier, London.

National Institute of Health and Care Excellence, 2006. Therapeutic Amnioinfusion for Oligohydramnios during Pregnancy (Excluding Labour). Available at: www.nice.org.uk/guidance/ipg192/documents/.

Okada, H., Tsuzuki, T., Murata, H., 2018. Decidualization of the human endometrium. Reprod. Med. Biol. 17 (3), 220–227.

Qazi, M., Saqib, N., Ahmed, A., Wagay, I., 2017. Therapeutic amnioinfusion in oligohydramnios during pregnancy (excluding labor). IJRCOG 6 (10), 4577–4582.

Rampersad, R., Cervar-Zivkovic, M., Nelson, M., 2011. Development and anatomy of the human placenta. In: Kay, H.K., Nelson M & Wang, Y. (Eds.), The Placenta, from Development to Disease. Wiley-Blackwell, Oxford.

Tal, R., Taylor, H.S., 2021. Endocrinology of pregnancy. In: Feingold, K.R., Anawalt, B., Blackman, M.R., Boyce, A., Chrousos, G., Corpas, E., et al. (Eds.), Endotext. MDText.com, South Dartmouth.

Turco, M.Y., Moffett, A., 2019. Development of the human placenta. Development 146 (22), dev163428.

Annotated recommended reading

Blackburn, S.T., 2018. Maternal, Fetal and Neonatal Physiology: A Clinical Perspective, fourth ed. Elsevier Saunders, Missouri.

This is an excellent reference book for the interested reader. It provides detailed and up-to-date evidence-based information on the placenta and membranes.

Johnson, M.H., 2018. Essential Reproduction, eighth ed. Wiley-Blackwell, Oxford.

This is an excellent book on the physiology of reproduction and describes events in an easily understood and well-researched style.

Moore, K., Persaud, T.V.N., Torchia, M., 2018. The Developing Human, eleventh ed. Elsevier, London.

The layout, diagrams and content of this book are excellent. It clearly describes the formation of the placenta, membranes and amniotic fluid.

13
Fetal Growth and Development

THOMAS McEWAN

Students and midwives need to have clear knowledge of fetal development during pregnancy. This knowledge can be used in practice to support assessment of fetal growth and wellbeing, interpret obstetric ultrasound reports and to offer pregnant women explanation and appropriate guidance on these findings.

Introduction

The general organizing principles of embryology, the development of systems and the structure and function of the placenta were previously discussed (see Chapters 9–11). From the beginning of the ninth week of intrauterine life, most of the organs are in place but may not yet be functional. The fetal period is mainly concerned with an increase in size and maturation of these systems.

The Fetal Period

Care must be taken to avoid confusion when calculating fetal age. Traditionally this has been calculated from the first day of the **last menstrual period** (LMP). After the use of ultrasound scanning, it is more common to calculate fetal age by using the estimated day of fertilization. The date of birth is about 266 days, or 38 weeks, after fertilization and 280 days, or about 40 weeks, from the first day of the LMP. **Post-fertilization age** is usually used when describing organ development, and this method will be used throughout this chapter.

Fetal Growth

Differentiation of tissues and organs formed during the embryonic period occurs during the fetal period (ninth week until birth) (Moore, Persaud & Torchia, 2020). Fetal growth is defined as 'an increase in size, which occurs by cell multiplication, increase in cell size and deposition of extracellular material' (Wolpert, Tickle & Arias, 2019). Apoptosis (cell death) is also important in determining overall growth rate.

Tissues may grow by:
- Cell proliferation or **hypertrophy**: increased cell numbers.
- Cell enlargement or **hyperplasia**: increased cell size.
- Accretion of extracellular material such as bone matrix.

From fertilization, during cleavage and blastula formation there is little growth and cells become smaller with each cleavage division. From weeks 9–24 there is remarkable growth, and then growth slows but remains constant from 30–36 weeks when it slows again (Johnson, 2018). In early pregnancy, growth is mainly by hyperplasia. This is followed by a period of simultaneous hyperplasia and hypertrophy (Cameron & Bogin, 2012). After 34 weeks, growth is mainly by hypertrophy (Blackburn, 2018). **Growth** and **maturation** of systems are directly linked to the ability of the fetus to survive after birth, a concept known as **viability.**

Control of Cell Growth and Proliferation

Growth factors and other **signalling proteins** play a key role in controlling cell growth and proliferation, and apoptosis (programmed cell death) is activated without these signals (Wolpert, Tickle & Arias, 2019). The mechanisms of embryonic cell division are poorly understood. Placental, fetal and maternal factors determine fetal growth.

TABLE 13.1   Fetal Development based on Weeks from Fertilization

Weeks	Developmental Feature
9	The fetal head measures half the crown–rump length
10	Intestinal cells have all re-entered the body cavity
12	Fetal length has more than doubled
	The upper limbs have attained their relative length in comparison to the trunk, but the lower limbs remain short
	The mature forms of the external genitalia appear
	There is a decrease in red cell formation in the liver and onset in the spleen
	The formation and excretion of urine begin
	The beginning of fetal muscle movement occurs
	The eyelids fuse
13–16	This is a period of very rapid growth
16	The head is now smaller in comparison to the trunk, and the lower limbs have reached their correct proportions
	The skeleton can be seen clearly on X-ray films
	The face is more human, with the eyes pointing anteriorly rather than laterally
	The external ears have moved to their positions on the sides of the head
17–20	Growth slows down
	Fetal movements are felt by the mother
	The skin is covered by vernix caseosa to protect it from amniotic fluid
	Lanugo has developed all over the body
	Head and eyebrow hair become visible
	Highly metabolic brown fat is formed
21–25	Surfactant production in the lungs begins
	Towards the end of this period survival becomes possible
	The skin lacks subcutaneous fat and is wrinkled
	The skin appears red because of blood capillaries just under the surface
	The fetus now has periods of sleep and activity and responds to sound
26–29	The lungs are capable of breathing and allowing gas exchange
	The nervous system controls rhythmic breathing movements and body temperature
	Intrauterine respiratory movements occur
	The eyes re-open
	Head and lanugo hair are well developed
	White, subcutaneous fat is laid down under the skin
	At 28 weeks, erythropoiesis ends in the spleen and begins in the bone marrow
30–34	The papillary light reflex is present
	Body fat expands to 8% of total body weight
	The skin is opaque and smooth
	From 32 weeks, most fetus es will survive
	Lanugo disappears from the face
	The fetus begins to store iron

TABLE 13.1	Fetal Development based on Weeks from Fertilization—cont'd
Weeks	**Developmental Feature**
35–38	The grasp is firm Most fetus es are plump
	At 36 weeks, head and abdominal circumferences are equal. Later the abdominal circumference becomes greater. Growth slows towards term.
	By 38 weeks, body fat is 16% of body weight
	Breast tissue is present in both sexes
	The testes are in the scrotum in males
	The nails reach the tips of the fingers
	Lanugo disappears from the body

From: Moore, K.L., Persaud, T.V.N., Torchia, M.G., 2020.

Key Events in the Fetal Stage of Development

Details of developmental stages are presented in Table 13.1. Dimensional variations increase with age, making the judgement of gestational age less accurate (Figs. 13.1 and 13.2). Viability is generally accepted as 24 weeks, but active treatment and resuscitation is reported from 22 weeks' gestation (Di Stefano et al., 2021).

Fetal Size

Before birth, the fetus is usually measured by sitting height or crown–rump length. Table 13.2 is based on post-fertilization age. Control of fetal size is discussed in Box 13.1.

Estimation of Fetal Age and Assessment of Fetal Growth

Growth Curves

A series of measurements can be plotted on a graph and used to calculate growth. Growth can be viewed as a motion through time (Cameron & Bogin, 2012), and if measurements are plotted at regular intervals, a *distance curve* is produced (Fig. 13.3). A distance curve is usually plotted when monitoring fetal growth. To show how the rate of growth alters over time, the speed or velocity of growth is plotted, generating a *velocity curve* (Fig. 13.4).

Maternal Weight and Fetal Growth

Maternal weight gain has traditionally been used to assess fetal well-being in pregnancy, and continued weight gain is thought to be a favourable sign. However, weight gain varies widely from weight loss to a gain of 23 kg or more. Many factors affect maternal weight gain, including the presence of oedema, maternal metabolic rate, dietary intake, gastrointestinal problems, smoking and the size of the fetus (Box 13.2).

Attempts to control maternal weight gain to reduce the size of the fetus and make delivery easier have had little effect on fetal size. The only components of maternal weight gain available for manipulation are maternal fat and extracellular fluid, and neither obesity nor oedema are influenced by regular weighing. An average weight gain appears to be about 12 kg and should be 2 kg in the first 20 weeks and 0.5 kg/week until term. Components of normal weight gain are shown in Table 13.3.

Poor weight gain has been associated with **intrauterine or fetal growth restriction** (IUGR/FGR) (Bendix, Miller & Winterhager, 2020), but is not a sensitive indicator, and babies with IUGR/FGR are delivered when weight gain has been normal. In addition, daily fluctuations in a woman's weight can be up to 1% of total bodyweight. Symphysis–uterine **fundal height** (SFH) is the most common way to assess fetal growth. The measurements are made in centimetres using a disposable tape measure from the upper border of the symphysis pubis to the top of the fundus. Once the top of the fundus is confirmed, the tape measure is held securely, turned over and the number of centimetres read (Johnson & Taylor, 2023). Errors may occur if the woman is too thin or obese or has too much or too little abdominal muscle tone. Breech presentation or transverse lie can also result in error. Fundal height can be plotted against a standard curve. A wide variation in the results was observed for predictive accuracy of SFH measurement during pregnancy. The results from a multicentre study show that it does not have good diagnostic value for predicting and ruling out small-for-gestational-age (SGA) babies (National Institute of Health and Care Excellence [NICE], 2021).

Ultrasound

The gestational age is calculated from the mother's LMP or taken from an early first- or second-trimester ultrasound scan (Box 13.3). Plotting of later measurements must be accurate

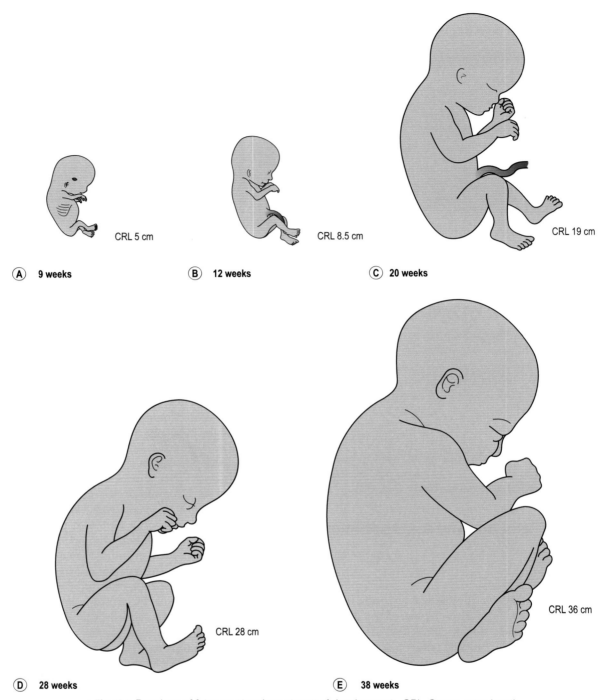

CRL 5 cm

(A) **9 weeks**

CRL 8.5 cm

(B) **12 weeks**

CRL 19 cm

(C) **20 weeks**

CRL 28 cm

(D) **28 weeks**

CRL 36 cm

(E) **38 weeks**

• **Fig. 13.1** Drawings of fetus es at various stages of development. *CRL*, Crown–rump length.

to avoid a wrong diagnosis. The success rate of ultrasound in detecting IUGR/FGR can be as high as 95%. Ultrasound measurements can also be plotted against a normal curve. Linear and non-linear measurements can be used.

Linear Measurements

Crown–rump length is used to estimate gestational age in the first trimester. If the crown–rump length is above 84 mm, the gestational age should be estimated using head circumference (HC) (NICE, 2021). The measurement between the two biparietal eminences is called the *biparietal diameter (BPD)* (Fig. 13.5). The correct position of the fetal head must be located (Fig. 13.6). This is a useful estimate of gestational age in the second trimester but is less accurate later in pregnancy. Femur length can also be used to assess gestational age.

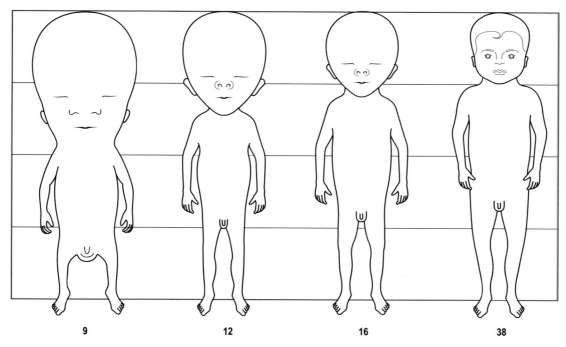

Fertilization (conception) age in weeks

• **Fig. 13.2** The changing proportions of the body during the fetal period. At 9 weeks, the head is about half the crown–rump length of the fetus . By 38 weeks, the circumferences of the head and the abdomen are approximately equal. After this, the circumference of the abdomen may be greater. All stages are drawn to the same total height.

TABLE 13.2	The Average Size of the Fetus Related to Weeks of Gestation	
Age (Weeks)	Crown–rump Length (mm)	Weight (g)
10	61	14
12	87	45
14	120	110
16	140	250
18	160	320
20	190	460
22	210	630
24	230	820
26	250	1000
28	270	1300
30	280	1700
32	300	2100
34	320	2500
36	340	2900
38	360	3400

Non-linear Measurements

Measurement of the HC is preferred in the third trimester when moulding of the head may alter the BPD. Abdominal circumference (AC) is measured at the level of the bifurcation of the hepatic vein in the centre of the fetal liver. A reduction of AC suggests a reduction in liver size due to depleted stores.

Ratios

- HC:AC compares the status of the brain to the liver. A raised ratio suggests IUGR/FGR.
- The femur:AC ratio compares the length of the femur, which is minimally affected by IUGR/FGR, to the AC. A raised ratio suggests IUGR/FGR.

Doppler Waveform Analysis

Measuring the velocity of blood in the umbilical cord using Doppler ultrasound has been suggested as an additional means of assessing fetal well-being (Chapter 14).

Multiple Pregnancies

Multiple pregnancy is the term used to describe the development of more than one fetus in utero at the same time. In spontaneous pregnancy, the presence of twins is about 1 in 100, but this increased to epidemic proportions in the 1990s with **assisted reproductive techniques** (Johnson, 2019). Because of the economic, social and ethical dilemmas affecting parents, policies in **ovum induction** and **in vitro fertilization** aim to reduce the number of fetus es returned to the uterus and so reduce the incidence of multiple pregnancy (Aurell et al., 2006).

Growth of the fetus is multifactorial, involving both genetic and environmental factors. Fetal growth involves the accumulation of protein early in development, reaching a maximum of 300 g by week 35. Fat deposition exceeds the amount of protein by week 38, most of which is subcutaneous. The human baby has the most subcutaneous fat of any animal which may be related to protecting brain growth. The relative amount of water in fetal tissues decreases. A large fetus may have difficulty at delivery, but if it remains too small, health can be compromised in childhood and later life. Fetal growth restriction is discussed in Chapter 14.

The mother adapts to fetal needs by increasing calorie intake and modifying metabolic activity, possibly in response to signals from the fetoplacental unit. The mother seems to be able to limit fetal growth. Maternal height is linked to uterine capacity, and small women appear to have small babies (mechanism is unclear). The placenta may limit the amount of nutrients transferred to the fetus in late pregnancy.

Additional maternal influences include parity. Primiparous women have smaller babies (less than 200 g) than multiparous women, and adolescents have smaller babies than mature mothers. This may be because of a first pregnancy on the uterine vascular bed, giving the analogy of elastic bands being easier to stretch after use (Gluckman & Hanson, 2005). The uterine blood vessels, small and tortuous before pregnancy, respond to placental oestrogens and progesterone by relaxing and dilating. This improves fetal nutrition and the baby grows larger. This may be seen in multiple pregnancies when each baby obtains less nutrition than a singleton baby and is therefore smaller. Fetal size may be constrained by the size of the intrauterine environment (Gluckman & Hanson, 2005).

Fetal growth may be determined by conflict between maternal and paternal genes (Abu-Amero et al., 2006; Haig, 2019; Wolpert, Tickle & Arias, 2019). The insulin-like growth factors IGF1 and IGF2 closely resemble the simple insulin molecule and appear to have a key role in embryonic and fetal growth. In humans, IGF2 is inherited on chromosome 11. The IGF2 gene inherited from the father makes a growth factor which helps the fetus to grow, whereas the maternal gene is programmed to be non-functional. This phenomenon is called **genomic imprinting** (i.e., expressed in a parent-specific manner regardless of Mendelian inheritance) (Wolpert, Tickle & Arias, 2019).

The fetus contributes to growth control through genetic inheritance and by sex (i.e., males grow larger than females). Synthesis of the IGFs increases throughout pregnancy. IGF1 is a major direct endocrine stimulus, whereas IGF2 may have a more indirect effect by stimulating placental growth and transport mechanisms (see Chapter 12).

Types of Twin Pregnancy
Dizygotic

About two-thirds of twin pregnancies are dizygotic (DZ) (binovular, non-identical or fraternal twins) which results from the release and fertilization of two separate ova by two separate sperm. Two babies develop who are genetically no more related than normal siblings but share the uterus at the same time. There is an inherited aspect so that the incidence of recurrence in families is three times that of the rest of the population. Also, this type of twinning varies between ethnic groups so that the incidence is 1 in 500 in Asians, 1

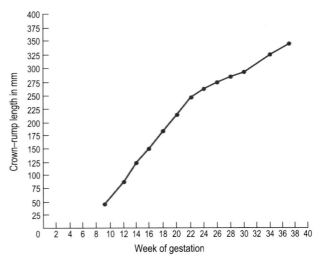

• **Fig. 13.3** An example of a distance curve using data from fetal crown–rump measurements.

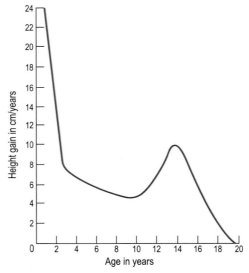

• **Fig. 13.4** An example of a velocity curve demonstrating the growth of the body from birth to age 18 years.

Maternal weight and height should be measured at the first antenatal appointment and the woman's BMI calculated and documented.

Repeated weighing during pregnancy should be confined to circumstances where clinical management may be influenced (NICE, 2021).

in 125 in White populations and as high as 1 in 20 in some African populations (Moore, Persaud & Torchia, 2020). DZ twins have separate placentas, two chorions and two amnions (dichorionic–diamniotic). They may be the same sex or different sexes. The incidence of congenital malformation is only slightly greater than normal.

TABLE 13.3	Distribution of Maternal Weight Gain in Pregnancy	
Component of Fetal Weight		**Gain (g)**
The fetus		3400
The placenta		600
The amniotic fluid		600
The uterus		900
The breasts		500
Fat stores		3500
Blood volume		1500
Extracellular fluid		1000
Total		12000

• BOX 13.3   Ultrasound Management

Pregnant women should be offered an early ultrasound scan between 11 weeks 2 days and 14 weeks 1 day to determine gestational age and detect multiple pregnancies. This ensures consistency of gestational age assessment and reduces the incidence of induction of labour for prolonged pregnancy (NICE, 2021).

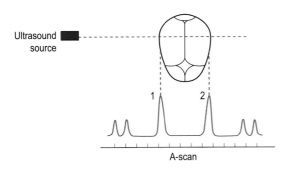

Ultrasound source

A-scan

• **Fig. 13.5** Measuring the biparietal diameter by ultrasound. 1 and 2 indicate the parietal eminences.

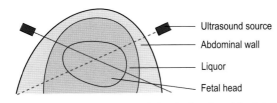

Ultrasound source
Abdominal wall
Liquor
Fetal head

• **Fig. 13.6** A diagram showing the abdominal wall and the fetal head.

Monozygotic

About one-third of twinning occurs when a single fertilized ovum divides into two separate fetus es. These are **monozygotic** (MZ) (uniovular or identical) twins. About one-third of MZ twins are **dichorionic** (each has its own chorion)

and two-thirds share one placenta and one chorion. In 95% of these, each baby has its own amnion (**monochorionic–diamniotic**). In the remaining 5%, the babies share one amnion (**monochorionic–monoamniotic**) (Fig. 13.7). About 1% of monoamniotic twins are conjoined (Siamese twins) (Landon et al., 2020; Sebire et al., 2000).

MZ twinning usually begins in the blastocyst at the end of the first week when the embryoblast divides into two embryonic primordia. If the embryonic disc does not divide completely or the adjacent embryonic discs fuse, conjoined twins may develop (Carlson, 2019; Moore, Persaud & Torchia, 2020).

MZ twins are identical in their genetic make-up, having developed from one fertilized ovum, and are always of the same sex, except in very rare abnormalities of the sex chromosomes. There is a connection between the two fetal circulations via the placenta. The high incidence of errors of development and of congenital malformations may be linked to the cause of the twinning. MZ twinning begins in the blastocyst, about the end of week 1. It results from the division of the **embryoblast** into two embryonic **primordia.**

The Incidence of Multiple Pregnancies

Since the advent of infertility treatment by stimulation of ovulation, multiple births have become more common. In naturally occurring pregnancies, twins occur in 1 in 90 pregnancies, triplets in about 1 in 90^2, quadruplets in 1 in 90^3 and quintuplets in 1 in 90^4 pregnancies (Moore, Persaud & Torchia, 2020). The differences in twinning rates result from variations in DZ twinning, and the incidence of MZ twinning is constant at 3.5 per 1000 across all nationalities. Other factors influencing the frequency of DZ twinning include:
- Maternal age (incidence increases with maternal age).
- Parity.
- Conception soon after discontinuing oral contraceptives; if these have been taken for more than 6 months and conception occurs within a month of discontinuation, the chances of a twin pregnancy double.

Ultrasound scanning has shown that the incidence of twin pregnancy at conception may be double the number of eventual twin births. One embryo may be reabsorbed (**vanishing twin syndrome**) or rarely remains between the membranes as a fetus papyraceous (paper fetus).

Triplets and Higher Order Pregnancies

Drugs to induce ovulation such as **clomifene citrate** have led to a 10% risk in pregnancies with multiple fetus es being conceived. In the UK, triplet births have doubled since 1989. The implications for maternity and neonatal care of these high-risk pregnancies are a cause for concern. The outcome of such pregnancies can be poor, and some centres have advocated fetal reduction to ensure survival of fewer fetus es, but there is a danger that all fetus es could be lost.

When the figures on fetal survival in triplets and higher order births are contrasted with selective feticide, it is difficult to support a decision to reduce fetal numbers if there

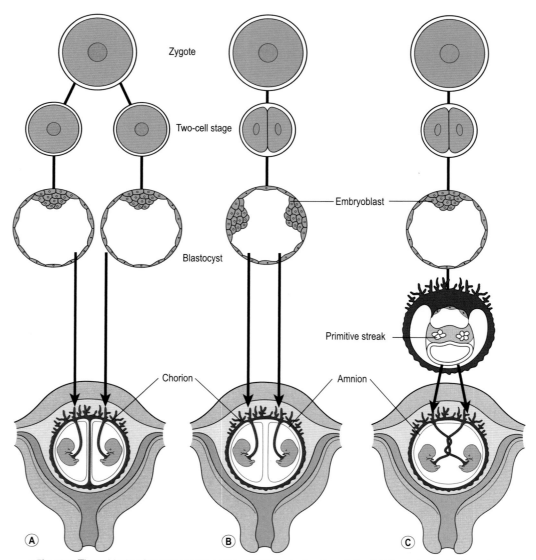

• **Fig. 13.7** Three kinds of monozygotic twins. (A) Dichorionic–diamniotic. (B) Monochorionic–diamniotic. (C) Monochorionic–monoamniotic.

are three or more fetus es. The acceptability of this option and willingness to undergo reduction in the number of fetus es by selective termination may not be acceptable to women, particularly couples with a history of infertility (Dodd, Dowswell & Crowther, 2015; Sebghati & Khalil, 2021).

Diagnosis of Twin Pregnancy

The earlier the diagnosis of twins is made, the more successful the outcome. Perinatal losses may be much larger when the diagnosis is made after 28 weeks. Since the development of routine ultrasound scanning, the incidence of undiagnosed twins at delivery is rare. However, not all midwives work in areas where access to scanning is easy or possible; therefore it is important to be able to diagnose a multiple pregnancy by clinical examination. A family history of twinning should alert the professional to the possibility, but vigilance is needed in all pregnancies.

Abdominal Examination

Inspection

This method is unlikely to diagnose twins before 20 weeks of pregnancy, but the uterus may appear larger than expected for gestational age. The uterus may look large and broad, and fetal movements may be obvious all over the abdomen.

Palpation

The fundal height may be greater than expected for the period of gestation. The presence of two fetal poles in the fundus may be an identifying feature. Location of three poles suggests the presence of at least twins. Multiple limbs may also be felt. A later clue is the apparent smallness of the fetal head in relation to the size of the uterus. Lateral palpation may find two fetal backs or the presence of fetal limbs on both sides of the uterus.

Auscultation

It has been stated that hearing two fetal hearts simultaneously with a difference of 10 bpm is diagnostic of twins.

Practically, this is difficult to achieve as the fetal heart of a singleton can be heard over a wide area.

Ultrasound

Ultrasound diagnosis of multiple pregnancy can be made as early as 5 weeks after the LMP. However, it may not be possible to confirm a twin pregnancy until after 12 weeks because of the likelihood of vanishing twin syndrome (Moore, Persaud & Torchia, 2020). Ultrasound diagnosis should be made to ascertain the number of placentas and types of membranes present. Diagnosis of monoamniotic twins is essential because of the higher risk of abnormalities so that management can be planned (Landon et al., 2020).

Complications of Pregnancy

Obstetric complications are more frequent in multiple births than in singleton births. These included pre-eclampsia, antepartum haemorrhage, anaemia, delivery by caesarean section, preterm delivery, admission of babies to neonatal intensive care units, postpartum haemorrhage and maternal infections. The incidence of complications increases with the number of fetus es present (Landon et al., 2020).

Fetal Problems
Abortion (Miscarriage)

Loss of pregnancy by abortion (miscarriage) is more common, possibly due to fetal abnormality in early pregnancy and overdistension of the uterus in later pregnancy.

Single Fetus Demise

Before 14 weeks, single fetal demise will probably cause no problems for the survivor. Later there may be transfer of **thromboplastin** released from the tissues of the dead twin. This may cause arterial occlusion, brain damage and renal cortical necrosis. A serious maternal problem is the onset of **disseminated intravascular coagulation** about 3 weeks after fetal death.

Congenital Malformations

Congenital malformations are more likely to occur in twin pregnancies. Although the incidence is about the same in MZ and DZ twins, abnormalities in DZ twins tend to be minor, whereas those in MZ twins tend to be multiple and lethal. The most common in all sets of twins are cleft lip and palate, central nervous system defects and cardiac defects. In MZ twins, conjoined twins and **fetal acardia** occur.

Monoamniotic Twins

When monoamniotic twins are present, the perinatal mortality is as high as 50%, mainly because of umbilical cord entanglement. Other causes of loss are **twin-to-twin transfusion syndrome (TTTS),** congenital abnormalities and preterm birth. Ultrasound scanning should be carried out regularly to diagnose any problems and plan management. The babies are best delivered by caesarean section to avoid cord entanglement.

Conjoined Twins

Conjoined twins occur in about 1% of MZ twin pregnancies (Fig. 13.8); this means about 1 in 900 twin pregnancies and 1 in 40,000 live births. In conjoined twins, 70% will be female, and the reason is unknown. Partial or complete duplication of just the upper or lower part of the body may occur with associated malformations (Spitz, Kiely & Pierro, 2018). Table 13.4 shows the different types of conjoined twins.

A diagnosis can be made by ultrasound, and suspicion should be raised in the following cases:
- Monoamniotic twins.
- Twins who face each other.
- The heads are at the same level and in the same plane.
- The thoracic cages are in close proximity.
- Both fetal heads are hyperextended.
- There is no change in fetal positions on a later scan.

Once the diagnosis is confirmed, delivery by caesarean section is planned, but the outcome is poor. About one-third of conjoined twins are stillborn, and another third die within 24 h. Surgical separation of conjoined twins is the only means by which independent lives can be achieved. The presence of shared organs may make it impossible to save both babies.

Acardiac Twinning

This is a malformation occurring in about 1% of MZ twins where one twin has no heart and the circulation for both is maintained by the heart of the second twin. The acardiac twin is non-viable, and circulatory overload may cause heart failure in the normal twin, giving a mortality rate of 35%.

Twin–Twin Transfusion Syndrome

TTTS affects between 15% and 35% of MZ twins. Vascular communications across the placenta occur between the fetus es, causing a circulatory imbalance. This results in **hypovolaemia, oliguria** and **oligohydramnios** in the donor twin, who is small, pale and anaemic. If anaemia is severe, the donor may develop **hydrops fetalis** and heart failure. **Hypervolaemia, polyuria** and **polyhydramnios** occur in the recipient, who is large and **polycythaemic** and may develop **circulatory overload** and **congestive cardiac failure** (Bamburg & Hecher, 2022; Moore, Persaud & Torchia, 2020). In a systematic review, Roberts et al. (2014) concluded that endoscopic laser coagulation of anastomotic vessels should be considered in the treatment of all stages of TTTS to improve neurodevelopmental outcomes. Fetal loss of up to 80% occurs without treatment. Prenatal diagnosis is made when the following conditions are present:
- Same-sex twins.
- Diamniotic-monochorionic membranes.
- A 20% difference in estimated fetal weights.
- A discrepancy in the amniotic fluid surrounding the fetus es.
- Fetal hydrops in one or both twins.

Attempts to treat the problem antenatally may reduce the mortality to 40%. These include bed rest and preterm delivery, **amnioreduction** (selective removal of amniotic fluid), occlusion of the vascular anastomoses by **laser coagulation**

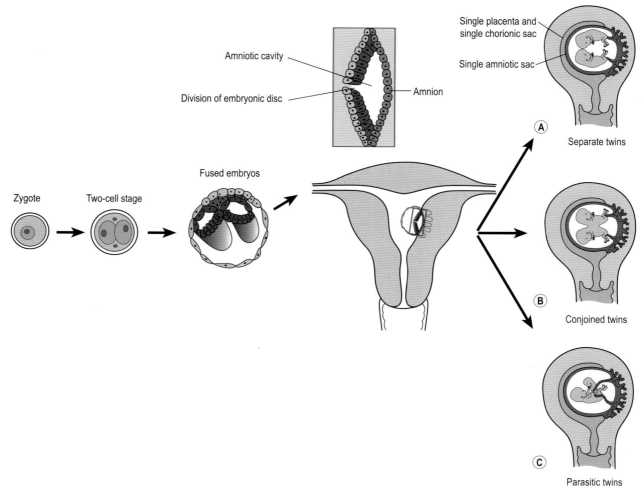

• **Fig. 13.8** Diagrams showing how some monozygotic (MZ) twins develop. This method of development is very uncommon. Division of the embryonic disc results in two embryos with one amniotic sac. (A) Complete division of the embryonic disc gives rise to twins. Such twins rarely survive because their umbilical cords are often so entangled that interruption of the blood supply to the fetus es occurs. (B, C) Incomplete division of the disc results in various types of conjoined twins.

TABLE 13.4	Classification of Conjoined Twins by the Site of Union	
Name	Percentage Occurrence	Description
Thoracopagus	40	Joined at the chest
Omphalopagus	35	Joined at the anterior abdominal wall
Pygopagus	18	Joined at the buttocks
Ischiopagus	6	Joined at the ischium
Craniopagus	2	Joined at the head

and selective ending of the life of one fetus and septostomy (creating a hole between the two chorionic membranes). Laser treatment is associated with fewer babies dying compared with amnioreduction (Bamberg & Hecher, 2022). If there is no expert available to perform laser surgery, then amnioreduction may need to be the method of choice.

Polyhydramnios

Polyhydramnios is associated with MZ twins and with fetal abnormality. Acute polyhydramnios occurs in mid-pregnancy and usually leads to abortion.

Intrauterine or Fetal Growth Restriction

Most twins show discordant growth, with one twin obtaining more nourishment than the other. This is a feature of placental mass and occurs more frequently in DZ twins. Genetic syndromes and TTTS may also result in discordant growth.

Maternal Problems

Accounts of the following maternal problems are detailed in other chapters.

Exacerbation of Minor Disorders

The presence of more than one fetus means a higher level of pregnancy hormones and more pressure from the growing uterus. This tends to exacerbate all minor disorders of pregnancy, notably morning sickness, nausea and heartburn (see Chapter 30).

Anaemia

The rate of anaemia in multiple pregnancy is about double that in singleton pregnancies. Both **iron deficiency** and **folic acid deficiency** occur. Early in pregnancy, iron is utilized in the growth of tissues, in particular the expansion of maternal plasma volume, with formation of extra maternal red blood cells. After 28 weeks, fetal demands further deplete the iron stores.

Pregnancy-Induced Hypertension

Hypertension is more common in women with a multiple pregnancy. Both hypertension and oedema may develop because of the increased blood volume but often respond to rest. A more worrying occurrence is the increased risk of pre-eclampsia with proteinuria, vasoconstriction and reduced blood volume (Landon et al., 2020).

Women are advised to take 75–150 mg of aspirin daily from 12 weeks until the birth of the babies if they have one or more of the following moderate risk factors for pre-eclampsia (NICE, 2019):

- Nulliparity.
- Age 40 years or older.
- Pregnancy interval of more than 10 years.
- Body mass index (BMI) of 35 kg/m² or more at first visit.
- Family history of pre-eclampsia.

Antepartum Haemorrhage

There is a significant increase in antepartum haemorrhage. **Placenta praevia** may occur because of the large placental site and **abruptio placentae** because of polyhydramnios. If the membranes rupture early, sudden extreme decrease in uterine size may detach the placenta.

Complications of Labour

Fetal Malpresentations

In a seminal study still relevant today, Farooqui, Grossman and Shannon (1973) found that at the presentation was vertex–vertex at the commencement of labour in 39.6% of twins, vertex–breech in 27.7%, and vertex–transverse, breech–breech, breech–vertex, breech–transverse and other combinations being equally distributed amongst the remaining 33.2% (Table 13.5). Effectively, these figures may not always be significant as after delivery of the first twin the lie, presentation and position of the second twin may change and must be assessed before proceeding with the delivery.

Locked Twins

Locked twins occur in 1 in 1000 twin labours. Typically, the babies will have presented in a breech–vertex pattern with the head of the first breech twin obstructed by the head of the second vertex twin. If diagnosed before the onset of labour, a situation that should be checked in every breech–vertex combination, an elective caesarean section should be performed.

If the body of the first baby has already been born, an attempt to free the head should be made. This may be successful as the babies are usually small; otherwise an emergency caesarean section is performed.

TABLE 13.5	Fetal Presentation in Twins by Percentage Occurrence	
Fetal Presentation	**Percentage**
Vertex–vertex	39.6
Vertex–breech	27.7
Vertex–transverse	7.2
Breech–breech	9
Breech–vertex	6.9
Breech–transverse	3.6
Other combinations	6.9

Umbilical Cord Problems

Problems affecting the umbilical cord are more common in multiple pregnancies. These include:

- The presence of a single umbilical artery.
- Cord prolapse.
- Velamentous insertion of the cord.
- Vasa praevia.
- Umbilical cord entanglement.

Preterm Onset of Labour

Labour may begin spontaneously before term or may be induced for maternal or fetal complications. It is unusual for a twin pregnancy to go beyond term. In a systematic review of hospital admission for bed rest in uncomplicated multiple pregnancies, Crowther & Han (2010) found no evidence that bed rest could prevent preterm birth or fetal mortality. However, the reviewers suggest that fetal growth may be improved.

Mode of Delivery

Many obstetricians believe that indications for a caesarean section should include **breech presentation** or **transverse lie** of the first twin. However, in 75% of twin pregnancies, the first twin presents by the vertex and there is no contraindication to vaginal delivery. The second twin should deliver easily as long as the lie is longitudinal. If the lie of the second twin is oblique or transverse, most can be easily converted to longitudinal lie by external cephalic version. Labour may be prolonged by poor uterine action because of uterine overdistension, which can be remedied by oxytocin infusion. Epidural analgesia is the first choice as it does not affect the fetus es and allows any unforeseen manipulative manoeuvres to be made. In cases where there are three or more babies in utero, delivery by caesarean section is probably advisable.

Postpartum Haemorrhage

Poor uterine tone and the presence of a large placental site predispose women giving birth to multiple fetus es to **postpartum haemorrhage**, a life-threatening condition, especially if the woman's haemoglobin level is low. Prevention of haemorrhage is a priority. An intravenous infusion of oxytocin should be available following appropriate management of the third stage.

Undiagnosed Twins

If the head of the baby appears small in contrast to the known size of the uterus before delivery or the baby itself appears small, a second twin should be suspected and the uterus palpated. If an oxytocic drug has already been given, delivery of the second twin needs to be quick, as its life may be in danger. The second baby may be asphyxiated and need active resuscitation.

Postnatal Care of Mother and Babies

Care of the Babies

After birth, once the babies are breathing well, care will depend on their size and maturity. **Premature** or SGA babies will need appropriate care. Some twins may not need any special care other than helping the mother to care for them, possibly in a neonatal transitional care environment. The babies may be breastfed if the mother wishes. Skin-to-skin contact should be initiated as soon as possible.

Care of the Mother

Involution of the uterus may be painful because of the increased muscle bulk, and analgesia should be offered. If the mother decides to breastfeed both babies, a balanced diet will be needed and appropriate rest between feeds. Anaemia should be treated, and postnatal exercises geared at improving muscle tone of the abdominal wall and pelvic floor encouraged.

Main Points

- Ultrasound scanning is more accurate to calculate the age of the fetus from the estimated day of fertilization.
- Continued maternal weight gain is associated with fetal growth, but this is also affected by many factors.
- Two-thirds of twin pregnancies are DZ. Babies are only as alike as any other two siblings. Ethnic origin, maternal age, parity and conception soon after discontinuing oral contraception influence the frequency of DZ twinning.
- About one-third of MZ twins are dichorionic and two-thirds share one placenta and chorion. In 95% of these, each baby has its own amnion, and in 5% the babies are monoamniotic.
- The earlier the diagnosis of twins is made, the more successful the outcome.
- Obstetric complications in twins include abortion, pre-eclampsia, antepartum haemorrhage, anaemia, caesarean section delivery, preterm delivery, low birthweight, stillbirth, postpartum haemorrhage and maternal infection.
- When monoamniotic twins are present, perinatal mortality can be as high as 50%, mainly because of umbilical cord entanglement, TTTS, congenital abnormalities, conjoined twins and preterm birth.
- The outcome for conjoined twins is poor. The presence of shared organs may make it impossible to save both babies.
- TTTS may be dealt with by amnioreduction, laser obliteration of the vascular anastomoses or septostomy.
- Most twins show discordant growth because one twin gets less nourishment. Genetic syndromes and TTTS may also result in discordant growth.
- If locked twins are diagnosed before the onset of labour, an elective caesarean section should be performed. If the body of the first twin has been born, an attempt at vaginal manipulation to free the head should be made. If unsuccessful, urgent caesarean section is necessary.
- In 75% of twin pregnancies, the first twin presents by the vertex and there is no contraindication to vaginal delivery.

References

Abu-Amero, S., Monk, D., Apostolidou, S., Stanier, P., Moore, G., 2006. Imprinted genes and their role in human fetal growth. Cytogenet. Genome. Res. 113 (1–4), 262–270.

Aurell, R., Tur, R., Torelló, M.J., Coroleu, B., Barri, P.N., 2006. Clinical strategies to avoid multiple pregnancies in assisted reproduction. Gynecol. Endocrinol. 22 (9), 473–478.

Bamberg, C., Hecher, K., 2022. Twin-to-twin transfusion syndrome: controversies in the diagnosis and management. Best Pract. Res. Clin. Obstet. Gynaecol. 84 (2022), 143–154.

Bendix, I., Miller, S.L., Winterhager, E., 2020. Causes and consequences of intrauterine growth restriction. Front. Endocrinol. 11, 205.

Blackburn, S.T., 2018. Maternal, Fetal and Neonatal Physiology: A Clinical Perspective, fifth ed. Elsevier, St. Louis.

Cameron, N., Bogin, B., 2012. Human Growth and Development, second ed. Elsevier, London.

Carlson, B.M., 2019. Human Embryology and Developmental Biology, sixth ed. Elsevier, St. Louis.

Crowther, C.A., Han, S., 2010. Hospitalisation and bed rest for multiple pregnancy. Cochrane Database Syst. Rev. 2010 (7), CD000110.

Di Stefano, L.M., Wood, K., Mactier, H., Bates, S.E., Wilkinson, D., 2021. Viability and thresholds for treatment of extremely preterm infants: survey of UK neonatal professionals. Arch. Dis. Child. Fetal Neonatal Ed. 106 (6), 596–602.

Dodd, J.M., Dowswell, T., Crowther, C.A., 2015. Reduction of the number of fetuses for women with a multiple pregnancy. Cochrane Database Syst. Rev. 2015 (11), CD003932.

Farooqui, M.O., Grossman, J.H., Shannon, R.A., 1973. A review of twin pregnancy and perinatal mortality. Obstetrical & Gynecological Survey 28 (2), 144–153.

Gluckman, P., Hanson, M., 2005. The Fetal Matrix: Evolution, Development and Disease. Cambridge University Press, Cambridge.

Haig, D., 2019. Cooperation and conflict in human pregnancy. Curr. Biol. 29 (11), 455–458.

Johnson, M.H., 2018. Essential Reproduction, eighth ed. Wiley-Blackwell, Oxford.

Johnson, M.H., 2019. A short history of in vitro fertilization (IVF). Int. J. Dev. Biol. 63 (3–4–5), 83–92.

Johnson, R., Taylor, W., 2023. Skills for Midwifery Practice, fifth ed. Elsevier, London.

Landon, M.B., Galan, H.L., Jauniaux, E.R., Driscoll, D.A., Berghella, V., Grobman, W.A., et al. 2020. Obstetrics: normal and Problem Pregnancies. Elsevier Health Sciences, Philadelphia.

Moore, K.L., Persaud, T.V.N., Torchia, M.G., 2020. The Developing Human: Clinically Oriented Embryology, eleventh ed. Elsevier Saunders, Philadelphia.

National Institute of Health and Care Excellence (NICE), 2019. Hypertension in Pregnancy: Diagnosis and Management. NICE, London.

National Institute of Health and Care Excellence (NICE), 2021. Antenatal Care. NICE, London.

Roberts, D., Neilson, J.P., Kilby, M.D., Gates, S., 2014. Interventions for the treatment of twin-twin transfusion syndrome. Cochrane Database Syst. Rev. 2014 (1), CD002073.

Sebghati, M., Khalil, A., 2021. Reduction of multiple pregnancy: counselling and techniques. Best Pract. Res. Clin. Obstet. Gynaecol. 70, 112–122.

Sebire, N.J., Souka, A., Skentou, H., Geerts, L., Nicolaides, K.H., 2000. First trimester diagnosis of monoamniotic twin pregnancies. Ultrasound Obstet. Gynecol. 16 (3), 223–225.

Spitz, L., Kiely, E., Pierro, A., 2018. Conjoined twins. In: Losty, P.D., Flake, A.W., Rintala, R.J., Hutson, J.M., Iwai, N. (Eds.), Rickham's Neonatal Surgery. Springer, London.

Wolpert, L., Tickle, T., Arias, A.M., 2019. Principles of Development, sixth ed. Oxford University Press, Oxford.

Annotated recommended reading

Moore, G.E., Ishida, M., Demetriou, C., Al-Olabi, L., Leon, L.J., Thomas, A.C., et al. 2015. The role and interaction of imprinted genes in human fetal growth. Philos Trans. R. Soc. Lond. B. Biol. Sci. 370 (1663), 20140074.

For those interested in genetic control of growth, this is a fascinating paper that explores the parent-of-origin effects.

Chassen, S.S., Zemski-Berry, K., Raymond-Whish, S., Driver, C., Hobbins, J.C., Powell, T.L., 2022. Altered cord blood lipid concentrations correlate with birth weight and Doppler velocimetry of fetal vessels in human fetal growth restriction pregnancies. Cells 11 (19), 3110.

A recent paper that explores the relationship between fetal growth restriction and lipid concentrations within cord blood.

14

Common Fetal Problems

THOMAS McEWAN

Students and midwives must have clear knowledge and understanding of common fetal problems. This is required to support appropriate risk assessment during pregnancy, the ability to support women to make informed choices on antenatal screening and the timely introduction of health improvement interventions.

Introduction

A selection of topics concerning risk and compromise to the fetus are covered in this chapter. The impact on the neonate of the following problems is discussed in Chapters 48–53.

Intrauterine or Fetal Growth Restriction

Before discussing **intrauterine or fetal growth restriction** (IUGR/FGR) (Bendix, Miller & Winterhager, 2020), it is useful to understand some definitions:
- A **low-birthweight baby** is a baby who weighs 2500 g or less at birth.
- A **very-low-birthweight baby** is a baby who weighs less than 1500 g at birth.
- A **small-for-gestational-age** (SGA) baby is one whose birthweight is below the 10th percentile for its gestational age but is not necessarily growth restricted.

- A **large-for-gestational-age** (LGA) baby is one whose birthweight is above the 90th percentile for gestational age.
- A **preterm infant** is a baby born before 37 completed weeks of pregnancy irrespective of the birthweight. A preterm infant may also be SGA or LGA.

IUGR/FGR can be defined as a rate of fetal growth less than the normal potential growth for that fetus at that gestational age (Priante et al., 2019). Incorrect classification of IUGR/FGR does not allow for fetuses that are small and healthy (i.e., constitutionally small), which may lead to inappropriate intervention during pregnancy.

Complications of IUGR/FGR

In the antepartum and intrapartum periods there is an increase in the number of stillbirths, oligohydramnios and fetal distress. Neonatal complications will be discussed in Section 4A. These include meconium aspiration syndrome, persistent fetal circulation, hypoglycaemia, hypocalcaemia, hyperviscosity syndrome and poor temperature control.

Factors Adversely Affecting Fetal Growth

Fetal growth depends on interacting factors such as genetic determinants, maternal health and nutrition, availability of growth substrates and an effective maternal blood supply to the placenta (Blackburn, 2018). The essential substrates are oxygen, glucose and amino acids. Any decrease in substrate availability due to pathological conditions affecting the mother, placenta and fetus will result in poor growth.

Fetal growth restriction may be **asymmetric** or **symmetric.** Asymmetric growth is when fetal weight is reduced out of proportion to length and head circumference and the fetus has little subcutaneous fat. The factors involved are usually maternal in origin. Symmetric growth restriction is due either to a congenital or genetic defect or to decreased growth potential in the fetus. The babies have the normal amount of subcutaneous fat for their size, and the head circumference and length are in proportion to the weight.

Maternal conditions include hypertension and renal disease, diabetes mellitus, severe cardiac disease, smoking and alcohol consumption, with fetoplacental problems ranging from chromosomal abnormalities and infection to placental morphology and site of implantation.

Maternal Malnutrition

Severe protein calorie malnutrition, especially in the second half of pregnancy, will reduce birthweight; babies born in the Dutch famine of 1944–1945 had a reduced birthweight in proportion to their length (De Rooij et al., 2022). There is also a suggestion that maternal malnutrition may have an epigenetic effect on the fetal genome with later consequences in adult life (Kitsiou-Tzeli & Tzeli, 2017; Wu et al., 2004).

Smoking

Maternal smoking has a clear association with the reduced overall growth of the fetus, significantly affecting brain, lung and kidney size and development, as identified on magnetic resonance imaging by Anblagan et al. (2013). They also identified smaller placental volumes in mothers who smoked within this study. Epigenetic consequences have also been identified in later child development (Nakamura, François & Lepeule, 2021).

Alcohol Consumption

The **fetal alcohol spectrum disorders (FASD)** describe a syndrome with a range of physical and neurological disorders due to maternal consumption of alcohol during pregnancy (Mukherjee, 2019; Riley, Infante & Warren, 2011). Alcohol has a low molecular weight and crosses the placental barrier. It is a known teratogen, and fetal damage has been associated with alcohol consumption in pregnancy. In a few women, alcohol-induced malnutrition will add to fetal problems. The characteristics of FASD are presented in Box 14.1.

Placental Insufficiency

In **placental insufficiency,** the placenta is usually small with a reduction in the number of stem and villous capillaries and reduced uteroplacental blood flow with incomplete penetration by trophoblastic cells (Zamir, Nelson & Gimosar, 2021). There appears to be a failure in vascular invasion of the myometrial spiral arteries with increased risk of morbidity and mortality. These findings are also present in maternal conditions such as pre-eclampsia (Nirupama et al., 2021).

Multiple Pregnancy

Poor fetal growth occurs in about 21% of twins, mainly due to abnormal placentation (see Chapter 13).

• BOX 14.1 Characteristic Features of FASD

- Deficient overall growth.
- Facial abnormalities, including small eyes and underdeveloped or absent philtrum.
- Musculoskeletal abnormalities, poor tone.
- Genitourinary abnormalities, including undescended testes and hypoplastic labia.
- Cardiac abnormalities with a high prevalence of atrial or ventricular septal defects.
- Signs of alcohol withdrawal.

Genetic Factors and Chromosomal Aberrations

There is a high prevalence of genetic and chromosome disorders amongst babies with IUGR/FGR (Freire et al., 2022), with an incidence of congenital abnormalities with IUGR/FGR of between 5–27% compared with 0.1–4% in babies with normal growth (Monier et al., 2021; Ott, 2001).

Diagnosis and Management of IUGR/FGR

Antenatal surveillance using customized fetal growth charts to record serial fundal height measurement is a relatively new tool in the detection of IUGR/FGR, with the use of ultrasound imaging to assess biometry and Doppler flow remaining a reliable and proven diagnostic approach (Figueras & Gardosi, 2011; Priante et al., 2019). Additionally, the shifting movement to the concept of fetal growth potential completes this revised approach to IUGR/FGR detection.

Delivery of the Baby

If the fetal condition necessitates delivery, consideration should be given to optimizing lung maturity and preventing intrapartum asphyxia. As such, the presence of clinicians skilled in resuscitation of the new-born is advisable.

Most of these babies now survive the neonatal period but they remain smaller than their age cohorts for several years. However, poor fetal growth increases the incidence of later complications that include hypertension and metabolic disorders (i.e., type 2 diabetes mellitus) (Priante et al., 2019).

Rhesus Isoimmunization and ABO Incompatibility

Rhesus Isoimmunization (RhD Incompatibility)

Readers should ensure they understand blood group inheritance before reading on. The fetus inherits a gene for the **rhesus factor** from each parent, and as rhesus D is a dominant gene if one or two genes are inherited, the baby will be rhesus positive (Rh+). Only if the baby inherits two recessive d genes will the blood group be rhesus negative (Rh−) (Fig. 14.1).

If the mother is Rh− and the fetus Rh+, **haemolysis** of fetal red cells may occur (Fig. 14.2) after antibody formation. This rarely affects the first baby as there are no spontaneous anti-D antibodies present in a woman's blood before her first pregnancy unless fetal red blood cells cross the placental barrier during that pregnancy, or she has been accidently transfused with Rh+ blood.

During pregnancy and labour there is normally no mixing of maternal and fetal circulations. However, when the placenta separates, the chorionic villi tear and there is a risk of **fetomaternal haemorrhage** (FMH); usually between 0.5–5 mL of fetal blood enters the maternal circulation. If the fetus is Rh+ the production of antibodies will be stimulated, and memory cells will mount a secondary response should the mother become pregnant with a second Rh+ baby. This process is called **isoimmunization**.

Spontaneous or therapeutic abortion, amniocentesis, antepartum haemorrhage or external cephalic version may lead to FMH and antibody formation. The problem arises in subsequent pregnancies because anti-D antibodies cross the placenta and haemolyze fetal red cells. Some protection occurs if the mother and fetus are ABO incompatible, as the naturally occurring anti-A or anti-B will destroy fetal red cells before the maternal immune system can respond to the rhesus factor.

Prevention of Maternal Isoimmunization

In the past, **haemolytic disease of the new-born** led to fetal or neonatal death from rhesus haemolytic disease, but this is now largely preventable if three conditions are met:

1. Rh+ blood should never be transfused if a woman's blood group is unknown.
2. Unnecessary risk of FMH should be avoided, for example, by placental localization before amniocentesis.

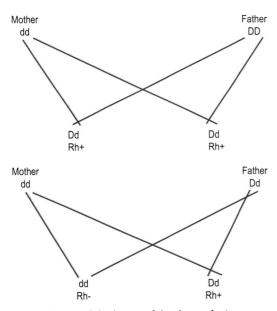

• **Fig. 14.1** Inheritance of the rhesus factor.

Abdominal palpation of women with an antepartum haemorrhage should be kept to a minimum.

3. If there is a risk of FMH, **anti-D immunoglobulin** (rhesus D antibodies) should be administered to the mother within 72 hours, with some protection offered with late administration up to 10 days post-exposure (Qureshi et al., 2014). The antibodies will coat and destroy any fetal red cells in the maternal circulation (Visser et al., 2021).

The number of fetal red cells in maternal blood may be estimated by means of a Kleihauer test and the required dose of anti-D immunoglobulin (Ig) calculated.

Antenatal Management: Anti-D Prophylaxis

Every pregnant woman has her blood tested for ABO and rhesus types early in pregnancy. Any Rh– women will be screened for RhD antibodies. If the test is negative, further screening will be carried out. It is now recommended that all non-sensitized women who are rhesus-D negative should be offered anti-D prophylaxis antenatally to prevent fetal rhesus isoimmunization from undetected FMH in pregnancy (National Institute of Health and Care Excellence [NICE], 2021).

Care at Delivery

Cord blood is taken for testing by using a syringe and needle directly into a placental vein to avoid the risk of contamination by maternal blood and Wharton jelly, which would make interpretation of the results difficult. The needle is removed before transferring the blood into a bottle to avoid haemolysis. Cord blood is tested for ABO and rhesus type, a **direct Coombs test** looks for maternal antibodies on fetal red cells and a haemoglobin estimate checks for haemolysis. If the mother has rhesus antibodies, the cord blood is also tested for serum bilirubin level. Overall management if rhesus antibodies are present during pregnancy is summarized in Box 14.2.

Rhesus Haemolytic Disease

All babies whose mothers have rhesus antibodies should be monitored closely until the results of the cord blood tests are known. Depending on the percentage of fetal red blood cells destroyed, this disease varies in severity from mild jaundice

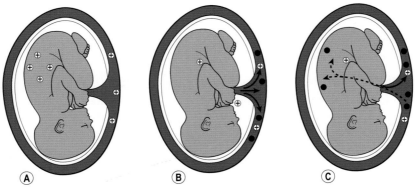

• **Fig. 14.2** Antibody formation. (A) Transfer of rhesus antigen (+) to the maternal circulation. (B) Antibody formation (●) in the rhesus-negative mother. (C) Transfer of the rhesus antibody to the fetus.

to severe intrauterine anaemia, fetal hydrops and stillbirth (Sinha, Miall & Jardine, 2017). In surviving babies with severe jaundice and anaemia, initial management should be performed with phototherapy, intravenous Ig, and immediate transfusion of packed cells as required. An exchange transfusion may be necessary to reduce bilirubin levels and risk of kernicterus if initial management has been unsuccessful (Wolf, Childers & Gray, 2020).

ABO Incompatibility

In this condition, the mother is blood group O and the baby either group AO or BO. Maternal blood contains unprovoked anti-A and anti-B antibodies even in the first pregnancy, and these cross over the placenta to haemolyze fetal red cells. The first child can be affected, but the jaundice, which appears in the first 24 hours, is usually mild. Treatment will depend on the rate of bilirubin rise in the neonate's blood.

Maternal Infection in Pregnancy

Microbes are small organisms that live in and on the human body. They can be divided into five major classes: **bacteria, viruses, algae, fungi** and **protozoa.** Some are helpful **commensal organisms** like the lactobacilli that increase vaginal acidity. However, many are **pathogens** causing serious infections against which the immune system develops defence mechanisms. Systemic infections may cause reproductive problems such as infertility and congenital defects, and some infections are specific to the genital tract. Some organisms that cause genital tract disease will be outlined, followed by systemic disorders that may damage the fetus.

Suppression of Cell-mediated Immunity

Although the maternal immune system is altered in pregnancy, most women are not immunocompromised. However, the suppression of cell-mediated immunity means that some infections are more severe, especially by viruses such as poliomyelitis and influenza, and **opportunistic pathogens** associated with HIV such as *Pneumocystis carinii* and *Toxoplasma gondii*. Pregnancy may also reactivate latent cytomegalovirus (CMV) and herpes.

Sexually Transmitted Diseases

The control of sexually transmitted diseases (STDs) is a difficult public health problem. In men they may cause few problems, but in women pelvic inflammatory disease (PID) and decreased fertility are frequently seen. Also, pregnant women may pass the STD to the fetus, resulting in birth defects or stillbirth (Wynn et al., 2020). About one-third of cases in developed countries affect teenagers because young people often have more than one sexual partner. Many STDs have no symptoms or vague non-specific symptoms, and social stigma means that people are less likely to seek treatment. The presence of a second disease often complicates treatment; for example asymptomatic chlamydial infection may remain after gonorrhoea has been treated.

Bacterial Infections

Four significant bacterial infections that may complicate pregnancy, and neonatal outcomes are presented in Box 14.3.

Viral Infections
Human Immunodeficiency Virus

HIV is a **retrovirus** which carries its genetic information as **ribonucleic acid** (RNA), unlike most organisms which contain deoxyribonucleic acid (DNA). Cells of the immune system (Chapter 29) containing **CD4 molecules** are its targets. These include T lymphocytes, monocytes and macrophages. On entering a cell, the viral RNA is converted to DNA and takes over the cell to produce more viruses. Modes of transmission are summarized in Box 14.4.

Factors that increase the risk of transmission include a high maternal viral load and a low CD4 count. Antiretroviral drugs may decrease the viral load and inhibit viral reproduction in the fetus, thus reducing the risk of mother-to-child transmission (MTCT).

As HIV infection may not be obvious at birth but present with recurrent infections and failure to thrive months or years later, it is difficult to assess the risk for MTCT. Studies show that there is a risk of transmission during breastfeeding, and it may be best in developed countries to advise women not to breastfeed. However, most cases occur in developing countries so the risk of transmission must be weighed against the risks of not breastfeeding where there is no access to clean water and sanitation. Additionally for this group, studies examining the prophylactic administration of antiretroviral therapy to prevent HIV transmission during breastfeeding suggest it markedly reduces the risk of transmission (Mehta & Grover, 2022).

TORCH Organisms and Pregnancy Risk

TORCH is a word derived from the first letters of a series of infections that can cross the placenta to affect the fetus. These are **toxoplasmosis, others, rubella, cytomegalovirus** and

• BOX 14.3   Significant Bacterial Infections with Implications for Pregnancy and the Baby

Gonorrhoea

This human disease is still one of the most widespread, and symptoms differ between men and women. In women the initial symptoms are mild vaginitis which may go unnoticed, whereas in men the organism causes a painful infection of the urethral canal. The organism can also cause a severe eye infection in neonates.

The causative organism, *Neisseria gonorrhoeae*, is easily killed outside the body and is transmitted by intimate bodily contact. Severe complications include pelvic inflammatory disease (PID) and damage to heart valves and joint tissues. Most cases respond to the antibiotics erythromycin, cefotaxime or ceftriaxone (Mehta & Grover, 2022).

Syphilis

Syphilis is more serious than gonorrhoea but better controlled as penicillin is very effective against the causative spirochaete *Treponema pallidum*. In those who are allergic to penicillin, erythromycin is advocated. The organism enters the body through a break in the skin or mucous membrane. In men, infection is usually on the penis, whereas in women it may be hidden in the vagina or on the cervix. In about 10% of cases the infection is extragenital, usually in the oral region. The disease can be transmitted across the placenta to cause congenital syphilis.

The organism multiplies within 2–6 weeks at the entry site to form a primary lesion or **chancre** which soon heals. It then spreads throughout the body and a **generalized skin rash** appears—the secondary stage. About 25% of people undergo a spontaneous cure, 25% remain symptomless although the organism is still present and 50% will develop the tertiary stage with possible fatal involvement of the cardiovascular and/or central nervous systems. Because symptoms are noticeable in both sexes, sufferers usually seek treatment. In the UK, pregnant women are screened for syphilis and offered treatment to prevent or treat fetal infection.

Chlamydia

Infection with the intracellular organism *Chlamydia trachomatis* is the most common sexually transmitted disease. There are various serotypes of this organism. One strain causes severe eye infections, but others can cause venereal diseases. Chlamydia is asymptomatic in about 80% of cases but can cause **non-gonococcal urethritis** in men and is the major cause of PID in women. In men, testicular swelling and prostate inflammation can occur; in women, fallopian tubes may be damaged or blocked by destruction of epithelial lining cells, leading to adhesions (Mehta & Grover, 2022). Infertility may result in both sexes.

Doxycycline and **quinolones** would be the antibiotics of choice but cannot be used in pregnancy due to their adverse effects. **Azithromycin** and **erythromycin** are good alternatives (Romero & Nygaard, 2015). Chlamydia is often present in people with gonorrhoea, and treatment to eradicate both organisms should be given.

Group B Streptococcus

Two in ten women in the UK may have rectal or vaginal carriage of **group B streptococcus (GBS)** at some time during their pregnancy. Maternal infection is asymptomatic, but the organism is the most common cause of overwhelming sepsis in neonates, with around 1 in 2000 infants developing early-onset GBS infection. Screening and treating these women is difficult because of recurrence of infection, but intrapartum antibiotic administration appears to reduce the risk of neonatal infection (Chan et al., 2022).

• BOX 14.4   HIV Transmission Types

Horizontal transmission includes sexual contact, infected blood contact with skin or mucous membrane lesions, or contamination via shared needles.

Vertical transmission refers to mother-to-child transmission (MTCT) prenatally, at time of delivery or postnatally through breastfeeding.

---

can be offered vaccination in the postnatal period. Those working with mothers and babies should also be screened and offered vaccination if needed.

Varicella

Varicella (chicken pox) is a childhood illness transmitted by respiratory droplets. If it occurs in pregnancy, a woman may develop **adult respiratory distress syndrome** with a mortality rate of up to 35%. Preterm labour is common, as is **herpes zoster** (shingles) (Mehta & Grover, 2022).

Fetal varicella syndrome with developmental abnormalities may occur if maternal infection is in the first trimester. This includes **low birthweight, eye lesions, undeveloped limbs, skin scars** and **psychomotor retardation**. Infection in the third trimester may cause neonatal infection with **pneumonitis, hepatitis** and **disseminated intravascular coagulation**. Varicella zoster immunoglobulin can be offered to women who have been in contact with chicken pox or shingles, as can acyclovir. Ultrasound to diagnose fetal abnormalities can be used.

Cytomegalovirus

This double-stranded DNA virus is a member of the herpesvirus family and is transmitted by contact with infected blood, saliva and urine or by sexual contact.

---

herpes. Most will cause congenital abnormality if acquired in the first trimester and neonatal infection, often affecting the lungs, liver, spleen and brain, if acquired later in pregnancy.

Rubella

In 1941, Sir Norman Gregg in Australia described an association between maternal rubella (German measles) and **congenital cataracts** (Gregg, 1941). Rubella infection during the first few weeks of pregnancy inhibits cell division in the embryonic eyes, ears, heart and brain. After the third month the most common defect is deafness. An infant born with congenital rubella is highly infectious and must be isolated from other women and infants (Winter & Moss, 2022) but not from their own mothers. Rubella vaccination of girls has been carried out in the UK, and levels of infection are reduced to a low level. Pregnant women are screened and

The varied demographic and population prevalence is between 40–100%, and seroprevalence in women of childbearing age is potentially 86% (Mehta & Grover, 2022). It is often asymptomatic, but there may be non-specific symptoms such as malaise and fever, usually in immunocompromised people. If the primary infection occurs in pregnancy, abortion, preterm labour, IUGR/FGR or fetal death may occur. The greatest risk to the fetus is in the first 20 weeks, although organs develop normally. However, damage to the fetal liver and nervous system may occur. If the baby is born with symptoms the prognosis is poor.

Toxoplasmosis

The causative organism is a protozoon, *T. gondii,* found in dog and cat faeces and in uncooked meat. Infection is usually asymptomatic and occurs in 1 in 500 pregnant women. About 36% of their babies will be affected. **Microcephaly, hydrocephaly** and **hepatosplenomegaly** may occur. Screening in pregnancy could be offered, and treatment is with **spiramycin.** Umbilical cord blood may be tested to see if the fetus is infected. Some women may consider termination of pregnancy.

Herpes Simplex

Maternal genital infection with type 1 or type 2 herpes simplex virus (HSV-1 and HSV-2) may lead to rare, but serious, neonatal infection and has a reported global incidence of approximately 10.3/100,000 live births (Looker et al., 2017). An infected baby may develop localized lesions, encephalitis or generalized herpes infection, including septicaemia, pneumonitis, **liver dysfunction** and **coagulopathy** (Mehta & Grover, 2022). This is a difficult problem as many women show no signs of clinical infection. The first diagnosis may be made on appearance of neonatal infection by clinical signs and viral isolation. Further detail for the management of birth options is summarized in Box 14.5.

Listeriosis

The food-borne pathogen *Listeria monocytogenes* is a bacterium found throughout the environment which may cause abortion, fetal disease or death. Cook–chill products have been implicated in the transmission of infection. Diagnosis in women or neonates is by culturing the organism from blood and/or cerebrospinal fluid, and it is susceptible to penicillin and erythromycin. Health education on safe preparation of food would help reduce the incidence of infection.

Hepatitis B (Serum Hepatitis)

The hepatitis B virus (HBV) is an important cause of morbidity and mortality worldwide. It can be transmitted sexually or parenterally through blood or blood products and by vertical transmission to the fetus. Other body fluids have been implicated in transmission, but blood is the main source of spread. This includes contamination of medical equipment and sharing of needles and syringes by drug addicts and needlestick injuries in health workers. Tattooing and acupuncture can also be risky activities.

As in many viruses, the structure includes a **central core** carrying the genetic material, an **outer envelope** and an **outer surface.** There are three sites that can stimulate antibody production: the **surface antigen** HBs Ag (formerly Australia antigen), the **envelope antigen** HBe Ag and the **core antigen** HBc Ag. Chronic hepatitis B (CHB) affects 65 million women of childbearing age globally (Joshi & Coffin, 2020). The risk factors for HIV are shared by HBV.

Antenatal screening of all pregnant women is recommended with treatment of the affected neonate and precautions taken by birth attendants. The presence of HBe Ag indicates that the disease is highly infectious, and there is a 25% risk of transmission to the baby. If women are HBe Ag positive or have had a late-pregnancy infection, the babies are given hepatitis B vaccine, with the first dose within 24 hours of birth, repeated at 1 month and 6 months of age to protect them against long-term dangers. If women have become infected during pregnancy or do not have HBe Ag present, the baby should receive **hepatitis B-specific immunoglobulin** at birth at a different site from the vaccination.

Hepatitis C

Hepatitis C virus (HCV) infection also causes viral hepatitis worldwide and is usually contracted through contact with infected blood. Vertical transmission is low, but higher rates may be seen in women who are HIV and HCV positive. There is no evidence to support transmission in breast milk.

SARS-CoV-2 (COVID-19)

This coronavirus resulted in the COVID-19 pandemic. Within the lungs, this infection leads to damage, inflammation and haemorrhage. The vascular leak that results may

---

> • **BOX 14.5** **Birthing Options with History of Herpes Simplex Infection**
>
> If the woman gives a history of infection, the mode of delivery should be discussed. The delivery method may be based on the clinical appearance of the genital tract at the onset of labour. If no active lesions are present, a vaginal delivery may be completed. However, if the woman presents with a primary episode at the time of delivery, a caesarean section should be recommended. In both cases, interventions that break the baby's skin, such as scalp electrode or fetal blood sampling, should be avoided. It is not clear whether intrapartum acyclovir reduces the risk of neonatal infection (Hammad & Konje, 2021).

provide the mechanism for dissemination into the blood-stream and spread to other organs (Moore & Suthar, 2021). A recent meta-analysis identified that 27% of COVID-19–positive pregnant women had adverse events including preterm birth and fetal malperfusion (Dubey et al., 2020). Some key management considerations are summarized in Box 14.6.

> ### • BOX 14.6 Key Management Considerations Following Birth for COVID-19
>
> Management of infected pregnant women will require multidisciplinary input. Optimal cord clamping at delivery can be performed with skin-to-skin and breastfeeding supported in positive cases with appropriate observation and precautions (Mehta & Grover, 2022).

Main Points

- Optimal birthweight depends on an interaction between fetal growth potential and intrauterine environment. Genetic determinants, maternal health and nutrition and availability of substrates interact to create fetal growth. Some fetuses may be small but healthy, making diagnosis of IUGR/FGR problematic.
- Associated maternal conditions include hypertension, cardiac disease, chronic renal disease, diabetes mellitus, smoking and alcohol abuse. Placental conditions include small placental size, inadequate implantation and placental infarcts.
- IUGR/FGR increases the risk of stillbirth, oligohydramnios and fetal distress. Neonatal complications include hypoglycaemia, hypocalcaemia and poor temperature control. Genetic and chromosomal disorders are common in babies with symmetric IUGR/FGR.
- Prophylactic antenatal administration of anti-D immunoglobulin is now routinely offered. Rhesus haemolysis of fetal red cells rarely affects the first baby, as there are no spontaneous anti-D antibodies. If the first fetus is Rh+, these may develop if an FMH occurs. Anti-immunoglobulin should be administered to the mother within 72 hours of any sensitizing event.
- Although naturally occurring anti-A antibodies and anti-B antibodies occur and first babies can be jaundiced within the first 24 hours, the jaundice is usually mild.
- Systemic infections may cause infertility or congenital defects during pregnancy. Because of the suppression of cell-mediated immunity, some infections, such as poliomyelitis and influenza, may be more severe with reactivation of CMV and herpes infections possible.
- If untreated, STDs such as gonorrhoea and syphilis can have long-term serious health consequences, and pregnant women may transmit the infection to the fetus causing birth defects or stillbirth.
- Infection with GBS is common and is most often responsible for overwhelming neonatal sepsis with a high mortality rate. Screening and treating women in pregnancy are difficult because of a high recurrence rate, but antibiotic treatment of labouring women may be useful.
- Women who are HIV positive may pass the virus across the placenta to the fetus or contaminate their baby during the birth process. A third way of transmission is via breastfeeding. Anti-retroviral drugs may decrease the viral load and inhibit viral reproduction in the fetus, thus reducing the risk of vertical transfer.
- TORCH organisms can cause fetal abnormality if acquired during the first trimester. If acquired later in pregnancy, neonatal infection may occur.
- Maternal genital infection with type 1 or type 2 herpes simplex virus may lead to serious neonatal infection. Delivery by caesarean section may not protect completely against neonatal infection because of transplacental infection.
- HBV is transmitted by blood and sexual intercourse and by vertical transmission to the fetus. Long-term infection can cause chronic hepatitis, liver cirrhosis and liver cancer. Antenatal screening ensures that vulnerable babies are treated.
- Hepatitis C is another blood-borne virus but is more difficult to transmit than HBV. There is no evidence to support transmission in breast milk.
- Management of COVID-19 infection in pregnancy requires multidisciplinary input.

References

Anblagan, D., Jones, N.W., Costigan, C., Parker, A.J., Allcock, K., Aleong, R., et al., 2013. Maternal smoking during pregnancy and fetal organ growth: a magnetic resonance imaging study. PLoS One 8 (6), e67223.

Bendix, I., Miller, S.L., Winterhager, E., 2020. Causes and consequences of intrauterine growth restriction. Front. Endocrinol. 11, 205.

Blackburn, S.T., 2018. Maternal, Fetal and Neonatal Physiology: A Clinical Perspective, fifth ed. Elsevier, St. Louis.

Chan, Y.T.V., Lau, S.Y.F., Hui, S.Y.A., Ma, T., Kong, C.W., Kwong, L.T., et al., 2022. Incidence of neonatal sepsis after universal antenatal culture–based screening of group B streptococcus and intrapartum antibiotics: a multicentre retrospective cohort study. Br. J. Obstet. Gynaecol. 130 (1), 1–8.

Deka, D., Sharma, K.A., Dadhwal, V., Singh, A., Kumar, G., Vanamail, P., 2013. Direct fetal intravenous immunoglobulin infusion as an adjunct to intrauterine fetal blood transfusion in rhesus-allommunized pregnancies: a pilot study. Fetal Diagn. Ther. 34 (3), 146–151.

De Rooij, S.R., Bleker, L.S., Painter, R.C., Ravelli, A.C., Roseboom, T.J., 2022. Lessons learned from 25 years of research into long term consequences of prenatal exposure to the Dutch famine 1944–45: the Dutch famine birth cohort. Int. J. Environ. Health Res. 32 (7), 1432–1446.

Dubey, P., Reddy, S.Y., Manuel, S., Dwivedi, A.K., 2020. Maternal and neonatal characteristics and outcomes among COVID-19 infected women: an updated systematic review and meta-analysis. Eur. J. Obstet. Gynecol. Reprod. Biol. 252, 490–501.

Figueras, F., Gardosi, J., 2011. Intrauterine growth restriction: new concepts in antenatal surveillance, diagnosis, and management. Am. J. Obstet. Gynecol. 204 (4), 288–300.

Freire, B.L., Homma, T.K., Lerario, A.M., Seo, G.H., Han, H., de Assis Funari, M.F., et al., 2022. High frequency of genetic/epigenetic disorders in short stature children born with very low birth weight. Am. J. Med. Genet. 188 (9), 2599–2604.

Gregg, N.McA., 1941. Congenital cataract following German measles in the mother. Trans. Opthalmol. Soc. Aust. 3, 35–46.

Hammad, W.A.B., Konje, J.C., 2021. Herpes simplex virus infection in pregnancy—an update. Eur. J. Obstet. Gynecol. Reprod. Biol. 259, 38–45.

Joshi, S.S., Coffin, C.S., 2020. Hepatitis B and pregnancy: virologic and immunologic characteristics. Hepatol. Commun. 4 (2), 157–171.

Kitsiou-Tzeli, S., Tzetis, M., 2017. Maternal epigenetics and fetal and neonatal growth. Curr. Opin. Endocrinol. Diabetes Obes. 24 (1), 43–46.

Looker, K.J., Magaret, A.S., May, M.T., Turner, K.M.E., Vickerman, P., Newman, L.M., et al., 2017. First estimates of the global and regional incidence of neonatal herpes infection. Lancet Global Health 5 (3), e300–e309.

Mehta, S., Grover, A. (Eds.), 2022. Infections and Pregnancy. Springer Nature, Singapore.

Monier, I., Receveur, A., Houfflin-Debarge, V., Goua, V., Castaigne, V., Jouannic, J.M., et al., 2021. Should prenatal chromosomal microarray analysis be offered for isolated fetal growth restriction? A French multicenter study. Am. J. Obstet. Gynecol. 225 (6), 676.e1–676.e15.

Moore, K.M., Suthar, M.S., 2021. Comprehensive analysis of COVID-19 during pregnancy. Biochem. Biophys. Res. Commun. 538, 180–186.

Mukherjee, R., 2019. FASD: the current situation in the UK. Adv. Dual. Diagnosis 12 (1/2), 1–5.

Nakamura, A., François, O., Lepeule, J., 2021. Epigenetic alterations of maternal tobacco smoking during pregnancy: a narrative review. Int. J. Environ. Res. Publ. Health 18 (10), 5083.

National Institute of Health and Care Excellence (NICE), 2021. Antenatal Care. Available at: https://www.nice.org.uk/guidance/ng201.

Nirupama, R., Divyashree, S., Janhavi, P., Muthukumar, S.P., Ravindra, P.V., 2021. Preeclampsia: pathophysiology and management. J Gynecol Obstet Hum Reprod 50 (2), 101975.

Ott, W.J., 2001. The ultrasonic diagnosis and evaluation of intrauterine growth restriction. Ultrasound Rev. Obstet. Gynecol. 1 (3), 205–215.

Priante, E., Verlato, G., Giordano, G., Stocchero, M., Visentin, S., Mardegan, V., et al., 2019. Intrauterine growth restriction: new insight from the metabolomic approach. Metabolites 9 (11), 267.

Qureshi, H., Massey, E., Kirwan, D., Davies, T., Robson, S., White, J., et al., 2014. BCSH guideline for the use of anti-D immunoglobulin for the prevention of haemolytic disease of the fetus and newborn. Transfus. Med. 24 (1), 8–20.

Romero, R., Nygaard, I., 2015. CDC updates guidelines for treating sexually transmitted diseases. Am. J. Obstet. Gynecol. 213 (2), 117–118.

Riley, E.P., Infante, M.A., Warren, K.R., 2011. Fetal alcohol spectrum disorders: an overview. Neuropsychol. Rev. 21 (2), 73–80.

Sacco, A., David, A.L., 2020. Advancing fetal therapy in the United Kingdom. Obstet. Gynaecol. Reprod. Med. 30 (3), 91–93.

Sinha, S., Miall, L., Jardine, L., 2017. Essential Neonatal Medicine, sixth ed. Wiley-Blackwell, West Sussex.

Visser, G.H.A., Thommesen, T., Di Renzo, G.C., Nassar, A.H., Spitalnik, S.L., FIGO Committee for Safe Motherhood, Newborn Health, 2021. FIGO/ICM guidelines for preventing Rhesus disease: a call to action. Int. J. Gynecol. Obstet. 152 (2), 144–147.

Winter, A.K., Moss, W.J., 2022. Rubella. Lancet 399 (10332), 1336–1346.

Wolf, M.F., Childers, J., Gray, K.D., 2020. Exchange transfusion safety and outcomes in neonatal hyperbilirubinemia. J. Perinatol. 40 (10), 1506–1512.

Wu, G., Bazer, F.W., Cudd, T.A., Meininger, C.J., Spencer, T.E., 2004. Maternal nutrition and fetal development. J. Nutr. 134 (9), 2169–2172.

Wynn, A., Bristow, C.C., Cristillo, A.D., Murphy, S.M., van den Broek, N., Muzny, C., et al., 2020. Sexually transmitted infections in pregnancy and reproductive health: proceedings of the STAR sexually transmitted infection clinical trial group programmatic meeting. Sex. Transm. Dis. 47 (1), 5–11.

Zamir, M., Nelson, D.M., Ginosar, Y., 2021. Hemodynamic consequences of incomplete uterine spiral artery transformation in human pregnancy, with implications for placental dysfunction and preeclampsia. J. Appl. Physiol. 130 (2), 457–465.

Annotated recommended reading

Kilpatrick, S.J., Cahill, A.G., 2020. Obstetrics: normal and Problem Pregnancies. Elsevier Health Sciences, Philadelphia.

This text provides a comprehensive account of obstetric conditions and management, including those discussed within this chapter, and includes detailed illustrations, searchable online content and material developed by internationally recognized experts.

Dashraath, P., Wong, J.L.J., Lim, M.X.K., 2020. Coronavirus disease 2019 (COVID-19) pandemic and pregnancy. Am. J. Obstet. Gynecol. 222 (6), 521–531.

This is an informative article providing a detailed examination of the impact of COVID 19 on pregnancy, the woman, the fetus and the newborn.

15

Congenital Anomalies

THOMAS McEWAN

CHAPTER CONTENTS

Congenital anomalies have varied origins, including genetic and environmental. However many are multifactorial and difficult to predict. This chapter outlines for students and midwives a selection of common anomalies with an overview of prenatal screening in pregnancy.

Introduction

Congenital anomalies can be defined as structural or functional anomalies that occur during intrauterine life. Also called birth defects, congenital disorders or congenital malformations, these conditions develop prenatally and may be identified before or at birth, or later in life. An estimated 6% of babies worldwide are born with a congenital anomaly, resulting in hundreds of thousands of associated deaths (World Health Organization [WHO, 2023]). However many congenital anomalies are minor and of no functional significance. The percentage of diagnosis increases as children develop and reaches 6% in 2-year-olds and 8% in 5-year-olds (Moore, Persaud & Torchia, 2019). Congenital anomalies that are present at birth may be visible, involving obvious changes in organs, or hidden, such as changes in protein molecules (e.g., haemoglobin or cell receptors).

Congenital anomalies can occur as single or multiple abnormalities and can result from a genetic or non-genetic cause (Table 15.1). This chapter will discuss major causes of congenital anomalies with examples that will be encountered in midwifery practice. Important key points are highlighted in information boxes for specific conditions. The chapter will conclude with an overview of screening methods used to detect anomalies in pregnancy.

General Causes of Congenital Anomalies

The major causes of congenital anomalies are (Moore, Persaud & Torchia, 2019):
- Unknown cause: 50–60%
- Multifactorial inheritance: 20–25%
- Chromosomal abnormalities: 6–7%
- Mutant genes: 7–8%
- Environmental agents: 7–10%

Genetic Causes

Fetal anomalies can sometimes be the result of chromosomal abnormalities or genetic mutation. An introduction to genetics is presented in Chapter 3 and the role of genes in embryogenesis in Chapter 8. Mutations may occur in the DNA of protein-encoding genes or in genes involved in the regulation of coding sequences. Genetic causes of congenital anomalies can be categorized as the result of chromosomal abnormalities, single gene disorders or multifactorial inheritance. Each of these is described, with examples that may be encountered in midwifery practice.

Chromosomal Abnormalities

Chromosomal abnormalities account for approximately 6% of all recognized congenital anomalies (Turnpenny, Ellard & Cleaver, 2021). They can be classified as numerical, mainly due to a non-disjunction event arising during the meiotic divisions that occur during gamete formation and leading to aneuploidy. Alternatively, they may be caused by a structural chromosomal aberration, such as a deletion, translocation or the formation of a ring chromosome that results from chromosome breakage and misrepair during meiosis. The most common human aneuploidy is trisomy

TABLE 15.1	Classification of Congenital Anomalies	
Single Abnormalities	**Genetic or Non-genetic Cause**	**Example**
Malformation	An inherent abnormality may occur in the development of an organ or part of an organ. Multifactorial or chromosomal factor.	Congenital heart abnormalities.
Disruption	External factors such as ischaemia, infection or trauma disturb development. Not usually genetic.	A band of amnion can become caught around a baby's forearm or fingers and disrupt further development.
Deformation	A normally developed structure can become deformed as a result of excessive pressure or force.	Dislocation of the hip and mild positional talipes.
Dysplasia	The organization of cells into tissues is abnormal.	Ectodermal dysplasia.
Multiple Abnormalities	**Chromosomal Abnormalities or Single Gene Mutations**	**Example**
Sequence	A single primary occurrence results in a cascade of events.	Potter sequence
Syndrome	A pattern of abnormalities, often with a known cause such as chromosome abnormalities or single gene defects.	Down syndrome
Association	Several malformations occurring together; not explained as a sequence or a syndrome.	VATER association (affecting many body systems)

From Turnpenny, P., Ellard, S., Cleaver, R., 2021. Emery's Elements of Medical Genetics, sixteenth ed. Elsevier, Edinburgh.

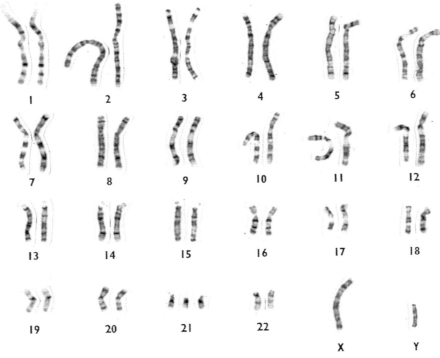

• **Fig. 15.1** A banded karyotype of Down syndrome (trisomy 21).

21, or Down syndrome, in which three copies of chromosome 21 are present in the cells of the infant (Fig. 15.1).

Other trisomic conditions include trisomy 18 (Edwards syndrome) and trisomy 13 (Patau syndrome). Furthermore, cases of triploidy, in which each chromosome is present three times, or tetraploidy, with a chromosome number of 92, may occasionally be encountered. Triploidy and tetraploidy are a frequent cause of early and late miscarriage, but some cases may survive to birth. Sex chromosome aneuploidy, where non-disjunction results in an abnormal sex chromosome constitution (e.g., Turner and Kleinfelter syndromes), may occur but is not as recognizable from the clinical features at birth.

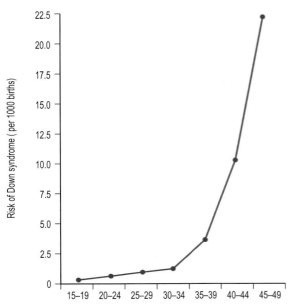

• **Fig. 15.2** The risk of Down syndrome at different maternal ages.

• BOX 15.1	Distinctive Features of Down Syndrome

A small head with flattened occiput and a broad flat nose.
A small mouth cavity with thick gum margins and protruding tongue.
Epicanthic folds.
Brushfield spots, which are white flecks seen in the iris.
Short hands with incurving little fingers.
A single palmar crease.
A wide deviation of the great toe with a plantar crease between the first and second toes.
Dry skin.
Hypotonic muscles.

Down Syndrome

First described by John Langdon Down in 1866, Down syndrome (or Down's syndrome in many countries) is one of the most common autosomal chromosome abnormalities (Antonarakis et al., 2020). The natural incidence of trisomy 21 is about 1 in 800 births but increases significantly with maternal age (Fig. 15.2) such that the incidence may rise as high as 1 in 40 births to older mothers. About 95% of cases of Down syndrome are caused by chromosome **non-disjunction,** but Robertsonian chromosomal **translocation** (for example, involving chromosomes 14 and 21) (Chapter 3), may occur in women of any age and may be inherited.

Congenital heart disorders are present in approximately 50% of infants born with Down syndrome, the most common being atrioventricular septal defects, ventricular septal defects and tetralogy of Fallot (Antonarakis et al., 2020). Distinctive features of Down syndrome are outlined in Box 15.1 (Fig. 15.3). The intellectual ability of affected children can vary. IQ scores can range from 30–70, with the average IQ around 50 for young adults (Turnpenny, Ellard & Cleaver, 2021). Additional complications include intestinal

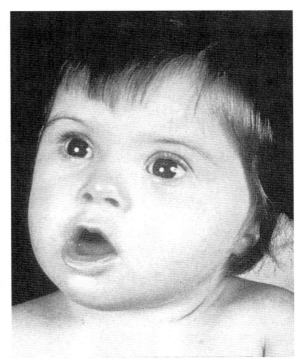

• **Fig. 15.3** Down syndrome.

anomalies such as duodenal atresia and an increased risk of Alzheimer's disease (Carlson, 2019). Some problems can be serious, but many can be treated or managed. With good healthcare, a person with trisomy 21 can expect to live to around 60 years (Snyder et al., 2020).

Single Gene Disorders

Single gene disorders are due to a mutation in the DNA of a single gene and can be classified according to whether the mutated allele is dominant or recessive and whether it occurs on an autosome or one of the sex chromosomes: autosomal-dominant disorders (e.g., Huntington's disease), autosomal-recessive disorders (e.g., cystic fibrosis) or sex-linked disorders (e.g., Duchenne muscular dystrophy). These account for 7–8% of congenital anomalies (Turnpenny, Ellard & Cleaver, 2021). It is important to determine whether the anomaly has a single-gene basis, as genetic counselling will be required due to the possible inheritability of the condition. Cystic fibrosis (CF) is a common example of a single-gene disorder that follows a direct pattern of Mendelian recessive inheritance (Chapter 3).

Cystic Fibrosis

CF is a recessive inherited disease of the **exocrine glands** with the production of thick mucus that obstructs the gastrointestinal tract, reproductive organs and the lungs. It is one of the most common autosomal-recessive disorders in individuals in western Europe with an incidence varying from 1 in 2500–3000. The incidence is lower in Southeastern Europeans and in African American and Asian American populations (Turnpenny, Ellard & Cleaver, 2021).

The causative gene is in the middle of the long arm of chromosome 7 and codes for the protein **cystic fibrosis transmembrane regulator** (CFTR). CFTR controls the passage of sodium and chloride ions across cell membranes, causing the cells and their secretions to contain less water. The resulting thick mucus obstructs the ducts of the pancreas and the lungs, impairing their structure and function. In the lung, secondary bacterial infection is common, with progressive involvement of the bronchial tree resulting in large cystic dilations of all bronchi.

Genetic marker analysis allows the prenatal diagnosis of CF and carriers of the mutant allele will be detected in over 70% of families with a history of CF. More than 1000 mutations of this gene have been found, not all of which cause severe disease. One that is present in about 70% of all mutations is called **Delta F508 (ΔF508)**. This is caused by the deletion of three bases in the DNA of the gene leading to the deletion of a phenylalanine amino acid at position 508 in the CFTR protein. There are now national newborn screening tests for CF in many countries (see Box 15.2). Modern treatments have increased life expectancy and include heart–lung transplantation. Because this disease is caused by the absence or defect of a single protein molecule, there is potential for gene-replacement therapy. In addition, CF is considered a prime candidate for gene therapy because the crucial target organs are so accessible, including the lungs (Turnpenny, Ellard & Cleaver, 2021). Originally, clinical trials focused on CFTR delivery via nebulizers using vectors such as adenovirus. However problems have been encountered with poor vector efficiency and inflammatory responses, particularly when adenovirus has been used as a vector (Turnpenny, Ellard & Cleaver, 2021). More recent research has shown modest improvement in lung function when the *CFTR* gene is delivered to the lungs within a cationic liposome (Alton et al., 2015). This provides optimism for CF management in the future, including the use of CFTR modulator therapies (Lopes-Pacheco, Pedemonte & Veit, 2021).

Multifactorial Inheritance

Multifactorial inheritance is responsible for 20–25% of congenital anomalies and results from a combination of genetic and environmental factors (Moore, Persaud & Torchia, 2019). Single major defects such as cleft lip, cleft palate and neural tube defects (NTDs) are examples of multifactorial inheritance but may also have a genetic or environmental cause (Moore, Persaud & Torchia, 2019).

Cleft Lip and Cleft Palate

Cleft lip and cleft palate occur in approximately 1.42 per 1000 live births and isolated cleft palate in 1 per 2000 live

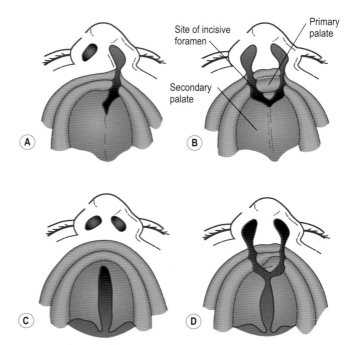

• **Fig. 15.4** Common varieties of cleft lip and palate.

births (Vyas et al., 2020). The cause of cleft lip and cleft palate is usually multifactorial. Clefts can occur in isolation or can be associated with some chromosomal syndromes (e.g., trisomy 13), or associated with the teratogenic effect of drugs (e.g., anticonvulsant medications) (Carlson, 2019). The primary and secondary palate begin to develop early in the sixth week of pregnancy (Moore, Persaud & Torchia, 2019). A cleft lip results when the maxillary and nasomedial processes fail to fuse, and a cleft palate when the palatal shelves fail to fuse (Carlson, 2019).

The extent of the cleft varies with each individual infant. A cleft lip can exist unilaterally or bilaterally. A cleft palate can exist in association with or in isolation from a cleft lip. Two groups of cleft lip and cleft palate exist: anterior and posterior cleft defects (Moore, Persaud & Torchia, 2019). Anterior cleft defects involve cleft lip and may include cleft of the alveolar portion of the maxilla to the incisive fossa. Posterior cleft defects involve clefts of the secondary palate, including the soft and hard palates to the incisive fossa (Fig. 15.4) (Moore, Persaud & Torchia, 2019). Many cases of cleft lip are diagnosed during prenatal screening, but some might not be diagnosed until birth. However delays in detection of cleft palate have been identified (Maraka et al., 2020; Royal College of Paediatrics and Child Health [RCPCH], 2014).

Neural Tube Defects

NTDs are the result of defective closure of the neural tube from about week 4 from conception (Turnpenny, Ellard & Cleaver, 2021). The cause of NTDs is multifactorial, as they can be associated with genetic, nutritional and environmental factors (Moore, Persaud & Torchia, 2019). Spinal cord defects such as spina bifida (Fig. 15.5) result from the embryonic neural arches failing to fuse. NTDs involve the

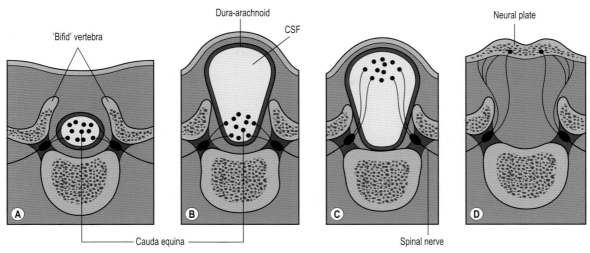

• **Fig. 15.5** Variants of spina bifida. (A) Spina bifida occulta. (B) Meningocele. (C) Meningomyelocele. (D) Myelocele.

tissues lying over the spinal cord, including the meninges, neural arches, muscles and skin (Moore, Persaud & Torchia, 2019). The severity of the defect can vary. With **spina bifida occulta** no external signs or clinical symptoms may exist. A **meningocele** contains meninges and cerebrospinal fluid (CSF) but no spinal cord. A **myelomeningocele** contains spinal cord, meninges and CSF (Lissauer et al., 2020) (Fig. 15.6). A myelomeningocele is associated with more disability than a meningocele. However, the impact on the infant depends on the location and the extent of the lesion (Moore, Persaud & Torchia, 2019).

Anencephaly can occur with the absence of a major portion of the brain, skull and scalp (Salari et al., 2022). One of the most lethal congenital anomalies, those babies who survive to birth will live for only a few hours. A study of 26 cases of anencephaly in the intrapartum period found that intrauterine deaths occurred in 23% (n = 6) before labour, 35% (n = 9) during labour and 42% (n = 11) of infants died in the neonatal period. The duration of survival ranged from 10 min to 8 days (median 55 min) (Obeidi et al., 2010). More recently, however, a case report described unassisted survival of an infant with anencephaly for 28 months (Dickman, Fletke & Redfern, 2016).

Preconception care and the importance of folic acid supplementation in the prevention of NTDs are important aspects of midwifery practice (Chapter 8). Research in the 1980s investigated folic acid supplementation on the prevention of NTDs.

There was clear evidence to recommend that folic acid supplementation be given to all women who were likely to become pregnant (Crider et al., 2022) (see Box 15.3).

Environmental Factors

The rate of new mutations can be increased by environmental factors such as microbial, biochemical and dietary factors; smoking; alcohol ingestion; radiation; and many

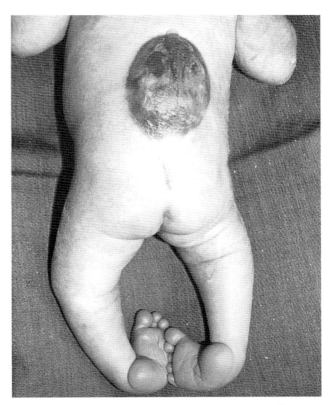

• **Fig. 15.6** Meningomyelocele with bilateral severe talipes.

• BOX 15.3 Folic Acid Supplementation

Folic acid is important for neural tube development in the fetus. Folic acid supplementation has been shown to reduce the incidence of neural tube defects.

chemicals. These may interfere with embryonic development at very precise times during organogenesis. Some factors such as the rubella virus are easily associated, but others, such as environmental pollution, are more difficult to ascertain (Chapter 8).

Teratogens

Teratology is the study of the causes, mechanisms and patterns of abnormal fetal development. Gregg's finding in 1941 that rubella virus caused a syndrome of abnormalities (Chapter 14) was the first clear evidence of **teratogenesis.** There is ongoing evidence that infection by the Zika virus in pregnancy can cause microcephaly and other fetal anomalies (Royal College of Obstetricians and Gynaecologists [RCOG] et al., 2019). The Zika virus is transmitted from the bite of the female *Aedes* mosquito. Transmission can also occur from a blood transfusion and from mother to fetus (Meaney-Delman et al., 2016). Sexual transmission has also occurred in a few cases. Women who are pregnant should seek travel advice to postpone travel to areas with active Zika transmission (RCOG et al., 2019).

The effects of the drug thalidomide between 1957 and 1962 further convinced scientists of the environmental effect on a fetus that up until the 1940s had been thought to be totally protected from the outside world. Malformation of a particular structure is usually caused only during the sensitive period of its development. If malformations occur during the first 2 weeks, they are usually so complex as to be fatal. Between 4 and 8 weeks when organogenesis is taking place, survival with major defect is likely (Moore, Persaud & Torchia, 2019). Maternal diabetes that is poorly controlled, particularly during the stage of organogenesis, is associated with an increased risk of congenital malformation (Wu et al., 2020). Women with diabetes are advised about the importance of maintaining good blood sugar control before conception and throughout pregnancy to reduce the risk of congenital malformation, stillbirth and neonatal death (National Institute of Health and Care Excellence [NICE], 2020).

Drugs

Medicinal drugs may be dispensed by practitioners or bought over the counter from a chemist. Recreational drugs such as cocaine and heroin may be bought illegally on the streets. These drugs may damage gametes or may prevent nutrient absorption such that essential nutrients are absent at crucial times (Table 15.2). **Thalidomide,** a drug taken for morning sickness around 1960, caused **major limb-reduction deformities** and other problems. Thalidomide is contraindicated in pregnancy and in women during childbearing years (Moore, Persaud & Torchia, 2019). Thalidomide continues to be used today to treat leprosy and multiple myeloma (Vargesson & Stephens, 2021). **Angiotensin-converting enzyme (ACE) inhibitors** and **angiotensin receptor blockers (ARBs)** are being used more commonly in women of childbearing age for the treatment of hypertension. However, prescribed contraception during treatment and improved preconceptual advice is necessary

TABLE 15.2	Drugs Known to Cause Fetal Anomalies
Drug	**Effect**
Thalidomide	Teratogenic risks
Warfarin	Congenital malformations. Placental, fetal or neonatal haemorrhage.
Valproate	Minor and major congenital malformations (neural tube defects) and long-term neurodevelopmental effects
Androgens	Masculinization in female fetus
Diethylstilbestrol	In first trimester associated with vaginal carcinoma, urogenital abnormalities and reduced fertility in female offspring; increased risk of hypospadias in male offspring
Cytotoxic drugs	Most cytotoxic drugs are teratogenic
Tetracycline	Discoloration of child's teeth

Information sourced from BNF 2022.

• BOX 15.4 Importance of Preconception Care

Preconception care is important for women and partners so that risks associated with known teratogens are reduced.

due to their teratogenic effects (Lovegrove, Robson and McGettigan, 2020) (Box 15.4).

Prenatal Screening for Congenital Anomalies

Detection of congenital anomalies can be achieved using prenatal diagnostics such as ultrasonography, tissue and blood sampling and non-invasive sampling techniques. The woman should be fully informed about the nature and purpose of screening, which can vary according to the trimester of pregnancy (Allen & Kean, 2020). It is important that parents receive information appropriately during screening, as this can be an anxious time (Nabhan & Aflaifel, 2015). Women's choice in accepting or refusing screening should be respected (Public Health England, 2022b). As a result of prenatal screening, couples may wish to continue with or terminate the pregnancy. Early diagnosis offers a chance to plan and prepare for either option. The dilemma for parents in choosing either option cannot be underestimated. Therefore information, support and understanding from health professionals are required at this time (Box 15.5).

Ultrasonography

Women are offered an **ultrasound scan** (USS) in pregnancy. The embryonic sac can be seen as early as 6 weeks

• BOX 15.5   Informed Consent for Prenatal Screening

Informed consent should be sought from the woman before prenatal screening, with appropriate access to counselling and support.

• CLINICAL APPLICATION 15.1   Combined and Quadruple Tests

The **combined screening test** is offered in the first trimester (between 10 and 14 weeks) to determine the risk of Down syndrome (trisomy 21), Edwards syndrome (trisomy 18) and Patau syndrome (trisomy 13) (Public Health England, 2022a). Combined screening consists of the nuchal translucency measurement (NT) by USS, blood tests (free beta human chorionic gonadotropin [hCG] and pregnancy-associated plasma protein A) and maternal age in addition to gestation age to calculate risk. NT measures a fluid-filled space at the back of the fetal neck (Gilmore, 2020). An increased NT is associated with genetic and structural abnormalities (Allen & Kean, 2020), but it is not used in isolation when calculating risk of fetal anomalies (Public Health England, 2022a).

A second-trimester **quadruple test** is available for women who miss the opportunity for the combined screening test or when the NT measurement has not been obtained. This only screens for trisomy 21. It uses age and the levels of four biochemical substances to calculate risk. These are hCG, unconjugated oestriol (uE_3), alpha-fetoprotein (AFP) and inhibin A. It has lower detection rates than the combined screening test, but it is the recommended option in the second trimester (Public Health England, 2022a). The level of AFP alone can be used to screen for open neural tube defects.

after conception (Allen & Kean, 2020). Real-time B-mode ultrasonography is most often used (Davis & Kallapur, 2020), and developments in ultrasound are ongoing. Detection of congenital anomalies is one of the many functions of USS. In the first trimester of pregnancy, USS may identify large fetal structural abnormalities, such as anencephaly. A second-trimester fetal anomaly ultrasound scan is offered between 18^{+0} and 20^{+6} weeks' gestation and screens for 11 conditions (Public Health England, 2022b). Further details on the combined and quadruple test are provided in Clinical Application 15.1.

Obtaining Fetal Tissue for Genetic Testing

All invasive techniques carry a risk of infection, haemorrhage and fetal loss. The risks must be weighed against the likelihood of fetal abnormality being present. Cells obtained by **amniocentesis** or **chorionic villus sampling** (CVS) can be used for **karyotyping** for chromosomal abnormalities such as Down syndrome, **genetic analysis** using gene probes as in cystic fibrosis and **sexing the embryo** if there is a family history of X-linked disorders such as Duchenne muscular dystrophy. **Enzyme assay** for

detection of inborn errors of metabolism is available in many disorders. These invasive tests should be carried out at a specialist centre.

Amniocentesis

A sample of amniotic fluid is withdrawn from the amniotic cavity through a transabdominal needle using ultrasound to avoid the placenta. This is usually carried out from about 15 completed weeks' gestation onwards (15^{+0}) (Navaratnam, Alfirevic & RCOG, 2021). Chromosomal or genetic analysis is undertaken on the sample obtained.

Chorionic Villus Sampling

This involves obtaining a small amount of placental tissue from the chorionic villi for chromosomal or genetic analysis. CVS is an invasive procedure that can be performed transvaginally or transabdominally under the continuous guidance of ultrasound (Navaratnam, Alfirevic & RCOG, 2021). The procedure is usually performed between 11^{+0} and 13^{+6} weeks' gestation (Public Health England, 2022b).

There is <0.5% chance of miscarriage with amniocentesis or CVS when performed by an appropriately trained operator (Navaratnam, Alfirevic & RCOG, 2021).

Fetal Blood Sampling

A needle is guided to the base of the umbilical cord using ultrasound visualization and a sample of fetal blood is removed (**cordocentesis**). The use of fetal blood sampling has declined because there are improved molecular and cytogenetic tests that allow more diagnoses to be made from chorionic villi or amniotic fluid. The most common indication for cordocentesis today is to determine fetal genetic, metabolic, haematological or infection status (Kunochova *et al.*, 2019; Santiago-Munoz, 2020).

Non-invasive Prenatal Testing

Fetal blood cells can be detected in maternal blood. This allows for DNA testing of the fetal blood cells from the mother's blood (Public Health England, 2022a). It can be offered where a higher chance result has been produced by the combined or quadruple test. It has been recommended for introduction by the UK National Screening Committee as an evaluative rollout (Public Health England, 2022a).

Conclusion

Congenital anomalies are numerous, and some of the more common ones are discussed in this chapter. Their causes are varied but generally can be classified as genetic, environmental, multifactorial and unknown. In some cases, knowing the cause can be preventative; in others it can result in timely detection and diagnosis. Several prenatal screening tools are available for the detection of congenital anomalies. The risks and benefits of these screening tools must be considered by healthcare practitioners in consultation with the woman.

Main Points

- Congenital anomalies account for severe illness during infancy and childhood and a significant proportion of infant deaths.
- The incidence of Down syndrome (trisomy 21) increases with maternal age and can reach 1 in 40. Screening in pregnancy uses a combination of advanced maternal age, ultrasonography and several biochemical tests on maternal serum. Fetal karyotyping can be carried out if strongly indicated.
- Modern treatments for CF have increased life expectancy and quality of life. Research into gene therapy for CF is focusing on effective ways to introduce healthy copies of the gene via nebulizers and more recently fat bubbles (cationic liposomes).
- Cleft lip and cleft palate result from multifactorial causes. Most cases of cleft lip are diagnosed during prenatal screening, but many are diagnosed at or following birth.
- Teratogens lead to genetic mutations. Drugs may be teratogenic and interfere with normal development.
- Detection of congenital anomalies can be achieved using prenatal screening, including ultrasonography, tissue and blood sampling and non-invasive sampling techniques.

References

Allen, K., Kean, L., 2020. Antenatal screening of the mother and fetus. In: Marshall, J.E., Raynor, M.D. (Eds.), Myles Textbook for Midwives, seventeenth ed. Elsevier, Edinburgh.

Alton EWFW, Armstrong DK, Ashby D, Bayfield KJ, Bilton D, Bloomfield EV, et al., Cystic Fibrosis Gene Therapy Consortium, 2015. Repeated nebulisation of non-viral CFTR gene therapy in patients with cystic fibrosis: a randomised, double-blind, placebo-controlled, phase 2b trial, Lancet Respir. Med., 3 (9), 684–691.

Antonarakis, S.E., Skotko, B.G., Rafii, M.S., Strydom, A., Pape, S.E., Bianchi, D.W., et al., 2020. Down syndrome. Nat. Rev. Dis. Prim. 6 (1), 1–20.

Carlson, B.M., 2019. Human Embryology and Developmental Biology, sixth ed. Elsevier Mosby, Philadelphia.

Crider, K.S., Qi, Y.P., Yeung, L.F., Mai, C.T., Head Zauche, L., Wang, A., et al., 2022. Folic acid and the prevention of birth defects: 30 years of opportunity and controversies. Annu. Rev. Nutr. 42, 423–452.

Davis, P., Kallapur, S., 2020. Perinatal ultrasound. In: Martin, R.J., Fanaroff, A.A., Walsh, M.C. (Eds.), Fanaroff & Martin's Neonatal-Perinatal Medicine: Diseases of the Fetus and Infant, eleventh ed. Elsevier, Philadelphia.

Dickman, H., Fletke, K., Redfern, R.E., 2016. Prolonged unassisted survival in an infant with anencephaly. BMJ Case Rep. 2016, bcr2016215986.

Gilmore, A., 2020. Genetic aspects of perinatal disease in perinatal diagnosis. In: Martin, R.J., Fanaroff, A.A., Walsh, M.C. (Eds.), Fanaroff & Martin's Neonatal-Perinatal Medicine: Diseases of the Fetus and Infant, eleventh ed. Elsevier, Philadelphia.

Joint Formulary Committee, 2022. BNF: 84: September 2022 – March 2023. Pharmaceutical Press, London.

Kunochova, I., Papcun, P., Krizko Jr., M., Gabor, M., Alfoldi, M., Ferianec, V., 2019. The value of cordocentesis in current management of intrauterine patient. Bratisl. Lek. Listy 120 (8), 563–565.

Lissauer, T., Fanaroff, A.A., Miall, L., Fanaroff, D. (Eds.), 2020. Neonatology at a Glance, fourth ed. Wiley-Blackwell, Oxford.

Lopes-Pacheco, M., Pedemonte, N., Veit, G., 2021. Discovery of CFTR modulators for the treatment of cystic fibrosis. Expert Opin. Drug Discov. 16 (8), 897–913.

Lovegrove, E., Robson, J., McGettigan, P., 2020. Pregnancy protection and pregnancies in women prescribed ACE inhibitors or ARBs: a cross-sectional study in primary care. Br. J. Gen. Pract. 70 (700), e778–e784.

Maraka, J., Butterworth, S., Sainsbury, D., Hodgkinson, P., 2020. Growth concerns in the early weeks of life: don't forget the palate. Br. Med. J. 371, m4255.

Meaney-Delman, D., Rasmussen, S.A., Staples, J.E., Oduyebo, T., Ellington, S.R., Petersen, E.E., et al., 2016. Zika virus and pregnancy. What obstetric health care providers need to know. Obstet. Gynecol. 127 (4), 642–648.

Moore, K.L., Persaud, T.V.N., Torchia, M.G., 2019. Before We Are Born: Essentials of Embryology and Birth Defects, tenth ed. Elsevier Saunders, Philadelphia.

Nabhan, A.F., Aflaifel, N., 2015. High feedback versus low feedback of prenatal ultrasound for reducing maternal anxiety and improving maternal health behaviour in pregnancy. Cochrane Database Syst. Rev. 2015 (8), CD007208.

National Institute of Health and Care Excellence (NICE), 2020. Diabetes in Pregnancy: Management from Preconception to the Postnatal period. Available at: https://www.nice.org.uk/guidance/ng3.

Navaratnam, K., Alfirevic, Z., Royal College of Obstetricians and Gynaecologists (RCOG), 2021. Amniocentesis and chorionic villus sampling: green-top Guideline no. 8. Br. J. Obstet. Gynaecol. 129 e1-e15.

Obeidi, N., Russell, N., Higgins, J.R., O'Donoghue, K., 2010. The natural history of anencephaly. Prenat. Diagn. 30 (4), 357–360.

Public Health England (PHE), 2022a. Screening for Down's Syndrome, Edwards' Syndrome and Patau's Syndrome. Available at: https://www.gov.uk/government/publications/fetal-anomaly-screening-programme-handbook/screening-for-downs-syndrome-edwards-syndrome-and-pataus-syndrome--3.

Public Health England (PHE), 2022b. Fetal Anomaly Screening Programme Handbook. Available at: https://www.gov.uk/government/publications/fetal-anomaly-screening-programme-handbook.

Royal College of Obstetricians and Gynaecologists (RCOG), Royal College of Medicine (RCM), Public Health England (PHE), Health Promoting Schools (HPS), 2019. Clinical Guidelines, Zika Virus Infection and Pregnancy: Information for Healthcare Professionals. Available at: https://www.rcog.org.uk/media/vzjln5ib/zika-virus-rcog-feb-2019.pdf.

Royal College of Paediatrics and Child Health (RCPCH), 2014. Palate Examination: Identification of Cleft Palate in the Newborn – Best Practice Guide. Available at: http://www.rcpch.ac.uk/improving-child-health/clinical-guidelines-and-standards/published-rcpch/inspection-neonatal-palate.

Salari, N., Fatahi, B., Fatahian, R., Mohammadi, P., Rahmani, A., Darvishi, N., et al., 2022. Global prevalence of congenital anencephaly: a comprehensive systematic review and meta-analysis. Reprod. Health 19 (1), 1–18.

Santiago-Munoz, P., 2020. Fetal blood sampling and transfusion. In: Queenan, J.T., Spong, C.Y., Lockwood, C.J. (Eds.), Protocols for High-Risk Pregnancies: An Evidence-Based Approach, seventh ed. Wiley-Blackwell, Oxford.

Snyder, H.M., Bain, L.J., Brickman, A.M., Carrillo, M.C., Esbensen, A.J., Espinosa, J.M., et al., 2020. Further understanding the connection between Alzheimer's disease and Down syndrome. Alzheimer's Dementia 16 (7), 1065–1077.

Turnpenny, P., Ellard, S., Cleaver, R., 2021. Emery's Elements of Medical Genetics, sixteenth ed. Elsevier, Edinburgh.

Vargesson, N., Stephens, T., 2021. Thalidomide: history, withdrawal, renaissance, and safety concerns. Expert Opin. Drug Saf. 20 (12), 1455–1457.

Vyas, T., Gupta, P., Kumar, S., Gupta, R., Gupta, T., Singh, H.P., 2020. Cleft of lip and palate: a review. J. Fam. Med. Prim. Care 9 (6), 2621–2625.

World Health Organization (WHO), 2022. Congenital Disorders. Available at: https://www.who.int/news-room/fact-sheets/detail/birth-defects.

World Health Organization (WHO), 2023. Congenital Disorders. Available at: https://www.who.int/health-topics/congenital-anomalies#tab=tab_1.

Wu, Y., Liu, B., Sun, Y., Du, Y., Santillan, M.K., Santillan, D.A., et al., 2020. Association of maternal prepregnancy diabetes and gestational diabetes mellitus with congenital anomalies of the newborn. Diabetes Care 43 (12), 2983–2990.

Annotated recommended reading

Kasper, E., Schneidereith, T.A., Lashley, F.R. (Eds.), 2016. Lashley's Essentials of Clinical Genetics in Nursing Practice, second ed. Springer, New York.

A great resource for practitioners who require knowledge for using genomics in their practice.

Moore, K.L., Persaud, T.V.N., Torchia, M.G., 2019. Before We Are Born: Essentials of Embryology and Birth Defects, tenth ed. Elsevier Saunders, Philadelphia.

This textbook clearly describes embryo development week by week and provides an excellent source for understanding the origin of congenital defects. The illustrations are excellent.

Public Health England (PHE), 2022. Fetal Anomaly Screening Programme Handbook. Available at: https://www.gov.uk/government/publications/fetal-anomaly-screening-programme-handbook.

Clear and detailed information provided on the fetal anomaly screening programme offered in England.

SECTION 2B

Pregnancy—The Mother

This section is about the numerous normal physiological adaptations women develop during pregnancy to compensate for the needs of the developing fetus. The adaptations are dynamic during pregnancy and can often have a profound and dramatic effect on the body systems. Firstly, it is essential that student midwives and midwives have sound knowledge and understanding of the anatomy and physiology of the non-pregnant body systems. Therefore, each of the key body systems are described in the non-pregnant healthy state. Thereafter, the physical and physiological adaptations brought about by pregnancy are detailed. These adaptations will become more meaningful to students and midwives in the context of the non-pregnant parameters. Related systems have been grouped as far as possible. The chapters also provide revision for nurses who enter the midwifery profession. The haematological system (Chapter 16) and the cardiovascular system (Chapter 17) are integral to the support of the growing fetus. Three other systems involved in gas exchange, acid–base control (pH) and fluid balance are the respiratory system (Chapter 18), the renal system (Chapter 19) and fluid balance (Chapter 20). Chapters 21–23 examine the organs of the digestive tract and nutrition, and Chapters 24 and 25 explore the musculoskeletal system. The relationship between the nervous, endocrine and immune systems provides much knowledge about human health. Chapters 26–29 present the systems related to the relatively new science of psychoneuroimmunology.

The everyday practice of student midwives and midwives must always be underpinned with detailed knowledge of the anatomy and physiology of the body systems and the physical and physiological changes and adaptations during each stage of pregnancy, childbirth and the puerperium. This knowledge will ensure there is appropriate recognition of any deviation from the norm and the appropriate safe management of the pregnant woman by the midwife through effective application of interventions and care.

16

The Haematological System—Physiology of the Blood

JEAN RANKIN

This chapter details the physiology of the blood, the cellular content, blood groups and haemostasis. Iron metabolism and the maternal haematological adaptations to pregnancy are detailed.

Blood as a Tissue

In small-cell organisms, the diffusion of substances is sufficient to maintain the metabolic needs of the cell. However, multicellular organisms need more advanced mechanisms other than diffusion to enable the transport of substances. During evolution this has been achieved through the cardiovascular system and the circulation of blood.

Blood is a fluid connective tissue that communicates between internal cells and the body surface and between the various specialized tissues and organs. In an adult human, blood will normally comprise 6–8% of body weight; this is 5–6 L in a man and 4–5 L in a woman.

If a sample of blood is placed in a test tube and prevented from clotting, the heavier cellular elements settle to the bottom and the plasma rises to the top. The **haematocrit,** or packed cell volume fraction, essentially represents the percentage of total blood volume occupied by erythrocytes. White blood cells (WBCs) and platelets form only 1%, settle on top of the red blood cells (RBCs) and can be seen between the two main layers as a thin cream-coloured layer called the **buffy coat.** The haematocrit averages 45% and the plasma averages 55% of the total volume. Table 16.1 details the properties and characteristic constituents of blood.

Functions of Blood

Blood has three general functions:
1. **Transportation:** Blood transports oxygen from the lungs to the cells and transports carbon dioxide from the cells to the lungs, nutrients from the gastrointestinal tract, hormones from endocrine glands and heat and waste products away from the cells.
2. **Regulation:** Blood is involved in the regulation of acid–base balance, body temperature and water content of cells.
3. **Protection:** Clotting factors in blood protect against excessive loss from the cardiovascular system. WBCs protect against disease by producing antibodies and performing phagocytosis.

TABLE 16.1	Properties and Characteristic Constituents of Blood	
Property	**Value**	
Specific gravity (relative to water)	1.05 (varies with body temperature)	
Viscosity (relative to water)	1.5–1.75 (cells contribute equally to viscosity)	
pH	7.35–7.45	
H+ concentration	35–45 nmol/L	

Characteristic constituents:
- Blood comprises 6–8% of adult bodyweight (i.e., 5–6 L for a man and 4–5 L for a woman).
- The haematocrit (packed cell volume fraction) averages 45% and plasma averages 55%.
- Erythrocytes (red blood cells or RBCs) make up >99% of the cellular component.
- White cells and platelets are present in <1% of the cellular component.

TABLE 16.2	Outline of Blood Constituents and Function
Constituent	**Function**
Water (90% of plasma volume)	Transport medium of nutrients, wastes, gases Heat distributor
Plasma protein—albumin	Transports many substances Large contribution to colloid oncotic pressure
Plasma protein globulins—α and β	Transport substances, involved in clotting
Plasma protein globulins—γ	Antibodies
Plasma protein—fibrinogen	Inactive precursor for fibrin
Electrolytes	Osmotic distribution of fluid between compartments

Constituents of Blood

Blood has a characteristic constituency of living cells suspended in a plasma matrix (Table 16.1). It is a sticky, viscous, dark red, opaque fluid consisting of 55% plasma and 45% cells. More than 99% of the cellular component consists of erythrocytes (RBCs). WBCs and platelets are present in small quantities. If blood is exposed to the air, it solidifies into a clot and exudes a clear fluid called *serum*.

Plasma

Plasma is the liquid portion of the blood which acts as the transport medium of substances being carried in the blood. Water comprises approximately 90% of the plasma volume, with the remainder containing protein (8%), inorganic ions (0.9%) and organic substances (1.1%). The characteristic straw colour of plasma is produced by bilirubin, the waste product of haemoglobin (Hb) breakdown. Table 16.2 outlines the constituents and function of plasma.

Serum is blood plasma without fibrinogen and other clotting factors. As protein molecules are too large to pass into the interstitial fluid at the capillary beds, there is a higher protein content in plasma than in interstitial fluid (i.e., 8% compared with 2%). Most of the protein that does pass into the interstitial fluid is taken up by the lymphatic system and returned to the blood. The main plasma proteins are presented in Table 16.3.

The functions of plasma proteins are to:
- Prevent fluid loss from blood to tissues by exerting colloid osmotic (**oncotic**) pressure. This is mainly due to the presence of the protein albumin. If plasma protein levels fall due to either reduced production or loss from the blood vessels, then osmotic pressure is also reduced. Fluids will then move into the tissues (oedema) and body

TABLE 16.3	Plasma Proteins	
Name	**Origin**	**% of total**
Albumin	Synthesized in the liver	60
Fibrinogen	Synthesized in the liver	4
Globulins α and β	Synthesized in the liver	36
Globulin γ	Synthesized in the immune system	Trace

cavities. This may occur in diseases of the liver and kidneys, burns, inflammation and allergic disorders.
- Transport bound substances to prevent them from being metabolized until they reach their target tissue: for instance, albumin binds bilirubin. Some substances can displace others and compete for binding sites. An example is displacement of bilirubin from albumin by aspirin or sulphonamides.
- Aid in clotting and fibrinolytic activities.
- Assist in prevention of infection: γ-globulins (also known as *immunoglobulins*—see Chapter 29) function as specific antibodies for specific protein antigens such as microbial agents and pollen.
- Help regulate acid–base balance by acting in buffering systems.
- Act as a protein reserve that forms part of the amino acid pool.
- Contribute about 50% to the total viscosity of blood.

Other proteins found in the blood in small quantities are hormones, enzymes and most of the clotting factors. There is also a series of plasma proteins called **complement** that assist in the inflammatory and immune mechanisms. Albumin is the smallest of the plasma proteins with a molecular

TABLE 16.4	Outline of the Cellular Constituents of Blood	
Constituent	**Function**	
Erythrocytes (red cells)	Oxygen and carbon dioxide transport	
Leucocytes (white cells)	Defence against micro-organisms	
Thrombocytes (platelets)	Haemostasis	

mass of 69,000 Da and is just too large to pass through the capillary walls in normal circumstances. If the glomerular capillaries in the kidney are damaged, albumin can be lost from the blood in large quantities.

The Cellular Components of Blood

Three major cell types are present in blood, each having a very different function: RBCs (**erythrocytes**), WBCs (**leucocytes**) and platelets (**thrombocytes**) (Table 16.4).

Under normal circumstances, the proportions of these cells remain constant within narrow limits. However, the body may adjust these levels to maintain health. A simple routine test can measure the cellular content of blood and is normally carried out as either part of health screening or to diagnose illness.

Haemopoiesis is the term used for blood cell formation. Embryonic blood cells appear in the bloodstream as early as the third week of development. All blood cell types are descended from a single type of bone marrow cell called a *pluripotent stem cell* or **haemocytoblast.** This is an undifferentiated cell capable of giving rise to the precursor of any of the blood cell types. These include the RBCs and megakaryocytes (leading to platelets). The pluripotent stem cells branch to form myeloid stem cells, which leads to the production of granulocytes and monocytes in the bone marrow (Fig. 16.1). Lymphoid stem cells leave the bone marrow to reside in the lymphoid tissues and produce lymphocytes. Each person has about 1500 g of red bone marrow in the body with the function of producing RBCs and WBCs.

Red Blood Cells

The major function of erythrocytes or RBCs is the carriage of oxygen from the lungs to all the cells of the body. Erythrocytes contain large amounts of Hb with which oxygen and carbon dioxide (to a lesser extent) reversibly combine. The shape and size of the erythrocytes are significant for this function. Erythrocytes are biconcave discs (circular and flattened, thinner in the middle than around the edge) and are approximately 7.5 μm in diameter. This shape provides a high surface-to-volume ratio well suited to the exchange of gases and allows the volume of the cell to readily alter with the osmotic shifts of water between cell and plasma. The plasma membrane is strong and conveniently pliant.

These characteristics allow the cells to become deformed as they squeeze through torturous and narrow capillary vessels whose diameter may be smaller than the RBC.

Erythrocytes are the main cellular contributor to blood viscosity. Therefore, any increase in RBC levels will also raise the viscosity of blood, which may occur in circumstances such as a slower flow of blood or a change in environment to an area of high altitude. Any subsequent decrease, such as is seen in normal pregnancy, will lower viscosity and blood will flow more rapidly.

Erythrocytes are completely dedicated to the transport of oxygen and carbon dioxide. Hb is the oxygen-carrying capacity of the erythrocytes. Hb also picks up about 20–25% of carbon dioxide returning from the tissues to form carbaminohaemoglobin. However, most of the carbon dioxide is in solution in the blood. Measurements of red cell count, volume and Hb content are routine and useful assessments in clinical practice (see Table 16.5).

Haemoglobin

Hb is a red-coloured pigment found in red cells. Hb is made up of the protein **globin** bound to the red **haem** pigment. Globin is rather complex. It consists of four polypeptide chains—two alpha (α) and two beta (β)—each bound to a ring-like haem group (Fig. 16.2). Each haem contains one iron ion (Fe^{2+}) that can combine reversibly with one oxygen molecule to form the bright red **oxyhaemoglobin** (HbO_2). The iron–oxygen interaction is very weak, and the two can be easily separated without any damage. Once the oxygen has been released in the tissues, it becomes darker red and is known as **deoxyhaemoglobin.**

Each Hb molecule can carry four molecules of oxygen. These are picked up one at a time, and each binding changes the configuration of globin and increases the affinity of the Hb molecule for oxygen. The binding of the first oxygen allows the second, third and fourth oxygen molecules to bind with increasing ease. This aspect of oxygen uptake will be examined in greater detail when considering respiration in Chapter 18.

The pigment haem is made up of ring-shaped organic molecules called **pyrrole rings.** Four of these join to form a larger ring, and the nitrogen atom of each pyrrole ring holds a ferrous iron atom centrally. At birth, fetal Hb (HbF) makes up two-thirds of Hb content and adult Hb (HbA) one-third. The adult ratio is established from the age of 5 years.

Formation of Erythrocytes

Mature RBCs develop from haemocytoblasts within the erythroid tissue in the bone marrow. After 3–5 days the cells pass into the circulation as cells called **reticulocytes** because they still contain rough endoplasmic reticulum and clumped ribosomes. These structures disappear when the cell is mature, which normally takes 4 days. Three or four mitotic cell divisions are involved so that each haemocytoblast gives rise to 8 or 16 red cells. Other organelles and the

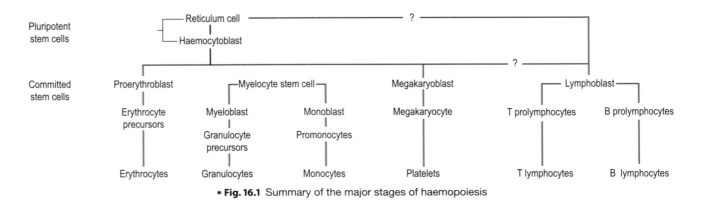

• **Fig. 16.1** Summary of the major stages of haemopoiesis

TABLE 16.5	**Red Cell Laboratory Values**		
Parameter			**Value**
Red cell (erythrocyte) count – number of red cells per litre, or cubic millilitre (mm³) of blood		Male:	4.5×10^{12}–6.5×10^{12}/L
			(4.5–6.5 million/mm³)
		Female:	3.8×10^{12}–5.8×10^{12}/L
			(3.8–5.8 million/mm³)
Packed cell volume (PCV, haematocrit) – the volume of red cells in 1 L or mm³ blood			0.40–0.55 L/L
Haemoglobin – the weight of Hb in whole blood, measured in g/100 mL blood		Male:	13–18 g/100 mL
		Female:	11.5–16.5 g/100 mL
		Infant:	14–20 g/100 mL
Mean cell Hb (MCH) – the average amount of haemoglobin per cell, measured in picograms (1 pg = 10^{-12} g)			27–32 pg/cell
Mean cell haemoglobin concentration (MCHC) – the weight of Hb in 100 mL red cells			30–35 g/100 mL red cells
Mean cell volume (MCV) – the volume of an average cell, measured in femtolitres (1 fL = 10^{-15} L)			80–96 fL
(Abbreviations in brackets are commonly used in laboratory reports)			

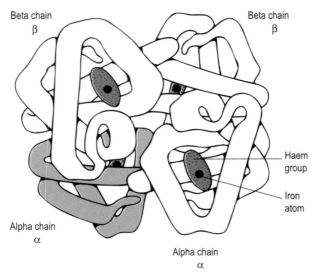

• **Fig. 16.2** The structure of haemoglobin. Haemoglobin is a protein with four subunits (two α polypeptides and two β polypeptides). Each subunit contains a haem group with an iron atom.

nucleus are extruded from the cell. There is a reduction in cell size and a change in cell shape. Reticulocytes normally comprise less than 2% of the red cells in the blood of an adult. The formation of erythrocytes is called **erythropoiesis.** Table 16.6 summarizes the necessary dietary substances.

The Lifespan of Red Cells

About 1% of erythrocytes are replaced daily. Production is stimulated by the hormone **erythropoietin,** which originates in the kidney. This is a glycoprotein produced when the kidney cells are hypoxic: for example, during haemorrhage, haemolytic crises, at altitude and following exercise. RBCs live for about 120 days and are finally ingested and destroyed by macrophages, mainly in the spleen. As the cells circulate, their plasma membrane becomes progressively more damaged until it ruptures. They are fragmented to produce protein and haem, which is mostly reclaimed in the body stores for reuse. The remainder of the haem portion is degraded and bilirubin is excreted as bile (Fig. 16.3).

TABLE 16.6	Dietary Substances Needed for Erythropoiesis	
Substance	**Utilization**	
Protein	Synthesis of the globin part of haemoglobin and for cellular proteins	
Iron	Contained in the haem portion of haemoglobin	
Vitamin B$_{12}$ (hydroxocobalamin)	Needed for DNA synthesis	
Folic acid	Needed for DNA synthesis	
Vitamin C (ascorbic acid)	Facilitates absorption of iron	

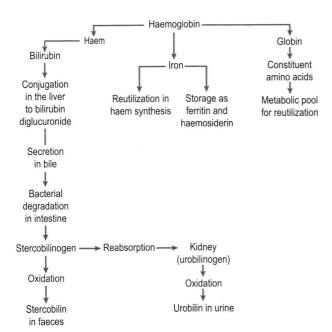

• **Fig. 16.3** A summary of haemoglobin breakdown.

Iron Metabolism

Absorption

A typical Western mixed diet usually contains about 14 mg of iron daily, but normally only 1–2 mg (5–10%) are absorbed. There are two distinct forms of absorption: iron attached to haem and inorganic iron. Iron attached to haem is found in the Hb and myoglobin protein found in animal products. It is absorbed more efficiently than non-haem iron and is not affected by factors affecting the absorption of non-haem iron. In most foods, iron is present in its ferric form and needs to be converted to ferrous iron to be absorbed.

Absorption is enhanced if reducing agents that can aid this conversion are available. Hydrochloric acid found in gastric juice performs this function, as can ascorbic acid (vitamin C). In grain foods, iron forms a complex with phytates, and only small amounts of soluble iron are available. The amount of iron absorbed depends on the rate of red cell production, the extent of iron stores, the content of the diet and if iron supplements are given. Intestinal absorption of iron is facilitated when there is erythroid hyperplasia, rapid turnover of iron and a high concentration of unsaturated transferrin, as occurs in pregnancy.

Serum Iron, Transferrin and Total Iron-binding Capacity

Non-pregnant women have a serum iron content of 13–27 μmol/L. This shows immense individual variability and fluctuates hourly, with the processes for change not fully understood. A low concentration of serum iron usually indicates iron-deficiency anaemia. The **total iron-binding capacity** (TIBC) is 45–72 μmol/L. A low concentration of TIBC is associated with iron-deficiency anaemia. **Transferrin** is the protein that specifically binds iron and is usually between 2.0 and 3.6 g/L. During pregnancy, there is a rise in transferrin by up to 70%. The TIBC is usually one-third saturated with iron and this also increases during pregnancy by up to 70%. The hormone oestrogen probably causes the change, as this is seen in women taking oestrogen-containing oral contraceptives. The TIBC returns to normal within 3 weeks following birth.

Serum Ferritin

Ferritin is a glycoprotein with a high molecular mass and is found in cells where it holds two-thirds of the iron store. It is also present in small amounts in the plasma at a wide range of 15–300 μg/L. It is stable, not affected by iron ingestion and is a good indicator of iron stores, especially in the lower range as in iron-deficiency anaemia in pregnancy.

Marrow Iron

Occasionally it is useful to examine bone marrow to assess iron stores. Marrow is taken by aspiration from the iliac crest. A stainable iron–protein complex called **haemosiderin** (like ferritin) may be seen. No stainable iron will be seen if the serum ferritin has fallen below 40 μg/L. In the absence of iron supplementation, no stainable iron is seen in 80% of women at term. Developing erythrocytes can also be examined for signs of iron deficiency. The presence of infection, especially urinary tract infection, can block the incorporation of iron into Hb as the microbes may utilize iron in their own metabolic processes.

Folate Metabolism

Vitamin B9 is water-soluble and comes in two forms: folate (natural) and folic acid (synthetic). Liver is a good source of folate, in addition to leafy green vegetables such as spinach and in mushrooms and oranges. Folic acid can be taken in the form of supplements. Both forms of vitamin B9 can be destroyed by prolonged boiling or by the addition of bicarbonate of soda to the cooking water. Some drugs act as anti-folate and folic acid antagonists and prevent their absorption. A typical Western diet contains 500–800 μg daily, and normal daily needs are 100–200 μg. This excess intake in the diet partly compensates for the loss in cooking.

Folates are absorbed in the duodenum and jejunum and then stored in the liver. Deficiency is more likely to be seen in the winter months when foods containing folic acid may be difficult to obtain. It is more common in poor and socially deprived groups. The metabolism of folic acid is the basis for cellular use of folate, and it is essential for cell growth and division. Tissue that is active in reproduction and growth is more dependent on the efficient turnover and supply of folate coenzymes, and during pregnancy folate metabolism is increased.

Blood Groups

RBCs, like all cells, have **glycoproteins** in their plasma membranes which are genetically coded for and therefore inherited. These can act as **antigens**, provoking an immune reaction if incompatible blood enters the circulation. These RBCs are then agglutinated and destroyed. Over 400 different antigens are found on the surface of RBCs. Some of these antigens cause a more vigorous reaction than others. The two most commonly problematic are those of the ABO system and the rhesus (Rh) system.

The ABO System

The ABO blood groups are based on the presence of two RBC antigens (known as **agglutinogens**) called *type A* and *type B.* These types are co-dominant (i.e., neither gene masks the presence of the other so that both proteins are expressed). A person inheriting both antigens will have blood group AB. If neither antigen is inherited, then blood group O arises. Four blood groups are possible depending on the surface antigens present on the red cells: A, B, AB and O.

A unique factor associated with the ABO system is the presence of preformed antibodies (known as **agglutinins**) in the plasma within 2 months of birth with no previous sensitization event. A baby cannot have antibodies against any antigen carried on its own RBCs or the cells would be destroyed. Therefore, a baby who has neither the A nor the B antigen on its RBCs will have both anti-A and anti-B antibodies in the serum. In contrast, a baby with the blood group AB will have neither antibody present in the serum. Those with blood group A will have anti-B antibodies, and those with blood group B will have anti-A antibodies.

The Rhesus (Rh) System

There are eight types of Rh antigens but only three are common. These are called the *C, D* and *E agglutinogens.* One gene codes for each type, and there are two alleles to each gene, giving CDE/cde as the full range of alleles. Rhesus D is by far the most clinically important antigen. The word *rhesus* is used because agglutinogen D was originally identified in rhesus monkeys.

About 85% of people in the Western world are rhesus positive (Rh+), which means they have the Rh agglutinogen on their RBCs, and 15% are rhesus negative (Rh–) and do not have this marker. In Japan 99.7% of people are Rh+ and only 0.3% are Rh–. Unlike the ABO system, there are no spontaneously occurring anti-Rh antibodies; these are only formed if there is a sensitization event with the presence of Rh+ RBCs in the circulation of a Rh– person. Issues associated with the Rh factor in pregnancy are discussed in Chapter 14.

White Cells

These cells are the **leucocytes** and can be referred to as *WBCs.* Taking all the types together, the average number of WBCs in the circulation is 5000–9000 per mm^3 (also reported as $5–9 \times 10^9$/L). These account for ≤1% of the cellular content of the blood. An increase in WBCs is called **leucocytosis** and a decrease is **leucopoenia.** The WBCs present in the blood represent only a small part of the body's total WBC content, as many of the cells are in the tissues.

The newborn baby has approximately double the WBC count of an adult, which decreases to reach adult levels by about 5–10 years of age. These cells are part of the immune defence system (see Chapter 29) and are protective against bacteria, viruses, parasites, toxins and tumour cells. Some white cells undergo **diapedesis.** This means that the cells can slip out of capillaries with an amoebic action in response to positive **chemotaxis** (chemical call).

Types of WBCs

Granulocytes (polymorphonuclear leucocytes) contain granules that have a lobed nucleus and substances that can fight infection in their cytoplasm. They are 10–14 μm in diameter. Granulocytes can be further divided into three groups, categorized by the size of their granules and uptake of Wright stain. All these granulocytes are phagocytic.

1. **Neutrophils** contain granules of varying sizes that stain violet because they take up both acidic red dyes and basic blue dyes. Neutrophils are the most common types of granulocytes, accounting for more than 50% of all WBCs. Neutrophils are chemically attracted to sites of inflammation and will ingest and destroy bacteria and some fungi.
2. **Eosinophils** have large granules which are stained red by acidic dyes. The nucleus usually has two lobes. Eosinophils make up about 1–4% of the WBC population. The most important role of this type of cell is to attack parasitic worms such as tapeworms and round worms. When such a worm enters the body, the eosinophils surround it and release enzymes from their granules onto the parasite's surface to digest it from the outside. Eosinophils are also involved in dealing with allergy attacks by destroying antigen–antibody complexes.

3. **Basophils** have large granules that take up a basic dye and stain blue-black. The nucleus usually has two or three lobes. These are the rarest of the WBCs, accounting for only 0.5% of the population. Their large granules contain histamine, which is an inflammatory substance that acts as a vasodilator and draws other WBCs to the site of inflammation. **Mast cells** are cells like basophils that are present in connective tissue. Both types of cells release histamine when they bind to immunoglobulin E (IgE). The immune system is discussed in Chapter 29.

The Production of Granulocytes

Granulocytes arise from myeloid precursor cells in the red bone marrow, a process that takes about 14 days. This time can be reduced considerably if cells are urgently required, such as when infection is present. There is also a pool of granulocyte cells in the bone marrow where there can be 50 cells for every granulocyte in the circulation. During **granulopoiesis,** there is progressive condensation and lobulation of the nucleus. Granules develop in the cell cytoplasm, and there is loss of organelles such as mitochondria.

Within 7 hours of reaching the circulation, half of the granulocytes will have left to meet tissue needs and will not return to the blood. The normal survival of these cells in the tissues is about 4–5 days. Dead cells are eliminated from the body in faeces and respiratory secretions. Dead neutrophils form the pus at infection sites.

Agranulocytes

These include lymphocytes and monocytes and do not contain visible cytoplasmic granules.

Lymphocytes

Lymphocytes are produced in the bone marrow, and immature cells migrate to the thymus and other lymphoid tissue to divide again and mature. These are round cells with large round nuclei and are the second most common type of leucocyte. Even though large numbers of lymphocytes exist in the body, only a small number are found in the circulation. Most lymphocytes are often present in lymphoid tissue and are involved in immune reactions.

Monocytes

Monocytes are large cells that are produced in the bone marrow. Mature cells spend about 30 hours in the blood and then migrate to the tissues where they develop into macrophages. Macrophages are also phagocytic, although they respond more slowly than neutrophils. They are also greatly involved in regulating the immune response by activating B and T lymphocytes (see Chapter 29).

Platelets

Platelets are small, non-nuclear cellular elements produced in the bone marrow. These are colourless discoid bodies

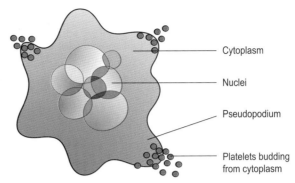

• **Fig. 16.4** Diagram of a megakaryocyte showing platelet budding.

- Cytoplasm
- Nuclei
- Pseudopodium
- Platelets budding from cytoplasm

and have a diameter of only 2–4 μm. The normal blood platelet count is between 150×10^9/L and 350×10^9/L (150,000–350,000/mm³).

Production of platelets (**thrombopoiesis**) occurs in the bone marrow. They are formed inside the cytoplasm of large cells called *megakaryocytes* and bud off from the cell surface (Fig. 16.4). Each megakaryocyte takes about 10 days to mature and produces about 4000 platelets. The lifespan of a platelet is 7–10 days and they are destroyed by macrophages, mainly in the spleen but also in the liver.

Platelets are complex and have many functions other than being involved in the clotting process of blood. They can phagocytose small particles such as viruses and immune complexes. They store and transport **histamine** and **serotonin** which are released when platelets are damaged. This affects the tone of smooth muscle in blood vessel walls. Platelets secrete **platelet-derived growth factor** (PDGF) which stimulates proliferation of smooth muscle walls to support healing after injury.

Haemostasis

If the endothelium of blood vessels is smooth and uninterrupted, blood flow is maintained. If a blood vessel is damaged, a series of reactions occurs to maintain haemostasis and minimize blood loss. The mechanism is fast, localized and carefully controlled. Many blood coagulation factors normally present in plasma are involved. Some substances involved in the blood clotting process are released from platelets and injured tissues. Haemostasis involves three phases: vascular spasm, platelet plug formation and coagulation of blood (Fig. 16.5). This is followed 30–60 min later by clot retraction and the removal of unnecessary clots by fibrinolysis.

Vascular Spasm

Vasoconstriction after injury is brought about by direct injury to vascular smooth muscle, compression of the vessel by extravasated blood, chemicals released by endothelial cells and platelets and reflexes triggered by pain receptors. A strongly constricted artery can significantly reduce blood loss for up to 30 min. This allows time for platelet plug formation

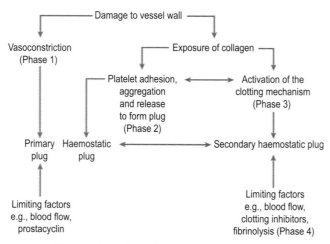

• **Fig. 16.5** An outline of the events of haemostasis.

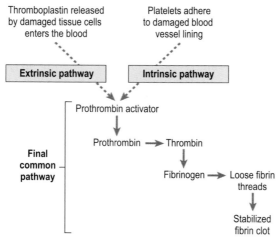

• **Fig. 16.6** Stages of blood clotting.

and blood clotting to occur. A blunt injury crushes tissue and is more efficient at causing vascular spasm than a sharp cut.

Formation of a Platelet Plug

Normally platelets do not stick to each other or to the endothelial lining of blood vessels. Damage to or disruption of the endothelium exposes underlying collagen fibres. This causes platelets to swell, form spiky processes and stick to the exposed area. Once the platelets have adhered to the endothelium, lipids in the platelet plasma membrane release a short-lived prostaglandin derivative called thromboxane A_2. Degranulation of platelets occurs and other chemicals are released. These are serotonin (enhances vascular spasm) and adenosine diphosphate to attract more platelets. Within 1 minute a platelet plug forms (Fig. 16.6). Prostacyclin (PGI_2) limits the process by confining platelet aggregation to the immediate area of damage.

Coagulation

There are three critical events in coagulation of blood:
1. Prothrombin activator is formed.

2. This converts the plasma protein prothrombin to thrombin.
3. Thrombin causes fibrinogen molecules to form a fibrin mesh. This traps blood cells and seals the hole in the blood vessel.

Over 30 different substances affect the process. There are factors that enhance clot formation, called **procoagulants** (see Table 16.7); those that inhibit clot formation are called **anticoagulants.** Most of the clotting factors, or procoagulants, are plasma proteins synthesized in the liver, except factors III and IV. The factors are released into the blood where they remain inert until the clotting cascade is triggered.

Clotting may be initiated by either of two pathways. These are the intrinsic and extrinsic pathways; both pathways are usually triggered by the same tissue-damaging events. The intrinsic pathway only initiates clotting of blood outside the body, whereas the extrinsic pathway initiates clotting of blood that has escaped into the tissues. Clot formation is normally complete within 3–6 min. The extrinsic pathway involves fewer steps and is more rapid than the intrinsic pathway. In severe trauma the extrinsic mechanism can clot blood within 15 s.

Clot Retraction and Fibrinolysis

After 30–60 min a platelet-induced process called **clot retraction** occurs. A contractile protein, **actomyosin,** works in the same way as it does in muscle cells. Serum is squeezed out, the clot is compacted and the torn edges of the blood vessel are drawn together. This is the beginning of healing. PDGF released by degranulation of the platelets stimulates smooth muscle and fibroblasts to divide and rebuild the muscle wall.

Unnecessary clots are removed by **fibrinolysis** to prevent occlusion of blood vessels. Yet another of the plasma proteins, **plasminogen,** is activated to produce plasmin which is a protein-digesting enzyme. Large amounts of plasminogen may be incorporated into a big clot but remain inactive, producing plasmin only as necessary. Plasminogen activators are released from endothelial cells when a clot is present. Factor VII and thrombin are potent plasminogen activators.

Factors Limiting Clot Growth or Formation

- Rapid removal of coagulation factors.
- Inhibitors of activated clotting factors.

Any tendency to clot in rapidly moving blood is usually unsuccessful because any activated clotting factors are diluted and washed away. **Heparin** is a natural anticoagulant normally contained in the granules of the leucocytes—mast cells and basophils. Endothelial cells also produce heparin. Small amounts released into the plasma normally prevent inappropriate blood coagulation.

Maternal Haematological Adaptations to Pregnancy

During pregnancy, the significant maternal changes noted in the haematologic system and haemostasis are essential

TABLE 16.7   **Procoagulant Factors**

Factor	Name	Function
I	Fibrinogen	Converted to fibrin mesh
II	Prothrombin	Converted to thrombin which converts fibrinogen to fibrin
III	Thromboplastin	Catalyses thrombin formation
IV	Calcium ions	Needed at all stages
V	Platelet accelerator	Affects both intrinsic and extrinsic methods
VI	No substance	
VII	Serum prothrombin conversion accelerator (SPCA)	Extrinsic pathway conversion
VIII	Antihaemophilic factor	Intrinsic mechanism (absence = haemophilia A)
IX	Plasma thromboplastin component (PTC, Christmas factor)	Intrinsic mechanism (absence = haemophilia B)
X	Stuart–Power factor	Both extrinsic and intrinsic pathways
XI	Plasma thromboplastin antecedent (PTA)	Intrinsic mechanism (absence = haemophilia C)
XII	Hageman factor	Intrinsic mechanism
XIII	Fibrin stabilizing factor (FSF)	Cross-links fibrin to make it insoluble

Vitamin K is essential for synthesis of factors II, V1I, IX and X.

for healthy development of the fetus and the protection of maternal homeostasis. These changes are critical as they support the woman to tolerate blood loss and the separation of the placenta from the uterine wall at delivery. However, these physiological adaptations also increase the risk for maternal complications such as thromboembolism, iron-deficiency anaemia and coagulopathies.

Blood Volume and Composition

Total blood volume is a combination of plasma and RBCs and is the most significant haematologic change to occur during pregnancy. The average increase in total blood volume during pregnancy is between 30% and 45% (approximately 1.5 L). Plasma volume and total RBC mass are under separate control and bear no fixed relation to one another (Antony et al., 2017). The increase in blood volume relates to an initial rapid increase in cardiac output as early as the sixth week of pregnancy and peaks between 32 and 34 weeks (Blackburn, 2018; Broughton Pipkin, 2018). Throughout uncomplicated pregnancy, plasma volume increases progressively. Plasma volume increases by approximately 45–50% (range 40–60%) or about 1200–1600 mL above non-pregnant values (Blackburn, 2018; Broughton Pipkin, 2018). In twin pregnancies, plasma volume increases up to 70% above non-pregnant values (Blackburn, 2018). The increase in plasma volume results in hypervolaemia, haemodilution and a fall in Hb level often referred to as **physiological anaemia** (Figs. 16.7–16.9). The aetiology of plasma expansion is thought to be related to the effects of

nitric oxide–mediated vasodilation on the renin–angiotensin–aldosterone system and subsequent sodium and water retention (Blackburn, 2018). The increase in plasma volume is positively correlated with the birthweight of the baby.

The benefits of hypervolaemia are to fulfil the extra demands on the circulation in pregnancy. For instance, the basal metabolic rate increases by 20% in pregnancy with the production of more heat. Blood flow to the skin is increased and this allows heat to be lost. The increased blood volume also helps maintain blood pressure when blood may be sequestered in the lower part of the body in the third trimester. This helps to safeguard the woman against haemorrhage at delivery. The decrease in viscosity with increase in cardiac force leads to a decreased resistance to blood flow, which is essential for placental perfusion.

Blood Cellular Components

The main changes in cellular components during pregnancy are summarized in Table 16.8. The increase in RBC content in a normal pregnancy has been difficult to ascertain because many women take iron supplements. The nature of the increase in RBC production is not fully understood, but there is a three-fold increase in erythropoietin in plasma in the second trimester (Blackburn, 2018).

The total WBC count rises slightly in pregnancy and is due to an increase in neutrophils with an elevation in mature leucocyte forms (Blackburn, 2018; Broughton Pipkin, 2018). The total WBC count increases sharply in labour with the count returning to normal by 4–7 postnatal days (Blackburn, 2018).

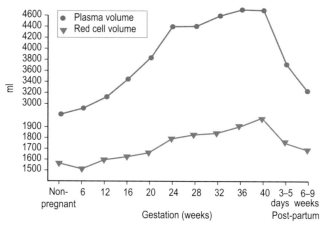

• **Fig. 16.7** Mean total plasma and red cell volume during normal pregnancy.

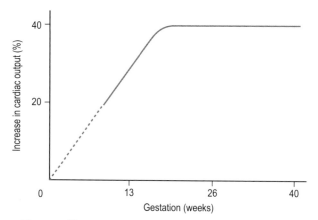

• **Fig. 16.8** Changes in cardiac output throughout pregnancy.

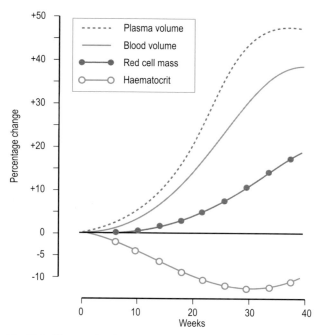

• **Fig. 16.9** Changes in plasma volume, blood volume, red cell mass and haematocrit during normal pregnancy.

Although the lymphocyte count remains unchanged in pregnancy with no change in circulating T cells and B cells, there is profound depression of cell-mediated immunity. This picture is also seen in women taking oral contraceptives (containing oestrogen). Oestrogen may increase the number of glycoproteins on the cell surface, leading to impaired response to stimuli. Human chorionic gonadotrophin from the placenta and prolactin from the anterior pituitary are known to suppress lymphocyte function. There is no apparent impairment to the production of immunoglobulins or to humoral-mediated immunity. The depression of cell-mediated immunity is essential to the survival of the fetus but may increase susceptibility to viral infections such as rubella, poliomyelitis and influenza. Worldwide, the increased susceptibility of women to malaria leads to an infected placenta with increased fetal mortality.

Iron Requirements during Pregnancy

To meet the expansion in RBC mass and the needs of the fetus and placenta, extra iron is needed in pregnancy. The total requirements are calculated as between 700–1400 mg throughout pregnancy. Table 16.9 presents an overview of the distribution of iron requirements in pregnancy. The needs can be met only by mobilizing iron stores in addition to achieving maximum absorption from dietary iron. Box 16.1 provides an overview of iron-deficiency anaemia and issues around supplementation in pregnancy.

Folate Metabolism in Pregnancy

Folates together with iron have a central role in the nutrition of pregnancy. Requirements for folates are increased in pregnancy to meet the needs of the growing fetus and placenta, and for the increased maternal tissues of the growing uterus and RBC mass. The placenta transports folates actively to the fetus even if maternal folate status is deficient. Maternal folate metabolism is altered early in pregnancy before fetal demands act directly.

Haemostasis in Pregnancy

The major changes occur in the haemostatic components of blood, and some of these are unique to pregnancy. Adaptations lead to a hypercoagulable state during pregnancy (Broughton Pipkin, 2018). Adequate haemostasis depends on a complex interaction between blood vessel wall, platelets, coagulation factors and fibrinolysis. In health, haemostasis has three main functions: to keep the circulating blood inside the vascular tree, to maintain the fluidity of blood and to arrest bleeding after injury to vessels.

The following changes are seen in pregnancy (Blackburn, 2018):

- Platelet count and volume are largely unchanged in most pregnancies although they may slightly decrease in relation to the haemodilution. Platelet reactivity is increased in the second and third trimesters and does not return to normal until about 12 weeks postpartum (Broughton Pipkin, 2018). There is a 20% decrease in platelets due to placental separation at delivery which gradually increases to non-pregnant values by 3–5 days after birth. No change in function has been reported.

TABLE 16.8   Changes in Blood Cellular Components during Pregnancy

| Component | Changes | | |
	Direction	Pattern	Basis for Change
RBCs	Increases by 20–30% (erythropoietin three-fold increase (plasma) in second trimester)	Slow, continuous and linear increase beginning in first trimester; may accelerate slightly in third trimester	Erythropoietin stimulated by HPL, progesterone and prolactin
Haematocrit (reduces in parallel with RBC decrease)	Decreases by 3–5% to 33.8% at term (range, 33–39%)	Decreases from second trimester (as plasma volume peaks). (PP – return to non-pregnant levels 4–6 weeks)	Haemodilution
Hb	Decreases by 2–10% to 12.1–12.5 g/dL (range, 11–13 g/dL) at term	If iron and folate are adequate, little change until week 16. Lowest values between 16 and 22 weeks with slow increase until term. (PP – returns to non-pregnant levels by 4–6 weeks)	Haemodilution; total body Hb increases by 65–150 g
Reticulocytes	Increases by 1–2%	Gradual increase to third trimester. (PP – returns to non-pregnant levels by 4–6 weeks)	Increased RBCs
WBCs: neutrophils	Increases by 8% to 5000–12,000/mm³ (up to 15,000/mm³ seen), mainly due to neutrophils	Increase primarily involves neutrophils and begins in second month. Peaks at 33 weeks. (PP – normal values in 4–7 days)	Oestrogen NB: Massive increase (four-fold) in labour and immediately after delivery
Eosinophils Basophils	Slight increase. Slight decrease.	Variable Variable	Haemodilution Haemodilution
Platelets	May decrease slightly but usually remain within range of normal values. Survival of platelets is reduced.	Variable. Platelet reactivity – increased in 2nd and 3rd trimesters. (PP – returns to normal around 12 weeks)	Major haemodynamic changes relating to clotting systems
ESR	Increases	Progressive	Increased plasma globulin and fibrinogen

ESR, Erythrocyte sedimentation rate; *Hb,* haemoglobin; *HPL,* human placental lactogen; *PP,* postpartum; *RBCs,* red blood cells; *WBCs,* white blood cells.
Based on Blackburn S.T., 2018. Maternal, Fetal and Neonatal Physiology: A Clinical Perspective, fifth ed. Elsevier, Philadelphia; Pipkin, B.F., 2018. Maternal physiology. In: D.K., Lees, C., Bourne, T.H., (Eds.) Textbook of Obstetrics and Gynaecology, ninth ed. Wiley-Blackwell, Oxford.

TABLE 16.9   The Distribution of the Extra Iron in Pregnancy

Tissue Usage	Requirements (mg)
Expansion of the red cell mass	570
Fetus	270–370
Placenta	35–100
Blood loss at delivery	100–250
Breastfeeding (6 months)	100–180
Loss from skin, faeces, urine	270

- Levels of coagulation factors VII, IX, X and XII increase at a slower pace. Factor VII may increase 10-fold (also seen in women taking oestrogen/progesterone contraceptives). From as early as the third month of gestation, there is a marked increase in plasma fibrinogen coagulation. The activity of factor VIII doubles. Plasma fibrinogen levels may also double in late pregnancy and labour due to increased synthesis.

- These changes are consistent with a continuous low-grade coagulation activity with fibrin deposition in the intervillous space of the placenta and in the walls of the spiral arteries supplying the placenta (see Chapter 12). As pregnancy progresses, a fibrin matrix replaces the smooth muscle and elastic lamina of the spiral arteries. This allows expansion of the lumen to accommodate an increase in blood volume and decrease the pressure of arterial blood flowing to the placenta. This hypercoagulability is advantageous after placental separation to help control blood loss and prevent haemorrhage. After delivery, a fibrin mesh very rapidly covers the placental site. The fibrinogen used represents up to 10% of the total circulating fibrinogen.

• BOX 16.1 Iron Deficiency Anaemia and Iron Supplementation in Pregnancy

Globally, anaemia affects 1.62 billion people, which corresponds to 24.8% of the population (World Health Organization (WHO), 2020a). Iron deficiency is the most common cause of anaemia, affecting approximately 500 million individuals worldwide, especially in low-income populations (WHO, 2015). During childbearing years, iron-deficiency anaemia has a higher incidence in women due to the loss of iron through pregnancy and menstruation. Globally the prevalence of anaemia is around 38% in women during pregnancy and around 39% in non-pregnant women, particularly in low- and middle-income countries. Worldwide, available data on the prevalence of postpartum anaemia is limited (WHO, 2016). In high-income countries the incidence of postpartum anaemia is 10–30%, with a higher incidence suggested in low- and middle-income countries (WHO, 2016). Anaemia in pregnancy is a public health problem in developing countries (Stephen et al., 2020; WHO, 2020b). During pregnancy, it is estimated that 75% of diagnosed anaemia arises from iron deficiency, with pregnant adolescents being at particular risk (Broughton Pipkin, 2018; WHO, 2022b). In the UK, the prevalence of anaemia was found to be 24% in a multicentre national study (Barroso et al., 2011) and anaemia was reported in 46% of women at booking or 28-week assessments in a two-centre English study (Nair et al., 2017). Approximately 50% of women commence pregnancy with insufficient iron stores to supply the increased maternal and fetal needs (WHO, 2001).

Causes of iron-deficiency anaemia are multifactorial and are broadly attributed to dietary deficiency, malabsorption and increased loss or requirements (National Institute of Health and Care Excellence (NICE), 2021). In pregnancy, iron deficiency is usually due to an imbalance of demand and supply, which becomes more significant with advancing pregnancy (Stephen et al., 2020). In the first trimester, the physiological expansion of plasma volume exceeds the increased production of red blood cells and haemoglobin (Hb). This causes haemodilution which contributes to the fall in Hb during pregnancy, although plasma volume levels out by the third trimester (Costantine, 2014). Anaemia is defined as Hb levels less than two standard deviations below the mean for a healthy matched population (WHO, 2020a).

There remains variation in the normal Hb values for pregnancy. The WHO (2008) defined anaemia in pregnancy as a Hb concentration of <11 g/dL (<110 g/L) and postpartum anaemia as Hb <10.0 g/dL (<100 g/L). According to recent UK guidelines, anaemia should be defined as Hb <110 g/L in the first trimester,

<105 g/L in the second and third trimesters and <100 g/L postpartum (2D) (Pavord et al., 2020).

Even relatively mild maternal anaemia is associated with increased placental weight/birthweight ratios and decreased birthweight (Broughton Pipkin, 2018). Many women in low- and middle-income countries have poor diets and are deficient in nutrients and micronutrients. This is a huge challenge in pregnancy when it is so important for normal functioning, growth and development of the pregnancy and fetus and maternal health (Pavord et al., 2020). However, inappropriate supplementation can itself be associated with pregnancy problems. NICE (2021) recommends that iron supplementation should be considered for pregnant women with Hb <110 g/L throughout pregnancy and for 3 months following correction of Hb levels.

Numerous studies have focused on interventions of supplementations to promote good health of the mother and fetus and prevent anaemia during pregnancy. Several large Cochrane reviews have been conducted with varying results. In a recent review (involving 17,771 women), Lassi et al. (2013) looked at the impact of providing folic acid supplementation during pregnancy. They found no conclusive evidence of benefit on pregnancy outcomes of folic acid supplementation during pregnancy. Peña-Rosas et al. (2015) reviewed the use of intermittent oral iron supplementation during pregnancy as an alternative to daily supplementation. Findings suggest that intermittent regimens may be a feasible alternative to daily iron supplementation among those pregnant women who are not anaemic and have adequate antenatal care. Keats et al. (2019) conducted a review of 20 trials (141,849 women) with 19 in low/middle-income countries and one UK trial. Findings provide a strong basis to guide the replacement of iron and folic acid with multiple-micronutrient supplements for pregnant women in low- and middle-income countries where multiple-micronutrient deficiencies are prevalent among women. Overall, women receiving multiple-micronutrient supplementation had fewer low-birthweight babies, small-for-gestational-age babies and stillbirths than women who received only iron, with or without folic acid.

NICE (2021) recommends that healthcare professionals should be aware that iron-deficiency anaemia in pregnancy is associated with increased risk of perinatal morbidity and mortality. It also has important potential implications for the future neurodevelopment of the infant (WHO, 2020b).

- Fibrinolytic activity decreases during pregnancy, remains low in labour and delivery and returns to normal as early as 1 hour after placental delivery. These changes help combat the hazards of haemorrhage at delivery.

Intrapartum and Immediate Postpartum Periods

The decrease in blood and plasma volume during the immediate postpartum period corresponds to the amount of blood loss with delivery (Blackburn, 2018). Blood volume loss at delivery varies (500 mL for singletons and 1000 mL for caesarean section or a multiple birth. However, blood losses can often be underestimated or overestimated (Blackburn, 2018). The normal response to blood loss in non-pregnant women is a reduction in

blood volume, which is compensated by vasoconstriction. Over the next few days, the blood volume expands back to near-normal values because of increased plasma volume. As a result, there is a fall in the haematocrit proportional to the blood loss. In the healthy pregnant woman, the response to blood loss is modified because of the hypervolaemia of pregnancy. After the acute blood loss at delivery, there is no compensatory increase in blood volume, which remains relatively stable. There is a gradual fall in plasma volume, primarily due to diuresis. The RBC mass increase during pregnancy gradually reduces to normal values as RBCs come to the end of their lifespan. The haematocrit gradually increases and blood volume returns to non-pregnant levels by 4–8 weeks postpartum.

Over the postpartum period, the woman continues to be at increased risk for thromboembolism.

Main Points

- Blood is a fluid connective tissue carrying oxygen and nutrients to the body cells and carbon dioxide and metabolic waste from the cells. Blood volume is about 5–6 L in a man and 4–5 L in a woman.
- The functions of blood are internal transport of substances for respiration, nutrition and excretion; maintenance of water, electrolyte and acid–base balance; metabolic regulation; protection against infection; protection from haemorrhage; and maintenance of body temperature.
- Blood consists of two components: 55% plasma and 45% cells.
- Plasma proteins prevent fluid loss, transport substances around the body, are involved in clotting and fibrinolytic activities, assist in prevention of infection, help regulate acid–base balance, act as a protein reserve and contribute half of total blood viscosity.
- *Haemopoiesis* is the term for blood cell formation (i.e., RBCs, WBCs and platelets). Erythrocytes are involved in the transport of gases to and from cells; leucocytes are involved in the defence of micro-organisms; and platelets have a key role in haemostasis.
- RBCs live for about 120 days.
- WBCs account for 1% of the blood's cellular content.
- Platelets are produced in the bone marrow. In the clotting process, they form a platelet plug.
- Haemostasis involves vascular spasm, platelet plug formation and blood coagulation.
- The ABO blood groups are based on the presence of two RBC antigens: type A and type B. The O blood group arises if neither antigen is inherited; if both are inherited, group AB results.

- Only three Rh antigens are common: C, D and E agglutinogens. Rhesus D is by far the most clinically important antigen.
- Total blood volume is a combination of plasma volume and RBC volume. The increase in blood volume during pregnancy relates to an increase in cardiac output.
- In pregnancy, increases are noted in RBC mass (or total volume of RBCs) and plasma volume. This difference results in hypervolaemia, haemodilution and a fall in Hb level, often referred to as *physiological anaemia*.
- The decrease in viscosity with increase in cardiac force leads to a decreased resistance to blood flow which is essential for placental perfusion.
- During pregnancy, major changes occur in the haemostatic components of blood leading to a hypercoagulable state.
- Haemostasis has three main functions: to keep the blood circulating, to maintain the fluidity of blood and to arrest bleeding after injury to vessels.
- RBCs increase during pregnancy to 20–30% of non-pregnant values.
- WBCs (neutrophils) increase during pregnancy by up to 8% with a slight increase in eosinophils and slight decrease in basophils.
- Continuing low-grade coagulopathy is a feature of normal pregnancy.
- Platelets may decrease slightly but remain within normal values.
- Erythrocyte sedimentation rate increases in pregnancy due to the increase in fibrinogen and other physiological changes.

References

Antony, K.M., Racusin, D.A., Agaard, K., Dildy III, G.A., 2017. Maternal physiology. In: Gabbe, S.G., Niebyl, J.R., Simpson, J.L., Landon, M.B., Galan, H.L., Jauniaux, E.R.M., et al., (Eds.), Obstetrics: Normal and Abnormal Pregnancies, seventh ed. Elsevier, Philadelphia.

Barroso, F., Allard, S., Kahan, B.C., Connolly, C., Smethurst, H., Choo, L., et al., 2011. Prevalence of maternal anaemia and its predictors: a multi-centre study. Eur. J. Obstet. Gynecol. Reprod. Biol. 159 (1), 99–105. https://doi.org/10.1016/j.ejogrb.2011.07.041.

Blackburn, S.T., 2018. Maternal, Fetal and Neonatal Physiology: A Clinical Perspective, fifth ed. Elsevier, Philadelphia.

Costantine, M.M., 2014. Physiologic and pharmacokinetic changes in pregnancy. Front. Pharmacol. 5, 65.

Keats, E.C., Haider, B.A., Tam, E., Bhutta, Z.A., 2019. Multiple-micronutrient supplementation for women during pregnancy. Cochrane Database Syst. Rev. 2019 (3), CD004905.

Lassi, Z.S., Salam, R.A., Haider, B.A., Bhutta, Z.A., 2013. Folic acid supplementation during pregnancy for maternal health and pregnancy outcomes. Cochrane Database Syst. Rev. 2013 (3), CD006896.

Nair, M., Churchill, D., Robinson, S., Nelson-Piercy, C., Stanworth, S.J., Knight, M., 2017. Association between maternal haemoglobin and stillbirth: a cohort study among a multi-ethnic population in England. Br. J. Haematol. 179 (5), 829–837.

National Institute of Health and Care Excellence (NICE), 2021. Clinical Knowledge Summaries: Anaemia - Iron Deficiency. Available at: https://cks.nice.org.uk/topics/anaemia-iron-deficiency/.

Pavord, S., Daru, J., Prasannan, N., Robinson, S., Stanworth, S., Girling, J., BSH Committee, 2020. UK guidelines on the management of iron deficiency in pregnancy. Br. J. Haematol. 188 (6), 819–830.

Peña-Rosas, J.P., De-Regil, L.M., Gomez Malave, H., Flores-Urrutia, M.C., Dowswell, T., 2015. Intermittent oral iron supplementation during pregnancy. Cochrane Database Syst. Rev. 2015 (10),CD009997.

Pipkin, B.F., 2018. Maternal physiology. In: Edmonds, D.K., Lees, C., Bourne, T.H. (Eds.), Dewhurst's Textbook of Obstetrics and Gynaecology, ninth ed. Wiley-Blackwell, Oxford.

Stephen, G., Mgongo, M., Hussein Hashim, T., Katanga, J., Stray-Pedersen, B., Msuya, S.E., 2020. Anaemia in pregnancy: prevalence, risk factors, and adverse perinatal outcomes in northern Tanzania. Anemia 2018,1846280.

World Health Organization (WHO), 2001. Prevention and Control of Iron Deficiency Anaemia in Women and Children: Report of the UNICEF/WHO Regional Consultation, Geneva, Switzerland 3-5 February 1999. WHO Press, Geneva.

World Health Organization (WHO), 2008. Treatment for Iron-Deficiency Anaemia in Pregnancy. WHO Press, Geneva.

World Health Organization (WHO), 2015. The Global Prevalence of Anaemia in 2011. WHO Press, Geneva.

World Health Organization (WHO), 2016. Iron Supplementation in Postpartum Women. WHO Press, Geneva. https://iris.who.int/handle/10665/249242.

World Health Organization (WHO), 2020a. Worldwide Prevalence of Anaemia 1993-2005. WHO Press, Geneva.

World Health Organization (WHO), 2020b. WHO Guidance Helps Detect Iron Deficiency and Protect Brain Development. WHO Press, Geneva.

Annotated recommended reading

Blackburn, S.T., 2018. Maternal, Fetal and Neonatal Physiology: A Clinical Perspective, fifth ed. Elsevier, Philadelphia.

This text provides a detailed description of the major changes that occur in the body systems during pregnancy. There is an extensive review of the literature of the haematological and cardiovascular system, extending from classical research studies to more recent research findings.

Tortora, G.J., Derrickson, B.H., 2020. Principles of Anatomy and Physiology, sixteenth ed. Wiley, Hoboken.

This textbook provides an in-depth description of human anatomy and physiology. The section on the blood is further detailed and well-illustrated.

Websites

Pavord, S., Daru, J., Prasannan, N., Robinson, S., Stanworth, S., Girling, J., BSH Committee, 2020. UK guidelines on the management of iron deficiency in pregnancy. Br. J. Haematol. 188 (6), 819–830. https://doi.org/10.1111/bjh.16221.

This site provides the most recent UK guidelines (2020) on the management of iron deficiency in pregnancy. The interested reader can obtain specific details of iron deficiency anaemia and treatment.

https://www.who.int/publications/i/item/9789240000124

This WHO site provides global, evidence-informed recommendations on the use of indicators for assessing a population's iron status and application of the use of ferritin concentrations for monitoring and evaluating iron interventions. The recommendations are intended for a wide audience, including health professionals, clinicians, researchers and public health policy-makers.

17

The Cardiovascular System

JEAN RANKIN

This chapter details the cardiovascular system. This includes the anatomy and physiology of the heart and the circulatory system. The maternal adaptations to the cardiovascular system during and following pregnancy are described.

Introduction

The cardiovascular system (CVS) consists of the heart and blood vessels. The system is designed to meet the crucial homeostatic needs of the cells and tissues by maintaining an adequate blood supply during varying physiological circumstances. For instance, blood can be preferentially directed to individual body systems as required. Flow increases to the muscles during exercise and to the gastro-intestinal system after food intake. Centres in the brain control the CVS, although local events and reflexes may modify the end result.

There are three main roles for the CVS:
1. Delivery of nutrients and oxygen.
2. Removal of metabolic waste and carbon dioxide.
3. Dissipation of heat from active tissues and redistribution of heat around the body.

Circulatory Pathways

Blood flows through a network of blood vessels extending between the heart and peripheral tissues. The circulation of blood can be subdivided into two distinct circuits, which both begin and end in the heart. The **pulmonary circulation** takes deoxygenated blood from the right side of the heart to the lungs and returns oxygenated blood from the lungs to the left side of the heart. The **systemic circulation** takes oxygenated blood from the left side of the heart to all the tissues and returns deoxygenated blood to the right side of the heart. Exchange of nutrients and metabolic waste products takes place in the systemic circulation. In a normal adult at rest, the amount of blood circulated through the heart is 5 L/min.

The force required to move blood around the body comes from the heart, which is essentially two separate pumps: the left side supplies the systemic circulation, and the right side supplies the pulmonary circulation. As a general principle, veins carry blood *to* the heart. Therefore, veins carry oxygenated blood in the pulmonary circulatory system and deoxygenated blood in the systemic veins (Fig. 17.1). Arteries carry blood *away* from the heart. Therefore, arteries carry deoxygenated blood in the pulmonary circulatory system and oxygenated blood in the systemic circulation.

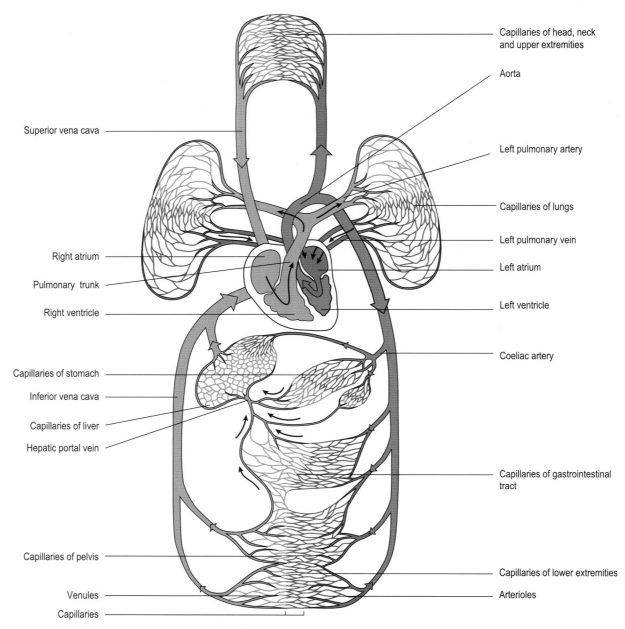

Capillaries of head, neck and upper extremities

Aorta

Left pulmonary artery

Capillaries of lungs

Left pulmonary vein

Left atrium

Left ventricle

Coeliac artery

Capillaries of gastrointestinal tract

Capillaries of lower extremities

Arterioles

Superior vena cava

Right atrium

Pulmonary trunk

Right ventricle

Capillaries of stomach

Inferior vena cava

Capillaries of liver

Hepatic portal vein

Capillaries of pelvis

Venules

Capillaries

• **Fig. 17.1** A general plan of the circulatory system.

Anatomy of the Heart

Description

The heart lies in the mediastinum of the thoracic cavity between the two lungs enclosed in their pleural sacs. It is positioned with two-thirds of its mass to the left of the body's midline. It is shaped like a blunt cone with its apex pointing downwards and to the left. The heart covers about 12–14 cm from the second to the fifth intercostal space. The base of the heart points upwards towards the right shoulder and is about 9 cm wide. The adult heart normally weighs about 300 g.

Layers

The myocardium, endocardium and pericardium make up the three layers of the heart.

The **myocardium,** or contractile wall of the heart, consists mainly of cardiac muscle. Connective tissue forms a dense fibrous network which reinforces the myocardium and anchors the muscle fibres. This network limits the spread of electrical action potentials to specific pathways.

The inner lining, or **endocardium,** consists of squamous epithelium resting on connective tissue. This also covers the valves and the tendons that hold them in place. It is continuous with the endothelial lining of the blood vessels entering the heart.

The heart is enclosed in a fibroserous sac called the **pericardium,** which protects it and anchors it to the large blood vessels, diaphragm and sternal wall. It has two layers: an outer fibrous layer and an inner serous pericardium. The serous pericardium is also composed of two layers: the outer parietal layer and the inner visceral layer

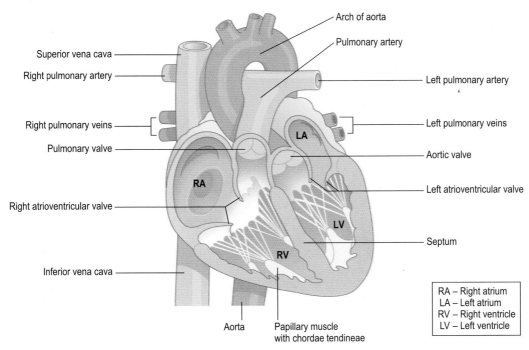

Superior vena cava

Right pulmonary artery

Right pulmonary veins

Pulmonary valve

RA

Right atrioventricular valve

Inferior vena cava

Aorta Papillary muscle with chordae tendineae

Arch of aorta

Pulmonary artery

Left pulmonary artery

Left pulmonary veins

LA

Aortic valve

Left atrioventricular valve

LV

Septum

RV

RA – Right atrium
LA – Left atrium
RV – Right ventricle
LV – Left ventricle

• **Fig. 17.2** The interior of the heart.

next to the myocardium called the **epicardium.** Between the visceral and parietal layers of the serous pericardium is the **pericardial cavity,** which is filled with **pericardial fluid.** This fluid provides a friction-free area within which the heart can pump.

Chambers and Valves

There are four **chambers** in the heart: two superior atria and two inferior ventricles (Fig. 17.2). The right ventricle forms most of the anterior surface of the heart, and the left and largest ventricle forms the apex and the inferior posterior aspect of the heart. These chambers are separated by valves and septa: the interatrial septum and the interventricular septum. The valves are attached to papillary muscles by the **chordae tendinae,** which anchor them in the closed position. The valves direct and control the flow of blood through the heart by opening as the associated chamber contracts and closing as the chamber relaxes. The valves ensure a one-way flow of blood through the heart.

The Atrioventricular Valves

The **tricuspid** valve separates the right atrium from the right ventricle. The **mitral** or **bicuspid** valve separates the left atrium from the left ventricle.

The Semilunar Valves

The **pulmonary** valve separates the right ventricle from the pulmonary artery. The **aortic** valve separates the left ventricle and the aorta.

The Coronary Circulation

Oxygen is carried to the cardiac muscle by the right and left coronary arteries, which originate from the aorta just beyond the aortic valve. The right coronary artery supplies the right atrium, right ventricle and portions of the left ventricle. The left coronary artery divides near its origin into:
- The left anterior descending branch, supplying the anterior part of the left ventricle and a small part of the right ventricle.
- The circumflex branch, which supplies blood to the left atrium and upper left ventricle.

Blood returns from the left side of the heart to the right atrium via the coronary sinus, and blood returns from the right side of the heart via small anterior cardiac veins.

Pulmonary and Systemic Circulations

The **pulmonary circulation** takes deoxygenated blood from the right atrium to the lungs via the pulmonary trunk, which divides into two pulmonary arteries with one directed to each lung. The arteries further subdivide until the capillary level where they unite into venules and then veins. Oxygenated blood is then returned to the left atrium from the lungs via four pulmonary veins. Fig. 17.3 shows the direction of blood flow through the heart.

In the **systemic circulation,** oxygenated blood leaves the left ventricle via the aorta and is diverted to all the tissues and cells around the body through smaller arteries and arterioles. At tissue level the blood reaches capillaries, merging with venules to form veins. These veins unite to return deoxygenated blood to the right atrium through two large

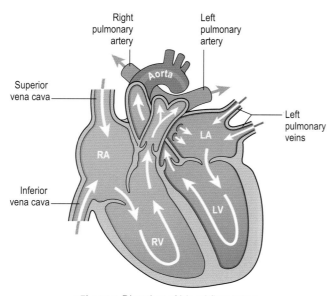

• **Fig. 17.3** Direction of blood flow taken.

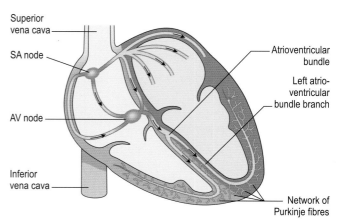

• **Fig. 17.4** The conducting system of the heart.

veins called the venae cavae: the inferior vena cava collects blood from the lower body, and the superior vena cava collects blood from the upper body.

Physiology of the Heart

Cardiac muscle combines properties of both skeletal and smooth muscle (see Chapter 25). It is striated like skeletal muscle, but the individual muscle cell membranes have very low electrical resistance. Structures called **intercalated discs** allow action potentials to pass easily from one cardiac muscle cell to another so that the muscle mass can function in unison. Intercalated discs contain anchoring units called **desmosomes** to hold the fibres together. Gap junctions between the muscle cells allow easy movement of ions to facilitate the spread of action potentials. The action potential is prolonged, allowing the electrical impulse to travel over the whole atrial and ventricular mass so that the cardiac muscle contracts as a unit. There is then a prolonged refractory period where the relaxation phase occurs, and no further contraction can begin. This is when the heart chambers refill with blood.

Both atria contract together, propelling blood into each ventricle. Both ventricles then contract together, propelling blood into the pulmonary and systemic circulations. As the atria contract, the ventricles are relaxed so they can fill up with blood. As the ventricles contract, the atria are relaxed and fill up with blood ready for the next cycle.

The Electrical Conducting System (Nodal System)

The electrical conducting system of the heart has the following components (Fig. 17.4):
- Sinoatrial (SA) node.
- Atrioventricular (AV) node.
- AV bundle of His.
- Left and right branch bundles.
- Purkinje fibres.

The **SA node,** located in the right atrium, initiates the action potential that causes contraction. It then spreads through both atria and enters the **AV node** at the base of the right atrium. This, plus the **bundle of His,** provides the only conduction link to the ventricles. There is a 0.1-s delay in conduction, allowing the atria to complete contracting and emptying their blood into the ventricles. The wave now spreads via the left and right branch bundles, which lie on either side of the interventricular septum, to the **Purkinje fibres** and the ventricular muscle. The spread is simultaneous, and there is coordinated contraction.

The Cardiac Cycle

The **cardiac cycle** is taken from the end of one contraction to the end of the next (Fig. 17.5). It produces two distinct sounds in a single beat, 'lub-dup'. The first heart sound is produced by the closure of the AV valves at the beginning of ventricular contraction, or **systole.** The second sound is produced by the closure of the semilunar valves at the beginning of ventricular relaxation, or **diastole.** The **heart rate** (HR) is the number of cycles or beats per minute (bpm). Each cardiac cycle lasts approximately 0.8 s with approximately 0.4 s being in systole and 0.4 s in diastole.

Control of the Heart Rate

Intrinsic Control

The intrinsic conduction system of the heart allows the heart muscle to beat on its own with no external control. The heart's electrical conduction system has **autorhythmicity.** The SA node acts as a pacemaker and in the absence of any nervous or hormonal influences initiates a rate of 100 bpm. Other parts of the conducting system also have autorhythmicity. The unopposed AV node can initiate a rate of 40–60 bpm, and the rest of the system will initiate a rate of 15–40 bpm.

Extrinsic Control

HR can also be externally influenced by the autonomic nervous system, hormones such as adrenaline (epinephrine), stretching the atria, temperature and drugs.

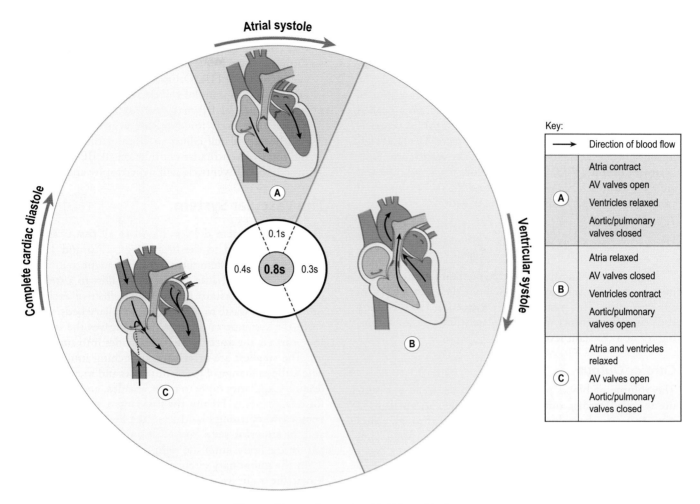

Atrial systole

Complete cardiac diastole

Ventricular systole

0.1s

0.4s **0.8s** 0.3s

Key:

	Direction of blood flow
Ⓐ	Atria contract AV valves open Ventricles relaxed Aortic/pulmonary valves closed
Ⓑ	Atria relaxed AV valves closed Ventricles contract Aortic/pulmonary valves open
Ⓒ	Atria and ventricles relaxed AV valves open Aortic/pulmonary valves closed

• **Fig. 17.5** The cardiac cycle. *AV*, Atrioventricular.

Nervous Control

In the medulla oblongata, the **cardiovascular centre (CVC)** receives input from baroreceptors, chemoreceptors and higher centres in the brain such as the cortex and hypothalamus. The CVC can be subdivided into the **cardiac centre,** affecting heart function, and the **vasomotor centre,** affecting blood vessels, but these probably function interactively. The CVC sends both sympathetic fibres and parasympathetic fibres (from the vagus nerve) to the heart (SA and AV nodes and myocardium) and blood vessels. Activity in these fibres is essential for controlling blood pressure (BP) (Table 17.1). The parasympathetic influence, dominant at rest, is sometimes known as the **vagal brake.** This explains why a normal resting HR averages 70 bpm compared with the unopposed SA node rate of 100 bpm.

Hormonal Control

Adrenaline (epinephrine) stimulates β_1 receptors in cardiac muscle and causes the HR to increase in response to stress. The hormones noradrenaline (norepinephrine) and thyroid hormone also enhance the effect of the sympathetic nervous system to increase HR.

TABLE 17.1	The Influence of the Autonomic Nervous System on the Heart and Blood Vessels	
	Sympathetic Stimulation	**Parasympathetic Stimulation**
Heart	Increases rate Increases strength of cardiac contraction	Reduces rate Reduces strength of cardiac contraction
Blood vessels (BVs)	Most BVs constrict Arteries supplying skeletal muscles and the brain dilate	Most BVs do not have parasympathetic blood supply

Stretch

Stretching of the atrial walls can be caused by increased venous return or increased blood volume. Atrial stretching can increase the HR by 10–15%. This is the **Bainbridge reflex** and occurs because the stretch receptors in the atrial walls send impulses to stimulate sympathetic output.

Stroke Volume

Excess blood also stretches the ventricles (**ventricular end-diastolic volume** (VEDV)). The more the ventricles are stretched before contraction, the greater the force of contraction and the greater the amount of blood leaving the heart. This is **Starling's law of the heart.** The amount of blood leaving each ventricle during one contraction is called the **stroke volume** (SV) and is normally 70 mL. A ventricle does not empty completely when it contracts. The blood left in the ventricle at the end of systole is the **ventricular end-systolic volume** (VESV). Typical values for an adult at rest are SV = 70 mL, VEDV = 135 mL and VESV = 65 mL, and can be represented by the following equation:

(Eqn. 17.1)

$$SV = VEDV - VESV$$

In good health, adding the atrial contents to the remaining blood in the ventricle brings about the extra VEDV of the next cycle. This increases the contraction force, causing the ventricle to empty more completely and thus maintaining SV at a constant level.

Cardiac Output

The volume of blood pumped by each ventricle per minute is called cardiac output (CO), usually expressed in L/min. It is also the volume of blood flowing through either the systemic or pulmonary circuit per minute. The CO is determined by multiplying the HR (the number of beats per minute (bpm)), by the stroke volume (blood ejected by each ventricle with each beat):

(Eqn. 17.2)

$$CO = HR \times SV$$

If each ventricle has a rate of 72 bpm and ejects 70 mL of blood with each beat, then the CO is 5.0 L/min as calculated in Equation (17.2):

$$CO = 72 \text{ bpm} \times 0.07 \text{ L} / \text{beat} = 5.0 \text{ L} / \text{min}$$

These are the approximate values for a healthy adult at rest. Because the total blood volume is also approximately 5 L, this means that essentially all the blood is pumped around the circuit once each minute. CO may reach 35 L/min in well-trained athletes during periods of strenuous exercise (i.e., total blood volume pumped around the circuit seven times a minute). Sedentary individuals can reach COs of 20–25 L/min. The difference between the CO at rest and the *potential* CO is called the **cardiac reserve.**

In response to being stretched, the atria secrete a hormone called **atrial natriuretic factor** or **atrial natriuretic peptide** (ANP). This is a potent diuretic that causes the kidney to excrete excess sodium and water, resulting in a decrease in blood volume and BP.

Other Influences

- Alterations in core body temperature influence HR: i.e., an increase in HR with an increase in temperature and a lowering of core temperature will decrease the HR. This latter is seen in people with hypothermia. Body temperature changes alter the rate of electrical discharge.
- Drugs such as isoprenaline or adrenaline (epinephrine) can increase the HR. Drugs acting as β-adrenergic blockers such as propranolol will decrease the HR.
- A raised arterial BP may decrease SV because the ventricles must exert force against a greater load. A normal heart will self-adjust to counter this by increasing the force of ventricular contraction. If BP is chronically raised, the left ventricle will hypertrophy and fail.

The Vascular System

The vascular system delivers blood to all tissues as needed and returns blood to the heart (Figs. 17.6 and 17.7). To achieve this, the system must be able to adapt to local needs. A change from pulsatile arterial blood flow to a steady capillary flow is necessary to allow the effective exchange of nutrients and waste to occur at the capillary beds.

In the systemic circulation, blood leaves the left side of the heart via the **aorta,** which subdivides into smaller arteries. The smallest are **arterioles,** branching into **capillaries** where the exchange of gases, nutrients and metabolic wastes occurs. Capillaries unite to form **venules,** and these unite to form larger veins. Finally, the two largest veins, the **inferior vena cava** returning blood from the lower part of the body and the **superior vena cava** returning blood from the upper part of the body, enter the right atrium of the heart.

In the pulmonary circulation, a single pulmonary artery leaves the right ventricle and divides into two branches, which deliver deoxygenated blood returning from the tissues to each lung for oxygenation. The division into smaller arteries, arterioles, capillaries, venules and veins is the same as in the systemic circulation. Four pulmonary veins deliver oxygenated blood back to the left atrium.

Structure of Blood Vessels

The structure of the blood vessels varies depending on their specific functions, but the walls of the blood vessels (except for capillaries) contain the same three layers of tissue (Fig. 17.8):

1. **Tunica intima** is the innermost layer, called the *endothelium,* which is a single layer of extremely flattened epithelial cells. A basement membrane and some connective and elastic tissue support this layer (which is only found in capillaries).
2. **Tunica media** is the middle layer and consists mainly of smooth muscle and elastic tissue. This is the layer that gives rise to the variation throughout the vascular system.
3. **Tunica adventitia** is the outer layer and is composed of fibrous connective tissue, collagen and fibroblasts.

The Arterial System
Elastic Arteries (Conducting Arteries)

Large arteries contain more elastic tissue and can passively expand and recoil to accommodate changes in blood volume. This allows blood to be kept under continuous pressure rather than starting and stopping with the pulsatile

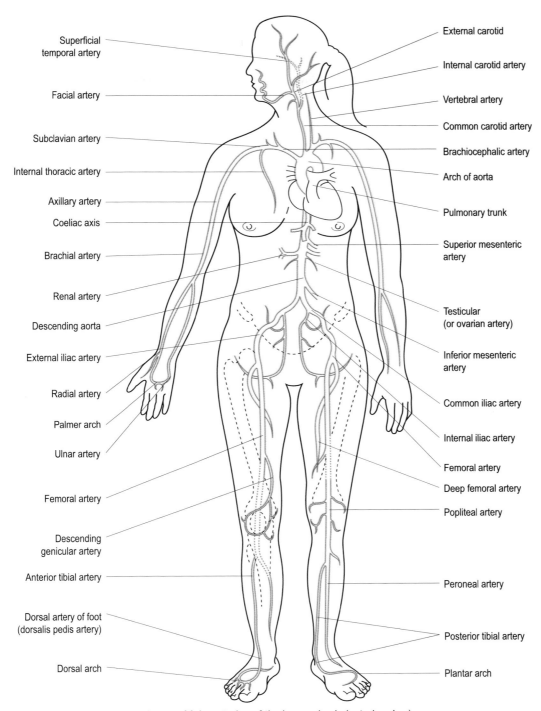

Superficial temporal artery

Facial artery

Subclavian artery

Internal thoracic artery

Axillary artery

Coeliac axis

Brachial artery

Renal artery

Descending aorta

External iliac artery

Radial artery

Palmer arch

Ulnar artery

Femoral artery

Descending genicular artery

Anterior tibial artery

Dorsal artery of foot (dorsalis pedis artery)

Dorsal arch

External carotid

Internal carotid artery

Vertebral artery

Common carotid artery

Brachiocephalic artery

Arch of aorta

Pulmonary trunk

Superior mesenteric artery

Testicular (or ovarian artery)

Inferior mesenteric artery

Common iliac artery

Internal iliac artery

Femoral artery

Deep femoral artery

Popliteal artery

Peroneal artery

Posterior tibial artery

Plantar arch

• **Fig. 17.6** Major arteries of the human body (anterior view).

heartbeat. When the heart contracts, blood is forced into the aorta and distends these vessels. When the heart rests, the large arteries return to their normal diameters. They have large diameters: that of the aorta is about 2.5 cm.

Muscular Arteries (Distributing Arteries)

These medium-sized arteries distribute blood to all tissues. They have an average diameter of about 0.4 cm and remain distensible so that resistance to flow is low. As they branch farther and become smaller, the amount of elastic tissue decreases and the smooth muscle component increases.

Arterioles

Arterioles are the smallest arteries, less than 0.3 cm in diameter, with a thicker wall mainly composed of muscle tissue in concentric layers. The total resistance to blood flow is mainly determined by the diameter of the arterioles. The **precapillary sphincters** are specialized regions near the junction between the terminal arterioles and the capillaries. They consist of smooth muscle fibres arranged in a circular manner around the vessels, controlling the amount of blood flowing into a capillary bed.

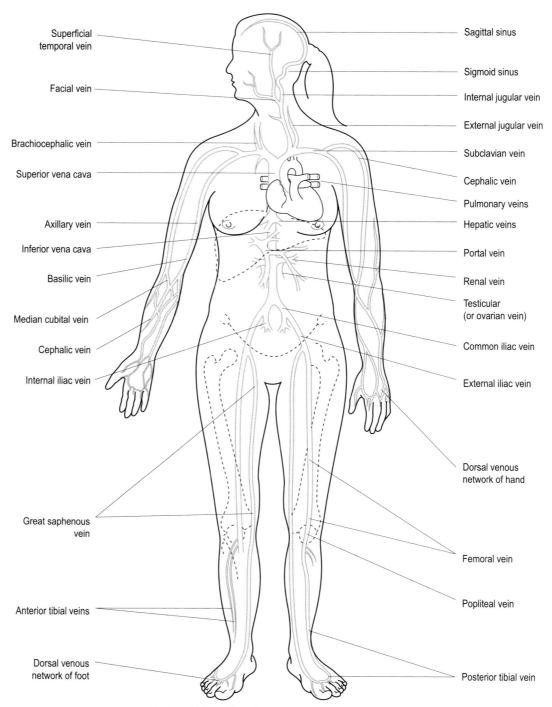

Superficial temporal vein

Facial vein

Brachiocephalic vein

Superior vena cava

Axillary vein

Inferior vena cava

Basilic vein

Median cubital vein

Cephalic vein

Internal iliac vein

Great saphenous vein

Anterior tibial veins

Dorsal venous network of foot

Sagittal sinus

Sigmoid sinus

Internal jugular vein

External jugular vein

Subclavian vein

Cephalic vein

Pulmonary veins

Hepatic veins

Portal vein

Renal vein

Testicular (or ovarian vein)

Common iliac vein

External iliac vein

Dorsal venous network of hand

Femoral vein

Popliteal vein

Posterior tibial vein

• **Fig. 17.7** Major veins of the human body (anterior view).

Capillaries

Capillaries form a dense network of very narrow short vessels with red blood cells passing through in single file. Capillaries are the exchange vessels where gases, nutrients and metabolic waste products pass between individual cells and the vascular system. Approximately 50 million capillaries are present in the body (only 25% may be patent at rest). Some modified, wider capillaries are known as **sinusoids.** They are found mainly in the liver, bone marrow, lymphoid tissues and endocrine organs. Blood flows slowly through sinusoids to allow modification of its content: for instance, in the liver when nutrients are extracted.

The Microcirculation

Each cell must have access to a capillary supply if it is to remain healthy. Substances need to travel a very short distance to enable adequate **diffusion.** Different tissues have varying amounts of capillaries, depending on their metabolic needs. There may also be **arteriovenous shunts,**

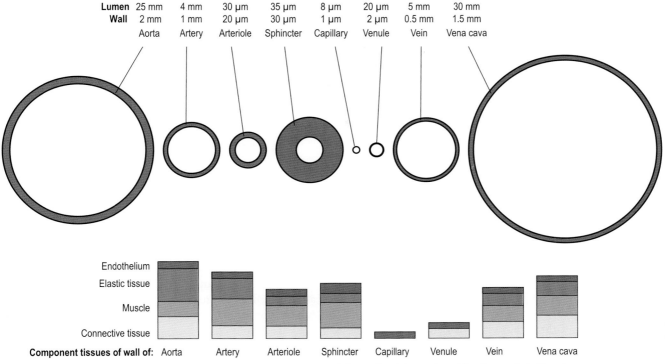

Lumen	25 mm	4 mm	30 μm	35 μm	8 μm	20 μm	5 mm	30 mm
Wall	2 mm	1 mm	20 μm	30 μm	1 μm	2 μm	0.5 mm	1.5 mm
	Aorta	Artery	Arteriole	Sphincter	Capillary	Venule	Vein	Vena cava

Endothelium
Elastic tissue
Muscle
Connective tissue
Component tissues of wall of: Aorta   Artery   Arteriole   Sphincter   Capillary   Venule   Vein   Vena cava

• **Fig. 17.8** The variations in size and components of the walls of the various blood vessels in the circulatory system.

connections between the arteries and veins that bypass the capillaries. Blood can flow rapidly through the shunts facilitating dissipation of heat from the body via the skin if needed.

The Venous System

Veins return blood from the capillary beds to the heart passively along a pressure gradient. As the veins become fewer and larger, resistance to flow decreases. Vein walls have the same three layers as arteries, but they are thinner and more distensible than arteries. Some veins, such as those in the legs, have folds in the endothelium which act as valves to ensure that blood flows in one direction towards the heart. These valves may be damaged if overstretched by high pressures (for instance, in pregnancy), and this may lead to oedema and varicose veins. The larger part of the circulating blood, about 60%, is contained in the venous system.

The Physiology of Circulation

Blood Vessel Diameter

Changes in blood vessel diameter regulate BP and blood flow to tissues. Altering the degree of smooth muscle contraction in the tunica media changes the blood vessel diameter. Increasing contraction of the circular muscle fibres reduces blood vessel diameter (**vasoconstriction**). When the muscle relaxes, the diameter increases (**vasodilation**). The smooth muscle of the blood vessel walls is normally in a state of contraction known as **vasomotor tone.** Control of the smooth muscle involves nervous and chemical factors.

Nervous Control

Sympathetic nerve fibres from the vasomotor centre innervate the smooth muscle in the tunica media with nerve discharge increasing muscle contraction and causing vasoconstriction. This increases total vascular resistance, increases venomotor tone and reduces venous capacity and venous return.

Chemical Control

Vascular smooth muscle is influenced by hormones and locally produced metabolites. Adrenaline (epinephrine) and noradrenaline (norepinephrine) cause vasoconstriction. Angiotensin II, formed by the action of renin (produced by the kidney) on angiotensinogen, is also a potent vasoconstrictor. Histamine and plasma kinins are released from inflamed local tissues and cause vasodilation of small vessels. Local prostaglandins may also be involved in vasodilation.

Endothelial-mediated Regulation

The endothelium produces a factor, **endothelial-derived relaxing factor**, that causes relaxation of vascular smooth muscle and vasodilation. Local chemical control becomes extremely important when there is a localized increase in metabolism. Local chemicals largely mediate control of circulation to the brain and the heart. A major factor is the level of oxygen in the blood. The blood flow to the skin is mainly under sympathetic nervous control.

Blood Pressure

The following facts about the nature of a fluid may help the reader to understand the concepts involved in BP.

Fluid Pressure

Hydrostatic pressure is the force a liquid exerts against the walls of its container. In the vascular system, this is the pressure the blood exerts on the blood vessel walls, which is called **blood pressure.** Pressure will also vary with the height of the liquid column and is related to gravity. In the standing position, the venous pressure in the feet is greater than that in the head. The distensibility of the container also influences hydrostatic pressure. This pressure is less in a distensible container compared with a rigid container. The heart generates a head of pressure that is highest in the aorta and falls throughout the vascular system along the path to the tissues.

Fluid Flow

The flow of a fluid through a vessel is determined by the pressure difference between the two ends of the vessel and the resistance to flow. **Resistance to flow** is a measure of the ease with which a fluid flows through a tube. In the vascular system, this is described as vascular resistance, but for practical purposes, most resistance is generated in the small peripheral vessels. This is referred to as **peripheral resistance** (PR). It is affected by:

- **Viscosity,** which is the thickness of a fluid. In blood, viscosity is affected by the ratio of red cells and plasma proteins to plasma fluid. Viscosity increases when there is an increase in cell content or a reduction in plasma fluid, such as in dehydration. An increase in plasma fluid will decrease viscosity. The greater the viscosity, the more force is required to move the fluid along the vessel.
- **Blood vessel length**—the longer the blood vessel, the greater the resistance to flow.
- **Arteriolar diameter**—small changes in diameter can lead to large changes in PR. The smaller the diameter, the greater the resistance.
- **The lining** also affects flow. A smooth lining in a blood vessel will create a smooth **laminar** flow, whilst a rough lining will cause a **turbulent** flow.

BP is the force exerted on the wall of a blood vessel by the blood it contains. It is measured in millimetres of mercury (mmHg). There are typical values for different parts of the vascular tree (i.e., arteries, capillaries, veins, etc.). These gradients facilitate blood flow around the systems. Pressures in the pulmonary circulation are lower than in the systemic circulation, but there is still a falling gradient from the right ventricle to the left atrium.

Venous Return

BP in the capillary beds is very low, so a mechanism is needed to ensure blood returns to the right atrium. BP in the venules is greater than that in the right atrium. Blood returning from the head is aided by gravity when in the upright position, and dizziness may occur due to a temporary reduction in brain blood supply if a person stands up too quickly. If venous return to the heart is impeded, CO will fall.

There are several mechanisms to ensure adequate blood flow:

- Increasing **venomotor tone** will reduce the capacity of the venous system.
- The **skeletal muscle pump**: contractions of the skeletal muscles, especially in the limbs, squeezes the veins and pushes the blood towards the heart. Venous valves prevent backflow most effectively when a person is walking. Standing still means the muscle pump cannot act and venous return is not as good (with the risk of fainting).
- The **respiratory pump**: as a person breathes in, pressure in the thorax and the right atrium is lowered, which increases the pressure gradient and assists venous return.

The arterial BP is of most value clinically because it ensures an adequate blood supply to the tissues. The main parameter affecting BP is the relationship between CO and PR. This can be represented by the following simple equation:

(Eqn. 17.3)

$$BP = CO \times PR$$

Arterial Blood Pressure

Arterial BP changes throughout the cardiac cycle. Contraction of the ventricles during systole ejects blood into the aorta and raises the arterial pressure. This is the **systolic pressure** and is determined by the stroke volume and the force of the contraction. Systolic pressure will be raised if the arterial walls are stiffer because the vessels cannot distend to accommodate the extra blood. As the heart relaxes during diastole, blood leaves the main arteries and BP falls. This is the **diastolic pressure,** which is affected by PR. Diastolic pressure, therefore, depends on the level of systolic pressure, the elasticity of the arteries and the viscosity of blood. If the HR is slow, diastolic pressure will fall as there is more time for extra blood to flow out of the artery. An increase in HR will raise the diastolic pressure.

Pulse Pressure and Mean Arterial Pressure

Each ventricular contraction initiates a pulse of pressure through the arteries. The difference between the systolic and diastolic pressure is called the **pulse pressure.** A typical BP would be 120/70 mmHg, giving a pulse pressure of 50 mmHg, i.e., $120 - 70 = 50$ mmHg.

An average or mean value for arterial pressure is useful as it represents the pressure driving the blood through the arteries. **Mean arterial pressure** (MAP) is more useful as a guide to tissue perfusion than the usual systolic/diastolic BP reading. It is estimated by:

(Eqn. 17.4)

$$MAP = \text{Diastolic pressure} + \text{one} - \text{third of the pulse pressure}$$

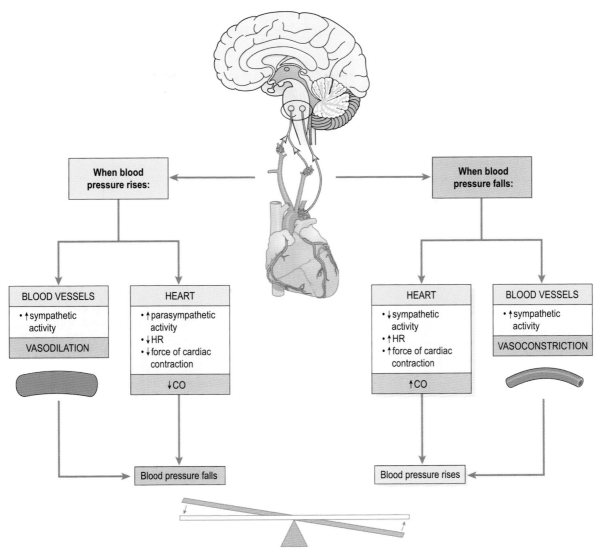

• **Fig. 17.9** The baroreceptor reflex. CO, Cardiac output; *HR*, heart rate.

For example, using Equation (17.4), a BP of 120/70 mmHg gives:

$$\text{MAP} = 70 + \left(\frac{1}{3} \text{ of } 50 \right) = 87 \text{ mmHg}$$

The Regulation of Blood Pressure

Neural, chemical and renal controls act to modify BP by influencing CO, PR and/or blood volume. Fig. 17.9 presents the baroreceptor reflex.

Neural System

The neural system can either alter blood distribution or maintain adequate systemic BP. The system operates by spinal reflex. The vasomotor centre sends sympathetic nerve impulses via vasomotor efferent fibres to the muscular walls of the arterial system and acts mainly on the arterioles. The more impulses from these neurons, the more constricted are the arterioles. The vasomotor centre activity is modified by baroreceptors and chemoreceptors.

Baroreceptors are situated in the tunica adventitia of the internal carotid artery (especially in the carotid sinus), the transverse section of the aortic arch and the largest vessels in the neck and thorax. These provide a short-term feedback mechanism responding to changes in posture and activity levels. Nerve fibres run from the baroreceptors via the glossopharyngeal cranial nerve (IX) and the vagal nerve (X). The nerve endings respond to stretching of the arterial wall. The normal action of these nerves on the CVC is inhibitory. They slow the HR and decrease the force of ventricular contraction, as well as causing arterial vasodilation.

Chemoreceptors are situated in the aortic arch and carotid bodies. They respond to a fall in blood oxygen or an

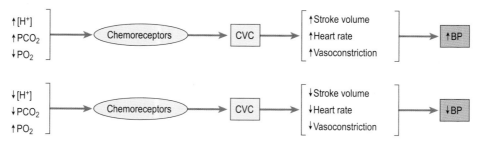

• **Fig. 17.10** The relationship between stimulation of chemoreceptors and arterial blood pressure. *BP*, Blood pressure; *CVC*, cardiovascular centre.

TABLE 17.2	Blood Pressure Values	
Age (years)	Systolic Blood Pressure (mmHg)	Diastolic Blood Pressure (mmHg)
Newborn	80	46
10	103	70
20	120	80
40	126	84
60	135	89

increase in blood acidity. The main effect is on the respiratory system, but in severe hypoxia they stimulate sympathetic activity, which increases HR and BP. Brain centres such as the cortex and the hypothalamus also affect BP. Fig. 17.10 shows the relationship between stimulation of chemoreceptors, CVC and arterial BP.

Chemical Control

Hormones from the adrenal medulla, namely adrenaline (epinephrine) and noradrenaline (norepinephrine), act to increase sympathetic activity (the flight or fight response). Antidiuretic hormone (from the posterior pituitary) is released into the circulation to retain fluid during pain and low BP. Some drugs such as morphine, alcohol and nicotine increase the blood volume by preventing renal excretion of fluid.

The Renal System

The kidneys respond to altered blood volume by altering the amount of urine excreted via the **renin–angiotensin mechanism** (see Chapters 19 and 20). A reduction in BP and kidney blood flow results in the excretion of renin by the kidney juxtaglomerular apparatus. Renin acts on angiotensinogen to release angiotensin I, which is then converted to angiotensin II by enzymes. Angiotensin II is a powerful vasoconstrictor and also triggers the release of aldosterone from the adrenal cortex to cause retention of sodium and increased excretion of potassium. Water is retained passively by the increased amount of sodium.

Blood Pressure Values

The range of BP values is highly variable between individuals and within an individual. This makes it difficult to quote normal BP for a population but easier for the typical value of an individual. Both physiological and genetic factors and a range of external influences can affect BP. It is more valuable to consider a normal range. Normal adult BP is between 90/60 mmHg and 140/90 mmHg (National Institute of Health and Care Excellence (NICE), 2022). BP readings from 250,000 healthy individuals presented in Table 17.2 illustrate the range.

The Formation of Tissue Fluid

In the tissues, blood contained in the capillaries is separated from both the interstitial fluid and intracellular fluid of the cells. Capillary walls consist of a single layer of endothelial cells resting on a basement membrane. Water and solutes diffuse to and from the blood and interstitial fluid. Although there is a high rate of substance diffusion between the two compartments, the fluid content of the plasma and the interstitial fluid changes very little. The volume of fluid moving out of the capillaries is equal to the amount returned. The hydrostatic pressure on each side of the capillary wall and the osmotic pressure of protein in the plasma and tissue fluid help to ensure this equilibrium.

Hydrostatic Pressure

Hydrostatic pressure is the force of water pushing against the cell membrane. In the vascular system it is generated by BP. In the capillaries, a hydrostatic pressure of 25 mmHg is sufficient to push water across the capillary membrane into the extracellular space. It is partly balanced by **osmotic pressure.** The excess water moves into the lymph system.

BP falls from the arteriolar end of the capillary to the venous end. Fluid, with its dissolved solutes, will also cross the capillary wall. It is forced out at the arteriolar end and returns in the blood at the venous end. Capillary hydrostatic pressure (HP_c) is higher at the arteriolar end (about 25–35 mmHg) than at the venous end (10–15 mmHg). Hydrostatic pressure in the interstitial space (HP_{if}) has usually been rated as 0

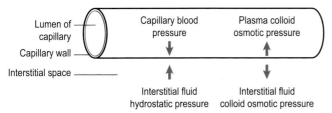

• Fig. 17.11 Forces affecting fluid movement across the capillary wall.

mmHg because there is very little fluid present. This is because most of it is drawn into the lymphatic system. This pressure may have a negative value of about –8 mmHg (Marieb & Hoehn, 2022). The net hydrostatic pressure is $HP_c – HP_{if}$.

Osmotic Pressure

Osmosis is the movement of water down a concentration gradient across a semipermeable membrane. The water moves from high water content to lower water content. Osmosis is directly related to hydrostatic pressure and solute concentration but not to particle size. Osmotic pressure is created by the presence of large non-diffusible substances in a fluid. In blood, this is provided by plasma proteins (mainly albumin molecules) that apply osmotic pressure if the water concentration surrounding them is lower than the water concentration on the opposite side of the capillary membrane. Capillary osmotic pressure (OP_c) is about 25 mmHg, whereas interstitial fluid, which contains few proteins, has a much lower pressure at $OP_{if} = 0.1–5$ mmHg. The net osmotic pressure is $OP_c – OP_{if}$. The forces affecting fluid movement across the capillary wall are shown in Fig. 17.11.

Fluid will leave the capillary where the net hydrostatic pressure is greater than the net osmotic pressure. Hydrostatic forces dominate at the arteriolar end at about 35 mmHg, whereas net osmotic pressure is about 25 mmHg (+10 mmHg). Osmotic pressure dominates at the venous end of the capillary with a net hydrostatic pressure of 13 mmHg and a net osmotic pressure of 23 mmHg (–10 mmHg). Therefore fluid is forced out of the circulation at the arteriolar end of the capillary beds and forced back in at the venous end.

Diffusion

Movement of substances always occurs along a concentration gradient, from high to low concentration. Oxygen and nutrients will pass from blood to the interstitial fluid and then to cells. Carbon dioxide and waste products of metabolism will flow from the cells into the capillary blood to be eliminated from the body.

Maternal Adaptations to Pregnancy

During pregnancy, physiologically significant but reversible changes occur in the maternal cardiovascular system (Blackburn, 2018). A series of adaptive mechanisms are activated early in pregnancy, possibly as early as 5 weeks. These changes are necessary to meet the extra maternal and fetal demands imposed by pregnancy (Coad, Pedley and Dunstall, 2019). The uteroplacental circulation allows the exchange of gases, nutrients and waste products between mother and fetus. The fetal requirements place an increased load on the CVS, added to by the increased circulating blood mass, placental circulatory system and gradual increase in bodyweight (Broughton Pipkin, 2018). Changes are normally tolerated well, but if CVS disease exists the changes could be hazardous for the mother and fetus. On the other hand, no change occurring could compromise fetal health, as there may be a possible link between low blood volume and poor fetal growth.

Haemodynamic Changes

The timing of the adaptive mechanisms and other changes in maternal physiology remains an enigma as to why the changes are initiated early in pregnancy before there is any physiological need for them. Current evidence suggests that the hormonal and immunological alterations act together very early to begin the process of haemodynamic adaptation. The most important haemodynamic changes during pregnancy include the increase in blood volume and CO and the decrease in PR (Broughton Pipkin, 2018). Other changes occur in the position and size of the heart, HR, stroke volume and distribution of blood flow (Blackburn, 2018). The major physiological changes that occur during pregnancy are outlined in Table 17.3. Changes in HR, CO and BP during pregnancy are presented in Fig. 17.12. The effects of the regional redistribution of blood flow are detailed in Box 17.1.

Size and Position of the Heart

As pregnancy progresses, the heart is pushed upwards by the elevation of the diaphragm and rotated forward so that the apex is moved upwards and laterally, appearing in the fourth rather than the fifth intercostal space. The heart volume increases from 70 to 80 mL (about 12%) between early and late pregnancy. There is little increase in wall thickness, and the increased venous filling increases the heart size rather than muscle hypertrophy.

All four chambers of the heart enlarge, with the most change noted in the left atrium (Blackburn, 2018). The increase in atrial size related to the increase in venous return has been associated with more production of ANP in pregnancy. ANP has a diuretic effect, and this helps cope with the increased blood volume of pregnancy. During pregnancy there is an enhanced myocardial performance with a slight increase in myometrial contractility, probably due to lengthening of the myocardial muscle fibres.

HR is the determinant of CO that has the widest range of values from rest to maximal exercise, providing the circulatory system with stability (Broughton Pipkin, 2018). HR rises synchronously so the CO begins to rise. As pregnancy progresses, a possible fall in baroreflex sensitivity results in HR variability

TABLE 17.3	Physiological Changes of Pregnancy on the Cardiovascular System		
Parameter	Modification	Magnitude	Time of Peak Increase or Decrease
Oxygen consumption (VO_2)	Increase	+20–30%	Term
Plasma	Increase	+40–60% (usually 45–0%)	32 weeks. By third trimester, PV has increased from its baseline by ~50% (first pregnancy) and 60% (subsequent pregnancies).
Red blood cells	Increase	+20–30%	30–32 weeks
Total body water	Increase	+6–8 L	Term
TPR SVR PVR	Decreases Decreases Decreases	−20–30% −20–25% Varies	All decrease in resistance starts in early pregnancy (~5–6 weeks) reaching lowest point (nadir) around mid-pregnancy.
Blood pressure (SVR × CO)*: Systolic Diastolic	Systolic–slight or no decrease Diastolic–decrease	10–15 mmHg	16–34 weeks 34 weeks
Myocardial contractility HR (*Chronotropism – increases HR*) SV (*Inotropism – increases contractility*)	Increase Increase by 10–15 bpm Increase	+0–20% +25–30%	28–32 weeks 16–24 weeks A fall in baroreflex sensitivity may be due to HR variability falling as pregnancy progresses. SV rises a later in first trimester.
CO (HR × SV)*	Increase	+30–50%	28–32 weeks (increases during labour)
Uteroplacental circulation	Increase	Greater than 1000%	Term

*Positional.

CO, Cardiac output; *HR*, heart rate; *PV*, plasma volume; *SV*, stroke volume; *SVR*, systemic vascular resistance; *TPR*, total peripheral resistance.
Adapted from: Blackburn, S.T., 2018; Pipkin, B.F., 2018.

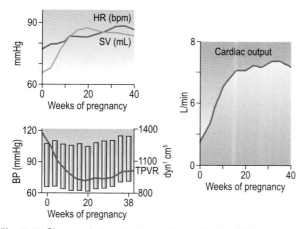

• **Fig. 17.12** Changes in heart rate, cardiac output and blood pressure during pregnancy. *BP*, Blood pressure; *HR*, heart rate; *SV*, stroke volume; *TPVR*, total peripheral vascular resistance.

falling. Stroke volume rises later in the first trimester. HR and SV together push the cardiac output up by 35–40% in a first pregnancy and by about 50% in subsequent pregnancies. Twin pregnancies have an earlier acceleration in HR with a maximum increase at term of 40% above non-pregnant levels and a greater increase in CO. The growing uterus provides the

primary influence on changes in CO with selected maternal positions. A change from the left lateral recumbent position to supine position can lead to a 25–30% decrease in CO (Bamber, 2003). In the supine position, the uterine mass compresses the inferior vena cava, leading to this decrease in CO (Higuchi et al., 2015). This syndrome, referred to as **supine hypotension,** is associated with acute haemodynamic changes including increased HR and stroke volume in response to reduced venous return and decreased output (Blackburn, 2018). There is somewhat less compression of the vena cava in the sitting position, and the most favourable position for venous return is the lateral recumbent position.

During the labour experience, forceful uterine contractions accompanied by pain and anxiety may result in significant haemodynamic changes and CVS activity. Changes result from the release of catecholamines and increased systemic vascular tone (Blackburn, 2018). These transient changes settle down following delivery. Most of the CVS changes noted during pregnancy have resolved by 6–8 weeks postpartum.

Control of Cardiovascular Changes

Control of CVS changes is partly hormonal, with increased circulating levels of oestrogen, progesterone and

• BOX 17.1   The Effects of Regional Distribution of Increased Blood Flow

Uterus

- Increased circulation of pregnancy targets the uterus. It is difficult to estimate blood flow to the placental site due to inaccessibility of the uterus and the complex blood supply.
- The uterine vascular bed is widely dilated so that oxygen consumption is dealt with by increases in extraction rather than increased blood flow.
- Both steroid hormones and the renin–angiotensin system may contribute to the uterine blood flow of pregnancy.

Kidneys

- Increase in blood flow in early pregnancy (approx. 400 mL/min above non-pregnant levels).
- This may fall towards the end of pregnancy (see Chapter 19).

Skin

- Blood flow to the skin, particularly that of the hands and feet, is greatly increased in pregnancy.
- Increased temperature in fingers and toes. Women feel warmer.

Liver

- Research evidence relating to increased blood flow through the liver is not clear. It may be due to the increased metabolic rate during pregnancy (see Chapter 23).

Breasts

- Increased mammary blood flow with increased temperature (see Chapter 54).

Peripheral Vasodilation

- Increased supply to the hands with increased fingernail growth.
- Increased supply to the nasal mucous membrane with increased nasal congestion. Nose bleeds may occur, as does increased snoring.
- Increased supply to hair affecting rate of hair growth.
- Non-pregnant women have 85% of hairs actively growing with 15% in resting stage before falling out.
- During pregnancy, women have 95% of hairs in the growing stage. By the end of pregnancy there is an increased number of over-aged hairs ready to fall out. This leads to the common anxiety of hair coming out 'in handfuls'.

• BOX 17.2   Exercise and the Cardiovascular System

Pregnancy is unique as it involves significant maternal anatomical and physiological adaptations. This situation raises questions in the ways pregnancy alters a woman's ability to exercise and to what extent exercise influences pregnancy and outcomes. Many studies have investigated the additional impact that exercise has on the changes normally occurring in the body during pregnancy. Physiological responses to exercise include a redistribution of blood, changes in cardiac output and stroke volume, increased oxygen consumption and alterations in venous pooling. Review of study findings indicate uterine blood flow is reduced by exercise, and evidence based on animal and human studies suggests that the fetus may experience transient hypoxia resulting in a reduction in the fetal heart rate during maternal exercise. Population data with self-reported exercise frequency and intensity have shown improved pregnancy outcomes, less gestational weight gain, fewer caesarean deliveries, less gestational diabetes and less pre-eclampsia (Newton & May, 2017).

Review of controlled trials indicated that regular aerobic exercise during pregnancy appears to improve (or maintain) physical fitness and body image (Kramer & McDonald, 2006); diet and/or exercise during pregnancy may prevent excessive weight gain during pregnancy (Muktabhant et al., 2015), whilst diet combined with exercise may help women lose weight after childbirth (Amorim-Adegboye & Linne, 2013). Further high-quality evidence is required to establish more convincing findings.

Regular physical activity in all phases of life, including pregnancy, promotes health benefits. To date, there is insufficient data of the physiological parameters to infer important maternal or fetal risks or benefits. The level of intensity associated with exercise suggests an important margin of safety is essential for pregnant women who are less healthy, i.e., overweight, unfit, or have mild hypertension or gestational diabetes. Available evidence supports a monitored stepwise increase in physical activity to decrease adverse pregnancy outcomes (Newton & May, 2017).

Based on current research, physical exercise and sport can be recommended during pregnancy so long as women are aware of the contraindications and follow guidelines for safe exercise (Mota and Bø, 2020; Royal College of Obstetricians and Gynaecologists (RCOG), 2017; World Health Organization (WHO), 2022). Women with uncomplicated pregnancies should be encouraged to engage in aerobic and strength-conditioning exercise before, during and after pregnancy.

prostaglandins, and partly mechanical, with changes of growth and development of organs necessitating increased blood supply. Vasodilation of peripheral blood vessels is the primary haemodynamic alteration, followed by increases in circulating blood volume and CO. An increase in physical activity levels has an impact on the CVS. Box 17.2 provides an overview of the current knowledge related to exercise during pregnancy.

Main Points

- The CVS has three main roles: delivery of nutrients and oxygen; removal of metabolic waste and carbon dioxide; and distribution of heat around the body. Blood flows in two distinct circuits: the pulmonary circulation and the systemic circulation.
- The myocardium (middle and contractile layer), endocardium (inner layer) and pericardium (outer layer) make up the three layers of the heart. The heart has four chambers, two superior atria and two inferior ventricles, separated by septa and valves. Valves direct and control the flow of blood through the heart.
- The cardiac cycle is taken from the end of one contraction to the end of the next and lasts 0.8 s. CO is about 5 L/min increasing to 35 L/min under extreme conditions.
- The structure of blood vessels depends on their specific functions. Muscle contraction will bring about vasoconstriction, and muscle relaxation causes vasodilation.
- The flow of a fluid through a vessel is determined by the pressure difference between the two ends of the vessel and the resistance to flow.
- BP (mmHg) is the force exerted on the wall of a blood vessel by its contained blood. The main parameter affecting BP is the relationship between CO and PR ($BP = CO \times PR$).
- Contraction of the ventricles during systole ejects blood into the aorta and pulmonary artery and raises the arterial pressure (systolic pressure).
- Neural, chemical and renal controls modify BP by influencing CO, PR and/or blood volume.
- In pregnancy, the maternal CVS changes to meet the demands of the fetus. The most important changes are increase in blood volume, increased CO and reduced PR.
- CO is increased by 30–50% during pregnancy, reaching peak levels between 28 and 32 weeks.
- The increased circulation of pregnancy mainly targets the uterus.
- Control of CVS changes is partly hormonal and partly mechanical, as changes in growth and development of organs necessitate increased blood supply.
- The woman's physiological response to exercise includes changes in CO, redistribution of blood, increased oxygen consumption and alterations in venous pooling.

References

Adegboye, A.R., Linne, Y.M., 2013. Diet or exercise, or both, for weight reduction in women after childbirth. Cochrane Database Syst. Rev. 2013 (7), CD005627.

Bamber, J.H., 2003. Aortacaval compression in pregnancy: the effect of changing the degree and direction of lateral tilt on maternal cardiac output. Anesth. Analg. 97 (1), 256–258.

Blackburn, S.T., 2018. Maternal, Fetal and Neonatal Physiology: A Clinical Perspective, fifth ed. Elsevier, Philadelphia.

Coad, J., Pedley, K., Dunstall, M., 2019. Anatomy and Physiology for Midwives, fourth ed. Elsevier, London.

Higuchi, H., Takagi, S., Zhang, K., Furui, I., Ozaki, M., 2015. Effect of lateral tilt angle on the volume of the abdominal aorta and inferior vena cava in pregnant and nonpregnant women determined by magnetic resonance imaging. Anesthesiology 122 (2), 286–293.

Kramer, M.S., McDonald, S.W., 2006. Aerobic exercise for women during pregnancy. Cochrane Database Syst. Rev. 2006 (3), CD000180.

Marieb, E.N., Hoehn, K., 2022. Human Anatomy and Physiology, twelfth ed. Pearson, Harlow.

Mota, P., Bø, K., 2020. ACOG Committee Opinion No. 804: physical activity and exercise during pregnancy and the postpartum period. Obstet. Gynecol. 137 (2), 376.

Muktabhant, B., Lawrie, T.A., Lumbiganon, P., Laopaiboon, M., 2015. Diet or exercise, or both, for preventing excessive weight gain in pregnancy. Cochrane Database Syst. Rev. 2015 (6), CD007145.

National Institute of Health and Care Excellence (NICE), 2022. Hypertension in Adults: Diagnosis and Management. Available at: nice.org.uk/guidance/ng136.

Newton, E.R., May, L., 2017. Adaptation of maternal-fetal physiology to exercise in pregnancy: the basis of guidelines for physical activity in pregnancy. Clin. Med. Insights Women's Health 10,1179562X17693224.

Pipkin, B.F., 2018. Maternal physiology. In: Edmonds, D.K., Lees, C., Bourne, T.H. (Eds.), Dewhurst's Textbook of Obstetrics and Gynaecology, ninth ed. Wiley-Blackwell, Oxford.

Royal College of Obstetricians and Gynaecologists (RCOG), 2017. Physical Activity during and Following Pregnancy. Available at: https://www.rcog.org.uk/for-the-public/browse-our-patient-information/physical-activity-and-pregnancy/.

World Health Organization (WHO), 2022. Physical Activity. Available at: who.int/news-room/fact-sheets/detail/physical-activity.

Annotated recommended reading

Blackburn, S.T., 2018. Maternal, Fetal and Neonatal Physiology: A Clinical Perspective, fifth ed. Elsevier, Philadelphia.

This book gives a more in-depth review of the adaptations to the cardiovascular system during pregnancy and following pregnancy.

Marieb, E.N., Hoehn, K., 2022. Human Anatomy and Physiology, twelfth ed. Pearson, Harlow.

This textbook presents a detailed overview of human anatomy and physiology. It is well illustrated with diagrams and pictures. Attention is given to the cardiovascular and haematological systems, homeostasis and the interrelationship with other body systems.

Websites

nice.org.uk/guidance/ng136.

This site provides up-to-date, hypertension-related evidence-based guidelines and good practice resources.

acog.org/womens-health/faqs/exercise-during-pregnancy.

assets.publishing.service.gov.uk/government/uploads/system/uploads/attachment_data/file/1054538/physical-activity-for-pregnant-women.pdf.

cdc.gov/physicalactivity/basics/pregnant-and-postpartum-women.html.

nhs.uk/pregnancy/keeping-well/exercise/.

rcog.org.uk/physical-activity-and-pregnancy/.

webmd.com/baby/exercise-during-pregnancy.

who.int/news-room/fact-sheets/detail/physical-activity.

These websites provide up-to-date evidence-based guidance and advice on physical activity during and following pregnancy.

18

Respiration

JEAN RANKIN

CHAPTER CONTENTS

This chapter details the anatomy and physiology of the respiratory system. This includes the control of ventilation and transport of gases. The maternal adaptations occurring during pregnancy are outlined.

Introduction

Respiration is the process by which the body exchanges gases with the atmosphere to provide for the changing needs of cell metabolism. Oxygen (O_2) is taken from the atmosphere and transported around the body in the blood to the tissues. Carbon dioxide (CO_2), produced as metabolic waste by the cells, is returned to the lungs and excreted into the air. Efficient respiration depends on the interactions of respiratory, cardiovascular and central nervous system functions that alter the rate and depth of respiration as needed. An adult utilizes about 250 mL of O_2 per minute, and this can be dramatically increased in severe exercise.

Anatomy of the Respiratory System

The respiratory system consists of the airways from the nasal passages to the pharynx and larynx, as well as the bronchi, bronchioles and alveoli of the lungs (Fig. 18.1). The chest structures necessary for moving air in and out of the lungs are part of the system. The respiratory system is normally divided into the upper and lower airways at the level of the cricoid cartilage.

The Upper Airways

The **nasal cavity** is a large, irregular-shaped cavity divided by a septum. Bony structures, called the **turbinates,** increase the surface area of the cavity, and it is lined with ciliated epithelium that warms, filters and moistens the incoming air. Air enters the upper pharynx through two internal nares.

The **pharynx** is a common passageway for water and food, as well as air. It is a funnel-shaped tube extending from the internal nares to the level of the cricoid cartilage. The auditory or **Eustachian tubes** open into the upper pharynx, and the mouth opens into the central portion or oropharynx. The tonsils and adenoids, which are organs of the lymphatic system, are found in the larynx. The oropharynx divides into the oesophagus, transporting food and water into the stomach, and the trachea, transporting air into the lungs.

The **larynx,** commonly called the *voice box,* is composed of pieces of cartilage connected by ligaments and moved by muscles. It is lined with mucous membrane continuous with the pharynx and trachea. In the larynx are the **vocal cords,** responsible for the production of sound, and between the vocal cords is the **glottis,** through which air passes. The

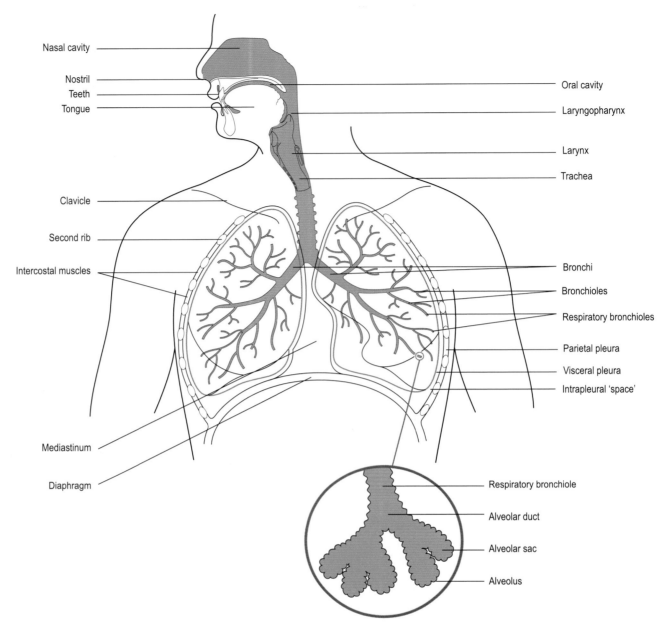

• **Fig. 18.1** Organization of the respiratory system.

epiglottis is a leaf-shaped piece of cartilage anchored to the thyroid cartilage. It moves up and down during swallowing to act as a cover for the glottis and prevent food and water from being inhaled into the larynx and lungs.

The Lower Respiratory Tract

The lower part of the airway is also called the **bronchial tree** (Fig. 18.2). The trachea is a cylindrical tube, 10–12 cm long, made up of 16–20 C-shaped cartilaginous rings joined together by fibrous and muscular tissue. This gives the trachea a firm structure to prevent collapse of the airway during inspiration. The trachea extends from the larynx to the level of the fifth vertebra, where it divides into the two **primary bronchi.** The right primary bronchus is wider and

shorter and more vertical than the left so that inhaled objects tend to enter the right lung rather than the left. The primary bronchi enter the lungs at the **hilum,** where the right bronchus goes on to divide into three—the right upper, middle and lower bronchi—to serve three lobes of the right lung. The left primary bronchus divides into two: the left upper and lower bronchi, to serve the two lobes of the left lung.

The lower branches of the airway, known as *bronchi,* still have cartilage in their structure. After this, they are known as **bronchioles** and have smooth muscle in their walls. The smooth muscle responds to stimuli by causing dilatation or constriction of the lumen of the bronchioles. This function is mainly under control of the autonomic nervous system, with sympathetic impulses causing bronchodilation and parasympathetic impulses causing bronchoconstriction. There

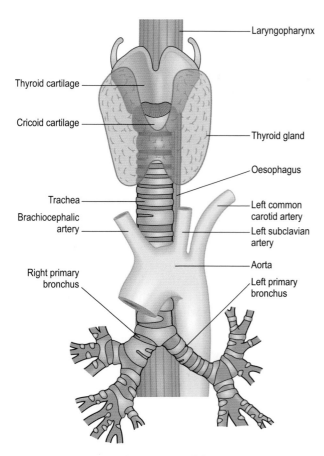

• **Fig. 18.2** Organization of the airways.

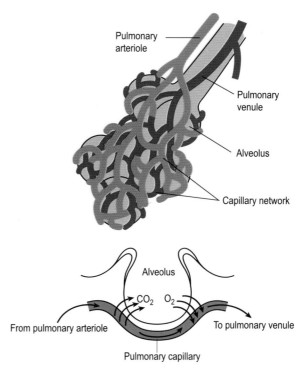

• **Fig. 18.3** Relationship between alveoli and blood vessels. Gas exchange can occur across the vast surface area provided by the dense network of capillaries.

are around 8–13 divisions from the trachea to the smallest bronchi and another 3–4 before the terminal bronchioles are reached. Each terminal bronchiole divides into about 50 respiratory bronchioles. About 200 sac-like **alveoli** are supplied with air by each respiratory bronchiole. Alveoli do not form part of the conducting zone of the respiratory system.

The Thoracic Cage

The thoracic cage forms the cavity and contains the two conical lungs and the heart. The organs are separated from each other by the mediastinum and its contents. Each lung is surrounded by a double-layered, fluid-filled sac called the **pleura,** which also attaches them to the inner surface of the thorax. The inner, or visceral, pleura covers the outer surface of the lung and is reflected back to become the outer or parietal pleura which is attached to the inner surface of the thoracic cavity.

Physiology of the Respiratory Tract

The Epithelial Lining

The upper airway protects the alveolar tissues by warming, filtering and moistening the air. It contains glands that secrete thick sticky mucus to trap particles and is ciliated to waft

excess mucus and foreign particles towards the pharynx where they can be swallowed. The cilia beat about 600–1000 times per minute. Large numbers of phagocytic cells will engulf and destroy debris and bacteria trapped by the mucus.

Reflex Mechanisms

Coughing is a forceful expiration reflex under the control of the respiratory centre in the medulla, which will expel irritant particles from the larynx. Air rushes out at a speed of 500 miles per hour instigated by messages from a sensitive part of the airway at the bifurcation of the trachea, called the **carina. Sneezing** is a similar reflex, instigated by irritation of the nasal mucosa. The **swallowing reflex** is extremely important for respiration. Particles of food or water can be inhaled into the larynx or lung in the absence of this reflex (e.g., unconscious or anaesthetized individuals).

Structure and Function of the Alveoli

The terminal bronchioles feed into respiratory bronchioles which branch into the alveolar ducts. These lead into alveolar sacs and the alveoli, where most gas exchange occurs (Fig. 18.3). The alveoli are expansions of the alveolar sacs, making the latter resemble bunches of grapes. Alveoli open into a common chamber called the **atrium** at the terminus of the alveolar duct. Around 300 million alveoli in the lungs provide an enormous area for gas exchange.

The alveolar wall (Fig. 18.4) consists of a single layer of flattened squamous epithelial cells called *type I cells.* The external surface of an alveolus has a few elastic fibres around

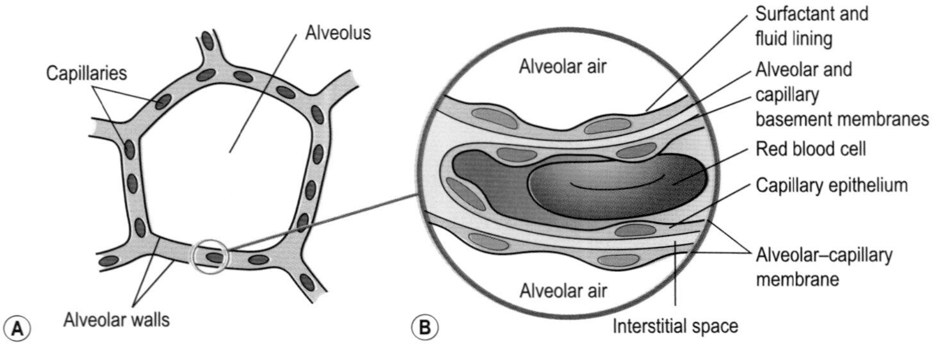

• **Fig. 18.4** (A) Cross-section of an alveolus. (B) Higher magnification showing histology of part of the alveolar–capillary membrane. The dense network of capillaries forms an almost continuous sheet of blood in the alveolar walls, providing a very efficient arrangement for gas exchange.

the opening. There is a dense network of pulmonary capillaries surrounding each alveolus, providing a continuous encircling sheet of blood. Each capillary wall is also only one cell thick so that the interstitial space between the alveolus and its capillary network, forming the air–blood interface, is extremely thin (0.2 μm, compared with the 7-μm diameter of an average red blood cell). This interface is called the **respiratory membrane** and has blood flowing on one side and gas on the other. Gas exchange occurs by simple diffusion across the respiratory membrane and depends on the existence of pressure gradients between the lungs and the atmosphere. The total surface area of alveoli in contact with capillaries is roughly the size of a tennis court. This extensive area and the thinness of the barrier permit the rapid exchange of large quantities of O_2 and CO_2 for diffusion.

Surfactant

In addition to the type I cells forming the alveolar wall, the alveolar epithelium contains cuboidal type II alveolar cells which secrete pulmonary surfactant. This is a phospholipid that helps keep the membrane moist and maintains the patency of the alveolus. Macrophages called *dust cells,* part of the defence system of the body, are also present in the lumen of the alveoli, mopping up bacteria, dust and other inhaled particles. The alveolar surface is usually sterile.

Blood Supply to the Lungs

The lungs act to oxygenate the blood, but they also need their own blood supply to maintain healthy tissue. The blood to be oxygenated reaches the lungs by branches of the pulmonary arteries, is re-oxygenated in the pulmonary capillary network surrounding the alveoli and returns to the heart via the pulmonary veins. The two left and one right bronchial arteries arising from the aorta provide the blood supplying the lung tissue with O_2. Venous return is by both bronchial veins and the pulmonary veins.

Nerve Supply to the Respiratory Muscles

The phrenic nerve to the diaphragm (originating in cervical nerves 3, 4 and 5) and the intercostal nerves to the intercostal muscles (originating in thoracic nerves 1–12) innervate the respiratory muscles. This is why severance of the spine above C3 results in total respiratory paralysis but, below that, diaphragmatic breathing can occur, although the intercostal muscles will be paralyzed.

The Physiology of Pulmonary Ventilation (Breathing)

The major function of the respiratory system is to supply the body with O_2 and dispose of CO_2 (Fig. 18.5). Four distinct events, collectively called *respiration,* must occur to perform this function:

1. **Pulmonary ventilation**—This process is called *breathing* and includes the movement of air in and out of the lungs.
2. **External respiration**—This involves the exchange of gases (O_2 loading and CO_2 unloading) between the pulmonary blood and alveoli.
3. **Respiratory gas transport**—O_2 and CO_2 must be transported to and from the lungs and body tissues via the bloodstream.
4. **Internal respiration**—This involves the process of gas exchange between the blood and the tissue cells in the body.

There are two phases to breathing: **inspiration,** or breathing in, and **expiration,** or breathing out. Mechanical factors and neural factors are involved in the control of respiratory rate. Atmospheric air contains about 21% O_2 and 79% nitrogen with traces of inert gases, CO_2 and water vapour. Alveolar air exchanges O_2 for CO_2 and water vapour.

Mechanical Factors

Under normal conditions and pressure gradients, O_2 passes from the alveolus into the blood and CO_2 from the blood into the alveolus. The movement of gases flowing from a high to a lower pressure down a gradient is said to occur by bulk flow. Air flows in and out of the lungs during breathing by bulk flow. Expansion of the thoracic cage by contraction of the respiratory muscles during inspiration increases lung volume and causes a temporary drop in the pressure in the

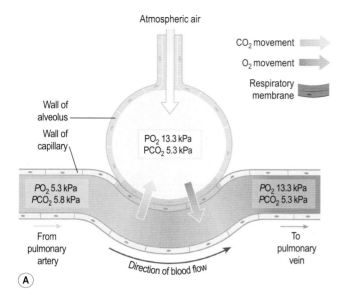

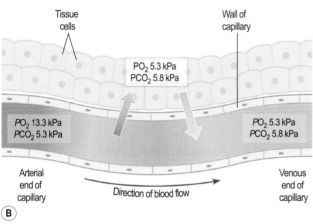

• **Fig. 18.5** Respiration. (A) Internal respiration. (B) External respiration.

alveoli. Atmospheric air flows in until pressure inside the lung is equal to the atmospheric pressure. Relaxation of the respiratory muscles causes expiration by reducing the volume of the thoracic cage, creating a temporary rise in pressure within the lung to above atmospheric pressure.

Inspiration

The diaphragm is the most important muscle of inspiration. It is a strong, dome-shaped sheet of muscle separating the thoracic and abdominal cavities from each other. The diaphragm flattens when it contracts. This change in shape presses down the abdominal contents and lifts the rib cage, enlarging the thoracic cavity both from top to bottom and from front to back. The external intercostal muscles are accessory muscles of respiration lying between the ribs. Normally these muscles play little part in this expansion of the rib cage, but they do help to stabilize it. During any need for extra O_2 such as during exercise or upper airway obstruction, the upper intercostal muscles along with other accessory muscles of respiration enlarge the rib cage to enhance lung expansion.

Expiration

Under resting conditions, expiration is a passive process brought about by the relaxation and elastic recoil of the diaphragm and intercostal muscles at the end of inspiration. The elastic lung returns to its original volume as air is pushed out of the lung (**functional residual capacity**) because the reduction in volume makes the alveolar pressure temporarily exceed atmospheric pressure. Active expiration may occur when the need for gas exchange increases under certain conditions such as during exercise or constriction of the airways.

Pulmonary Ventilation

Respiratory Parameters

Respiratory volumes and respiratory capacities can be described and measured using a spirograph. The following measurements are given for the average healthy adult.

Respiratory Volumes

- **Tidal volume** (TV) is the volume of air entering and leaving the lungs during a single breath. The TV during normal quiet breathing averages 500 mL for males and 400 mL for females.
- **Inspiratory reserve volume** (IRV) is the maximum amount of air that can be increased above the TV value during the deepest inspiration. Volumes differ significantly by sex: males average 3200 mL and females average 1900 mL.
- **Expiratory reserve volume** (ERV) is the maximum amount of air that can be voluntarily expelled after a normal quiet respiratory cycle. This averages 1200 mL for males and 700 mL for females.
- **Residual volume** (RV) is the volume of air remaining in the lungs at the end of maximal active expiration and is typically 1200 mL in males and 1100 mL in females.

Respiratory Capacities

- **Total lung capacity** (TLC) is the amount of air in the lungs at the end of a maximum inspiration. It includes TV + IRV + ERV + RV and averages 6100 mL in males and less in females (4200 mL) because of their smaller size.
- **Vital capacity** (VC) is total capacity minus RV and is typically 80% of TLC. This averages 4800 mL in males and 3100 mL in females.
- **Inspiratory capacity** (IC) is the maximum volume of air that can be inspired after a normal expiration. It is the sum of the TV and the IRV and averages 3700 mL for males and 2300 mL for females.
- **Functional residual capacity** (FRC) is the amount of air remaining in the lungs after a normal expiration. It is the sum of the ERV and the RV and averages 2200 mL in males and 1800 mL in females.

Minute Volume

The total volume of air exchanged with the atmosphere in 1 min is called the **minute volume** or **pulmonary ventilation.**

This volume depends on TV and respiratory rate and varies considerably in different states of health and according to age. An average TV in a resting adult is about 500 mL with a respiratory rate of 12 breaths per minute (Marieb & Hoehn, 2022). Therefore, pulmonary ventilation would be 6000 mL/min. Of this, about 150 mL of each breath is trapped in the **dead space** above the respiratory tissue and is breathed out with its composition unchanged.

Alveolar Ventilation

The volume of fresh air entering the alveoli each minute is called the **alveolar ventilation.** The calculation from the parameters mentioned earlier is as follows:

$$\text{Respiratory rate} \times (\text{Tidal volume} - \text{Dead space})$$
$$= \text{Alveolar ventilation}$$

For example, for the values given earlier:

$$12 \times (500 - 150) = 4200 \text{ mL/min}$$

Shallow rapid breathing is not as efficient as slower, deeper respiration because of the greater proportion of each breath wasted in the dead space.

Transport of Gases Around the Body

Gas Exchange in Tissues

Gas exchange in the tissues occurs at the capillary level. The constant usage of O_2 and production of CO_2 by the cells creates the necessary pressure gradients (see Chapter 16). O_2 is not very soluble in water and must therefore be carried around the blood in association with haemoglobin. CO_2 is about 20 times more soluble than O_2 and readily dissolves in water to form carbonic acid.

Transport of Oxygen

About 99% of O_2 in the blood is bound to haemoglobin. A small quantity of O_2 is also dissolved in the blood. This helps to determine the partial pressure of O_2 in the blood (PO_2) and maintain the pressure gradients, as the bound O_2 is not free to exert pressure. The O_2 content of the blood is determined partly by the haemoglobin level, but the hydrogen ion content of the blood also plays its part. As more O_2 is available, the PO_2 rises and haemoglobin will take it up. At a certain PO_2 when O_2 content is equal to O_2 capacity, the haemoglobin will be unable to take up any more O_2 and is said to be **fully** or **100% saturated.**

Partial Pressure Gradients and Gas Diffusion

The partial pressure gradient needed for the diffusion of O_2 is steep. For instance, the PO_2 of pulmonary blood is only 40 mmHg (5.3 kPa), whereas the PO_2 in the alveoli is 100 mmHg (13.3 kPa). O_2 diffuses from the alveoli into

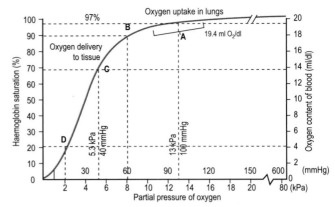

• **Fig. 18.6** The oxygen–haemoglobin dissociation curve. This applies when pH is 7.4, partial pressure of CO_2 is 40 mmHg (5.3 kPa) and blood is at 37°C. The total blood oxygen content is shown, assuming a haemoglobin concentration of 15 g/dL (i.e., O_2 capacity of 20 mL/dL).

the pulmonary capillary blood until there is equilibrium, with a PO_2 of 100 mmHg (13.3 kPa) on both sides of the respiratory membrane. CO_2 moves in the opposite direction down a much shallower gradient from about 45 mmHg (6.1 kPa) to 40 mmHg (5.3 kPa) with equilibrium at 40 mmHg (5.3 kPa). Although the gradients are so different, both gases are exchanged equally well because CO_2 has solubility in plasma and alveolar fluid 20 times that of O_2.

The Oxygen Dissociation Curve

The O_2–haemoglobin dissociation curve demonstrates the equilibrium between O_2 and haemoglobin (Fig. 18.6). The curve relates the partial pressure of O_2 to the percentage of haemoglobin that is saturated. There are two aspects of the curve that must be considered: its shape and position. The shape of the curve is sigmoid (S-shaped), indicating that at higher levels (less than 50 mmHg) the curve flattens and an increase in PO_2 produces little increase in saturation. The upper range is the PO_2 range in which O_2 binds to haemoglobin in the lungs. At low PO_2 levels, the curve is steep and small changes in PO_2 result in large changes in haemoglobin saturation. In this range, O_2 is released from haemoglobin and cellular activities occur. A small drop in PO_2 here allows a large amount of O_2 to be unloaded to the tissues.

Although each of the four haem groups in a haemoglobin molecule can take up a molecule of O_2, they vary in their affinity. The first haem group in the molecule to take up O_2 does so with difficulty but also holds on to its O_2 tightly. This association changes the shape of the haemoglobin molecule so that the second and third haem molecules take up O_2 readily for a relatively small increase in PO_2 as O_2 saturation goes from 25% to 75%. This is shown on the graph as the steep part of the sigmoid curve. The fourth haem group takes up O_2 more slowly and only at high PO_2. The unloading of O_2 at the tissues is also efficient, with the unloading of one molecule facilitating the unloading of the next. The binding and dissociation of O_2 to haemoglobin comprise a typical reversible reaction.

Factors Influencing the Oxygen–Haemoglobin Dissociation Curve

The position of the curve depends on the O_2 affinity for the haemoglobin molecules. The affinity of haemoglobin for O_2 must be sufficient to oxygenate the blood during its movement through the pulmonary circulation. However, it must be weak enough to allow release of the O_2 to tissues. Several factors can influence the affinity of haemoglobin for O_2 at any given PO_2. These include factors that move the O_2 dissociation curve to the right or to the left. A shift to the right implies a lowered affinity and enhances O_2 unloading. A shift to the left indicates that O_2 is more tightly bound to haemoglobin and unloading is inhibited.

Increase in Carbon Dioxide

An increase in CO_2 will reduce the ability of haemoglobin to bind O_2. This reduced affinity for O_2 in the presence of increased CO_2 is called the **Bohr effect.** Blood entering the tissues with a PCO_2 of 46 mmHg (6.1 kPa) will release more of its O_2 than blood with a PCO_2 of 40 mmHg (5.3 kPa). This will shift the O_2 dissociation curve to the right.

Increase in Hydrogen Ions

The O_2 dissociation curve moves to the right when the blood becomes acidic. As acidity increases in the blood, as occurs with the addition of lactic acid to the extra CO_2 during anaerobic cell metabolism in exercise, O_2 release to the tissues is facilitated by the presence of extra hydrogen ions.

Increase in 2,3-Diphosphoglycerate

This substance is a product of red blood cell metabolism and binds reversibly to haemoglobin, reducing its affinity for O_2. As the red blood cells reach the tissues, 2,3-diphosphoglycerate (2,3-DPG) is produced in more quantity and O_2 release is facilitated by moving the dissociation curve to the right.

Increase in Temperature

Local elevation of temperature due to muscle cell metabolism in exercise or other actively metabolizing cells will enhance the release of O_2 from red blood cells. This moves the dissociation curve to the right.

The effects are reversed in the lung where the extra CO_2 is blown off and the local temperature is cooler. Haemoglobin, therefore, has a higher affinity for O_2 in the pulmonary capillaries – an appropriate effect!

Carbon Monoxide

Carbon monoxide (CO) poisoning is a unique type of hypoxemic hypoxia and a leading cause of death from fire (Marieb & Hoehn, 2022). CO and O_2 compete for the same binding site on haemoglobin, but the affinity of haemoglobin for CO is 240 times greater than that of O_2. The product of haemoglobin with CO is carboxyhaemoglobin. Even small amounts of CO will block the uptake of O_2 and shift the O_2 dissociation curve to the left. The amount of O_2 in the blood is reduced, and the cells die from O_2 deprivation. CO is odourless, colourless and tasteless and is produced during the incomplete combustion of carbon products.

Transport of Carbon Dioxide

There are three ways in which CO_2 is carried around the blood:

- Five percent is carried in simple solution.
- Five percent is carried in combination with the globin rather than the haem part of haemoglobin as carbaminohaemoglobin.
- Ninety percent is transported as hydrogen carbonate (bicarbonate) ions.

Bicarbonate Ions

As the cells metabolize, they constantly produce CO_2 so that the PCO_2 of intracellular fluid is always greater than that of the blood in the tissue capillaries. This creates the pressure gradient for the removal of CO_2 from the tissues into the plasma. A small quantity will dissolve in the plasma to give carbonic acid (see Eqn. 18.1). This is a reversible reaction:

(Eqn. 18.1)

$$CO_2 + H_2O \rightleftharpoons H_2CO_3$$

An enzyme called **carbonic anhydrase** can catalyse (speed up) this reaction. The rapid production of carbonic acid mops up the CO_2, keeping the red blood cell PCO_2 low. This ensures maintenance of the pressure gradient along which the CO_2 flows.

As is characteristic of acids, the carbonic acid in the red blood cell quickly ionizes (dissociates) into hydrogen (H^+) and bicarbonate (HCO_3^-) ions, another reversible reaction:

(Eqn. 18.2)

$$CO_2 + H_2O \rightleftharpoons H_2CO_3 \rightleftharpoons H^+ + HCO_3^-$$

The Chloride Shift

HCO_3^- ions can readily pass out of the red blood cell into the plasma, unlike the H^+ ions, so that the HCO_3^- ions, but not the H^+ ions, can pass down a concentration gradient into the plasma. HCO_3^- ions are much more soluble in blood than CO_2. This movement out of the cell of HCO_3^- ions leaves the erythrocyte with a more positive electrical charge than the plasma and creates an electrical gradient down which chloride ions (Cl^-), the main plasma anion (**anions** are negatively charged ions and **cations** are positively charged ions), can diffuse into the red blood cell to restore electrical neutrality. This is known as the **chloride shift.**

Hydrogen Ions, Carbon Dioxide and the Acid–Base Balance

Most of the accumulated H^+ ions inside the red blood cell become bound to haemoglobin, as reduced haemoglobin has an affinity for them. This action of haemoglobin acts as a buffer, which neutralizes the released H^+ ions to prevent any rise in acidity within the red blood cell. The increased affinity for the uptake of CO_2 and H^+ ions that follows the removal of O_2 is called the **Haldane effect.** The Bohr and Haldane effects work together to facilitate O_2 release and the uptake of CO_2 and H^+ ions by red blood cells at the tissue level. During exercise, much larger amounts of CO_2 are produced by the tissues, but the increase in alveolar ventilation and in cardiac output ensures that arterial PCO_2 remains constant between 37 mmHg (4.9 kPa) and 43 mmHg (5.7 kPa).

The reactions are reversed once the blood reaches the lungs because of the reversed pressure gradients caused by the presence of atmospheric air in the alveoli. Here, CO_2 leaves the red blood cell to enter the plasma and crosses into the alveoli, and the freed H^+ ions combine with HCO_3^- ions to form H_2CO_3, which then separates into CO_2 and H_2O (see Eqn. 18.2), generating more CO_2 to diffuse out to the alveoli. This reaction is also catalysed by carbonic anhydrase.

As the HCO_3^- ions within the red blood cell are used up to generate CO_2, there is a shift inside the cell to a positive electrical charge, and plasma HCO_3^- ions and Cl^- ions now move back into the cell to restore electrical neutrality once more. This is a major pathway through which acid is removed from the body to maintain the acid–base balance: about 200 mL/min are removed from the tissues and eliminated from the lungs. O_2 now crosses from the alveoli into the plasma and then to the red blood cell to bind to haemoglobin.

Chapter 20 covers fluid and electrolyte balance and the maintenance of pH, including the role of the respiratory system in this process.

Control of Ventilation

Breathing, like the beating of the heart, must occur in a continuous rhythmic cycle to provide oxygen for the cells. The control of breathing is complex. The respiratory muscles, unlike cardiac muscle with its intrinsic pacemaker, are skeletal muscles and must receive nervous stimulation from the brain to make them contract. In normal circumstances, respiration is an involuntary act. The control of rhythmic breathing originates in the respiratory centre in the medulla.

Medullary Respiratory Centres

The Dorsal Respiratory Group

The pace-setting nucleus within the medulla oblongata is called the **inspiratory centre** or dorsal respiratory group (DRG). There is a second nucleus called the **expiratory centre** or ventral respiratory group, but its function is not well understood. Two other centres that influence the respiratory centre (higher in the brainstem in the pons) are the

pneumotaxic centre, which sends out inhibitory impulses to the DRG to prevent overinflation of the lungs, and the **apneustic centre,** which continuously stimulates the DRG to prolong inspiration. The pneumotaxic centre normally inhibits the apneustic centre. There is also a voluntary pathway of control by the cerebral cortex with descending pathways to the respiratory centre.

The Respiratory Cycle

Descending neurons from the respiratory centre terminate on the motor neurons controlling the respiratory muscles. As inspiration starts, there is a rapid increase in the number of nerve impulses from the DRG travelling along the phrenic and intercostal nerves to arrive at the respiratory muscles. The force of inspiration gradually increases and thoracic expansion occurs. At the end of inspiration, the DRG becomes dormant and there is a sudden reduction in the number of impulses, resulting in relaxation of the respiratory muscles and passive elastic recoil of the thoracic cage and lungs. Inspiration lasts about 2 s and expiration about 3 s. This cycle is repeated about 12–18 times per minute, but the level of ventilation is continuously adapted to changes in bodily requirements or atmospheric conditions so that adequate oxygenation is maintained.

Factors Influencing the Rate and Depth of Breathing

Multiple factors are involved in the regulation of respiration. These include neural, mechanical and chemical events and are best summarized in a diagram (Fig. 18.7).

Voluntary Control of Breathing

Voluntary control of the rate and rhythm of respiration (e.g., hyperventilation or breath-holding) is limited by the chemical stimuli that such efforts induce. Complex control of the respiratory system is necessary during speech and singing, as well as playing a musical wind instrument. Response to emotional states with laughing and crying also change respiratory patterns. When nerve impulses are sent to the vocal cords, simultaneous impulses are sent to the respiratory centre to control the flow of air between the vocal cords. Mental states influence respiratory rhythm: mental alertness and wakefulness have a stimulating effect, and sleep, sedatives, alcohol and some anaesthetics have an inhibitory effect.

Chemoreceptor Effects

Both peripheral and central chemoreceptors can respond to small changes in arterial PO_2 and PCO_2 to affect the rate and rhythm of respiration. **Peripheral chemoreceptors** are situated in the carotid bodies and other vascular structures around the aortic arch. These receptors respond to chemical changes in the blood. They sense the levels of PO_2, PCO_2 and H^+ ions and relay the information to the respiratory centre.

The response to O_2 levels depends primarily on these peripheral chemoreceptors. The response to excessive levels

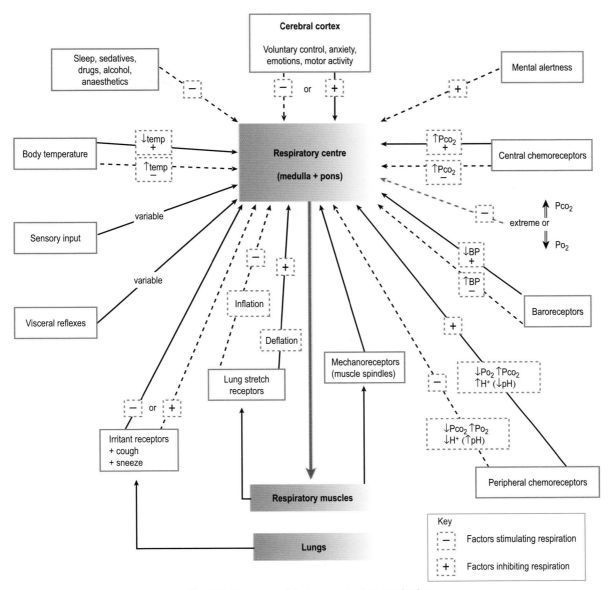

• **Fig. 18.7** Summary of factors controlling respiration.

of CO_2 (**hypercapnia**) depends on **central chemoreceptors** situated under the surface of the medulla. It is probable that, with a rise in arterial PCO_2, CO_2 crosses the blood–brain barrier from the cerebral blood vessels into the cerebrospinal fluid (CSF). This CSF bathes the central chemoreceptors and hydrogen ions are released (as in Eqn. 18.2). These hydrogen ions stimulate the central chemoreceptors, sending excitatory messages to the respiratory centre to increase the rate of respiration. A fall in PCO_2 will inhibit respiration.

The Hering–Breuer Reflex

Stretch receptors are present in the visceral pleura and in the conducting passages in the lungs and are stimulated if the lungs are overinflated. Inhibitory impulses are sent by these receptors via the vagus nerve to the medullary inspiratory centre, resulting in the termination of inspiration so that expiration can occur. The stretch receptors quiet down as

the lungs recoil so that inspiration can begin again. This is called the **inflation** or **Hering–Breuer** reflex.

Maternal Adaptations to Pregnancy

Pregnancy is associated with significant changes in the respiratory system in lung volume and ventilation. The anatomical and functional changes during pregnancy are needed to meet the increased metabolic needs for O_2 of the maternal body and foetoplacental unit (Fig. 18.8). The changes occur very early in pregnancy due to hormonal and biochemical influences, even before the growing uterus impairs ventilation.

Upper Respiratory Tract Changes

The mucosa of the nasopharynx becomes more hyperaemic and oedematous during pregnancy with hypersecretion of

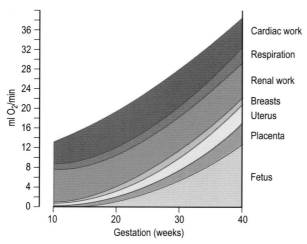

• **Fig. 18.8** Partition of the increased oxygen consumption in pregnancy among the organs concerned.

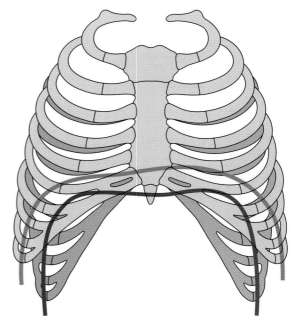

• **Fig. 18.9** The rib cage in pregnancy and in the non-pregnant state showing the increased subcostal angle, the increased transverse diameter and the raised diaphragm in pregnancy.

mucus due to the increase in circulating oestrogen. This may result in marked nasal stuffiness, epistaxis and polyposis of the nose and nasal sinuses. Vascular dilation can cause laryngeal changes with oedema of the vocal cords which may lead to hoarseness and a persistent cough (Coad, Pedley & Dunstall, 2019).

Anatomical Changes

Changes in the thorax occur early in pregnancy and in advance of the increasing size of the uterus. The muscles and cartilage of the thorax relax, creating anatomical changes in the shape of the chest which have implications for respiratory function (Fig. 18.9). The diaphragm becomes raised by a maximum of 4 cm, and the transverse diameter of the chest increases by 2 cm. The subcostal angle widens from the normal 68 degrees to 103 degrees in late pregnancy (Blackburn, 2018; Coad, Pedley & Dunstall, 2019). Breathing during pregnancy is more thoracic than abdominal (Coad, Pedley & Dunstall, 2019).

Biochemical Changes
Carbon Dioxide

Progesterone sensitizes the medulla oblongata to PCO_2 and so stimulates some overbreathing in the luteal phase and pregnancy (Broughton Pipkin, 2018). Overbreathing causes CO_2 to be washed out of the lungs so that the alveolar and arterial CO_2 concentration is lower than in a non-pregnant woman. Progesterone also causes an increase in carbonic anhydrase in red blood cells, which in turn facilitates CO_2 transfer, tending to decrease PCO_2 even without the presence of a change in ventilation. The resulting mild respiratory alkalosis is essential to create the gas gradients for exchange across the placenta.

Progesterone may contribute to airway resistance decreasing by relaxing the smooth muscles of the bronchioles (up to 50%). This will reduce the work of breathing and facilitate a greater airway flow in pregnancy. Prostaglandins may also influence the smooth muscle in the lung tissue, with PGF_{2a} acting as a bronchoconstrictor and PGE_1 and PGE_2 acting as bronchodilators (Blackburn, 2018). Table 18.1 provides a summary of the changes in respiration. Dyspnoea and the effects of smoking on pregnancy outcomes are outlined in Clinical Application 18.1.

Oxygen

Posture affects alveolar O_2 levels: a supine position in late pregnancy results in lower alveolar O_2 pressure than when in a sitting position (Blackburn, 2018). During pregnancy, maternal O_2 consumption at rest and during exercise is increased compared with a non-pregnant female proportionate to the growing tissue mass of pregnancy.

Pregnancy causes less stress to the respiratory system than to the cardiovascular system. Therefore, women with respiratory disease are less likely to show deterioration in their condition than those with cardiac disease.

Postpartum Changes

The changes in the respiratory system rapidly return to normal after delivery. This is initiated by the fall in progesterone levels and the reduction in intra-abdominal pressure. A rise in PCO_2 is seen within 48 h of delivery. Overall, anatomical changes and ventilation parameters return to normal between 1–3 weeks after delivery (Blackburn, 2018).

TABLE 18.1   Changes in the Respiratory System in Pregnancy

Parameter	Change in Pregnancy
Pulmonary ventilation (minute ventilation) Total air taken in 1 min (= TV × RR) Typical non-pregnant values: 4800–6000 mL	40% increase (in parallel with TV) Due to progesterone on respiratory mechanisms in the brainstem
Respiratory rate (RR) Number of breaths per minute Typical non-pregnant value: 12 bpm	Mainly unchanged/slight increase to 15 bpm Ventilation increases during pregnancy by the woman deepening her respirations and not by breathing more frequently.
Tidal volume (TV) Volume of normal breath at rest Typical non-pregnant value: 500 mL	Increases ~200 mL (>40%) in first trimester
Inspiratory reserve volume (IRV) Volume of air inspired above resting tidal volume Typical non-pregnant value: ~1900 mL	Unchanged
Expiratory reserve volume (ERV) Volume of air expired in addition to tidal volume Typical non-pregnant value: 1200 mL	Reduces progressively from early pregnancy to ~1100 mL
Residual volume (RV) Volume left in lungs after max. expiration Typical non-pregnant value: 1100 mL	Decreases progressively
Total lung capacity (TLC) Maximum volume in lungs (= TV + IRV + ERV + dead space)	Remains unchanged
Vital capacity (VC) Total amount of gas that can be moved in and out of the lungs (= TLC − RV) Typical non-pregnant value: 3100 mL	Increases 100–200 mL in late pregnancy
Inspiratory capacity Total inspired ability (= IRC + TV) Typical non-pregnant value: 2400 mL	Increases to ~2600 mL at term
Functional residual capacity (FRC) Volume remaining in the lungs after a resting breath (= ERV + RV) Typical non-pregnant value: 2300 mL	Decreases progressively to 1800 mL; increases mixing efficiency
Oxygen consumption	Increases by ~16% due to increasing maternal and fetal demands
Alveolar ventilation	Increases by 50% Results in a physiological change to overbreathing

Based on: Blackburn, S.T., 2018; Pipkin, B.F., 2018.

• CLINICAL APPLICATION 18.1   Dyspnoea and the Effects of Smoking on Pregnancy Outcomes

Dyspnoea

During pregnancy, ventilation increases by the woman deepening her respirations and not by breathing more frequently. The major influence leading to the physiological need to overbreathe is central respiratory control along with anatomical changes and alterations in lung volumes. The woman may complain of feeling uncomfortable due to dyspnoea and 'shortness of breath'. This is not always related to exercise but is more likely to be present when sitting down rather than when walking about.

Smoking

Smoking is a key public health issue and remains the leading modifiable risk factor for poor birth outcomes, including stillbirth, miscarriage and pre-term birth (Mund et al., 2013; Royal College of Physicians (RCP), 2018). It also increases the risk of children developing several respiratory conditions, attention and hyperactivity difficulties, learning difficulties, problems of the ear, nose and throat, obesity and diabetes (Kovess et al., 2015; RCP, 2018).

Evidence clearly suggests that cigarette smoking has harmful effects on the respiratory and cardiovascular systems. In particular, it interferes with O_2 exchange at the cellular level in the alveoli. This can be detrimental for maternal–fetal gas exchange during pregnancy, restricting O_2 to the fetus and causing an increased heart rate and exposure to harmful toxins (Marufu et al., 2015).

Both men and women planning to start a family need to stop smoking for the health and safety of the mother and baby (Action on Smoking and Health (ASH), 2021). The effects of smoking on human reproduction are discussed in Chapter 7.

Smoking during pregnancy is a health inequality associated with complications in pregnancy and serious long-term health implications for both mothers and their babies (Chamberlain et al., 2017). There are large variations in maternal smoking rates depending on age, geography, socio-economic status and ethnicity. Women from disadvantaged backgrounds are more likely to smoke before pregnancy, less likely to quit during pregnancy and, among those who quit, more likely to resume after childbirth.

Main Points

- Respiration enables the exchange of gases between the body and the atmosphere.
- The respiratory system consists of the airways from the nasal passages to the alveoli of the lungs, providing an enormous area for gas exchange. Pulmonary surfactant keeps the membrane moist and maintains the patency of the alveolus.
- Inspiration and expiration are the two phases of breathing. Mechanical and neural factors are involved in the control of respiration rate.
- The relationship between haemoglobin saturation and PO_2 is called the *O$_2$ dissociation curve*. In situations where this curve moves to the right, this enhances the unloading of O_2 to the cells. In contrast, if the curve moves to the left, this inhibits O_2 transfer.
- The control of breathing involves the respiratory centre in the medulla and neural, mechanical and chemical events.

- In pregnancy, changes in the respiratory system are brought about by hormonal and biochemical influences, as well as by the mechanical effect of the enlarging uterus.
- The diaphragm is pushed upwards, and the transverse diameter of the chest increases. Breathing changes from abdominal to thoracic.
- Inspiratory capacity increases progressively throughout pregnancy. Ventilation during pregnancy increases by the woman deepening her respirations and not by breathing more.
- Smoking has harmful effects on the respiratory and cardiovascular systems. In particular, it interferes with O_2 exchange at the cellular level in the alveoli and can restrict O_2 to the fetus.
- Smoking is associated with adverse pregnancy and birth outcomes.

References

Action on Smoking and Health (ASH), 2021. Smoking, Pregnancy and Fertility. Available at: ash.org.uk/uploads/Smoking-Reproduction.pdf.

Blackburn, S.T., 2018. Maternal, Fetal and Neonatal Physiology: A Clinical Perspective, fifth ed. Elsevier, Philadelphia.

Chamberlain, C., O'Mara-Eves, A., Porter, J., Coleman, T., Perlen, S.M., Thomas, J., et al. 2017. Psychological interventions for supporting women to stop smoking in pregnancy. Cochrane Database Syst. Rev. 2017 (2), CD001055.

Coad, J., Pedley, K., Dunstall, M., 2019. Anatomy and Physiology for Midwives, fourth ed. Elsevier, London.

Kovess, V., Keyes, K.M., Hamilton, A., Pez, O., Bitfoi, A., Koç, C., et al. 2015. Maternal smoking and offspring inattention and hyperactivity: results from a cross-national European survey. Eur. Child Adolesc. Psychiatr. 24 (8), 919–929.

Marieb, E.N., Hoehn, K., 2022. Human Anatomy and Physiology, twelfth ed. Pearson, Harlow.

Mund, M., Louwen, F., Klingelhoefer, D., Gerber, A., 2013. Smoking and pregnancy- a review on the first major environmental risk factor of the unborn. Int. J. Environ. Res. Publ. Health 10 (12), 6485–6499.

Marufu, T.C., Ahankari, A., Coleman, T., Lewis, S., 2015. Maternal smoking and the risk of still birth: systematic review and meta-analysis. BMC Publ. Health 15 (1), 239.

Pipkin, B.F., 2018. Maternal physiology. In: Edmonds, D.K., Lees, C., Bourne, T.H. (Eds.), Dewhurst's Textbook of Obstetrics and Gynaecology, ninth ed. Wiley-Blackwell: Oxford.

Royal College of Physicians (RCP), 2018. Hiding in plain Sight: Treating Tobacco Dependency in the NHS. RCP, London.

Annotated recommended reading

Blackburn, S.T., 2018. Maternal, Fetal and Neonatal Physiology: A Clinical Perspective, fifth ed. Elsevier, Philadelphia.

This book provides a detailed summary of the physiological changes in the maternal respiratory system during pregnancy.

Tortora, G.J., Derrickson, B.H., 2020. Principles of Anatomy and Physiology, sixteenth ed. Wiley, Hoboken.

This textbook provides an in-depth description of human anatomy and physiology. The section on 'respiration' is well illustrated and provided in more detail.

ash.org.uk/uploads/Smoking-Reproduction.pdf.

This publication provides up-to-date evidence and information on the adverse effects of smoking on reproduction.

19

The Renal Tract

JEAN RANKIN

This chapter details the anatomy and physiology of the renal tract and the production of urine. The maternal adaptations during and following pregnancy are described.

Introduction

The kidneys play a critical role in maintenance of **homeostasis** within the internal environment. Chapter 20 details fluid and electrolyte balance and regulation to integrate the roles of the respiratory and renal systems and the renin and the angiotensin–aldosterone system.

Kidney Functions

The kidneys have a critical role in regulating the volume and composition of body fluids in the maintenance of **homeostasis.** In addition to this regulatory function, the kidneys have a major role in **excretion,** the removal of organic waste products from body fluids and **elimination,** the discharge of waste products into the environment. Box 19.1 provides a further breakdown of all key renal functions.

Anatomy of the Kidney

The kidneys are paired, compact organs situated on either side of the vertebral column between the twelfth thoracic and third lumbar vertebrae. Situated behind the peritoneum, they are attached to the posterior abdominal wall by adipose tissue. An adult kidney is bean-shaped with a convex lateral surface and concave medial surface. A cleft in the medial surface is called the **hilum** and leads to a space within the kidney called the **renal sinus.** The hilum is the site of entry and exit of structures that include the ureters, renal blood vessels, lymphatics and nerves. Each kidney is about 10 cm long, 6.5 cm wide, 3 cm thick and weighs about 100 g (Coad, Pedley & Dunstall, 2019). The adrenal gland sits on top of the kidney. The right kidney is slightly lower, probably due to the liver.

Structure

Kidneys are embedded in and held in position by a mass of fat (**adipose capsule**). A sheath of dense fibrous connective tissue, the **renal fasci,** encloses and anchors the kidney, adrenal gland and renal fat. The outer fibrous capsule (**renal capsule**) closely surrounds the kidney and provides a preventive barrier to infections. Beneath this capsule lie three distinct regions: the outer **cortex,** the **medulla** and the inner **renal pelvis** (Fig. 19.1).

> **• BOX 19.1 Functions of the Kidneys**
>
> - Regulation of water balance, pH (acid–base balance) and inorganic ion balance (potassium, sodium and calcium).
> - Regulation of blood pressure (renin–angiotensin, through production of enzyme renin).
> - Regulation of volume and chemical makeup of the blood.
> - Control of formation of red blood cells (via erythropoietin).
> - Excretion of metabolic and nitrogenous waste products (urea from protein, uric acid from nucleic acids, creatinine from muscle creatine and haemoglobin breakdown) and removal of toxic chemicals (drugs, pesticides and food additives).
> - Secretion of hormones, including erythropoietin, vitamin D3 (1,25-dihydroxycholecatciferol, also called calcitriol) and prostaglandins.
> - Gluconeogenesis (formation of glucose from amino acids and other precursors).
> - Conversion of vitamin D to its active form.
> *The body excretes toxins, metabolic wastes and excess ions through the formation and excretion of urine.*

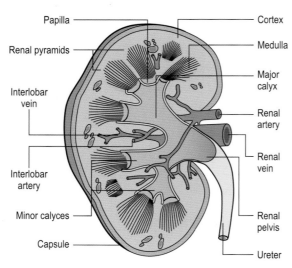

• **Fig. 19.1** Longitudinal section of the kidney.

- The **cortex** is a reddish-brown layer of tissue immediately below the capsule and outside the renal pyramids.
- The medulla, the innermost layer, consists of pale conical-shaped striations called **medullary** or **renal pyramids.** Urine formed within the kidney passes through the renal papilla at the apex of a pyramid into a **minor calyx.** The pyramids have a striped appearance (consisting of bundles of microscopic tubules).
- The **renal pelvis** is a flat funnel-shaped structure that narrows when it leaves the kidney and continues as the ureter to the bladder. It is formed by the combination of two or three major calyces (several minor calyces open into a major calyx).

The renal columns are extensions of cortical tissue separating the pyramids. Each medullary pyramid and its cap of cortical tissue is known as a **lobe** of the kidney (between 8–18 lobes in a kidney). Urine produced flows continuously from the papillae into the calyces and ureters. The walls of the calyces, renal pelvis and ureters are lined with transitional epithelium and contain smooth muscle. Peristalsis, the intrinsic contraction of this smooth muscle, propels urine through the calyces, renal pelvis and ureters to the bladder for storage and excretion via the urethra.

Microscopic Structure of the Kidney

Each kidney contains over 1 million nephrons (i.e., functional units of the kidney) and a fewer number of collecting ducts. Urine is transported via the collecting ducts through the pyramids to the calyces (giving pyramids the striped appearance) and are supported by connective tissue containing blood, lymph vessels and nerves (Fig. 19.2).

Each nephron consists of a renal tubule and a tuft of blood vessel capillaries called the **glomerulus.** The tubule is closed (blind end) at one end and joins the collecting duct at the other end. The closed end is enlarged and indented to form a cup-shaped glomerular capsule (**Bowman's capsule**).

Bowman's capsule is a network of tiny arterial capillaries called the **glomerulus** which resembles a coiled tuft

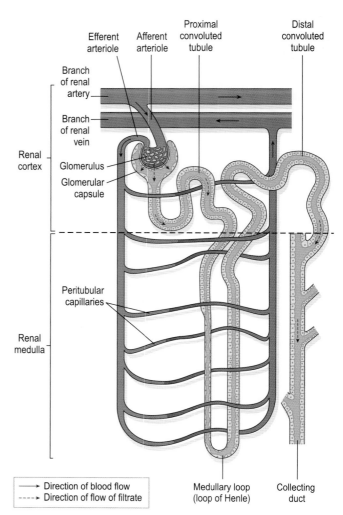

| → Direction of blood flow |
| ----> Direction of flow of filtrate |

• **Fig. 19.2** A nephron and associated blood vessels.

(Fig. 19.3). The capillary endothelium of the glomerulus is porous, allowing large quantities of solute-rich fluid to pass from the blood into the glomerular capsule. This fluid, called the **filtrate,** is processed by renal tubules to form urine. The capsule and glomerulus are known as a **renal corpuscle** and are situated in the renal cortex. The structure comprising the capillary endothelium, basement membrane and podocytic epithelium constitutes the selective filtration barrier.

Continuing from the capsule, the remainder of the renal tubule of the nephron is about 3 cm long and is described in three regions (Figs. 19.2 and 19.4).

1. The **proximal convoluted tubule** extends about 16 mm through the cortex. This region is lined by large columnar epithelial cells with a brush border of microvilli on their internal surface for solute reabsorption.
2. The **loop of Henle** (medullary loop) has a descending and an ascending limb. The thin-walled descending limb extends from the proximal convoluted tubule, dips down into the medulla, makes a U-turn and moves back into the cortex by the thick-walled ascending limb.

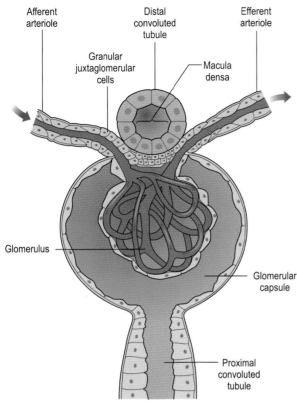

• **Fig. 19.3** A glomerular body.

3. The **distal convoluted tubule,** continuous with the loop of Henle, is comparatively short (about 4–8 mm) and leads into the **collecting ducts,** which fuse together as they approach the renal pelvis to form papillary ducts. These ducts open at the tips of the medullary papillae to discharge urine into calyces and the renal pelvis. The first part of the distal tubule folds back to bring it nearer to the granular cells of the afferent arteriole (this part of the tubule is called the **macula densa**). Both the granular cells and macula densa form the **juxtaglomerular apparatus.** This apparatus has important roles secreting renin (via granular cells) and monitoring (via macula densa cells) the sodium chloride concentration of fluids passing through.

The kidneys receive about 25% of the cardiac output (more than any other organ). Every nephron is closely associated with two capillary beds forming the microvasculature of the nephron: the glomerulus and the peritubular capillary bed. After entering the hilum, the renal artery divides into smaller arteries and arterioles. In the cortex, an afferent arteriole enters each glomerular capsule and subdivides into a cluster of tiny arterial capillaries, forming the glomerulus. The glomerular capillary bed is adapted for filtration. The efferent arteriole leads away from the glomerulus. The glomerulus is unlike any other capillary bed because it is fed and drained by arterioles. The efferent arteriole divides into a second peritubular capillary network, which is adapted for

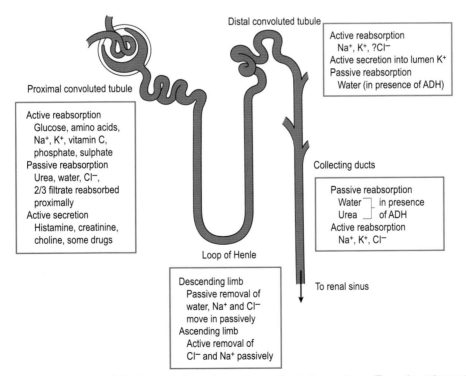

• **Fig. 19.4** Regional specialization in reabsorption and secretion in the nephron. Throughout the nephron, exchange of Na^+ for H^+, HCO_3^- reabsorption and NH_2 secretion occur.

reabsorption due to low-pressure porous capillaries. These wrap around the remainder of the tubule and bloodstream, allowing exchange between the fluid and blood. This maintains the local supply of oxygen and nutrients and removes waste products. Venous blood drained from this capillary bed eventually leaves the kidney via the renal vein (empties into the inferior vena cava).

The walls of the glomerulus and the glomerular capsule consist of a single layer of flattened epithelial cells. The glomerular walls are more permeable than those of other capillaries. The remainder of the nephron and the collecting ducts are formed by a single layer of simple squamous epithelium.

Renal blood vessels are supplied with a rich supply of sympathetic and only a few parasympathetic nerves. Stimulation of these nerves causes vasoconstriction, reduced renal blood flow, reduced glomerular filtration rate (GFR) and release of renin from the juxtaglomerular apparatus. The kidneys also have some sensory nerve fibres allowing the sensation of pain. These fibres are stimulated by distension of the renal capsule in such situations as bleeding, inflammation or obstruction by renal calculi. Ischaemia may also cause pain.

The Role of Blood Pressure

Blood pressure (BP) within the glomerular capillary bed is very high for two reasons:
1. Arterioles are high-resistance vessels.
2. The afferent arteriole has a much larger diameter than the efferent arteriole.

This high pressure forces fluids and solutes out of the glomerular blood along its entire length into Bowman's capsule. About 99% of this filtrate is reabsorbed into blood in the peritubular capillary beds. Blood flowing into the renal circulation encounters high resistance, first in the afferent and then in the efferent arterioles. Renal BP declines from 95 mmHg in the renal arteries to 8 mmHg in the renal veins. The resistance of afferent arterioles protects the kidney from large fluctuations in the systemic BP. Resistance in efferent arterioles maintains the high glomerular pressure and reduces hydrostatic pressure in the peritubular arteries to facilitate reabsorption.

Renal Function

The Production of Urine

In an adult, about 180 L of plasma are filtered every day and 99% of the filtrate is reabsorbed by the nephrons. This results in the production of about 1.5 L of urine per day. Fluid intake, diet and extrarenal fluid losses will affect the amount of urine produced (Marieb & Hoehn, 2022). Box 19.2 provides an outline of physiological factors related to renal function. Three processes are involved in the formation of urine:
- Filtration.
- Selective reabsorption.
- Secretion.

• BOX 19.2 **Physiological Factors Related to Renal Function (see Chapter 20)**

Electrolytes are solutes that are electrically charged and dissociate into their constituent ions in solution. Electrolytes are polarized into those carrying a positive charge (cations) and those carrying a negative charge (anions). They are in both extracellular fluid (ECF) and intracellular fluid (ICF). In ECF, sodium is the cation (Na^+) and chloride is the main anion (Cl^-). In ICF, potassium is the cation (K^+) and protein the anion.

Diffusion is the movement of a solute molecule down a concentration gradient across a permeable membrane. This movement depends on the electrical potential across the membrane, the particle size, lipid solubility and water solubility.

Osmosis is movement of water down a concentration gradient across a semipermeable membrane from a high water content to a lower one. The membrane must be more permeable to water than to the solutes, and there must be a greater concentration of solutes in the destination solution for water to move easily. Osmosis is directly related to hydrostatic pressure and solute concentration but not to particle size. For example, in plasma the protein albumin is smaller but more concentrated than the protein globulin; therefore, albumin exerts the greater osmotic force for drawing fluid back from the extracellular fluid into the intravascular compartment.

Oncotic pressure is the overall osmotic effect of the plasma proteins, sometimes called *colloid osmotic pressure.*

Hydrostatic pressure is the mechanical force of water pushing against cell membranes. It is generated by blood pressure in the vascular system. In the capillaries, a hydrostatic pressure of 25 mmHg is sufficient to push water across the capillary membrane into the extracellular space. It is partly balanced by osmotic pressure. The excess water moves into the lymph system.

The amount of hydrostatic pressure needed to oppose the osmotic pressure of the solution depends on the type and thickness of the plasma membrane, size of the molecules, concentration of the molecules on the gradient and solubility of the molecules. An example is the movement of water in the glomerulus of the kidney.

Glomerular Filtration

Filtration is a largely passive, non-selective process in which fluids and solutes are forced through a membrane (i.e., filtrate) by hydrostatic pressure (Marieb & Hoehn, 2022). The passage of water and solutes across the semipermeable membrane of the glomerulus is similar to that in other capillary beds, moving down a pressure gradient. However, the glomerular filtration membrane is thousands of times more permeable to water and solutes, and glomerular pressure is much higher than normal capillary BP. There is a high net filtration pressure.

Filtration takes place because there is a difference between the BP in the glomerulus and the pressure of the filtrate in the glomerular capsule (see Box 19.3). This results in 180 L/day of filtrate compared with the 4 L/day formed by all other capillary beds combined. Unlike other capillary beds, movement is only one way, from the capillary into the glomerulus. The **GFR** is the volume of plasma filtered through the glomeruli in 1 min (normally 125 mL/min).

• BOX 19.3 Pressures for Glomerular Filtration (Example)

The efferent arteriole is narrower than the afferent arteriole, and a capillary hydrostatic pressure of about 55 mmHg (7.3 kPa) builds up in the glomerulus. This hydrostatic pressure is opposed by the osmotic pressure of the blood, provided mainly by plasma proteins, about 30 mmHg (4 kPa) and the filtrate hydrostatic pressure of about 15 mmHg (2 kPa) in the glomerular capsule. Based on these values, the net filtration pressure is:

$$55 - (30 + 15) = 10 \text{ mmHg}$$

or

$$7.3 - (4 + 2) = 1.3 \text{ kPa}$$

• BOX 19.4 Blood Constituents of Glomerular Filtrate and Glomerular Capillaries

Constituents in Glomerular Filtrate

- Water
- Glucose
- Amino acids
- Mineral salts
- Hormones (some)
- Ketoacids
- Creatinine
- Urea
- Uric acid
- Some drugs (small)

Constituents Remaining in Glomerular Capillaries

- Erythrocytes
- Platelets
- Leucocytes
- Plasma proteins
- Some drugs (large)

Water and other small molecules easily pass through (although they may be reabsorbed later). Blood cells, plasma proteins and other larger molecules are prevented from passing through by the capillary pores, and these larger molecules remain in the capillaries. The filtrate in the glomerulus is similar in composition to plasma (important exceptions are blood cells and plasma proteins) (see Box 19.4). Regulation of glomerular filtration is outlined in Box 19.5.

Tubular Reabsorption and Secretion

During the second stage of urine production, the filtrate is greatly modified as it moves along the tubule. Most reabsorption occurs in the proximal tubule where two-thirds of the filtrate is removed. The walls of the proximal tubule are lined with microvilli to increase the surface area for absorption. Fig. 19.4 shows regional specialization in reabsorption and secretion by the nephron.

Vital solutes such as glucose, amino acids and electrolytes are reabsorbed together with water. They pass from the lumen of the nephron, across the epithelial layer, into the peritubular capillary network. A few substances are secreted into the filtrate from the peritubular capillaries. Mechanisms for reabsorption from the nephron may be active or passive (see Box 19.6).

• BOX 19.5 Regulation of Glomerular Filtration

Intrinsic Control by Autoregulation

The kidney can control its own blood supply over a wide range of arterial blood pressure (BP), from 80–180 mmHg. This intrinsic system is called **autoregulation** and depends on alterations in the diameter of afferent and efferent arterioles in response to a systemic BP change. Factors involved may include:
- The myogenic mechanism—tendency of vascular smooth muscle to contract when stretched.
- A tubuloglomerular feedback mechanism directed by the macula densa cells and solute concentration.
- The renin–angiotensin mechanism and renal vasoconstriction (see Box 19.7).
- Prostaglandin E_2 and renal vasodilation.

Extrinsic Control by Sympathetic Nervous System Stimulation

Adrenaline (epinephrine) from the adrenal medulla is released into the blood when the body is stressed. This causes strong constriction of afferent arterioles and inhibits filtrate formation. Blood can be shunted to the brain and muscles at the expense of the kidneys. The juxtaglomerular cells are also stimulated to release renin, which activates angiotensin II to raise systemic BP by generalized vasoconstriction. If there is a less intensive response, afferent and efferent arterioles are constricted to the same extent. This restricts blood flow out of the glomerulus, as well as into it, and the glomerular filtration rate declines only slightly.

Hormones Influencing Selective Reabsorption

- Aldosterone is secreted by the adrenal cortex. It increases reabsorption of sodium and water and the excretion of potassium. Secretion is regulated through a negative feedback system (Fig. 19.5). See Box 19.7 for the renin–angiotensin–aldosterone system.
- Antidiuretic hormone (ADH) is secreted by the posterior pituitary gland. It increases the permeability of the distal convoluted tubules and collecting tubules, increasing water reabsorption. Secretion is controlled by a negative feedback system (Fig. 19.6).
- Atrial natriuretic peptide (ANP) is secreted by the atria of the heart in response to stretching of the atrial wall when blood volume is increased. It decreases reabsorption of sodium and water from the proximal convoluted tubules and collecting ducts. Secretion is regulated by a negative feedback system (Fig. 19.7).
- Parathyroid hormone is secreted by the parathyroid glands and, together with calcitonin from the thyroid gland, regulates reabsorption of calcium and phosphate from the distal collecting tubules so that normal blood levels are maintained. Parathyroid hormones increase the blood calcium level, and calcitonin lowers it.

Tubular secretion is an important mechanism in clearing the blood of unwanted substances. Urine is therefore composed of both filtered and secreted substances. Secreted substances include hydrogen ions, ammonia and drug metabolites. Drugs are secreted into the tubules, such as penicillin and undesirable substances such as urea or excess potassium ions. Tubular secretion of hydrogen ions [H^+] is important in monitoring normal blood pH (see Box 19.8).

• BOX 19.6 Transport Mechanisms in the Nephron

Active transfer

This is uphill movement of solutes against an unfavourable chemical or electrical gradient. Solutes move from a low to a high chemical concentration or electrical potential. Energy in the form of adenosine triphosphate (ATP) is used.

Sodium is actively transported bound to a carrier protein. About 80% of energy is used in the transport of sodium ions. Substances actively reabsorbed include glucose, amino acids, lactate, vitamins and most ions. Many are co-transported bound to the sodium carrier complex.

There is a transport maximum depending on the number of carriers available in the renal tubule. When the maximum is exceeded, any surplus substance will be excreted in the urine (e.g., glycosuria).

Passive transfer
(i.e., diffusion, facilitated diffusion and osmosis)

This is movement of non-electrolytes and ions across cell membranes according to prevailing chemical or electrical gradients. Solutes move downhill from an area of high to low chemical concentration or electrical potential (see Chapter 2). No energy is directly used.

Na^+ is moved from the tubule to the peritubular capillaries and creates an electrical gradient that favours the transfer of anions such as HCO_3^- and HCl^- so that electrical neutrality is restored in plasma and filtrate. Na^+ movement establishes a strong osmotic gradient, and water moves from the lumen of the tubule into peritubular capillaries. This movement increases the concentration of solutes in filtrate and follows their concentration gradients out of the tubules. This is called **solvent drag.**

Non-reabsorbed substances

Substances are not reabsorbed because they:
- Lack carriers.
- Are not lipid soluble and cannot diffuse through cell membranes.
- Are too large to pass through plasma membrane pores in the tubular cells. Substances include the end products of protein and nucleic acid metabolism: urea, creatinine and uric acid. Urea is a small molecule and about 45% is reabsorbed, but creatinine is not reabsorbed at all; it is a useful substance to measure when assessing glomerular filtration rate and glomerular function.

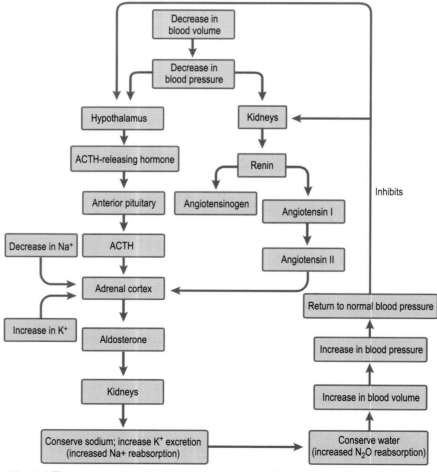

• **Fig. 19.5** The renin–angiotensin–aldosterone system. *ACTH*, Adrenocorticotropic hormone.

• BOX 19.7 The Renin–Angiotensin–Aldosterone System (Fig. 19.5)

When renal blood flow is reduced or blood sodium (Na^+) levels fall, the enzyme renin is produced by the juxtaglomerular apparatus (kidney). Renin converts the plasma protein angiotensinogen, produced by the liver, to inactive angiotensin I. Angiotensin-converting enzyme formed in small quantities in the lungs, proximal kidney tubule and other tissues converts angiotensin I to angiotensin II. This now stimulates secretion of aldosterone. Angiotensin II causes vasoconstriction and increases blood pressure, closing the negative feedback loop.

Renin, produced by the juxtaglomerular apparatus (kidney), stimulates production of the inactive blood peptide angiotensin I. This is converted into active angiotensin II acting as a hormone to stimulate the secretion of aldosterone and cause vasoconstriction.

Aldosterone (from the adrenal cortex) regulates Na^+. Na^+ with associated ions (chloride (Cl^-) and bicarbonate (HCO_3^-)), regulate osmotic forces and water balance. Na^+ also works with potassium (K^+) to maintain neurotransmission, regulate acid–base balance (via sodium bicarbonate) and participate in membrane reactions.

Na^+ concentration is maintained within a narrow range (136–145 mEq/L), primarily via renal tubular reabsorption. Daily intake of Na^+ averages 6 g, but only 500 mg are needed. If Na^+ is taken in excess, a combination of aldosterone and neural and renal mechanisms (via the renin–angiotensin system) work together to control the balance.

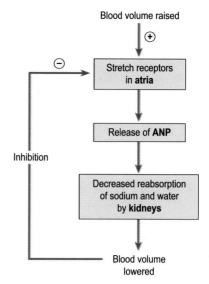

• **Fig. 19.7** Negative feedback regulation of secretion of atrial natriuretic peptide (ANP).

• BOX 19.8 pH and Acid–Base Balance

pH is a measure of the **hydrogen ion concentration** [H^+]. It is the negative logarithm of the hydrogen ions in solution on a scale of 1–14. There is a 10-fold change in hydrogen ion concentration from one pH unit to the next. It is negative because as hydrogen decreases, the pH value increases.

- Low pH values with more hydrogen ions result in an acidic solution.
- High pH values with a low hydrogen ion concentration result in an alkaline solution.
- pH of 7 is neutral.
- Acid body fluids: gastric juices (pH 1–3) and urine (pH 5–6).
- Most other body fluids are just alkaline with a pH between 7 and 8.
  Many pathological conditions disturb the acid–base balance.

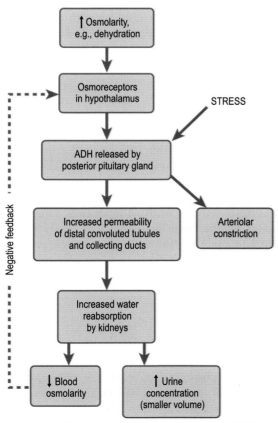

• **Fig. 19.6** The action of antidiuretic hormone (ADH).

Regulation of Urine Concentration and Volume

The role of the kidney in maintaining fluid and electrolyte balance and regulating pH is discussed in Chapter 20. Briefly, an important function of the kidney is to keep the solute load of the body constant by regulating urine concentration and volume. This is accomplished by a function called the **countercurrent exchange** (i.e., **s**omething flows in opposite directions through adjacent channels). In this case, the loop of Henle and adjacent blood vessels, the **vasa recta**, are involved. The capillaries of the vasa recta are long, hairpin-shaped blood vessels that run parallel to the loops of Henle. Blood flows slower due to the hairpin shape, which helps maintain the osmotic gradient required for water reabsorption.

The descending limb is quite impermeable to solutes and permeable to water. Water passes out of the filtrate into interstitial fluid by osmosis along the descending loop, and the solute load becomes concentrated. The ascending limb is impermeable to water and actively transports sodium into the surrounding interstitial fluid. The concentration of solutes in the filtrate as it enters the ascending limb is very high. Sodium is pumped out of the lumen into the interstitial fluid. The urine becomes more dilute and becomes hypotonic with respect to plasma.

The two loops are close enough to influence each other's activity. Water diffusing out of the descending limb produces the salty filtrate that the ascending limb uses to raise the osmolarity of the medullary interstitial fluid. The more salt the ascending limb extrudes, the saltier the filtrate in the descending limb becomes. This positive feedback mechanism is referred to as a **countercurrent multiplier.**

The collecting tubules add to the osmolality of the renal medulla by allowing urea to leak out into the interstitial space. The vasa recta are freely permeable to both water and salt and provide another countercurrent exchange to regulate the content of the interstitial fluid while still maintaining the gradient established by the loop of Henle. Blood moving down the descending limb of the vasa recta gains solutes and loses water, whereas in the ascending limb the blood loses solutes and gains water.

Formation of Concentrated Urine

Because water follows the osmotic gradients established by salt concentration, sodium and water balance are interrelated. Water balance is mainly regulated by ADH (Fig. 19.6). The secretion is initiated by an increase in plasma osmolality, by a decrease in blood volume and by a lowered BP. If blood volume decreases, volume receptors (located in right and left atria and thoracic vessels) and baroreceptors (located in aorta, pulmonary arteries and carotid sinus) stimulate release of ADH. With release, water absorption increases plasma volume and urine concentration is increased. This is called **facultative water reabsorption.** The amount of urine excreted is reduced and its concentration is increased. Table 19.1 describes the composition of urine.

The Lower Urinary Tract

The Ureters

The structural changes occurring in the lower urinary tract are important. The two ureters are hollow muscular tubes (Fig. 19.8). Urine that is secreted into the renal pelvis drains down through the ureters to be stored in the bladder.

Structure

The walls of the ureters are composed of the following layers:
1. A lining layer of mucous membrane in longitudinal folds.

TABLE 19.1	Composition of Urine	
Characteristics	**Normal Range (Approx. Values)**	
pH	4.5–8 (average 6.0)	
Specific gravity	1.010–1.030	
Osmotic concentration (osmolarity)	855–1335 mOsm/L	
Water content	93–97%	
Volume	Varies depending on intake but usually 1000–1500 mL/day	
Colour	Clear pale straw (dilute) Dark brown (very concentrated) Clear (in babies)	
Odour	Varies with composition	
Bacterial content	None (sterile)	
Urea: 2%	Uric acid, creatinine, ammonia sodium, potassium: 2%	Chlorides, phosphates, sulphates, oxalases: 2%

2. A fibrous tissue layer containing elastic fibres on which the epithelium rests.
3. A smooth muscle layer consisting of three sets of fibres: a weak inner layer of longitudinal fibres, a middle layer of circular fibres and an outer well-defined longitudinal layer.
4. A coat of fibrous connective tissue.

Situation and Size

The ureters lie outside and behind the peritoneum throughout their length. They extend from the renal pelvis to the posterior wall of the urinary bladder, crossing the pelvic brim anterior to the sacroiliac joints. The ureters run through the pelvic fascia and pass through special tunnels in the cardinal ligaments. They enter the posterior bladder wall in front of the cervix and run at an oblique angle for about 20 mm, which prevents the back flow of urine. They open into the cavity of the bladder at the posterior lateral angles of the **trigone.** In an adult, the ureter is about 30 cm long and 3 mm in diameter.

Blood Supply, Lymphatic Drainage and Nerve Supply

Blood supply is from the common iliac, internal iliac, uterine and vesical arteries, and drainage is by corresponding veins. Lymphatic drainage is to internal, external and common iliac nodes. The nerve supply is via aortic, renal and hypogastric plexi.

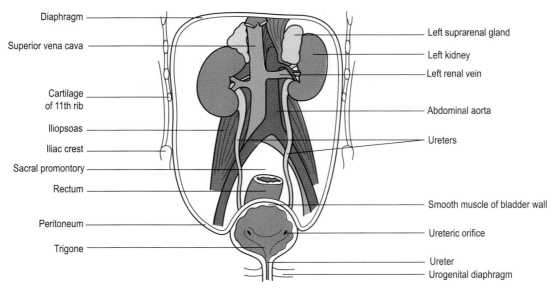

Diaphragm

Superior vena cava

Cartilage
of 11th rib

Iliopsoas

Iliac crest

Sacral promontory

Rectum

Peritoneum

Trigone

Left suprarenal gland

Left kidney

Left renal vein

Abdominal aorta

Ureters

Smooth muscle of bladder wall

Ureteric orifice

Ureter

Urogenital diaphragm

• **Fig. 19.8** Anatomy of the lower urinary tract.

The Bladder

The bladder is a hollow, distensible muscular organ acting as a reservoir for storage of urine. It is roughly pyramidal when empty and lies in the pelvis. It has a posterior base, or **trigone** (resting on the vagina), and an anterior apex. In a healthy adult, the capacity of the bladder when full is normally 500 mL (300–700 mL). It then becomes globular and expands upwards and forwards into the abdomen when full. Box 19.9 outlines the process of micturition.

The trigone of the bladder is triangular, and each side measures 2.5 cm. The two ureteric orifices are situated on either side of the base of the trigone, and the apex is formed by the internal meatus of the urethra. This region may be called the **bladder neck.**

Structure

The structures of the bladder walls are as follows:
1. A lining of transitional epithelium resting on a layer of **areolar tissue.** The lining, except for the trigone, is thrown into folds, or rugae, to allow it to distend. Over the trigone the epithelium is firmly bound to the muscle.
2. Three coats of smooth muscle (inner longitudinal, middle circular and outer longitudinal) called the **detrusor muscle.** This contracts to expel urine during micturition. Around the internal meatus, the circular muscle is thickened to form the **internal sphincter** of the bladder. This thickened muscle is in a state of sustained contraction except during micturition. There is a special arrangement of muscle fibres in the trigone. Fibres run between the ureteric openings and form a band known as the **interureteric ridge.** Muscle fibres running from each ureteric opening to the urethral orifice are also raised into ridges.
3. The upper surface of the bladder is covered by peritoneum reflected off the uterus to form the **uterovesical**

• BOX 19.9   The Physiology of Micturition

Micturition needs coordination of autonomic and somatic nerves. Motor and sensory sympathetic and parasympathetic nerves pass to and from the bladder. Sympathetic fibres play a minor role. When the bladder contains ~300 mL of urine, stretch receptors are stimulated and sensory parasympathetic nerves convey sensations of fullness to the basal ganglia, reticular formation and cortical centres of the brain. The individual senses this but can voluntarily postpone voiding until convenient.

The bladder empties by the muscle wall contracting, the internal sphincter opening (action of Bell's muscles) and voluntary relaxation of the external sphincter. Increased pressure in the pelvic cavity due to lowering of the diaphragm and contraction of the abdominal muscles assists with emptying. The external sphincter tone is affected by psychological stimuli (e.g., waking or leaving home) and external stimuli (e.g., running water), and any factor increasing intra-abdominal and intra-vesicular pressures (e.g., laughter or coughing) in excess of the urethral closing pressure can result in incontinence.

The centre for reflex control of micturition, situated in the second to fourth sacral segments of the spinal cord, activates when the bladder contains about ~500–600 mL when micturition cannot be avoided any longer. Nerve impulses from the cerebral cortex increase parasympathetic activity and decrease sympathetic activity, causing relaxation of the internal sphincter and contraction of the detrusor muscle. The external sphincter is relaxed, intra-abdominal pressure is raised and expulsion of urine occurs. Cortical control of micturition is learned in infancy and usually achieved around 2 years of age.

pouch. Its remaining surfaces are covered by visceral pelvic fascia.

Ligaments

There are five ligaments attached:
• A fibrous band called the **urachus** runs from the apex of bladder to the umbilicus.

- Two **lateral ligaments** pass from the bladder to side walls of the pelvis.
- Two **pubovesical ligaments** attach the bladder neck anteriorly to the pubic bones. They form part of the pubocervical ligaments of the uterus.

Relations

- Anterior: pubic bones are separated from the bladder by a space filled with fatty tissue called the **cave of Retzius.**
- Posterior: cervix and ureters.
- Lateral: lateral ligaments of the bladder and the side walls of the pelvis.
- Superior: body of the uterus and the intestines lying in the uterovesical pouch.
- Inferior: upper half of the anterior vaginal wall and the levator ani muscles.

Blood Supply, Lymphatic Drainage and Nerve Supply

Blood supply is from the superior and inferior vesical arteries and drainage is by corresponding veins. Lymphatic drainage is to the external iliac and obturator nodes. Nerve supply is via sympathetic and parasympathetic fibres of the autonomic system.

The Urethra

The female urethra is a narrow tube about 4 cm long passing from the internal meatus of the bladder to the vestibule where it opens externally. It runs embedded in the lower half of the anterior vaginal wall. The internal sphincter surrounds it as it leaves the bladder. As it passes between the levator ani muscles, it is enclosed by bands of striated muscle known as the **membranous sphincter** of the urethra, which is under voluntary control.

Structure

The walls of the urethra consist of the following layers:
1. The lumen is thrown into small longitudinal folds and is lined by transitional epithelium in the upper half and squamous epithelium in the lower half. It is normally closed.
2. A layer of vascular connective tissue.
3. An inner longitudinal layer of smooth muscle.
4. An outer circular layer of smooth muscle.

Several small crypts open into the urethra at its lowest point. The two largest are **Skene's ducts** and correspond to the prostate gland in the male.

Blood Supply, Lymphatic Drainage and Nerve Supply

Blood supply is via inferior vesical and pudendal arteries, and drainage is by corresponding veins. Lymphatic drainage is to internal iliac nodes. Nerve supply to the internal sphincter is from the sympathetic system, and the voluntary control of the membranous sphincter is via sympathetic and parasympathetic fibres of the autonomic system.

Maternal Adaptations to Pregnancy

During pregnancy, the renal system undergoes structural and functional changes, with many structural changes persisting well into the postpartum period. The main physiological changes of pregnancy are sodium retention and increased extracellular volume. Parameters used to assess normal renal function become altered, and this makes it difficult to assess against normal reference parameters.

The Prenatal Period

The maternal kidneys must act as the primary excretory organ for fetal waste besides dealing with the increased intravascular and extracellular volume and metabolic waste products. As in many of the widespread physiological adaptations to pregnancy, renal changes are related to the effects of progesterone on smooth muscle, pressure from the enlarging uterus and cardiovascular alterations such as increased cardiac output and increased blood volume (Blackburn, 2018).

Structural Changes—The Renal Tract

A summary of the main structural changes in the renal tract is presented in Table 19.2. The dilatation of the renal calyces, renal pelvis and ureters is the predominant structural change noted. This change begins in the early weeks of pregnancy, reaching maximal by the middle of

TABLE 19.2	The Structural Changes in the Renal Tract in Pregnancy
Organ	**Change**
Kidneys	Enlarge and the length may increase by 1.5 cm mainly due to increased blood flow, vascular volume and increase in interstitial space.
Glomerular size	Increases with no change in the number of cells. The microscopic structure of the kidney is the same in the pregnant and non-pregnant woman.
Renal calyces, renal pelvis, ureters	Dilatation (most striking change), elongation, increased muscle tone, decreased peristalsis. Elongated ureters become tortuous in later pregnancy, becoming displaced laterally by the uterus. Urine in ureters hold 25 times more and contain as much as 300 mL.
Bladder	Mucosa becomes oedematous and hyperaemic (tortuous blood vessels) with incompetence of vesicoureteral sphincter.
	Decreased bladder tone, bladder capacity increases to 1 L (i.e., doubles by term). Bladder becomes displaced anteriorly and superiorly by end of the second trimester.

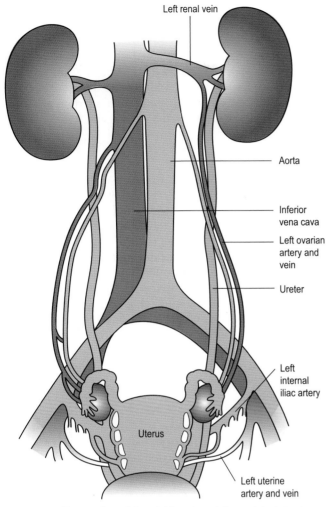

Left renal vein

Aorta

Inferior vena cava

Left ovarian artery and vein

Ureter

Left internal iliac artery

Uterus

Left uterine artery and vein

• **Fig. 19.9** Obstruction of the right ureter at the pelvic brim by an enlarged ovarian vein. Note that the ovarian vein enters the vena cava by several trunks and that the pelvic portion of the ureter is normal.

the second trimester. Changes are mainly seen in that portion of the ureters above the pelvic brim as the portion of ureters below the pelvic brim does not usually enlarge (Fig. 19.9). This may be because the connective tissue surrounding the ureters hypertrophies and prevents the hormonally induced dilatation. The diameter of the lumen of the ureter increases, there is hypertrophy of the smooth muscle of ureters, there is an increase in muscle tone and there is no decrease in peristalsis. The changes greatly increase the risk of urinary tract infection, and hyperaemia makes the structures more vulnerable to trauma and infection.

Oestrogenic influences cause the trigone in the bladder to become hyperplastic with hypertrophy of the bladder musculature. The decrease in bladder tone leads to incompetence of the vesicoureteral sphincters, and there may be reflux of urine (Blackburn, 2018). This may be increased by the displacement of the bladder and of the terminal ureters. Box 19.10 outlines the possible causes of physiological hydroureter and hydronephrosis.

• **BOX 19.10** Physiological Hydroureter and Hydronephrosis

The cause of physiological hydroureter (dilatation of ureters) and hydronephrosis (dilatation of the renal pelvis) in pregnancy remains unclear. The external compression of ureters against the pelvic brim by the growing uterus is likely to be the main factor. Growing blood vessels (such as iliac arteries and venous plexi) may add to the compression effect.

Dilatation is more prominent in primigravidae where the firmer abdominal wall does not permit the uterus to expand anteriorly. In 85% of women, the right ureter is more dilatated than the left. The possible cause is the dextrorotation of the growing uterus due to the presence of the sigmoid colon in the left quadrant of the pelvis. Increased urine flow in pregnancy may cause a small amount of dilatation.

TABLE 19.3 Physiological Changes in the Renal Tract in Pregnancy

Organ	Change
Renal blood flow	Significant increase 35–60% (end of first trimester), slight decrease until end of pregnancy
Glomerular capillaries	Vasodilation in afferent and efferent capillaries
Glomerular filtration rate	Increases 40–50% (i.e., greater proportion of renal blood filtered)
Tubular function	Increased reabsorption of solutes
	Increased excretion of glucose, protein, amino acids, urea, uric acid, water-soluble vitamins, calcium, hydrogen ions, phosphorus
	Retention of sodium and water
Renin–angiotensin–aldosterone system	Increase in all components
	Resistance to pressor effects of angiotensin II
Glucose	Urinary glucose values increase (10-fold)
Amino acids	Protein excretion increases (varies daily)

Changes in Renal Physiology

The physiological changes in pregnancy are summarized in Table 19.3. Alterations are due to the significantly increased blood volume and cardiac output in addition to the decreased renal vascular resistance brought about by the relaxing effects of progesterone. The increase in GFR begins shortly after conception and peaks at 9–16 weeks before stabilizing. The early second-trimester level is maintained until term. Values for GFR may reach more than 150 mL/min. The volume of urine produced in 24 hours is 25% higher during pregnancy.

No single cause has been identified for the increase in GFR in pregnancy, although it is related to the increased blood flow. The decreased plasma oncotic pressure present because of the reduced concentration of plasma proteins due to haemodilution also increases GFR, and there is involvement of hormones. Prolactin release from the pituitary gland has been found to induce changes in GFR in rats and is probably implicated in the human response to pregnancy. Prostaglandins may cause the renal vasodilation of pregnancy, accommodating the increase in blood plasma volume and renal blood flow.

The rise in GFR increases the amount of fluid and solutes present within the tubules by 50–100%. Tubular reabsorption must increase to prevent the loss of sodium, chloride, glucose, potassium and water. However, tubular reabsorption rate and clearance may not accommodate the increased load, and substances such as amino acids and glucose are excreted (Pipkin, 2018). This leads to glycosuria commonly occurring in pregnancy. There is a reduced ability of the tubules to reabsorb glucose in proportion to the amount in the filtrate (fractional reabsorption), possibly due to the changes in pregnancy steroid hormones. The changes are possibly due to the increased plasma levels of oestrogen and progesterone, and a similar effect is seen in some women taking the oral contraceptive pill.

Proteinuria is also more common during pregnancy with the extra excretion of amino acids. A value of 1+ on a protein labstick is not abnormal, and protein excretion up to 300 mg/day can be accepted. Protein excretion does not correlate with the severity of renal disease and may not indicate progressive deterioration of the disease. However, proteinuria associated with hypertension is serious and associated with increased risk to the woman and fetus.

The Postnatal Period

During the postnatal period, there is a rapid and sustained loss of sodium and diuresis, especially within the first 5 days. The first day is associated with a marked glomerular hyperfiltration (+41%) with the GFR at 2 weeks postnatal remaining moderately elevated (+20%) above non-pregnant levels. A normal urine output during this time may be up to 3000 mL with voiding of 500–1000 mL at any one micturition. By the end of the first week, urinary excretion of calcium, phosphate, vitamins, glucose and other solutes returns to normal, but it may take up to 3 weeks to achieve normal fluid and electrolyte balance. Structural changes described earlier may take up to 3 months to disappear, although structures return to normal in 6–8 weeks in most women.

Main Points

- The kidneys play a critical role in maintenance of internal homeostasis by regulating the volume and composition of the body fluids.
- Each kidney contains over 1 million nephrons (functioning units). Each nephron consists of a renal tubule and a tuft of blood vessel capillaries (glomerulus) within Bowman's capsule.
- Three processes are involved in urine formation: filtration, selective reabsorption and secretion.
- About 25% of cardiac output supplies the kidneys each minute.
- In an adult, ~180 L of plasma are filtered every day. About 99% of the filtrate is reabsorbed in the nephrons. Adults produce ~1.5 L of urine daily.
- Filtration is a passive, non-selective process in which fluids and solutes are forced through a membrane by hydrostatic pressure. The GFR is the volume of plasma filtered through each glomerulus in 1 min (~120 mL/min).
- Water, glucose, amino acids and creatinine are examples of constituents in the glomerular filtrate.
- Blood cells and plasma proteins are constituents remaining in the glomerular capillaries.
- Urine production is greatly modified as it moves along the tubule. Most reabsorption occurs in the proximal tubule (two-thirds of filtrate are removed). Vital solutes such as glucose, amino acids and electrolytes are reabsorbed together with water.

- Transport across the nephron may be active or passive.
- Urine is composed of filtered and secreted substances. Secreted substances include hydrogen ions, ammonia and drug metabolites.
- Water balance is mainly regulated by ADH.
- Sodium is regulated by aldosterone from the adrenal cortex.
- The renal system undergoes structural and functional changes during pregnancy.
- Kidneys enlarge due to increased blood flow, vascular volume and interstitial space. Ureters elongate, become more tortuous and are displaced laterally by the growing uterus. They may hold ~25 times more urine.
- Bladder capacity doubles by term to ~1000 mL (non-pregnant ~500 mL).
- Renal blood flow increases by 60% by the end of the first trimester then slightly decreases until birth. GFR increases by 50% in pregnancy (peaks at 9–16 weeks).
- Urinary glucose values may rise ~10-fold during pregnancy. Proteinuria is more common during pregnancy along with the extra excretion of amino acids.
- After birth there is a rapid and sustained loss of sodium and a diuresis (between days 2 and 5). It may take 3 weeks to achieve normal fluid and electrolyte balance. Structural changes may take 3 months to disappear (~6–8 weeks).

References

Blackburn, S.T., 2018. Maternal, Fetal and Neonatal Physiology: A Clinical Perspective, fifth ed. Elsevier, Philadelphia.

Coad, J., Pedley, K., Dunstall, M., 2019. Anatomy and Physiology for Midwives, fourth ed. Elsevier, London.

Marieb, E.N., Hoehn, K., 2022. Human Anatomy and Physiology, twelfth ed. Pearson, Harlow.

Pipkin, B.F., 2018. Maternal physiology. In: Edmonds, D.K., Lees, C., Bourne, T.H. (Eds.), Dewhurst's Textbook of Obstetrics and Gynaecology, ninth ed. Wiley-Blackwell: Oxford.

Annotated recommended reading

Blackburn, S.T., 2018. Maternal, Fetal and Neonatal Physiology: A Clinical Perspective, fifth ed. Elsevier, Philadelphia.

This textbook provides a detailed description of the major changes in the body systems during pregnancy and after childbirth.

Marieb, E.N., Hoehn, K., 2022. Human Anatomy and Physiology, twelfth ed. Pearson, Harlow.

This textbook provides an excellent account of the renal and related systems with detailed figures.

20

Fluid, Electrolyte and Acid–Base Balance

JEAN RANKIN

CHAPTER CONTENTS

This chapter steps outside of individual systems and examines the integration of systems in the control of fluid, electrolyte and acid–base balance in the body. Students and midwives need to have sound knowledge and understanding of this important aspect of life and the implications for pregnant women.

Introduction

Cell function depends on the maintenance of a stable environment through the continuous supply of nutrients, removal of waste and homeostasis of the surrounding fluids. Therefore, it is essential that fluid, electrolyte and acid–base balance of the extracellular fluids (ECF) are kept within a narrow range. For instance, changes in the composition of electrolytes can affect the electrical potentials of neurons. Changes in pH can also disrupt cellular enzyme systems. Cells depend on a continuous supply of nutrients and removal of metabolic wastes and various organs are involved in co-ordinating fluid balance.

Fluid and Electrolytes

Body Water Content

The total body water (TBW) of adults of average build is ~40 L (~60% of body weight). This ratio varies depending on age, sex, bodyweight and relative amount of body fat (Marieb & Hoehn, 2022). Most of the TBW is found inside the cells (~70% or 28 L of the average 40 L). The remaining 30% (12 L) is extracellular, of which the majority is interstitial fluid (IF) bathing the cells and a smaller percentage is found in plasma (Fig. 20.1). Further detail of fluid compartments is provided in Table 20.1.

Solutes: Electrolytes and Non-electrolytes

Water is the universal solvent and contains a variety of solutes. These can be broadly divided into electrolytes and non-electrolytes. The **non-electrolytes'** bonds (usually covalent bonds) prevent them from dissociating into their component particles in solution. These are mainly organic molecules such as glucose, lipids, creatinine and urea. **Electrolytes** are chemical compounds that dissociate into ions in water and are charged particles capable of conducting an electric current. Electrolytes include inorganic salts, both inorganic and organic acids and bases and some proteins.

All dissolved solutes contribute to the osmotic activity of a fluid. Electrolytes have the greatest osmotic power because each molecule can dissociate into at least two ions. An example is sodium chloride (NaCl):

(Eqn. 20.1)
$$NaCl \rightarrow Na^+ + Cl^-$$

Electrolytes have more ability to cause fluid shifts because water moves along osmotic gradients from areas of lesser osmolality to areas of greater osmolality. Table 20.2 provides the composition between intracellular fluids (ICF) and extracellular compartments.

Movement of Fluid Between Compartments

Water Movement Between Plasma and Interstitial Fluid

Distribution of water, and the movement of nutrients and waste products between plasma in the capillary and the interstitial space, occurs because of changes in hydrostatic pressure and osmotic forces between arterial and venous ends of the capillary network. The capillary membrane is semipermeable and allows interchange of fluids and solutes between the intravascular and IF compartments.

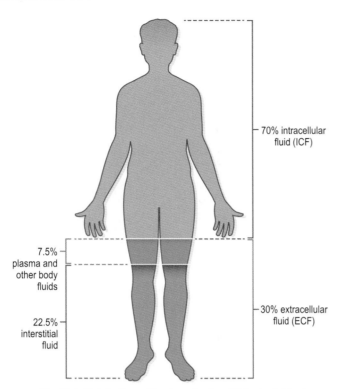

70% intracellular fluid (ICF)

7.5% plasma and other body fluids

30% extracellular fluid (ECF)

22.5% interstitial fluid

• **Fig. 20.1** Distribution of body water in a 70-kg individual.

Net filtration (Starling's hypothesis) is the movement of fluid back and forth across the capillary wall. The major forces of filtration are within the capillary. Net filtration is the balance between forces favouring filtration (e.g., capillary hydrostatic pressure (blood pressure (BP)) and interstitial oncotic pressure), and forces opposing filtration, such as plasma oncotic pressure. As plasma flows from the arterial to the venous end of the capillary, BP falls, reducing the hydrostatic pressure. Oncotic pressure remains constant. At the arterial end of the capillary, hydrostatic pressure exceeds oncotic pressure and fluid is forced out into the interstitial space. At the venous end of the capillary, oncotic pressure exceeds hydrostatic pressure and fluid is drawn back into the capillary (Marieb & Hoehn, 2022).

Water Movement Between ICF and Extracellular Compartments

This water movement between compartments is a function of **osmosis.** Water moves freely across cell membranes so that the osmolality of TBW is normally at equilibrium. The ICF balance is maintained by active transport of ions out of the cell and interstitial hydrostatic pressure. Movements of respiratory gases, nutrients and wastes are unidirectional. Water intake must balance water loss. Table 20.3 summarizes the normal daily water balance in a healthy adult and the fluid-regulation mechanisms. Clinical Application 20.1 presents disorders of water balance and clinical considerations.

Disorders of Water Balance

Oedema is the accumulation of fluid within the interstitial space. It involves fluid distribution and does not necessarily indicate excess intake. Oedema may be accompanied by signs of dehydration if fluid becomes sequestered (locked) within a compartment. Factors may cause increased fluid flow out of the plasma or hinder its return. Three major contributors to oedema include:

1. **Increased capillary hydrostatic pressure** from venous obstruction such as in thrombophlebitis, hepatic obstruction, tight clothing or prolonged standing.
2. **Reduced plasma oncotic pressure** follows the loss of plasma proteins found in renal failure, diminished production of plasma proteins found in liver disease or protein malnutrition.
3. **Increased capillary membrane permeability** is associated with inflammatory or immune reactions. Burns, crush injuries, cancer and allergy also produce this effect. If the lymphatic system is blocked, then proteins and fluids accumulate in the interstitial spaces causing localized lymphoedema. This blockage can be caused by infection, inflammation, lymphatic cancer or surgical removal.

Clinical Considerations

Oedema may be generalized or localized and is associated with weight gain, swelling of the tissues and puffiness. Clothing may feel tight. Movement may be limited, and blood flow may be restricted. Wounds tend to heal more slowly, and the risk of pressure sores and wound infections is increased. The sequestered fluid is not available for metabolic processes, and dehydration may occur, e.g., after burns. Hypovolaemic shock may occur. Person-centred treatment may include elevation of affected limbs, support stockings, avoiding prolonged standing, reducing salt intake and prescribing diuretics.

Electrolyte Balance

Electrolytes include salts, acids and bases. Salts are the main electrolytes and are involved in many physiological processes. The four main electrolytes are sodium (Na^+), potassium (K^+), calcium (Ca^{2+}) and magnesium (Mg^{2+}). Salts are obtained from food and, to a lesser extent, in drinking water. Small amounts of salts may be released during metabolism. An example is the release of phosphate during the breakdown of nucleic acids.

A major problem for humans is their preference for salty food, a possible acquired taste. Equally, this may be an innate factor to replenish salts lost in perspiration, including faeces and urine. If depleted of salt, then perspiration will be more dilute.

The role of Sodium in Fluid and Electrolyte Balance

Salts containing sodium account for at least 90% of solutes in ECF. Regulating the balance between sodium intake and output is a major function of the kidneys. Na^+, the most abundant ECF cation, is the main cause of osmotic pressure. As Na^+ does not easily cross the cell membrane, it is ideal for controlling

TABLE 20.1	Distribution, Main Functions and Variations of Body Fluid Compartments	
Intracellular fluid (ICF) (approx. 70%)	Fluid in body cells.	
	Different compositions from ECF.	
	Controlled by cell itself because of selective uptake and discharge mechanisms in the cell membrane.	
	Water passes freely in both directions across the cell membrane.	
Extracellular fluid (ECF) (approx. 30%)	Fluid divided into interstitial fluid (between cells) and plasma (inside vascular system).	
	Special types of ECF (separate from interstitial fluid and plasma) include lymph, transcellular fluid (secreted by cells), cerebrospinal fluid, sweat, intestinal, intraocular fluid, urine and for lubrication purposes, synovial, pleural, peritoneal and pericardial. These are considered ECF due to similar composition.	
	Bathes all cells (except outer layer of skin).	
	Provides a medium through which substances diffuse from cells to blood.	
	Closely regulated through homeostatic mechanisms.	
Variations	• Infants contain approximately 73% of water (lower bone mass and body fat). • Men contain more water than women (extra amount of body fat leads to a reduction in water content, i.e., female adipose tissue and lower muscle mass). • Obese people contain less water proportionate to body weight (fat is least hydrated of all body tissues). • Older people contain less water as fat content is increased and muscle content is decreased. Kidney ages and is less able to concentrate urine and more fluid is lost in urine. Other losses of body fluid can be life-threatening in the elderly.	

TABLE 20.2	Pattern of Electrolytes in the ECF and ICF	
Extracellular fluid (ECF)	Sodium (Na^+) – most abundant cation	
	Chloride (Cl^-) – major anion	
Intracellular fluid (ICF)	Potassium (K^+) is the most abundant cation	
	Phosphate (HPO_4^-) is a major anion	

Except for the high protein content of plasma, all ECF has a similar composition.
Balance in concentrations of Na^+ (ECF) and K^+ (ICF) reflects activity of the **sodium pump** (see Chapter 2).

ECF volume and water distribution in the body. Because water follows salt, a change in Na^+ content will be followed by a change in water content of a fluid compartment. Blood volume and BP are linked to Na^+ balance, and there is a regulatory effect by the hormone aldosterone (see Chapter 19).

Aldosterone

The release of aldosterone, produced by the cortical cells of adrenal glands, is mediated by the production of renin by the juxtaglomerular apparatus of the kidney (see Fig. 19.5). In brief, renin catalyses a series of reactions leading to the activation of angiotensin II, causing aldosterone release. Normally, without the influence of aldosterone, approximately 75% of sodium in the renal filtrate is reabsorbed in the proximal tubules of the nephrons of the kidneys.

If aldosterone levels are high, most remaining Na^+ is reabsorbed in the distal tubules and collecting ducts. If the permeability of tubules has been increased by antidiuretic hormone (ADH, also known as *arginine vasopressin*), water will passively follow Na^+. This results in Na^+ and water retention. When aldosterone release is inhibited, there will be little reabsorption of Na^+ beyond the proximal tubules. Urinary excretion of large amounts of Na^+ will always result in the excretion of large amounts of water. Aldosterone allows large amounts of Na^+-free water to be excreted in times of Na^+ depletion. Like all hormones, aldosterone has a slow effect, taking hours or days to alter fluid compartments.

Other influences on fluid and electrolyte balance include the cardiovascular system baroreceptors, the regulation of ADH and the influence of atrial natriuretic factor (see Chapters 17 and 19). Oestrogens and glucocorticoids also play a part in enhancing tubular reabsorption of sodium.

Regulation of Potassium Balance

K^+, the main cation in ICF, is necessary for normal neuromuscular functioning and other processes (e.g., protein synthesis). K^+ is toxic, especially to heart muscle. Both **hyperkalaemia** (excess K^+) and **hypokalaemia** (K^+ depletion) can cause abnormalities of cardiac rhythm and even cardiac arrest. K^+ also acts as a part of the buffer system controlling the pH of body fluids. Shifts of hydrogen ions (H^+) into and out of cells are compensated by shifts of K^+ in the opposite direction to maintain cation balance.

Renal mechanisms maintain K^+ and Na^+ balance. However, Na^+ loss or retention is controlled to meet the specific needs of the body, whereas K^+ loss is constant. Most K^+ is reabsorbed by the proximal tubule, but about 10–15% is lost in urine despite any changes in the body.

Tubular Cell Secretion of Potassium

The amount of K^+ secreted into the lumen of the tubule can be changed. When ECF levels of K^+ are low, K^+ leaves the cells. The kidneys then conserve K^+ by reducing the amount secreted into the tubule. Three factors altering the rate and amount of K^+ secretion are the intracellular K^+ content of the tubule cells, aldosterone levels and pH of the ECF.

Tubule Cell Potassium

If a high K^+ load is taken on, there is an increase in K^+ in the ECF and then in the ICF. This triggers the tubule cell to secrete K^+ into the lumen of the proximal tubule of the nephron. The reverse effect occurs with a low K^+ intake. Low ECF levels of K^+ result in low levels of K^+ in ICF, and the tubule cells reduce their secretion of K^+.

Aldosterone

Aldosterone helps regulate both Na^+ and K^+ ions by keeping Na^+ and releasing K^+ from the body. To maintain electrolyte balance, there is a one-for-one exchange of Na^+ for K^+ in the collecting tubules of the kidney, and for each Na^+ absorbed, a K^+ is secreted. Therefore, as plasma Na^+ levels rise, K^+ levels fall. The adrenal cortex, also sensitive to high levels of potassium, will react by releasing aldosterone.

pH of the ECF

The excretion of both K^+ and H^+ is linked to the reabsorption of Na^+ ions. They are co-transported with Na^+ and compete for places. If the pH of blood begins to fall, the secretion of H^+ increases and K^+ secretion falls. Box 20.1 presents the regulation of calcium and magnesium, and Clinical Application 20.2 outlines the alterations in electrolyte balance and clinical considerations.

TABLE 20.3	Normal Daily Water Intake and Output and Regulation Mechanisms		
Intake	Amount (mL)	Output	Amount (mL)
Drinking	1400–1800	Urine	1400–1800
Water in food	700–1000	Faeces	100
Water of oxidation	300–400	Skin	300–500
		Lungs	600–800
Total	2400–3200		2400–3200

Regulation of Water Intake

Main mechanism is 'thirst' (poorly understood). The thirst centre in the hypothalamus responds to either a drop in plasma volume or an increase in plasma osmolarity. Salivary glands probably make us drink fluids. Glands obtain their fluid from blood, and less saliva produced will dry the mouth. Fluid intake will quench thirst immediately even before blood volumes are affected.

Regulation of Water Output

Water is often lost from the body in ways that cannot be avoided. These are the **obligatory water losses** and include the insensible loss of water from lungs and via skin. Because a large amount of perspiration is lost daily, especially in hot climates, humans are a riverine species (i.e., most settlements before piped water were next to a river). Water in faeces is included in the loss. Kidneys must excrete an absolute minimum of 500 mL of urine per 24 hours even when urine is concentrated to the maximum level.

• CLINICAL APPLICATION 20.2 Alterations in Electrolyte Balance and Clinical Considerations

Alterations in Sodium, Chloride and Water Balance

Alterations can be classified as isotonic, hypertonic and hypotonic (Table 20.4).

Isotonic – same solute concentrations in all fluid compartments. Cell volume remains stable.

Hypertonic – a high solute concentration and low water concentration compared to body fluids.

Hypotonic – a low solute concentration and high water concentration compared to body fluids.

Isotonic Alterations

Depletion of fluids causes contraction of extracellular fluid (ECF) volume with weight loss, dry skin and mucous membranes; decreased urinary output and symptoms of hypovolaemia: rapid heart rate, flattened neck veins and normal or decreased BP.

Excesses of fluids are usually due to over-administration of intravenous fluids, hypersecretion of aldosterone or the effect of drugs such as cortisone. There will be weight gain and a decrease in haematocrit and plasma proteins. Neck veins distend and BP increases. Tissue oedema results from increased capillary hydrostatic pressure. If excess is severe, then pulmonary oedema and heart failure may result.

Hypertonic Alterations

Hypertonicity results from excess Na^+ (**hypernatraemia**) or depleted water (**dehydration**). Hypernatraemia (serum Na^+ concentration >145 mEq/L) is rarely due to dietary excess. Causes include inappropriate use of hypertonic saline solution (i.e., sodium bicarbonate to correct acidosis) and medical conditions, hyperaldosteronism and Cushing syndrome with oversecretion of adrenocorticotrophic hormone.

Dehydration occurs when water cannot be ingested to address thirst. Pathological causes include fever, respiratory infections, diabetes insipidus, diabetes mellitus, profuse sweating and diarrhoea. Clinical manifestations include thirst, dry skin and mucous membranes, elevated temperature, weight loss and often concentrated urine (except in diabetes insipidus). Isotonic salt-free solutions (e.g., 5% dextrose) are given in both hypernatraemia and water loss until plasma serum concentration returns to normal. Plain water *cannot* be given (increases intracellular fluid and causes cell lysis).

Hypotonic Alterations

Common causes are sodium deficiency (**hyponatraemia**) and water excess (**water intoxication**). Hyponatraemia develops when the plasma Na^+ concentration falls below 135 mEq/L. It is rarely caused by low intake and often caused by vomiting, diarrhoea, gastrointestinal suctioning and burns. Hyperglycaemia increases ECF osmolality and pulls fluid from the plasma into the tissues.

Dilutional hyponatraemia results from excess water through over-intake in thirsty people. Pathological conditions include reduced urinary output (e.g., oliguric renal failure, congestive cardiac failure and liver cirrhosis). Clinical manifestations include neurological symptoms like lethargy, confusion, apprehension, nausea, headache, convulsions and coma. For severe symptoms, small doses of hypertonic saline are given with caution. Oedema may develop with dilutional hyponatraemia. Appropriate intravenous solutions are given with fluid restrictions. A summary of hypertonicity and hypotonicity is presented in Table 20.5.

• BOX 20.1 Regulation of Calcium and Magnesium Balance

In the body, 99% of **calcium** content is found in bones. Ionic calcium found in extracellular fluid is extremely important for normal blood clotting, membrane permeability and secretory behaviour (Marieb & Hoehn, 2022). Calcium is like potassium and sodium in that it has a large effect on neuromuscular excitability: hypocalcaemia increases excitability and leads to muscle tetany, whereas hypercalcaemia inhibits muscle cells and neurons leading to cardiac arrhythmias.

Calcium is extremely well regulated and is balanced by the interaction of two hormones: **parathyroid hormone** (PTH) and **calcitonin**. PTH is released by the parathyroid glands situated on the posterior aspect of the thyroid gland. Calcitonin is produced by the parafollicular cells of the thyroid gland.

PTH acts to release calcium into the blood from the bones. It also stimulates the small intestine to absorb calcium by causing the kidneys to transform **vitamin D** into its active form. Activated vitamin D is necessary for intestinal absorption of calcium. PTH increases calcium reabsorption by the kidneys, while also decreasing phosphate reabsorption. Declining plasma levels of calcium stimulate the release of PTH.

Calcitonin encourages deposition of calcium salts in bone tissue and inhibits bone reabsorption. Although an antagonist of PTH, it has a small role in calcium homeostasis.

Regulation of Magnesium Balance

Magnesium is an essential activator of coenzymes needed in carbohydrate and protein metabolism. It is also implicated in neuromuscular functioning. About 50% of magnesium is in the skeleton with the remainder found intracellularly (i.e., heart, skeletal muscle and liver). The mechanism of magnesium balance remains unclear, but renal tubules are probably involved.

TABLE 20.4 Changes in Tonicity

Tonicity	Mechanism
Isotonic (iso-osmolar) imbalance	Gain or loss of extracellular fluid (ECF) results in a concentration equivalent to a 0.9% NaCl solution (normal saline) with no shrinkage or swelling of cells.
Hypertonic (hyperosmolar) imbalance	An imbalance with an ECF concentration greater than 0.9% salt solution due either to water loss or solute gain. Cells shrink as fluid moves out of them into the ECF.
Hypotonic (hypo-osmolar) imbalance	An imbalance with an ECF concentration of less than 0.9% salt solution due to either water gain or solute loss. Cells gain water from ECF and swell.

TABLE 20.5 Summary of Hypertonicity and Hypotonicity

Hypertonicity		
Sodium excess	Water normal	Hypervolaemia
Sodium normal	Water deficit	Hypernatraemia
Hypotonicity		
Sodium deficit	Water normal	Hypovolaemia
Sodium normal	Water deficit	Hypervolaemia

TABLE 20.6 pH Values in Fluid Compartments

Arterial blood	pH is normally 7.4
Venous blood	pH of 7.35
Interstitial fluid	pH of 7.35
Inside the cell	pH is 7.0

Acidosis occurs when arterial blood pH falls below 7.35.
The fall in pH is due to the presence of acid metabolites.
Alkalosis occurs when arterial blood pH is over 7.45.

Acid–Base Balance

Almost all biochemical reactions in the body are influenced by the pH of their fluid environment. The acid–base balance of body fluids is crucial to many biochemical reactions. There is a slight difference in pH between fluid compartments (see Table 20.6).

Chemical buffers tie up excess acids and bases as a temporary measure but cannot excrete them from the body. The lungs can dispose of carbonic acid (H_2CO_3) by excreting carbon dioxide (CO_2). However, the kidneys dispose of metabolic or fixed acids generated by cellular metabolism. These include phosphoric acid, uric acid and ketone bodies, the causes of metabolic acidosis. Also, only the kidneys have the power to regulate blood levels of alkaline substances. Therefore, the kidneys are the main regulators of acid–base status and act slowly and steadily to regulate the large acid–base imbalances occurring due to diet, metabolism or disease. Their most important mechanisms are the regulation of H^+ ions and the conservation or generation of bicarbonate (HCO_3^-) ions. The three chemical buffer systems are detailed in Box 20.2.

The Role of the Kidney in Acid–Base Balance
Regulation of Hydrogen Ion Secretion

Cells in the tubule cells and collecting ducts respond directly to the pH of the ECF. They alter their H^+ secretion as needed to restore balance. The secreted ions are obtained from the dissociation of carbonic acid, H_2CO_3 (carbon dioxide + water), within tubule cells, and for each H^+ ion secreted into the lumen, one Na^+ ion is reabsorbed into the tubule cell from the filtrate. This maintains the electrochemical balance. The rate of H^+ secretion varies directly with CO_2 levels in the ECF. The kidneys respond to alterations in blood pH because CO_2 levels in blood are directly associated with blood pH.

Conservation of Filtered Bicarbonate Ions

HCO_3^- ions are an important part of the carbonate buffer system. To maintain the **alkaline reserve** (available HCO_3^- ions) to act in the buffer system, the kidneys must replenish stores of HCO_3^- as necessary. The tubule cells are almost impermeable to HCO_3^- ions and cannot reabsorb them from the filtrate. However, they can shunt HCO_3^- ions generated within them into peritubular blood. Dissociation of one molecule of H_2CO_3 inside the tubule cell releases one HCO_3^- ion and one H^+ ion.

One-to-one exchange of HCO_3^- ions depends on the number of H^+ ions secreted by the tubule cells. For each filtered HCO_3^- ion that is lost from the body, another one is generated from the dissociation of H_2CO_3 in the tubule cells. When large amounts of H^+ are secreted, equally large amounts of HCO_3^- enter the peritubular blood.

Respiratory Regulation of Hydrogen Ions

Respiration and CO_2 transport have an important effect on the pH of the body. The acidity of blood and body fluids is determined by H^+ ion concentration, or $[H^+]$; H^+ ions are the most highly reactive cations in the body. The intake and production of H^+ ions vary according to diet, energy output, disease and some drugs. To maintain homeostasis, it is essential to both buffer these ions in body fluids and excrete them from the body via lungs and kidneys.

These three mechanisms are brought into effect sequentially. Chemical buffers act within a fraction of a second and are the first line of defence against a change in pH (see Box 20.2). Respiratory rate is adjusted in 2–3 min. The kidneys are the most efficient regulator, but it may take hours for the kidney to bring about a change in blood pH.

Excretion of Hydrogen Ions by the Lungs

Any increase in PCO_2 and $[H^+]$ with a consequent fall in pH will be sensed by the central and peripheral chemoreceptors. A rapid rise in alveolar ventilation occurs resulting in the reaction speeding up:

(Eqn. 20.2)

$$H^+ + HCO_3^- \rightleftharpoons H_2CO_3 \rightleftharpoons CO_2 + H_2O$$

This leads to rapid excretion of excess CO_2 and H^+ ions. The reverse situation will occur with any decrease in PCO_2 and $[H^+]$, with a consequent rise in pH leading to a decrease in respiratory effort. These two mechanisms form an efficient response to short-term chemical changes in blood. The

---

• BOX 20.2 Chemical Buffer Systems

Buffer systems minimize changes in pH. Acids are proton donors (release free H^+ ions into solution). Bases are proton acceptors mopping up free H^+ ions from solution. Chemical buffers minimize pH changes by binding to H^+ ions when fluid becomes more acidic (i.e., reduced pH). They release H^+ ions when fluid becomes more alkaline (increase pH). Three major buffer systems work together, including the:
1. Bicarbonate (carbonate) buffer system.
2. Phosphate buffer system.
3 Protein buffer system.

The Bicarbonate Buffer System

In solution, strong acids dissociate into component molecules and release H^+ ions, and strong alkalis dissociate to release hydroxyl (OH^-) ions. The bicarbonate (HCO_3^-) buffer system is important in both extracellular fluid (ECF) and intracellular fluid (ICF). It is a mixture of carbonic acid (H_2CO_3) and its salt, sodium bicarbonate ($NaHCO_3$), in the same solution. H_2CO_3, a weak acid, does not dissociate to release H^+ ions in neutral or acidic solutions. However, in a buffered solution with a stronger acid (e.g., hydrochloric acid), HCO_3^- ions of the salt will tie up H^+ ions released by the stronger acid to form more H_2CO_3:

(Eqn. 20.3)

$$HCl + NaHCO_3 \rightarrow H_2CO_3 + NaCl$$

Similarly, if a strong base such as sodium hydroxide (NaOH) is added to a buffered solution, the weak base, $NaHCO_3$, will *not* dissociate to release OH^- ions, but H_2CO_3 will be forced to dissociate and release H^+ ions to mop up OH^- ions released by the strong alkali to form water (H_2O):

(Eqn. 20.4)

$$NaOH + H_2CO_3 \rightarrow NaHCO_3 + H_2O$$

In these examples, the result will drive the pH of the solution back to a biologically acceptable level. Potassium bicarbonate or magnesium bicarbonate acts as a buffer within cells where there is little sodium present. The HCO_3^- ion concentration in ECF is normally about 25 mEq/L. The concentration of H_2CO_3 is about one-twentieth that of HCO_3^-. It is freely available from cellular respiration and is subject to respiratory control.

The Phosphate Buffer System

The phosphate (HPO_4^-) buffer system is almost identical to the HCO_3^- buffer system with the control of H^+ ions occurring in a similar manner. HPO_4^- ions replace HCO_3^- ions in the equations. It is a very effective buffer in ICF and in urine, where phosphate concentrations are high.

The Protein Buffer System

The body's most abundant and powerful source of buffers is proteins (in plasma and cells). At least 75% of the buffering power of body fluid resides within cells, and most reflect the buffering activity of intracellular proteins. Some amino acids have side groups called *organic acid* or **carboxyl groups** (–COOH), which release H^+ ions. Other amino acid side chains can accept H^+ ions. An exposed NH_2 group can bind H^+ to form NH_3 or release it as needed. This type of molecule is **amphoteric**. Haemoglobin in red cells is an excellent example of a protein that acts as an intracellular buffer.

kidneys play the main role in long-term control of pH and acid–base balance.

Box 20.3 presents the abnormalities of acid–base balance and clinical considerations.

Maternal Adaptations in Childbearing

Pregnancy

To meet the needs of the fetus and her own metabolic changes, a woman's body retains fluids and electrolytes. Renal processes are modified and a new balance is achieved, especially in sodium and water homeostasis (Blackburn, 2018). This adaptation is achieved by the ADH and the renin–angiotensin–aldosterone system. Changes in pregnancy affecting acid–base balance are detailed in Box 20.4.

Changes in Labour and Following Birth

In the intrapartum period, the renin–angiotensin–aldosterone system is altered with an elevation of the components resulting in fluid retention. This mechanism is thought to assist uteroplacental blood flow during labour (Blackburn, 2018). Labouring women on intravenous fluids may suffer from water intoxication if given too much, especially if oxytocin is administered, as this has an antidiuretic effect. This may produce symptoms of agitation and delirium, although most women will cope with over-enthusiastic fluid administration in labour (see Chapter 37). A decrease in glomerular filtration rate (GFR) and decrease in Na^+ excretion with an increase in vasoconstriction complicate the use of general anaesthesia. This effect may be further complicated if the woman is stressed. Accurate documentation of fluid balance is essential.

• BOX 20.3 Abnormalities of Acid–Base Balance

Severe acidosis will depress the central nervous system (CNS). If not corrected, the individual will go into a coma, shortly followed by death.

Alkalosis overexcites the CNS, resulting in muscle tetany, extreme nervousness and convulsions.

Other body systems will try to compensate for the imbalance. Death may occur due to respiratory arrest.

- **Respiratory acidosis** develops when the respiratory system cannot eliminate all the CO_2 generated by peripheral tissues.
  Clinical implication: Respiratory rate is normally depressed (causes the acidosis). Caused by any condition that impairs lung ventilation and gas exchange (e.g., rapid shallow breathing, narcotic or barbiturate overdose).

  Metabolic acidosis develops in the following situations:
- The most widespread cause is the production of many fixed or organic acids. This results in released H^+ overloading the carbonic acid–bicarbonate buffer system and reduction in pH levels.
- The less common cause is an impaired ability to excrete H^+ ions at the kidneys (e.g., glomerulonephritis).
- After severe bicarbonate loss (e.g., severe diarrhoea).
  Clinical implication: Respiratory compensation involves increased respiratory rate and depth due to stimulation of the respiratory centres by high levels of H^+ ions. Respiration blows off as much CO_2 as possible to reduce blood pH (e.g., during starvation, untreated diabetes mellitus, prolonged tissue hypoxia).

- **Respiratory alkalosis** develops when respiratory activity lowers plasma CO_2 to below-normal levels, a condition called *hypocapnia*. Always caused by hyperventilation whatever the triggering factor.
- **Metabolic alkalosis** occurs when HCO_3^- concentrations become elevated. Caused by vomiting of acid gastric contents, diuretics that cause salt loss and severe constipation.
  Clinical implication: Respiratory compensation involves slow, shallow breathing, allowing CO_2 to accumulate in blood.

• BOX 20.4 Changes During Pregnancy

Sodium

- Increase in the glomerular filtration rate (GFR) results in an increase of up to 50% in filtered sodium. Tubular reabsorption increases so that 99% of the filtered sodium is reabsorbed.
- Sodium retention is the highest in the last 8 weeks of pregnancy when ~60% of retained sodium is utilized by the fetus. The remainder is distributed in maternal blood and extracellular fluid (ECF).
- Multiple factors influence maintenance of sodium retention during pregnancy:
  - Antidiuretic hormone (ADH) and the renin–angiotensin–aldosterone system.
  - Decrease in plasma albumin.
  - Vasodilatory effects of prostaglandins.
  - Effects of the pregnancy hormones human placental lactogen and oestrogen.
- Water accumulation is directly proportional to sodium retention.

Renin–Angiotensin–Aldosterone System

- Increases in components of the renin–angiotensin–aldosterone system and decreases in response to the vasoconstrictor effects of angiotensin II are brought about by oestrogens, progesterone and prostaglandins, and alterations in sodium processing.
- Plasma renin activity increases during the first trimester and remains elevated until delivery.
- Renin release is stimulated by oestrogens.
- Progesterone stimulates renal sodium loss, causing release of renin and aldosterone.
- Angiotensinogen levels double by 8–10 weeks, increase two- to three-fold by 20 weeks and peak at 30–32 weeks (Blackburn, 2018). This is due to the effect of oestrogen on the liver (which manufactures plasma protein).
- Plasma aldosterone levels significantly increase by 8 weeks and reach levels four to six times higher than non-pregnant levels by the third trimester (Blackburn, 2018).

Continued

• BOX 20.4 **Changes During Pregnancy—cont'd**

- Angiotensin II, a potent vasopressor, rises during pregnancy. However, blood pressure actually decreases because of the reduced peripheral vascular resistance.

Water

- About 7 L of fluid is accumulated over non-pregnant levels to meet the needs of the fetus and altered maternal metabolism.
- About 75% of weight gain is due to accumulation of fluid in ECF.
- Interstitial fluid increases by about 1.5 L (as early as 6 weeks and peaks at 30 weeks). This increase occurs despite decreases in plasma osmolality and colloid osmotic pressure.
- Vasodilation, brought about by oestrogen and progesterone, enables the vascular system to accommodate more blood volume. This is probably a major cause as increased volume is retained without stimulating ADH production.
- Thirst and urine output remain in balance.

Antidiuretic Hormone

- Early in pregnancy plasma osmolality decreases, in particular, the decreased solute load.
- ADH secretion and its effect on reabsorption of water remain similar to non-pregnant levels.
- Osmotic threshold is reset so that ADH release occurs at the lower plasma osmolality. This allows the vascular tree to accommodate more fluid volume with a lower osmolarity due to the haemodilution of pregnancy.

- The main influence on osmoregulation may be human chorionic gonadotrophin (hCG). Circulating hCG levels decrease the thresholds for thirst and the secretion of ADH.

Acid–Base Regulation

- Plasma hydrogen ion concentration [H^+] decreases by 2–4 mmol/L in early pregnancy with change sustained until term.
- Blood is slightly more alkaline (pH change to 7.44 from a non-pregnant value of 7.4).
- Plasma bicarbonate concentration decreases. This mild alkalaemia may be respiratory in origin as women normally hyperventilate in pregnancy, reducing their arterial PCO_2 by about 25% (Johnson, 2018).
- Renal bicarbonate reabsorption and H^+ excretion are unchanged.
- Blood changes, especially the reduction in plasma CO_2 level, disadvantage the pregnant woman if significant metabolic acidosis develops such as in diabetic ketoacidosis or acute renal failure.

Potassium and Calcium Excretion

- Selective retention of potassium is mostly used by the fetus.
- Urinary calcium excretion increases, possibly to combat high levels of circulating 1,25-dihydroxyvitamin D (calcitriol), which increases absorption of calcium in intestines.
- Serum calcium levels are raised, and renal calcium reabsorption is reduced.

The Postnatal Period

Urinary excretion of electrolytes and glucose normally returns to normal after 1–2 weeks. There is marked diuresis with loss of Na^+ and water for up to 21 days or earlier depending on reaching prepregnancy levels (Blackburn, 2018). It may take 3 weeks to achieve normal fluid and electrolyte balance, with renal blood flow and GFR usually returning to normal by 6 weeks (see Chapter 19).

Main Points

- Cell function depends on a stable environment. Fluid, electrolyte and acid–base balances of ECF must be kept within a narrow range.
- Water can be found in the ICF (fluid inside cells) and ECF (IF and plasma).
- In an adult, total body water accounts for ~40 L (~60% of bodyweight).
- Water is the universal solvent, containing a variety of solutes.
- Electrolytes have the greatest ability to cause fluid shifts.
- Movement of water, nutrients and waste products across the capillary membrane is due to changes in hydrostatic pressure and osmotic forces between the arterial and venous ends of the capillary network.
- Oedema is the accumulation of fluid within the interstitial space.
- Electrolytes include salts, acids and bases. Salts are the main electrolytes (from food and water).
- Baroreceptors, ADH and atrial natriuretic factor influence fluid and electrolyte balance.

- K^+, the main cation in ICF, is necessary for normal neuromuscular functioning and other processes (e.g., protein synthesis).
- Aldosterone helps regulate K^+ and Na^+ ions. As plasma Na^+ levels rise, K^+ levels fall.
- If blood pH begins to fall, then the secretion of H^+ increases and K^+ secretion falls.
- Ca^{2+} (found in ECF) is important for normal blood clotting, membrane permeability and secretory behaviour.
- Small pH changes in the body could disrupt metabolic processes, resulting in death.
- The pH of arterial blood is normally 7.4, with venous blood being pH 7.35.
- Chemical buffers neutralize excess acids and bases.
- Respiration and CO_2 transport have an important effect on the acid–base status of the body.
- [H^+] determines the acidity of blood and body fluids. It is essential to buffer these ions to maintain homeostasis.

- Chemical buffers act in less than a second and are the first line of defence against changes in pH.
- Three chemical buffer systems work together: the bicarbonate, phosphate and protein buffer systems.
- Severe acidosis depresses the CNS. The individual will go into a coma and death will follow if not corrected.
- Alkalosis overexcites the CNS, resulting in muscle tetany, extreme nervousness and convulsions. Death may occur due to respiratory arrest.
- Acidosis occurs when arterial blood falls below pH 7.35.
- Alkalosis occurs when arterial blood pH is over 7.45.
- Respiratory acidosis results from any condition that impairs lung ventilation and gas exchange.
- Metabolic acidosis is caused by severe diarrhoea, untreated diabetes mellitus or starvation.
- Respiratory alkalosis is always caused by hyperventilation.
- Metabolic alkalosis is caused by vomiting gastric acid content, some diuretics or severe constipation.
- The pregnant woman's body retains fluids and electrolytes, and renal processes modify to achieve a new balance, especially in Na^+ and water.

- Changes in renal processes are due to ADH and the renin–angiotensin–aldosterone system.
- Pregnant women accumulate ~7 L more water, and ~75% of weight gain is due to accumulation of ECF fluid.
- The plasma $[H^+]$ decreases early in pregnancy and the change is sustained until term. This makes blood slightly more alkaline (pH changes to 7.44 from 7.4 non-pregnant value). Plasma HCO_3^- levels also decrease. Mild alkalaemia may be respiratory in origin as pregnant women hyperventilate.
- Urinary Ca^{2+} excretion increases, serum Ca^{2+} levels are raised and renal Ca^{2+} reabsorption is reduced.
- During labour and delivery, the renin–angiotensin–aldosterone system is altered with an increase in components (causes fluid retention).
- Labouring women on intravenous therapy may suffer from water intoxication (especially with oxytocin; i.e., antidiuretic effect).
- Postpartum, normal levels are attained around 1–2 weeks postpartum for urinary excretion of electrolytes and glucose and at 6 weeks for renal blood flow and GFR. There is diuresis with Na^+ and water loss until prepregnancy levels are reached by 3 weeks.

References

Blackburn, S.T., 2018. Maternal, Fetal and Neonatal Physiology: A Clinical Perspective, fifth ed. Elsevier, Philadelphia.

Johnson, M.H., 2018. Essential Reproduction, eighth ed. Wiley-Blackwell, Oxford.

Marieb, E.N., Hoehn, K., 2022. Human Anatomy and Physiology, twelfth ed. Pearson, Harlow.

Annotated recommended reading

Blackburn, S.T., 2018. Maternal, Fetal and Neonatal Physiology: A Clinical Perspective, fifth ed. Elsevier, Philadelphia.

This textbook provides a detailed description of the major changes that occur in the body systems during pregnancy. There is an extensive review of the literature, extending from classical research studies to more recent research findings.

Marieb, E.N., Hoehn, K., 2022. Human Anatomy and Physiology, twelfth ed. Pearson, Harlow.

This textbook presents a detailed overview of the maintenance of fluid balance. Attention is given to the nature of the structure and function of body systems, their interrelationships and homeostasis.

21

The Gastrointestinal Tract

LYNSAY MATTHEWS

CHAPTER CONTENTS

This chapter details the anatomy, functions and control of the gastrointestinal tract (aka the alimentary canal), focusing on the mouth, stomach and small and large intestines. The significant maternal adaptations occurring during pregnancy are discussed.

Introduction

A healthy digestive system is essential for growth, repair and energy production in the body. These processes need raw materials converted in the digestive system from the food we eat. The organs of the digestive system can be divided into two main groups: the gastrointestinal tract (GI tract) and the accessory digestive organs (teeth, tongue, salivary glands, liver, gall bladder and pancreas). The accessory organs will be discussed fully in Chapter 22 followed by nutrition in Chapter 23.

Anatomy of the Gastrointestinal Tract

The adult GI tract is a continuous, coiled fibromuscular tube of variable diameter about 4.5 m long. It is open to the external environment at both ends and extends from the mouth to the anus. It varies in structure and function throughout its length. The organs of the GI tract are the mouth, pharynx, oesophagus, stomach, small intestine and large intestine (Fig. 21.1). Readers are referred to a textbook such as Tortora & Derrickson (2020) for detailed anatomy. A brief description is given next.

The basic structure of the GI tract is the same throughout its course. From the oesophagus to the anal canal, the walls of every organ consist of the same four basic layers (Fig. 21.2):

1. The **mucosal layer** is innermost and lines the tract. This layer is variable along the length of the tube depending on the required function. The lumen is lined with stratified epithelial cells from which mucus-secreting cells develop. The turnover rate for the epithelial cells is high because of the amount of frictional damage. The epithelial cells are supported by a sheet of connective tissue called the **lamina propria,** and beneath that is a thin layer of smooth muscle called the **muscularis mucosae.** The mucosal layer also contains patches of lymphoid tissue which defend the tract against micro-organisms.

2. The **submucosa** consists of loose connective tissue that supports blood vessels, lymphatics and nerves. The nerve fibres are called the **submucosal** or **Meissner's plexus.**

3. The **muscularis layer** is formed of smooth involuntary muscle fibres, bound together in sheets called **fasciculi.** There are two sheets: an inner circular layer and an outer longitudinal layer. In the stomach, there is an additional

oblique layer. Between the two layers of muscle fibres is a network of nerve fibres called the **myenteric** or **Auerbach's plexus.** The muscle fibres respond rhythmically to stimulation by the autonomic nervous system and some hormones.

4. The **adventitia** or **serosa** (visceral peritoneum) is the outermost protective layer and is formed of connective tissue and squamous, serous epithelium. It is continuous with the mesentery of the abdominal cavity and supports blood vessels and nerves.

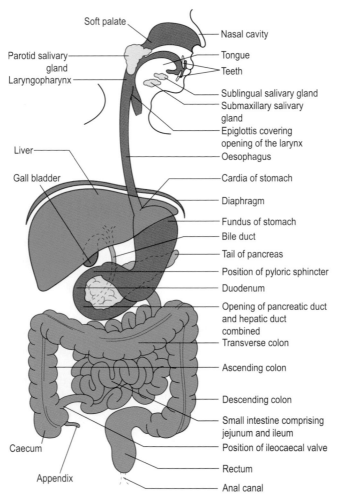

• **Fig. 21.1** Diagrammatic representation of the gastrointestinal tract.

Soft palate
Nasal cavity
Parotid salivary gland
Tongue
Teeth
Laryngopharynx
Sublingual salivary gland
Submaxillary salivary gland
Epiglottis covering opening of the larynx
Liver
Oesophagus
Gall bladder
Cardia of stomach
Diaphragm
Fundus of stomach
Bile duct
Tail of pancreas
Position of pyloric sphincter
Duodenum
Opening of pancreatic duct and hepatic duct combined
Transverse colon
Ascending colon
Descending colon
Small intestine comprising jejunum and ileum
Caecum
Position of ileocaecal valve
Rectum
Appendix
Anal canal

The Peritoneum

Most of the digestive organs lie in the abdominopelvic cavity. All body cavities contain friction-reducing serous membranes. The peritoneum of the abdominopelvic cavity is the largest of these membranes. The **visceral peritoneum** covers the external surface of most of the digestive organs and is continuous with the **parietal peritoneum** that lines the walls of the abdominopelvic cavity. Between the two layers is the **peritoneal cavity** containing fluid secreted by the serous membranes.

The Mesentery

Connecting the visceral and parietal layers of the peritoneum is a fused double layer of peritoneum called the **mesentery.** This helps support the organs, blood vessels, lymphatics and nerves. It also stores fat and prevents infection and inflammation by walling off areas of infection and inflammation. Another fold of peritoneum, the **lesser omentum,** runs from the liver to the stomach. The **greater omentum** is a fold of peritoneum that hangs in front of the intestines and is reflected off the stomach. In most places, the mesentery is attached to the posterior abdominal wall.

Blood Supply

Branches of the abdominal aorta serve the digestive organs and the special hepatic portal circulation. These include the hepatic, splenic and left gastric branches of the coeliac trunk which supply the liver, spleen and stomach. They also include the superior and inferior mesenteric arteries supplying the small and large intestines. The hepatic portal circulation collects nutrient-rich venous blood from the digestive organs and takes it to the liver (as discussed in Chapter 22).

Control of the Gastrointestinal Tract

Autonomic Nervous System

Nerve fibres from the **autonomic nervous system** (ANS) control the function of the GI tract via the submucosal and myenteric nerve plexi. In the submucosal plexus, **parasympathetic** nerve fibres synapse with ganglion cells present in the submucosa. Postganglionic fibres, accompanied by some **sympathetic** fibres, leave the ganglion cells and send impulses to the glands and smooth muscle of the tract.

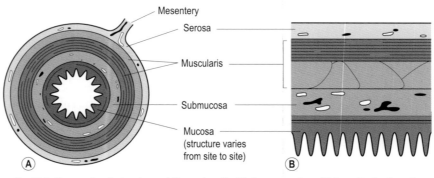

Mesentery
Serosa
Muscularis
Submucosa
Mucosa (structure varies from site to site)

• **Fig. 21.2** Generalized structure of the gut wall. (A) Cross-section. (B) Longitudinal section.

In the myenteric plexus, parasympathetic nerve fibres synapse with ganglion cells in the muscularis layer. Postganglionic fibres leave the ganglion cells and send impulses to the smooth muscle. Sympathetic fibres also supply the muscle. Both plexi run the length of the gut and receive both sympathetic and parasympathetic nerve fibres. The two plexi are connected, and activity in one can affect the other. Stimulation at the upper end of the GI tract can be transmitted to more distal parts; for instance, entry of food into the oesophagus stimulates secretion of gastric and intestinal enzymes.

Parasympathetic activity leads to an increase in both the motility and secretory functions of the tract. It also relaxes the gut sphincters. The **vagus nerve,** which is the 10th cranial nerve, is the source of parasympathetic supply to the oesophagus, stomach, pancreas, bile duct, small intestine and proximal colon. The parasympathetic supply to the distal colon is via the nervi erigentes from the sacral outflow.

In contrast, **sympathetic activity** leads to a decrease in blood supply to the gut with a decrease in secretions and gut motility. There is a contraction of the gut sphincters. As in other parts of the body, there are two types of catecholamine receptors in the gut: **α and β$_2$ receptors.** Note that β$_1$ receptors are present only in cardiac muscle. Stimulation of α receptors causes contraction of the smooth muscle of the GI tract, whereas stimulation of β$_2$ receptors causes relaxation.

Regulatory Chemicals

Two chemicals produced by the tract help in neural regulation. These are substance P and serotonin:
1. **Substance P,** a small peptide of only 11 amino acids, is found in high concentrations in the gut. It acts like a neurotransmitter and is referred to as a *regulatory peptide* or *neuropeptide.* It is involved in the conduction of pain impulses but also brings about vasodilation and contraction of non-vascular smooth muscle.
2. **Serotonin** (5-hydroxytryptamine or 5-HT) is synthesized in the myenteric plexus and may also act as a substance for interneuronal transmission.

Functions of the Gastrointestinal Tract

The role of the GI tract is to alter food so that it can be utilized by the body cells. This is achieved through six individual processes, each of which is discussed throughout the remainder of this chapter:
1. Ingestion.
2. Propulsion.
3. Mastication.
4. Mechanical and chemical digestion.
5. Absorption.
6. Elimination of non-usable residues as faeces.

The Mouth

Ingestion and mastication take place in the mouth. Food is mixed with saliva, broken into small pieces by the teeth and propelled backwards into the oesophagus by the tongue.

The tongue allows us to taste food. On its superior surface are numerous peg-like projections called **papillae.** These contain most of the 10,000 taste buds, which allow differentiation between four taste modalities: sweet, sour, salty and bitter. All taste buds have the potential for recognizing the four tastes, although particular ones are associated with one taste. The four tastes result in different neural firing patterns, which are interpreted in the cerebral cortex. Taste is aided by the sense of smell, which sends impulses to the brain via the **olfactory nerve.** This is why inflammation and hypersecretion of the nasal mucosa, which may occur in pregnancy, will result in a loss or alteration of taste.

Saliva

The salivary glands and the production of saliva are discussed more fully in Chapter 22. The three pairs of salivary glands—the **parotid, submaxillary** and **sublingual** glands—produce 1.5 L of saliva daily, consisting of 99% water and a pH range of 5.4–7.6 (Waugh & Grant, 2018). Saliva contains the digestive enzyme **α-amylase** which acts upon cooked starch to convert **polysaccharides** into **disaccharides.** It helps form the bolus of partly broken-up food ready to swallow. Saliva is produced in response to the thought, sight or smell of food or the presence of food in the mouth.

The ingested and masticated food is propelled down the oesophagus into the stomach for further digestion. The process is called **deglutition.** The tongue contracts and presses the bolus of food against the hard palate in the roof of the mouth. It then arches backwards and the bolus of food is propelled into the oropharynx.

The Stomach

Chemical breakdown of food by the secretion of enzymes begins in the stomach and is completed in the small intestine. The stomach is approximately 25 cm long and lies in the left side of the abdominal cavity partly hidden by the diaphragm and liver. It is continuous with the oesophagus above and the duodenum below. When empty, it is J-shaped. Its mucosal layer has folds (**rugae**) which allow distension. The rugae are further folded, providing a large absorptive surface, and contain millions of deep **gastric pits** with microscopic gastric glands that produce gastric juice.

Functions of the Stomach

- A reservoir for food.
- Production of the intrinsic factor.
- Gastric absorption.
- A churn to mix food.
- Secretion of mucus, hormones and gastric juice.

A Reservoir for Food

At rest, the stomach's capacity is approximately 50 mL, but with receptive relaxation, the muscles of the stomach wall can allow distension of up to 1.5 L. Under exceptional circumstances, the stomach can hold 4 L of content. The pyloric sphincter controls the rate of food transfer to the small intestine.

Production of the Intrinsic Factor

The **intrinsic factor** is a glycoprotein necessary for the absorption of **vitamin B$_{12}$** (cyanocobalamin) produced by the gastric parietal cells, which also produce gastric acid. Intrinsic factor binds to vitamin B$_{12}$ in the small intestine to form a complex which is transferred into the blood. Vitamin B$_{12}$ is required for the maintenance of healthy myelin sheaths around the nerves and formation of red blood cells in the bone marrow. Lack of vitamin B$_{12}$ may lead to **megaloblastic anaemia.** The resulting **pernicious anaemia** may lead to degeneration of the spinal cord.

Gastric Absorption

Food that has reached the stomach is only partly broken down there. Many of the molecules are still too large to be absorbed. There are also no carrier systems present in the gastric mucosa. Water and some drugs such as aspirin (acetylsalicylic acid) can be absorbed from the stomach. Absorption of aspirin lowers intracellular pH and may cause damage, leading to gastric irritation and bleeding.

A Churn to Mix Food

The stomach converts food to a thick soup consistency by mixing it with gastric secretions. This also dilutes the food and makes it compatible with the extracellular fluid in the duodenum. The semiliquid, formed by waves of peristalsis of the smooth muscle in the stomach wall, is called **chyme.**

Secretion of Mucus

Mucus is produced by cells of deep gastric glands in both the cardiac and pyloric sphincters. It adheres to the gastric mucosa to protect the stomach from being digested by the gastric enzyme **pepsin.** The layer of mucus that protects the mucosa must be 1 mm thick.

Secretion of Hormones

Enteroendocrine cells release a variety of hormones which influence target organs in the digestive system. These include gastrin, serotonin, cholecystokinin, somatostatin and endorphins. Histamine, produced by circulating mast cells and basophils, increases gastric acid secretion by binding to histamine receptors (H$_2$ receptors) on the gastric parietal cells (Table 21.1).

Secretion of Gastric Juice

There are 2–3 L of gastric juice produced daily. It is a mixture of secretions from two types of cells present in the gastric pits. The gastric pit cells are:

1. **Parietal or oxyntic cells,** which secrete **hydrochloric acid** (HCl) and the intrinsic factor.
2. **Chief or zymogen cells,** which secrete the enzymes.

There are about 1 billion parietal cells in the gastric pits of an adult stomach. Hydrogen ions (H$^+$) are secreted into the lumen of the stomach against a concentration gradient. Carbon dioxide (CO$_2$) diffuses into the parietal cells from arterial blood and combines with water to form carbonic acid (H$_2$CO$_3$). Equal numbers of H$^+$ ions (formed by the dissociation of H$_2$CO$_3$ into H+ and bicarbonate ions (HCO$_3^-$)) and chloride ions (Cl$^-$) are secreted into the lumen of the gastric pits. They form HCl, which is then diluted by water. Histamine or the hormone gastrin stimulates the secretion of HCl into the lumen of the stomach.

The functions of gastric acid are:
- Inactivation of salivary amylase.
- Bacteriostasis (to prevent growth of bacteria).
- Alteration of the molecular structure of ingested proteins to tenderize them.
- Curdling of milk.
- Conversion of pepsinogen to pepsin.

Children produce an enzyme called **rennin** which acts on the milk protein **casein** and converts it into curds.

The chief cells produce a pepsinogen-rich secretion. When gastric pH is lower than 5.5, pepsinogen is converted into pepsin by HCl. Pepsin converts proteins to polypeptides by breaking the bonds between specific amino acids. Once chyme leaves the stomach, the pH returns to alkaline and pepsin's activity ceases.

Control of Gastric Juice Secretion

Gastric juice secretion is controlled by both neural and hormonal mechanisms.

Neural Control

There are two phases in the neural control of gastric juice secretion, although the two work interdependently. The **cephalic phase** is an anticipatory conditioned reflex to the sight, smell or thought of food. This phase is mediated by the vagus nerve, which stimulates both parietal and chief cells. The **gastric phase** is mediated by stretch receptors and chemoreceptors. Stretch receptors in the stomach wall respond to distension by food. Chemoreceptors respond to the presence of protein molecules within the stomach. Impulses from these two types of receptors are sent to the submucosal plexus where they synapse with parasympathetic neurons. Excitatory impulses are then dispatched to the parietal cells (which secrete HCl and intrinsic factor).

Hormonal Control

Hormonal influences contribute most to the gastric phase of secretion. Throughout, the gut regulatory hormones called **peptides** are active. Many of them are also found in the central nervous system, and alternative names for them are *neurohormones, neuropeptides* or *neurotransmitters*. The term **gastrin** refers to a group of similar hormones produced by **G cells** in the lateral walls of the gastric glands in the antrum of the stomach. They are a major influence on gastric juice secretion. A small amount of gastrin is produced

TABLE 21.1   Hormones That Aid Digestion

Hormone	Stimulus	Target Organ	Effect
Gastrin	Presence of food in the stomach	Stomach	Increased gastric gland secretions, most effect on hydrochloric acid (HCl) production
		Small intestine	Causes contraction of intestinal muscle
		Ileocaecal valve	Relaxes valve
		Large intestine	Stimulates mass movements
Serotonin	Food in stomach	Stomach	Inhibits gastric acid secretion Increases peristalsis
Histamine	Food in stomach	Stomach	Release of HCl
Somatostatin	Food in stomach	Stomach	Inhibits gastric secretion, motility, emptying
	Sympathetic nerve stimulus	Pancreas	Inhibits secretion
		Small intestine	Inhibits GI blood flow and intestinal absorption
		Gall bladder	Inhibits contraction and bile release
Secretin	Acidic or irritant chyme, partially digested fats and proteins	Stomach	Inhibits gastric secretion and motility during gastric phase
		Pancreas	Increases bicarbonate-rich pancreatic juice Potentiates CCK action
		Liver	Increases bile output
Cholecystokinin (CCK)	Fatty chyme or partially digested proteins	Liver/pancreas	Potentiates secretin action
		Gall bladder	Increases enzyme-rich output
		Sphincter of Oddi	Stimulates contraction with expulsion of bile Relaxes to allow bile and pancreatic juice to enter duodenum
Gastric inhibitory peptide	Fatty and/or glucose-containing chyme	Stomach	Inhibits gastric gland secretion and motility during gastric phase Stimulates insulin production in response to a meal
Ghrelin	Absence of food in the stomach	Brain	Relays information to the brain, when needing fed. Increases appetite
Intestinal gastrin	Acidic/partly digested food in duodenum	Stomach	Stimulates gallbladder, pancreas and motility
		Small intestine	Causes contraction of intestinal muscle
		Ileocaecal valve	Relaxes valve
		Large intestine	Stimulates mass movements

by the duodenal mucosa, sometimes referred to as a third or **intestinal phase** of gastric juice secretion. The production of gastrin is stimulated by food in the stomach, particularly by partially digested proteins and caffeine.

P cells throughout the GI tract secrete **bombesin,** the gastrin-releasing peptide. Gastrin enters the gastric circulatory capillaries and the systemic circulation. It has the following actions:

- Stimulates the production of gastric acid by the parietal cells by the release of histamine.
- Has a minor role in stimulating the production of pepsinogen by chief cells.
- Stimulates the growth of the gastric and intestinal mucosa.

- Causes enhanced contraction of the cardiac sphincter to prevent gastric reflux.
- Stimulates the secretion of insulin and glucagon in the pancreas.

Control of Gastric Motility

Increase in Gastric Motility

Stomach contractions empty the stomach and compress, knead and mix the food with gastric juice to produce chyme. Waves of peristalsis pass from the cardiac sphincter to the pylorus about three times a minute. The more liquid parts of chyme pass through the pylorus into the small intestine, whereas the more solid parts are sent back to the body of the stomach for further gastric mixing. The regulatory peptide **motilin** increases gastric motility. It is produced by cells in the duodenum and jejunum in response to the entry of acid chyme.

Carbohydrates and liquids leave the stomach fastest, followed by proteins and fats. The **enterogastric reflex** is initiated when the products of protein digestion, together with the acid, enter the duodenum, resulting in a slowing of gastric motility. Gastric emptying usually takes 4–5 h, during which the antrum, pylorus and duodenal cap contract in sequence. This is the gastric pump mechanism, which results in squirts of chyme entering the duodenum.

Inhibition of Gastric Motility

When glucose and fats enter the duodenum, a regulatory peptide called **gastric inhibitory peptide** (GIP) is secreted by the **K cells** of the duodenal and jejunal mucosa. GIP, also known as *glucose-dependent insulin-releasing peptide,* decreases gastric secretion and motility and stimulates the secretion of insulin. **Vasoactive intestinal polypeptide,** produced in the **D cells** of the duodenum and colon, also inhibits gastric motility by acting as a smooth muscle relaxant. It also stimulates the intestinal secretion of electrolytes.

The Small Intestine

The Structure of the Small Intestine

The small intestine is the main digestion organ. It is here that food digestion is completed and absorption of nutrients and most of the water from the chyme take place. It is a long coiled tube, about 6 m long, that extends from the pyloric sphincter to the ileocaecal valve. Its diameter is only 2.5 cm.

There are three sections of the small intestine:
1. The duodenum lies mainly behind the peritoneum. It is C-shaped, approximately 25 cm long and surrounds the head of the pancreas.
2. The jejunum, 250 cm long, makes up about 40% of the remainder of the small intestine.
3. The ileum, 360 cm long, makes up the other 60% and joins the large intestine at the ileocaecal valve. Protective lymph nodes called **Peyer's patches** are present in the ileum.

The Duodenum

Salivary amylase begins the digestion of cooked starch into maltose and dextrins. Pepsin begins the breakdown of proteins into polypeptides. There is no secretion of enzymes by the duodenum, although it does secrete hormones. The duodenum receives the secretions of the pancreas and liver via the pancreatic duct and common bile duct (Fig. 21.3) after they join at the ampulla of Vater, at the sphincter of Oddi. These secretions are alkaline (pH of about 8) and produce a rapid change in pH from the acidity of the stomach to the alkalinity of the duodenum. Enzymes are pH-sensitive and function within a narrow range. The first few centimetres of the duodenum are called the **duodenal cap.** The tissue is

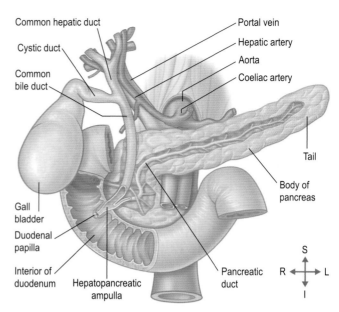

• **Fig. 21.3** The pancreas in relation to the duodenum and biliary tract. Part of the anterior wall of the duodenum has been removed.

protected from the acid chyme by a large number of mucus-secreting **Brunne's glands.**

Extrinsic Pancreatic Secretions

The exocrine function of the pancreas is achieved by secretions from **acinar cells** and plays a major role in digestion. The production of enzymes is discussed more fully in Chapter 22. The enzymes are secreted into the pancreatic duct and the duodenum. The three proteolytic enzymes are:

1. **Trypsinogen,** which is in an inactive form to safeguard the gut from autodigestion.
2. **Trypsin,** which is formed from trypsinogen in a reaction catalysed by the enzyme enterokinase (enteropeptidase). Trypsin completes the breakdown of proteins into amino acids.
3. **Carboxypeptidase,** which acts on peptides.
   Other enzymes are:
   • Pancreatic amylase, which converts starch to maltose.
   • Pancreatic lipase, which breaks down triglycerides into three fatty acids and glycerol.
   • Ribonuclease (RNase), which breaks down RNA.
   • Deoxyribonuclease (DNase), which acts on DNA to release free nucleotides.

Control of Pancreatic Juice Secretion

The hormone **secretin** results in the secretion of the watery component, rich in bicarbonate but low in enzymes. Another hormone, **cholecystokinin** (CCK), causes the release of the enzymes. Stimulation of pancreatic juice secretion can be divided into a cephalic phase, with vagal control brought about by the sight, smell or thought of food or the presence of food in the mouth, and a gastric phase stimulated by the release of gastrin.

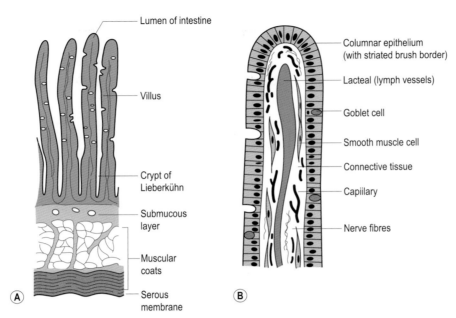

• **Fig. 21.4** (A) Villi in the small intestine. (B) A single villus.

CCK causes:
- Stimulation of enzyme-rich pancreatic secretion.
- Augmentation of the activity of secretin.
- Slowing of gastric emptying and inhibition of gastric secretion.
- Stimulation of enterokinase secretion.
- Stimulation of glucagon secretion.
- Stimulation of intestinal motility.
- Contraction of the gall bladder for the release of bile.

Bile

Bile is produced by the liver and stored in the gall bladder. It contains no digestive enzymes but emulsifies fats so that the fat-soluble vitamins and iron can be absorbed. Its production, content and function are discussed more fully in Chapter 22. The control of bile secretion also involves neural and hormonal factors. CCK is the major controller, causing contraction of the gall bladder and relaxation of the sphincter of Oddi. Once the gall bladder is empty, further flow of bile into the duodenum occurs directly from the liver. Vagus nerve stimulation will bring about a similar action. About 97% of bile salts are reabsorbed into the portal circulation and returned to the liver.

Intestinal Juice

The process of digestion is completed by mucus-rich juices secreted by the duodenum and jejunum. **Lieberkühn glands** in the jejunum and ileum secrete most of the watery juice. The nutrients are absorbed into the circulating blood through small finger-like projections on the surface of the small intestine called **villi**. They are covered by a layer of mucus to prevent autodigestion.

Intestinal Enzymes

These enzymes are produced by enterocytes in the villi and break down food particles into an absorbable form. Proteins are broken down into amino acids. Fats are broken down to form fatty acids and glycerol. Carbohydrates are broken down into monosaccharides: **glucose, fructose** and **galactose.** The enzymes are:
- Aminopeptidases: act on peptides.
- Dipeptidases: act on dipeptides.
- Maltase: converts maltose to glucose.
- Lactase: converts lactose to glucose and galactose.
- Sucrase: converts sucrose into glucose and fructose.

The Villi

Visible folding of the mucosa and submucosa forms **plicae circularis** (circular folds) which increase the surface area of the small intestine. The addition of villi and microvilli dramatically increases the surface area to 600 times that of a simple tube of the same size, giving a surface area of 200 m². Between the villi are small pits called the **crypts of Lieberkühn** where the mucus-secreting glands are situated. Villi have an external covering of simple columnar epithelium continuous with the crypts (Fig. 21.4). They have a central lacteal containing lymph, which empties into the local lymphatic circulation. There is a capillary blood supply linked to both hepatic and portal veins.

Two other types of cells are associated with the villi: **goblet cells** that secrete mucus are situated mainly in the crypts, and **enterocytes** are tall columnar cells involved in digestion and absorption. Enterocytes have many mitochondria to provide the energy for enzyme secretion and nutrient absorption. They have a high rate of mitosis, and those at the tip of the villi are replaced every 30 h.

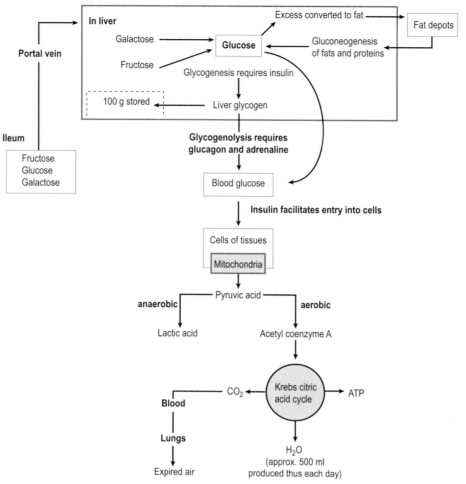

• **Fig. 21.5** Metabolic pathways for glucose.

Absorption

Lymphocytes and plasma cells are situated at intervals between the enterocytes. The plasma cells secrete **immunoglobulin A** to protect the gut from pathogens. There are also cells in the intestinal wall secreting 5-hydroxytryptamine, which may increase intestinal motility.

Absorption

There are 8–9 L of water and 1 kg of nutrients absorbed daily across the gut wall. The transport of nutrients can be either active or passive. **Active transport** requires energy and is usually against a concentration gradient. Most such substances require carrier molecules, including vitamin B_{12}, iron, sodium ions, glucose, galactose and amino acids. Water follows passively along an osmotic gradient. **Passive transport** requires no energy, depending on the direction of concentration and electrical gradients. It includes water, lipids, drugs and some electrolytes and vitamins. Some substances passively cross the gut wall membrane, with the help of carrier molecules, by **facilitated diffusion.**

Nutrients and Minerals
Monosaccharides

About 500 g of monosaccharides are absorbed daily. Galactose and glucose pass into the villous capillaries and then to the hepatic portal vein. A high concentration of sodium ions on the surface of the enterocytes facilitates the active transport of these molecules. Glucose and sodium ions share the same carrier molecule. The sodium concentration in the enterocyte is low so that sodium moves into the cell along a concentration gradient accompanied by glucose. Fructose has a different carrier molecule, and its transport is not influenced by sodium.

Monosaccharides are transported to the liver where galactose and fructose are converted to glucose (Fig. 21.5). Some of the glucose is converted to glycogen (**glycogenesis**) under the influence of insulin. About 100 g of glucose are stored in the liver, sufficient to maintain blood glucose levels for 24 hours. Some glycogen, approximately 400 g, is stored in skeletal muscle to provide energy for muscle action. The liver converts any glucose that is surplus to the body's needs into adipose tissue.

Blood glucose is maintained normally at a level of 4–7 mmol/L (72–126 mg/dL) (Diabetes UK, 2023). When the glucose level falls, liver glycogen is broken down (**glycogenolysis**) to release glucose. This occurs under the influence of glucagon and adrenaline (epinephrine). Once glycogen stores in the liver are depleted, the liver manufactures glucose from amino acids and glycerol (**gluconeogenesis**).

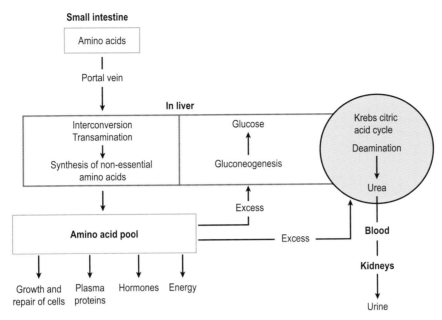

• **Fig. 21.6** Metabolic pathways for amino acids.

When circulating glucose arrives at the tissues, the cells take it up by facilitated diffusion, under the influence of insulin. In the **mitochondria** of the cells, glucose is oxidized to form energy in the **Krebs** or **citric acid cycle.** The glucose is converted to pyruvic acid, which in turn is converted to acetyl coenzyme A, usually referred to as **acetyl CoA** in a process requiring oxygen (i.e., aerobic). Acetyl CoA enters the Krebs cycle to undergo changes mediated by enzymes. The process of oxidation forms the energy-storage molecule adenosine triphosphate, along with water and CO_2. If there is insufficient oxygen to convert pyruvic acid to acetyl CoA, lactic acid is formed (see Chapter 23).

Amino Acids

In an adult, approximately 200 g of amino acids are absorbed daily from the ileum, of which 50 g/day are needed for tissue growth and repair and to maintain nitrogen balance. The mechanism for absorption of amino acids is not fully understood but might involve sodium and may depend on whether the amino acid is acidic, basic or neutral.

Amino acids cannot be stored by the body. Instead, they are absorbed into the blood where they can be removed as necessary (Fig. 21.6). However, the liver can interconvert amino acids by utilizing the eight essential amino acids to synthesize the non-essential amino acids. The process of **deamination** in the liver breaks down any excess amino acids. The nitrogen portion is converted into urea, which enters the blood and is excreted by the kidney.

Fats

About 80 g of fat are absorbed daily, mainly in the duodenum. The products of fat digestion (fatty acids and glycerol) are insoluble in water. Instead, bile salts and phospholipids help convert them into small water-soluble molecules known as **micelles.** The contents of the micelles are discharged onto the microvilli and enter the enterocytes by passive diffusion. Short-chain fatty acids enter the capillary network and travel in the hepatic portal vein as free fatty acids. Longer chain fatty acids are resynthesized in the enterocyte to become triglycerides coated with a layer of lipoprotein, cholesterol and phospholipid. These complexes enter the central lacteals to form **chyle,** which enters the lymphatic system and then the bloodstream. Faeces typically contain less than 20% fat for a healthy diet.

Bile salts, steroid hormones and cell membranes are formed from cholesterol. Cholesterol is found in the blood, mainly as lipoproteins (i.e., in combination with a protein carrier). There are three types:

1. High-density lipoproteins (HDLs).
2. Low-density lipoproteins (LDLs).
3. Very low-density lipoproteins (VLDLs).

Cholesterol (in the form of LDLs and VLDLs) is laid down in arterial walls as atheromatous plaques. HDLs are colloquially referred to as 'happy lipids' as they offer protection against ischaemic heart disease. An increased ratio of HDLs to LDLs and VLDLs has been shown in vegetarians, in those whose fat intake is largely unsaturated and in those who take regular exercise. The ratio is reduced in those who smoke cigarettes.

Fat can be utilized by the body to form energy, and any excess fat is stored as adipose tissue. When fat stores are needed for energy production, they are mobilized under the influence of growth hormones or cortisol and taken to the liver. Here the triglycerides are broken down into free fatty acids and glycerol. The fatty acids are converted to acetyl CoA in the presence of oxygen and glucose, and these enter the Krebs citric acid cycle (Fig. 21.7). If glucose is not available, acetyl CoA metabolism is deranged, forming the

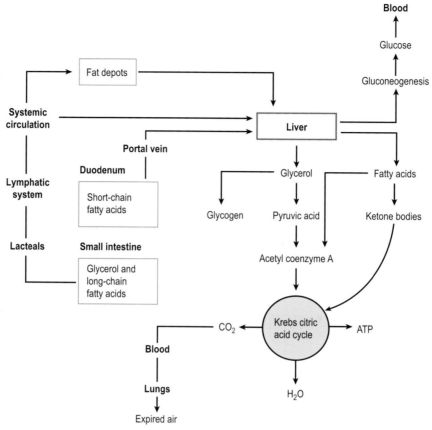

• **Fig. 21.7** Metabolic pathways for fats.

ketone bodies acetoacetic acid and β-hydroxybutyric acid. These can be oxidized to release energy, but they also accumulate in the blood, causing metabolic acidosis.

Sodium, Potassium and Water

About 2 L of fluid are ingested daily. A further 8–9 L of fluid are added to the gut during the production of digestive juices. Only 50–200 mL are lost in the faeces, the rest being absorbed from both the small and large intestine at a rate of 200–400 mL/min. The jejunum, ileum and colon actively reabsorb sodium ions, which are followed passively by chloride and water. Some potassium is actively secreted into the gut and reabsorbed from the ileum and colon along a concentration gradient.

Vitamins

The **water-soluble vitamins** (C and eight different B complexes), except vitamin B_{12} (absorbed as a complex with the intrinsic factor in the terminal ileum), are passively absorbed with water. The **fat-soluble vitamins** (A, D, E and K) enter the enterocytes in the micelles. Bile and lipase are necessary for their absorption.

Most calcium is absorbed in the upper part of the small intestine under the influence of parathyroid hormone and calcitonin. This active process is facilitated by vitamin D.

Iron

In developed countries, about 15–20 mg of iron is ingested daily, mostly as ferric salts, but only 5–10% is absorbed into the blood. There is a daily loss of 1 mg/day from desquamation of the skin and in the faeces. Women lose about 25 mg each month during menstruation. Iron is more readily absorbed in the ferrous form. The ferric form is reduced to the ferrous form by gastric juice and vitamin C.

Iron is actively absorbed in the upper part of the small intestine and is stored in the enterocytes when their cellular stores are low. The enterocytes discharge iron into the bloodstream when serum levels fall. Iron travels in the blood bound to **apoferritin,** which is known as **ferritin** when iron is bound to it. About 70% of iron in the body is in haemoglobin and 3% in myoglobin in muscle protein. The rest is stored in the liver as ferritin or as **haemosiderin.** Iron is used by the body to make the oxygen-carrying proteins haemoglobin and myoglobin. Iron also forms part of many other proteins in the body.

The Large Intestine

The adult large intestine is about 1.5 m long, consisting of the caecum, appendix, colon and rectum (Fig. 21.8). It has a diameter of 5–6 cm and can store large quantities of food residues. The large intestine has no villi and a much smaller

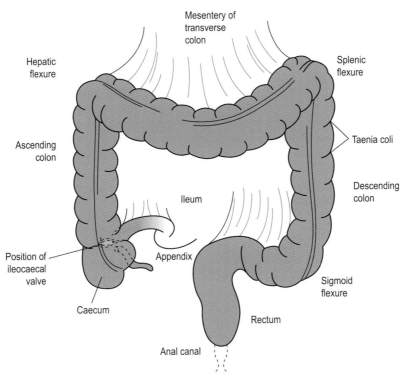

• **Fig. 21.8** The large intestine.

internal surface than the small intestine. The colon differs from the generalized structure of the GI tract; the longitudinal muscle bands are incomplete and the wall is gathered into three longitudinal bands, the **taeniae coli.** These bands are shorter than the remaining colon, so that when the circular muscles contract the wall pouches outwards into **haustrations** (buckets). The filling and emptying of the haustrations help to mix the colonic contents. Patches of lymphoid tissue are scattered throughout the length of the large intestine, protecting against pathogens.

About 1 L of porridge-like chyme enters the large intestine daily through the ileocaecal valve. This valve, normally closed because of back pressure from the colon's contents, opens in response to peristaltic waves. The caecum relaxes and the ileocaecal valve opens, a reflex called the **gastrocolic reflex.** The colonic peristalsis that follows fills the rectum with faeces, resulting in the urge to defecate.

The **caecum,** a blind pouch between the ileocaecal valve and the colon, is about 7 cm long. This has no known function in humans, although it is involved in cellulose digestion in herbivores. The **vermiform appendix,** a worm-like sac projecting from the end of the caecum, contains lymphoid tissue and enlarges in the presence of infection or inflammation (appendicitis). If an enlarged appendix ruptures, faecal material and bacteria enter the abdominal cavity, leading to peritonitis.

The Colon

The large intestine is divided anatomically into three regions:

1. The **ascending colon,** about 15 cm long, commences at the caecum and extends upwards on the right of the abdominal cavity as far as the lower border of the liver.
2. The **transverse colon,** 30–60 cm long, begins at the hepatic flexure and traverses the abdominal cavity below the liver and stomach.
3. The **descending colon,** about 25 cm long, descends along the left side of the abdominal cavity. The sigmoid (S-shaped) colon, about 40 cm long, is a continuation of the descending colon and empties into the rectum.

The large intestine has five functions:

1. Storage of unabsorbed food residues before defecation. About 70% of food residues are excreted within 72 hours of ingestion, but the remainder may stay in the colon for 1 week. Non-absorbable dietary fibre gives bulk to the faeces.
2. Absorption of water, electrolytes and some vitamins. Sodium is actively reabsorbed into the hepatic portal vein, followed passively by water and chloride. The amount of water reabsorbed depends on how long the residue remains in the colon. In constipation the residue may stay in the colon for several days, resulting in removal of most of the water.
3. Synthesis of vitamin K and some B vitamins—thiamine, folic acid and riboflavin—by commensal colonic bacteria. Bacterial fermentation of food residues results in the formation of flatus, which consists of nitrogen, CO_2, hydrogen, methane and hydrogen sulphide. Between 500–700 mL of flatus is produced daily depending on the type of food eaten; legumes lead to an increase in flatus production.

4. Secretion of mucus, which acts as a lubricant for elimination of faeces. The mucus contains bicarbonate, which impacts the pH of the large intestine as it moves from ascending colon (pH around 5.5) to descending colon (pH around 8.0).
5. Secretion of potassium ions.

Movements of the Colon

Contraction of the circular muscle fibres occurs about once every 30 min. This causes **segmentation,** a non-propulsive movement in the colon, which mixes the colonic contents and facilitates absorption. **Peristalsis** moves the faeces towards the rectum. The final propulsion towards the rectum is called **mass movement.**

The Rectum

The rectum is a muscular tube about 15 cm long. It is capable of great distension but is usually empty until just before defecation. The sudden distension of the rectal walls brought about by mass movement results in the urge to defecate. The rectum opens to the exterior by the anal canal, which has both internal and external sphincters.

The Anal Canal

The anal canal is about 3 cm long and begins where the rectum perforates the levator ani muscle of the pelvic floor. It has a sphincter at both ends. The **internal anal sphincter** is composed of smooth muscle fibres and is not under voluntary control. When nerve fibres from the sympathetic system are stimulated, the muscle fibres in the internal anal sphincter contract. Fibres from the parasympathetic system inhibit contractions and the sphincter relaxes. The **external anal sphincter** is made up of striated voluntary muscle and is supplied by fibres from the pudendal nerve. The sphincter is under conscious control from about 18 months of age. Damage to the sphincter or its nerve supply may occur in childbirth, resulting in incontinence of faeces.

Two superficial venous plexi, the haemorrhoidal veins, are associated with the anal canal. These may become distended, resulting in varicosities or haemorrhoids.

Defecation

Afferent nerve impulses travel to the sacral spinal cord when faeces enter the rectum. Impulses then travel back from the spinal cord in a reflex arc to the terminal ileum and anal sphincter to allow defecation. The cerebral cortex receives nerve messages, which allow inhibition of the spinal reflex arc if it is not convenient to defecate. Defecation is usually assisted by voluntary effort, which raises intra-abdominal pressure. A deep breath is taken and is expired against a closed glottis. This is called the **Valsalva manoeuvre.** The levator ani muscles contract and the pressure in the rectum is raised to about 200 mmHg (26 kPa). The anal sphincters relax and the contents of the rectum are expelled. During straining there is a sharp rise in blood pressure followed by a sudden fall.

Faeces

About 100–150 g of faeces are eliminated each day, consisting of 30–50 g solids and 70–100 g water. The solid portion consists mainly of cellulose, shed epithelial cells, bacteria, some salts and stercobilin, which gives it the brown colour. The characteristic odour of faeces is caused by bacterial breakdown of amines.

Maternal Adaptations to Pregnancy

The GI system undergoes significant changes during pregnancy to support the nutritional demands of the mother and fetus. The related alterations are often accompanied by upsets of the GI function, which are probably the most common cause of complaint by pregnant women. These minor disorders are discussed in Chapter 30.

The Mouth

Pregnant women usually find that they have an increased appetite and cravings or aversions for certain food. Some experience **pica,** which is a craving for non-food substances. Specific changes in food consumption and food habits are strongly influenced by cultural and economic factors and may also change to meet the needs of the fetus. Progesterone is a known appetite stimulant bringing about changes in appetite which closely follow the hormonal changes during the menstrual cycle. During pregnancy, alterations in the balance of oestrogen, progesterone, glucagon and insulin contribute to the changes in food intake.

The Gums and Teeth

The gums may become swollen and spongy and bleed easily. This results from oedema due to the effects of oestrogen on blood flow and the consistency of connective tissue. Oedema causes an increase in gingivitis and periodontal disease. This is often more extreme with increased maternal age and parity and where there are pre-existing dental problems. About 5% of pregnant women will develop an **epulis** (pregnancy tumour), which is a friable growth or hyperplasia of the gum usually found on the palatal side of the maxillary gingiva. It may bleed or interfere with chewing and will usually regress after delivery, although occasionally excision of the growth may be necessary.

Although dentists and women believe that pregnancy damages teeth, there is no evidence to suggest that demineralization of teeth occurs during pregnancy. The calcium needs of the fetus are drawn from maternal stores (skeleton) and not from maternal teeth. Changes in saliva and the nausea and vomiting of pregnancy may increase the risk of caries during pregnancy. There is growing evidence to suggest poor dental health is associated with adverse pregnancy outcomes such as preterm birth and low birthweight (Nannan, Xiaoping & Ying, 2022).

Saliva

Ptyalism, or excess salivation, may occur due to a reluctance of women to swallow because of associated nausea. There is no evidence to suggest that more saliva is actually produced. Ptyalism is often a particular problem in Afro-Caribbean women. Ganglion-blocking drugs may be required if ptyalism becomes a major problem. There is uncertainty as to the changes in the pH of saliva. It is more likely that the pH drops and saliva becomes more acidic in pregnancy.

The Oesophagus

Heartburn affects up to 80% of women by the third trimester (Phupong & Hanprasertpong, 2015). It is probably due to reflux oesophagitis caused by progesterone relaxing the cardiac sphincter between the oesophagus and stomach. The competence of the sphincter is impaired and regurgitation of gastric acid is more likely. This may not be the only cause, as acid reflux has also been found to be present in 40% of people with no heartburn. There is an increased risk of **hiatus hernia** where the cardiac sphincter is displaced into the thorax. Displacement of the sphincter has probably a minor role to play in heartburn and the more likely factor to be considered is the strength of the sphincter.

The Stomach

Acid Secretion

The effect of pregnancy on gastric acid secretion is unclear. There may be a tendency for secretions to decrease during pregnancy, beginning in the early weeks and becoming even less in late pregnancy. This may explain why a peptic ulcer is rarely detected in pregnancy and why those women with an ulcer have remission during pregnancy, with symptoms returning by the third month after delivery (Kelly & Savides, 2018).

Emptying Time

Gastric muscle tone and motility are reduced during pregnancy due to progesterone. However, low levels of circulating motilin have been found during pregnancy. This results in delay in emptying, which is probably associated with the lower secretion rate of gastric juices. The digestion time for solid food is prolonged, although watery food is digested and passed on to the small intestine with little delay. Drinks containing high levels of glucose, such as those administered in glucose tolerance tests, have a high osmotic effect, and gastric emptying is delayed in hyperosmotic foods. The reduced activity of the gastric muscle may exaggerate the effect and result in nausea. During labour, reduced stomach motility leads to a delay in emptying and a risk of acid aspiration.

The Small Intestine

Even though metabolism is anabolic during pregnancy, there is no increase in the absorption of food. Any increased nutrition must come from increased intake. There is facilitated absorption of nutrients such as iron and calcium. The prepregnant levels of calcium absorption (20–25%) increase early in pregnancy to 50% absorption by mid-pregnancy and thereafter remain stable (Ryan & Kovacs, 2021). Phosphate and magnesium absorption is assumed to follow calcium in terms of intestinal absorption. The transit time of food and waste products through the intestine is prolonged due to reduced mobility and a decrease in the tone of the intestinal musculature because of progesterone (Blackburn, 2018).

The Large Intestine

The colon shares in the general relaxation of smooth muscle found throughout the body. Constipation is a common complaint during pregnancy and is made worse by the prolonged transit time of waste materials and the resulting increased absorption of water in the colon. Increased flatulence may also occur.

Main Points

- The GI tract extends from the mouth to the anus. It consists of the mouth, pharynx, oesophagus, stomach, small intestine and large intestine.
- The GI tract undertakes six processes: ingestion, propulsion, mastication, digestion, absorption and elimination.
- The function of the GI tract is controlled by the ANS. Parasympathetic activity increases both the motility and secretory functions of the tract and relaxes the gut sphincters. Sympathetic activity decreases blood supply to the gut, secretions and gut motility.
- Digestion of food begins in the stomach and is completed in the small intestine.
- Saliva contains the digestive enzyme salivary amylase, which acts upon starch to convert polysaccharides into disaccharides.
- Gastric acid inactivates salivary amylase, alters the molecular structure of ingested proteins to tenderize them, curdles milk and converts pepsinogen to pepsin.
- Pepsin converts proteins to polypeptides.
- The small intestine is composed of the duodenum, the jejunum and the ileum. This is where absorption of nutrients and most of the water takes place.
- Pancreatic juice contains three proteolytic enzymes: trypsinogen, trypsin and carboxypeptidase.
- Bile emulsifies fats so that fat-soluble vitamins and iron can be absorbed.
- CCK controls bile release, causing contraction of the gall bladder and relaxation of the sphincter of Oddi.
- About 2 L of fluid are ingested daily. A further 8–9 L of fluid are added to the gut during the production of digestive juices. Only 50–200 mL are lost in the faeces, with the rest being absorbed from both the small and large intestines.
- Most calcium is absorbed in the upper part of the small intestine under the influence of parathyroid hormone and calcitonin. The process is facilitated by vitamin D.

- The large intestine consists of the caecum, appendix, colon and rectum.
- The colon absorbs most of the remaining water and electrolytes, synthesizes vitamin K and some B vitamins, secretes mucus and acts as a lubricant for elimination of faeces.
- Sudden distension of the rectum results in the urge to defecate. About 100–150 g of faeces are eliminated each day.
- Pregnant women usually find that they have an increased appetite and food consumption, craving for certain foods and avoidance of others. Pica is a craving for non-food substances. The gums may become swollen and spongy in pregnancy and bleed easily.
- Constipation is a common symptom of pregnancy. Gastric muscle tone and motility are reduced due to progesterone.
- Although the metabolism of pregnant women is anabolic, food absorption does not increase. Any increased nutrition must come from increased intake. Iron and calcium appear to be absorbed more readily.

References

Blackburn, S.T., 2018. Maternal, Fetal and Neonatal Physiology: A Clinical Perspective, fifth ed. Elsevier, Philadelphia.

Diabetes UK, 2023. A guide to diabetes. Available at: https://www.diabetes.org.uk/

Kelly, T.F., Savides, T.J., 2018. Gastrointestinal disease in pregnancy. In: Creasy, R.K. (Ed.), Maternal–fetal Medicine: Principles and Practice, eighth ed. Elsevier, Philadelphia.

Nannan, M., Xiaoping, L., Ying, J., 2022. Periodontal disease in pregnancy and adverse pregnancy outcomes: progress in related mechanisms and management strategies. Front. Med. 9, 963956.

Phupong, V., Hanprasertpong, T., 2015. Interventions for heartburn in pregnancy. Cochrane Database Syst. Rev. 2015 (9), CD011379.

Ryan, B.A., Kovacs, C.S., 2021. Maternal and fetal vitamin D and their roles in mineral homeostasis and fetal bone development. J. Endocrinol. Invest. 44 (4), 643–659.

Tortora, G.J., Derrickson, B.H., 2020. Principles of Anatomy and Physiology, sixteenth ed. Wiley, Hoboken.

Waugh, A., Grant, A., 2018. Ross & Wilson Anatomy and Physiology in Health and Fitness, thirteenth ed. Elsevier, London.

Annotated recommended reading

Blackburn, S.T., 2018. Maternal, Fetal and Neonatal Physiology: A Clinical Perspective, fifth ed. Elsevier, Philadelphia.

This text provides a detailed description of the major changes that occur in the body systems during pregnancy. There is an extensive review of the literature, extending from classical research studies to more recent research findings.

Sherwood, L., 2015. Human Physiology: From Cells to Systems, ninth ed. Cengage, Boston.

This textbook provides in-depth information on the physiology of the GI tract relevant for undergraduates in the healthcare profession.

22

The Accessory Digestive Organs

LYNSAY MATTHEWS

CHAPTER CONTENTS

This chapter discusses the contribution of the salivary glands, the pancreas and the liver to the process of digestion. The role of the liver in detoxification of drugs and ingested substances and the limitations to the protective role of the placenta are also described.

Introduction

The alimentary system contains not only the gastrointestinal tract discussed in Chapter 21 but also the accessory organs for digestion. Although it is artificial to separate these accessory organs from the wider system, the reader may find this easier. If required, readers are referred to the selection of referenced textbooks for more in-depth detail.

The Salivary Glands

Saliva aids speech, chewing and swallowing. There are three pairs of salivary glands: the parotid, submaxillary and sublingual glands. The **parotid glands** are the largest pair and are situated by the angle of the jaw. These glands produce a watery solution forming 25% of the daily saliva secretion. The **submaxillary glands** lie below the upper jaw and produce thicker saliva which forms 70% of the total daily output. The **sublingual glands** lie under the tongue on the floor of the mouth and produce only 5% of the daily output. Their solution is rich in glycoproteins, called *mucins,* which are primarily responsible for the lubricating action of saliva. Salivary glands produce 1–1.5 L of saliva each day. Saliva consists of 99.5% water and 0.5% solutes and has a pH value of around 7.0.

The Functions of Saliva

- It cleanses the mouth. Saliva contains lysozyme and the immunoglobulin IgA as a defence against micro-organisms.
- It provides oral comfort, reducing friction and allowing speech.
- It ensures that food is in solution so that the taste buds can recognize the contained chemicals.
- It facilitates the formation of a bolus of partly broken-up food ready to swallow. The mucins present in saliva help to mould and lubricate the bolus.
- It contains a digestive enzyme, salivary or α-amylase (formerly known as *ptyalin*), which acts upon starch to convert polysaccharides into disaccharides.

Control of Saliva Production

The secretion of saliva is controlled primarily by a parasympathetic supply from the facial (VII cranial) nerve and the glossopharyngeal (IX cranial) nerve. Normally, parasympathetic stimulation produces continuous moderate watery amounts of saliva. In contrast, sympathetic activity produces a sparse viscid secretion and the dry mouth most of us experience during times of stress (or after the administration of atropine or hyoscine, which block receptor sites for the neurotransmitter acetylcholine).

Saliva is produced as a conditioned reflex in response to the cerebral perception of the thought, sight or smell of food. The presence of food in the mouth will also lead to saliva production via an unconditioned reflex. The process of deglutition propels the food into the stomach for the next stage of digestion.

The Pancreas

The pancreas is a gland lying just below the stomach that has both endocrine and exocrine functions. It is a soft, friable, pink gland and is 'tadpole'-shaped, with a head surrounded by the C-shaped loop of the duodenum and a tail which extends towards the right side of the abdomen. Most of the pancreas is retroperitoneal. Through the centre of the pancreas runs the **pancreatic duct,** which fuses with the common bile duct just before it enters the duodenum at the hepatopancreatic ampulla.

Exocrine Functions of the Pancreas

Within the pancreas are the acini, which are clusters of cells surrounding small ducts. These provide the exocrine function and play a major role in digestion. The cells form and store zymogen granules, consisting of a wide range of digestive enzymes that act on all nutrients. The enzymes are secreted into the pancreatic duct and then into the duodenum.

Pancreatic Juice

The pancreatic enzymes were briefly mentioned in Chapter 21. About 1.5–2 L of pancreatic juice are secreted daily with a pH of 8–8.4. A mixture of two types of secretions is produced, containing a copious watery solution and a scanty solution rich in enzymes. The profuse watery solution contains the ions hydrogen carbonate (bicarbonate), sodium, potassium, calcium, magnesium, chloride, sulphate, phosphate and some albumin and globulin proteins. The enzyme-rich secretion contains the three proteolytic enzymes trypsinogen, trypsin and carboxypeptidase. Enzyme activity is summarized in Fig. 22.1. Other enzymes

are pancreatic amylase, pancreatic lipase, ribonuclease and deoxyribonuclease.

Control of Pancreatic Juice Secretion

The hormones secretin and cholecystokinin (CCK) were introduced in Chapter 21. Secretin is in the duodenum and upper jejunum when acid chyme enters the duodenum. Secretin enters the venous systemic circulation and arrives back at the pancreas via the pancreatic artery. Its presence results in the secretion of the watery component, which is rich in bicarbonate but low in enzymes.

CCK is secreted by the columnar cells of the duodenum and jejunum in response to the presence of the products of protein and fat digestion. CCK also circulates and returns to the pancreas via the pancreatic artery. Its presence causes release of the enzyme-rich secretion. CCK has many important functions:

- Stimulation of the enzyme-rich pancreatic secretion.
- Augmentation of the activity of secretion.
- The slowing of gastric emptying and inhibition of gastric secretion.
- Stimulation of the secretion of enterokinase.
- Stimulation of glucagon secretion.
- Stimulation of motility of the small intestine and colon.
- Contraction of the gall bladder with the release of bile.

Endocrine Functions of the Pancreas

Scattered among the acinar cells are approximately a million pancreatic islets (also called **islets of Langerhans**). These are tiny cell clusters that make up 1% of the pancreas and produce pancreatic hormones. There are two types of cells: the **α cells,** which synthesize glucagon, and the **β cells,** which produce insulin. The normal human pancreas produces about 40 international units of insulin in 24 hours. The other cells produce **somatostatin,** which acts to suppress islet cell hormone production. A hormone called **amylin** appears to be an insulin antagonist.

Glucagon

Glucagon is a short polypeptide of 29 amino acids. It is a potent hormone causing the release of millions of glucose molecules into the blood (Marieb & Hoehn, 2022).

Glucagon acts mainly in the liver to promote:

- Glycogenolysis (the breakdown of glycogen to glucose).
- Lipolysis.
- Gluconeogenesis (the formation of glucose from fatty acids and amino acids).

The liver releases glucose into the bloodstream, raising the blood sugar level. There is a fall in serum amino acid levels as the liver then takes up amino acids to synthesize new glucose molecules.

Falling blood sugar levels stimulate secretion of glucagon from α cells. Increasing amino acid levels also stimulates glucagon release. Glucagon release is suppressed by increasing blood sugar levels and by somatostatin.

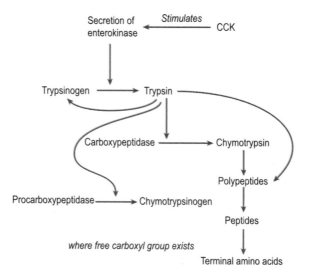

• **Fig. 22.1** Summary of activity of the pancreatic proteolytic enzymes. *CCK,* Cholecystokinin.

TABLE 22.1	The Effects of Insulin on Foods			
On Glucose	**On Fat**	**On Protein**	**On Electrolytes**
Removes glucose from the blood stream and moves it into cells Stimulates glycogen synthesis Inhibits glycogen breakdown Inhibits gluconeogenesis	Increases uptake of fatty acids from the blood Increases synthesis of triglycerides Inhibits triglyceride breakdown	Stimulates uptake of amino acids for protein synthesis	Increases the permeability of many cells to potassium, magnesium and phosphate ions

Insulin

Insulin is also a small polypeptide consisting of 51 amino acids. It begins as the middle part of a larger polypeptide chain called **proinsulin.** Enzymes cut the amino acid bonds to release the insulin just before it is secreted from the β cell. Insulin affects the metabolism of fat and protein as well as glucose (Table 22.1).

Production of Insulin

Insulin production is stimulated by the presence of glucose, amino acids and fatty acids in the blood and by hyperglycaemic agents such as glucagon, adrenaline (epinephrine), growth hormone, thyroxine and glucocorticoids. Insulin production is inhibited by somatostatin. Insulin binds firmly to a receptor site on the cell membrane. It appears to modify cellular activity without entering the cell. The presence of calcium is necessary for its functioning. A high-carbohydrate diet leads to increased sensitivity of tissues to insulin, and this may be due to a rise in the number of insulin receptors in the cell walls.

The Role of Insulin at the Cellular Level

Insulin assists entry of glucose into muscle, connective tissue and white blood cells. It does not facilitate entry of glucose into liver, kidney and brain cells. Those cells have easy access to glucose regardless of insulin. Insulin counters any metabolic activity that would increase plasma glucose levels such as glycogenolysis and gluconeogenesis. These last effects are probably due to insulin inhibition of glucagon. Once glucose has entered the cells, insulin triggers enzyme activity which:
- Catalyses the oxidation of glucose to produce adenosine triphosphate.
- Joins glucose molecules together to form glycogen.
- Converts glucose to fat, particularly in adipose tissue.

These processes are discussed more in Chapter 23.

The Liver and Gall Bladder

The liver is one of the body's most important organs. It is one of the accessory organs and is associated with the small intestine. Although it has many metabolic roles (see Chapter 23), its only digestive function is to secrete **bile,** which it stores in the gall bladder and discharges into the duodenum. Bile acts on fats to emulsify them (i.e., break them up into tiny particles) so that they are more accessible to digestive enzymes.

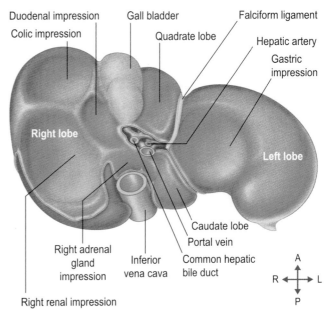

• **Fig. 22.2** The liver Inferior view (turned up to show the posterior surface).

Anatomy

The liver is a very large gland and weighs on average 1.4 kg. It is in the abdominal cavity under the diaphragm, extending more to the right of the midline than the left, obscuring the stomach. It lies totally protected by the rib cage. The liver has four lobes:
1. The right lobe, which is the largest.
2. The smaller left lobe.
3. The caudate lobe, which is the posterior lobe.
4. The quadrate lobe, which lies inferior to the left lobe.

The right lobe is the largest and is separated from the left lobe by a deep fissure. The right and left lobes are also separated by the **falciform ligament,** a cord of mesentery which suspends the liver from the diaphragm and the anterior abdominal wall. A fibrous remnant of the left umbilical vein, called the **ligamentum teres,** runs along the free edge of the falciform ligament. The superior aspect of the liver, or bare area, is fused to the diaphragm, and the remainder of the organ is enclosed in visceral peritoneum. The lesser omentum anchors the liver to the lesser curvature of the stomach. Fig. 22.2 shows an inferior view of the liver, identifying the lobes and blood supply.

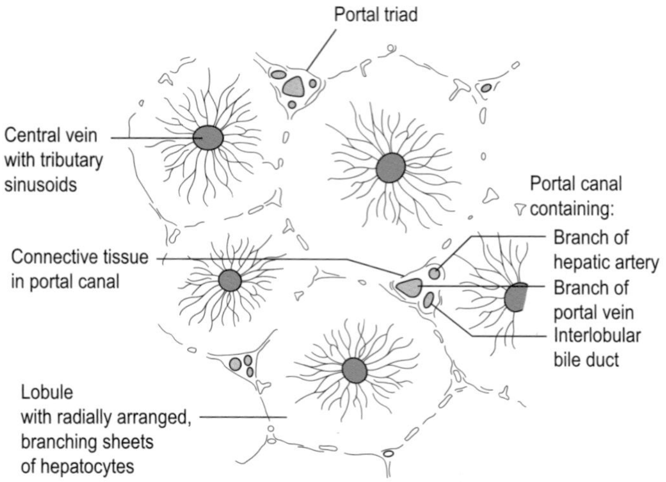

Portal triad

Central vein
with tributary
sinusoids

Connective tissue
in portal canal

Portal canal
▽ containing:

Branch of
hepatic artery

Branch of
portal vein

Interlobular
bile duct

Lobule
with radially arranged,
branching sheets
of hepatocytes

• **Fig. 22.3** The general features of the liver lobules at low magnification, showing the portal triad.

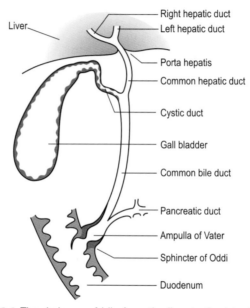

Liver

Right hepatic duct

Left hepatic duct

Porta hepatis

Common hepatic duct

Cystic duct

Gall bladder

Common bile duct

Pancreatic duct

Ampulla of Vater

Sphincter of Oddi

Duodenum

• **Fig. 22.4** The drainage of bile from the liver to the intestine (the biliary tract).

Microscopic Anatomy

The liver is composed of small units called *liver lobules*. Lobules are small hexagonal cylinders consisting of plates of **hepatocytes** (epithelial liver cells) (Fig. 22.3). The hepatocytes produce bile, process blood-borne nutrients and play an important role in detoxification (see later). The hepatocytes radiate outwards from a central vein running along the longitudinal axis of each lobule. At each of the six corners of a lobule is a **portal triad** (Fig. 22.4). The three structures present in a triad are:

1. A branch of the hepatic artery, supplying arterial blood to the liver.
2. A branch of the hepatic portal vein, carrying nutrient-rich blood from the digestive tract.
3. A bile duct.

The hepatic artery and the hepatic portal vein enter the liver at the **porta hepatis.** Between the hepatocyte plates are enlarged capillaries called **sinusoids.** Blood percolates

through the sinusoids from both the hepatic artery and the hepatic portal vein and is collected up into the central veins. Inside the sinusoids are the **Kupffer cells,** hepatic macrophages which remove debris such as worn-out blood cells and bacteria from the blood.

Digestive Functions of the Liver

The liver produces bile and enzymes that detoxify the many noxious substances arriving at the liver via the bloodstream.

The Production of Bile

Bile produced by the hepatocytes flows into tiny channels called **bile canaliculi** and enters the bile duct branches in the portal triads. Collectively, the hepatocytes produce as much as 1000 mL (1 L) of bile daily. More is produced if a fatty meal is eaten. Blood and bile flow in opposite directions in the liver lobules. The bile flows into the hepatic duct and, if needed by the digestive system, flows into the duodenum. If no bile is needed, the sphincter of Oddi is tightly closed and bile flows through the cystic duct to be stored in the gall bladder (Fig. 22.4).

The gall bladder is a thin-walled muscular bag about 10 cm long, situated in a fossa on the inferior surface of the liver's right lobe. It stores secreted bile and concentrates it by absorbing water and ions. When empty, its walls are thrown into rugae to allow for distension. When the muscular wall contracts, bile is ejected into the cystic duct, leading to the common bile duct.

Bile contains no digestive enzymes, and its chief role is to emulsify fats so that they and the fat-soluble vitamins and iron can be absorbed. Bile is a viscous fluid and is green-yellow to brown in colour. It contains 97% water, 0.7% bile salts, mucin and bicarbonate. Also present in bile are fatty acids, lecithin, inorganic salts, alkaline phosphatase and the excretory products of steroid-based hormones. Bile is alkaline with a pH of 7.0–8.0.

Bile Salts

Bile salts are formed from the steroids cholic acid and deoxycholic acid, which are manufactured in the liver from cholesterol. In the liver, cholic acid is **conjugated** (joined together with the elimination of water) with the amino acids taurine and glycine to form taurocholic acid and glycocholic acid. The bile acids form salts with sodium and potassium.

The functions of the bile salts are to:
- Deodorize faeces.
- Activate lipase and proteolytic enzymes in the duodenum.
- Reduce the surface tension of fat droplets (which helps emulsify them).

Bile salts combine with lipids, lecithin and cholesterol to form water-soluble micelles which allow fat to be more easily absorbed. If bile salts are absent, about 25% of ingested fat will be lost in the stools. These stools will be bulky and have an offensive odour.

Bile Pigments

Bile pigments make up 0.2% of the composition of bile. They are produced from the breakdown of red blood cells and are mainly **bilirubin** with a small amount of **biliverdin.** The pigments are taken to the liver bound to plasma albumin where they are conjugated with glucuronic acid in the presence of the enzyme glucuronic transferase. This forms the water-soluble bilirubin diglucuronide which enters bile to give it the golden colour. In the gut stercobilinogen is formed and, after conversion by bacterial action, is excreted as stercobilin. Some stercobilinogen is absorbed by the bloodstream and excreted as urobilinogen by the kidneys.

Control of Bile Secretion

As with other secretions into the gastrointestinal tract, the control of bile secretion involves neural and hormonal factors. CCK is the major controller, causing contraction of the gall bladder and relaxation of the sphincter of Oddi. Once the gall bladder has emptied its contents, further flow of bile into the duodenum occurs directly from the liver. Vagus nerve stimulation brings about a similar action. About 97% of bile salts are reabsorbed into the portal circulation and returned to the liver (after their passage through the intestine). This is called the **enterohepatic circulation of bile salts.** The production of bile by the liver depends on the blood level of bile salts. High blood levels of bile salts stimulate the liver cells to secrete more bile.

Detoxification of Ingested Material

A second important function of the liver is the detoxification of ingested substances. Systems have evolved to protect humans from ingested poisons found especially in plants (see Chapter 8). This involves detoxification by enzymes and subsequent excretion of the by-products by the liver. Any alteration in liver or kidney function may reduce the ability of the body to handle harmful chemicals. Many drugs are naturally occurring chemicals, and even those synthesized in the laboratory will have similar chemical structures to naturally occurring substances.

The Role of the Liver in Metabolism

The liver processes nearly every type of nutrient absorbed from the digestive tract. It also plays a major part in controlling plasma cholesterol levels. The hepatocytes carry out

at least 500 metabolic functions. It would take a textbook devoted to the topic to begin to explore all the functions of the liver. That is why the liver is such an important organ. Major metabolic roles include:
- Packaging fatty acids into forms that can be stored and transported.
- Synthesizing plasma proteins.
- Synthesizing non-essential amino acids.
- Converting ammonia from the deamination of amino acids to urea for excretion.
- Storing glucose as glycogen.
- Regulating blood sugar level by glycogenolysis and gluconeogenesis.
- Storing vitamins.
- Conserving iron from the breakdown of red blood cells.
- Detoxifying substances such as alcohol and drugs.

The Absorption, Distribution and Fate of Drugs

There are two main ways of describing drugs in the body:
1. **Pharmacokinetics,** which is concerned with the way the body handles drugs.
2. **Pharmacodynamics,** which is concerned with the effect drugs have on the body function (Ritter et al., 2018).

Drugs are often given to patients because of a need to support a failing system or organ. Examples are the administration of insulin when the pancreas is unable to make sufficient insulin of its own in type 1 (and some cases of type 2) diabetes or the use of antibiotics to support the immune system in bacterial invasion. Drugs may also be used to control a function: for example, the administration of the contraceptive pill to control reproductive function. Drugs usually have the following attributes:
- They bind to protein targets.
- They exert chemical influences on one or more cellular components.
- They may affect one or more tissues.
- They may have agonist or antagonist effects.

The protein targets of drugs may be enzymes in metabolic reactions, carrier molecules on cell membranes, receptor molecules on cell membranes or ion channels in cell membranes (Ritter et al., 2018).

Drug Disposition

Drug disposition is the process of drug molecule behaviour in the body. There are four stages:
1. Absorption from the site of administration.
2. Distribution within the body (translocation).
3. Metabolic alteration.
4. Excretion from the body.

Absorption

Absorption is the passage of a drug from the site of administration into the plasma. Except for some topical applications and some inhaled substances, most drugs must enter the plasma to travel to target tissues. Drugs are absorbed at different rates from sites, and some may be unsuitable for some routes.

Distribution Within the Body (Translocation)

There are two main phases in drug distribution. The first is **bulk flow transfer,** which is the transport of drugs around the body by the circulatory system. Some drugs may be transported freely in solution, but many are carried around the blood attached to a carrier molecule such as plasma albumin. The second phase at the cellular level is **diffusional transfer.** This describes the carriage of drugs into the cells in a specific tissue. Diffusional transfer may be by:

- Diffusion through the lipid cell membrane.
- Diffusion through aqueous pores which traverse the lipid membrane.
- Combination with a carrier molecule to ferry the drug across the membrane.
- Pinocytosis to engulf the substance.

There is controversy as to whether aqueous pores exist; if they do, they are probably too small to allow entry of most molecules. Pinocytosis, where a piece of cell membrane surrounds the substance and draws it into the cell, concerns large biological molecules only.

Diffusion Through the Lipid Membrane

This is one of the most important pharmacokinetic characteristics of a drug. Fat-soluble drugs diffuse across capillary walls and through cell membranes easily. Other determinants of diffusion include the pH of body fluids (acids and alkalis neutralize each other to precipitate salt and water) and ionization (drugs that are strongly ionized are not lipid-soluble and may not be able to enter cells unaided).

Carrier Mediation

Many drugs have specialized transport mechanisms to regulate entry and exit from cells. This usually involves a carrier molecule incorporated into the cell membrane. In facilitated diffusion, energy is not needed. In contrast, active transport requires energy. Some pharmaceutical effects are the result of interference with carrier protein function.

Drug Metabolism in the Liver

Drugs pass through the liver several times while they are in the circulation. Metabolic alteration of drug molecules involves two kinds of biochemical reactions brought about by liver enzymes:

1. **Phase 1 reactions,** which may result in a more active or toxic metabolite of the drug, involve:
   a. Oxidation—adding oxygen or removing hydrogen.
   b. Reduction—adding hydrogen or removing oxygen.
   c. Hydrolysis—splitting of the molecule into separate parts by water.
2. **Phase 2 reactions** involve conjugation by liver enzymes, resulting in a water-soluble, inactive product ready for excretion.

Excretion of Drugs

Drugs are mainly excreted by the kidney, but may also be excreted in expired air, perspiration, faeces and breastmilk. In pregnancy, they may cross the placental barrier to the fetus . In the kidney, there are three processes for excretion of drugs:

1. **Glomerular filtration**: if drugs are free in the plasma (i.e., not bound to plasma proteins) and if their molecular weight is below 20,000 Da.
2. **Active tubular secretion/reabsorption**: independent carrier systems are present in the proximal tubule for non-lipid-soluble drugs or ionized drugs (one for acids and one for bases).
3. **Passive diffusion across the tubular epithelium**: diffusion of lipid-soluble drugs occurs across the tubular and capillary cell membranes in the distal and collecting tubules.

Drugs that are hydrophilic and poorly lipid soluble, such as antibiotics, do not enter cells readily. They have a lower density volume and are readily excreted by the kidney. Lipid-soluble drugs are readily reabsorbed in the renal tubule and need breaking down to water-soluble by-products, usually in the liver, to be excreted.

Maternal Adaptations to Pregnancy

The Pancreas

There is a slight decrease in serum amylase and lipase, although this seems to have no significance. The alterations in glucose metabolism, due to increasing insulin resistance, are much more significant. This may be enough to precipitate gestational diabetes in susceptible women. Glucose metabolism is discussed in Chapter 23 and diabetes in pregnancy in Chapter 35.

The Gall Bladder

The decrease in muscle tone and motility of the gall bladder during pregnancy is probably due to the effects of progesterone on smooth musculature. As a result, the volume is increased and the emptying rate is decreased. An increased fasting volume is probably due to decreased water absorption by the mucosa of the gall bladder. This change is due to reduced activity of the cell wall sodium pump, which is a function of the increased circulating oestrogens. Alterations in gall bladder tone lead to retention of bile salts, leading to pruritus (itchiness of the skin) (Blackburn, 2018). Pregnancy may predispose to gall stones, but there is little empirical evidence to support this belief.

The Liver

As pregnancy progresses, the liver is displaced superiorly, posteriorly and anteriorly by the growing uterus. Although there is no change in blood flow to the liver, there may be a reduction in the proportion of cardiac output to the liver of about 30% (Blackburn, 2018).

The production of plasma proteins, bilirubin, serum enzymes and serum lipids is altered by the liver. Some changes arise from the presence of oestrogen and some from haemodilution. These changes show up on liver function tests. However, results need to be interpreted in relation to pregnancy; for example, reference ranges for alanine and aspartate transaminases, bilirubin and alkaline phosphatase are different in pregnancy (Guarino, Cossiga & Morisco, 2020). Many changes are reversible and resolve after labour and delivery. Some do not require further investigation, such as isolated raised alkaline phosphatase, palmar erythema or spider naevi.

Some liver function changes are, however, harmful to either the mother or fetus . Abnormal liver function tests associated with signs and symptoms should result in referral to secondary care. Pruritus, jaundice and upper abdominal pain are associated with the most common pregnancy-related liver problems. Referral should also be considered with raised serum bile acids, hypertension or proteinuria.

Pruritus is a common complaint affecting around 25% of pregnant women. In most cases it is benign. However, in association with abnormal liver function tests, certain complications should be considered. For example, **intrahepatic cholestasis,** which affects approximately 0.7% of pregnancies in the UK, is associated with increased rates of intra-uterine death, fetal hypoxia and preterm labour (Guarino, Cossiga & Morisco, 2020).

An important point about pregnancy-related liver problems is that they should resolve spontaneously after delivery. Women who exhibit ongoing abnormal liver function after delivery should be investigated further for underlying disease.

Pharmacokinetics and Pregnancy

Health professionals who prescribe drugs must consider the likelihood of a woman being pregnant or lactating (Schaefer, Peters & Miller, 2014). Drugs taken in early pregnancy may be teratogenic, a prime example being the tragedy of thalidomide in the 1960s (Blackburn, 2018). Drugs given in late pregnancy may cause behavioural anomalies in children. Many women are unaware of the danger of taking over-the-counter drugs. Taking drugs during pregnancy may be essential for some women; their life and the life of the fetus may be endangered if the drugs are discontinued, even though the drugs may be involved in causing abnormalities in the fetus . An example would be the use of Epanutin (phenytoin) in epilepsy, which may cause oral deformities.

Modification of Pharmacokinetics

Ingestion

Nausea and vomiting may cause rejection of the drug. Some women will not comply with taking medicines during pregnancy.

Absorption

Most drugs are taken orally and are absorbed by the stomach and small intestine. Gastric motility is reduced throughout pregnancy and especially in labour. This slows down absorption of some drugs but may increase absorption of others.

Most common drugs show little change from normal. Taking antacid preparations will lead to the absorption of some drugs being reduced.

Distribution

Increased extracellular fluid and body fat may alter the compartmental distribution of drugs. The fetus is considered to be a compartment and, although probably resistant to bolus doses, may be at risk in long-term drug therapy.

Protein Binding

Many drugs circulate around the body bound to plasma proteins, especially albumin, which is reduced in pregnancy. There is an increase in some specific proteins such as transferrin and thyroid-binding hormone. Some drugs which bind to α_1 acid glycoprotein are more likely to cross the placenta.

Elimination

Drugs that act within the central nervous system or within cells are lipid-soluble. These cannot be effectively excreted without conjugation to water-soluble by-products in the liver. The kidney will excrete those drugs excreted by the renal tubules. The role of the placenta as a barrier to drugs is discussed in Box 22.1.

• BOX 22.1 The Placenta and Fetus

Almost all drug reactions carried out by the liver have been identified in placental tissue. To date, no studies have been carried out in vivo. This means we cannot trust the placenta to protect the fetus from the effect of drugs. The main trophoblastic layer in the placenta is a syncytium, covered by a continuous lipid membrane. This membrane acts in a similar way to the blood–brain barrier so that lipid substances of low molecular weight (below 1000 Da) can readily diffuse across the membrane. Water-soluble molecules of up to 100 MW can also diffuse easily, but charged ionic molecules cannot pass unless they are bound to a carrier protein (Schaefer, Peters & Miller, 2014). Therefore, drugs that affect the central nervous system will readily cross the placental barrier.

Other drugs such as barbiturates, non-steroidal anti-inflammatory agents, warfarin and anticonvulsants are weak acids, whereas narcotics, local anaesthetics, beta-blockers or beta stimulants are weak bases. These act as non-ionic substances and will cross the placental barrier slowly. Polar drugs such as penicillins and cephalosporins are transferred so slowly that the fetus has no problem eliminating the drugs faster than they are transferred. Heparin is a large molecule and cannot cross the placenta. The fetus and neonate have a reduced ability to handle drugs because of immaturity of liver enzyme systems.

Maternal elimination of polar non-lipid drugs is much faster during pregnancy. This means that the dose requirements of some drugs, such as anticonvulsants, may rise during pregnancy. Some of these drugs cannot cross the placental barrier, whereas others are excreted rapidly by the fetus and pose no problem. Some drugs such as anticonvulsants build up slowly in the fetus and may cause malformations. Maternal breakdown of lipid-soluble drugs is slower in pregnancy. These drugs readily cross the placenta into fetal tissues and may be excreted very slowly (Blackburn, 2018).

Main Points

- There are three salivary glands: the parotid, submaxillary and sublingual glands. Saliva contains lysozyme and the immunoglobulin IgA to defend against micro-organisms. Salivary or α amylase acts upon starch to convert polysaccharides into disaccharides.
- Parasympathetic supply produces continuous watery saliva via a conditioned reflex in response to the perception of the thought, sight or smell of food.
- The pancreas has both endocrine and exocrine functions. About 1% of the pancreas consists of the islet of Langerhans cells. The α cells synthesize glucagon, which promotes glycogenolysis, lipolysis and gluconeogenesis. The β cells produce insulin, which stimulates glucose utilization, glycogen synthesis, inhibition of glycogen breakdown and inhibition of gluconeogenesis. It also assists the entry of glucose into muscle, connective tissue and white blood cells. The δ cells produce somatostatin, which acts to suppress islet cell hormone production.
- The hepatocytes in the liver produce bile, process blood-borne nutrients and have a key role in detoxification. The liver processes nearly every type of nutrient absorbed from the digestive tract.
- Bile salts are manufactured in the liver. Bile pigments are produced from the breakdown of red blood cells.
- The control of bile secretion involves neural and hormonal factors. CCK is the major controller, causing contraction of the gall bladder and relaxation of the sphincter of Oddi. High blood levels of bile salts stimulate the liver cells to secrete more bile. When no bile is needed, the sphincter of Oddi is tightly closed and bile flows through the cystic duct to be stored in the gall bladder.
- Changes to the accessory digestive system during pregnancy may result in increased insulin resistance, pruritis (itching) or less common complications such as intrahepatic cholestasis.
- Increased extracellular fluid and body fat during pregnancy may alter the compartmental distribution of drugs. Many drugs circulate around the body bound to plasma proteins, especially albumin. Some drugs are likely to cross the placenta.
- Almost all drug reactions carried out by the liver have been identified in placental tissue. The fetus and neonate have a reduced ability to handle drugs because of immaturity of liver enzyme systems.
- Maternal elimination of polar non-lipid drugs is much faster during pregnancy, as the kidney excretes them. Maternal breakdown of lipid-soluble drugs is slower in pregnancy. These drugs readily cross the placenta into fetal tissues and may be excreted very slowly.

References

Blackburn, S.T., 2018. Maternal, Fetal and Neonatal Physiology: A Clinical Perspective, fifth ed. Elsevier, Philadelphia.

Guarino, M., Cossiga, V., Morisco, F., 2020. The interpretation of liver function tests in pregnancy. Best Pract. Res. Clin. Gastroenterol. 44–45, 101667.

Marieb, E.N., Hoehn, K., 2022. Human Anatomy and Physiology, twelfth ed. Pearson, Harlow.

Ritter, J.M., Flower, R.S., Henderson, G., Loke, Y.K., MacEwan, D., Rang, H., 2018. Rang & Dale's Pharmacology, ninth ed. Elsevier, Edinburgh.

Schaefer, C., Peters, P.W.J., Miller, R.K., 2014. Drugs During Pregnancy and Lactation: Treatment Options and Risk Assessment, third ed. Elsevier, London.

Annotated recommended reading

Marieb, E.N., Hoehn, K., 2022. Human Anatomy and Physiology, twelfth ed. Pearson, Harlow.

This textbook presents a detailed overview of human anatomy and physiology related to the gastrointestinal tract and accessory organs. It is well illustrated with diagrams and pictures.

Ritter, J.M., Flower, R.S., Henderson, G., Loke, Y.K., MacEwan, D., Rang, H., 2018. Rang & Dale's Pharmacology, ninth ed. Elsevier, Edinburgh.

This textbook presents a detailed overview of pharmacokinetics for information about drugs, how they affect the body and how the body handles drugs.

23

Nutrition and Metabolism During Pregnancy

HORI SOLTANI AND FRANKIE FAIR

CHAPTER CONTENTS

This chapter discusses the principles of general nutrition. This includes a brief overview of basic nutrition physiology and biochemistry and general food groups, energy nutrients and metabolism. In addition, pregnancy-specific nutritional requirements and metabolic adaptation are detailed. Students and midwives need to have confidence in their knowledge base to provide appropriate nutritional advice and guidance.

Introduction

Adequate nutrition during pregnancy has both short- and long-term impacts on the well-being of the mother and her growing fetus . Nutritional advice for pregnant women includes careful consideration of dietary quality and quantity as needed. Some health professionals do not feel confident giving nutritional advice to their clients (Dieterich & Demirci, 2020).

Nutrition

Nutrients are utilized by the body for tissue growth, maintenance and repair. They can be divided into six categories: the three major nutrients (macronutrients) are carbohydrates, lipids and proteins, and micronutrients including vitamins and minerals, which are required in small amounts. Additionally, water makes up approximately 60% of the adult body and is considered a vital nutrient due to its role as a solvent and because of its necessity for optimal health.

Food Groups

Four food groups provide a balanced diet. The types and a general guide on daily food choices are:
1. Potato, bread, cereal, rice and pasta: base meals on these and choose whole grains where possible.
2. Fruits and vegetables: at least five portions every day.
3. Beans, pulses, fish, eggs, meat and other proteins: 2–3 servings.
4. Dairy products, milk, cheese, yoghurt and alternatives: have some dairy in lower fat and lower sugar options.

Public Health England (2016) has combined these groups alongside a fifth group—oils and spreads—into an 'Eatwell' guide showing quantities of each source required in relation to each other for health benefits (Fig. 23.1). Foods high in fat, sugar or salt are no longer a part of this plate, representing the need to remove overall intake of these items to achieve a healthier lifestyle.

Macronutrients

The different types of macronutrients including carbohydrates, lipids and proteins as well as their function and metabolism pathways are briefly described.

Carbohydrates

Carbohydrates are the main source of energy in our food, although other macronutrients can also be metabolized to

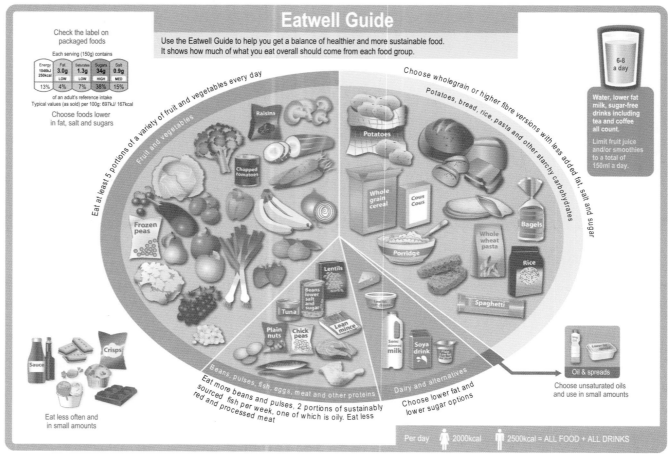

• **Fig. 23.1** A schematic presentation of a balanced diet, including various food categories.

• BOX 23.1 Three Types of Carbohydrates

1. Monosaccharides (single sugars):
   a. Glucose, which is the ultimate example (corn syrup, processed foods).
   b. Fructose (fruits, honey).
   c. Galactose (milk).
2. Disaccharides (double sugars) – some of the most common ones are:
   a. Sucrose: glucose + fructose (sugar).
   b. Lactose: glucose + galactose (milk).
   c. Maltose: glucose + glucose (commercial malt product of starch breakdown).
3. Polysaccharides (multiple sugars or complex carbohydrates) – some of the most common ones are:
   a. Starch (grains, legumes, root vegetables).
   b. Glycogen (liver and muscle meats).
   c. Cellulose which forms a large part of dietary fibre (whole grains, fruits, vegetables, seeds and nuts).

---

yield energy. The three types of carbohydrates are summarized in Box 23.1.

Carbohydrates play a fundamental role in the physiology of the body. For example, glucose is the ultimate common refined body fuel that is oxidized in cells to give energy. For normal functioning, it is important to maintain a certain range of glucose in the blood between 4.0–7.8 mmol/L. Cellulose, a form of plant carbohydrate (dietary fibre) unable to be processed by the human digestive system, provides roughage to increase the bulk of faeces, thus facilitating defecation. Dietary fibres have a role in the management of serum lipid and glucose levels (Reynolds, Akerman & Mann, 2020). They help to prevent and manage chronic diseases such as diabetes and cardiovascular disease.

Carbohydrate Metabolism

The Krebs (Tricarboxylic Acid or Citric Acid) Cycle. Glucose circulating in blood is taken up by cells through facilitated diffusion under the influence of insulin. It is taken to the cells' mitochondria where it is oxidized to form energy via the Krebs cycle (Figs. 23.2 and 23.3). A series of reactions called *glycolysis* break glucose, a 6-carbon molecule, down into two 3-carbon molecules, pyruvic acid.

Pyruvic acid reacts with coenzyme A (a derivative of a B complex vitamin, pantothenic acid) to form acetyl coenzyme A (acetyl CoA). Acetyl CoA is a 2-carbon molecule, with the additional carbon atom from pyruvic acid combining with oxygen to form carbon dioxide. Acetyl CoA enters the Krebs cycle, also known as the citric acid cycle, to undergo changes mediated by the enzyme adenosine triphosphate (ATP), with water and carbon dioxide formed in the process of oxidation.

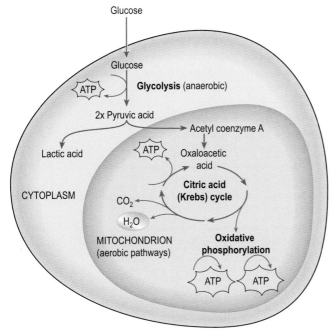

• **Fig. 23.2** Oxidation of glucose.

Each glucose molecule produces two pyruvic acid molecules, allowing two turns of the Krebs cycle. The Krebs cycle consists of a series of eight separate biochemical reactions. Excess carbon atoms unite with oxygen to produce carbon dioxide. Surplus hydrogen atoms are combined with nicotinamide adenine dinucleotide (NAD) and flavin adenine dinucleotide (FAD), converting them into NADH and FADH$_2$, respectively.

Adenosine Triphosphate Synthesis. Energy is stored in food, in carbon–hydrogen bonds, but cells cannot use energy in this form. They must convert it into the high-energy phosphate bonds of ATP (Hall & Hall, 2020). ATP consists of two high-energy phosphate bonds. When a bond between adenosine (a nucleotide) and a phosphate group in ATP is split, large amounts of energy are released and adenosine diphosphate (ADP) plus an inorganic phosphate molecule (P$_i$) is formed. Some energy produced is in the form of heat which helps maintain the temperature of the body. This can be written as:

$$\text{Splitting by hydrolysis: ATP} \rightarrow \text{ADP} + \text{P}_i + \text{energy}$$

Cellular Respiration

Aerobic Cellular Respiration. The main role of the Krebs cycle is to prepare NADH and FADH$_2$ for entry into the electron transport system (respiratory chain) in the inner mitochondrial membrane. Electron transfer molecules are mostly brightly coloured, protein-bound,

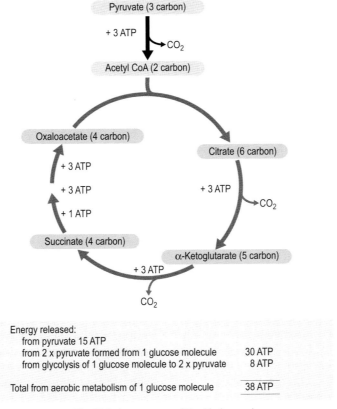

Energy released:
from pyruvate 15 ATP
from 2 x pyruvate formed from 1 glucose molecule   30 ATP
from glycolysis of 1 glucose molecule to 2 x pyruvate   8 ATP

Total from aerobic metabolism of 1 glucose molecule   38 ATP

• **Fig. 23.3** A summary of the Krebs cycle.

iron-containing pigments called *cytochromes.* As high-energy electrons pass though the electron transport system they release energy, which is used to increase the concentration of hydrogen ions in the intermembrane space. This creates an electrochemical proton gradient across the mitochondrial inner membrane, which is a source of potential energy. Hydrogen ions flow back across the membrane down their concentration gradient through a protein called ATP synthetase. This provides the energy required to attach a phosphate group to ADP to create ATP. NAD and FAD are released to capture more hydrogen and begin the energy transfer again. At the end of this chain, electrons combine with two hydrogen ions and inspired oxygen, creating a water molecule (Silverthorn, 2018). The theoretical total production of ATP from oxidation of one glucose molecule is 38 molecules; however due to inefficiencies, the observed ATP yield is closer to 30.

This process using oxygen and phosphate is called *oxidative phosphorylation* or *aerobic respiration* (Marieb & Hoehn, 2022).

Anaerobic Cellular Respiration. If no oxygen is available, oxidation of glucose cannot take place. In this instance, two molecules of ATP are synthesized for each glucose molecule during glycolysis, but the process cannot proceed further. This is called *substrate-level phosphorylation* (Marieb & Hoehn, 2022). The energy remains trapped in the molecules of pyruvic acid, and lactic acid is formed (anaerobic respiration). An oxygen debt arises and metabolic acidosis is created. When oxygen is available, the lactic acid is gradually converted to pyruvic acid and fed into the Krebs cycle (Hall & Hall, 2020).

Lipids

Fats provide the highest-density source of energy for the body (Brown, 2018). Carbohydrates can be converted to fat and stored in the adipose tissue. *Lipid* is the chemical name for fats and fat-related compounds. The most common source of lipids is triglycerides, which are made up of fatty acids and glycerol. Fatty acids are a refined fuel form which is preferred by some cells (e.g., heart muscle) over glucose.

Fatty acids consist of carbon, hydrogen and oxygen atoms. Lipids containing fatty acids that are filled with as much hydrogen as they can take are called *saturated fats.* Saturated fats are mainly in animal fats such as meat and dairy products. Monounsaturated fats contain fatty acids with one double bond between adjacent carbon atoms (Brown, 2018). The main sources of such fats are olive oils and canola oil, which is derived from rapeseed. Finally, lipids made mainly from unsaturated fatty acids with two or more places unfilled with hydrogen are called *polyunsaturated.* These fatty acids are found in vegetable oil and oily fish.

Humans can synthesize saturated and monounsaturated fatty acids, but there are some that the liver cannot make. These include omega-3 (alpha-linoleic acid (ALA)) and omega-6 (linoleic acid (LA)) which are essential fatty acids and so must be included in dietary intake. Arachidonic, eicosapentaenoic and docosahexaenoic acids (DHA) which are synthesized from LA and ALA, can also become essential fatty acids if the supply of LA and ALA is limited.

Body Fat Stores and Functions

Body fat is mainly stored subcutaneously (under the skin) and retroperitoneally (around the abdominal organs). It is continually interchanged with fats circulating in the bloodstream and metabolized for use as fuel. It is recommended that fat intake should range from 20–35% of total calories (Brown, 2018). Fats are essential for many of the body's functions:

- They are a source of energy.
- Triglycerides provide the major fuel for energy for hepatocytes and skeletal muscle.
- They are involved in the absorption of fat-soluble vitamins.
- Fats are involved in cell metabolism; combinations of lipids and protein, called *lipoproteins,* carry lipids in the blood to cells.
- Phospholipids are a component of cell membranes.
- Phospholipids are a component of myelin sheaths that surround larger nerves, so they are involved in nerve impulse transmission.
- Fatty deposits act as protective cushions for the vital organs such as eyes and kidneys.
- Fats provide an insulating layer under the skin.
- Prostaglandins, which play a role in smooth muscle contraction and inflammatory responses, are formed from LA.

Lipid Metabolism

In glucose shortage, fat stores are mobilized under the influence of adrenaline, noradrenaline, growth hormones or cortisol. They are taken to the liver where the triglycerides are broken down into free fatty acids and glycerol which are released into the blood. The breakdown of fat (lipolysis) provides 9 kcal/g of energy, which is twice that obtained from the metabolism of glucose or protein (4 kcal/g).

Glycerol is converted to an intermediate product of glycolysis called *glyceraldehyde 3-phosphate.* In the presence of oxygen and glucose, oxidation of fatty acids releases pyruvic acid which is fused to coenzyme A to form acetyl CoA, which enters the Krebs cycle. If no glucose is available (e.g., in starvation, diabetes mellitus, some slimming diets or hyperemesis gravidarum), metabolism of a large amount of fat may occur, acetyl CoA accumulates and the liver converts the molecules to ketone bodies (i.e., acetoacetic acid and β-hydroxybutyric acid), which accumulate in the blood. These can be oxidized to release energy, but metabolic acidosis will occur. Fatty acids cannot be used for gluconeogenesis (glucose synthesis) because they enter the cycle beyond the pyruvic acid stage when the changes are irreversible.

Cholesterol

Cholesterol forms part of every human cell. It belongs to the steroid family and has a key role as a structural component of cell membranes. Cholesterol also helps to make and metabolize hormones and bile acids, which promote the digestion and absorption of fats, and cholesterol is needed to produce vitamin D from sunlight (Brown, 2018). Cholesterol is found in the blood—mainly in combination with a protein carrier—as lipoproteins, of which there are three types:

1. High-density lipoproteins (HDLs).
2. Low-density lipoproteins (LDLs).
3. Very low-density lipoproteins (VLDLs).

Cholesterol is found in animal foods, mainly egg yolk and organ meats such as kidneys and liver. Even with no dietary intake, cholesterol is synthesized in the liver.

High circulating levels of cholesterol in the form of LDLs are linked to atheromatous plaques being laid down in arterial walls. A high ratio of HDLs to LDLs and VLDLs may offer protection against ischaemic heart disease (Hall & Hall, 2020). The ratio of HDLs to LDLs and VLDLs is increased in vegetarians, people whose fat intake is largely unsaturated and who take regular exercise, and it is reduced in smokers.

Proteins

Animals (including humans) can synthesize protein from amino acids. Twenty amino acids are present within the human body, of which the body can synthesize ten de novo. The amino acids that the body cannot make or cannot make in sufficient amounts are called *essential* or *semi-essential amino acids.* Human dietary sources of amino acids and proteins are plants or other animals. The best source of essential amino acids is animal products. Plants can synthesize amino acids from carbon dioxide, water and nitrogen.

Protein foods with all essential amino acids such as eggs, meat and milk (particularly human breastmilk) are said to have a high biological value. Protein foods from plant sources tend to have a lower biological value. However, strict vegetarians can obtain all the essential amino acids by varying their diet carefully, as the proteins in a mixture of plant sources—for instance, cereals and legumes—complement each other, and when combined they contain all the essential amino acids.

The Functions of Proteins

Amino acids can be used to synthesize proteins or can be converted to glucose to provide energy. These functions depend on adequacy of calorie intake, nitrogen balance (balance between protein synthesis and protein breakdown) and the influence of hormones. Anabolic hormones such as growth hormone and sex hormones encourage protein synthesis, and the glucocorticoids produced in stress enhance protein breakdown and the conversion of amino acids to glucose. Proteins are needed by the body for:

- The formation of new tissue, so they are essential for growth, recovery from injury, pregnancy and lactation.
- The manufacture of enzymes, hormones and antibodies.
- Structural proteins such, collagen and elastin in connective tissue and keratin in skin.
- Muscle protein that causes contraction.
- Transport molecules such as haemoglobin.
- The control of osmotic pressure between body fluid compartments.
- Plasma proteins acting as buffers to maintain acid–base balance.
- Blood clot formation.
- Gluconeogenesis once glucose stores are depleted.

The amount of protein needed in the diet is influenced by age, size, metabolic rate and nitrogen balance. The Dietary Reference Intake for protein is 0.8 g/kg bodyweight, which is equivalent to 45 g (female)–56 g (male) daily for an average sedentary person (Public Health England, 2016).

Amino Acids

Amino acids cannot be stored by the body. They are either converted into protein within cells or the liver can interconvert amino acids by utilizing the essential amino acids to synthesize the non-essential amino acids through a process called *transamination.* Any excess amino acids are broken down by a process of deamination in the liver. The nitrogen of amino acids is converted into urea, which enters the blood and is excreted by the kidneys.

Micronutrients

A brief overview of major micronutrients including various types of vitamins and minerals and their functions are described below.

Vitamins

Vitamins are needed in small amounts for growth and health (Marieb & Hoehn, 2022). They mainly function as coenzymes to assist in the catalysis of metabolism in the body. The human body is unable to synthesize most vitamins apart from vitamin K, vitamin D and some of the B vitamins. There are two types of vitamins: the fat-soluble vitamins (A, D, E and K), which are absorbed bound to digested lipids, and the water-soluble vitamins (most of the B complex and vitamin C), absorbed with water from the gastrointestinal tract. A normal varied diet should provide them all. Excessive intake can create as many health problems as insufficient intake. Box 23.2 provides further details of the vitamins.

Minerals, Trace Elements and Water

Minerals and trace elements known as *micronutrients* are inorganic elements that are widely distributed in nature. The mineral content of the human body is very similar to that of the Earth. There are seven minerals that the human body requires in greater amounts: calcium, phosphorus,

• BOX 23.2 The Vitamins

Fat-soluble Vitamins

Vitamin A

Vitamin A is available in two forms: β-carotene and the active form, retinol. β-Carotene is found in plant food (e.g., carrots and deep-green leafy vegetables such as broccoli and spinach) and retinol in animal food sources (fish liver oils, egg yolk, liver and dairy products). There is uncertainty over the teratogenic effect of dietary vitamin A; however synthetic retinoids such as those used to treat acne when taken in early pregnancy can cause birth defects including problems with the ears, eyes, brain and heart (Brown, 2018).

Deficiency

Vitamin A is an antioxidant. Its absorption is impeded by alcohol consumption. Severe deficiencies may lead to blindness, skin disorders, impaired immunity and gastrointestinal disorders. Dietary vitamin A deficiency during pregnancy is associated with fetal malformations including of the lungs, urinary tract and heart (Brown, 2018).

Vitamin D

The vitamin D sterol hormone precursor from animal products is 7-dehydrocholesterol and ergosterol from plants. After ingestion, both are absorbed in the small intestine with the aid of bile and transported to the skin. In skin, 7-dehydrocholesterol is changed by the action of ultraviolet light to an intermediate product, vitamin D_3 (cholecalciferol), and ergosterol is converted to vitamin D_2 (ergocalciferol). Cholecalciferol is then modified by the liver, followed by the kidneys, to produce physiologically active vitamin D_3 (calcitriol, 1,25-dihydroxycholecalciferol). Vitamin D is stored in adipose cells and is heat- and light-stable. Dietary sources of vitamin D are fish liver oils, egg/egg yolk, liver and fortified milk. Laxatives and antacids may inhibit gut absorption.

Deficiency

Vitamin D activates absorption of calcium and promotes bone mineralization. Deficiency may cause diseases such as rickets in children and osteomalacia in adults. Reduced levels of vitamin D have also been associated with increased blood clots. There may be poor muscle tone, restlessness and irritability.

Vitamin E (Tocopherol)

Vitamin E is chemically related to sex hormones. Vitamin E is found in vegetable oils, margarine, whole grains (wheat germ oil), nuts, seeds and green leafy vegetables. It is unstable in oxygen and destroyed by food processing. Its absorption is reduced by the contraceptive pill.

Deficiency

In vitamin E deficiency, cell membranes are more in danger of oxidation and breakdown. Vitamin E is an antioxidant and may prevent against cancer. It may also cause neurological symptoms, as it is involved in repairing myelin, the protective fat covering the long axons of nerve cells. Vitamin E may have a role in reproduction, with deficiency reducing fertility and resulting in spontaneous abortion. Vitamin E deficiency can particularly occur in premature infants, as vitamin E stores normally build up in the last month or two of fetal life. It is particularly associated with increased risk of haemolytic anaemia in preterm infants.

Vitamin K (Coagulation Vitamin)

Different forms of vitamin K include vitamin K_1 (phylloquinone), the dietary form found in green leafy vegetables (and small amounts in fruit, meat, dairy products and cereal), and vitamin K_2 (menaquinone), mainly produced by intestinal bacteria but also present in some dairy products and meat products. The vitamin is stored in small amounts in the liver but is rapidly metabolized and excreted.

Deficiency

Vitamin K has a role in blood clotting. In severe deficiency, easy bruising and bleeding occur due to prolonged clotting time. Deficiency can occur because of anticoagulant or antibiotic therapy.

Water-soluble Vitamins

Vitamin C (Ascorbic Acid)

Humans obtain vitamin C from fruits and vegetables, particularly citrus fruits, strawberries, tomatoes and fresh potatoes. It decomposes rapidly when dissolved in water, with heat, light and alkalis increasing decomposition. Food containing vitamin C should therefore be cooked with minimum water for brief periods and kept covered. It is not stored in a single tissue but is distributed throughout body tissues. Sufficient vitamin C is present in human breastmilk (with a balanced diet) but little exists in cow's milk, and so it is added to formula milk.

Pollution, industrial toxins, smoking, alcoholism, overcooking and poor food storage can interfere with absorption, as can some drugs such as aspirin, anticoagulants, antibiotics, diuretics, cortisone, the contraceptive pill and antidepressants (Jewell, 2017).

Deficiency

Vitamin C is an antioxidant and helps maintain body tissues (e.g., collagen), especially blood vessel walls. Its deficiency can cause scurvy which is associated with bruising and haemorrhage. Deficiency is also linked to poor resistance to bacterial infections, poor wound healing, persistent anaemia and gum disease.

Vitamin B_1 (Thiamine)

B vitamins are mostly coenzymes involved in the metabolism of carbohydrate, fat and proteins and in tissue building. They can be stored in small amounts (a continuous supply is necessary); excess is eliminated in urine. Vitamin B_1 is fairly unstable, being destroyed by alkalis and high temperature. Its requirement depends on carbohydrate and energy intake. The recommended dietary allowance (RDA) for adults is 0.5 mg/1000 kcal daily, with slightly increased intake recommended during pregnancy and lactation. Vitamin B_1 is found in lean meat, liver, whole grains, nuts and legumes. Its absorption in the small intestine is reduced by alcohol, coffee and food additives and its content is food is reduced by overcooking, as it is lost in cooking water.

Deficiency

Because it is involved in energy and glucose metabolism, deficiency of thiamine can affect the gastrointestinal (deficiency of hydrochloric acid), nervous, cardiovascular and musculoskeletal systems. Its deficiency causes the disease beri-beri (Sinhalese for *I can't, I can't*) with pain, weakness, degeneration of muscles and inability to perform coordinated movements. Thiamine deficiency causes Wernicke–Korsakoff syndrome, which occurs in people with long-term nutrient malabsorption or in alcoholics. Its symptoms include poor memory, confusion, double vision, apathy and ataxia.

Vitamin B_2 (Riboflavin)

This vitamin contains the sugar ribose and is heat-stable but photosensitive. Vitamin B_2 is mainly found in milk in addition to lean meat, yeast, liver, eggs, fortified cereals and nuts. Absorption is reduced by the contraceptive pill and some antibiotics.

Deficiency

Poor wound healing and cracks in the lips, corners of mouth and tongue are typical signs of vitamin B_2 deficiency. Riboflavin

• BOX 23.2   The Vitamins—cont'd

is photosensitive, so attention for the symptoms of riboflavin deficiency should be given to infants receiving phototherapy treatment.

Vitamin B₃ (Niacin)

Niacin exists in two common forms: nicotinic acid and nicotinamide, which are simple, stable organic compounds. It is found in any proteinaceous food: meat, peanuts, dry beans and peas. The body synthesizes niacin easily from the amino acid tryptophan. Niacin's absorption is reduced by alcohol, coffee, antibiotics and antitubercular drugs.

Deficiency

Vitamin B₃ deficiency causes the disease pellagra with headache, weight loss, loss of appetite and, later, soreness and redness of the lips and tongue, vomiting, diarrhoea and skin ulceration. Neurological symptoms may also occur.

Vitamin B₆ (Pyridoxine)

This vitamin is stable to heat but sensitive to alkalis and light. The RDA is 1.3 mg/day, increasing to 1.9 mg/day in pregnancy and 2.0 mg/day during lactation. Large amounts (>1000 mg/day) can be toxic. Vitamin B₆ is found in chickpeas, fortified cereals, meat, liver, fish and some non-citrus fruit. Its absorption is reduced by alcohol, antibiotics and antitubercular drugs.

Deficiency

Vitamin B₆ is important for the nervous system and neurotransmitter synthesis, amino acid metabolism, conversion of tryptophan to niacin and red blood cell production. Vitamin B₆ deficiency may cause anaemia, dermatitis and depression, as well as exacerbate premenstrual depression in adults and cause convulsions, irritability, vomiting and abdominal pain in infants.

Vitamin B₁₂ (Cyanocobalamin)

This vitamin is complex and contains cobalt. It is heat-stable but inactivated by acids and alkalis. Vitamin B₁₂ is found mainly in meat, fish, dairy products and eggs. It is found in some seaweeds and some is synthesized by intestinal bacteria.

Deficiency

Vitamin B₁₂ is necessary for brain and nerve cell development and myelin sheath maintenance around nerve cells. It is also involved in the formation of DNA and in its absence, erythrocytes do not divide. Stores in the liver are sufficient to last 3–5 years in normal health. Vitamin B₁₂ deficiency causes pernicious anaemia and neurological symptoms. Vegans and vegetarians may have diets deficient in vitamin B₁₂.

Folic Acid

Folic acid is not a stable vitamin, so considerable losses occur in cooking. Small amounts are stored in the liver, but most is excreted in urine. It is toxic in excessive amounts. Folic acid is in food sources such as liver, yeast, eggs, whole grains, deep-green vegetables and nuts. It is also synthesized in the gut by enteric bacteria. Absorption is hindered by alcohol and drugs that are folic acid antagonists such as anticonvulsants and sulphonamides.

Importance

Folic acid is essential for the formation of red blood cells. It is necessary for the health of the nervous system, and it facilitates the metabolism of proteins with the help of vitamins B₁₂ and C.

Deficiency

Perinatal supplementation of folic acid is believed to have a strong protective effect against neural tube defects (De-Regil et al., 2015) (see Chapters 15 and 33).

---

potassium, sulphur, sodium, chloride and magnesium. The remaining 18 elements, called *trace elements,* include iron, iodine and zinc and are no less important, but they occur in very small amounts. Iron (in haemoglobin) is discussed in Chapter 16, sodium and potassium in Chapter 20 and calcium and phosphorus (in bone) in Chapter 24.

Generally, minerals and trace elements (4% of total bodyweight) function as structural and catalyst substances. These include regulation of fluid balance and acid–base balance, transmission of action along nerves, bone formation and contraction of muscle fibres. They are also important as components of enzymes and hormones essential for energy metabolism and functioning of the immune system.

Regulation of Food Intake and Energy Balance

Energy is produced from oxidation of macronutrients in the body and is essential to maintain life. When energy intake and energy output are balanced, bodyweight remains stable. Obesity occurs when energy intake exceeds energy output. This is, however, more complicated than a straightforward equation. Genetic and environmental factors are believed to have a role in causing obesity. Body mechanisms appear to control intake which enable most people to maintain a steady weight.

Nutritional States

There are two nutritional states: the absorptive state when nutrients are being eaten and absorbed by the digestive tract and the postabsorptive state when the gastrointestinal tract is empty and energy requirements are met by breakdown of body stores. The absorptive state lasts for about 4 hours after a reasonable meal has been eaten. If three meals a day are eaten, there is a balance between the two states, each occupying about half of a 24-hour period. Insulin directs the events of the absorptive state, mainly by its control of blood glucose levels.

The body can be maintained in the postabsorptive state for days or weeks in a famine or during illness, as long as sufficient water is taken. Glucose is made available to cells by glycogenolysis in the liver. Muscle glycogen cannot be broken down to glucose because it lacks the enzymes. It is partly oxidized to pyruvic acid or, in anaerobic conditions, to lactic acid. The hormone glucagon is released when blood sugars become too low. Glucagon targets the liver and adipose tissue to enable glucose to be released into the blood.

Total Energy Expenditure

The total energy requirements in the body are to support three main energy uses: the basal metabolic rate (BMR) or resting metabolic rate (RMR) (BMR and RMR are sometimes used interchangeably, although they are slightly different measurements), the thermic effect of food and variable amounts of physical activities.

Metabolic Rate

BMR is the amount of energy required for the body's internal organs to maintain resting activities; it is measured after an overnight fast in a normal environmental temperature. In general, the younger the person, the higher the BMR, and males have a higher BMR than females because of the ratio of metabolically active muscle to the metabolically sluggish fatty tissue. Factors that positively influence BMR are lean body mass, growth, fever, disease and cold climate. BMR makes the largest contribution to total energy expenditure (about 60–70%).

The Effect of Food Intake and Body Heat Production

The ingestion of food stimulates metabolism and requires energy to meet the needs of the processes involved: digestion, absorption and transport of nutrients. This is called the *thermic effect of food* and comprises 10–15% of total energy expenditure.

Regulation of Body Temperature

The body temperature of humans is usually maintained within a range of 36.1–37.8°C independently of external environment or internal heat production. A rise in body temperature increases enzyme activity, and most adults will have convulsions when their temperature reaches 41°C and die if their temperature exceeds 43°C. The body's core (organs within the body cavities) has the highest temperature and the shell (heat loss surface of the skin) has the lowest temperature. Rectal temperature is nearer to the core temperature than oral temperature. The hypothalamus is the major heat-regulating centre.

Body Composition and Bodyweight

Body composition is mainly divided into two compartments: lean mass and fat mass. Other more detailed models classify the body into three, four or five compartments (including lean, fat, water, mineral mass (bones) and glycogen stores). For practical reasons, anthropometric measures such as body mass index are often used for defining nutritional status, but body composition indicators could be more informative in relation to health outcomes. For example, excessive fat and its central distribution can lead to metabolic abnormalities. Central obesity (accumulation of excess fat around the abdomen and upper body) is related to chronic illnesses such as diabetes and cardiovascular diseases.

Maternal Adaptation to Pregnancy

Nutrition

Maternal nutrition is essential for the health of the mother and baby with long-term health and developmental implications for the child. Available evidence suggests a relationship between poor and inappropriate nutrition and a higher incidence of perinatal morbidity and mortality (Marshall et al., 2022). Fetal growth and well-being appear to be compromised with poor maternal nutrition (both undernutrition and obesity) leading to increased risk of low-birthweight (LBW) babies, babies small for gestational age and preterm birth, as well as babies large for gestational age and macrosomia, with long-term negative health impacts such as chronic childhood and adult diseases (Marshall et al., 2022). The implications of LBW in the causation of adult diabetes mellitus and hypertension were postulated by Barker (1992; 2003) and is supported by recent evidence (Knop et al., 2018; Zhao et al., 2018). Nutrition in pregnancy is of particular importance in low- and middle-income countries where there are high levels of malnutrition before and during pregnancy; in some cases over half of the population gain inadequate weight during pregnancy (Soltani et al., 2017). There is evidence that in countries where women are most at risk of undernutrition, micronutrient supplementation can reduce the risk of fetal growth restriction and LBW (Oh, Keats & Bhutta, 2020). In some countries, inappropriate nutrition acts as a double-edged sword as both growing obesity and undernutrition put mothers and babies at higher risks of adverse pregnancy outcomes. Appropriate nutritional advice and support to prevent obesity and/or undernutrition prior to and throughout pregnancy are essential to optimize maternal and neonatal health (Marshall et al., 2022).

Specific Requirements of Pregnancy

During pregnancy, maternal weight and body composition change significantly and include the products of conception, increased blood volume, growing uterine and breast tissue. There are additional nutritional requirements to meet the increase in maternal tissue and fetal needs. Other factors that influence nutritional requirements during pregnancy include age and inter-pregnancy spacing.

Energy

Factors influencing energy needs during pregnancy include metabolic cost, pre-pregnancy weight, level of activity and the stage of pregnancy. The average total energy cost of pregnancy is estimated to be about 70,000 kcal for a woman with a pre-pregnancy weight of 60 kg and fat deposition of 2–2.4 kg during pregnancy. The UK dietary reference value (DRV) for extra energy requirement in pregnancy is 200 kcal/day, but only during the last trimester (National

Institute of Health and Care Excellence (NICE), 2010). This recommendation varies in different countries: e.g., 340 kcal/day during the second and 453 kcal/day in the third trimester in the United States (Rasmussen & Yaktine, 2009). These are guidelines, and the actual requirements depend on the individual basis: e.g., size, activity, age and the woman's original nutritional status.

Protein

The quality of protein intake depends on the type and quantity of food eaten and the conditions under which it is eaten. For example, if the total energy supplied by the diet is so low that gluconeogenesis utilizes amino acids to provide energy, the ability to construct new tissue will be reduced. The daily reference intake for protein increases from 0.80 g/kg per day prior to pregnancy to 1.1 g/kg per day for an average pregnant woman (Institute of Medicine, 2005). This equates to 14.7–16.1% of total energy coming from protein during pregnancy (Mousa, Naqash & Lim, 2019). A review found inconsistent evidence around the benefits to fetal growth when mothers receive protein supplementation during pregnancy (Mousa, Naqash & Lim, 2019). However, most women in developed countries already eat more protein than is needed for health.

Carbohydrates and Fats

There is little need to increase glucose or fats for energy, but the absorption of fat-soluble vitamins must be considered when advising women about diet in pregnancy. During pregnancy women should have adequate dietary intakes of essential fatty acids and their longer derivatives, omega-6 (mainly arachidonic acid) and omega-3s (mainly DHA). Dietary fat intake in pregnancy and lactation, particularly long-chain fatty acids and DHA, has a vital role in brain, cognitive and visual development of the growing baby (Mun et al., 2019). In addition, increased consumption of omega-3 reduces the rate of premature birth (Ciesielski, Bartlett & Williams, 2019) and increases birthweight (Zhao et al., 2021). Dietary fat intake recommendations for pregnant and lactating women are the same as for the general population, including an average intake of 200 mg DHA/day. This can be achieved by consuming one or two portions of oily fish (tuna—fresh not canned, salmon and mackerel) per week. Caution should be applied by avoiding large predatory fish which are more likely to be contaminated with pollutants such as methylmercury.

Vitamins

In developed countries, there is usually no need for vitamin supplementation for healthy women with a balanced diet. However, supplementation may be necessary in women with restricted dietary intake or previous gastrointestinal surgery, especially ileostomy. Folic acid, for example, is essential for supporting rapid cell growth and is particularly important in the prevention of neural tube defects (De-Regil et al., 2015). There have been efforts to add folic acid to basic foods to ensure compliance with intake, especially before conception (see Chapter 33). Reference values for some of the vitamins are summarized next.

Vitamin A

The DRV for retinol during pregnancy is an extra 70 μg/day (Mousa, Naqash & Lim, 2019). However because of the teratogenic effects of excessive retinol, vitamin A supplements are not advised in pregnancy in developed countries where vitamin A deficiency is rare.

Vitamin D

Pregnant and lactating women, especially teenagers, vegans or darker-skinned women, are at high risk of vitamin D deficiency. They are therefore recommended to take a daily supplement of 10–15 μg vitamin D (Scientific Advisory Committee on Nutrition, 2016).

Thiamine, Riboflavin and Folate

The need for thiamine increases with increased energy requirements. The average increment for riboflavin intake is 0.3 mg/day throughout pregnancy. NICE (2014) recommends 400 μg/day of folic acid prior to conception and for the first 12 weeks of pregnancy. This is in addition to eating foods rich in folates (e.g., citrus fruits, dark-green leafy vegetables, nuts and liver) or fortified with folic acid.

Vitamin C

To ensure sufficient maternal stores of vitamin C, an increment of 10 mg/day during pregnancy is recommended.

Calcium

The adult average requirement for calcium is 1 g/day (Mousa, Naqash & Lim, 2019). No increment is established for pregnancy because calcium absorption increases and maternal stores meet the requirement. However, for teenage pregnant mothers, calcium-rich diets are advisable to meet their own growth and pregnancy requirements.

Iron

The iron requirement nearly doubles in pregnancy but may be met by utilizing maternal stores, cessation of menstrual losses and increased absorption. No extra iron is therefore required in healthy women with a balanced diet (see Chapter 16).

Metabolism

The addition of a new endocrine organ (placenta) and increased endocrine activity have major influences on maternal metabolism to allow provision of nutrients for fetal growth. Human chorionic gonadotrophin (hCG), human placental lactogen (hPL), oestrogen and progesterone affect metabolism, some by reducing insulin sensitivity (or increasing insulin resistance).

Plasma T_3 (triiodothyronine) and T_4 (thyroxine) are increased, leading to a physiological state of hyperthyroidism (see Chapter 35). Increased maternal insulin plasma levels, alongside a state of maternal insulin resistance, ensures availability of glucose for placental uptake and fetal utilization. The changes in glucose tolerance and insulin levels during pregnancy make it a diabetogenic condition. Women who have predisposing factors such as obesity may develop gestational diabetes.

The BMR rises during pregnancy, reflecting increased oxygen demands of the fetus , placenta and mother. Metabolism of carbohydrate, protein and fat alters, with a major shift in the fuel sources: fat becomes the maternal fuel, while glucose becomes the major fetal fuel (Brown, 2018). Approximately 45–65% of daily energy requirements during pregnancy are derived from carbohydrates, 10–35% from protein and the remainder from fat (Danielewicz et al., 2017). Maternal metabolic adjustments vary depending on fetal size and therefore energy demand, as well as maternal metabolic and nutritional status. For example, to meet the extra energy required in late pregnancy, maternal fat stores are mobilized as well as alterations occurring in maternal physical activity and food consumption (Clarke, Gatford & Young, 2021).

Carbohydrates

Blood glucose levels are generally 10–20% lower than in the non-pregnant state. This decrease leads to lower insulin levels in the postabsorptive state and a tendency towards ketosis. As pregnancy progresses, there is less peripheral use of glucose by the mother because of increasing insulin antagonism (blockage of cellular uptake), making glucose more readily available to the fetus . Insulin resistance is thought to be due to a decrease in sensitivity of cell receptors because of hPL, progesterone and cortisol. In response, the pancreatic β islet cells undergo hyperplasia and hypertrophy to produce increased insulin during meals. The changes associated with each hormone are listed briefly:

- Progesterone helps increase insulin secretion, decrease peripheral insulin usage and increase insulin levels after meals.
- Oestrogen increases the level of plasma cortisol, which is an insulin antagonist, stimulates β-cell hyperplasia and enhances peripheral glucose usage.
- Cortisol depletes hepatic glycogen stores through glycogenolysis and increases hepatic glucose production.
- The role of hPL is not very clear, but it is biologically similar to growth hormone, and it correlates with fetal and placental weight. Plasma levels increase as pregnancy progresses, and it is higher in multiple pregnancies. hPL antagonizes insulin to increase glucose availability and increases the synthesis and availability of lipids which can be used as an alternative fuel to glucose.

Proteins

Pregnancy is an anabolic state with significant nitrogen retention, especially in late pregnancy. Protein metabolism changes gradually through pregnancy to reduce nitrogen excretion and achieve nitrogen conservation for fetal growth (Brown, 2018). Concentrations of plasma amino acids are reduced in early pregnancy because they are transported across the placenta against the concentration gradient, with reduced plasma amino acid levels persisting through the later stages of gestation (Manta-Vogli et al., 2020). Additionally, a 50% expansion of plasma volume and changes in hormone levels cause a reduction of biochemical substances such as plasma albumin and haemoglobin. Due to the key role of amino acids in supporting essential metabolic processes (e.g., gluconeogenesis), providing precursors for hormones and regulating gene expression and immunity, they are essential for pregnancy, which involves rapid placental and fetal development and enormous physiological changes in the mother. To ensure healthy pregnancy outcomes, it is crucial to not only provide adequate total protein in quantity but also attention should be given to the quality and composition of the special amino acids due to the competition amongst amino acids and its negative impact on fetal growth (Manta-Vogli et al., 2020). Appropriate nutritional advice for a diet balanced in protein, energy and amino acids as well as other macro- and micronutrients is paramount for all pregnant mothers, particularly for those who are vegan or vegetarian and especially if they are from economically deprived backgrounds (Manta-Vogli et al., 2020).

Lipids

Every aspect of lipid metabolism changes in pregnancy. During the first two trimesters, triglyceride synthesis and fat storage (lipogenesis) increase, mediated by the increase in insulin production and enhanced by progesterone. Most fat storage occurs in the first half of pregnancy. Fat gain accounts for approximately 3.5 kg of the total weight gain in pregnancy, with most of this fat gained in the second trimester (Perales, Nagpal & Barakat, 2019).

There is a steady increase in plasma lipids throughout pregnancy, with the highest levels in the third trimester (Brown, 2018), reflecting increased maternal insulin resistance (Grimes & Wild, 2018). Lipolysis increases during the third trimester, probably due to increased hPL. Ketogenesis in the liver accelerates due to increased oxidation of free fatty acids for conversion into energy. Fats therefore act as an alternative source of energy, conserving glucose for the fetus . In the last trimester, when glucose transfer to the fetus is maximal, there is also decreased lipogenesis in adipose tissue, tipping the balance in the direction of lipolysis (Murray & Hendley, 2020). Blood cholesterol increases steadily as pregnancy progresses and stays stationary for the last few weeks before delivery. This is unrelated to diet.

Changes in the Absorptive and Postabsorptive States

During the absorptive state, ingested nutrients are digested and absorbed by the gastrointestinal tract. The absorptive state in pregnancy is characterized by relative hyperinsulinaemia and hyperglycaemia due to reduced liver uptake. There is also hypertriglyceridaemia and increased lipogenesis due to the conversion of glucose to fat for storage.

In the postabsorptive or fasting state, energy must be supplied from the body stores, with most coming from the catabolism of fat. Fat and protein synthesis are decreased and catabolism exceeds anabolism. The central nervous system has no alternative but to use available glucose; however other organs move to produce energy from lipids. Triglycerides are broken down and fed into the Krebs cycle, producing ketone bodies. If these accumulate, ketoacidosis will occur. After an overnight fast, maternal plasma glucose falls significantly below that of a non-pregnant woman because of impaired gluconeogenesis and extra demand by the fetus . Gluconeogenesis and circulating free fatty acids are decreased. The reduced gluconeogenesis capacity preserves maternal muscle mass.

Maternal Weight Gain and Body Composition

Although the total amount of gestational weight gain varies between women, the weight of the fetus accounts for about 27% of the total (Triunfo & Lanzone, 2015). The additional components of gestational weight gain include maternal fat stores at 27% (which are deposited onto the hips, back and thighs); blood volume and extracellular fluid at 23%; placenta, amniotic fluid and uterus at 20%; and increased breast tissue weight at 3% (Triunfo & Lanzone, 2015). The recommended weight gain for mothers whose body mass index is within the normal range is 11.5–16 kg for a full-term pregnancy (Rasmussen & Yaktine, 2009). It is however suggested that regional body mass index categories should be considered when applying gestational weight gain recommendations; for example, in Asian women (Goldstein et al., 2018).

Maternal pre-pregnancy weight, socioeconomic status, genetic factors and gestational weight gain have all been shown to influence infant birthweight. A wide range of gestational weight gains, from weight loss to gains of 30 kg, are reported during pregnancy. A greater incidence of poor outcome is associated with the extremes of this range. A higher risk of small-for-gestational-age infants is reported in women with low net-weight gains during pregnancy (Santos et al., 2019). High net-weight gains during pregnancy are also problematic as they lead to increased birthweight (Santos et al., 2019), as well as increased risk of a pregnancy complicated by pre-eclampsia, caesarean birth and retained maternal weight after birth. Most excess weight is lost within the first 3 months after birth; however postpartum women retain, on average, 2.2 kg of fat mass over the mean pre-pregnancy value (Abduljalil et al., 2012). Factors that influence postpartum weight loss are maternal age, pre-pregnancy weight, gestational weight gain, the mother's desired weight and length of lactation. For example, women gaining weight within the recommended range have approximately 3 kg less postpartum weight retention 3 years after birth (Brown, 2018).

It is not advisable to encourage weight loss or the use of restrictive diets during pregnancy (NICE, 2010; Marshall et al., 2022). Nonetheless, a modest reduction in energy intake for some women is unlikely to have any adverse effect on the birthweight, yet it may prevent the problem of excessive weight gain by the woman. Physical activity and nutritional interventions have been shown to reduce gestational weight gain. However among women with overweight or obesity, current evidence has found no clear benefit of this small reduction in weight gain on maternal or infant health outcomes (Fair & Soltani, 2021). Pregnant women are currently recommended to have a healthy balanced diet including vegetables, fruits, whole grains, nuts, legumes, fish, monounsaturated oils and fibre to achieve optimum pregnancy outcomes, while avoiding diets with high levels of simple sugars and processed foods (Marshall et al., 2022).

Main Points

- There are about 50 essential nutrients that cannot be manufactured by the body and must be provided in the diet.
- Four food groups provide a balanced diet: grains or potatoes, fruits, vegetables, meat, fish and milk products.
- The best source of essential amino acids is animal products. Plant proteins are nutritionally incomplete, being low in one or more essential amino acids.
- Vitamins may be fat-soluble or water-soluble. Their main role is as coenzymes to assist in catalysis of biochemical processes in the body.
- Body cells convert ingested food into the high-energy phosphate bonds of ATP. Glucose is taken up by cells via facilitated diffusion under the influence of insulin. Glucose is oxidized in the mitochondria to form energy through the Krebs cycle.
- Excess fat is stored as adipose tissue. When needed for energy production, fat is mobilized under the influence of adrenaline, noradrenaline, growth hormones or cortisol, taken to the liver and broken down into free fatty acids and glycerol and then released into the blood.
- Cholesterol, combined with a protein carrier such as lipoprotein, exists as three types: HDLs, LDLs and VLDLs. The ratio of HDLs to LDLs and VLDLs is increased in those whose fat intake is largely unsaturated and who take regular exercise and is reduced in cigarette smokers.
- Around 50 g of protein per day is needed to maintain nitrogen balance and provide for growth and repair of tissues.
- In pregnancy, increased nutrients, particularly protein, are needed to meet increased maternal and fetal demands, although reducing energy expenditure without increased intake may be sufficient. In women with restricted dietary intake or those with ileostomy, vitamin supplementation may be necessary.
- Folic acid deficiency is implicated in the cause of neural tube defects.

- As pregnancy progresses, increasing insulin antagonism results in less peripheral maternal glucose use, allowing increased glucose availability for the fetus .
- In pregnancy, serum amino acid and protein levels are decreased because of placental uptake, increased insulin and gluconeogenesis. Nitrogen excretion is reduced to achieve nitrogen conservation for fetal growth.
- During the first half of pregnancy, fat storage increases due to increased insulin production and progesterone.

During the third trimester, lipolysis increases. Fats act as an alternative energy source to conserve glucose for the fetus.

- The central nervous system can only use available glucose, but other organs move to produce energy from lipids.
- A wide range of weight loss to a weight gain of 30 kg is reported during pregnancy. A greater incidence of poor outcome is associated with the extremes of this range.

References

Abduljalil, K., Furness, P., Johnson, T.N., Rostami-Hodjegan, A., Soltani, H., 2012. Anatomical, physiological and metabolic changes with gestational age during normal pregnancy: a database for parameters required in physiologically based pharmacokinetic modelling. Clin. Pharmacokinet. 51 (6), 365–396.

Barker, D.J.P., 1992. Fetal and Infant Origins of Adult Disease. BMJ Books, London.

Barker, D.J.P., 2003. The Best Start in Life. Century, London.

Brown, J.E., 2018. Nutrition through the Life Cycle, seventh ed. Cengage Learning, Boston.

Ciesielski, T.H., Bartlett, J., Williams, S.M., 2019. Omega-3 polyunsaturated fatty acid intake norms and preterm birth rate: a cross-sectional analysis of 184 countries. BMJ Open 9 (4), e027249.

Clarke, G.S., Gatford, K.L., Young, R.L., 2021. Maternal adaptations to food intake across pregnancy: central and peripheral mechanisms. Obesity 29 (11), 1813–1824.

Danielewicz, H., Myszczyszyn, G., Dębińska, A., Myszkal, A., Boznański, A., Hirnle, L., 2017. Diet in pregnancy – more than food. Eur. J. Pediatr. 176, 1573–1579.

De-Regil, L.M., Peña-Rosas, J.P., Fernández-Gaxiola, A.C., Rayco-Solon, P., 2015. Effects and safety of periconceptional oral folate supplementation for preventing birth defects. Cochrane Database Syst. Rev. 2015 (12), CD007950.

Dieterich, R., Demirci, J., 2020. Communication practices of healthcare professionals when caring for overweight/obese pregnant women: a scoping review. Patient. Educ. Couns. 103 (10), 1902–1912.

Fair, F.J., Soltani, H., 2021. A meta-review of systematic reviews of lifestyle interventions for reducing gestational weight gain in women with overweight or obesity. Obes. Rev. 22 (5), e13199.

Goldstein, R.F., Abell, S.K., Ranasinha, S., Misso, M.L., Boyle, J.A., Harrison, C.L., et al., 2018. Gestational weight gain across continents and ethnicity: systematic review and meta-analysis of maternal and infant outcomes in more than one million women. BMC Med. 16 (1), 153.

Grimes, S.B., Wild, R., 2018. 'Effect of pregnancy on lipid metabolism and lipoprotein levels'. In: Feingold, K.R., Anawalt, B., Blackman, M.R., Boyce, A., Chrousos, G., Corpas, E., et al., (Eds.), Endotext [Internet]. MDText.com, South Dartmouth.

Hall, J.E., Hall, M.E. (Eds.), 2020. Guyton and Hall Textbook of Medical Physiology, fourteenth ed. Elsevier, Philadelphia.

Institute of Medicine, 2005. Dietary Reference Intakes: Energy, Carbohydrate, Fiber, Fat, Fatty Acids, Cholesterol, Protein and Amino Acids. National Academies Press, Washington, DC.

Jewell, K., 2017. 'Nutrition,' in Macdonald S. In: Johnson, G. (Ed.), Mayes Midwifery, fifteenth ed. Elsevier, London.

Knop, M.R., Geng, T.T., Gorny, A.W., Ding, R., Li, C., Ley, S.H., et al., 2018. Birth weight and risk of type 2 diabetes mellitus, cardiovascular disease, and hypertension in adults: a meta-analysis

of 7 646 267 participants from 135 studies. J. Am. Heart Assoc. 7 (23), e008870.

Manta-Vogli, P.D., Schulpis, K.H., Dotsikas, Y., Loukas, Y.L., 2020. The significant role of amino acids during pregnancy: nutritional support. J. Matern. Fetal Neonatal Med. 33 (2), 334–340.

Marieb, E.N., Hoehn, K., 2022. Human Anatomy and Physiology, twelfth ed. Pearson, Harlow.

Marshall, N.E., Abrams, B., Barbour, L.A., Catalano, P., Christian, P., Friedman, J.E., et al., 2022. The importance of nutrition in pregnancy and lactation: lifelong consequences. Am. J. Obstet. Gynecol. 226 (5), 607–632.

Mousa, A., Naqash, A., Lim, S., 2019. Macronutrient and micronutrient intake during pregnancy: an overview of recent evidence. Nutrients 11 (2), 443.

Mun, J.G., Legette, L.L., Ikonte, C.J., Mitmesser, S.H., 2019. Choline and DHA in maternal and infant nutrition: synergistic implications in brain and eye health. Nutrients 11 (5), 1125.

Murray, I., Hendley, J., 2020. 'Changes and Adaptation in Pregnancy'. In: Marshall, J.E., Raynor, M.D. (Eds.), Myles' Textbook for Midwives, seventeenth ed. Elsevier, London.

National Institute of Health and Care Excellence (NICE), 2010. Weight Management before, during and after Pregnancy. NICE, London.

National Institute of Health and Care Excellence (NICE), 2014. Maternal and Child Nutrition. NICE, London.

Oh, C., Keats, E.C., Bhutta, Z.A., 2020. Vitamin and mineral supplementation during pregnancy on maternal, birth, child health and development outcomes in low- and middle-income countries: a systematic review and meta-analysis. Nutrients 12 (2), 491.

Perales, M., Nagpal, T.S., Barakat, R., 2019. 'Physiological changes during pregnancy: main adaptations, discomforts, and implications for physical activity'. In: Santos-Rocha, R. (Ed.), Exercise and Sporting Activity during Pregnancy: Evidence Based Guidelines. Springer, Cham.

Public Health England, 2016. The Eatwell Guide. Available at https://www.gov.uk/government/publications/the-eatwell-guide.

Rasmussen, K.M., Yaktine, A.L., 2009. Weight Gain during Pregnancy: Reexamining the Guidelines. National Academies Press, Washington, DC.

Reynolds, A.N., Akerman, A.P., Mann, J., 2020. Dietary fibre and whole grains in diabetes management: systematic review and meta-analyses. PLoS Med. 17 (3), e1003053.

Santos, S., Voerman, E., Amiano, P., Barros, H., Beilin, LJ., Bergström, A., et al., 2019. Impact of maternal body mass index and gestational weight gain on pregnancy complications: an individual participant data meta-analysis of European, North American and Australian cohorts. Br., J., Obstet. Gynaecol. 126 8, 984–995.

Scientific Advisory Committee on Nutrition, 2016. Vitamin D and Health. Available at https://www.gov.uk/government/publications/sacn-vitamin-d-and-health-report.

Silverthorn, D.U., 2018. Human Physiology: An Integrative Approach, eighth ed. Pearson, Harlow.

Soltani, H., Lipoeto, N.I., Fair, F.J., Kilner, K., Yusrawati, Y., 2017. Pre-pregnancy body mass index and gestational weight gain and their effects on pregnancy and birth outcomes: a cohort study in West Sumatra, Indonesia. BMC Wom. Health 17 (1), 102.

Triunfo, S., Lanzone, A., 2015. Impact of maternal under nutrition on obstetric outcomes. J. Endocrinol. Invest. 38 (1), 31–38.

Zhao, H., Song, A., Zhang, Y., Zhen, Y., Song, G., Ma, H., 2018. The association between birthweight and the risk of type 2 diabetes mellitus: a systematic review and meta-analysis. Endocr. J. 65 (9), 923–933.

Zhao, R., Gao, Q., Wang, S., Yang, X., Hao, L., 2021. The effect of maternal seafood consumption on perinatal outcomes: a systematic review and dose-response meta-analysis. Crit. Rev. Food. Sci. Nutr. 61 (21), 3504–3517.

Annotated recommended reading

Barker, D.J.P., 2003. The Best Start in Life. Century, London.

This easy-to-read book develops Barker's theory on the effects of pregnancy on the fetus in causing disease in later life and is suitable for practitioners and prospective parents.

Hall, J.E., Hall, M.E. (Eds.), 2020. Guyton and Hall Textbook of Medical Physiology, fourteenth ed. Elsevier, Philadelphia.

Chapters 68–74 provide an excellent detailed account of metabolism. However pregnancy metabolic changes are not discussed in any detail.

Marshall, N.E., Abrams, B., Barbour, L.A., Catalano, P., Christian, P., Friedman, J.E., et al., 2022. The importance of nutrition in pregnancy and lactation: lifelong consequences. Am. J. Obstet. Gynecol. 226 (5), 607–632.

This is a good review article of the importance of nutrition during the childbearing cycle, with the scientific basis for current recommendations provided.

24

The Nature of Bone—The Female Pelvis and Fetal Skull

JEAN RANKIN AND AISHAH AHMAD

CHAPTER CONTENTS

This chapter focuses on the general structure and function of bone, calcium and phosphorus metabolism. A detailed description of the pelvis and fetal skull is provided. Knowledge of the anatomy of the normal female pelvis and fetal skull is key to effective midwifery and obstetric practice. Maternal positions in labour are introduced.

Introduction

Successful childbearing depends on the relationship between the size and shape of the maternal pelvis and key fetal diameters. Related knowledge of the maternal pelvis and fetal skull is essential to provide optimal care during pregnancy and labour and manage deviations from normal.

The Nature of Bone: Function and Structure

Functions of Bone

Bone is a highly vascular, constantly changing, hard mineralized connective tissue that contains depositions of calcium and phosphorus (Waugh & Grant, 2018). It performs important functions for the body, including:
- Support and protection of the soft organs.
- Movement by acting as anchorage for muscles and levers.
- Storage of fat.
- Large reservoir of calcium and phosphorus.
- Storage of smaller amounts of potassium, sulphur, magnesium and copper.
- Blood cell formation.

Structure of Bone

Bone is a living matrix consisting of three basic components:
i) An organic matrix of **collagen** known as **osteoid,** a cartilage-like material differing from cartilage in that calcium salts are readily deposited in it.
ii) A **mineral matrix** of calcium and phosphorus.
iii) **Bone cells** which include **osteoblasts, osteoclasts** and **osteocytes.**

Calcium (Ca^{2+}), the most common mineral in the body, and phosphorus are present in the bone as crystals of **hydroxyapatite** $(Ca_3(PO_4)_2)_3 \cdot Ca(OH)_2$, attached to collagen fibres. This results in the hardness and strength of bone. Remodelling of bone is a continuous process as osteoblasts deposit new bone and osteoclasts reabsorb it. Calcium and phosphorus are slowly exchanged between bone and extracellular fluid (ECF). Bone can be divided into **compact** (lamellar) bone and **spongy** (trabecular) bone (Waugh & Grant, 2018).

Bone Cells

- **Osteoblasts** are present on all bone surfaces in single layers next to the unmineralized osteoid of newly forming bone. Osteoblasts synthesize and secrete the constituents of the organic matrix and promote mineralization.

- **Osteocytes** are derived from osteoblasts that have become trapped in lacunae. These cells maintain the bone matrix, and if they die the surrounding matrix is absorbed.
- **Osteoclasts** reabsorb bone and are found on or near surfaces undergoing erosion. They are derived from monocytes and may have developed separately from osteoblasts. Osteoclasts contain both proteolytic enzymes and acids such as lactic acid and citric acid which remove the organic and mineral matrix.

Compact Bone

Compact bone forms the outer rim or cortex of all bones and consists of **osteons** or **Haversian systems** (Fig. 24.1). There is a central Haversian canal oriented to the long axis of the bone. Running at right angles to the long axis of the bone are secondary canals called perforating or **Volkmann's canals** which carry nerves, blood vessels and lymphatic vessels. Around the central canal are concentric hollow tubes of bone called **lamellae.** Each lamella has small concavities at the junctions with others called **lacunae** which contain the spider-shaped osteocytes. Hair-like canals called **canaliculi** connect the lacunae and the central canal, linking all the osteocytes in an osteon together. This facilitates the exchange of nutrients and the removal of waste products. Anatomical features of a long bone are shown in Fig. 24.2.

Spongy Bone

Spongy bone contains far fewer Haversian systems and is made up of a lattice of **trabeculae** with red or fatty bone marrow filling the cavities. Trabeculae are only a few cell layers thick and contain irregularly arranged lamellae and osteocytes connected by canaliculi. There are no osteons present. Nutrients arrive at the osteocytes by diffusing through narrow spaces between bony spicules. The tiny struts of bone are arranged to combat the stress placed on the bone during activity.

Periosteum and Endosteum

Most bones have a tough outer covering of fibrous connective tissue, the **periosteum,** which does not cover the articular surfaces of joints (Waugh & Grant, 2018). The periosteum transmits blood vessels and acts as an attachment surface for ligaments and muscles. It is supplied abundantly with nerve fibres. Beneath this is a layer of osteoblasts. Lining the marrow cavity is the **endosteum,** a layer of tissue containing the osteoblasts and osteoclasts.

Calcium and Phosphorus Metabolism

An adult body has about 1000 g of calcium, of which the skeleton contains 99%, leaving only 10 g available for other cellular processes. The small amount of calcium found in body fluids and cells plays an important part in metabolic processes and is maintained within narrow limits. Phosphorus is also crucial to body function, of which the skeleton contains 85%.

Functions of Calcium

Calcium is an intracellular and extracellular ion with many functions. It is present in ECF in two forms: half is bound to the proteins albumin and globulin and half is in a free ionized form (Ca^{2+}), which is important in many cell activities, including:

- Nerve and muscle function.
- Hormonal actions.
- Blood clotting.
- Cell motility.
- When bound to the protein **calmodulin**, it acts as a secondary messenger between an environmental stimulus and cell function by modulating enzyme response.

Functions of Phosphorus

Phosphorus in the form of phosphates plays a large role in cellular function:

- As a component of nucleic acids.
- By regulating energy storage as adenosine triphosphate.

Hormonal Control of Calcium and Phosphorus Metabolism

Regulation of calcium balance is closely associated with the regulation of phosphate. Continuous exchange of calcium takes place between different sites (calcium pools) in the body. Three hormones control calcium and phosphorus metabolism by maintaining the concentration of calcium in ECF. These hormones are **parathyroid hormone** (PTH), **vitamin D** and **calcitonin.** Plasma inorganic phosphate is more loosely controlled than calcium.

If there is no change in the amount of skeletal calcium, the ECF calcium level depends on the balance between calcium absorption in the gut and its excretion in urine and faeces. About 50% of the calcium in the blood passing through bone capillaries is exchanged in a single passage. About 300 mmol of calcium is involved in calcium exchange between blood and bone every day.

Parathyroid Hormone

Four parathyroid glands are embedded in the thyroid gland and secrete PTH. This PTH increases the concentration of Ca^{2+} in blood and depresses plasma phosphate concentration by acting on bone and kidneys. PTH increases osteocyte reabsorption of bone with a rapid release of calcium and phosphorus into the blood. Calcium reabsorption in the kidney tubules is increased, but the excretion of phosphate is increased. This results in a rise in plasma calcium and a fall in plasma phosphate. PTH activity is directly related to serum calcium concentration. When plasma calcium level rises, PTH production falls, resulting in calcium deposition in bone, and vice versa.

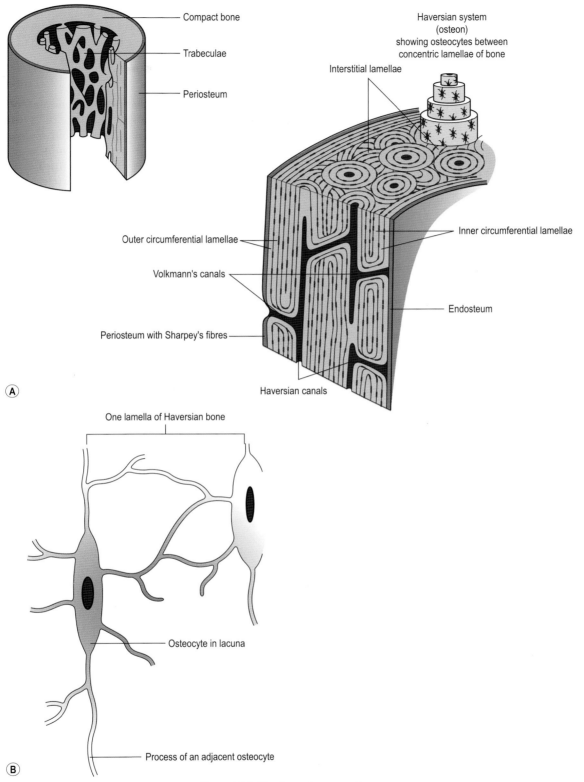

Compact bone

Trabeculae

Periosteum

Haversian system
(osteon)
showing osteocytes between
concentric lamellae of bone

Interstitial lamellae

Outer circumferential lamellae

Volkmann's canals

Periosteum with Sharpey's fibres

Inner circumferential lamellae

Endosteum

Haversian canals

(A)

One lamella of Haversian bone

Osteocyte in lacuna

Process of an adjacent osteocyte

(B)

• **Figure 24.1** Structure of compact bone.

Vitamin D

The D vitamins are steroid substances formed from **ergosterol** in plants and **7-dehydrocholesterol** in animals. Ultraviolet radiation modifies these to **ergocalciferol** (vitamin D$_2$) and **cholecalciferol** (vitamin D$_3$). Humans can either ingest vitamin D from plants and animals or manufacture it by the action of sunlight on the skin to form cholecalciferol. Vitamin D has to be further metabolized by adding hydroxyl groups before it can become active. The liver first converts it to **25-hydroxycholecalciferol,** and the kidney produces

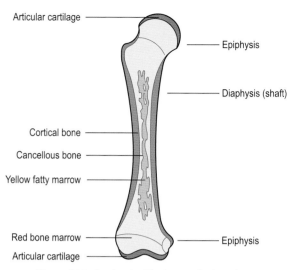

Articular cartilage

Epiphysis

Diaphysis (shaft)

Cortical bone

Cancellous bone

Yellow fatty marrow

Red bone marrow

Articular cartilage

Epiphysis

• **Figure 24.2** Anatomical features of a long bone.

the active form **1,25-dihydroxycholecalciferol** (calcitriol) in response to PTH stimulation. Calcitriol is released into the circulation and transported to its target organs of the intestine, bone and kidneys (Waugh & Grant, 2018).

Calcitonin

Calcitonin is secreted by the **parafollicular cells (clear or C cells)** of the thyroid gland. Its main effect is opposite to PTH, causing a fall in plasma calcium and phosphate concentrations. This hormone may play a part in skeletal growth in children but appears to have no role in adults other than in pregnant women. Calcitonin secretion is directly related to plasma calcium concentration.

The Pelvic Girdle

The pelvic girdle offers an attachment for the lower limbs and supports the pelvis and, to some extent, the abdominal organs. In an upright posture, the pelvic girdle transmits the weight of the trunk to the legs, so the sacroiliac joints must be strong and stable (Farthing, 2018). The size, shape and rigidity of the pelvic girdle are related directly to bipedal locomotion, and the human pelvis compared with other primates is short, squat and basin-shaped (Trevathan, 2017).

The gynaecoid pelvis is adapted for giving birth to a comparatively large-headed baby, but **mechanisms of labour** are necessary to facilitate the descent of the head through the pelvis. These include passive alterations to fetal position and moulding of the fetal skull.

Pelvic Bones

The pelvis is made up of four irregularly shaped bones: **two** innominate **bones** forming the lateral and anterior walls, and the **sacrum** and **coccyx** forming the posterior wall. Each innominate bone consists of three fused bones: the **ilium, ischium** and **pubis** (Farthing, 2018). These are

formed as cartilage in the fetus, and their ossification centres begin to fuse at puberty and are completed about age 25. The description of these bones is mirrored to the left and right of the pelvis.

The Ilium

The ilium has an upper flat plate of bone and forms part of the acetabulum below (Figs. 24.3 and 24.4). The external part of the plate of bone is curved and has a roughened surface for attachment of the **gluteal muscles** which form the buttocks. The inner surface forms the **iliac fossa** which is smooth and concave. The **iliacus muscle,** forming a platform on which the abdominal organs rest, originates from this surface. The upper ridge of the ilium is called the **iliac crest** and is S-shaped. The muscles of the abdominal wall have attachments to this surface.

At the anterior end of the iliac crest is the **anterior superior iliac** spine, which can be identified under the skin. At the posterior end is the **posterior superior iliac spine,** marked externally by a dimple at the level of the second sacral vertebra. Two **inferior iliac spines,** anterior and posterior, can be found below the superior spines. The lower margin of the ilium forms two-fifths of the acetabulum where it fuses with the ischium and pubis. Behind the acetabulum, the ilium forms the **greater sciatic notch,** through which nerves from the sacral plexus pass. Above the greater sciatic notch is the area of the ilium which articulates with the sacrum at the **sacroiliac joint.**

The Ischium

The ischium forms the lowest aspect of the innominate bone. The upper part forms two-fifths of the acetabulum, where it fuses with the ilium and pubis. Below the acetabulum, a thick buttress of bone called the **ischial tuberosity** takes the weight of the seated body. The **hamstring muscles** of the thigh arise from this bone. Passing upwards and inwards from the ischial tuberosity, a shaft of ischium meets the **inferior ramus of the pubic bone** to form the **pubic arch.**

The ischium also forms the lower border of the **obturator foramen,** a large opening in the lower part of the innominate bone below the acetabulum (Farthing, 2018). The ischial spine (an important landmark on vaginal examination) can be found protruding from the posterior edge about 5 cm above the tuberosity. The ischial spine separates the **greater sciatic notch** from the **lesser sciatic notch.**

The Pubis

This square-shaped bone forms the anterior aspect of the innominate bone. The two pubic bones articulate medially to form a joint called the **symphysis pubis.** Laterally, the **superior ramus of the pubic bone** forms one-fifth of the acetabulum. The superior ramus also forms the upper boundary of the obturator foramen. The inferior ramus passes downwards and outwards to join the ischium and form the pubic arch. The upper surface of the pubis forms the **pubic crest** ending laterally in the **pubic tubercle.**

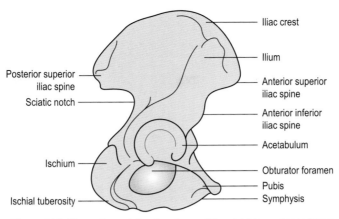

• **Figure 24.3** The outer or lateral surface of the right innominate bone.

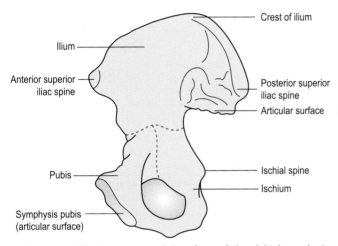

• **Figure 24.4** The inner or medial surface of the right innominate bone.

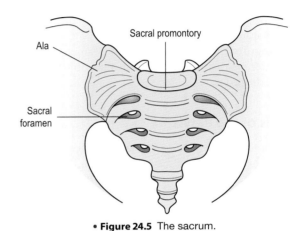

• **Figure 24.5** The sacrum.

The Sacrum

The sacrum is a shield-shaped mass of bone formed from five fused sacral vertebrae (Fig. 24.5). It articulates with the two innominate bones at the sacroiliac joints. The anterior surface is smooth and concave, both from above downwards and from side to side, forming the **hollow of the sacrum.** The first sacral vertebra overhangs the sacral hollow, and the central point of this projection is called the **sacral promontory** (Farthing, 2018). Through the centre of the bone, sacral and coccygeal nerves pass into the **sacral canal.**

Four pairs of **foramina** (openings) are present anteriorly between the five fused sacral vertebrae where sacral nerves exit to form the **sacral plexus.** Posterior branches of the sacral nerves pass through eight small foramina to supply the skin of the buttocks and the muscles of the lower back. On its upper surface, a smooth oval area forms an articular surface for the fifth lumbar vertebra to form the **lumbosacral joint.** Lateral masses of bone on either side of the sacrum are called the **wings of the sacrum** or **sacral alae.**

The Coccyx

This small triangular bone with its base uppermost is made of four fused coccygeal vertebrae. The first coccygeal vertebra articulates with the lower end of the sacrum to form the sacrococcygeal joint. The rudimentary vertebrae forming the rest of the coccyx are smooth on their inner surface and support the rectum. The external anal sphincter is attached to the lowest point.

Pelvic Joints

There are four pelvic joints: one symphysis pubis, two sacroiliac and one sacrococcygeal joint (Farthing, 2018):

- The **symphysis pubis** consists of an oval disc of fibrocartilage about 4 cm long lying between the two pubic bones. The joint is reinforced by ligaments crossing from one pubic bone to the other.
- The **sacroiliac joints** are synovial joints with a cavity filled with synovial fluid, a capsule formed of the synovial membrane and tough external supporting ligaments. Very strong posterior ligaments transmit the weight of the trunk, head and arms to the legs. Movement of these joints is slight but increases in range during pregnancy when relaxin softens the ligaments.

- The **sacrococcygeal joint** lies between the sacrum and coccyx. There is sometimes a small synovial joint cavity present. Slight movement can occur backwards, and this is increased greatly when the baby's head passes through the pelvis in labour.

Pelvic Ligaments

Besides the ligaments supporting the pelvic joints, there are three other pairs of ligaments:
- The **sacrotuberous ligament** crosses from the posterior superior iliac spine and the lateral borders of the sacrum and coccyx to the ischial tuberosity. It bridges the greater and lesser sciatic notches.
- The **sacrospinous ligament** passes in front of the sacrotuberous ligament from the side of the sacrum and coccyx, crosses the greater sciatic notch and attaches to the ischial spine.
- The **inguinal ligament** (Poupart's ligament) runs from the anterior superior iliac spine to the pubic tubercle and forms the groin.

Regions of the Pelvis

There is a clear line of bone called the **pelvic brim** which separates the upper flare of the iliac fossae. This is the **false pelvis.** The **true pelvis** arises from the basin-shaped part of the pelvis and has a cavity and outlet through which the fetus passes during birth.

The Pelvic Brim

Landmarks are identifiable on the pelvic brim (inlet), and important measurements are made between them. In the normal **gynaecoid (female) pelvis,** the brim is oval-shaped with the anteroposterior diameter reduced by the sacral promontory. Starting at the centre of the sacral promontory and tracing the brim round to the symphysis pubis, the landmarks are identified in Fig. 24.6.

If a piece of paper is placed across the landmarks, an imaginary flat surface is formed. This is called a **plane,** and the concept is also applied to the cavity and outlet. The **pelvic diameters** are measured from landmarks across the planes.

The Pelvic Cavity

The cavity is that part of the pelvis between the brim and the outlet. It is a **curved canal** with a short anterior surface measuring 4.5 cm, formed by the inner aspect of the pubic bones and symphysis pubis and a longer posterior surface measuring 12 cm formed by the hollow of the sacrum. The lateral walls are formed from the greater sciatic notch, the inner surface of part of the ilium, the body of the ischium and the obturator foramen. The plane of the pelvic cavity is taken from the midpoint of the symphysis pubis anteriorly to the junction of the second and third sacral vertebrae posteriorly.

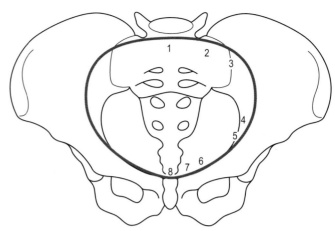

- **Figure 24.6** The pelvic brim. 1, Sacral promontory; 2, sacral ala; 3, sacroiliac joint; 4, iliopectineal line; 5, iliopectineal eminence; 6, superior pubic ramus; 7, body of pubic bone; 8, symphysis pubis.

The Pelvic Outlet

Two pelvic outlets are described: the **anatomical** and the **obstetric outlets.** The anatomical outlet is traced from the lower border of the symphysis pubis along the pubic arch to the inner border of the ischial tuberosity and along the sacrotuberous ligament to the tip of the coccyx. It varies in size during labour because of the range of backwards tilting of the coccyx in different women. The obstetric outlet has more practical significance as it includes the constricted lower portion of the true pelvis, through which the fetus must navigate. The obstetrical outlet, a more useful landmark, includes the following structures:
- The lower border of the symphysis pubis.
- A line passing along the pubis, obturator foramen and ischium to the ischial spine.
- The sacrospinous ligament.
- The lower border of the sacrum.

The plane of the outlet is an imaginary flat surface between these structures which is occupied by the muscles of the pelvic floor (Chapter 25).

Pelvic Dimensions (Diameters)

Measurements are taken of the planes of the brim, cavity and outlet, using the landmarks described earlier, in three directions: anteroposterior, oblique and transverse. Table 24.1 gives the average measurements for a gynaecoid pelvis.

The Brim

The four principal diameters of the brim include: the anteroposterior diameter, the transverse diameter and the two oblique diameters. Three conjugate diameters can be measured: the anatomical (true) conjugate, the obstetric conjugate and the internal or diagonal conjugate (Fig. 24.7).
- The smallest diameter of the brim is the **anteroposterior diameter** which is measured from the upper border of the symphysis pubis to the midpoint of the sacral

TABLE 24.1	Pelvic Measurements (Gynaecoid Pelvis)		
	Anteroposterior	**Oblique**	**Transverse**
Brim	11 cm	12 cm	13 cm
Cavity	12 cm	12 cm	12 cm
Outlet	13 cm	12 cm	11 cm

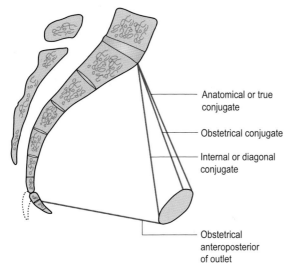

• **Figure 24.7** Median section of the pelvis showing anteroposterior diameters.

Labels: Anatomical or true conjugate; Obstetrical conjugate; Internal or diagonal conjugate; Obstetrical anteroposterior of outlet

promontory. This is the **anatomical conjugate,** which measures 12 cm. However, this is not available for accommodating the fetal head. If the measurement is taken from the inner border of the symphysis pubis to the sacral promontory, the measurement is 11 cm; this is the **obstetric conjugate.** The obstetric conjugate represents the shortest anteroposterior diameter of the birth canal. As such, it reflects the capacity of the pelvic inlet to allow the passage and the engagement of the fetal head (Kibuka et al., 2021). This is of clinical significance for midwives. The **diagonal conjugate,** measured during the pelvic assessment, is taken from the lower border of the symphysis pubis to the sacral promontory and measures 13 cm (Fig. 24.7). It is normally difficult to measure because its length exceeds the reach of most people. If the sacral promontory is reached, the obstetric conjugate is calculated by subtracting 2 cm.

• The two **oblique diameters** are taken from one sacroiliac joint to the opposite iliopectineal eminence. They are right and left after the corresponding sacroiliac joint. All the oblique diameters of the pelvis are 12 cm.

• The **transverse diameter** is taken between points on the iliopectineal lines that are farther apart and measures 13 cm. The descending colon passes the left sacroiliac joint and may limit the space available for the passage of the fetus.

• The **sacrocotyloid diameter** is a brim measurement taken from the sacral promontory to the iliopectineal eminence. It measures 9.5 cm. In an occipitoposterior presentation, the fetal parietal eminences may become caught in this diameter, causing the head to extend.

The Cavity

• The cavity is considered circular in diameter, and the measurements taken through its plane are 12 cm.

The Obstetric Outlet

• The outlet is diamond-shaped with its longer diameter being anteroposterior. This is measured from the lower border of the symphysis pubis to the sacrococcygeal joint and is 13 cm.

• The oblique diameter has no fixed points but is between the obturator foramen and the opposite sacrospinous ligament. The oblique diameter is 12 cm.

• The transverse diameter is measured between the two ischial spines and is 11 cm.

Pelvic Inclination

When a person stands up, the pelvic basin is tilted with the plane of the brim forming an angle of 60 degrees to the horizontal. If the reader stands facing and pressed up against a vertical surface, the two points touching that vertical surface are the pubic bones and the anterior superior iliac spines. The plane of the cavity forms an angle of 30 degrees, and that of the outlet is 15 degrees (Fig. 24.8).

Three other angles are important indicators of pelvic size, all of which should measure at least 90 degrees:

1. The subpubic angle of the pubic arch.
2. The sacral angle lying between the plane of the brim and the anterior surface of the first sacral vertebra.
3. The greater sciatic notch.

Axes of the Pelvic Canal

If imaginary lines are drawn at right angles through the pelvic planes, axes can be created. If these lines are joined together, a curve called the **curve of Carus** can be traced because each plane is at a different angle to the horizon. This unique feature of the human pelvis is the price paid for an upright posture, as it makes delivery of the fetus more difficult. Instead of an easy journey through a straight pelvic canal, the fetus must be moved passively by mechanisms to overcome the changing curves and diameters (Figs. 24.9 and 24.10).

Basic Types of Pelves

Four basic types of pelves are described according to the shape of the brim and other features (Fig. 24.11 and Table 24.2). These types are gynaecoid, android, anthropoid and platypelloid. Although gynaecoid is cited as the ideal pelvis for childbearing, many pelves cannot be classified as easily as they contain features of different types. The size of the pelvis in relation to the fetus is now considered to be more important than a slight abnormality of shape. There is an expression that 'the fetal head is the best pelvimeter'.

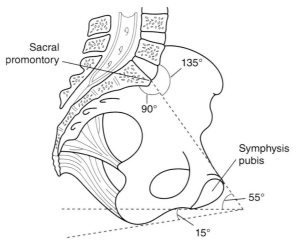

• **Figure 24.8** The pelvis, showing the degrees of inclination. Inclination of the pelvic brim to the horizontal, 55 degrees; inclination of the pelvic outlet to the horizontal, 15 degrees; angle of pelvic inclination, 135 degrees; inclination of the sacrum, 90 degrees.

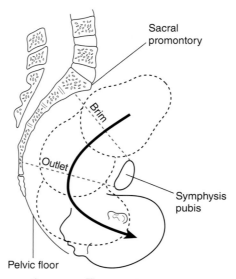

• **Figure 24.9** The axis of the birth canal.

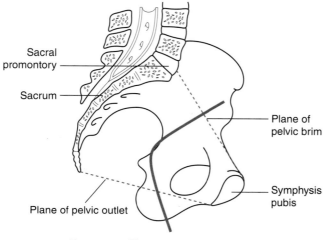

• **Figure 24.10** The curve of the birth canal.

Maternal Positions in Labour

Maternal birth positions refer to the posture a women may assume during labour and birth. Maternal posture alters the skeletal, muscle and ligature components of the pelvis to create space for the fetus, which in turn aids negotiation of the maternal pelvis (Kibuka et al., 2021). As the diameters of the fixed bony structures are known, it is understood that altering maternal posture may aid movement and create some changes to internal space, increasing or in certain positions reducing access within the pelvis. Therefore, discussion around maternal positions must not solely consider increasing space but instead access to the available space, namely at the pelvic inlet and obstetric outlet. Box 24.1 summarizes the evidence available on maternal positions in labour. Further research is required in this area and the impact on the pelvis.

Maternal Physiological Adaptations in Pregnancy

Calcium and Phosphorus Metabolism in Pregnancy
Calcium

Maternal calcium metabolism is altered during pregnancy to meet fetal needs for skeletal mineralization, especially in the third trimester (Blackburn, 2018). Absorption and urinary excretion are increased. Maternal serum levels begin to fall shortly after fertilization and reach their lowest levels from 30 weeks of pregnancy. These changes are reversible following birth and cessation of lactation. Although bone mineral density falls during lactation, prolonged breastfeeding does not lead to permanent osteoporosis.

The fetal plasma calcium level exceeds maternal levels, suggesting that the mineral is actively transported across the placenta. Calcitonin and PTH cannot cross the placenta so the fetus must manufacture its own. The placenta can transfer vitamin D to the fetus and synthesize vitamin D. During pregnancy, maternal calcium, phosphorus and magnesium levels fall due to increased production of PTH, calcitonin and vitamin D. Calcium storage may increase in preparation for lactation, but an increase in dietary calcium does not increase bone density. Any increase in bone calcium due to human placental lactogen is counterbalanced by oestrogen causing decreased reabsorption.

Diet

These changes are independent of calcium intake, and supplements are unnecessary in countries where dietary intake is adequate. Supplementation may be needed in adolescents and where dietary insufficiency is suspected. The total extra calcium needed by term is about 25–30 g. Some foods such as those containing excessive fats, phytates (found in some vegetables) and oxalates interfere with the absorption of calcium by forming calcium salts in the intestine. High sodium intake may also interfere with calcium absorption (Blackburn, 2018).

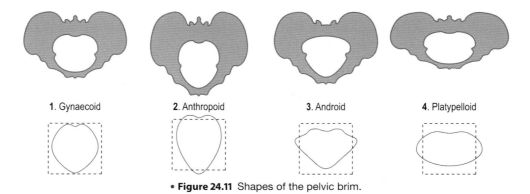

1. Gynaecoid   2. Anthropoid   3. Android   4. Platypelloid

• **Figure 24.11** Shapes of the pelvic brim.

TABLE 24.2	Variants of the Pelvic Structure				
Feature of Pelvis	Brim	Forepelvis	Shape of Cavity	Ischial Spines	Pubic Diameter
Gynaecoid	Rounded	Large	Shallow	Blunt	90 degrees
Anthropoid	Oval	Large	Deep	Not prominent	Wide or normal
Android	Heart-shaped	Narrow	Funnel	Prominent	<90 degrees
Platypelloid	Kidney-shaped	Flat	Shallow	Blunt	>90 degrees

Vitamin D

Levels of active vitamin D (calcitriol) show a small rise by 10 weeks of pregnancy, although staying within normal limits. They rise above normal in the last few weeks. However there is little elevation in either intact PTH or calcitonin levels. Intestinal absorption of vitamin D is enhanced throughout pregnancy.

Diet

An increased intake of vitamin D is needed to ensure maternal and fetal needs for calcium are met, and 400 IU/day is advised. Supplementation is advisable if dietary intake is poor or there is poor exposure to sunlight. Milk is an excellent source of calcium, phosphorus and vitamin D. Women who cannot drink milk should eat cheese, yogurt, sardines, wholegrain foods or green leafy vegetables.

Box 24.2 provides information on rickets and osteomalacia.

Phosphorus and Magnesium

Serum inorganic phosphate and magnesium levels fall slightly until 30 weeks and return to non-pregnant levels by term. These changes are related to haemodilution.

Diet

Although phosphorus is essential during pregnancy, high intake levels limit calcium absorption, whereas high plasma levels increase urinary excretion of calcium. Processed meats, snack foods and cola drinks all have high phosphorus but low calcium levels.

The Fetal Skull

Fetal head geometry plays an important role in the mechanics of childbirth during the second stage of labour (Yan et al., 2015). The shape and size of the human pelvis create difficulties in birthing, compounded further by the large size of the fetal brain which constitutes approximately 10% of the total birthweight. The brain continues to grow at fetal rates for the next 20 months to reach 1000 g. As such, evolutionary changes have developed to facilitate birth, including:
- Rapid brain growth after birth.
- Flexion of the fetal head on its neck so that the narrowest diameters pass through the pelvis.
- Moulding of the skull bones to change the shape from ovoid to cylindrical.

Anatomy of the Skull

The fetal skull is ovoid-shaped and the bones can be divided into the vault, the face and the base. The vault extends from the orbital ridges to the base of the occiput and contains the brain, which rests on the base of the skull. For measurement and categorizing presentations, the fetal skull is divided into regions of face, brow, vertex and occiput (Fig. 24.12):
- The **face** extends from the chin to the orbital ridges.
- The **brow** or **sinciput** is the area of the two frontal bones, extending from the orbital ridges to the anterior fontanelle.
- The **vertex** is bounded by the anterior fontanelle, the posterior fontanelle and the two parietal eminences.
- The **occiput** is the area over the occipital bone, extending from the posterior fontanelle to the nape of neck.

The biomechanical mechanisms of the position adopted for labour and birth are associated with pelvic dimensions, intrauterine pressure, moulding of the fetal head and progression of fetal head angle through the birth canal (Kibuka et al., 2021). The two main maternal positions during childbirth are upright and horizontal positions. These positions are based on the angle made by the horizontal plane and the line linking the midpoints of the third and fifth lumbar vertebrae. The upright position is considered when the spine is vertical and >45 degrees and horizontal when <45 degrees.

Maternal birthing positions introduced focus on the maternal pelvis (see Chapters 37 and 39). When considering the pelvic outlet, the negotiation of space is pivotal during the active first and second stages of labour. Upright birth positions are associated with improved birth outcomes. Two systematic reviews of studies involving primigravid and multigravid women in labour demonstrated the following key points (Lawrence et al., 2013; Gupta et al., 2017).

Lawrence et al. (2013) conducted a systematic review (25 studies) with 5218 women looking at the positions adopted in the first stage of labour in relation to maternal, neonatal and labour outcomes.

Main findings:
- Walking and upright positions reduce both the duration of labour and the risk of caesarean birth.
- Women were less likely to have an epidural and less chance of babies admitted to the neonatal unit.

In a systematic review of 32 studies (9015 women), Gupta et al. (2017) reviewed a range of maternal upright and lying positions adopted in labour to determine any associated benefits and risks.

Main findings (upright position group):
- All women adopting the upright position were associated with a reduction in duration of second stage.
- A reduction in episiotomy rates and assisted births was also noted.

For upright posture, there was blood loss greater than 500 mL (this may be due to greater accuracy of estimation) and a possible increased risk of second-degree tears.

The discussion around increased second-degree perineal trauma may relate to the directed pressure of the presenting part when the mother assumes certain positions. The directed pressure on the perineal body is greater in certain maternal positions. This specifically relates to the association between the perineum and the lower maternal limbs.

It is recommended that women in labour should be informed of the benefits of upright positions and encouraged and assisted to assume optimal positions. Chapter 37 presents a range of maternal positions adopted in labour to promote optimal fetal descent through the pelvis. Other maternal positions adopted can reduce the birthing angle and compromise the space available in the pelvis.

Bones: The Vault

Five main bones make up the vault with two others helping to form the lateral walls: the squamous (flattened) portion

Malabsorption of calcium is usually caused by a deficiency in vitamin D due to a low intake. This is sometimes combined with low exposure to sunlight. Vitamin D deficiency is not only associated with a wide range of health conditions but has a classic role in the prevention of bone diseases of **rickets** (in childhood) and **osteomalacia** (in adulthood). In these diseases, the bones are poorly ossified and soft and become deformed. Distortion of the pelvis may occur, leading to severe problems in childbirth associated with birth by caesarean section.

Vitamin D deficiency may result from low vitamin D intake, relatively high adiposity, sun exposure avoidance and wearing a covered dress style for cultural reasons. Midwives need to be vigilant about women presenting during pregnancy with vitamin D deficiency (**hypovitaminosis D**). There is a clear need for urgent public health action to address this vitamin D deficiency epidemic in South Asian women living in Western countries (Darling, 2020).

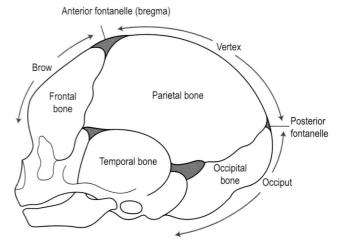

• **Figure 24.12** The bones, fontanelles and regions of the fetal skull.

of the temporal bones. Each bone is named for the portion of the brain lying beneath it:
- Two frontal bones whose ossification centres are indicated by the frontal bosses.
- Two parietal bones whose ossification centres are indicated by the parietal eminences.
- Two squamous portions of the temporal bones.
- One occipital bone whose ossification centre is indicated by the occipital protuberance.

Ossification is incomplete at birth, and membranous sutures remain between the bones and membranous fontanelles where two or more sutures meet. These membranous areas facilitate moulding of the fetal skull during birth and provide landmarks that can be identified during vaginal examination (Fig. 24.13).

The Sutures

- The **frontal** suture lies between the two frontal bones.
- The **sagittal** suture runs from the anterior to the posterior fontanelle, uniting the two parietal bones.

- The **lambdoidal** suture (resembling the Greek letter lambda—λ) lies between the posterior edges of the parietal bones and the occipital bone.
- The **coronal** suture separates the posterior edges of the two frontal bones from the anterior edges of the two parietal bones.

The Fontanelles

There are two main fontanelles (Figs. 24.12 and 24.13):
- The **anterior** fontanelle or **bregma** is diamond-shaped and formed at the junction of four sutures: the frontal, parietal and two halves of the coronal sutures. It measures 2.5 cm across by 3 cm long and is not fully closed by ossification until 18 months of age.
- The **posterior** fontanelle or **lambda** is much smaller and triangular-shaped and formed at the junction of three sutures: the sagittal suture and the two halves of

the lambdoidal suture. It closes by the sixth week after birth.

In addition, there are four minor fontanelles on the sidewalls of the vault. There are two temporal fontanelles at the ends of the coronal suture and two mastoid fontanelles at the ends of the lambdoidal suture (shaded in Fig. 24.12). These are not of any significance in childbearing.

Bones: The Base

The fused bones of the base of the skull are perforated by the foramen magnum which allows passage of the spinal cord leading from the brain.

Diameters of the Fetal Skull

Measurements of the skull are used to assess its size in relation to the maternal pelvis. Longitudinal diameters are taken between key landmarks so that the diameters presenting at the pelvis in different degrees of flexion or extension can be estimated (Figs. 24.14 and 24.15):

1. The **suboccipitobregmatic** is measured from the nape of neck to the centre of the anterior fontanelle. It is 9.5 cm and presents when the head is fully flexed.
2. The **suboccipitofrontal** is measured from the nape of neck to the centre of the frontal suture. It is 10 cm and presents when the head is almost completely flexed.
3. The **occipitofrontal** is measured from the glabella (bridge of the nose) to the occipital protuberance. It is 11.5 cm and presents when the head is deflexed, as in an occipitoposterior position.
4. The **mentovertical** is measured from the point of the chin to the highest point on the vertex. It is 13.5 cm and presents when the head is midway between flexion and extension in a brow presentation.
5. The **submentovertical** is measured from the junction of the chin with the neck to the highest point on the vertex. It is 11.5 cm and presents when the head is not fully extended in a face presentation.

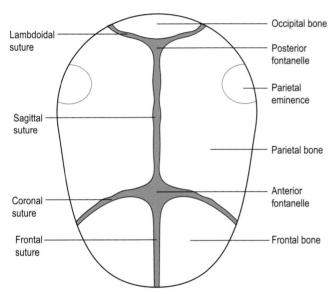

Lambdoidal suture
Occipital bone
Posterior fontanelle
Parietal eminence
Sagittal suture
Parietal bone
Anterior fontanelle
Coronal suture
Frontal suture
Frontal bone

• **Figure 24.13** The fetal skull, showing the bones, fontanelles and sutures.

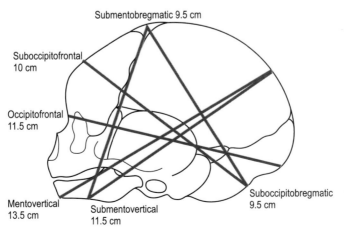

Submentobregmatic 9.5 cm
Suboccipitofrontal 10 cm
Occipitofrontal 11.5 cm
Mentovertical 13.5 cm
Submentovertical 11.5 cm
Suboccipitobregmatic 9.5 cm

• **Figure 24.14** The diameters of the fetal skull.

6. The **submentobregmatic** is measured from the junction of the chin with the neck to the midpoint of the anterior fontanelle. It is 9.5 cm and presents when the head is fully extended in a face presentation.

Transverse diameters are also taken:

1. The **biparietal** is measured between the parietal eminences. It is 9.5 cm and is the widest transverse diameter.
2. The **bitemporal** is measured between the widest aspects of the coronal suture. It is 8 cm.
3. The **bimastoid** is measured between the mastoid processes. It is 7.5 cm.

Circumferences of the skull are:

• The **suboccipitobregmatic**: 33 cm presents when the head is well flexed. The head engages, fits well onto the cervix and labour should progress easily.

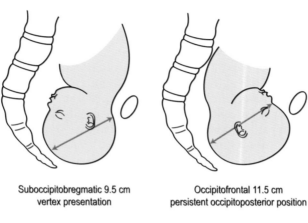

Suboccipitobregmatic 9.5 cm
vertex presentation

Occipitofrontal 11.5 cm
persistent occipitoposterior position

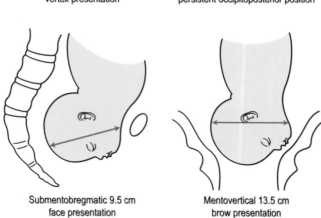

Submentobregmatic 9.5 cm
face presentation

Mentovertical 13.5 cm
brow presentation

• **Figure 24.15** The diameters of the fetal skull in relation to the maternal pelvis.

• The **occipitofrontal**: 35 cm presents when the head is deflexed. Engagement is delayed, the membranes may rupture early and labour may be difficult.
• The **mentovertical**: 39 cm presents when the head is midway between flexion and extension. The head cannot descend into the pelvis unless it completes extension and labour is obstructed.

Moulding

Moulding of the fetal skull results in a change in shape (but not size) of the vault brought about by the pressures of the pelvis and pelvic floor during labour. The diameters, which are compressed, reduce in size by at least 0.5 cm, whereas those at right angles to them are elongated (Table 24.3). The sutures and fontanelles allow an overlap of the bones in a typical way:

• The frontal bones are pushed under the anterior edge of the parietal bones.
• The occipital bone is pushed under the posterior part of the parietal bones.
• The medial edge of the leading parietal bone is pushed under the other parietal bone.

Moulding (Fig. 24.16), if too rapid or too extreme, may compress the brain, risking intracranial damage.

Caput Succedaneum

During labour, especially after rupture of the membranes, the fetal head is pressed against the dilating cervix. In cephalic presentations, venous return of the scalp circulation is impeded and oedema forms in the loose tissues to a varying degree, thus forming a **caput succedaneum** (Fig. 24.17) (see Chapter 53).

External Features of the Fetal Skull

The fetal scalp consists of five layers:

1. The **pericranium** covers the outer surface of the bones and is firmly attached to the edges of the bones. Bleeding may occur between the bone and the pericranium to form a swelling called a **cephalhaematoma** (see Chapter 53). The size of the haematoma is limited by the attachment of the pericranium to that of the bone over which it forms.

TABLE 24.3	Involvement of Diameters of the Fetal Skull in Moulding	
Presentation	**Diameters Increased**	**Diameter Decreased**
Vertex	Suboccipitobregmatic biparietal	Mentovertical
Brow	Mentovertical biparietal	Suboccipitobregmatic
Face	Submentobregmatic biparietal	Occipitofrontal
Occipitoposterior	Occipitofrontal biparietal	Submentobregmatic

2. A loose layer of **areolar tissue** that permits limited movement of the scalp over the skull.
3. A layer of **tendon** known as the **galea** that is attached to the frontalis muscle anteriorly and the occipitalis muscle posteriorly.
4. A layer of **subcutaneous tissue** containing blood vessels and hair follicles. This is the part of the scalp affected by the caput succedaneum (see Fig. 24.17).
5. The **skin.**

Internal Structures of the Fetal Skull

The Meninges

The brain is surrounded by three membranes. From the inside out, these are:

1. The **pia mater,** which is very delicate and has many tiny blood vessels closely applied to the surface of the brain.

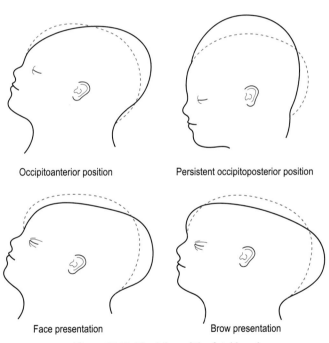

Occipitoanterior position

Persistent occipitoposterior position

Face presentation

Brow presentation

• **Figure 24.16** Moulding of the fetal head.

2. The **arachnoid mater,** which forms a loose brain covering and is attached to the pia mater by thread-like extensions which cross the subarachnoid space containing cerebrospinal fluid.
3. The outer, tough **dura mater,** which is a double-layered membrane, lines the skull with its periosteal layer and is reflected onto the surface of the brain as the meningeal layer, extending inwards to form septa that anchor the brain to the skull and limit movement.

Sinuses and Venous Drainage

There are two main folds of the dura mater. The **falx cerebri** is a double fold forming a partition between the two cerebral hemispheres. It is attached to the skull following the line of the frontal and sagittal sutures from the root of the nose to the internal aspect of the occipital protuberance. Its lower edge is unattached and sickle-shaped.

The **tentorium cerebelli** lies horizontally, separating the cerebrum from the cerebellum. It is at right angles to the falx cerebri and is horseshoe-shaped. Each side of the horseshoe is attached laterally to the sphenoid bone and along the inner surface of the petrous portion of the temporal bone. It meets the falx at the inner aspect of the occipital protuberance. The brainstem passes in front of this junction of the two folds of the dura mater.

Venous drainage is by channels in the dural folds called sinuses (Fig. 24.18):

1. The **superior longitudinal sinus** (sagittal) runs along the upper border of the falx cerebri.
2. The **inferior longitudinal sinus** (sagittal) runs along the lower border of the falx cerebri.
3. The **straight sinus** is a continuation of the inferior longitudinal sinus which runs posteriorly to join the superior longitudinal sinus.
4. The **great vein of Galen** joins the straight sinus at the junction with the inferior longitudinal sinus.
5. From the confluence of sinuses, the **lateral sinuses** pass along the line of attachment of the tentorium cerebelli and emerge from the skull to become the internal **jugular veins** of the neck.

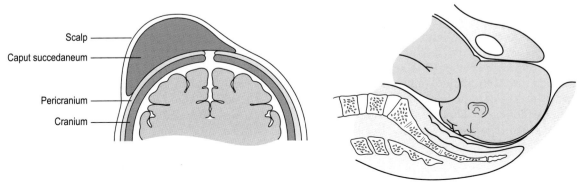

Scalp

Caput succedaneum

Pericranium

Cranium

• **Figure 24.17** Caput succedaneum.

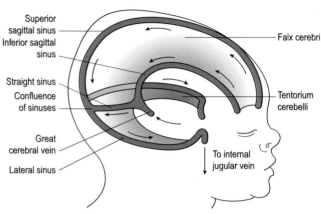

• **Figure 24.18** Internal structures of the fetal skull.

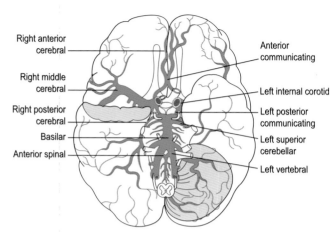

• **Figure 24.19** Arterial blood supply to the brain, including the circle of Willis.

When moulding is abnormal these membranes and sinuses may be torn, especially at the junction of the two folds of the dura. The tentorium is most likely to be damaged, and bleeding involves the great vein of Galen, the straight sinus and the inferior longitudinal sinus.

Blood Supply to the Brain

The arterial blood supply is by two **internal carotid arteries** and **two vertebral arteries.** The internal carotid arteries give off pairs of **anterior, middle** and **posterior cerebral arteries.** Each vertebral artery gives off a branch that supplies the **cerebellum** and **medulla oblongata** before uniting with its partner to form the **basilar artery.** The basilar artery gives off two pairs of arteries to the cerebellum and upper brainstem before dividing into two terminal branches that link up with the ends of the internal carotid arteries. The intercommunicating arteries at the base of the brain are called the *circle of Willis* (Fig. 24.19).

Main Points

- Bone is a connective tissue consisting of an organic matrix called *osteoid,* a mineral matrix of calcium and phosphorus, and bone cells. Bone can be divided into compact bone and spongy bone.
- Most bones have a tough outer periosteum and a cavity lining of endosteum. The endosteum contains osteoblasts, osteoclasts and their precursor cells.
- Osteoblasts synthesize bone and promote mineralization of the cortex. Osteoclasts contain enzymes that remove both organic and mineral matrix.
- The skeleton contains 99% of the calcium and 85% of the phosphorus present in the body. PTH, vitamin D and calcitonin are three hormones controlling calcium and phosphorus metabolism.
- The pelvic girdle provides attachment for the lower limbs and support for the abdominal organs.
- The pelvis is made up of two innominate bones, one sacrum and one coccyx. Each innominate bone consists of three fused bones: the ilium, ischium and pubis.
- The four pelvic joints are the symphysis pubis, two sacroiliac joints and the sacrococcygeal joint.
- The pelvic brim separates the upper flare of the iliac fossae known as the *false pelvis* above the brim from the basin-shaped true pelvis below the brim. The true pelvis forms the birth canal.

- Measurements are taken of the planes of the pelvic brim, cavity and outlet in three directions: anteroposterior, oblique and transverse.
- There are four basic pelvic types: gynaecoid, android, anthropoid and platypelloid.
- Maternal calcium metabolism alters to meet fetal needs for calcium and phosphorus for skeletal mineralization.
- Adequate calcium, phosphorus and vitamin D are essential in pregnancy.
- The bones of the fetal skull are divided into vault, face and base. The face and base are laid down in cartilage and are almost completely ossified by term. The vault is composed of flat bones which develop from membranes.
- The fetal skull is divided into regions of face, brow, vertex and occiput.
- Vault ossification is incomplete at birth so that membranous sutures and fontanelles remain between the bones. This allows the change in shape, called *moulding,* to occur.
- The brain is surrounded by three meninges: the pia mater, the arachnoid mater and the dura mater.
- The arterial blood supply to the brain is from two internal carotid arteries and two vertebral arteries with the intercommunicating arteries at the base of the brain known as the *circle of Willis.*

References

Blackburn, S.T., 2018. Maternal, Fetal and Neonatal Physiology: A Clinical Perspective, fourth ed. Saunders, Philadelphia.

Darling, A., 2020. South Asian populations: an unrecognised epidemic. Proc. Nutr. Soc. 79 (3), 259–271.

Farthing, A., 2018. Clinical anatomy of the pelvis and reproductive tract. In: Edmonds, D.K., Lees, C., Bourne, T.H. (Eds.), Dewhurst's Textbook of Obstetrics and Gynaecology, ninth ed. Wiley-Blackwell, Oxford.

Gupta, J.K., Sood, A., Hofmeyr, G.J., Vogel, J.P., 2017. Position in the second stage of labour for women without epidural anaesthesia. Cochrane Database Syst. Rev. 2017 (5), CD002006.

Kibuka, M., Price, A., Onakpoya, I, Tierney, S., Clarke, M., 2021. Evaluating the effects of maternal positions in childbirth: an overview of Cochrane Systematic Reviews. Eur. J. Midwifery. 5, 1–14.

Lawrence, A., Lewis, L., Hofmeyr, G.J., Styles, C., 2013. Maternal positions and mobility during first stage labour. Cochrane Database Syst. Rev. 2013 (10), CD003934.

Trevathan, W.R., 2017. Human Birth: An Evolutionary Perspective. Routledge, London.

Waugh, A., Grant, A., 2018. Ross & Wilson Anatomy and Physiology in Health and Fitness, thirteenth ed. Elsevier, London.

Yan, X., Kruger, J.A., Nielsen, P.M., Nash, M.P., 2015. Effects of fetal head shape variation on the second stage of labour. J. Biomech. 48 (9), 1593–1599.

Annotated recommended reading

Di Pasquo, E., Volpe, N., Labadini, C., et al., 2021. Antepartum evaluation of the obstetric conjugate at transabdominal 2D ultrasound: a feasibility study. Acta Obstet. Gynecol. Scand. 100. 1917–1923.

Study findings have demonstrated that among pregnant women at term gestation, sonographic measurement of the obstetric conjugate is feasible and reproducible. Antepartum assessment of maternal pelvimetry may improve the prediction of obstructed labour.

Marani, E., Koch, W. (Eds.), 2014. The Pelvis: Structure, Gender and Society. Springer, London.

A comprehensive text that explores the pelvis within many contexts and across several disciplines. This text is not yet updated but the content remains relevant. The interested reader is directed to the chapters on 'Construction Plan of the Bony Pelvis' and 'The Birth Canal' as particularly relevant to support the discussions within this chapter.

Yan, X., Kruger, J.A., Nielsen, P.M., Nash, M.P., 2015. Effects of fetal head shape variation on the second stage of labour. J. Biomech. 48 (9), 1593–1599.

A fascinating study detailing the important role that fetal head geometry plays in the mechanics of childbirth. Based on data collected and simulations created from computed tomography and magnetic resonance imaging scans undertaken of both newborn skulls and maternal pelves.

25

Muscle–The Pelvic Floor and the Uterus

LYNSAY MATTHEWS AND JEAN RANKIN

This chapter describes the nature of muscles in relation to muscle types, structure and physiology. The individual muscles of the pelvic floor, uterus and cervix are detailed. Students and midwives will use this knowledge to avoid or alleviate any related complications.

Introduction

Muscle makes up almost half of the body's mass and is specialized tissue which generates force resulting in movement. It can transform chemical energy from adenosine triphosphate (ATP) into mechanical energy.

Skeletal, smooth and cardiac are the three basic muscle types. Each muscle type differs in terms of structure, contractile properties and control mechanisms. Most skeletal muscle is attached to bone and is responsible for supporting and moving the skeleton. Smooth muscle is found in the walls of the viscera of the gastrointestinal, genitourinary and respiratory tracts. The specialized cardiac muscle propels blood throughout the body. Despite significant differences, each muscle type has a similar force-generating mechanism. All muscle cells are elongated and referred to as *fibres,* and all muscle cells contain two kinds of protein filaments: **actin** and **myosin.** The functions and properties of muscle are presented in Box 25.1.

Skeletal Muscle

Skeletal muscles have the longest muscle fibres and are attached to and cover the bony skeleton. One striking feature of the skeletal muscle fibres is obvious bands, or **striations,** hence the term **striated muscle.** Another term used for skeletal muscle is **voluntary,** as this muscle type is under voluntary control. Skeletal muscle can contract rapidly but tires easily and must be rested after short bursts of activity. Each skeletal muscle is a discrete organ made up of multiple muscle fibres. Other tissues found in muscles include connective tissue, blood vessels and nerve fibres. Muscle fibres are gathered into functional units by a network of fibrous connective tissue. This connective tissue condenses into the **tendons**, forming the muscular origins and insertions onto bone.

The activity of skeletal muscle depends on its rich blood supply and nerve supply. In contrast to other muscle types which contract without nerve stimulation, each skeletal muscle fibre is supplied with a nerve ending. The blood supply is essential to deliver the large amounts of oxygen and nutrients and to remove equally large amounts of metabolic waste. The smaller blood vessels are long and winding, which permits the changes in muscle length to occur. Box 25.2 presents an overview of the microscopic structure of skeletal muscle (Figs. 25.1 & 25.2) and the process of skeletal muscle contraction (Figs. 25.3 & 25.4).

The Pelvic Floor

The bony pelvis protects the pelvic organs, and the **pelvic floor** holds the organs in position. The pelvic floor is primarily composed of soft tissues which fill the outlet of the pelvis. The strong, funnel-shaped diaphragm of skeletal muscles attached to the pelvic walls are the most important. The posterior part of the diaphragm of pelvic muscles lies higher than the anterior part. Through it passes the urethra, vagina and anal canal (Fig. 25.5).

Four Functions

- Produce movement.
- Maintain posture.
- Stabilize joints.
- Generate heat.

Four Properties

- Excitability: ability to receive and respond to a stimulus.
- Contractility: ability to shorten when stimulated.
- Extensibility: ability to be stretched or extended beyond its resting length.
- Elasticity: ability of a muscle to recoil back to its resting length.

The pelvic floor consists of six layers of tissue as follows, from the inside outwards:

1. Pelvic peritoneum.
2. Visceral layer of pelvic fascia thickened to form pelvic ligaments which support the uterus.
3. **Deep muscles** encased in the fascia.
4. **Superficial muscles** encased in the fascia.
5. Subcutaneous fat.
6. Skin.

The nomenclature for pelvic muscles varies across journals and textbooks. The common names used to identify the same muscle are included.

Superficial Muscles

Superficial muscles (perineal muscles) lie external to the deep muscles and provide additional strength—similar

Skeletal muscle is composed of different structures of decreasing size. The main muscle body is made up of many **muscle fibres**. In turn these are composed of bundles of **myofibrils** made of smaller contractile units called **sarcomeres**, each containing **myofilaments** composed of proteins called **actin** and **myosin** (Fig. 25.1).

Muscle fibres can be huge with lengths varying from a few millimetres to 300 mm (1 ft) and diameters between 10 and 100 μm (10× other body cells). Each muscle fibre is a **syncytium** (fusion of many cells) formed during embryonic development. The **sarcolemma** (plasma membrane) has multiple oval nuclei, and **sarcoplasm** (cytoplasm) contains large amounts of stored glycogen and a unique oxygen-binding protein called **myoglobin**, similar to haemoglobin. Endoplasmic reticulum is referred to as the **sarcoplasmic reticulum** (Marieb & Hoehn, 2022).

Myofibrils form 80% of the cellular content. Myofibrils have alternate dark or **A bands** and light or **I bands** (striped appearance). The **A** band is interrupted in the mid-section by the highly refractive **H zone** (H stands for *helle,* bright). Each H zone is bisected by a dark line called the **M line**. The I bands have a midline interruption called the **Z line** (Fig. 25.2).

Sarcomere extends from one Z line to the next. A bands are formed of thick **myosin** filaments. Proteins **actin**, **troponin** and **tropomyosin** form the thin filaments, running the length of the I band and overlapping the thick filaments. In resting muscle, the orientation of tropomyosin blocks the myosin-binding sites on actin, preventing the formation of cross-bridges.

Process of Muscle Contraction

Most evidence supports the **sliding-filament theory** which explains how increasing the amount of overlap during contraction is brought about by the thin filaments sliding past the thick ones. The cross-bridges of the sarcomeres act simultaneously as a ratchet to pull the thin filaments towards the centre of the sarcomeres and shortening the muscle cell. The myosin heads 'walk up' the actin filaments step by step from one binding site to the next (Fig. 25.3). Ca^{2+} is needed for this process. As Ca^{2+} is removed by the sarcoplasmic reticulum, the contraction comes to an end and the muscle cell relaxes (Hall & Hall, 2020).

Regulation of Contraction

Skeletal muscle fibres are innervated by large, myelinated nerve fibres that contract in response to nerve stimulation,

resulting in an **action potential** (AP) along the sarcolemma (Hall & Hall, 2020). This electrical event causes a rise in intracellular Ca^{2+} ion levels, triggering the contraction at the *neuromuscular junction* or **motor endplate** (Fig. 25.4). The plasma membrane of the axonal ending does not touch the muscle fibre; between them is a small fluid-filled extracellular space called the **synaptic cleft**. The AP is transmitted across the space by the release of the neurotransmitter substance **acetylcholine (ACh)** from small membranous sacs in the axon terminal called **synaptic vesicles**.

When a nerve impulse reaches the end of an axon, **voltage-regulated calcium channels** open and Ca^{2+} flows in from the extracellular fluid (ECF). Ca^{2+} causes some synaptic vesicles to fuse with the plasma membrane and release ACh into the synaptic cleft. This process is called **exocytosis**. ACh diffuses across the synaptic cleft and attaches itself to ACh receptors on the sarcolemma. All plasma membranes are polarized with a **voltage gradient** across the membrane (membrane potential). The inside of the cell is negative. This attachment of ACh molecules opens chemically regulated ion gates. The positively charged sodium ion (Na^+) passes from its higher concentration in the ECF fluid down a gradient into the cell, leading to a slight decrease in the negative potential. This is called **depolarization** and allows an AP to be generated and to pass in all directions across the sarcolemma. **Repolarization** of the sarcolemma occurs after the wave of muscle AP when sodium channels close and potassium channels open. After the release of ACh and binding to the ACh receptors, it is quickly destroyed by the enzyme **acetylcholinesterase**. This prevents the contraction lasting longer than the stimulus requires.

Excitation–contraction coupling is the process involving the generation of an AP followed by activation of the contractile mechanism in the myofibrils (Hall & Hall, 2020). The energy released from ATP fuels muscle contraction. As APs continue to arrive, the process is repeated many times, allowing sustained muscle contraction. Ca^{2+} ions are continuously released and taken up by troponin which requires energy from ATP. As muscles store very little ATP, more needs to be regenerated for the contraction to continue (Martini, Nath & Bartholomew, 2018). This occurs in three ways: by the interaction of adenosine diphosphate with creatine phosphate, by aerobic respiration or by lactic acid fermentation.

to the webbing beneath the cushion on some chairs (Fig. 25.6). Superficial muscles consist of the:

- Ischiocavernosus.
- Bulbospongiosus (*also known as bulbocavernosus*).
- Transverse perinei (*also known as puboperineal*).
- External anal sphincter.

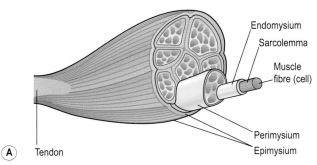

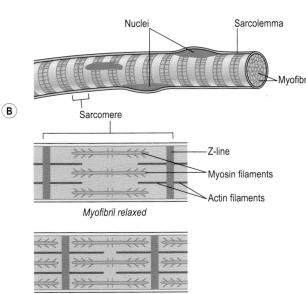

• **Fig. 25.1** Intracellular tubular systems.

- External urethral meatus, sometimes called the *membranous sphincter of the urethra.*

The origin and function of the superficial pelvic floor muscles are described in Table 25.1.

The superficial muscles do not form a continuous sheet and gaps are filled with other tissues. Anteriorly is the **triangular ligament** (or **urogenital diaphragm**) which is a strong, muscular membrane external and inferior to the pelvic diaphragm. It occupies the area between the symphysis pubis and ischial tuberosities, bounded by the ischiocavernosus and the transverse perinei. It consists of two layers of fascia. The triangular ligament stretches across the **pubic arch,** supporting the bladder neck. Posteriorly, the gap is filled with fat and is bounded by the gluteus maximus muscle, the sacrotuberous ligament and the transverse perinei. This area of space is known as the **ischiorectal fossa.**

Deep Pelvic Floor Muscles

The deep pelvic floor muscles are situated above the superficial muscles and are about 5 cm deep. Deep muscles called **levator ani** are the largest and most important muscles of the pelvic floor. The levator ani muscles raise or elevate the anus. They are collectively termed *coccygeus muscles* because they insert around the coccyx. Together with the fascia covering their surfaces, these muscles are referred to as the *pelvic diaphragm.* The arrangement of these muscles (pelvic diaphragm) gives the appearance of a funnel or sling suspended from its attachments on the pelvic wall (Fig. 25.7). These muscles are *vital* to the control of bladder and bowel function.

The levator ani is conventionally described in three pairs of deep muscles:

1. Pubococcygeus.
2. Iliococcygeus.
3. Ischiococcygeus.

The origin of the deep pelvic floor muscles is described in Table 25.2. Their function and clinical implications are presented in Box 25.3.

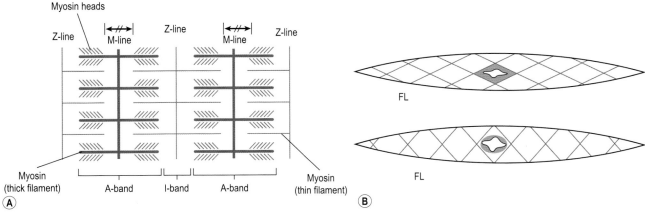

• **Fig. 25.2** Striated (A) and smooth (B) fibres. *A,* Actin; *FL,* filaments; *M,* myosin.

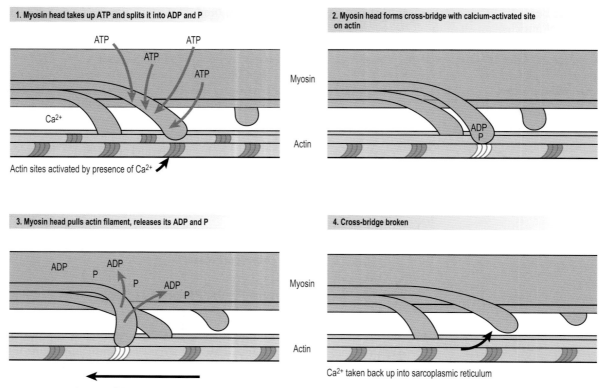

1. Myosin head takes up ATP and splits it into ADP and P

ATP ATP ATP ATP

Myosin

Ca²⁺

Actin

Actin sites activated by presence of Ca²⁺

2. Myosin head forms cross-bridge with calcium-activated site on actin

ADP P

3. Myosin head pulls actin filament, releases its ADP and P

ADP P ADP P ADP P

Myosin

Actin

4. Cross-bridge broken

Myosin

Actin

Ca²⁺ taken back up into sarcoplasmic reticulum

• **Fig. 25.3** Diagrammatic representation of the sliding-filament theory showing how the thick filaments of skeletal muscle move relative to one another as cross-bridges are formed and broken.

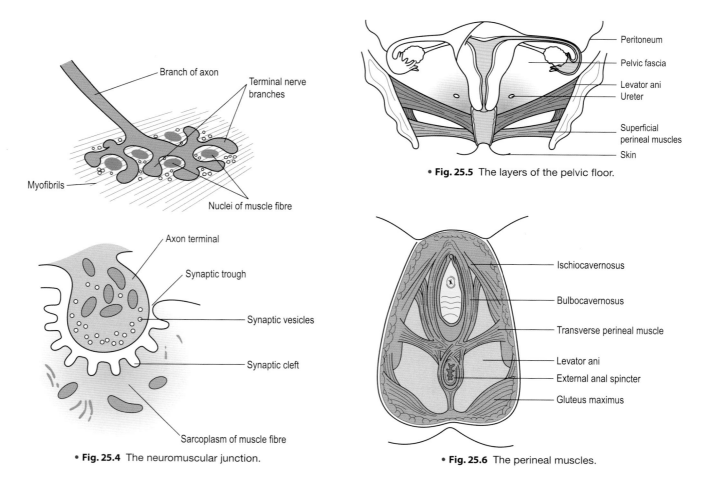

Branch of axon

Terminal nerve branches

Myofibrils

Nuclei of muscle fibre

• **Fig. 25.4** The neuromuscular junction.

Axon terminal

Synaptic trough

Synaptic vesicles

Synaptic cleft

Sarcoplasm of muscle fibre

Peritoneum

Pelvic fascia

Levator ani
Ureter

Superficial perineal muscles

Skin

• **Fig. 25.5** The layers of the pelvic floor.

Ischiocavernosus

Bulbocavernosus

Transverse perineal muscle

Levator ani

External anal spincter

Gluteus maximus

• **Fig. 25.6** The perineal muscles.

TABLE 25.1	Superficial Pelvic Floor Muscles	
Superficial Muscle	**Origin**	**Function**
Ischiocavernosus	This muscle runs from each ischial tuberosity along the pubic arch to the corpora cavernosa of the clitoris. The muscle is elongated, broader at the middle than the ends. Fibres also interweave with the membranous sphincter of the urethra.	In conjunction with the bulbospongiosus (or bulbocavernosus) muscle, it helps maintain clitoral erection.
Bulbospongiosus (also known as bulbocavernosus)	Fibres arise in the centre of the perineum, and fibres pass on either side of the vagina and urethra, encircling them both, to insert into the corpora cavernosa (body) of the clitoris just under the pubic arch.	Responsible for the erection of the clitoris and contraction of the vaginal walls.
Transverse perinei (also known as puboperineal)	One narrow slip of muscle arises from the inner surface of each **ischial tuberosity** of the pelvis and passes transversely to meet its fellow, inserting into the **perineal body**. Some fibres pass posteriorly to blend with the anal sphincter.	Fixates the perineal body (central tendon of perineum), supports the pelvic floor and expels the last drops of urine.
External anal sphincter (EAS)	This circle of muscle surrounds the anus formed by the merging of muscle fibres from deep and superficial layers. The sphincter muscle adheres posterolaterally to the perineal body and is attached behind the anus to the coccyx.	During childbirth: Injuries to the anal sphincter are collectively referred to as referred to as obstetric anal sphincter injuries (Hinshaw & Arulkumaran, 2018). See Chapter 39 for further classification.
External urinary meatus	The membranous sphincter of the urethra is composed of muscle fibres passing above and below the urethra and attached to the pubic bones.	This is a weak sphincter of the urethra although it is not a true sphincter (i.e., not circular in shape). It is not an important muscle and acts to close the urethra.

Blood Supply, Lymphatic Drainage and Nerve Supply

Arterial supply is by branches of the two internal iliac arteries, and drainage is by corresponding veins. Lymph drainage is widespread, both laterally and medially. The pelvic floor muscles are under voluntary control. The nerve supply is by branches of the pudendal nerve via the sacral plexus.

The Perineum

The perineum is the region below the pelvic diaphragm and corresponds to the outlet of the pelvis. The shape is described as either lozenge- or rhomboid-shaped. The perineum is bounded anteriorly by the pubic arch, laterally by the ischiopubic rami, ischial tuberosities and sacrotuberous ligaments and posteriorly by the apex of the coccyx. This central area is located by drawing an arbitrary line transversely between the ischial tuberosities. This divides the perineum into two triangular sections which do not lie on the same plane: the urogenital triangle and the anal triangle.

The Urogenital Triangle

The urogenital triangle lies anterior and contains the external urogenital organs. It is tilted down and back. This triangle also contains the superficial perineal fascia, the perineal anterior muscles and sphincters (Fig. 25.7A). It is bound anteriorly and laterally by the pubic symphysis and the ischiopubic rami. Innervation is derived from the branches of the pudendal nerve.

The Anal Triangle

The anal triangle lies posterior and contains the anal canal, anal sphincters, the ischioanal fossae and the rectovaginal septum. This triangle is tilted down and forward. The rectum terminates in the canal (Fig. 25.8). Anteriorly, the perineal body separates the anal canal from the vagina. Posteriorly, the anal canal is attached to the coccyx by the anococcygeal ligament. This is a midline fibromuscular between the coccyx and the external anal sphincter (posterior). Within the ischioanal fossae, loose adipose tissue surrounds the anus posteriorly and laterally. This is a potential pathway for the spread of puerperal sepsis from one side to the other. The pudendal nerves pass over the ischial spines at this point. These can be accessed for injection of local anaesthesia into the pudendal nerve at site. Anteriorly, the perineal body separates the anal canal from the vagina.

Anal Sphincter Complex

This complex contains the external anal sphincter and the internal anal sphincter. These are separated by the conjoint longitudinal coat (Fig. 25.8A).

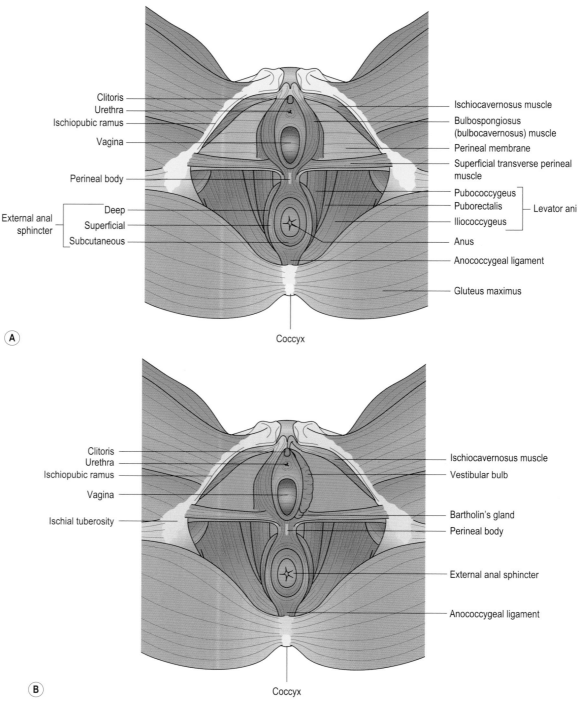

• **Fig. 25.7** Muscles of the pelvic diaphragm. (A) Diagram of the perineum demonstrating the superficial muscles of the perineum. The superficial transverse perineal muscle, the bulbospongiosus and the ischio-cavernosus form a triangle on either side of the perineum with a floor formed by the perineal membrane. (B) The left bulbospongiosus muscle has been removed to demonstrate the vestibular bulb and the Bartholin's gland.

• The external anal sphincter consists of striated muscle and appears red in colour. The external anal sphincter is normally under tonic contraction. Therefore, it tends to retract if this muscle is completely torn. Any defect can lead to urgency and/or faecal incontinence. The sphincter in females is shorter anteriorly. This becomes clinically relevant for assessment of anal sphincter injuries (Table 25.1).

• The internal anal sphincter is a thickened continuation of the circular smooth muscle of the bowel. It is pale and terminates with a well-defined rounded edge 6–8 mm above the anal margin. Any defect in this sphincter can lead to passive soiling of stools and flatus incontinence.

• The longitudinal layer is situated between the external and internal anal sphincters. It consists of a fibromuscular

TABLE 25.2	Deep Pelvic Floor Muscles	
Deep Muscle	**Origin**	**Function**
Pubococcygeus (most medial muscles)	Fibres arise from the inner border of the body of the pubis and the white line of the fascia (arcus tendineus fasciae). Fibres sweep posteriorly in three bands: 1. A central band of fibres surrounding the urethra. 2. Some fibres form a U-shaped loop around the vagina and insert into the lateral and posterior vaginal walls in the perineum. 3. Other fibres loop around the anus and insert into the lateral and posterior walls of the anal canal and the coccyx.	Supports and maintains the position of the pelvic viscera. Resists increased intra-abdominal pressure during forced expiration, vomiting, coughing, urination and defaecation; constricts the anus, urethra and vagina. During childbirth: • Supports the fetal head. • Muscles may be injured because of difficult childbirth or trauma (e.g., episiotomy).
Iliococcygeus	Fibres arise from the inner border of the white line of fascia on the iliac bone and from the ischial spines. Fibres run to the coccyx, some crossing over in the perineal body.	Supports and maintains the position of the pelvic viscera. Resists increased intra-abdominal pressure during forced expiration, vomiting, coughing, urination and defaecation. Pulls the coccyx anteriorly after defaecation or childbirth. During childbirth: • Muscles may be injured as a result of difficult childbirth or trauma (e.g., episiotomy).
Ischiococcygeus	Fibres arise from each ischial spine. Inserts into the upper edge of the coccyx and lower border of the sacrum.	Stabilizes the sacroiliac and sacrococcygeal joints of the pelvis. Flexes the coccygeal joints.

layer, the conjoint coat and the intersphincter space with its connective tissues (Fig. 25.8B).

- Innervation of the anal sphincter complex is derived from branches of the pudendal nerves.
- Anorectum blood supply is mainly provided from the superior and inferior haemorrhoidal arteries. The lower anal canal and the external anal sphincter drain via the inferior branch of the pudendal vein and the internal iliac vein. The anorectum has a rich network of lymphatic plexuses.

The ischial fossae (previously known as the ischiorectal fossa) extends around the anal canal. Anteriorly, it is bound by the perineal membrane and medially by the external anal sphincter complex (level of anal canal). Superiorly it is bound by the fascia of the levator ani muscle.

The Perineal Body

The perineal body is critical for maintaining the integrity of the pelvic floor, especially in females. It is the central point between the urogenital and the anal triangles of the perineum. The apex is uppermost and is the central point of the pelvic floor. The perineal body is a fibro-muscular structure of interlacing muscle fibres from the bulbospongiosus, superficial transverse perineal and external anal sphincter muscles.

Smooth Muscle

Smooth muscle has two characteristics: it lacks the cross-striated banding pattern found in skeletal and cardiac fibres, and the nerve supply is derived from the autonomic division

of the nervous system rather than the somatic division. Hence, the muscle is described as smooth, **non-striated** and **involuntary** and is often referred to as **visceral muscle** (Marieb & Hoen, 2022).

Smooth muscle has special features including:

- Less vigorous contractile response to being stretched so that distension of a hollow organ can occur without provoking expulsive contractions.
- Ability to change more in length and create more tension than skeletal muscle.
- Ability to divide—hyperplasia.
- Secretion of the connective tissue proteins collagen and elastin.

Box 25.4 presents an overview of the microscopic structure of smooth muscle and muscle contraction.

Uterine Muscle During Pregnancy

The **uterus** is unique among smooth muscular organs in that it undergoes profound, largely reversible changes during pregnancy. Like most other smooth muscle, the uterus is spontaneously contractile. When required, it can perform considerable muscular feats to expel its contents such as during menstruation and childbirth. At other times it is prevented from contracting and must remain quiescent to allow the development and growth of the fetus and placenta during pregnancy.

The uterus is expected to follow a predicted rate of growth during pregnancy. However this is only a reliable indicator of gestational age in the first 20 weeks of pregnancy.

• BOX 25.3 Pelvic Floor: Functions and Implications for Childbirth

Functions

Effective functioning is dependent on the integrity of the muscle fibres and the maintenance of muscle tone. The functions of the pelvic floor include:

- Supports and maintains the anatomical position of the internal female reproductive organs, bladder and intestine.
- Supports the weight of the abdominal and pelvic organs.
- Maintains optimal intra-abdominal pressure.
- Allows voluntary control of defaecation and micturition.
- Facilitates the movements of the fetus through the birth canal.
- Enables flexion of the sacrum and coccyx.

Implications for Childbirth

The sling-like arrangement of the gutter-shaped pelvic floor muscles and the resistance generated have an essential role as the fetus negotiates the pelvic cavity in labour. Childbirth is facilitated by the pelvic floor resisting descent of the fetal head and shoulders and forcing the fetus to rotate forward in the presence of strong regular uterine contractions.

Clinical Implications

Many women experience trauma to their pelvic floor during childbirth. Any trauma involving neurological damage can negatively impact the function of the internal bladder sphincter causing urgency of micturition. This urgency to void urine is increased by the degree of weakness in the sphincter and the amount of urine in the bladder. Pelvic floor muscle training during the antenatal and postnatal periods may prevent the problem of urinary incontinence. If persistent, the range of treatment options include a variety of surgical procedures, pharmacological treatment and modification to behaviour and lifestyle.

Loss of integrity and trauma to the pelvic floor is often associated with childbearing. Reproductive anomalies involving pelvic organ prolapse (POP) may occur with negative impact on the woman's quality of life. POP is defined as the downward displacement of pelvic organs from their original position into or beyond the vagina (Slack, 2018).

Uterovaginal Prolapse

Prolapse of the pelvic organs may cause women much anxiety, embarrassment and discomfort. There may be urinary and faecal incontinence (Khullar, 2018; Slack, 2018). Symptoms may also occur with ageing due to loss of muscle tone and withdrawal of oestrogen, prolonged immobility due to muscle atrophy and congenital weakness of the muscles. This includes uterine prolapse, which is downward displacement of the uterus to varying degrees. **Procidentia** is rare and is total prolapse of the uterus outside the body.

Vaginal Prolapse: Anterior Wall

A **cystocele** is a herniation of the bladder. This is often symptomless and may present with bladder irritation or a feeling of a lump in the vagina. If large, this may lead to a collection of residual urine, infection and pyelonephritis.

A **urethrocele** is a displacement of the urethra with loss of the acute angle between it and the bladder. This angle helps maintain continence so the result may be urinary stress incontinence (i.e., involuntary loss of small amounts of urine during coughing, sneezing or any other activity that increases intra-abdominal pressure) (Khullar, 2018).

Vaginal Prolapse: Posterior Wall

A **rectocele** is a prolapse of the posterior middle vaginal wall, allowing herniation of the rectum. This may be symptomless unless very large, when faeces become lodged in the herniated sac. Defaecation will be difficult unless digital pressure is applied on the vaginal side of the sac. An **enterocele** is a herniation higher in the vagina and on vaginal examination will not be palpable.

Dyspareunia (Painful Sexual Intercourse)

This may occur depending on the degree of prolapse (Wylie, 2018).

Treatment of Reproductive Anomalies

Treatment is usually by surgical repair. In a few women, such as those who refuse surgery or are too ill or frail, insertion of a ring pessary may be the treatment of choice.

Prevention of Prolapse

The midwife can take action to minimize the risk:

- Attempt to avoid pushing until full dilatation of the cervix.
- Prevent birth of the baby before full dilatation of the cervix.
- Ensure that the second stage is not prolonged without obvious progress.
- Avoid fundal pressure to deliver the placenta.
- Ensure careful repair of any perineal trauma.
- Ensure early ambulation of the woman.
- Encourage pelvic floor exercises in during pregnancy and in the puerperium.

Routine measurement of fundal height, using the umbilicus and xiphisternum as useful landmarks, is used to assess fetal growth. The main part of uterine growth during the second half of pregnancy is almost entirely due to hypertrophy (increase in size), where the growth of the fetus acts as a powerful stimulator for the growth of the contractile proteins of the myometrium. Table 25.3 presents the changes in the uterus during pregnancy.

Hormonal Influences on the Uterus in Pregnancy

Oestrogen and progesterone, initially from the corpus luteum and then the placenta, are the hormones mainly responsible for influencing the uterus. Oestrogen promotes the growth of muscle fibres, and progesterone maintains the quiescence of the myometrium. In particular, the interaction of these hormones has a growth-promoting effect and increases uterine muscle compliance.

Actions of Oestrogen and Progesterone on Target Cells

The hormones probably enter the target cell by passive diffusion across the cell membrane and then bind to specific receptor proteins present in the cellular cytoplasm. The complex formed between the steroid and the receptor is transferred to the nucleus where gene function is regulated. The hormone oestradiol stimulates RNA synthesis. The RNA is transferred to the cytoplasm where it is responsible for the synthesis of new proteins. The role of progesterone

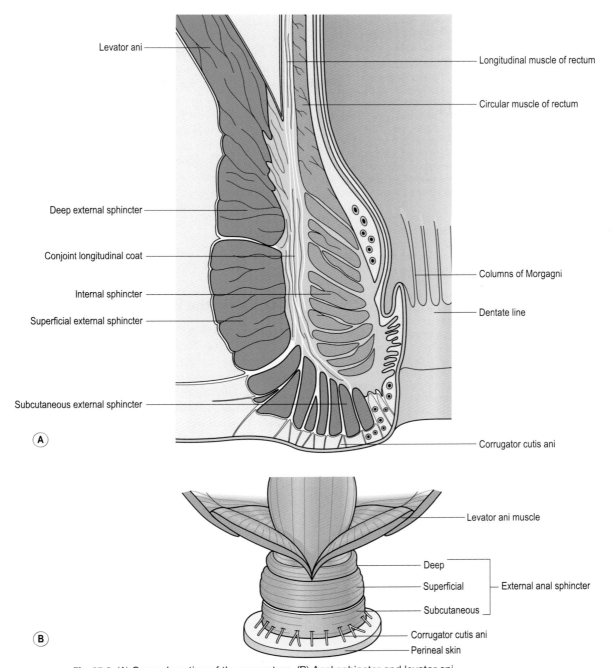

Levator ani

Longitudinal muscle of rectum

Circular muscle of rectum

Deep external sphincter

Conjoint longitudinal coat

Internal sphincter

Superficial external sphincter

Columns of Morgagni

Dentate line

Subcutaneous external sphincter

(A)

Corrugator cutis ani

Levator ani muscle

Deep
Superficial — External anal sphincter
Subcutaneous

Corrugator cutis ani
Perineal skin

(B)

• **Fig. 25.8** (A) Coronal section of the anorectum. (B) Anal sphincter and levator ani.

is less well understood. It may be responsible for increasing membrane resting potential in pregnancy so that muscle fibre contractions are less likely to occur.

The Uterus at Term

The uterus at term is generally described as having two main structural compartments: the **upper uterine segment** (UUS) and the **lower uterine segment** (LUS). The body and fundus of the uterus form the UUS with the isthmus and cervix forming the LUS. There is a gradual fall in the smooth muscle content from the fundus to the cervix. The muscle content of the cervix is estimated to be 10%, and the functional significance of this cervical muscle is not understood. The physiological mechanisms regulating these functions are becoming clearer. The pathophysiology remains uncertain, for example, in the **incompetent cervix.** Box 25.5 describes the layers of the uterus and Box 25.6 presents uterine blood flow and innervation.

Cervical Changes

In line with the gradual build-up of uterine activity in pregnancy, changes take place in the cervix. Its function changes

Smooth muscle fibres are small, spindle-shaped cells with a central nucleus. They have no striations, have a large surface area to allow Ca^{2+} ions to enter the cells easily and notably fewer myosin fibres than actin fibres. The myosin heads are arranged along the myosin fibre length so that each myosin fibre is attached to many actin fibres. The fibres are arranged in a spiral around the muscle cell and can change their lengths much more than skeletal muscle fibres. The fibres are arranged in two (or more) sheets, usually at right angles to each other. For instance, the body of the uterus has three layers: an outer, mainly longitudinal layer; an oblique middle layer; and an inner (mainly circular) layer.

Smooth muscle, like skeletal muscle, uses cross-bridge movements between actin and myosin filaments to generate force and Ca^{2+} ions to control cross-bridge activity. However, differences between the two types of muscles are noted in the organization of the contractile filaments and in the excitation–contraction coupling process.

Contraction in smooth muscle is slow, sustained and resistant to fatigue. There are no clear neuromuscular junctions. The innervating fibres have bulbous varicosities and release their neurotransmitter substance directly onto many fibres. This allows a slow, **synchronized contraction** of the whole muscle sheet. Action potentials are transmitted from cell to cell until the whole muscle sheet is contracting. Some fibres act as **pacemaker cells** to set the contractile pace for the whole muscle sheet. Both the rate and intensity of smooth muscle contraction can be modified by neural and chemical stimuli.

Ca^{2+} triggers the onset of contractions, and ATP provides the energy. Smooth muscle fibres take 30 times longer to contract and relax than skeletal muscle fibres. The same muscle tension can be maintained for long periods at less than 1% of the energy cost of skeletal muscle.

from a firm structure to an elastic tissue which can stretch to a diameter of 10 cm or more during labour and then almost return to its original state. During pregnancy the cervix increases in mass, water content and vascularity (Blackburn, 2018). It remains 2.5 cm long throughout pregnancy until effacement begins. Cervical softening occurs early in pregnancy. **Effacement,** or shortening of the cervix, and its gradual inclusion in the LUS occur in the last few weeks of pregnancy. Tension exerted by the outer longitudinal muscle fibres of the fundus may contribute to the process of effacement.

Dramatic changes need to occur in the cervix at the time of delivery to allow uterine contractions to influence dilatation of the cervix. The changes involve the degradation of the collagen content by enzymes such as **collagenase** and **elastase.** Changes also occur in the proteoglycans ground substance matrix which attracts water, and smooth muscle fibres which become more stretchable (Blackburn, 2018). Oestrogen causes increased vascularity, and the cervix appears purple when viewed through a speculum.

Myometrial contractions have little effect on the ripening of the cervix, which usually occurs before the onset of labour. Hormonal control of cervical ripening may involve multiple changes in oestrogen, progesterone, relaxin and

prostaglandins and seems to correlate well with a gradual rise in circulating oestrogens. PGE_2 and $PGF_{2\alpha}$ have a localized action on cervical softening that is independent of uterine activity. PGE_2 is used to improve the cervical state before induction of labour (Blackburn, 2018). However there is much variation in individual women in the changes in the cervix outlined earlier. Labour may begin in some women when the cervix is long, firm, uneffaced and undilatated. In others, the cervix may be soft, effaced and partly dilatated for some weeks before the onset of labour.

The cervix also acts as an efficient barrier to infection. Under the influence of progesterone, the mucus secreted by the endocervical cells becomes thicker and more viscous. It forms a cervical plug called the **operculum** which prevents ascending infection.

Muscle fibres in the cervix are mainly circular, with only a few longitudinal fibres.

Changes in the Vagina in Pregnancy

Oestrogen produces changes in both the muscle layer and the epithelium. There is hypertrophy of the muscle layer, and changes in the surrounding connective tissue allow the vagina to become more elastic. This elasticity allows the vagina to distend during the second stage of labour. There is marked desquamation of the superficial cells of the epithelium. This gives rise to an increased amount of normal vaginal discharge, called **leucorrhoea** (named because of the white colour).

The epithelial cells also have an increased glycogen content, and interaction with Döderlein's bacillus produces a more acidic environment, protecting against many micro-organisms. Unfortunately, this means an increased susceptibility to the organism *Candida albicans,* which causes moniliasis, or thrush (see Chapter 6). There is increased vascularity, with the vagina appearing to be reddish-purple in colour. This change in pregnancy is referred to as **Jacquemier's sign.** The increased vascularity of the pelvic organs gives rise to another sign of pregnancy called **Osiander's sign.** This sign refers to the increased pulsation in the lateral vaginal fornices.

Uterine Activity in Pregnancy

In smooth muscle, myosin-containing thick filaments interact with the actin-containing thin filaments and the energy source is ATP. There are no clear neuromuscular junctions. The innervating neurons release their neurotransmitter substance directly onto many fibres, resulting in a slow, synchronized contraction of the whole muscle sheet. As pregnancy progresses, the timing and speed of the myometrial action potentials change and the muscle cells increase their content of contractile proteins, gap junctions, sarcoplasmic reticulum and mitochondria. The uterus at term appears to have enhanced communication between cells, and action potentials can spread across the entire uterus in only 2–3 s.

<table>
TABLE 25.3
</table>

TABLE 25.3 Changes in the Uterus During Pregnancy

Non-pregnant Uterus	Pregnant	Comment
Shape: Pear-shaped	Globular until 20 weeks, pear-shaped or cylindrical until term	The upper part enlarges after implantation due to oestrogen
Position: Pelvic organ anteverted and anteflexed	12 weeks—no longer a pelvic organ Upright and often inclines to and rotates to the right	Abdominal organ after 12 weeks Typically inclines and rotates to the right due to the colon on the left side of the pelvic cavity; known as the *right obliquity of the uterus.* This increases with pregnancy
Uterine wall 10 mm	Thickened to 25 mm by 3–4 months By term has thinned to 5 and 10 mm	
Lower uterus 7 mm	The lower part of the uterus consisting of the isthmus; softens and elongates to 25 mm by about 10 weeks	This is the beginning of the differentiation of the lower uterine segment (LUS) Hegar sign: softening/compressibility of lower uterine segment, occurs at 6 weeks' gestation
Size: 7.5 cm in length, 5 cm in width and 2.5 cm deep	Term • 20 cm long, 25 cm wide and 22.5 cm deep	
Weight: 40–70 g	1100–1200 g by term	Up to a 20-fold increase
Muscle fibres	Early pregnancy • Growth of fibres • More compliant Term • Muscle fibres increase three-fold in diameter and 10-fold in length	Due to hyperplasia Under influence of oestrogen and independent of fetal growth If the fetus embeds outside of the uterus (ectopic gestation), this early growth would still occur

Level of the Uterus on Fundal Palpation:

12 weeks: just above the symphysis pubis
20 weeks: approaching level or just below the level of the umbilicus
24 weeks: at level of the umbilicus (if not just above level)

30 weeks: at midway between the umbilicus and xiphisternum
36 weeks: xiphisternum (maximum height)
The LUS is identified but is not complete

>36 weeks: fundal height may now reduce as presenting part of the fetus enters the pelvis
Due to softening of pelvic floor tissues + good uterine tone and further formation of the LUS; 'lightening' to laypeople

The Role of Pacemakers in Uterine Activity

Some fibres may act as pacemaker cells to set the contractile pace for the whole sheet. Cells near the cornua may likely initiate contractions. However specific pacemaker cells have not been identified and all myometrial cells have this property, not only those within the fundus. Neural and chemical stimuli can modify both the rate and intensity of smooth muscle contraction. Contraction in smooth muscle is slow, sustained and resistant to fatigue. The action potential is conducted from the cell membrane down the sarcoplasmic reticulum so that there is a rapid release of calcium (Ca^{2+}) deep in the cell.

In pregnancy, uterine activity gradually evolves, with activity seen as early as 7 weeks with high frequency (about two contractions per minute) but very low intensity (about 1–1.5 kPa) (Blackburn, 2018). This pattern continues until about 20 weeks when uterine contractions increase in both frequency and amplitude until term. These tend to occur more rapidly in the last 6–8 weeks of pregnancy. This is facilitated by the development of gap junctions within the myometrium where the plasma membranes of adjacent cells are closely applied, which act as areas of low resistance so that conduction of electrical impulses can spread rapidly from one cell to another. They are important in the spread of action potentials and the development of the coordinated uterine activity that is seen in efficient labour.

Gap Junctions

The appearance of gap junctions seems to depend on changes in the levels of oestrogen, progesterone and prostaglandins occurring in late pregnancy. Their appearance may be necessary to allow the development of effective uterine contractions in labour. Low-frequency but

• BOX 25.5 Layers of the Uterus

The Decidua

The **endometrium** thickens during pregnancy, becoming richer and more vascular in the upper part of the body of the uterus and the fundus, the normal site for implantation. During pregnancy, it is termed the **decidua** (sheds at the end of pregnancy). The decidua is thinner and less vascular in the lower pole of the uterus. The decidua provides the blastocyst with a glycogen-rich environment until the placenta can fulfil its functions. As the zygote embeds, the following changes occur in the endometrium (decidua) due to increased progesterone production by the corpus luteum:

- This layer hypertrophies to become 6–8 mm thick.
- Stroma become more vascular and oedematous and the functional layer becomes organized into two distinct areas:
  - Stroma cells enlarge and become closely packed together to form the compact layer. Known as **decidual cells,** they become polygonal in shape because of the pressure they exert on each other.
  - Tubular glands become dilatated and more tortuous in their deeper parts, with the lumen becoming packed with secretion. This dilatation below the compact layer is known as the *spongy* or *cavernous layer* due to its appearance.
- The basal layer remains unchanged.

The Myometrium

The myometrium forms the predominant part of the uterine wall, and the detailed arrangement of muscular tissue is highly effective. The two basic properties of this layer are contractility (ability to lengthen and shorten) and elasticity (ability to grow and stretch). Elasticity is essential for the uterus to accommodate the enlarging uterine contents, maintain uterine tonus and permit involution after birth (Blackburn, 2018). The muscle fibres become more differentiated and organized to fulfil their roles in labour and evacuation of the uterine contents (Figs 25.9 and 25.10). The myometrium is composed of at least three interdigitating muscle layers: an outer, a middle and an inner layer, with each layer performing a different function. These three layers become clearly defined as the uterine muscle undergoes initial hyperplasia (development of new fibres) and subsequent hypertrophy (increase in length and thickness of existing muscle fibres).

- Middle layer – involved with the expulsion of the fetus and the control of bleeding after delivery of the placenta. This layer forms the bulk of the organ and is composed of obliquely interdigitating strands of muscle fibres forming a network around blood vessels. The muscle fibres are often described as being mesh-like, crisscrossed or figure of eight-shaped (Fig. 25.10).
- Outer layer – contracts and retracts during labour. The outer is composed mainly of longitudinal fibres with some circular fibres.
- Inner layer – involved in distension of the LUS and dilatation of the cervix during labour. The inner layer contains mainly circular fibres, which are more evident around the cornua and LUS and cervix.

The outer and inner layers contain both longitudinal and circular fibres with structural studies indicating these layers may be continuous.

Muscle cells are grouped into bundles with thin sheets of connective tissue, including collagen, elastic fibres, fibroblasts and mast cells. The collagenous connective tissue serves two functions: supporting the muscle fibres and transmitting the tension developed by smooth muscle contraction.

The Perimetrium

This outer layer of the peritoneum is loosely applied and does cover the uterus. It drapes over the bladder anteriorly to form a fold called the *uterovesical pouch* and posteriorly it drapes over the rectum to form the pouch of Douglas. This layer forms the broad ligament, thus maintaining the anatomical position of the uterus and allowing unrestricted uterine growth during pregnancy (Blackburn, 2018; Coad, Pedley & Dunstall, 2019; Garfield & Yallampalli, 2008; Romanini, 2008).

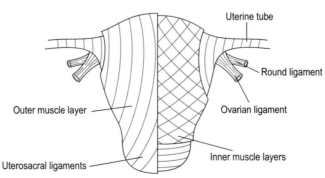

• **Fig. 25.9** The outer and inner layers of uterine muscle.

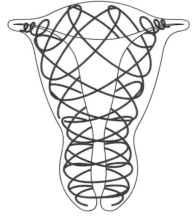

• **Fig. 25.10** The spiral arrangement of the uterine muscle fibres.

high-pressure **Braxton Hicks contractions** are perceived by the mother. These may be as strong as labour contractions but are not painful and the cervix does not dilatate. Box 25.7 outlines uterine sensitivity to oxytocin and prostaglandins.

• BOX 25.6 Uterus During Pregnancy: Blood Flow and Innervation

The uterine blood supply is derived mainly from the uterine artery, a branch of the anterior division of the internal iliac artery (Farthing, 2020). **Increased uterine blood flow** occurs due to increased vessel diameter and lowered resistance.

Prostacyclin (PGI_2) is produced by pregnant and non-pregnant myometrium and placental blood vessels. PGI_2 acts as a potent vasodilator to inhibit platelet aggregation and protect the vascular epithelium. During labour, PGI_2 has a key role in maintaining blood flow to the placenta and the uterus. Unlike other prostaglandins, PGI_2 has little effect on uterine contractibility.

Innervation

The uterus is innervated by both the sympathetic and parasympathetic fibres of the autonomic nervous system. The uterus is poorly innervated with a low density of nerves to smooth muscle compared with other smooth muscle cells. Labour will occur even if complete spinal transection is present. Innervation physiology is unknown, and the central nervous system connections are probably not essential to the onset and progress of labour.

Sympathetic Fibres

Preganglionic fibres leave the spinal cord and enter a chain of ganglia running alongside the spinal column from the T1–L5 vertebrae. In the ganglia, they synapse with postganglionic fibres that synapse with the target organ. The uterus is unusual, as the preganglionic fibres leaving T10–T12 run directly to the uterus to synapse with the postganglionic fibres. Preganglionic fibres release acetylcholine into the synapse from their endings, and postganglionic fibres release noradrenaline (norepinephrine) onto the target organ from their terminals.

There are two types of adrenergic receptors in target organs: α receptors (normally excitatory) and β fibres (normally inhibitory). There are two types of β receptors: $β_1$ and $β_2$. $β_1$ receptors are cardio specific and are excitatory, whereas $β_2$ receptors are present in the uterus and are inhibitory. Drugs inhibit uterine contractions in preterm labour (National Institute of Health and Care Excellence (NICE), 2022). However, usage will excite cardiac muscle, causing a rise in pulse rate, leading to increased cardiac output and blood pressure. Beta-blocking agents will enhance uterine activity (Bigelow et al., 2021).

Parasympathetic Fibres

Parasympathetic innervation to the pelvis is through the sacral outflow from S2–S4. The preganglionic fibres end in or near the target organs and synapse with short postganglionic fibres. The neurotransmitter in both preganglionic and postganglionic fibres is acetylcholine. Fibres innervate the uterus synapse in two nerve plexi on either side of the pouch of Douglas. These are the **paracervical plexi** (Lee–Frankenhäuser's plexi).

• BOX 25.7 Sensitivity to Oxytocin and Prostaglandins

Oxytocin and prostaglandins are used to induce labour. Sensitivity to oxytocin is dependent on both gestational age and the level of spontaneous uterine activity.
- Up to 30 weeks' gestation: the uterus is very insensitive to oxytocin, and it is necessary to give very high infusion rates of oxytocin to stimulate uterine activity.
- After 30 weeks' gestation: the uterus will respond to much smaller concentrations of oxytocin.

- By 40 weeks as little as 4 mU/min will cause uterine activity, similar to that seen in spontaneous labour.
  In contrast to this variable response, prostaglandins E_2 and $F_{2α}$ will induce uterine contractions at any gestational age. Therefore, prostaglandins are probably the final mediator of uterine contractions.
  (NICE, 2021)

Main Points

- The three basic muscle types are skeletal, smooth and cardiac muscle.
- Functions of muscle are the production of movement, maintenance of posture, stabilization of joints and the generation of heat.
- Properties of muscle are excitability, contractility, extensibility and elasticity.
- Skeletal muscles are attached to and cover bones. Fibres have obvious bands or striations and muscles rapidly and tire easily.
- All muscle cells contain two kinds of protein filaments: actin and myosin.
- Muscles contract via the sliding-filament theory in response to nerve stimulation, resulting in an action potential being sent along the sarcolemma.
- The pelvic floor is formed by the soft tissues (six layers) which fill the outlet of the pelvis. The most important tissue is the strong, funnel-shaped diaphragm of skeletal muscle attached to the pelvic walls. Through it passes the urethra, vagina and anal canals.
- The pelvic floor supports the abdominal and pelvic organs, maintains intra-abdominal pressure, enables defaecation and micturition, facilitates the fetus through the birth canal and enables flexion of the sacrum and coccyx.
- The perineal body is a wedge-shaped mass of muscular and fibrous tissue situated between the vaginal and anal canals.
- The superficial muscles lie external to the deep muscles and provide additional strength.
- The major muscles of the pelvic floor are the deep muscles called the *levator ani*. These muscles are vital for bladder and bowel function.
- Prolapse of the pelvic organs with the possibility of urinary and faecal incontinence may cause physical and emotional discomfort for women.

- Smooth muscle is non-striated, is involuntary and is referred to as *visceral muscle*. Contractions are slow and sustained. Innervating fibres release their neurotransmitter substance directly onto many fibres, allowing slow, synchronized contraction of the whole muscle sheet.
- Smooth muscle fibres in the uterus undergo hyperplasia in early pregnancy, but the main part of uterine growth is due to hypertrophy.
- Uterine growth is a reliable indicator of fetal gestation in the first 20 weeks.
- The uterus at term has two main structural compartments: the UUS formed of the body and fundus and the LUS formed of the isthmus and cervix.
- The smooth muscle fibres of the myometrium are arranged in two (or more) sheets, usually at right angles to each other. The three muscle layers are: an outer layer with mainly longitudinal fibres, a middle oblique layer and an inner layer with mainly circular fibres.
- Under the influence of oestrogen, the muscle layer in the vagina hypertrophies and the surrounding connective tissue becomes more elastic, allowing distension during the second stage of labour. Increased desquamation of superficial epithelial cells leads to leucorrhoea.
- Contraction of uterine smooth muscle involves the whole muscle sheet to contract slowly and synchronously. Some fibres may act as pacemaker cells.
- Sensitivity to oxytocin and prostaglandins depends on gestational age and the level of spontaneous uterine activity. Prostaglandins are probably the final mediator of uterine contractions.

References

Bigelow, C.A., Pan, S., Overbey, J.R., Stone, J., 2021. Propranolol for Induction of Labor in Nulliparas trial a double-blind, randomized, placebo-controlled trial. Am. J. Obstet. Gynecol. MFM 3 (2), 100301.

Blackburn, S.T., 2018. Maternal, Fetal and Neonatal Physiology: A Clinical Perspective, fifth ed. Elsevier, Philadelphia.

Coad, J., Pedley, K., Dunstall, M., 2019. Anatomy and Physiology for Midwives, fourth ed. Elsevier, London.

Farthing, A., 2018. Clinical anatomy of the pelvis and reproductive tract. In: Edmonds, D.K., Lees, C., Bourne, T.H. (Eds.), Dewhurst's Textbook of Obstetrics and Gynaecology, ninth ed. Wiley-Blackwell, Oxford.

Garfield, R.E., Yallampalli, C., 2008. Structure and function of uterine muscle. In: Chard, T., Grudzinskas, J.G. (Eds.), The Uterus, third ed. Cambridge University Press, Cambridge.

Hall, J.E., Hall, M.E., 2020. Excitation of skeletal muscle: neuromuscular transmission and excitation–contraction coupling. In: Guyton and Hall Textbook of Medical Physiology, fourteenth ed. Saunders, London.

Hinshaw, K., Arulkumaran, S., 2018. Malpresentation, malposition, cephalopelvic disproportion and obstetric procedures. In: Edmonds, D.K., Lees, C., Bourne, T.H. (Eds.), Dewhurst's Textbook of Obstetrics and Gynaecology, ninth ed. Wiley-Blackwell, Oxford.

Khullar, V., 2018. Urinary incontinence. In: Edmonds, D.K., Lees, C., Bourne, T.H. (Eds.), Dewhurst's Textbook of Obstetrics and Gynaecology, ninth ed. Wiley-Blackwell, Oxford.

Marieb, E.N., Hoehn, K., 2022. Human Anatomy and Physiology, twelfth ed. Pearson, Harlow.

Martini, F.H., Nath, J.L., Bartholomew, E., 2018. Fundamentals of Anatomy and Physiology, eleventh ed. Pearson, New York.

National Institute of Health and Care Excellence (NICE), 2021. Inducing Labour. Available at: www.nice.org.uk/guidance/ng207.

National Institute of Health and Care Excellence (NICE), 2022. Preterm Labour and Birth. Available at: www.nice.org.uk/guidance/ng25.

Radzimińska, A., Strączyńska, A., Weber-Rajek, M., Styczyńska, H., Strojek, K., Piekorz, Z., 2018. The impact of pelvic floor muscle training on the quality of life of women with urinary incontinence: a systematic literature review. Clin. Interv. Aging 13, 957–965.

Romanini, C., 2008. Measurement of uterine contractions. In: Chard, T., Grudzinskas, J.G. (Eds.), The Uterus, third ed. Cambridge University Press, Cambridge.

Slack, M., 2018. Uterovaginal prolapse. In: Edmonds, D.K., Lees, C., Bourne, T.H. (Eds.), Dewhurst's Textbook of Obstetrics and Gynaecology, ninth ed. Wiley-Blackwell, Oxford.

Wylie, K.R., 2018. Sexual dysfunction. In: Edmonds, D.K., Lees, C., Bourne, T.H. (Eds.), Dewhurst's Textbook of Obstetrics and Gynaecology, ninth ed. Wiley-Blackwell, Oxford.

Annotated recommended reading

Blackburn, S.T., 2018. Maternal, Fetal and Neonatal Physiology: A Clinical Perspective, fifth ed. Elsevier, Philadelphia.

This detailed evidence-based textbook is ideal for the reader interested in further understanding the changes occurring in the reproductive system during pregnancy and childbirth.

Edmonds DK Lees, C., Bourne, T., 2018. Dewhurst's Textbook of Obstetrics and Gynaecology, ninth ed. Wiley-Blackwell, Oxford.

This edited book provides specific chapters on sexual dysfunction, genital tract complications and urinary incontinence.

26

The Central Nervous System

LYNSAY MATTHEWS

The nervous system controls the function of every body system, thought, action and emotion. It is only possible to give a brief outline of this complex system. This chapter concentrates on the central nervous system.

Introduction

The human nervous system is the most complex and intricate of the evolved world. It works closely with the endocrine system to maintain homeostasis of all the body's processes (i.e., the ability of a system to maintain itself close to a fixed point). The ability to respond to environmental changes depends on rapid communication between the two systems. The nervous system transmits electrical signals and the endocrine system secretes hormones.

Organization of the Nervous System

The **central nervous system** (CNS) consists of the **brain** and **spinal cord.** It has an integration function, receiving messages from and sending messages to all parts of the body via the **peripheral nervous system** (PNS). The PNS is divided into (i) the **somatic nervous system** (SNS), which enables the voluntary control of muscle action and conveys special sensory input; and (ii) the **autonomic nervous system** (ANS), which enables the involuntary control of smooth muscle, cardiac muscle and glands of the viscera, and conveys sensory input from visceral organs. The ANS can be further subdivided into the **sympathetic nervous system** (which typically 'speeds up' processes)**, parasympathetic nervous system** (which typically 'slows down' processes) and **enteric nervous system**, which, controls only the gastrointestinal tract (Fig. 26.1).

Neuroanatomy

Nervous tissue is made up of two cell types: **neurons** (responsible for multiple functions) (Fig. 26.2) and a group of cell types collectively known as **neuroglia** (responsible for protection, nourishment and support of the neurons).

Neurons

The structural units of the nervous system are **neurons.** They are responsible for the many functions of the nervous system, including muscle action, hormone secretions, memory, sensing and thinking. These specialized cells have the following characteristics (Marieb & Hoehn, 2022).

- They have processes (extensions) called *axons* and *dendrites* that communicate with other cells.
- They conduct messages by nerve impulses from one body part to another.
- They are extremely long-lived but cannot undergo mitosis and divide.
- They have a very high metabolic rate, needing continuous glucose and oxygen.
- They cannot survive more than a few minutes without oxygen.

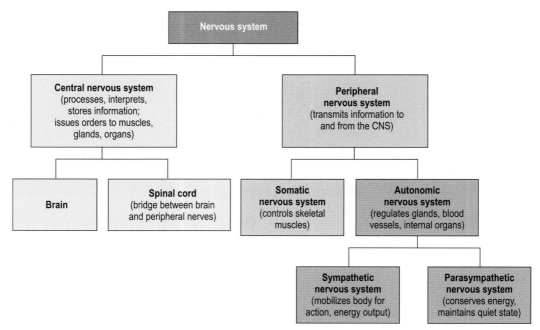

• **Fig. 26.1** Structure of the nervous system.

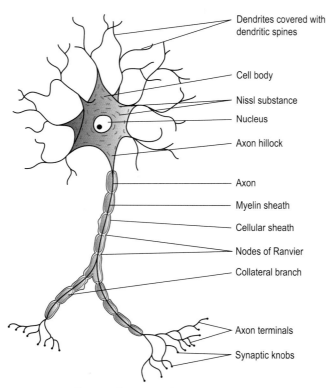

• **Fig. 26.2** Structure of a whole nerve fibre.

Structure of Neurons

The Cell Body

Each neuron has a cell body (**soma**) with a large spherical nucleus. **Neurotransmitters** (NTs) are synthesized in the soma. Most neuronal cell bodies are in the CNS, where they are clustered together in groups called **nuclei.** The few neuronal cell bodies in the PNS (Chapter 27) are called **ganglia.**

Dendrites

Dendrites are short, diffusely branching extensions which receive messages from other cells at **synapses** by conducting electrical signals called **graded potentials** towards and into the cell body. Dendrites are the input part of the neuron, and there may be hundreds clustering close to the cell body. They provide an enormous surface area for reception of signals from other cells.

Axons

The axon is another process (i.e., extension) of the neuron. It conducts messages to other cells (e.g., another neuron, muscle fibre, etc.) by electrical nerve impulses and NTs. Each neuron has only one axon arising from the **axon hillock** on the cell body. The axon is the same diameter along its length, and some are over 1 m long (such as those travelling from the spine to the foot). Axons may give off branches called **axon collaterals** and usually have terminal branches ending in **synaptic knobs** or **boutons.** Axons contain **microtubules** and **microfilaments** that transport substances to the cell body (**anterograde**) and from the cell body (**retrograde**).

Myelin Sheaths

Larger nerve fibres are covered in a white, fatty segmented coat called the **myelin sheath.** This protects and insulates fibres, increasing the rate of impulse transmission. Messages can be

TABLE 26.1	Classification of Neurons	
Structural Classification		
Multipolar neurons	The most common type. They have at least three processes, usually multiple dendrites and one axon.	
Bipolar neurons	These are rare and are found in special sense organs such as the retina or in the olfactory mucosa. They have two processes—an axon and one dendrite.	
Unipolar neurons	Found in the ganglia of the peripheral nervous system where they act as sensory neurons. They have a single, very short process (formed by fusion of the dendrites and axon).	
Functional Classification		
Motor neurons	Carry impulses away from the central nervous system (CNS; aka efferent) to control effector organs such as the muscles or glands.	
Sensory neurons	Carry impulses to the CNS (aka afferent) and often have very long dendritic branches that gather impulses from the periphery such as the ends of the toes and fingers.	
Association neurons	Often called *interneurons*. They carry signals between motor and sensory neurons in complex networks.	

transmitted up to 100 times more rapidly than in unmyelinated fibres. Myelin sheaths in the PNS are formed by **Schwann cells** which wrap themselves around the axon. Schwann cell protoplasm is squeezed out of the cell to leave the axon wrapped in a multi-layered membrane. The external portion is called the **neurolemma** or Schwann sheath. Adjacent Schwann cells along the axon do not touch, and the gaps between them, which occur at regular intervals, are called the **nodes of Ranvier.** Axon collaterals can only emerge at these nodes.

The myelin sheaths of the CNS are produced by cells called **oligodendrocytes.** Myelinated fibres form the white matter in the brain and spinal cord, and the cell bodies form the grey matter. Cell bodies are outside the white matter in the brain and inside the white matter in the spinal cord.

Classification of Neurons

Neurons may be classified structurally (**multipolar, bipolar** or **unipolar**) or functionally (**motor, sensory** or **association neurons**) (Table 26.1).

Neuroglia

Neuroglial cells support, nourish and protect neurons, outnumbering them in a ratio of 5:1. Because there are billions of neurons in the brain, the number of neuroglial cells is enormous. These cells are subdivided into four basic types (Mtui, Gruener & Dockery 2020):

1. **Astrocytes** are star-shaped cells with long, fine processes arising from their bodies. They have one process against a neuron, and their other processes lie close to capillary walls.
2. **Oligodendrocytes** in the CNS and Schwann cells in the PNS are smaller than astrocytes and have fewer processes. They form myelin sheaths around nerve fibres.
3. **Ependyma** form a continuous layer of cells lining the ventricles of the brain and spinal cord central canal. They help to produce cerebrospinal fluid (CSF).
4. **Microglia** are small cells which are part of the immune system, acting as macrophages.

The Structure of a Nerve

The axons from single neurons are bound together to form **nerves.** Nerves may contain **afferent fibres** (to the CNS), **efferent fibres** (from the CNS) or both when they are called **mixed nerves.** Each separate nerve fibre is embedded in a fibrous connective tissue sheath called the **endoneurium.** These are bound into groups by a connective tissue sheath called the **perineurium.** The complete nerve is surrounded by the **epineurium.** Each nerve has an arterial blood supply and venous drainage.

Neurophysiology

The Nerve Impulse

Both nerve fibres and muscle fibres are excitable tissues which conduct electrical signals. When a neuron is stimulated, an electrical impulse is sent along the axon (Fig. 26.3). Bodies are electrically neutral (i.e., their positive and negative charges are equal). Potential electrical energy is called **voltage,** which is measured in volts (V) or millivolts (mV). The flow of electricity from one point to another is called a **current.** Substances that hinder the flow are said to provide **resistance.** Ions, which are electrically charged particles, provide the currents and usually flow through an aqueous solution across a plasma membrane. Plasma membranes are studded with proteinaceous ion channels.

Polarization

When a membrane is resting, its potential is **polarized** (i.e., the inside has a different electrical potential from the interstitial fluid). The resting potential of neurons averages –70 mV. This is maintained by the distribution of negative and positive ions. Inside the cell, the positive ion is potassium and the negative ion is protein. In the interstitial fluid, the positive ion is sodium and the negative ion is chloride.

The Role of Sodium Ions

When the cell is stimulated, sodium channels open in the membrane and sodium ions rush into the cell, changing the membrane potential to +40 mV. This is called **depolarization.** The **action potential** is the sum of all negative and

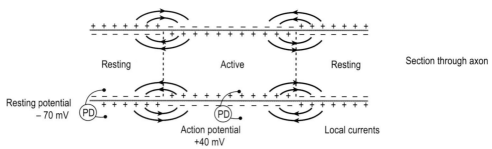

Section through axon

Resting   Active   Resting

Resting potential
– 70 mV

Action potential
+40 mV

Local currents

Local currents conduct the impulse to adjacent resting segments of the axon

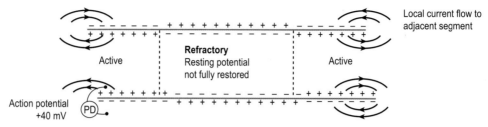

Local current flow to
adjacent segment

Refractory
Resting potential
not fully restored

Active   Active

Action potential
+40 mV

Action potentials now arise in adjacent segments of the axon without loss of amplitude

• **Fig. 26.3** Propagation of an action potential along a nerve fibre. *PD*, Potential difference.

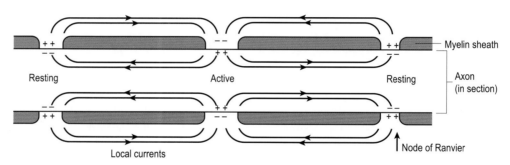

Myelin sheath

Axon
(in section)

Resting   Active   Resting

Node of Ranvier

Local currents

• **Fig. 26.4** Saltatory conduction in a myelinated nerve fibre. Local currents conduct the impulse from node to node. The action potential is regenerated at each node of Ranvier.

positive charges stimulating the cell and proceeds down the axon in a wave. Behind the wave, the cell pumps three sodium ions out in exchange for two potassium ions. The membrane potential falls to –90 mV (hyperpolarization) and then recovers.

The period of hyperpolarization is called the **refractory period** during which the cell cannot generate an action potential. Depolarization increases the chance of a nerve impulse being generated, but hyperpolarization decreases it. Firing of a neuron is an 'all-or-nothing' phenomenon, occurring only if the potential reaches a threshold. The size of an action potential is the same; strong stimuli result in more impulses, not stronger impulses.

Saltatory Conduction of the Impulse

Nerve fibres can be classified according to the speed of conduction of the action potential. The larger the nerve, the more rapidly it conducts impulses. Myelinated nerves conduct impulses more rapidly than unmyelinated nerves. The

myelin sheath is leaky at the **nodes of Ranvier**. The electrical current flows smoothly along each section of the sheath between nodes of Ranvier; however the impulse seems to jump from node to node by generating an action potential. This is called **saltatory conduction** (Fig. 26.4). In a non-myelinated nerve, new action potentials must generate across each adjacent section of the nerve membrane.

Classification of Nerves by Speed of Conduction

Nerve fibres can be classified as follows:
- Group A fibres are myelinated and can conduct impulses at up to 120 m/s. They are further subdivided into α, β, γ and δ (alpha, beta, gamma and delta) fibres.
- Group B fibres are myelinated. They are all preganglionic fibres of the ANS.
- Group C fibres are non-myelinated and conduct impulses as slowly as 1 m/s.

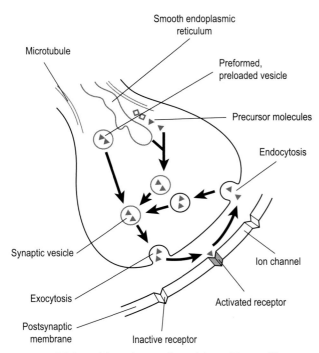

• **Fig. 26.5** Origin and fate of synaptic vesicle and transmitter-receptor binding.

The Synapse

Synapses are junctions between neurons and another cell (e.g., another neuron, a gland or a muscle) (Fig. 26.5). Synapses enable transfer of information between one cell and another. They may be electrical or chemical (Mtui, Gruener & Dockery (2020)). The presynaptic neuron conducts impulses towards the synapse, and the postsynaptic neuron transmits information away from the synapse.

Electrical Synapses

Electrical synapses synchronize interconnected neurons. They are rare in the adult but much more common in the embryo, gradually being replaced by chemical synapses. They are responsible for stereotypical movements such as the jerky movements of the eyes. They remain abundant in some nervous tissues such as cardiac and smooth muscle. They work via protein channels, which connect the cytoplasm of adjacent neurons, providing electrical pathways through which ions can flow from one neuron to another. Communication between cells is extremely rapid.

Chemical Synapses

The synaptic cleft is a fluid-filled space between the neuron and its target cell into which NTs are released from the presynaptic membrane. These open and shut ion channels in the postsynaptic membrane. The electrical message of the action potential is conducted chemically across the gap. This is a reversible change, and the NT is removed. Enzymes that degrade the NT are released into the synaptic cleft; the NT

is taken up by the presynaptic membrane and then diffuses away from the synapse.

Neurotransmitters

NTs help neurons communicate messages and regulate body activities and states (Marieb & Hoehn, 2022). Over 100 different chemicals act as NTs. They are classified according to chemical structure (Box 26.2).

The Brain

The average adult brain weighs 1500 g and is slightly heavier in men than in women. The extra size does not influence function. Although the brain is described as a single organ (Figs. 26.6 and 26.7), individual parts perform discrete functions. The brain can be subdivided into four main parts:
1. The cerebral hemispheres.
2. The diencephalon comprising the thalamus and hypothalamus.
3. The brainstem comprising the midbrain, pons and medulla.
4. The cerebellum.

The Cerebral Hemispheres

The two **cerebral hemispheres** form 85% of the weight of the brain and sit like an umbrella over the **diencephalon** and **brainstem.** The neurons have their cell bodies outermost forming the **grey matter,** or cortex, and their fibres innermost forming the **white matter.** The cortex is thrown into elevated ridges called **gyri,** separated by shallow grooves called **sulci.** This vastly increases the surface area of the cerebral cortex with most of it hidden from view in the walls of the sulci. The deepest grooves are called **fissures** and form important landmarks. There is a **midline sagittal fissure** (a midline longitudinal fissure) and the **transverse fissure** (which separates the cerebral hemispheres from the cerebellum).

Each hemisphere is divided into six main lobes. Four of these are the **frontal, parietal, occipital** and **temporal** lobes. The other two lobes are buried in the hemispheres and are the **insula,** revealed if the frontal and temporal lobes are eased apart, and the **limbic lobe,** which can be seen if the brain is divided along the mid-sagittal fissure.

The Cerebral Cortex
Structure

The cerebral cortex is also called the **pallium** (shell) and varies in thickness from 2–4 mm. It has a good blood supply via a dense capillary bed. The cortex contains about 50 billion neurons and is arranged in both a **laminar** (layered) and a **columnar** manner. There are three basic cell types: pyramidal, spiny stellate and smooth stellate cells (Table 26.2). There is an excellent chapter on the cerebral cortex in Mtui, Gruener & Dockery (2020).

• BOX 26.1 Elements of the Limbic System

The Cingulate Gyrus

The cingulate gyrus involves part of the cortex and part of the limbic system. The cingulate gyrus receives fibres from the parahippocampal gyrus, the temporal lobe, the thalamus and visual and tactile areas of the cortex. Its function is the emotional interpretation of pain and vision.

The Hippocampus

The hippocampus is situated in the temporal lobe, has a complex three-dimensional trumpet shape and is called Ammon's horn. It communicates with the neocortex, the thalamus and other subcortical regions. Its functions include memory, learning, spatial awareness and cognitive mapping. The hippocampi of London taxi drivers were found to be significantly enlarged whilst they were 'learning' the routes.

The Amygdala

The amygdalae (Greek for *almond*) are a group of paired nuclei in the temporal lobes. They are the focal point between incoming sensory systems and outgoing effector systems responsible for emotion and are linked to all sensory association areas of the cortex. They seem to be involved in the strength of emotion, especially in childhood. Irrational states of fear are generated (such as phobias and anxiety states with no conscious recall of why the fear is felt). This includes the physiological reactions of flight or fight (Mtui, Gruener & Dockery, 2020).

The Hypothalamus

This structure is involved in homeostasis and survival. Despite its small size—only 4 g—the hypothalamus contains centres involved in the regulation of food intake, water intake, sleep–wake cycles, sexual behaviour and defence against attack. The hypothalamus controls the output of anterior pituitary hormones by producing releasing and inhibiting factors. It also synthesizes the two posterior pituitary hormones, antidiuretic hormone and oxytocin.

The Thalamus

The thalamus is the largest nuclear mass in the nervous system and consists of a pair of organs joined in the midline of the centre of the brain. It has been likened to a traffic conductor. The thalami contain multiple nuclei, each with a specific function. These include hearing, vision, memory, cognition, judgement and mood.

The Insula

The insula lies deep within the brain. The anterior insula is a cortical centre for pain. The posterior insula is continuous with the entorhinal cortex and the amygdala and may be involved in the emotional response to pain. The central region is continuous with the frontoparietal and temporal cortex and may have a language rather than a limbic function (Mtui, Gruener & Dockery, 2020).

The Septum

The connections of the septum lie central to the brain. Fibres are received from the amygdala, olfactory tract, hippocampus and brainstem. Fibres from the septum connect with the hypothalamus, brainstem and hippocampus. The septum controls sensations of pleasure and well-being and is also involved in memory.

• BOX 26.2 Different Types of Neurotransmitters

Acetylcholine

Acetylcholine (ACh) was the first neurotransmitter (NT) to be identified and is one of the most well-known. Although it is the main NT released at neuromuscular junctions in the peripheral nervous system, it can also be used by some neurons in the central nervous system. ACh is synthesized and stored within synaptic vesicles in the presence of the enzyme choline acetyltransferase. Acetic acid is bound to coenzyme A to form acetyl CoA. This compound combines with choline and the coenzyme is released.

Choline Acetyltransferase

$$AcetylCoA + choline \rightarrow ACh + CoA$$

The released ACh binds to the postsynaptic membrane and is degraded to acetic acid and choline by the enzyme acetylcholinesterase. The released choline is captured by the presynaptic membrane and used to synthesize more ACh.

The Biogenic Amines

Five other NTs arise from the biogenic amine group. These include three catecholamines (dopamine, noradrenaline [norepinephrine] and adrenaline [epinephrine]), and two indolamines (serotonin [5-hydroxytryptamine] and histamine). Catecholamines are synthesized from the amino acid tyrosine in a common pathway. Neurons produce only the enzymes needed for a specific NT. The common pathway is:

$$Tyrosine \rightarrow L-Dopa$$
$$\rightarrow Dopamine \rightarrow Noradrenaline \rightarrow Adrenaline$$

Serotonin is synthesized from tyrosine by a different pathway. Histamine is synthesized from the amino acid histidine. NTs are widely distributed in the brain and are involved in emotional behaviour and in regulation of the body clock.

Amino Acids

The most important amino acids involved in neurotransmission are γ-aminobutyric acid (GABA) and glutamate.

Peptides

The neuropeptides include any molecules with diverse effects. These include the endorphins and encephalins involved in pain perception (Chapter 38).

The Laminae

In the neocortex, which forms 90% of the brain, there are six well-organized laminae. These are:

1. The molecular layer which contains the tips of the apical dendrites of pyramidal cells.
2. The outer granular layer which contains small pyramidal and stellate cells.
3. The outer pyramidal layer which contains medium-sized pyramidal cells and stellate cells.
4. The inner granular layer which contains stellate cells receiving afferents from the thalami.
5. The inner pyramidal layer which contains large pyramidal cells which project to the corpus striatum, brainstem and spinal cord.
6. The fusiform layer which contains modified pyramidal cells which project to the thalamus.

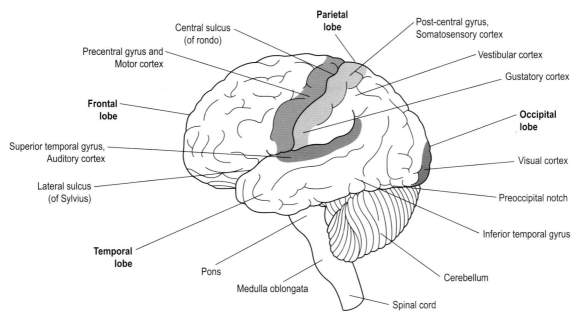

• **Fig. 26.6** Lateral aspect of the human brain.

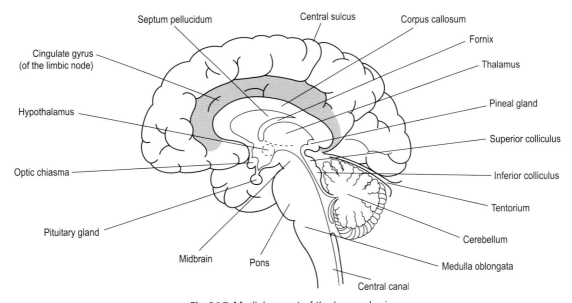

• **Fig. 26.7** Medial aspect of the human brain.

Columnar Organization

The neurons are arranged functionally in columns of 50–100 μm in diameter. These columns only respond to very specific stimuli from very specific body areas. They are the functional units or modules of the cortex.

Function

The **cerebral cortex** enables conscious behaviour such as perception, communication, memory, understanding, appreciation and initiation of voluntary movements. It can be divided into three functional areas:

1. The **primary sensory area,** which receives stimuli from the periphery of the body.
2. The **primary motor area,** which sends out impulses to control the periphery.
3. The **association areas.**

Sensory areas are posterior and motor areas are anterior to the central sulcus. This same arrangement occurs in the spinal cord columns with sensory fibres posterior and motor areas anterior.

The association areas integrate diverse information. These include the **prefrontal cortex** concerned with intellect; the **diffuse gnostic area,** which contributes memory of

TABLE 26.2	Types of Cells within the Cerebral Cortex
Pyramidal cells	Excitatory and use **glutamate** as their neurotransmitter. Diameter: 20–30 μm in laminae II and III (see later) to 60 μm in lamina V. **Giant cells of Betz** situated in the motor cortex are 80–100 μm in diameter.
Spiny stellate cells	Mainly excitatory. They have spiny dendrites. Receive most of the afferent input from the thalamus and form glutamatergic synapses on pyramidal cells.
Smooth stellate cells	Inhibitory. They have non-spiny dendrites. Receive collateral branches from pyramidal cells and form GABAergic synapses on other pyramidal cells.

sensation and emotional response; and the two main **language areas**, Broca's and Wernicke's areas, usually in the left hemisphere.

Prefrontal Cortex

The prefrontal cortex is concerned with higher mental functions such as abstract thinking, decision making, social behaviour and anticipating the effects of actions. It has two-way connections with the cortex on the same side of the brain (**ipsilateral**) (except the primary motor and sensory areas), the cortex on the opposite side of the brain (**contralateral**), the thalamus and the hypothalamus (Mtui, Gruener & Dockery 2020).

Sensory Cortex

Thalamic nerve fibres project to the sensory areas of the cerebral cortex. Nerves coming into the spinal cord from the body's periphery maintain **somatic organization** so that a representation of the body is organized in the sensory cortex. The size of an area of sensory cortex given over to input from the body depends on its innervation (e.g., sensitive parts of the body, such as the tongue, lips, fingers and toes, are represented as very large!). This results in a peculiarly shaped **homunculus.**

The Control of Movement

Motor Cortex

Movement of the body by skeletal muscles is controlled by input from the SNS. Motor control can be divided into three neural systems:

1. The **pyramidal system,** a fast and usually direct descending pathway from the cortex.
2. The **extrapyramidal system** with multiple synapses involving many brain structures of which the basal ganglia are the most important.
3. The **cerebellum.**

The extrapyramidal system is very important, with the 'intention to act' created by the integration of widespread neural impulses. Efferent fibres from the motor cortex project to the **basal ganglia,** the **thalamus,** the **red nucleus,** the **lateral reticular formation** and the **spinal cord** in a topographically organized manner. The red nucleus lies between the substantia nigra and the aqueduct of Sylvius. It is oval-shaped and involved in the control of limb flexion.

The Basal Ganglia

The basal ganglia are the most important structure in the extrapyramidal system. They consist of large nuclei lying laterally to the thalamus. These are the **globus pallidus,** the **pars compacta** (including the **substantia nigra**) and the **striatum** (including the **caudate nucleus** and the **putamen**), which is the largest subcortical mass of cells in the brain. Motor activity is strongly influenced by the basal ganglia which constitute the main extrapyramidal control. Four circuits have been demonstrated (Mtui, Gruener & Dockery 2020):

1. A motor loop concerned with learned movements.
2. A cognitive loop concerned with motor intentions.
3. A limbic loop concerned with the emotional aspects of movement.
4. An oculomotor loop concerned with voluntary saccades.

The Cerebellum

This large brain structure lies beneath the occipital lobes and is separated from them by a fold of dura mater called the *tentorium cerebelli*. The **cerebellum** is bilaterally symmetrical, divided by a midline structure called the **vermis.** There are no interhemispheric nerve fibres; therefore messages are not relayed between the two halves. The cerebellum monitors the strength and execution of movements. Its function is entirely inhibitory and controlled by the NT γ-aminobutyric acid (GABA).

The Limbic System

The **limbic system** is concerned with emotional (affective) feelings. It consists of nuclei and fibres located on the medial aspect of each cerebral hemisphere. Its structures encircle the upper part of the brainstem (limbus means *ring*) and include the **cingulate gyrus,** the **parahippocampal gyrus,** the **hippocampus** and the **amygdala,** the **hypothalamus,** part of the **thalamus,** the **insula** and the **septum** (described in Box 26.1)**.** It is closely related to the **reticular formation (RF).** The limbic system interacts with higher brain centres and facilitates a close relationship between cognition and emotion.

The Medulla Oblongata and Pons

The **medulla oblongata** is the conical-shaped lower part of the brainstem that blends into the spinal cord at the level of the **foramen magnum.** The central canal of the spinal cord broadens out in the medulla to form the **fourth ventricle.** The medulla functions as an **autonomic reflex centre,** maintaining homeostasis. Its nuclei include the **cardiac,** vasomotor and **respiratory centres** and nuclei that control vomiting, swallowing, coughing and sneezing.

The **pons** forms a bulbous structure between the medulla and midbrain and acts as part of the anterior wall of the **third ventricle.** It is a bridge of nerve fibres running between the spinal cord and higher brain centres. The transverse fibres of the pons belong to the giant **corticopontocerebellar pathway** which runs from one cerebral cortex to the contralateral cerebellar hemisphere.

The Reticular Formation

The RF is an old part of the brain, sometimes called the **reptilian brain.** It is important in autonomic and reflex activities. It extends through the medulla, pons and midbrain and is closely related to the olfactory and limbic systems. Its neurons have long, branching dendrites, and its fibres run in three columns: the main column or midline raphe, the medial nuclear group and the lateral nuclear group.

The **reticular activating system** is part of the RF, making multiple synapses throughout the brainstem. It is involved in the level of consciousness, alertness and the sleep–wake cycle (see Clinical Application 26.1). RF neurons maintain homeostasis by controlling the cardiac, vasomotor, respiratory, vomiting, swallowing, coughing and sneezing centres in the medulla. The RF is linked to many other brain centres, demonstrated by its list of functions:

1. Pattern generation and patterned cranial nerve activities.
2. Posture and locomotion.
3. Salivation and lacrimation.
4. Bladder control.
5. Involvement in circulation, respiration and blood pressure control.
6. Conveys both somatic and visceral sensory information to the cerebellum.
7. Sleeping and waking, attention, mood and arousal.

Protection of the Brain

Nervous tissue is very delicate, and neurons can be injured by even a slight pressure. Outwardly, the brain is protected by the bony skull and the **three meninges** (Chapter 24).

The Ventricles

Four fluid-filled ventricles help to cushion and protect the brain (Fig. 26.8): the two **lateral ventricles** and the **third** and **fourth ventricles.** The ventricles are continuous with each other and with the central canal of the spinal cord via the aqueduct of Sylvius. The hollow chambers are filled with **CSF** and lined by ependymal cells. Three apertures in the wall of the fourth ventricle connect the ventricles to the fluid-filled **subarachnoid space** (Chapter 24) surrounding the brain.

Tufts of capillaries called **choroid plexi** hang from the roof of each ventricle and manufacture CSF, which moves freely though the ventricles and into the central canal of the spinal cord (Fig. 26.9). Most of the CSF enters the

subarachnoid space, bathing the outer surface of the brain and spinal cord and returning to the blood via the **arachnoid** villi to the **dural sinuses.** An obstruction to the flow will result in CSF accumulating in the ventricles and putting pressure on the brain. In a neonate, the skull bones are not fused. A collection of fluid in the ventricles therefore causes skull enlargement (**hydrocephalus**).

The Blood–Brain Barrier

The blood–brain barrier ensures that the brain's internal environment remains stable. It selectively allows substances needed by the brain such as glucose, amino acids and some electrolytes to cross by facilitated diffusion whilst keeping toxic chemicals within the capillary network. Blood-borne

Conscious awareness allows the nervous system to interact deliberately with the environment. The neural processes that underlie altered states of consciousness, even the sleep–wake cycle, are not well understood. Dark and light cycles (circadian rhythms) are known to play a role in the sleep–wake cycle. Clinically, disruptions to circadian rhythm sleep–wake cycles are associated with depressive disorders (Hertenstein et al., 2019).

Several areas of the brain are involved in sleep, including the raphe nuclei in the pons and medulla, which spread locally in the brainstem reticular formation to the thalamus, hypothalamus and limbic system and cortex. The neurotransmitters serotonin (stimulates waking) and acetylcholine (helps in sleep onset), as well as other substances, may be involved in causing sleep.

Patterns of sleep can be studied by measuring the electrical activity of the brain by means of an electroencephalogram (EEG). Normal sleep consists of two types: **slow-wave sleep** and **rapid eye movement** (REM) sleep. In the normal waking state there are rapid, low-amplitude waves. The onset of sleep is accompanied by slow, high-amplitude waves due to the synchronization of many neurons (slow-wave sleep). This lasts for about 90 min before being replaced by REM sleep when dreams occur. These two phases alternate several times during a normal night's sleep. REM occurs in phases of 5–30 min and has several characteristics (Hall & Hall, 2020):

- It is associated with active dreaming and active body muscle movements.
- Muscle tone throughout the body is severely depressed indicating inhibition of spinal muscle control areas.
- Despite inhibition of the peripheral muscles, irregular muscle movements occur.
- Heart and respiratory rates become irregular when a person dreams.
- The person is more difficult to arouse, but they usually awake spontaneously, from REM sleep.
- The brain is highly active, and overall brain metabolism may be increased by as much as 20%. EEG brain waves are similar to those of wakefulness which is the source of the name *paradoxical sleep.*

Sleep may have two purposes: it may be restorative, a necessary part of replenishing energy and restoring tissues; or it may be protective to ensure safety for a daytime species relying on sight. REM sleep may allow the integration of the day's events into long-term memory, promoting learning, species-typical reprogramming or brain development.

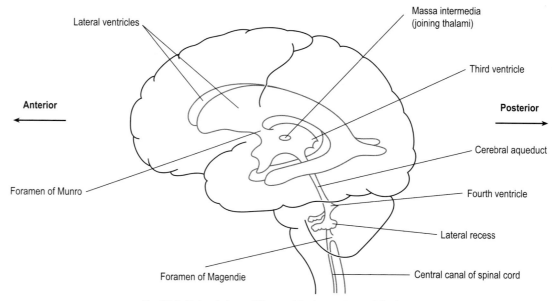

• **Fig. 26.8** Lateral view of the ventricular system of the brain.

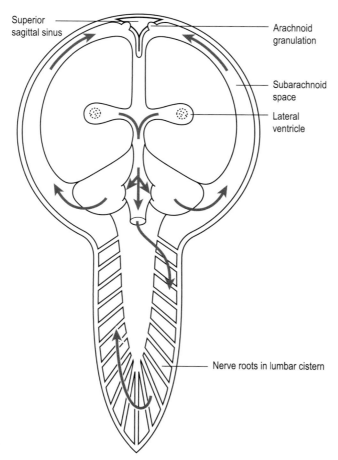

• **Fig. 26.9** Circulation of cerebrospinal fluid.

substances within the brain's capillaries are separated from the extracellular space and neurons by:

- A continuous endothelial capillary wall with tight junctions.

- A thick basal lamina surrounding the external face of the capillary.
- The bulbous feet of astrocytes clinging to the capillaries and signalling them to keep tight junctions.

The Cranial Nerves

Twelve pairs of cranial nerves are associated with the brain. The first two pairs originate from the forebrain and the rest from the brainstem. The 12 cranial nerves are outlined in Table 26.3.

The Spinal Cord

Knowledge of spinal cord anatomy is important because of the use of epidural analgesia in childbirth (Chapter 38). The spinal cord is enclosed within the vertebral column and extends from the **foramen magnum** of the skull to the level of the first **lumbar vertebra**. It is about 48 cm long and 1.8 cm thick and carries ascending and descending nerve pathways (Fig. 26.10).

Like the brain, the spinal cord is protected by bone, CSF and meninges. The dura mater is a single layer only and is unattached to the bony walls of the vertebral column. Between the bones and dural sheath is the **epidural space** filled with fat and blood vessels. The subarachnoid space between the pia and arachnoid maters is filled with CSF.

The Spinal Nerves

Thirty-one pairs of spinal nerves arise from the spinal cord and leave the vertebral column by the **intervertebral foramina** to target specific body areas (Mtui, Gruener & Dockery 2020). The vertebral column is divided into four segments, each with a different number of vertebrae: the **cervical** vertebrae (C1–C7), the **thoracic** vertebrae (T1–T12), the

TABLE 26.3	The 12 Cranial Nerves	
Cranial Nerve	Specific Name	Function
I	Olfactory	Sense of smell
II	Optic	Vision
III	Oculomotor	Moves four of the external eye muscles
IV	Trochlear	Moves one of the external eye muscles
V	Trigeminal	Facial sensation and motor fibres for chewing
VI	Abducens	Moves one of the external eye muscles
VII	Facial	Controls muscles of facial expression
VIII	Vestibulocochlear	Hearing and balance
IX	Glossopharyngeal	Innervates the tongue and pharynx
X	Vagus	Innervates thoracic and abdominal viscera
XI	Accessory	Assists the vagus nerve
XII	Hypoglossal	Controls the muscles of the tongue

lumbar vertebrae (L1–L5) and the **sacral** vertebrae (S1–S5) (Fig. 26.11). Each segment of the spinal cord is defined by a pair of spinal nerves. Each receives and conducts sensory information from a specific body area called a **dermatome** (Fig. 26.11).

Inferiorly, the spinal cord ends in a cone-shaped structure, the **conus medullaris.** The nerve roots fan outwards and downwards to exit through relevant vertebrae. This collection of nerve roots is called the **cauda equinae** ('horse's tail'). A fibrous extension of the pia, the **filum terminale,** runs downwards to attach to the posterior surface of the coccyx.

A Cross-section of the Spinal Cord
The Grey Matter and Spinal Roots

The grey matter of the cord consists of neuronal cell bodies, their unmyelinated processes and neuroglia. It is central to the white matter and looks like a letter H. There are two posterior or dorsal horns which contain interneurons and two anterior or ventral horns which house the cell bodies of somatic motor neurons (Fig. 26.12). The ventral roots of the spinal cord contain somatic motor neuron axons on their way to skeletal muscles. Afferent fibres of the peripheral sensory nerves form the dorsal roots of the spinal cord. Their cell bodies are in the dorsal root ganglion, an enlargement of the dorsal root. The dorsal and ventral roots are short and fuse to form the spinal nerves.

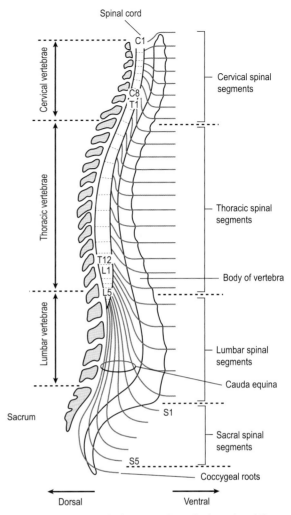

• **Fig. 26.10** The relationship between the spinal cord and the vertebral column.

The White Matter

The white matter of the spinal cord is composed of myelinated and unmyelinated nerve fibres running in three directions:
1. Ascending tracts of sensory inputs going to the higher centres.
2. Descending tracts of motor outputs coming from the brain.
3. Across from one side of the spinal cord to the other. These will be discussed in detail in Chapter 27.

Adaptation to Pregnancy

The following short list of changes can occur during pregnancy, mainly due to altered output from the endocrine system (see Clinical Application 26.2 for more information):
• CNS changes.
• Sleep disturbances.
• Alterations in sensation.

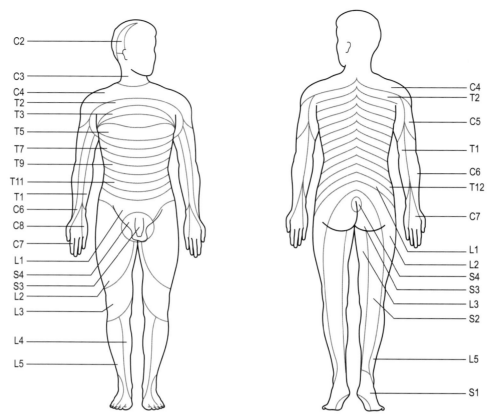

• **Fig. 26.11** Adult dermatome pattern.

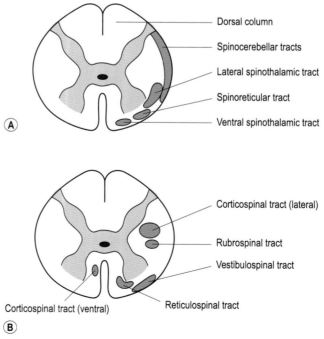

• **Fig. 26.12** Major nerve tracts of the spinal cord. (A) Ascending nerve tracts. (B) Descending nerve tracts.

• CLINICAL APPLICATION 26.2   Central Nervous System-Related Adaptations During Pregnancy

Central nervous system (CNS) changes	Pregnancy hormones affect the CNS, but the phenomenon is not well understood.
	Reduced cognitive ability, with difficulty in concentration and poor memory being top of the list.
	Size of woman's brain shrinks during pregnancy and may take at least 2 years to return to normal following delivery (Hoekzema et al., 2017).
Sleep disturbances	Sleep patterns change during pregnancy and in the postpartum period (Sedov et al., 2018 believes).
	Rapid eye movement sleep increases from 25 weeks' gestation, decreasing to non-pregnant levels by term.
	There is a corresponding decrease in slow-wave sleep, which returns to normal immediately after delivery.
	Increased sleep time and napping during first trimester.
	Increased night wakening in later trimesters due to nocturia, dyspnoea, heartburn, nasal congestion, muscle aches and anxiety.
	In late pregnancy, many factors contribute to poor sleep such as a full bladder, muscle discomfort and anxiety.
Alterations in sensation	Changes in the ear, nose and larynx occur because of changes in fluid dynamics and vascular permeability (due to oestrogen).
	Congestion and hyperaemia of the nasal mucosa causes nasal stuffiness and rhinorrhoea, which may lead to nose bleeds or to loss of sleep.
	Laryngeal changes may result in voice changes or persistent cough.
	A reduction in the sense of smell may lead to altered taste sensations and a change in food preference. There may also be nausea and food aversions, especially for foods that taste bitter. These aversions are believed to be protective as bitter foods are often poisonous or teratogenic.

Main Points

- The CNS receives and sends messages to all parts of the body via the PNS. It communicates by rapid transmission of electrical signals.
- The ANS innervates smooth muscle, cardiac muscle and glands of the viscera. It is subdivided into the sympathetic, parasympathetic and enteric systems.
- Nervous tissue consists of neurons and the neuroglia. Neurons provide a function (e.g., hearing, thinking), and neuroglia provide them with support, nourishment and protection.
- Neurons have axons and dendrites which communicate with other cells by electrical impulses and NTs.
- Large nerve fibres are covered in a protective myelin sheath which increases impulse transmission rate up to 100 times faster than unmyelinated fibres.
- The brain weighs about 1500 g and can be subdivided into two cerebral hemispheres, the diencephalon (thalamus and hypothalamus), the brainstem (midbrain, pons and medulla oblongata) and the cerebellum.
- Each cerebral hemisphere consists of a frontal, parietal, occipital, temporal, insula and limbic lobe. The cerebral cortex is divided into the primary sensory area, the primary motor area and the association areas.
- The limbic system links with higher brain centres, forming a close relationship between cognition and emotion.

- The hypothalamus is involved in homeostasis and survival. It controls the output of anterior pituitary hormones and synthesizes the posterior pituitary hormones.
- Functions of the thalamic nuclei include hearing, vision, memory, cognition, judgement and mood. The insula is involved in olfaction, taste and autonomic reflexes. The functions of the septum are sensations of pleasure, wellbeing and memory.
- The pons is a bridge formed of nerve fibres running between the spinal cord and higher brain centres.
- The RF is involved in the level of consciousness and alertness.
- The pia, arachnoid and dura mater protect the brain and spinal cord, protect blood vessels, enclose venous sinuses and contain CSF.
- The four ventricles are filled with CSF and are continuous with each other and with the central canal of the spinal cord via the aqueduct of Sylvius.
- The blood–brain barrier ensures that the brain's internal environment remains stable. It is selective. Substances needed by the brain cross over by facilitated diffusion whilst toxic chemicals are kept within the capillaries.
- There are 12 pairs of cranial nerves. The first two pairs arise in the forebrain and the rest in the brainstem. All but the vagus nerve target structures in the head and

neck. The vagus nerve innervates thoracic and abdominal viscera.

- The spinal cord carries ascending and descending nerve pathways. The vertebral column is divided into segments, and each segment conducts sensory information from a specific body part called a *dermatome*.
- The spinal cord ends in the conus medullaris and a collection of nerve roots called the *cauda equina*, which fan

outwards and downwards to attach to the posterior surface of the coccyx.

- Several changes occur in the CNS during pregnancy: women report difficulty in concentration and poor memory, sleep patterns change, they experience congestion and hyperaemia of the nasal mucosa, and research shows that the brain shrinks during pregnancy and may not return to normal until at least 2 years postpartum.

References

Hall, J.E., Hall, M.E., 2020. Guyton & Hall Textbook of Medical Physiology, fourteenth ed. Elsevier, Philadelphia.

Hertenstein, E., Feige, B., Gmeiner, T., Kienzler, C., Spiegelhalder, K., Johann, A., et al., 2019. Insomnia as a predictor of mental disorders: a systematic review and meta-analysis. Sleep Med. Rev. 43, 96–105.

Hoekzema, E., Barba-Müller, E., Pozzobon, C., Picado, M., Lucco, F., García-García, D., et al., 2017. Pregnancy leads to long-lasting changes in human brain structure. Nat. Neurosci. 20 (2), 287–296.

Marieb, E.N., Hoehn, K., 2022. Human Anatomy and Physiology, twelfth ed. Pearson, Harlow.

Mtui, E., Gruener, G., Dockery, P., 2020. Fitzgerald's Clinical Neuroanatomy and Neuroscience, eighth ed. Elsevier, Philadelphia.

Sedov, I.D., Cameron, E.E., Madigan, S., Tomfohr-Madsen, L.M., 2018. Sleep quality during pregnancy: a meta-analysis. Sleep Med. Rev. 38, 168–176.

Annotated recommended reading

Hoekzema, E., Barba-Müller, E., Pozzobon, C., Picado, M., Lucco, F., García-García, D., et al., 2017. Pregnancy leads to long-lasting changes in human brain structure. Nature Neuroscience, 20 (2), 287–296.

This interesting reference reports on a prospective study focusing on the effects of pregnancy on the human brain which are virtually unknown. Findings provide the first evidence that pregnancy confers long-lasting changes in a woman's brain.

Marieb, E.N., Hoehn, K., 2022. Human Anatomy and Physiology, twelfth ed. Pearson, Harlow.

This general anatomy and physiology textbook is ideal for the student of nursing and midwifery. Although not applied to reproduction in any depth, it has succinct and easy-to-follow explanations on the anatomy and physiology of the nervous system.

Mtui, E., Gruener, G., Dockery, P., 2020. Fitzgerald's Clinical Neuroanatomy and Neuroscience, eighth ed. Elsevier, Philadelphia.

This is a well-laid-out and detailed but easy-to-read textbook on the human nervous system. The format is full of interesting diagrams, and the headings make the book content easy to find and follow.

27

The Peripheral and Autonomic Nervous Systems

LYNSAY MATTHEWS

CHAPTER CONTENTS

This chapter focuses on describing the peripheral and autonomic nervous systems. In addition, the columns of the spinal cord are outlined to help students and midwives understand nerve pathways to the brain.

The Peripheral Nervous System

The **peripheral nervous system** (PNS) detects changes in the body's external or internal environments. Sensory receptors code them into nerve impulses and pass the information back to the central nervous system (CNS) so that appropriate action can occur. Some messages are not passed to the brain; they influence reflex actions at the level of the spinal cord or brainstem. The PNS includes all neural structures outside the brain and spinal cord (i.e., sensory receptors), peripheral nerves and associated ganglia and efferent motor endings (Marieb & Hoehn, 2022). For ease of understanding of **nerve pathways** to the brain, the spinal cord columns have been included in this chapter.

Ascending Sensory Tracts

Categories of Sensation

There are two kinds of sensations (Fig. 27.1): **conscious** sensations perceived at the level of the cortex and **non-conscious** sensations that are not. Conscious sensation can be divided into **exteroception** and **proprioception.** Exteroception involves messages from the outside world perceived in the cerebral cortex. Sensations may originate in body surface receptors or in telereceptors of the special senses such as vision or hearing. **Proprioceptors** in the locomotor system and the inner ear labyrinth inform the brain of the position when stationary (**position sense**) and during movement (**kinaesthetic sense**).

Non-conscious sensation is divided into two kinds: non-conscious proprioception affecting the cerebellum. This involves messages essential for smooth muscle coordination received through spinocerebellar pathways and brainstem. The second kind, enteroception, refers to non-conscious signals from visceral reflexes (Mtui, Gruener & Dockery, 2020).

Somatic Sensory Perception

Two major pathways are involved in somatic perception sensations: the **posterior column–medial lemniscal pathway** and the **spinothalamic pathway** (Fig. 27.2). There are common features:
- All contain first-order, second-order and third-order sensory neurons.
- Cell bodies of the first-order neurons are in the posterior root ganglia.
- Cell bodies of the second-order neurons are on the same side of the CNS grey matter as first-order neurons.
- Second-order axons cross the midline to ascend and terminate in the thalamus.
- Third-order neurons project to the somatosensory cortex.
- Both pathways are somatotopic, representing the body parts in an orderly fashion up to the sensory cortex.
- Both pathways can be modulated, either by inhibition or stimulation by other neurons.

The Posterior Column–Medial Lemniscal Pathway

First-order nerve fibres enter the dorsal columns of the spinal cord without synapsing. They are usually large **A fibres** with conduction velocities of ~70 m/s. As nerve fibres from higher levels in the cord are added, they take up lateral positions so that the higher the level of origin is, the more lateral the position of the fibre in the column. Fibres of second-order neurons at the level of the brainstem cross the midline to be projected to the thalamus. Crossing over is why one side of the brain controls the opposite (contralateral) side of the body. Cells in the sensory relay nucleus of the thalamus are third-order neurons and project their fibres to the **somatosensory cortex.**

Chief functions of this pathway are conscious proprioception and discriminatory touch. These provide the parietal lobe with an instantaneous report of our body position both at rest and when moving. Disturbances of this pathway cause demyelinating diseases such as multiple sclerosis.

The Spinothalamic Tract

The **dorsal root fibres** of this pathway tend to be the smaller **A-δ** or unmyelinated **C fibres** with slow conduction velocity. Dorsal root fibres enter the spinal cord and may ascend or descend a few segments before synapsing with cells of the dorsal horn in the **substantia gelatinosa.** Dorsal horn second-order fibres ascend or descend a few segments before crossing over the midline to ascend in the spinothalamic tract. These fibres terminate on thalamic third-order neurons whose fibres synapse on cells of the sensory cortex. The role of this pathway is the perception of heat, cold and touch on the opposite side of the body. The role of the substantia gelatinosa in the gate control theory of pain perception is discussed in Chapter 38.

Somatosensory Receptors

Sensory receptors are mostly adapted nerve fibre endings that respond to environmental changes. Sensory afferent nerves arising from the body are grouped together as the

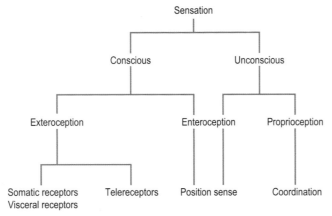

• **Fig. 27.1** Categories of sensation.

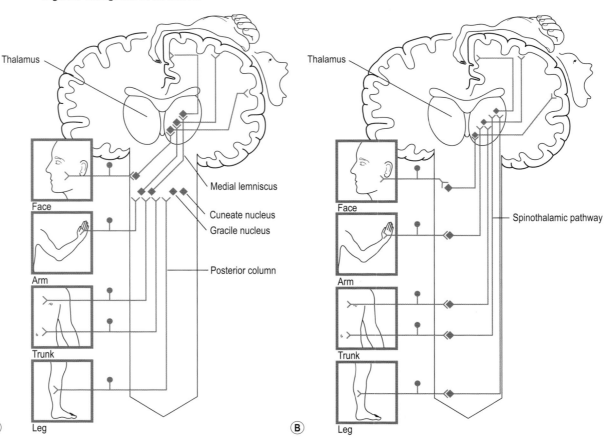

• **Fig. 27.2** Basic plans of (A) the posterior column–medial lemniscal pathway and (B) the spinothalamic pathway.

somatosensory system and include sensation from the skin, muscles, joints and viscera. The special senses are not included in this textbook (refer to Marieb & Hoehn, 2022). There are five different somatosensory receptors (Table 27.1).

Descending Motor Pathways

The descending tracts carry efferent messages from the brain down the spinal cord and are divided into four main pathways:
1. Corticospinal (pyramidal).
2. Reticulospinal (extrapyramidal).
3. Vestibulospinal.
4. Tectospinal.

The Corticospinal Tract

The corticospinal tract (Fig. 27.3) is the major motor pathway involved with voluntary movement. It contains ~1 million nerve fibres, more than 60% of which originate in the primary motor cortex. The tract descends through the internal capsule to the brainstem. It continues through the pons to the medulla oblongata where about 80% of fibres decussate (cross over to the other side of the body). The fibres, arranged somatotopically, synapse with interneurons or directly with anterior horn neurons.

The Reticulospinal Tract

The reticulospinal tract is partially crossed and originates in the reticular formation of the pons and medulla. It is involved in two kinds of motor behaviour: locomotion (where it controls bilateral rhythmicity) and postural control.

The Vestibulospinal Tract

The vestibulospinal tract is an uncrossed paired pathway originating in the vestibular nucleus of the medulla oblongata. It maintains balance when the head is tilted to one side.

The Tectospinal Tract

The tectospinal tract is a crossed pathway descending from the tectum of the midbrain to the medial part of the anterior horn at the cervical and upper thoracic levels. It orients the head and trunk towards visual or auditory stimuli in reptiles and may have a similar function in humans.

Upper and Lower Motor Neurons

Neurons of the motor cortex are called the *pyramidal cells* because of the shape of their bodies. They are referred to as the *upper motor neurons*. The anterior horn neurons whose axons leave the cord to innervate skeletal muscles are called the *lower motor neurons*. Damage to upper motor neurons causes floppy paralysis with loss of tendon reflexes. Damage to lower motor neurons causes weakness and wasting of muscles. Motor neuron disease is characterized by progressive degeneration of both upper and lower motor neurons (Mtui, Gruener & Dockery, 2020).

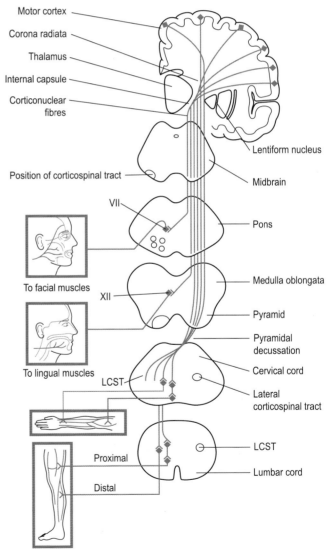

• **Fig. 27.3** Corticospinal tract viewed from the front. At the spinal cord level, only the lateral corticospinal tract is shown. *LCST*, Lateral corticospinal tract; *VII*, nucleus of facial nerve; *XII*, hypoglossal nucleus.

TABLE 27.1	Types of Somatosensory Receptors	
Receptor	**Responds to …**
Mechanoreceptors	Touch, pressure, vibrations and stretch
Thermoreceptors	Temperature change
Photoreceptors	Light
Chemoreceptors	Smell, taste and changes in blood chemistry
Nociceptors	Pain

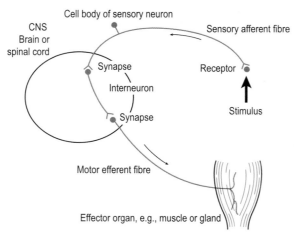

• **Fig. 27.4** The component structures of a reflex arc.

Reflex Activity

A reflex is a rapid, predictable, unlearned involuntary response to a stimulus. Some reflex activity is protective, such as rapid removal of the body from noxious stimuli such as heat. Other reflexes which control visceral activities occur without any awareness of change. Some reflexes are learned, such as driving a car. Many reflexes can be modified by learning and conscious effort.

The Reflex Arc

Reflexes occur over specific neural paths called **reflex arcs** (Fig. 27.4). These have five main components:
1. Receptor at the site where the stimulus occurs.
2. Sensory neuron which takes the message to the CNS.
3. Integration centre within the CNS, which may be a single synapse or may involve a chain of interneurons.
4. Motor neuron which conducts efferent impulses from the integration centre to an effector organ.
5. Effector which may be a gland or muscle fibre and acts to complete the reflex action. Reflexes may be somatic or autonomic. Somatic reflexes can be tested to confirm normal neural function.

Spinal Reflexes

Many spinal reflexes occur with little or no brain input:
• Stretch and deep tendon reflexes, where the messages from the proprioceptors in the muscles and joints are transmitted to the cerebellum and cerebral cortex. These allow normal muscle tone and activity to be maintained.
• The flexor reflex causes automatic withdrawal from painful stimuli.
• The crossed extensor reflex consists of an ipsilateral withdrawal reflex and a contralateral extensor reflex (important in maintaining balance).
• Superficial reflexes can be elicited by gentle stroking of the body. Examples include the plantar reflex (downward curl of the toes in response to stroking sole of foot) and

Babinski's reflex (extension of toes occurs in infants <1 year old).

The Autonomic Nervous System

The **autonomic** (self-regulating) nervous system, or ANS, is responsible for maintaining the stability of the body's internal environment. ANS stimulation does not occur voluntarily; the individual may be conscious of the effects (e.g., increase in heart rate). Motor neurons innervate smooth muscle, cardiac muscle and glands, making adjustments in response to messages from viscera sent to the CNS. Systemic changes brought about by the ANS include adjusting:
• Shunting (redirection) of blood to other areas.
• Heart rate.
• Blood pressure (BP).
• Respiratory rate.
• Body temperature.
• Stomach secretions.

The Role of the Two Divisions

There are differences between the somatic and ANS in their pathways and neurotransmitters (NTs). The ANS is divided into two arms: the sympathetic system (Fig. 27.5), which prepares the body for emergency action, and the parasympathetic system (Fig. 27.6), which counterbalances the sympathetic system and has a calming effect, allowing general body maintenance and the conservation of energy to occur. There is usually a dynamic interaction between the two systems maximizing homeostasis.

The Sympathetic Nervous System

The sympathetic nervous system is so called because it acts in sympathy with emotions. It is sometimes referred to as the *'fight-or-flight' system* and is activated if we are excited or in a threatening situation. Heart and respiratory rates increase, the skin becomes cold and sweaty, and the eye pupils dilate. Visceral blood vessels are constricted and digestion ceases. Blood is shunted to the heart and skeletal muscles, and the liver releases glucose into the blood to provide cells with energy.

The Parasympathetic Nervous System

The parasympathetic division is active when the systems are unstressed. It is often referred to as the *'rest-and-digest' system* and is active during digestion of food and elimination of waste. BP, heart and respiratory rates are low. The skin is warm as skeletal muscles do not need extra blood supply. Eye pupils are constricted and the lenses adjusted for close vision.

Anatomy of the Autonomic Nervous System

The motor unit of the ANS is a two-neuron chain:
• The first neuron is the **preganglionic neuron.** Its cell body is found in the brain or spinal column.
• The first neuron synapses with the second motor neuron, or **postganglionic neuron,** which has its cell body in the autonomic ganglion outside the CNS. The postganglionic neuron extends to the target tissue.

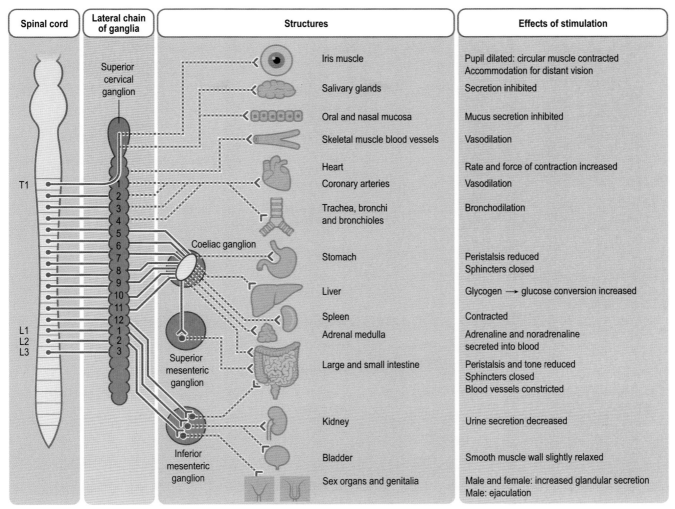

Spinal cord	Lateral chain of ganglia	Structures	Effects of stimulation
	Superior cervical ganglion	Iris muscle	Pupil dilated: circular muscle contracted Accommodation for distant vision
		Salivary glands	Secretion inhibited
		Oral and nasal mucosa	Mucus secretion inhibited
		Skeletal muscle blood vessels	Vasodilation
		Heart Coronary arteries	Rate and force of contraction increased Vasodilation
		Trachea, bronchi and bronchioles	Bronchodilation
	Coeliac ganglion	Stomach	Peristalsis reduced Sphincters closed
		Liver	Glycogen → glucose conversion increased
		Spleen	Contracted
		Adrenal medulla	Adrenaline and noradrenaline secreted into blood
	Superior mesenteric ganglion	Large and small intestine	Peristalsis and tone reduced Sphincters closed Blood vessels constricted
		Kidney	Urine secretion decreased
	Inferior mesenteric ganglion	Bladder	Smooth muscle wall slightly relaxed
		Sex organs and genitalia	Male and female: increased glandular secretion Male: ejaculation

• **Fig. 27.5** The sympathetic outflow, the main structures supplied and the effects of stimulation. Solid purple lines, preganglionic fibres; broken purple lines, postganglionic fibres. There are right and left lateral chains of ganglia.

Preganglionic neurons are thin and lightly myelinated, whereas postganglionic neurons are even thinner and unmyelinated. Both types of fibres may run with somatic nerves in spinal or cranial nerves.

Differences Between the Two Divisions

- Parasympathetic fibres emerge from the brain and sacral spinal cord (craniosacral division), whereas sympathetic fibres originate in the thoracolumbar region of the spinal cord.
- The parasympathetic division has long preganglionic fibres and short postganglionic fibres. The sympathetic division has short preganglionic fibres and long postganglionic fibres.
- Parasympathetic ganglia are in terminal ganglia within or close to the target organs. Sympathetic ganglia lie close to the spinal cord.

Sympathetic Division

The sympathetic division is more complex because it innervates more organs. Sympathetic activity tends to inhibit the activity of visceral organs, some body wall structures such as sweat glands and the smooth muscles (hair-raising muscles, erector pili). All arteries and veins are innervated by sympathetic fibres.

Preganglionic Fibres

Preganglionic fibres arise from cell bodies of neurons in the **thoracolumbar division** of the T1–L2 spinal cord segments. The presence of these preganglionic sympathetic neurons produces the lateral horns (visceral motor horns of the spinal cord). Fibres leave the cord via the ventral root and pass through a myelinated white ramus communicans to enter the appropriate paravertebral (chain) ganglion forming part of the sympathetic chain. Two sympathetic chains flank the spinal column. Fibres arising from the thoracolumbar region innervate 23 pairs of **ganglia** running from neck to pelvis:

- Three cervical.
- Eleven thoracic.
- Four lumbar.
- Four sacral.
- One coccygeal.

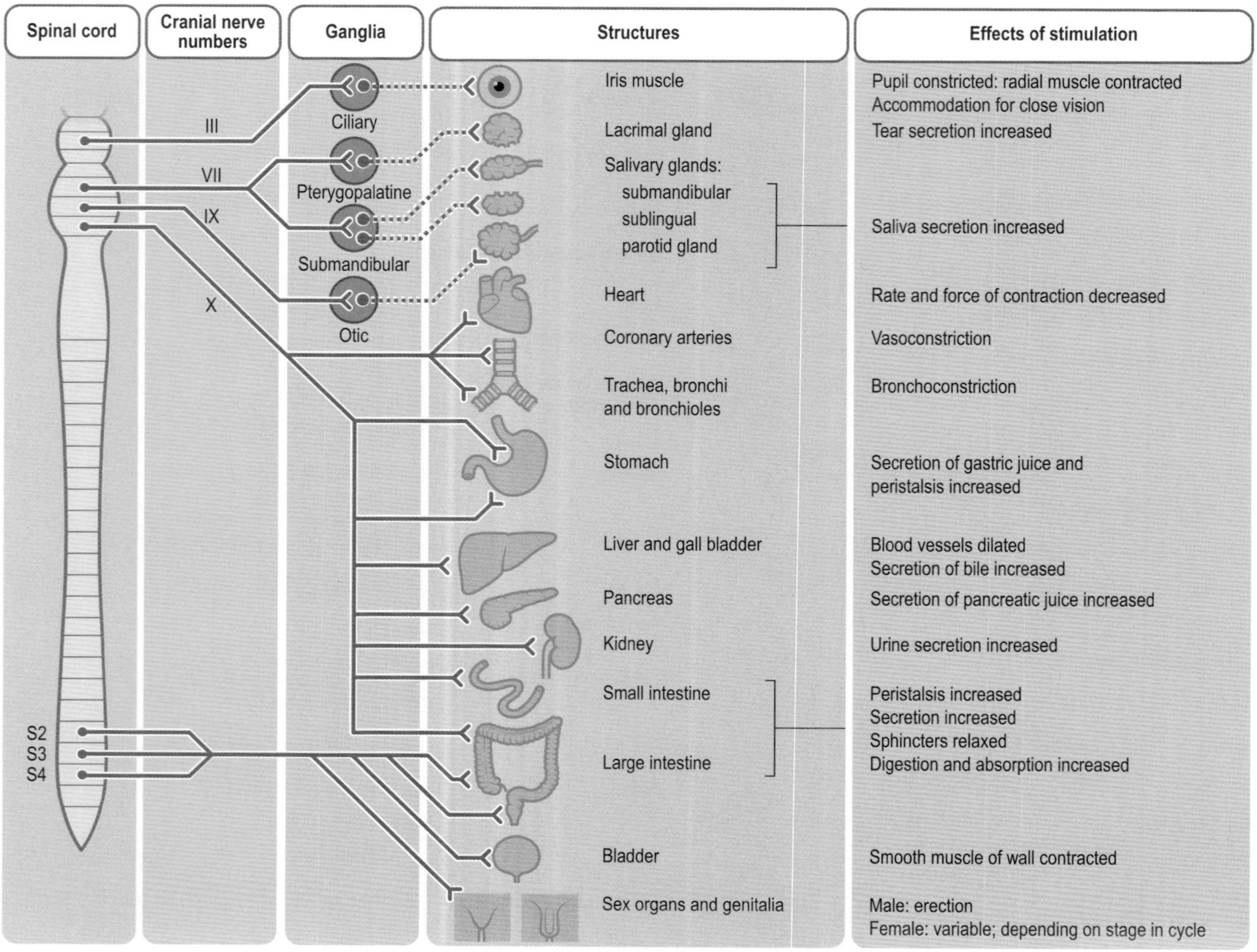

Spinal cord	Cranial nerve numbers	Ganglia	Structures	Effects of stimulation
	III	Ciliary	Iris muscle	Pupil constricted: radial muscle contracted / Accommodation for close vision
	VII	Pterygopalatine	Lacrimal gland	Tear secretion increased
	IX	Submandibular	Salivary glands: submandibular / sublingual / parotid gland	Saliva secretion increased
	X	Otic	Heart	Rate and force of contraction decreased
			Coronary arteries	Vasoconstriction
			Trachea, bronchi and bronchioles	Bronchoconstriction
			Stomach	Secretion of gastric juice and peristalsis increased
			Liver and gall bladder	Blood vessels dilated / Secretion of bile increased
			Pancreas	Secretion of pancreatic juice increased
			Kidney	Urine secretion increased
			Small intestine	Peristalsis increased / Secretion increased / Sphincters relaxed / Digestion and absorption increased
S2 / S3 / S4			Large intestine	
			Bladder	Smooth muscle of wall contracted
			Sex organs and genitalia	Male: erection / Female: variable; depending on stage in cycle

• **Fig. 27.6** The parasympathetic outflow, the main structures supplied and the effects of stimulation. Solid blue lines, preganglionic fibres; broken blue lines, postganglionic fibres. Where there are no broken lines, the postganglionic neuron is in the wall of the structure.

A preganglionic fibre reaching a paravertebral ganglion may:
- Synapse with a postganglionic neuron in the same ganglion.
- Ascend or descend within the sympathetic chain to synapse in another ganglion.

Fibres from T5–L2 pass through the ganglion and emerge as preganglionic **splanchnic nerves** (Mtui, Gruener & Dockery, 2020).

The splanchnic nerves—thoracic, lumbar and sacral—contribute to **nerve plexi** such as the aortic abdominal plexus, coeliac plexus, superior and inferior mesenteric plexi and hypogastric plexus. From these, postganglionic fibres fan out to reach their target organs (Table 27.2).

Postganglionic Fibres

From the synapse, postganglionic axons join the spinal nerves by non-myelinated branches called the **grey rami communicantes.** They are then distributed to sweat glands and smooth muscle of hair roots and blood vessels. Some postganglionic fibres travelling in the thoracic splanchnic

nerves synapse with adrenal medullary cells and are stimulated to produce adrenaline (epinephrine) and noradrenaline (norepinephrine).

Parasympathetic Division

The Cranial Outflow

Cranial parasympathetic preganglionic fibres run in several cranial nerves:
- Oculomotor nerve parasympathetic fibres innervate smooth muscle within the eye, causing the pupils to constrict and the lenses to shorten and thicken for near vision.
- Facial nerve parasympathetic fibres stimulate large glands in the head: the lacrimal and nasal glands and the submandibular and sublingual salivary glands.
- Glossopharyngeal parasympathetic fibres activate the parotid salivary glands.
- Vagus nerve parasympathetic activity accounts for 90% of preganglionic nerve activity. Axons synapse on intramural (within walls) ganglia of target organs—for example, organs in the thorax and abdomen.

TABLE 27.2	Segmental Sympathetic Supply to the Organs
Organ	**Spinal Cord Segment**
Head and neck + heart	T1–T5
Bronchi and lungs	T2–T4
Upper limb	T2–T5
Oesophagus	T5–T6
Stomach, spleen, pancreas	T6–T10
Liver	T7–T9
Small intestine	T9–T10
Kidney and reproductive organs	T10–L1
Lower limb	T10–L2
Large intestine, bladder, ureters	T11–L2

The Sacral Outflow

The sacral outflow arises from neurons in the lateral grey matter of sacral spinal cord segments S2–S4. Their axons run in the ventral roots of the spinal cord and branch off to form the splanchnic nerves contributing to the inferior and hypogastric ganglia. Most postganglionic fibres synapse in intramural ganglia in the distal half of the large intestine, urinary bladder, ureters and reproductive organs.

Visceral Sensory Neurons

Although the ANS is considered a motor system, there are **visceral pain afferents** in autonomic nerves which travel with somatic pain fibres. Visceral pain is caused by mechanisms such as inflammation, smooth muscle spasm and ischaemia. It is usually vague and deep seated and often accompanied by sweating and nausea. As it increases in severity, pain perception is referred to the somatic structures innervated from the same embryonic segmental level or dermatome (e.g., pain in labour).

Physiology of the Autonomic Nervous System

The terminal NT differs between sympathetic and parasympathetic nerves. NTs are molecules that help neurons communicate messages and regulate body activities and states (Marieb & Hoehn, 2022). The major NTs of the ANS are acetylcholine (ACh) and noradrenaline (norepinephrine).

ACh is released by all preganglionic axons and by the postganglionic axons of the parasympathetic system. ACh-releasing fibres are called **cholinergic fibres.** Most sympathetic postganglionic fibres release noradrenaline and are called **adrenergic fibres.** Exceptions are sympathetic postganglionic fibres innervating sweat glands, some skeletal muscle blood vessels and external genitalia which release ACh. ACh and

noradrenaline do not consistently produce excitation or inhibition on their target tissues. The response of visceral effectors depends on the type of receptor to which the NTs attach; there are at least two receptors for both NTs.

Cholinergic Receptors

Two types of ACh-binding receptors are given names associated with the drugs that bind to them, mimicking their effects. They are **nicotinic receptors** (binds nicotine) and **muscarinic receptors** (muscarine, a mushroom poison).

Site of Nicotinic Receptors
- Motor end plates of skeletal muscle cells (somatic targets).
- All postganglionic neurons, both sympathetic and parasympathetic.
- The hormone-producing cells of the adrenal medulla.
  The effect of ACh binding to nicotinic receptors is always excitatory.

Site of Muscarinic Receptors
- All cells stimulated by postganglionic cholinergic fibres targeted by the parasympathetic system.
- A few sympathetic targets such as the sweat glands and some blood vessels of skeletal muscles.
  The effect of ACh binding to muscarinic receptors may be excitatory or inhibitory depending on the target organ.

Adrenergic Receptors

There are two major classes of adrenergic receptors: alpha (α) and beta (β). In general, adrenaline binding to α receptors is excitatory, whereas binding to β receptors is inhibitory. There are medically important exceptions. Binding of adrenaline to β receptors of cardiac muscle induces vigorous activity in the heart. This is due to both α and β receptors having subclasses: α_1 and α_2 and β_1 and β_2 (Marieb & Hoehn, 2022).

Interactions of the Autonomic Divisions

Most visceral organs that receive innervation have dual innervation (i.e., sympathetic and parasympathetic). If both divisions are partially active, as is normal, a dynamic antagonism is present, allowing precise control of visceral activity. Antagonistic effects are seen on the activity of the heart and respiratory and gastrointestinal organs (i.e., fight-or-flight versus rest-and-digest modes).

Sympathetic and Parasympathetic Tone

The vascular system is innervated by sympathetic fibres which control BP, even at rest. The partial constriction of blood vessels maintaining vasomotor tone is under sympathetic control. If blood flow needs increasing, sympathetic impulses increase, vessels constrict and BP rises. If BP needs decreasing, impulses decrease, smooth muscle relaxes and vessels dilate. However, the heart, along with the gastrointestinal tract and urinary tract, is dominated by parasympathetic effects. The smooth muscles of these organs exhibit parasympathetic tone. The sympathetic division overrides this parasympathetic tone during stress.

Effects Unique to the Sympathetic Division

Some physiological functions are not under parasympathetic influences and are controlled by the sympathetic division. These include:

- Control of the adrenal medulla.
- Sweat glands.
- Erector pili muscles.
- Production of rennin by the kidney.
- Thermoregulatory response to heat.
- Mobilization of glucose and fats for fuel.

Control of Autonomic Functioning

Several levels in the CNS contribute to regulation of the ANS. These include controls in the brainstem modified by the hypothalamus and cerebral cortex.

Brainstem Controls

Most sensory impulses causing autonomic reflexes arrive in the brainstem via afferents from the vagus nerve. Centres in the medulla influenced include the cardiac, vasomotor and respiratory centres, and those controlling gastrointestinal activities. Control of micturition and defecation are reflexes that can be overcome by conscious control.

Hypothalamic Controls

Signals from the hypothalamus can affect the autonomic centres in the brainstem. It co-ordinates heart activity, BP, body temperature, water balance, endocrine activity, emotional states such as rage or pleasure and biological drives such as hunger and thirst. It can influence and be influenced by higher cortical centres. The hypothalamus is the main integration centre for the ANS, and the brainstem can be thought of as a relay station. Medial and anterior hypothalamic regions direct parasympathetic activities, whereas the posterior and lateral areas direct sympathetic functions.

Cortical Controls

Signals from the cerebrum can influence the activities of most of the brainstem autonomic control centres (Hall & Hall, 2020). Research areas include meditation, biofeedback, neuropsychoimmunity and psychosomatic illness.

Adaptation to Pregnancy

Changes in the functioning of the PNS and ANS are related to changes in the endocrine system during pregnancy. Chapter 54 describes neurohormonal reflexes in lactation. The role of the sympathetic system in the stress response is important for understanding uterine muscle activity and cervical dilatation in labour.

Main Points

- The PNS passes information about changes in the external and internal environment back to the CNS so that appropriate action can be taken. Sensory afferent nerves include sensation from skin, muscles, joints and viscera.
- Descending tracts carry efferent messages from the brain down the spinal cord.
- Pyramidal cells of the motor cortex are upper motor neurons. Anterior horn neuron axons leaving the cord to innervate skeletal muscles are lower motor neurons.
- Reflexes occur over reflex arcs and may be somatic or autonomic. Many spinal reflexes occur with little or no brain input.
- The ANS maintains stability of the body's internal environment. Motor neurons innervate smooth muscle, cardiac muscle and glands, making functional adjustments in response to visceral messages sent to the CNS.
- The ANS is divided into the (1) sympathetic nervous system (prepares the body for emergency action) and (2) parasympathetic system (calming effect). The dynamic interaction aims to maximize homeostasis.
- Sympathetic activity tends to inhibit the activity of visceral organs. Sympathetic fibres innervate sweat glands, smooth muscle fibres (e.g., erector pili) and blood vessels.
- Visceral pain afferents in autonomic nerves respond to ischaemia, distension, smooth muscle spasm and inflammation.
- Most visceral organs are innervated by both sympathetic and parasympathetic fibres.
- NTs of the ANS are ACh and noradrenaline. Ach is released by all preganglionic axons and by parasympathetic postganglionic axons.
- Most sympathetic postganglionic fibres are adrenergic.
- The sympathetic division controls vasomotor tone by partial constriction of blood vessels. The heart, gastrointestinal tract and urinary tract are dominated by parasympathetic impulses.
- The brainstem, hypothalamus and cerebral cortex in the CNS contribute to regulation of the ANS.

References

Hall, J.E., Hall, M.E., 2020. Guyton & Hall Textbook of Medical Physiology, fourteenth ed. Elsevier, Philadelphia.

Marieb, E.N., Hoehn, K., 2022. Human Anatomy and Physiology, twelfth ed. Pearson, Harlow.

Mtui, E., Gruener, G., Dockery, P., 2020. Fitzgerald's Clinical Neuroanatomy and Neuroscience, eighth ed. Elsevier, Philadelphia.

Annotated recommended reading

Marieb, E.N., Hoehn, K., 2022. Human Anatomy and Physiology, twelfth ed. Pearson, Harlow.

This is still one of the best general anatomy and physiology textbooks. Although not applied to reproduction, it has succinct explanations on the anatomy and physiology of the nervous system.

Mtui, E., Gruener, G., Dockery, P., 2020. Fitzgerald's Clinical Neuroanatomy and Neuroscience, eighth ed. Elsevier, Philadelphia.

This is a well-laid-out and easy-to-read textbook on the human nervous system. The format is full of interesting diagrams, and the headings make the book content easy to find and follow.

28

The Endocrine System

LYNSAY MATTHEWS

CHAPTER CONTENTS

This chapter discusses the endocrine system. The endocrine glands are detailed in relation to type, regulation, function and action in the body. The changes in the endocrine system during pregnancy are outlined.

Introduction

In the body, the nervous system (Chapters 26 and 27) is the rapid controller, whereas the endocrine system provides a much slower control and precise adjustment. The endocrine system facilitates the body's adaptation to external environmental changes by co-ordinating the internal physiology and modifying cell function. The endocrine system consists of glands widely separated from each other with no physical connections (Fig. 28.1). The endocrine glands are groups of secretory cells surrounded by an extensive network that facilitates diffusion of **hormones** (chemical messengers) from the secretory cell. These are usually secreted directly into the bloodstream where they are carried to target tissues and organs to influence cell growth and metabolism. This chapter will describe the role of the hypothalamus and focus on a selection of endocrine glands

and hormones. **Note the terminology**: endocrine glands secrete directly into the bloodstream, whereas exocrine glands (e.g., liver) secrete into ducts and channels.

The Hypothalamus

The **hypothalamus** controls the function of the **endocrine glands.** It provides a major link between the nervous and endocrine systems. As a **neuroendocrine** organ, the hypothalamus produces both releasing and inhibiting hormones influencing the production of anterior pituitary gland hormones.

Endocrine Glands and Hormones

Endocrine glands include the **thyroid, parathyroid, adrenal** and **pineal** glands. Other organs produce hormones, including the **pancreas** (Chapter 22), **ovaries** (Chapter 4), **testes** (Chapter 5) and **placenta** (Chapter 12). Functions of endocrine glands include reproduction, growth and development, mobilization of body defences against stress, maintenance of fluid and electrolyte balance, blood nutrient content, regulation of cell metabolism and energy balance. Tissue response to hormones varies and may take only a few seconds or days.

Hormones may be collected into distinct endocrine glands or found as single cells within organs; for example, the gastrointestinal tract. They affect tissues by binding to specific receptors on the surface of target cells. Some hormones act locally and are secreted into the extracellular fluid without entering the bloodstream. They affect adjacent cells of a different type (**paracrine**) or of the same cell type (**autocrine**).

Types of Hormones

Hormones can be divided into three groups based on their chemical structure: amino-acid derivatives, peptide hormones and steroid hormones (Table 28.1).

Overview of Hormone Action

Hormones only influence cells with specific receptors in their plasma membranes. This influence can involve a few tissues; for example, **adrenocorticotrophic hormone** can only influence certain adrenal cortical cells, whereas others such as thyroxine are essential for all cell metabolism.

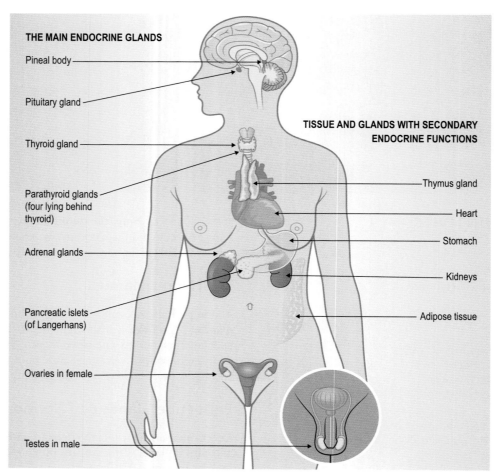

THE MAIN ENDOCRINE GLANDS

Pineal body

Pituitary gland

Thyroid gland

Parathyroid glands
(four lying behind
thyroid)

Adrenal glands

Pancreatic islets
(of Langerhans)

Ovaries in female

Testes in male

TISSUE AND GLANDS WITH SECONDARY
ENDOCRINE FUNCTIONS

Thymus gland

Heart

Stomach

Kidneys

Adipose tissue

• **Fig. 28.1** Positions of the endocrine glands.

TABLE 28.1	**Three Types of Hormones**
Type of Hormone	**Name of Hormones**
Amino-acid derivatives (from tyrosine)	Adrenaline (epinephrine) Noradrenaline (norepinephrine) Dopamine Thyroxine Triiodothyronine
Peptides (chains of amino acids)	Parathyroid hormone Oxytocin Vasopressin Insulin Anterior pituitary gland glycoprotein hormones (e.g., gonadotrophins, follicle-stimulating hormone and luteinizing hormone) Gastrointestinal hormones (e.g., secretin and gastrin)
Steroid hormones (derived from cholesterol)	Cortisone Aldosterone Testosterone Progesterone Oestrogen

When the hormone arrives at its target cell it binds to a specific receptor, where it influences chemical or metabolic reactions inside the cell (for lipid-based hormones) or on the cell membrane (for peptide hormones).

Hormones increase or decrease cellular activity by producing one or more of the following:

1. Changes in cell membrane permeability and/or electrical potential.
2. Enzyme synthesis, activation or deactivation.
3. Induction of secretory activity.
4. Stimulation of mitotic cell division.

Control of Hormone Release

The level of a hormone in the blood is variable and self-regulating within its normal range. It is affected by a negative and/or positive feedback mechanism.

The synthesis and release of hormones depend on inhibition by **negative feedback.** This may be controlled either indirectly through the release of hormones by the hypothalamus and the anterior pituitary (e.g., steroid and thyroid hormones) or directly by blood levels of the stimulus (e.g., insulin and glucagon). Hormone secretion is triggered by a stimulus and blood levels rise until they reach the required

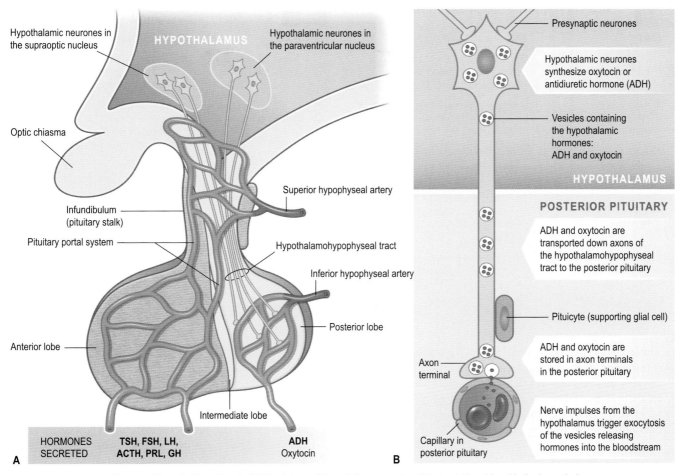

• **Fig. 28.2** The pituitary gland. (A) The lobes of the pituitary gland and their relationship with the hypothalamus. (B) Synthesis and storage of antidiuretic hormone (ADH) and oxytocin. *ACTH*, Adrenocorticotrophic hormone; *FSH*, follicle-stimulating hormone; *GH*, growth hormone; *LH*, luteinizing hormone; *PRL*, prolactin (lactogenic hormone); *TSH*, thyroid-stimulating hormone.

level when further hormone release is inhibited. This maintains blood levels within a narrow range. Stimuli can be hormonal, humeral or neural:

- **Hormonal stimulus**: hypothalamic releasing and inhibiting hormones regulate the pituitary gland hormones, some of which in induce other glands to secrete their hormones.
- **Humeral stimulus**: changing blood levels of ions and nutrients; for example, the production of parathyroid hormone is prompted by decreasing blood calcium levels.
- **Neural stimuli**: for example, the release of catecholamines by the sympathetic nervous system in response to stress.

Positive feedback mechanism is amplification of the stimulus and increasing release of the hormone until a particular process is complete and the stimulus ceases (e.g., release of oxytocin during labour).

The Pituitary Gland

The pituitary gland lies in the **hypophyseal fossa** of the sphenoid bone below the **hypothalamus.** It is attached to it by a **stalk** called the **infundibulum.** It has two lobes (Fig. 28.2):

- The posterior lobe (**neurohypophysis**), consisting of nerve fibres and neuroglia, is a downward growth of the hypothalamus. It does not manufacture hormones but stores hypothalamic hormones for release as required.
- The anterior lobe (**adenohypophysis**), composed of glandular tissue, manufactures and releases its own hormones.

The gland has a rich blood supply derived from the internal carotid artery via superior and inferior hypophyseal branches. Venous drainage is into the dural venous sinuses. The gland is susceptible to blood loss, particularly in pregnancy.

The Pituitary–Hypothalamic Axis

A nerve bundle called the hypothalamic–hypophyseal tract runs through the infundibulum (Fig. 28.2). The tract neurons are situated in two groups of nuclei in the hypothalamus:

1. The first group of nuclei secretes the posterior pituitary hormones: **oxytocin** from the hypothalamic paraventricular nuclei and **antidiuretic hormone** (ADH) from the supraoptic nuclei.

TABLE 28.2	Actions of Hypothalamic Neurohormones
Name	**Major Function(s)**
Thyrotrophin-releasing hormone (TRH)	Stimulates release of thyroid-stimulating hormone (TSH) and prolactin (PRL)
Gonadotrophin-releasing hormone (GnRH)	Stimulates release of luteinizing hormone (LH) and follicle-stimulating hormone (FSH)
Growth hormone-releasing hormone (GHRH)	Stimulates release of growth hormone (GH)
Growth hormone-release inhibiting hormone (somatostatin, SMS)	Inhibits release of GH, gastrin, vasoactive intestinal peptide, glucagons, insulin, TSH and PRL
Corticotropin-releasing hormone (CRH)	Stimulates release of adrenocorticotrophic hormone (ACTH)
Dopamine (DA)	Inhibits release of PRL

TABLE 28.3	Actions of Hormones Secreted by the Anterior Pituitary Gland
Name	**Major Function(s)**
Thyroid-stimulating hormone (TSH)	Stimulates growth and activity of the thyroid gland and controls production and secretion of T3 and T4
Growth hormone (GH)	Stimulates growth of tissues, especially bone and muscle, and helps regulate metabolism
Prolactin (PRL)	Stimulates milk production and growth of breast tissue
Adrenocorticotrophic hormone (ACTH)	Stimulates the adrenal cortex to produce and secrete glucocorticoids
Follicle-stimulating hormone (FSH)	Stimulates maturation of ovarian follicles and secretion of oestrogen by the ovaries and stimulates production of sperm in the testes
Luteinizing hormone (LH)	Stimulates ovulation and secretion of progesterone by the corpus luteum and stimulates secretion of testosterone by the testes

2. The second group, the hypothalamic–hypophyseal nuclei, is responsible for anterior pituitary function. There is no direct neural connection between the adenohypophysis and the hypothalamus. The vascular hypophyseal portal system carries hypothalamic releasing and inhibiting hormones to the anterior pituitary lobe.

Regulation of Function

Several hypothalamic neurohormones regulate anterior pituitary function. They have short half-lives in the circulation and act rapidly on specific anterior pituitary cells (Table 28.2).

Anterior Pituitary Hormones

The anterior lobe of the pituitary is called the *master endocrine gland* because of its control of other glands. There are six anterior pituitary hormones, four of which regulate hormonal functioning of other glands (Table 28.3). Abnormal levels of hormones can result in a variety of outcomes, demonstrated by growth hormone and prolactin below.

Growth Hormone

Growth hormone (GH) stimulates cells to grow and divide. It promotes growth of bone, soft tissue and viscera. Indirectly it promotes clonal expansion of newly differentiated cells mediated by **insulin-like growth factors** (IGF-1 and IGF-2). The amount secreted daily declines with age, and GH has a diurnal cycle, with the highest levels occurring during sleep. This is why sleep is important in recovery from illness and injury. It is anabolic and stimulates protein synthesis, facilitates the use of fats for fuel and conserves glucose.

Two hypothalamic hormones with antagonistic effects regulate production of GH: GH-releasing hormone and GH-inhibiting hormone (somatostatin). Hypersecretion of GH in childhood results in **gigantism** (reaching a height of 2.4 m). After cessation of longitudinal growth, enlargement of bony areas of the hands, feet and face occurs (**acromegaly**). Hyposecretion of GH in children leads to **pituitary dwarfism.** Body proportions are normal, but the maximum height is 1.2 m.

Prolactin

Prolactin (PRL) is similar to GH. The only known effect is the stimulation of breast milk production (Chapter 54). PRL is regulated by the negative control of dopamine (DA) in men and non-lactating women. Prolactin levels are influenced by the effect of oestrogen on the breast. The release of PRL just before menstruation accounts for premenstrual breast swelling and tenderness but no milk is produced. Hypersecretion of PRL causes inappropriate lactation (**galactorrhoea**) and is seen in both sexes, mostly due to an anterior pituitary gland tumour. Women will have amenorrhoea, and men may become impotent.

Posterior Pituitary Hormones
Oxytocin

Oxytocin is a strong stimulator of uterine contraction and is important in childbirth. Oxytocin is released during the final stage of labour due to the stretching of the lower genital tract, a phenomenon known as **Ferguson's reflex** (Chapters 36 and 39). It is also secreted after birth as a response to suckling.

Antidiuretic Hormone

ADH inhibits urine formation by influencing the renal tubules to reabsorb more water (Chapters 19 and 20). Less urine is produced and blood volume rises. Hypothalamic osmoreceptors monitor the solute concentration in blood and, if too much is detected, they send excitatory messages to the ADH-secreting neurons in the hypothalamus. ADH release is also stimulated by pain, low blood pressure (BP) and drugs such as nicotine, morphine and barbiturates. If blood loss is severe, enormous amounts of ADH are released, causing vasoconstriction and a rise in BP. ADH is sometimes called *vasopressin.*

Alcohol ingestion inhibits ADH production, causing diuresis. This accounts for thirst and dry mouth. Drinking large amounts of water will also suppress ADH release (Chapter 19). ADH production is similar in pregnant and non-pregnant women, but osmoreceptors are reset in pregnancy to accommodate increased blood volume.

Anterior Pituitary Changes During Pregnancy

The pituitary gland changes in pregnancy. In non-pregnant women, it is about 20% heavier than in men. During pregnancy, its weight increases by 30% in first pregnancies and 50% in subsequent pregnancies, almost entirely due to an increase in the number of prolactin-secreting cells (**lactotrophs**). The enhanced blood supply makes the pituitary gland more vulnerable to vasospasm, which may lead to **Sheehan's syndrome** (see Clinical Application 28.1). The number of GH-producing cells falls, probably due to the presence of human placental lactogen. GH returns to normal within a few weeks of delivery.

• CLINICAL APPLICATION 28.1 **Sheehan's Syndrome**

The oxygen demands of pregnancy result in increased circulation and increase in the size of the anterior pituitary gland. The unique blood supply to the pituitary gland makes it vulnerable to a reduction in arterial blood supply if there is vasospasm of the superior hypophyseal artery, leading to swelling and necrosis of the gland. This results in **Sheenan's syndrome** (or anterior pituitary necrosis), with symptoms caused by loss of the anterior pituitary hormones. One of the earliest signs is failure to lactate (due to prolactin deficiency), followed by amenorrhoea (due to loss of the gonadotrophic hormones).

Sheehan's syndrome is associated with a sudden decrease in blood volume or a localized bleed disrupting the hypophyseal portal system. Although rare, it is most associated with severe and prolonged obstetric shock, usually after haemorrhage during labour (Hinson, Raven & Chew, 2022). The activity of the thyroid and adrenal glands gradually diminishes, and the woman becomes lethargic and feels cold. Hair and skin become coarser. Genitalia and breasts atrophy, and the woman suffers loss of libido. Adequate and prompt treatment of obstetric shock will prevent the syndrome from developing. If the diagnosis is not made, the woman may die. Treatment is by total hormone replacement. The posterior gland is not involved because it has a separate blood supply.

During pregnancy, the fetoplacental hormones greatly influence the pituitary gland and the secretion of follicle-stimulating hormone (FSH) and luteinizing hormone (LH) are inhibited, possibly due to human chorionic gonadotrophin (hCG) release. Pregnancy hyperprolactinaemia also contributes to the fall in gonadotrophic secretion. Anterior pituitary hormone production changes in the puerperium to accommodate lactation.

The Thyroid Gland

The thyroid gland lies in front of the trachea and below the larynx. It has two lateral lobes joined by a medial isthmus. It is the largest adult endocrine gland, weighing 10–20 g. It concentrates **iodine** from the bloodstream to synthesize hormones. This gland produces two thyroid hormones: **thyroxine,** or T_4, and **triiodothyronine,** or T_3. Another group of cells, the **parafollicular cells,** produce the hormone **calcitonin.**

Thyroid-Stimulating Hormone (TSH)

Thyrotrophin-releasing hormone (TRH) influences the secretion of TSH from the anterior pituitary gland. The concentration of TSH in the circulating blood is the major factor controlling the rate of thyroid hormone release. TSH stimulates growth and activity of the thyroid gland, which secretes thyroxine (T_4; binds four iodine atoms) and triiodothyronine (T_3; binds three iodine atoms). The structure of the two hormones is similar, each consisting of two linked tyrosine molecules.

Release is lowest in the early evening and highest during the night. Secretion is regulated by a negative feedback system so that T_3 blood levels are maintained within a narrow limit (Fig. 28.3). When the blood level of thyroid hormones is high, then secretion is reduced. The opposite occurs when the blood level of thyroid hormones is low—then the secretion is increased.

Functions of Thyroid Hormones

In the adult, ~1 mg/week of dietary iodine is required for the manufacture of the thyroid hormones. Thyroid hormones affect most cells except the tissues of the brain, spleen, testes, uterus and the thyroid gland itself. They are essential for maintenance of normal metabolism by increasing the **basal metabolic rate.** Abnormalities of thyroid function are discussed in Chapter 35.

Changes in the Thyroid Gland During Pregnancy

Adaptations during pregnancy mimic hyperthyroidism (Blackburn, 2018). Overall thyroid function remains normal during pregnancy with only a small number of women exhibiting signs associated with an overactive thyroid gland, including thyroid hyperplasia or goitre. Although TSH levels remain within normal range, there is a reduced secretion in the first trimester, returning to normal for the remainder

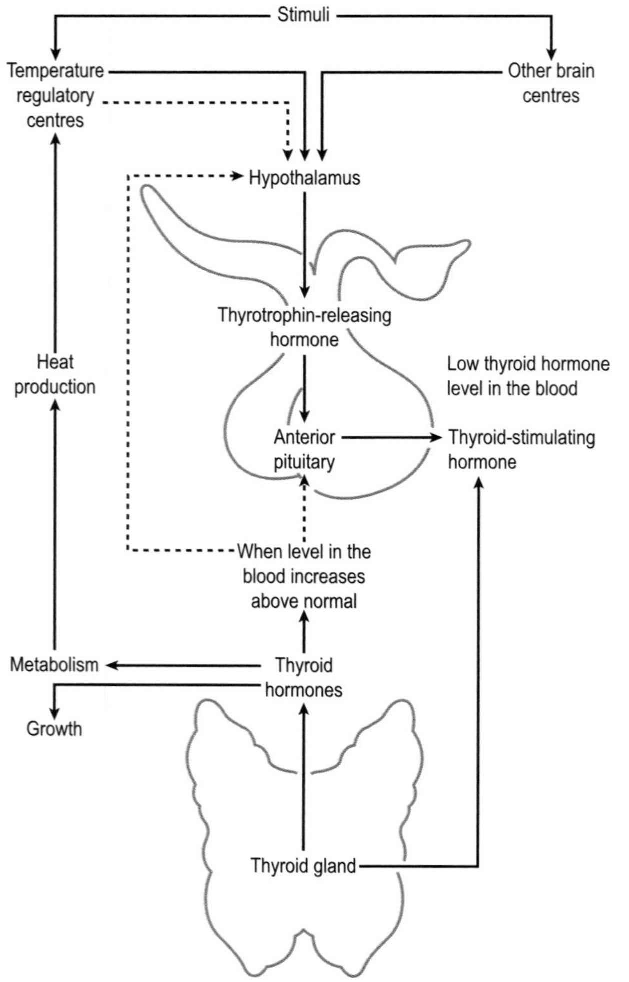

• **Fig. 28.3** The regulation of thyroid hormone secretion by negative feedback.

of pregnancy. During pregnancy, a balance is achieved by alterations in the metabolism of iodine. Renal iodide clearance doubles, plasma inorganic iodide falls and thyroid clearance of iodide trebles. The absolute uptake of iodine remains within normal limits. From 12 weeks, there is an increase in plasma thyroxine-binding globulin (TBG) and free thyroxine. The ability of TBG to bind doubles. Basal metabolic rate increases by 25% from 4 months. The changes revert to normal in the puerperium but may take 12 weeks.

These alterations have been linked with nausea and vomiting in early pregnancy, especially with hyperemesis gravidarum. hCG is similar in structure to TSH. When hCG peaks in pregnancy it is matched by a corresponding fall in TSH. hCG levels are high in hyperemesis and there is an increase in T_4 and T_3. Thyroid function reverts to normal for pregnancy when vomiting stops (Moleti et al., 2019).

The Adrenal Glands

The two adrenal (suprarenal) glands are situated on the upper pole of each kidney. The glands are composed of two parts, each with different structure and functions. The outer part is the cortex (essential to life), and the inner part is the medulla (not essential to life).

The inner medulla (reddish-brown in colour) is functionally part of the sympathetic nervous system. The outer cortex forms 80–90% of each gland and is derived from embryonic mesoderm similar to the ovary and testis. It is yellow due to its high lipid content.

The Adrenal Cortex

The cortex produces three groups of steroid hormones (from cholesterol), collectively called **adrenocorticoids.** The groups are mineralocorticoids, glucocorticoids and sex hormones (androgens).

The Mineralocorticoids

Mineralocorticoids regulate the amount of water and electrolytes in extracellular fluid by affecting sodium and potassium concentrations. **Aldosterone** is the main mineralocorticoid and is involved in maintaining water and electrolyte balance (see Chapters 19 and 20). Sodium balance is regulated by stimulating kidney tubule reabsorption of sodium ions from urine and returning them to the blood. Aldosterone also helps sodium reabsorption from perspiration, saliva or gastric juice. Potassium, hydrogen, bicarbonate and chloride ions are coupled to sodium regulation, and water follows sodium passively.

Four mechanisms help regulate the secretion of aldosterone (Fig. 28.4):
1. The renin–angiotensin mechanism.
2. Rising potassium and low levels of sodium in blood.
3. Release of atrial natriuretic factor by the heart as BP rises.
4. Decreasing blood volume and BP causes the hypothalamus to release corticotrophin-releasing factor (CRH), which increases adrenocorticotropic hormone (ACTH) production, leading to increases in aldosterone production.

The Glucocorticoids

Glucocorticoids include **cortisol** (hydrocortisone), **cortisone** and **corticosterone.** Only cortisol is secreted in significant amounts in humans. Commonly these are collectively known as *steroids.* They are essential for life, regulating metabolism and having a dramatic response to help the body through stress (Fig. 28.5). The control of glucocorticoid secretion is by feedback mechanism. CRH from the hypothalamus causes ACTH release by the anterior pituitary gland, which causes the release of cortisol.

Cortisol affects the metabolism of most cells by converting the intermittent intake of food to a steady level of plasma glucose by stimulating **gluconeogenesis,** the mobilization of fatty acids and the breakdown of proteins.

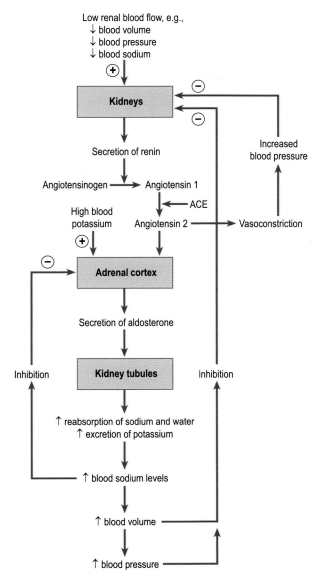

Fig. 28.4 Negative feedback regulation of aldosterone secretion.

Labels in figure:
Low renal blood flow, e.g.,
↓ blood volume
↓ blood pressure
↓ blood sodium
(+)
Kidneys
(−)
(−)
Increased blood pressure
Secretion of renin
Angiotensinogen → Angiotensin 1
ACE
High blood potassium
(+)
Angiotensin 2 → Vasoconstriction
(−)
Adrenal cortex
Secretion of aldosterone
Inhibition
Kidney tubules
Inhibition
↑ reabsorption of sodium and water
↑ excretion of potassium
↑ blood sodium levels
↑ blood volume
↑ blood pressure

Other functions of cortisol include:
- Reducing inflammation after injury.
- Enhancing the vasoconstrictive effects of noradrenaline.
- Increasing BP and circulatory efficiency.
- Maintenance of fluid balance by preventing the shift of water into tissue cells.

Sex Hormones

The main sex hormones (gonadocorticoids) secreted are the androgens with small amounts of oestrogen and progesterone. In adult women, adrenal androgens are thought to be responsible for libido. Adrenal oestrogens may replace ovarian oestrogens after menopause. Some women experience physical and psychological symptoms in response to fluctuating levels of sex hormones. These are outlined in Clinical Application 28.2.

CLINICAL APPLICATION 28.2 — Premenstrual Syndrome and Premenstrual Dysphoric Disorder

Women experience fluctuating levels of sex hormones throughout the menstrual cycle. Oestrogen rises sharply around the time of ovulation (approximately day 14), followed by a rise in progesterone throughout the luteal phase (approximately days 15–28), before returning to baseline levels at the onset of menstruation. Some women experience a negative reaction to these fluctuating levels.

Mild to moderate physical and emotional symptoms are collectively referred to as **premenstrual syndrome** (PMS). Approximately 3 in 4 women experience symptoms of PMS in their lifetime (Green et al., 2017). Physical symptoms include bloating, breast tenderness, headaches or clumsiness. Psychological symptoms may include mood swings, irritability or weepiness. Although unpleasant, symptoms typically do not impact on everyday life and do not require medical management.

One in twenty women, however, experience severe and life-impacting symptoms, known as **premenstrual dysphoric disorder (PMDD)**. This is classed as a DSM-5 mood disorder and is characterized by debilitating psychological symptoms in the luteal phase of the menstrual cycle. Some, but not all, women with PMDD experience resolution of their symptoms during pregnancy (and breastfeeding), only for them to return with their postpartum menstrual cycle. It is therefore important for students and midwives to be aware of the symptoms, which may overlap with other pregnancy-related disorders such as postpartum depression or postpartum psychosis.

- Symptoms include depressed mood, hopelessness, feeling 'out of control' or overwhelmed, feelings of worthlessness and guilt, anger or irritability, interpersonal conflict, mood swings, rejection sensitivity, anxiety, difficulty in concentration, decreased interest, lethargy, hypersomnia or insomnia. Almost 3 in 4 women with PMDD experience suicidal ideation or thoughts of self-harm, and 1 in 3 attempt suicide (Eisenlohr-Moul et al., 2022). Although psychological symptoms are at the core of PMDD, women may also experience physical symptoms including bloating, breast tenderness or weight gain.

Information and guidelines for health professionals are provided by the International Association of Premenstrual Disorders (www.iapmd.org).

The Role of the Fetal Cortex

In a full-term fetus , the adrenal gland is 20–30 times larger in relation to other organs than in an adult (Blackburn, 2018). It regresses after birth to reach normal proportions by 1 year. The fetal cortex appears to produce mainly **dehydroepiandosterone sulphate,** which is the substrate for placental oestrogen synthesis. The fetal adrenals cannot synthesize glucocorticoids. These may be obtained from the mother or made by the placenta for:

- Surfactant production.
- Development of the hypothalamic–pituitary axis.
- Changes in placental structure and amniotic fluid composition during development.
- Initiation of fetal endocrine changes in the fetus and mother (possible factor in onset of labour).
- The development of liver enzymes.
- Induction of thymic gland reduction.

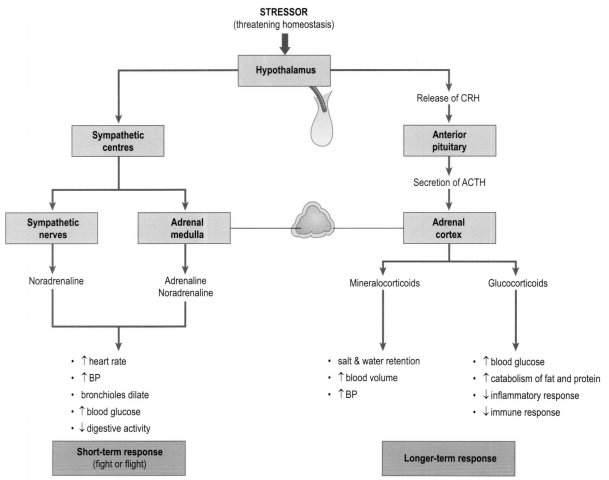

STRESSOR
(threatening homeostasis)

Hypothalamus

Release of CRH

Sympathetic
centres

Anterior
pituitary

Secretion of ACTH

Sympathetic
nerves

Adrenal
medulla

Adrenal
cortex

Noradrenaline

Adrenaline
Noradrenaline

Mineralocorticoids

Glucocorticoids

- ↑ heart rate
- ↑ BP
- bronchioles dilate
- ↑ blood glucose
- ↓ digestive activity

- salt & water retention
- ↑ blood volume
- ↑ BP

- ↑ blood glucose
- ↑ catabolism of fat and protein
- ↓ inflammatory response
- ↓ immune response

Short-term response
(fight or flight)

Longer-term response

• **Figure 28.5** Response to stressors that threaten homeostasis.

The Adrenal Medulla

Chromaffin cells produce the hormones adrenaline (epinephrine) and noradrenaline (norepinephrine), known collectively as the **catecholamines.** About 80% of production is adrenaline. Sympathetic nerve endings stimulate the adrenal medulla to produce the fight-or-flight response (Fig. 28.5). Adrenaline stimulates the heart and metabolic activity, whereas noradrenaline affects peripheral vasoconstriction and BP. Catecholamines produce short-term responses. During short-term stress, the main effects of the sympathetic nervous system are a rise in blood sugar levels and constriction of blood vessels. The heart beats faster, BP rises and blood is diverted to the brain and skeletal muscles.

Changes in the Adrenal Gland During Pregnancy

Cortical Function

ACTH plasma concentrations rise progressively during pregnancy, associated with a doubling of plasma cortisol, but remain within non-pregnant range. Normally, a rise in plasma cortisol would suppress ACTH production but the feedback mechanism appears to change during pregnancy.

The placenta may contribute to the increase in ACTH. The myometrium and decidua convert cortisone to cortisol, resulting in a local cortisol concentration of nine times normal. This may contribute to immunological protection of the fetus .

Cortisol

There is a steady rise in plasma cortisol due to a doubling of cortisol-binding globulin (also called *transcortin*). Free plasma cortisol is increased with loss of diurnal variation so that there is a greater maternal tissue exposure to it, especially in late pregnancy. The cushingoid appearance of pregnancy (with striae gravidarum, impaired carbohydrate tolerance and hypertension) may be due to the excess cortisol. There is increased cortisol production in labour, probably due to stress.

Aldosterone

There is an increase in renin substrate due to the higher oestrogen level. Excretion of sodium and chloride is increased in response to the presence of progesterone. Alterations in the renin–angiotensin mechanisms lead to increased aldosterone production, which enhances the reabsorption of sodium to maintain balance.

The Pineal Gland

The minute pineal gland hangs from the third ventricle. Neural connections between the retina and the pineal gland allow a light-regulated diurnal secretion of the hormone melatonin from its pinealocytes. This is highest during the night and lowest about noon. Melatonin causes the hypothalamus to inhibit gonadotrophin-releasing hormone. It also causes daily variations in temperature, sleep and appetite. The gland tends to atrophy after puberty and becomes calcified in later life.

Main Points

- The hypothalamus controls the function of the endocrine glands. It produces releasing and inhibiting hormones to influence the production of anterior pituitary hormones.
- Hormones are classified into three groups: amino-acid derivatives, peptide hormones and steroid hormones.
- Hormones can only influence cells with specific receptors.
- The level of a hormone in blood is variable and self-regulating within its normal range. The synthesis and release of hormones depend on inhibition by negative feedback.
- Fetoplacental hormones influence the pituitary gland, inhibiting the secretion of FSH and LH. Hyperprolactinaemia also contributes to the fall in gonadotrophin secretion.
- Hormone production by the anterior pituitary changes in the puerperium to accommodate lactation.
- ACTH plasma concentration rises during pregnancy and is associated with doubling of plasma cortisol. The placenta may contribute to the increase in ACTH.
- During pregnancy the size of the anterior pituitary gland increases due to an increase in PRL-secreting cells. Enhanced blood supply makes the gland vulnerable to vasospasm with a risk of Sheehan's syndrome.
- ADH production is similar in pregnant and non-pregnant women, but osmoreceptors are reset to accommodate the extra blood volume of pregnancy. ADH regulation is an example of a negative feedback mechanism.
- The release of oxytocin during labour is an example of a positive feedback mechanism.
- The thyroid gland synthesizes the hormones thyroxine (T_4) and triiodothyronine (T_3). Its parafollicular cells produce the hormone calcitonin. Thyroid hormones affect most cells and are essential for maintenance of normal metabolic functions.
- Thyroid function remains normal during pregnancy. The basal metabolic rate increases by 25% from 4 months.
- The adrenal cortex produces three groups of steroid hormones: mineralocorticoids, glucocorticoids and sex hormones (androgens).
- Aldosterone regulates the sodium balance through the reabsorption of sodium ions from urine in the renal tubules and returning them to blood.
- Cortisol reduces inflammation, enhances vasoconstrictive effects of noradrenaline, increases BP and maintains fluid balance.
- In severe stress, the output of glucocorticoids rises dramatically to help the body through the crisis. Sympathetic nerve endings stimulate the adrenal medulla to produce the fight-or-flight response. Adrenaline stimulates the heart and metabolic activity, whereas noradrenaline affects peripheral vasoconstriction and BP.
- The cushingoid appearance of pregnancy with striae gravidarum, impaired carbohydrate tolerance and hypertension may be due to excess cortisol. Increased cortisol production in labour is probably due to stress.
- Excretion of sodium and chloride is increased in response to the presence of progesterone. Alterations in the renin–angiotensin mechanisms lead to increased aldosterone production, enhancing reabsorption of sodium.
- The pineal gland secretes melatonin, which causes the hypothalamus to inhibit gonadotrophin-releasing hormone. It causes daily variations in temperature, sleep and appetite.

References

Blackburn, S.T., 2018. Maternal, Fetal and Neonatal Physiology: A Clinical Perspective, fifth ed. Elsevier, Philadelphia.

Eisenlohr-Moul, T., Divine, M., Schmalenberger, K., Murphy, L., Buchert, B., Wagner-Schuman, M., et al. 2022. Prevalence of lifetime self-injurious thoughts and behaviors in a global sample of 599 patients reporting prospectively confirmed diagnosis with premenstrual dysphoric disorder. BMC Psychiatr. 22 (1), 199.

Green, L.J., O'Brien, P.M.S., Panay, N., Craig, M., on behalf of the Royal College of Obstetricians and Gynaecologists, 2017. Management of premenstrual syndrome. BJOG 124, e73–e105.

Hinson, J., Raven, P., Chew, S., 2022. The Endocrine System: Basic Science and Clinical Conditions, third ed. Elsevier, Philadelphia.

Moleti, M., Di Mauro, M., Sturniolo, G., Russo, M., 2019. Hyperthyroidism in the pregnant woman: maternal and fetal aspects. J. Clin. Transl. Endocrinol. 16, 100190.

Annotated recommended reading

Martini, F.H., Nath, J.L., Bartholomew, E., 2018. Fundamentals of Anatomy & Physiology, eleventh ed. Pearson Global, New York.

This physiology textbook is very detailed in relation to the endocrine system. It will provide the reader with a fuller explanation of the hormones than is provided within this chapter.

Useful Website

www.iapmd.org.

This is the website for the International Association for Premenstrual Disorders. It provides a lifeline of support, information, and resources for women and individuals assigned female at birth (AFAB) with Premenstrual Dysphoric Disorder (PMDD) and Premenstrual Exacerbation (PME). It is also an informative resource for professionals.

29

The Immune System

LYNSAY MATTHEWS

CHAPTER CONTENTS

The immune system is an intricate and complex system designed to protect us from the external environment. This chapter describes the divisions and cells of the immune system and different mechanisms of immune response, followed by an outline of the immune system during pregnancy.

Introduction

The immune system protects us from environmental factors such as micro-organisms, irritants and abnormal cells. Pathogens such as viruses, bacteria and fungi constantly invade the body, both on its surface and internally (Male et al., 2020). Larger organisms such as worms are parasitic, obtaining their food from our metabolic processes. Many micro-organisms cannot harm healthy individuals but may cause death if the immune system is defective.

From a global perspective, factors complicating infection include intercontinental travel, which makes the transfer of deadly organisms more rapid, and developing problems such as resistant strains of bacteria, for example, methicillin-resistant *Staphylococcus aureus* and *Clostridium difficile*.

Divisions of the Immune System

The immune system recognizes pathogens and mounts an immune response to eliminate them. Because there are many pathogens, a wide variety of immune responses is needed and there are three lines of defence. The first two, **surface barriers** and the **inflammatory response,** are non-specific (**innate**). The third is a specific response (**acquired, adaptive**) to a particular foreign protein. Innate (non-specific) immunity prevents entry of many pathogens and acts rapidly to destroy those that manage to cross the barriers. Acquired (specific) immunity acts against a particular invader. This defence mechanism takes longer to mobilize but is highly effective. The two categories of immune response are interdependent and work together to either destroy the invader or reduce its harmful effects (Fig. 29.1).

Cells of the Immune System

Immune responses are mediated by a variety of cells and the soluble molecules they secrete. Leucocytes (white blood cells) are protective against bacteria, viruses, parasites, toxins and tumour cells. Most leucocytes are in the tissues, and there is a wide variation in the blood count as cells enter and leave the circulation from hour to hour. All leucocytes are produced in the bone marrow from **haematopoietic stem cells** (Male et al., 2020).

Types of Leucocytes

Several types of leucocytes are distinguished by their shape, appearance and function. **Granulocytes** (polymorphonuclear leucocytes) have granules in their cytoplasm which contain substances that fight infection. They are divided into three groups by the size of their granules: **neutrophils, eosinophils** and **basophils.** All are **phagocytic,** engulfing and destroying foreign proteins. **Agranulocytes,** which include **lymphocytes** and **monocytes,** do not contain granules. **Natural killer cells** (NK cells) are a specialized type of large, granular lymphocyte.

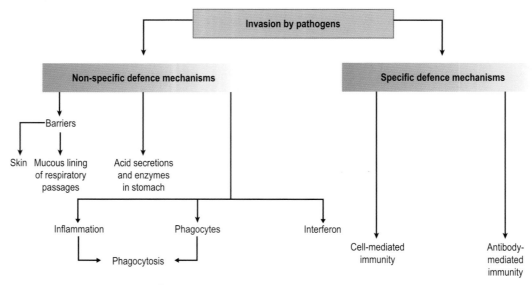

• **Fig. 29.1** Summary of specific and non-specific defence mechanisms.

Granulocytes

1. Neutrophils account for more than 50% of granulocytes and have the most lobular nuclei. They migrate to inflammation sites and are short-lived cells that engulf foreign material such as bacteria, destroy it and die.
2. Eosinophils make up 1–4% of leucocytes. They attack parasitic worms by surrounding them and releasing granular enzymes onto the parasite's surface to digest it from the outside. Eosinophils also deal with allergens by destroying antigen–antibody complexes.
3. Basophils account for only 0.5% of white cells. Their granules contain histamine, an inflammatory substance that acts as a vasodilator and draws other white cells to an inflammation site.

The Production of Granulocytes

The process of **granulopoiesis** normally takes ~14 days but will be considerably reduced if needed by cells. Within 7 hours of reaching the circulation, half of the granulocytes will have migrated into tissue and will not return. They survive ~5 days and are eliminated in faeces and respiratory secretions and form pus at infection sites. For every granulocyte in blood, there are 50 in bone marrow.

NK cells are present in blood and lymph, and account for 15% of blood lymphocytes. They only react to specific virus-infected or tumour cells. NK cells react against cells which do not express **major histocompatibility complex (MHC) class 1 molecules,** an important factor in the immunology of pregnancy.

Agranulocytes

Lymphocytes are the second most common type of leucocyte. Large numbers exist in the body, mostly in **lymphoid tissue.** They recirculate between blood and lymph and are subdivided into small and large lymphocytes.

There are two types of lymphocytes: **T** and **B lymphocytes.** Some lymphocytes leave bone marrow and migrate to the **thymus gland** where they will become T cells. They are selected so that they will not attack **self-antigens** present on the surface of an individual's cells. B cells were first identified in the **bursa of Fabricius,** a pocket of lymphoid tissue associated with the digestive tract in birds. T cells are involved in cell-mediated immunity and account for 80% of the lymphocytes found in blood. B cells are involved in humoral immunity and produce antibodies.

Monocytes are large cells produced in bone marrow from **myeloid progenitors.** Mature cells spend about 30 hours in the blood and then migrate to tissues where they develop into phagocytic **macrophages** (giant eaters). Macrophages regulate the immune response by presenting antigens to activate B and T cells.

Non-specific Responses

These can be divided into surface barriers, such as skin and mucous membranes, and cellular and chemical defences.

Surface barriers include:

- Intact healthy skin (with sebum and sweat).
- Intact mucous membranes lining the organs.
- Acidic secretions (e.g., in the vagina, gastric juices and urine).
- Sticky mucus to trap organisms.
- Ciliated cells that sweep particles towards the outside.
- Lysozyme, an enzyme that destroys bacteria, in saliva and tears.

Phagocytes

If intact surfaces are breached, cellular and chemical non-specific mechanisms are triggered. In most cases, phagocytic cells (Fig. 29.2) are involved. These are amoeba-like and

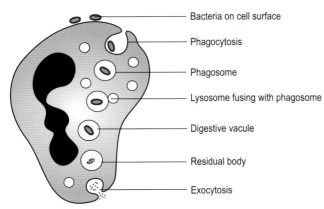

Bacteria on cell surface

Phagocytosis

Phagosome

Lysosome fusing with phagosome

Digestive vacule

Residual body

Exocytosis

• **Fig. 29.2** Diagram of a neutrophil undergoing phagocytosis.

travel through tissue spaces in search of invading organisms or other debris to engulf and destroy.

Macrophages are the main phagocytic cells and are long lived. Neutrophils become phagocytic if an infection is present and are destroyed during phagocytosis. Both cells destroy microbes by producing **free radicals.** Neutrophils produce antibiotic-like chemicals called **defensins. Complement proteins** and antibodies coat foreign proteins and provide binding sites for phagocyte attachment, a process called **opsonization.**

Inflammation

Inflammation is a physiological and localized response when there is tissue damage due to trauma or invasion by microorganisms. The response prevents the spread of damaging substances to nearby tissues, disposes of cell debris and pathogens and allows repair to begin. There are **four cardinal signs** of inflammation: heat, redness, swelling and pain. Depending on the site and type of tissue damage, chemicals are released into the extracellular fluid by injured cells, phagocytes, lymphocytes, mast cells and blood proteins. Four major plasma enzyme systems involved in the control of inflammation are (Male et al., 2020):

1. The clotting system.
2. The fibrinolytic system.
3. The kinin system.
4. The complement system.

The most important molecules are **histamine, kinins, prostaglandins, complement** and **lymphokines.** They induce vasodilation of localized small blood vessels, causing heat and redness. Capillary wall permeability increases, allowing a fluid exudate containing clotting factors and antibodies to seep into the tissue spaces and cause oedema and swelling. Clotting proteins form a **fibrin mesh** limiting the spread of harmful agents and acting as scaffolding for tissue repair. Pain results from pressure on local nerve endings, release of bacterial toxins, lack of cellular nutrition and the effects of prostaglandins and kinins. Loss of function may occur to aid healing.

The damaged area is first invaded by phagocytes. Rapid release of neutrophils by the bone marrow is caused by **leucocyte-inducing factors** so that the number of neutrophils

in the bloodstream can quadruple in a few hours. These cells are attracted to the injury site by chemicals called **chemotactic agents.** At the site, the cells cling on to capillary walls (**margination**) and squeeze through them (**diapedesis**) to the site where they devour bacteria, toxins and dead tissue. Monocytes now enter the tissue, swell and mature into macrophages.

If the infection is severe, pus is produced (from dead neutrophils, living and dead pathogens and damaged tissue cells). An abscess forms if this becomes walled off by collagen fibres. Some bacteria like *Tuberculosis bacillus* are resistant to digestion by macrophages because of their waxy outer coat and remain alive inside the macrophage. Infectious **granulomas** develop which have a central core of infected macrophages surrounded by uninfected macrophages and an outer fibrous capsule. Individuals become ill if resistance to infection is reduced.

Fever

Fever is an elevation of the body temperature in response to chemicals called **pyrogens** (e.g., **interleukins**). High fevers are dangerous because they inactivate enzymes and disrupt cellular metabolic processes. Mild-to-moderate fevers are helpful for stimulating the immune system and speeding up both metabolic rate of tissue and defensive actions to aid repair (Male et al., 2020). Antibacterial responses include the sequestering of zinc and iron in the liver and spleen to prevent their use as nutrients by bacteria.

Complement

Complement is a system of ~30 antimicrobial plasma proteins constituting ~10% of total plasma proteins. The term refers to the fact that this system complements the action of antibodies. They normally circulate in the blood in an inactive state. Their functions are (Male et al., 2020):

- Control of inflammatory reactions.
- Chemotaxis.
- Clearance of immune complexes.
- Cellular inactivation.
- Antimicrobial defence.
- Development of antibody responses.

Activation of the complement system (important proteins are **C1–C9**) releases chemical mediators, increasing the inflammatory response and enhancing the specific immune system. Complement can be activated by three pathways which activate C3, causing it to split into two fragments, C3a and C3b:

1. The **classical pathway** (Fig. 29.3) is activated by the formation of antigen–antibody complexes (most active and effective).
2. The **lectin pathway** is similar but activated by bacterial carbohydrates.
3. The evolutionary older alternative pathway provides non-specific immunity and is triggered by the presence of microbial pathogens.

An orderly **cascade** of complement protein activation occurs. C3b binds to the target cell's surface, resulting in the insertion of a group of complement proteins called the

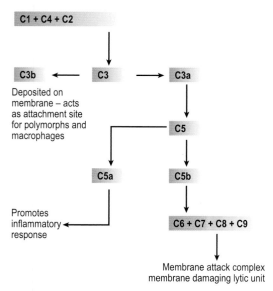

C1 + C4 + C2

C3b ← C3 → C3a

Deposited on membrane – acts as attachment site for polymorphs and macrophages

C5

C5a   C5b

Promotes inflammatory response

C6 + C7 + C8 + C9

Membrane attack complex membrane damaging lytic unit

• **Fig. 29.3** Simplified complement pathway.

membrane attack complex into the bacterial cell wall, punching a hole and allowing solutes to leak from the cell, which destroys it.

Specific Defence: the Immune System
Tissues of the Lymphatic System

The lymphatic system consists of two parts: a network of lymphatic vessels and lymphoid organs and tissues throughout the body. Organs and tissues are divided into **primary lymphoid organs,** such as the bone marrow and thymus gland where B and T cells mature, and the **peripheral lymphoid system** where they spend most of their active lives (Fig. 29.4). The peripheral lymphoid system includes encapsulated organs such as the spleen, tonsils and lymph nodes. Unencapsulated lymphoid tissue is found associated with mucosal surfaces in the gut, lungs and urogenital tract. Tissues of the lymphatic system are outlined in Box 29.1.

The Immune Response

Immunity can be active or passive. Active immunity is naturally acquired when the body is exposed to infection. Passive immunity can be naturally or artificially acquired (see Clinical Application 29.1).

Three important aspects of the immune response include:
1. It is antigen specific—directed against particular pathogens or foreign substances.
2. It is systemic—not restricted to the initial site of infection.
3. It has memory—recognizes and responds to an antigen from previous invasion.

Immunity can be divided into two types. **Humoral immunity,** or **antibody-mediated immunity,** is provided by the presence of antibodies in body fluids (humours). **Cellular immunity,** or **cell-mediated immunity,** is when

---

• BOX 29.1   Tissues of the Lymphatic System

Lymph Nodes

The immune response takes place in the lymphatic system. The kidney-shaped **lymph nodes** (Fig. 29.5) filter lymph, consisting of a radial network of fibres with embedded lymphocytes. The inner medulla contains macrophages, T cells, B cells and plasma cells. B cells are concentrated in primary and secondary follicles in the cortex. Cells at the centre of a follicle divide, whereas those at the periphery produce antibodies. T cells are found in the paracortical area.

Macrophages are fixed in lymphoid organs, whereas lymphocytes also circulate in the body. Lymph capillaries pick up pathogens and other foreign protein. Immune cells in lymph nodes are protective locally; for instance the tonsils combat organisms invading the nasal and oral cavities.

The Spleen

The **spleen,** the largest lymphoid organ, is located on the left of the body below the diaphragm. It is composed of venous sinuses and reticular connective tissue forming the **red pulp** where removal of ageing and defective red cells, cellular debris and micro-organisms takes place. Areas of reticular fibres with attached lymphocytes called the **white pulp** provide sites for lymphocyte proliferation. The spleen stores products from broken-down red cells and platelets.

The Thymus Gland

This bilobed gland, found in the mediastinum of thorax, is more active during childhood. It is organized into lobules. Within each lobule, lymphoid cells (**thymocytes**) are arranged in an outer cortex and inner medulla. The cortex contains immature cells, and the medulla contains densely packed, more mature cells. During adolescence, it decreases in size and atrophies. The thymus is involved in the differentiation of T lymphocytes. Embryonic stem cells migrate from bone marrow to the thymus, where they mature and differentiate.

Lymphatic Vessels

An extensive network of lymphatic vessels connects tissues to lymphoid organs. Lymphatic capillaries are like blood capillaries. Their cell wall endothelium does not lie on a basement membrane. They join to make larger vessels containing walls with smooth muscle and one-way valves. The flow of lymph is ensured by skeletal muscle contraction and negative intrathoracic pressure. Unlike veins, lymphatic vessels contract rhythmically to help lymph flow.

Lymph

Lymph originates as plasma which leaks from blood capillaries. It transports water and small molecules. Dietary fat is absorbed as triglycerides from the small intestinal villi.

Up to 4 L of lymph accumulates over 24 hours and is returned to blood into the large neck veins via the thoracic duct, which arises anterior to the second lumbar vertebra as an enlarged sac called the *cisterna chyli*. It drains the lower limbs, digestive system, left arm and left side of thorax, neck and head. The smaller right lymphatic duct accepts lymph from the right arm and right side of the thorax, neck and head.

---

lymphocytes attack an invader directly (Fig. 29.6). Three cell types are involved in the immune response:
1. B lymphocytes produce antibodies and are responsible for humoral-mediated immunity.

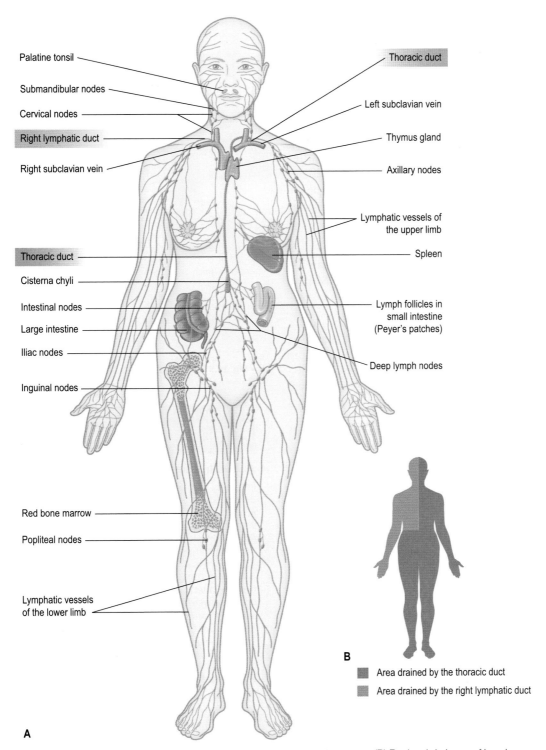

• Fig. 29.4 The lymphatic system. (A) Major parts of the lymphatic system. (B) Regional drainage of lymph.

2. T lymphocytes are involved in cell-mediated immunity.
3. Macrophages support two sets of lymphocytes.

The Humoral Immune Response

Recognition of a foreign antigen (non-self molecule) is the basis for specific adaptive immunity. Two different molecule types are involved: antibodies (immunoglobulins [Igs]) and T-cell antigen receptors. First encounter between an invading antigen and an immunocompetent lymphocyte involves the activation of a B cell and collaboration of T cells. Foreign antigens are molecules such as proteins, nucleic acids, lipids and large polysaccharides. A small antigen area called an **epitope** is recognized by a small area on a B-lymphocyte cell membrane receptor called the **antigen-binding site.**

Pollen grains and micro-organisms are the strongest antigens. Small molecules such as peptides, nucleotides and hormones are not immunogenic but may form protein complexes to cause allergies. These are **haptens** and include drugs, detergents, plant products and industrial pollutants. The immune system responds by producing antibodies (Fig. 29.7).

Antibodies

Antibodies, also called **Igs**, are a group of glycoproteins present in blood and tissue fluid. Some are present on the surface of B cells, where they act as receptors for specific antigens. Others, secreted by activated B cells and cloned antibody-forming cells after an encounter with a specific antigen, are free in the blood and lymph.

Antibody Classes

There are five classes of Igs, each given a letter from the Greek alphabet: IgG (gamma, **γ**), IgA (alpha, α), IgM (mu, μ), IgD (delta, δ) and IgE (epsilon, ε) (Table 29.1).

Antibody Functioning

Antibodies do not destroy antigens directly but inactivate them and tag them for other parts of the immune system to destroy by forming **antigen–antibody complexes.** Destruction is accomplished by mechanisms including complement fixation, neutralization, agglutination and precipitation. The first two of these are most important:

- **Complement fixation** is the main protection against cellular agents such as bacteria. When antibodies bind to a target cell, their shape changes to expose complement-binding sites on their constant regions. This triggers the complement cascade.
- **Neutralization** is when antibodies block specific sites on viruses or chemicals secreted by bacteria (exotoxins). This prevents them from binding to cells. Phagocytes destroy the resulting complexes.
- **Agglutination** of cell-bound antigens occurs because antibodies have more than one binding site and molecules have more than one antigenic site. Large lattices are formed by cross-linkage of immune complexes.
- **Precipitation** is a similar mechanism whereby soluble molecules are cross-linked into large complexes that settle out of solution. The large complexes formed by agglutination or precipitation are engulfed by phagocytes.

Cell-mediated Immune Response

T Lymphocytes

T lymphocytes form the basis for cellular immunity. There are two major groups of T cells: **cytotoxic T cells (T_C or killer cells)** and T_H cells or **helper T cells** (Fig. 29.8). All T cells have glycoproteins on their cell surfaces. These are **CD4** and **CD8 surface receptor molecules** (CD means *cluster of differentiation*). Generally, T_H cells have CD4 proteins and are known as *T4 cells;* T_C cells have CD8 molecules on their cell surfaces and are known as *T8 cells.* Both CD4 and CD8 cells can suppress immune responses (Male et al., 2020).

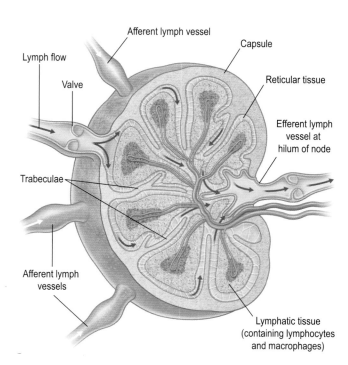

• **Fig. 29.5** Section through a lymph node. Arrows indicate the direction of lymph flow.

Active Immunity

Immunity to infectious diseases is naturally acquired when B cells produce antibodies against a bacterium or virus during an infection. Evidence of the naturally occurring immunity response was recently demonstrated during the COVID-19 pandemic (Sotgia & Lisanti, 2020).

Symptoms of disease may cause serious illness or death. This is where vaccines play an important role. The word *vaccine* is derived from the Latin for cow—*vacca*. Most vaccines contain dead or attenuated (weakened) pathogens which challenge the immune system without producing symptoms. This first came about when Edward Jenner noticed that people who caught cowpox were unaffected by smallpox (Sotgia & Lisanti, 2020). This technique is now used on a massive scale: protection against infectious diseases by raising antibodies.

Passive Immunity

Passive immunity can also be naturally or artificially acquired. Antibodies are not produced by the immune system but are obtained from another source. Protection against a disease is limited to the natural lifespan of the acquired antibody (usually 2–3 weeks). Naturally occurring passive immunity is acquired by the fetus through transfer of maternal IgG across the placenta and by the breastfed baby in breastmilk. Injection of immune serum such as γ-globulin can offer passive immunity to a person needing short-term protection from a pathogen they have been in contact with, such as hepatitis virus.

A further group of T lymphocytes identified, but not well understood, are **suppressor T (T_S) cells**. These can suppress both CD4 and CD8 cells by limiting the ability

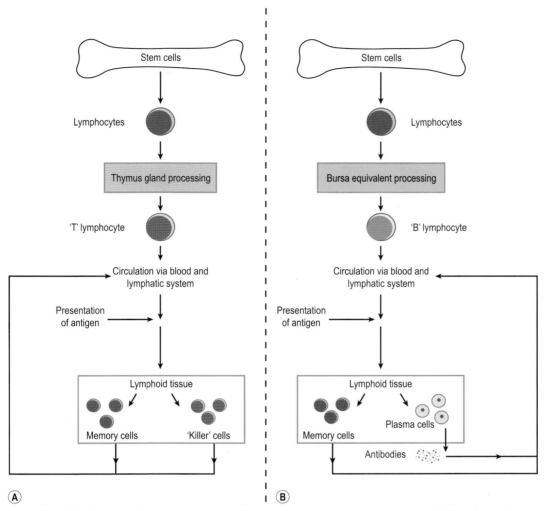

• **Fig. 29.6** Summary of the development of (A) the cell-mediated immune system and (B) the humoral immune system. Diagram summarizing the formation and protective function of the humoral immune system.

of the immune system to attack its own tissues, a process called *immune tolerance.* T_S cells are classified with T_H cells as regulatory T cells. It is believed that during the processing of T cells (via thymus and bone marrow), most of the clones capable of damaging a person's own tissues are destroyed before they can colonize the tissues.

The T-cell Antigen Receptor

T cells are distinguished by the type of T-cell antigen receptor (TCR) on their cell surface. The TCR recognizes antigen fragments bound and presented by specialist antigen-presenting molecules. They do not recognize free antigen—that is the antibody's role. **Class I** and **class II** molecules of the **MHC** are the most important. TCRs and antibodies are structurally related and both reproduce by cloning.

T-cell Differentiation: the MHC

For selection and cloning of T cells, there must be a double recognition of **antiself** (the antigen) and **self.** Every cell has surface proteins identifying it as self-coded for by the MHC, a very large gene complex. This provides the basis of

human uniqueness as genes can be combined in millions of ways. Only identical twins have identical MHC proteins, making tissue transplants difficult.

Two main classes of MHC protein important in T-cell activation are MHC class I and MHC class II. MHC I proteins are present on most body cells to enable self-recognition, but MHC II proteins are found only on surfaces of mature B cells, macrophages and some T cells. MHC cells are shaped like a hammock so that antigenic fragments to be displayed sit inside them, forming a self–antiself complex. T_H and T_C cells prefer different classes of MHC protein, a phenomenon called *MHC restriction.*

- T_H cells bind only to complexes that include MHC II proteins on the surfaces of macrophages.
- T_C cells are activated by complexes that include MHC I proteins on any cell.

Immunologic Surveillance

T cells crawl over other cells searching for antigens, a process called **immunologic surveillance.** When the T cell is activated by binding to the self–antiself complex, it

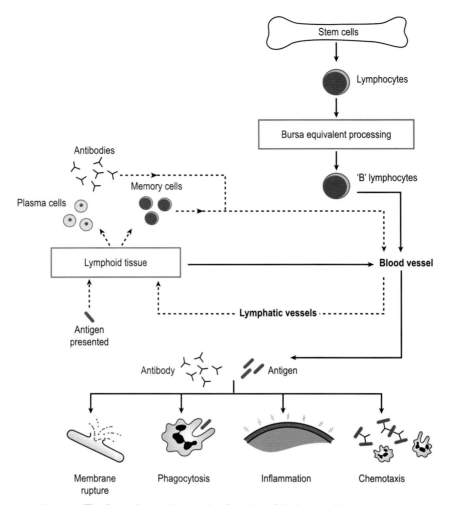

• **Fig. 29.7** The formation and protective function of the humoral immune system.

enlarges and forms a clone. Some, as with B cells, are left as memory cells. T_C cells act mainly against virus-infected cells but can kill cells invaded by some bacteria such as *T. bacillus*. T_H cells stimulate the proliferation of other B and T cells by releasing a **lymphokine** called **interleukin II.** Some T cells release lymphokines that inhibit the activated B and T cells, ensuring that the immune response is ended after the successful destruction of an antigen. Most T-cell activity consists of T_C cells attacking cells infected by micro-organisms or cancerous cells. They will also attack transplanted tissue.

The immune system cells release chemicals called *cyto-kines* (from cells) to stimulate each other. These soluble gly-coproteins fall into different categories: for example, they are called *lymphokines* when released from lymphocytes. Lymphokines enhance immune system cellular activity.

Cytokines

The principal sets of cytokines are (Male et al., 2020):
- **Interferons** (IFNs) limit spread of viral infections. They are produced by certain T cells early in a viral infection and may be the first line of resistance.

- They diffuse to nearby cells and stimulate them to pro-duce proteins that inhibit viral replication. αIFNs are produced by most white cells, and γIFNs are produced by lymphocytes. NK cells produce γIFNs, which can activate macrophages.
- **Interleukins** are a large group (>30 found so far). They are produced mainly by T cells and mainly direct other immune system cells to divide and differentiate.
- **Colony-stimulating factors** are primarily involved in directing the division and differentiation of bone mar-row stem cells.
- **Chemokines** are chemotactic cytokines directing cell movement around the body: for example, movement of immune cells out of blood and into tissues.
- **Tumour necrosis factors** mediate inflammation and cytotoxic reactions.

The Brain's Immune System

White cells secrete substances capable of killing neurons. These are prevented from entering the brain by the blood–brain barrier unless blood vessels are damaged. Microglia can

TABLE 29.1	Classification of Immunoglobulins
Immunoglobulin (Ig)	**Characteristics**
Gamma (γ)	IgG is produced in large quantities during the secondary response; diffuses through blood vessel walls and is the major class of antibody found in tissue fluids. IgG activates the classical complement pathway. It crosses the placenta to confer passive immunity to the fetus and is found in colostrum and breastmilk.
Alpha (α)	IgA protects the body's exposed surfaces against bacteria and fungi. Found in organ-lining mucous membrane secretions and in watery secretions such as tears, saliva and perspiration.
Mu (μ)	IgM is a large antibody found mainly in serum. The first and most abundant antibody secreted during the primary response. It binds to multiple antigens, causing them to agglutinate so that they are recognized by phagocytes. IgM is a potent trigger of the classical complement pathway.
Delta (δ)	IgD is mainly found attached to B cells.
Epsilon (ε)	IgE precipitates inflammatory reactions around parasites. Mainly bound to surfaces of basophils and mast cells (skin, lungs and mucous membranes). IgE is implicated in allergy and hypersensitivity reactions.

become phagocytic and are cells attacked by HIV attacks in the brain; their activation is implicated in AIDS dementia.

Physiological Changes in Pregnancy

During pregnancy, the immune system undergoes minor alterations in both primary and secondary defence mechanisms. The fetus is antigenically unique, and it is a mystery why it is not rejected as foreign tissue. The changes may help to protect the fetus but also increase the severity of autoimmune diseases (Blackburn, 2018).

White Cell Count

Total white cell count (WCC) rises early in pregnancy, mainly due to an increase in neutrophils and probably caused by circulating oestrogen. This increase peaks at 30 weeks, and a plateau is maintained until labour when there is a further rise, returning to a normal value by the sixth postnatal day. A slight rise only in eosinophils is seen with a sharp fall during labour. These are absent at delivery but return to normal values by the third postnatal day. Basophil and monocyte counts appear to remain unchanged.

Cell-mediated Immunity

Although lymphocyte count remains unchanged in pregnancy, there is a change in cell-mediated immunity. T_H cells decline in relation to T_C cells able to suppress the immune response, possibly due to pregnancy hormones. These changes are insufficient to prevent fetal rejection, so other mechanisms must also be present. Both maternal and fetoplacental mechanisms likely prevent fetal rejection.

Immunology of the Fetoplacental Unit

The fetoplacental unit is an **allograft** (foreign tissue from the same species) with different MHC cell surface receptors. Paternal antigens are expressed on fetal cells as early as the eight-cell stage. If the skin of a newborn baby is grafted onto the mother, she rejects it as foreign. In fact, there is an immunological rejection response to the fetus seen in the blood of pregnant women (Johnson, 2018). Alternative explanations have been explored, including a possible local immune regulation in the uterus due to high levels of circulating pregnancy hormones such as progesterone, corticosteroids and/or human chorionic gonadotrophin.

In summary, fetal protection from maternal immune response may depend on (Johnson, 2018):

- An antigenically unique trophoblast forming the front-line defences, possibly via local depression of immune reactivity. The fetal membranes separate the fetus (including blood) from the mother. The trophoblast at the fetal–maternal interface may be important in protecting the fetus from the maternal immune system by preventing maternal immune cells and antibodies from entering the fetal circulation. This does not fully explain, however, as some trophoblastic cells break away and enter the maternal circulation via the spiral arteries and provoke antibody formation.
- Special populations of NK cells in the decidua recognizing specific human leucocyte antigens (HLAs) on invading trophoblastic cells and via paracrine mechanisms regulating invasion and maternal immune resistance.
- A complete (or in humans, a highly selective) barrier in the transmission of immune cells or antibodies from mother to fetus. Although the placental barrier is effective against most cells and antibodies, IgG crosses to the fetus to protect it against any maternal infectious diseases with antibodies. Other antibodies such as rhesus may cross the placental barrier. The rhesus antigen exists as a cell surface antigen and is never found as a free molecule. Because red blood cells are too large to cross the placental barrier, there is no possibility of raising fetal antibodies unless maternal red cells escape into the fetal circulation, usually at delivery.
- Properties of fetal antigens mopping up any aggressive immune cells or antibodies before they can cause extensive damage to fetal tissues.

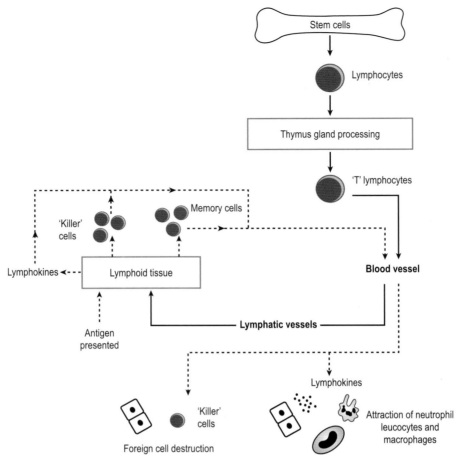

• **Fig. 29.8** The formation and protective function of the cell-mediated immune system.

The Immunology of Breastmilk

Colostrum and breastmilk during the first week after birth contain enormous quantities of immunoglobulin capable of reacting against many micro-organisms. There is protection against bacteria causing gastroenteritis in the neonate (see Chapter 54).

Autoimmune Disorders

There may be improvement, deterioration or no change in the status of **autoimmune disorders** during pregnancy. Both T cells and autoantigens (self cells) are needed to allow production of **autoantibodies.** The resulting immune complexes activate the complement system and mediate phagocytosis and an inflammatory response.

Pregnancy changes in the immune system are exactly opposite to the previously mentioned events so that women with an autoimmune disorder should experience relief from symptoms. Most women with **rheumatoid arthritis** improve during pregnancy.

However, women with **systemic lupus erythematosus** (SLE), particularly those with renal involvement, may have an exacerbation of their condition, affecting the fetus and neonate adversely. SLE is also associated with an increase in abortion and stillbirth (Wu et al., 2018).

Maternal Antibodies and the Fetus

The fetus of a woman with autoimmune disease may develop transient autoimmune symptoms. In **Graves' disease,** a thyroid-stimulating immunoglobulin crosses the placenta and may cause neonatal hyperthyroidism (see Chapter 35). **Myasthenia gravis** is associated with an antibody against acetylcholine receptors, resulting in profound muscle weakness. These antibodies can cross the placenta to produce transient myasthenia gravis in about 15% of neonates.

Main Points

- The immune system protects us from environmental factors such as micro-organisms, irritants and abnormal cells.
- Innate (non-specific) immunity prevents entry of many pathogens, acting rapidly to destroy those that manage to cross the barriers. Examples include intact healthy skin, mucous membranes, acidic secretions, etc.
- Acquired (specific) immunity acts against a particular invader. This defence mechanism takes longer to mobilize but is highly effective (e.g., peripheral lymphoid system).
- The lymphatic system consists of (i) primary lymphoid organs, where B cells and T cells differentiate and mature; and (ii) the peripheral lymphoid system, which includes encapsulated organs (e.g., spleen) and unencapsulated lymphoid tissue (e.g., tonsils).
- Specific immunity is divided into (i) humoral immunity or antibody-mediated immunity, which is provided by the presence of antibodies in body fluids (humours); and (ii) cellular immunity or cell-mediated immunity, where lymphocytes attack an invader directly.
- The five classes of antibodies each have a specific function: IgG provides passive immunity to the fetus; IgA protects the body's exposed surfaces; IgM is a potent trigger of complement pathway; IgD is found attached to β cells; and IgE precipitates inflammatory reactions.
- T lymphocytes form the basis for cellular immunity. Two major groups of T cells are cytotoxic T cells (T_C or killer cells) and T_H cells, or helper T cells. Both types of cells suppress immune responses.
- Most T-cell activity consists of T_C cells, which attack cells infected by micro-organisms or cancerous cells. They will also attack transplanted tissue.

- HIV attacks microglia in the brain and is implicated in AIDS dementia.
- During pregnancy, the immune system undergoes minor alterations in both primary and secondary defence mechanisms. Total WCC rises early in pregnancy, mainly due to an increase in neutrophils. There is a change in cell-mediated immunity. T_H cells decline in relation to T_C cells able to suppress the immune response, possibly due to pregnancy hormones.
- Fetal protection may be due to:
  - An antigenically unique trophoblast forming the front-line defences, possibly via local depression of immune reactivity.
  - Special populations of NK cells in the decidua recognizing specific HLAs on invading trophoblastic cells.
  - A complete (or in humans, a highly selective) barrier in the transmission of immune cells or antibodies from mother to fetus.
  - Properties of fetal antigens mopping up any aggressive immune cells or antibodies before they can cause extensive damage to fetal tissues.
- Colostrum and breastmilk in the first week contain high levels of immunoglobulins capable of reacting against many micro-organisms, particularly those that cause gastroenteritis.
- Active immunity to infectious diseases can be acquired during an infection.
- Passive immunity is acquired by the fetus by placental transfer of maternal IgG and by breastfed babies via antibodies in breastmilk.
- There is possible improvement, deterioration or no change in the status of autoimmune disorders during pregnancy.

References

Blackburn, S.T., 2018. Maternal, Fetal and Neonatal Physiology: A Clinical Perspective, fifth ed. Elsevier, Philadelphia.

Johnson, M.H., 2018. Essential Reproduction, eighth ed. Oxford, Wiley-Blackwell.

Male, D., Peebles, S., Male, V., 2020. Immunology, ninth ed. Elsevier, London.

Sotgia, F., Lisanti, M.P., 2020. Using the common cold virus as a naturally occurring vaccine to prevent COVID-19: lessons from Edward Jenner. Aging 12 (19), 18797–18803.

Wu, J., Ma, J., Bao, C., Di, W., Zhang, W.H., 2018. Pregnancy outcomes among Chinese women with and without systemic lupus erythematosus: a retrospective cohort study. BMJ Open. 8 (4), e020909.

Annotated recommended reading

Johnson, M.H., 2018. Essential Reproduction, eighth ed. Oxford, Wiley-Blackwell.

This book provides an excellent presentation of the possible reasons why the maternal immune system changes during pregnancy.

Kendall, M.D., 2011. Dying to Live: How Our Bodies Fight Disease, second ed. Cambridge University Press, Cambridge.

Although there is no recent update, this popular book presents the many levels of complexity of this subject in a manner that reduces the complexity without losing content.

Sotgia, F., Lisanti, M.P., 2020. Using the common cold virus as a naturally occurring vaccine to prevent COVID-19: lessons from Edward Jenner. Aging 12 (19), 18797–18803.

This is an interesting study showing evidence of cross-reactive immunity, to both SARS-CoV-2 and the common cold coronaviruses.

Pregnancy–The Problems

Although pregnancy is a normal physiological function, some women may develop illnesses independent of their pregnancy. Some minor health problems are caused by the pregnancy but are not life-threatening. These minor problems are discussed in Chapter 30. In addition, Chapter 30 now introduces the outcomes of the recent MBRRACE-UK enquiries into maternal deaths. A summary of the key messages is provided for practitioners involved in the care of women during and following pregnancy. In addition, there is a focus on related risk factors for pregnancy and childbirth highlighted in the MBRRACE report. Maternal deaths and risk factors will be referred to in several related chapters.

Long-term maternal health problems such as diabetes mellitus can be significantly influenced by pregnancy. Other conditions such as hypertensive disorders may be precipitated in some women by the pregnancy itself. Chapters 31–35 detail selected common pathological states relevant to the pregnant woman. Chapter 31 examines the possible causes and management of bleeding in pregnancy. Chapters 32–35 utilize a systems approach with each disorder discussed in depth including management in terms of diagnosis and treatment.

30

Minor Disorders of Pregnancy and Risk Factors

JEAN RANKIN AND THOMAS McEWAN

CHAPTER CONTENTS

This chapter first describes the common minor disorders often experienced by women during pregnancy. An overview of the key risk factors disadvantaging pregnant women is then provided. Risk factors result in adverse pregnancy, birth and maternal outcomes and are crucial to highlight to students and midwives.

Introduction

'*Minor disorders of pregnancy*' is the collective term referring to the range of inconvenient but not life-threatening symptoms often experienced by women during pregnancy. On occasion, the minor disorder may suddenly become a more serious maternal illness. Therefore, the midwife must pay attention to any signs noted or symptoms reported. This vigilance enables the midwife to offer the woman safe advice on alleviating the symptoms or appropriate referral as required.

Maintenance of Pregnancy

Once the blastocyst is present in the uterine cavity then the maternal physiological recognition of pregnancy begins. The development of the embryo and the placenta are described in Chapters 9–12. The corpus luteum normally regresses around 14 days if a fertilized ovum does not reach the uterus. The maintenance of the **corpus luteum of pregnancy** is attributed to the production of **human chorionic gonadotropin** (hCG) by the cells of the **syncytiotrophoblast** as they invade the endometrium. This is secreted into maternal blood and taken to the ovary where it augments the action of **luteinizing hormone** (from the anterior pituitary gland) to continue production of **progesterone** from the corpus luteum. The corpus luteum maintains pregnancy by secreting steroid hormones, mainly progesterone, until the placenta can take over the major role in early pregnancy (Johnson, 2018).

The hormone hCG can be identified in the blood 6–7 days post-fertilization and before the first missed period. The widely available **immunological pregnancy tests** are highly efficient at detecting the excretion of this hormone in the urine. There is no further ovulation, and endocrine production is changed to maintain the pregnancy.

Another important mechanism in maintaining early pregnancy is the suppression of **prostaglandin** concentrations in decidual tissue. In the menstrual cycle these play a role in **luteolysis,** the breakdown of the corpus luteum. Prostaglandin concentrations in early pregnancy are lower than in the endometrium during the menstrual cycle. This reduction in prostaglandin production is due to a substance that inhibits the biosynthesis of arachidonic acid, their precursor substance. The hormone **relaxin,** a small polypeptide, is produced by the luteal cells of the corpus luteum, with the levels peaking between 8–12 weeks and reducing by 20% as pregnancy progresses (Blackburn, 2018). This hormone inhibits myometrial activity and may play a role in the maintenance of early pregnancy (Fig. 30.1).

Minor Disorders of Pregnancy

The minor disorders occur because of physiological adaptation of the woman's body to pregnancy. This can be due to the effect of progesterone and other hormones on the smooth muscle and connective tissue. The common minor disorders are presented in relation to incidence, aetiology and management.

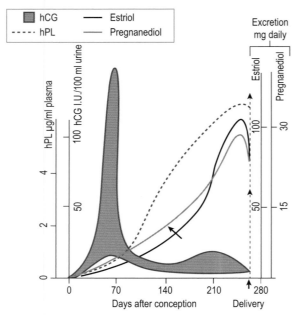

• **Fig. 30.1** Changes in hormone levels during pregnancy. *hCG*, Human chorionic gonadotropin; *hPL*, human placental lactogen.

The Digestive System

Nausea and Vomiting

Nausea and vomiting is a troublesome complaint experienced by 70–90% of pregnant women (Blackburn, 2018). The aetiology is not fully understood, although many theories have been proposed with insufficient evidence to be definitive. These include endocrinologic, mechanical, metabolic, genetic, allergic and psychosomatic aetiologies (Blackburn, 2018). It is more likely to result from a combination of metabolic and endocrine factors, with many being placental in origin (Patil et al., 2012).

Hormonal theories relate to the rapidly increasing and high levels of oestrogen, hCG and possibly thyroxine. Whilst evidence to date remains inconclusive, there is support for the hormonal basis. Findings from studies documenting nausea in women taking oestrogen medications or combined oral contraceptive pills have similarities with timing and the symptoms experienced in pregnancy.

Another possibility is that morning sickness is **adaptive** in an evolutionary sense, and nausea and food aversions minimize fetal exposure to toxins during the period of **organogenesis** (Blackburn, 2018; Patil et al., 2012). Women are inclined to eat bland food without strong odours and flavours. This avoids the ingestion of spicy plant toxins and foods produced by bacterial and fungal decomposition.

Clinical Application 30.1 provides further information on the management of nausea and vomiting.

• **CLINICAL APPLICATION 30.1**   **Nausea and Vomiting**

Nausea and vomiting can affect daily functioning and quality of life and cause pregnant women significant worry and upset. Therefore, the condition needs to be considered within this context and must not be ignored or dismissed as being a common symptom of physiological pregnancy. Although commonly referred to as *morning sickness,* many women feel nauseous with dry retching but may not vomit. Other women can vomit at any time of day. Very occasionally, the symptoms persist for the entire pregnancy (Crafter & Gordon, 2020).

Duration: the onset begins early in pregnancy around the 4th week. It usually persists until the 12th–16th week (Blackburn, 2018). Mild to moderate symptoms are usually resolved before 16–20 weeks' gestation (National Institute of Health and Care Excellence [NICE], 2021).

Management
- Reassurance that this condition is common and is likely to be resolved by 16–20 weeks' gestation.
- A wide range of pharmacological options are used in current practice – e.g., antiemetics, antihistamines (NICE, 2021).
- Discuss advantages and disadvantages of pharmacological options (NICE, 2021).
- Current evidence does not support the use of corticosteroids as a treatment for severe nausea and vomiting. However these may be used in cases of severe nausea and vomiting (NICE, 2021).
- Non-pharmacological measures supported – ginger (mild to moderate episodes), wrist acupressure (moderate to severe episodes) (NICE, 2021).
- Light snacks instead of heavy meals.
- Carbohydrate snack at bedtime.
- If vomiting persists or becomes severe, a medical practitioner needs to be consulted as a few women will develop severe vomiting known as **hyperemesis gravidarum** (see Chapter 34). Treatment involves intravenous therapy as an inpatient.

Further high-quality evidence is needed to confirm the effectiveness of interventions for nausea and vomiting in early pregnancy (Matthews et al., 2015).

Heartburn

Heartburn (**reflux oesophagitis with retrosternal burning**) arises from reflux of gastric acids into the lower oesophagus (Blackburn, 2018). The main cause is the relaxing effect of progesterone on the smooth muscle of the sphincter between the stomach and the lower oesophagus (Blackburn, 2018). In the non-pregnant woman, sphincter tone increases in response to raised intragastric pressure to prevent reflux. This ability is greatly diminished in pregnancy as peristaltic activity is slowed and gastric-emptying time is lengthened. Pressure from the growing uterus increases the intragastric pressure. Along with the flattening of the hemi-diaphragm, this distorts the shape of the stomach and decreases the angle at the gastrojejunal junction (Blackburn, 2018). The tendency towards reflux is increased by the decreased gastrointestinal muscle tone

• CLINICAL APPLICATION 30.2 Heartburn

Heartburn during pregnancy can be extremely uncomfortable and can negatively affect women's experience of pregnancy and their quality of life. About 25% of women complain of heartburn in the first trimester. Over the course of pregnancy, 80% of women report experiencing heartburn, which tends to be more problematic after 30 weeks and usually disappears after birth (Blackburn, 2018).

Management

- Offer general lifestyle and diet information for non-pregnant individuals (NICE, 2019).
- Prevent reflux by offering advice to sleep in a more upright position. Using additional pillows may help at night.
- Advise to eat small frequent meals, eat bland food and avoid spicy food.
- Avoid foods that reduce lower oesophageal sphincter pressure – e.g., alcohol, chocolate, caffeine (Blackburn, 2018).
- Antacids may be taken after meals and at bedtime only under medical supervision (Blackburn, 2018).

• CLINICAL APPLICATION 30.3 Maintaining Regular Bowel Activity

Constipation occurs in 10–30% of pregnant women and tends to be more severe in the first and third trimesters. The development of haemorrhoids may in turn lead to increased constipation because of a fear of pain. A poor diet and women disregarding the need to defecate adds to the problem. Oral iron therapy may also contribute to the problem for some women. Some recommendations are:
- Increase roughage in the form of fruits, vegetables and grains.
- Adequate fluid intake – both hot and cold liquids.
- Light exercise during pregnancy with early ambulation after birth.
- Use stool softeners.
- Mild laxative, monitor use and side effects.

(Blackburn, 2018; NICE, 2021)

and the relaxation of the cardiac sphincter. The anatomical changes may cause the sphincter to become incompetent, causing a **temporary hiatus hernia** (Coad, Pedley & Dunstall, 2019). Clinical Application 30.2 provides information and management.

Ptyalism

Saliva becomes more acidic during pregnancy with alterations in electrolyte content and micro-organism load but does not usually increase in volume (Blackburn, 2018). Ptyalism is excess salivation caused by the difficulty in swallowing saliva when experiencing nausea and vomiting in early pregnancy (Blackburn, 2018). If severe, it may lead to loss of fluids and electrolytes and dehydration. Similar advice as for morning sickness may help. It may also accompany heartburn.

This disorder, more common in women with an Afro-Caribbean background, is excess salivation and is the equivalent of morning sickness (Blackburn, 2018). In some cases, the woman must continuously wipe saliva from her mouth. It is referred to as *spitting* and is a sign of pregnancy, particularly in the West Indies.

Pica

Pica is the medical term for the ingestion of non-nutritive substances such as coal, washing starch, soap and toothpaste. This condition is also associated with pregnancy, although the prevalence remains unknown. A meta-analysis of 70 studies worldwide estimated the aggregated prevalence around 27% during pregnancy and postpartum (Fawcett, Fawcett & Mazmanian, 2016). Metabolic changes and hormones have been implicated. Research findings have not substantiated the belief that craving occurs because of fetal needs for certain minerals.

Constipation

Constipation is a common disorder of pregnancy. It primarily occurs from alterations to water transport and reabsorption from the large intestine (Blackburn, 2018). The increased production of progesterone in pregnancy causes relaxation and reduced peristalsis in the smooth muscle of the digestive tract. This increases the transit time of food through the intestine and a longer time for water to be absorbed in the large intestine. Other predisposing factors include compression of the rectosigmoid area by the enlarging uterus and changes in dietary habits and activity (Blackburn, 2018). See Clinical Application 30.3 for guidance on maintaining regular bowel activity.

Skin

Anterior pituitary production of **melanocyte-stimulating hormone** is increased by the progesterone and oestrogen levels of pregnancy. This increases skin pigmentation in pregnancy, possibly leading to a condition called **chloasma,** or 'pregnancy mask', typically found on the face. **Palmar erythema** may be seen due to increased circulation, and the palms may feel hot. The skin changes very common to all are the **striae gravidarum** of pregnancy due to the rupturing of small amounts of tissue under the skin caused by stretching of the skin layers. Women are advised to wear supportive clothing for the breast and abdomen (Blackburn, 2018). Although pink in pregnancy, as the skin returns to normal, the striae become mauve and less noticeable over time. Pruritus, or itching of the skin, can be a nuisance to the woman. Many women suffer from physiological pruritus in pregnancy, particularly over the abdomen as it grows and stretches. Cold compresses, oatmeal baths and topical creams such as calamine lotion can be soothing (Blackburn, 2018). Pruritus only becomes a problem when the liver enzymes are raised and **cholestasis of pregnancy** is suspected (Crafter & Gordon, 2020).

The Cardiovascular System

Fainting

The effect of progesterone on smooth muscle increases the incidence of fainting in pregnancy. Although the increase in circulating blood volume partly compensates, there is decreased vascular resistance. This alters the blood pressure and the venous return, permitting the pooling of blood in the lower extremities. Standing erect for long periods and the increased vasodilatation by being too warm may precipitate fainting.

In later pregnancy, **supine hypotension** can be problematic. This leads to the symptoms of nausea, weakness, light-headedness, dizziness or syncope (Blackburn, 2018). It is caused by the gravid uterus pressing on the inferior vena cava, preventing venous return to the heart and thus reducing cardiac output. It is easily prevented or reversed by avoiding the total supine position or turning the woman quickly onto her side if she begins to feel faint.

Varicosities

Varicosities (**varicose veins**) occur as an outcome of the relaxing effect of progesterone on the smooth muscle of the walls of the veins. They develop in around 40% of pregnant women. Varicosities mainly occur in the legs, but may also appear in the pelvic vessels, vulva and anal area with haemorrhoid formation (Blackburn, 2018). They are commonly found in the lower limbs as circulation becomes sluggish and the veins dilate, reducing valvular efficiency. The situation is exacerbated by pressure from the growing uterus, causing pelvic congestion and poor venous return and weight gain in the woman. Varicose veins of the leg can be made more bearable with the use of support tights applied in the morning and gentle walking to maintain circulation. Where possible, women should sit with their legs elevated and uncrossed.

Haemorrhoids occur as an outcome of the relaxing effect of progesterone on the veins of the anus, the reduction of venous return by the growing uterus and the incidence of constipation. They can be helped by the prevention and treatment of constipation (Blackburn, 2018). If needed, topical applications can be suggested and medical advice sought. As haemorrhoids often disappear after birth and because of the alteration in venous tone, surgery would not be performed in pregnancy.

Vulval varicosities, although rare, are very painful. A sanitary pad or sometimes a panty girdle may give support. Lying down will help prevent congestion in the area. Care must be taken during birth, as there is a risk of haemorrhage from the distended veins, especially if these are cut during an episiotomy.

The Musculoskeletal System

Backache and Pelvic Girdle Pain

Backache and lumbopelvic pain are common during pregnancy with the prevalence ranging between 50–70%.

• CLINICAL APPLICATION 30.4 **Pelvic Girdle Pain (PGP)**

PGP usually starts around 28 weeks' gestation. It is experienced by 1 in 5 women when walking, climbing stairs or changing position (Brook et al., 2017). Considering all pregnancies, PGP is deemed serious in 14–22%, of which 5–8% of women are complicated with severe pain and disability. Serious PGP is present in 7% of women postpartum.

Common signs and symptoms include difficulty walking (waddling gait), pain on weight bearing on one leg, pain and/or difficulty in straddle movements, clicking or grinding in the pelvic area, limited and painful hip abduction, difficulty lying in some positions and pain during normal activities of daily life (POGP, 2015).

Early diagnosis of PGP, advice and treatment can relieve pain safely during or after pregnancy. Based on current evidence, NICE (2021) recommends offering analgesics and providing information about lifestyle and health changes. Some hospitals have access to physiotherapy services to refer women for advice and guidance.

An appropriate plan for both pregnancy and care in labour should be developed and recorded. Relevant up-to-date advice and guidance are provided:

- Sitting – A comfortable chair is essential to support the back and thighs. The woman should sit well back. A small cushion may be required to support the lumbar spine.
- Standing – Backache will be prevented by standing tall with the abdomen and buttocks tucked in and the weight evenly distributed on both legs. Flat shoes are advised.
- Lying – Lying in the lateral position is preferred to the supine position. Good mattress support is essential. The woman needs to be advised to take care when changing position from lying down to sitting up to avoid strain on the back and abdominal muscles. Arms should be used to push up into a sitting position. Care is also required when rising from the examination couch. Advise the woman to roll onto her side and allow her legs to fall over the side of the couch, as this will reduce strain on the back.
- Lifting or dragging heavy objects should be avoided.
- Women need to adopt the best position at home and at work. Labour and birth – the birth plan needs to take account of safe and comfortable positions, analgesia and alternative positions for birth.

Differentiating the cause of back pain is essential to enable appropriate advice and treatment to be provided. Although the causes are multifactorial, postural changes result in lumbar lordosis with overstretched abdominal muscles and strained back muscles (Royal College of Obstetricians and Gynaecologists [RCOG], 2022). The relaxing effect of progesterone and relaxin on the pelvic ligaments may make the intervertebral joints unstable resulting in **pelvic girdle pain** (PGP), formerly referred to as symphysis pubic dysfunction (Crafter & Gordon, 2020). PGP refers to the collection of signs and symptoms of discomfort and pain in the pelvis and lower back (lumbopelvic) area, including musculoskeletal pain radiating to the upper thighs and perineum (Pelvic Obstetric & Gynaecological Physiotherapy [POGP], 2015). Normally the pelvic joints work together and move slightly. With relaxation, the distribution of pregnancy weight and changes to posture then the joints can move unevenly, leading to the pelvic girdle becoming less stable and painful (RCOG, 2022). Clinical Application 30.4 provides further information on PGP and guidance on minimizing pain.

The Nervous System

Carpal Tunnel Syndrome

Women who develop **carpal tunnel syndrome** (CTS) complain of numbness and tingling, often called *pins and needles,* in their fingers and hands. This is most likely to be present in the morning but can occur at any time of day. The cause is fluid retention and swelling of connective tissue which entraps or compresses the median nerve as it runs through the carpal tunnel in the wrist. It is more prominent in the dominant hand and usually occurs in the second and third trimesters (Blackburn, 2018). The woman may need to wear a splint at night and elevate the hand to prevent fluid collecting in the night. Occasionally the doctor may prescribe diuretics. This disorder is usually resolved by 3 months postpartum (Blackburn, 2018).

Fatigue

During pregnancy, fatigue is a physiological, psychological and potentially pathological condition of decreased energy (Bossuah, 2017). Many women experience fatigue in the first and third trimesters of pregnancy with a reduction in the second trimester. Lethargy and fatigue are often regarded as being normal for women to experience during pregnancy and the postpartum period. Women tend not to discuss fatigue with their midwife. However, fatigue has been associated with depression and nausea and causes an inability to carry out mental and physical tasks. Therefore, it is important for the midwife to distinguish normal maternal fatigue from clinical manifestation and advise women on self-care measures and when to seek medical care.

The physiological and psychological changes experienced in the early weeks of pregnancy can affect women's feelings about themselves. As sleep patterns change during the menstrual cycle, it would be anticipated that this would happen in pregnancy. Although sleep quality is reduced during pregnancy, it is not associated with changing hormone levels (Haufe and Leeners, 2023). Sleep is impacted by physiological factors including gastro-oesophageal reflux, musculoskeletal discomfort or nocturnal micturition. Health professionals need to be aware that sleep quality could reduce during pregnancy (Sedov et al., 2018).

The Genitourinary System

Frequency of Micturition

Urinary frequency is a troublesome disorder for women during pregnancy (Murray & Hendley, 2020). Frequency begins in the first trimester before the size of the uterus causes pressure on the bladder. The primary cause is the effects of hormonal changes, hypervolaemia and increased

---

• CLINICAL APPLICATION 30.5   Genitourinary Issues and Guidance

During pregnancy, urinary frequency (>7 daytime voidings) occurs in around 80% of women (Blackburn, 2018). Other common urinary issues include nocturia, dependent oedema, risk of urinary tract infections and difficulty in passing urine postpartum.

Urinary Frequency and Nocturia

- Restrict fluids in the evening by increasing fluid intake earlier in the day to ensure adequate intake.
- Encourage to void when there is sensation to reduce urine accumulation.
- Limit the intake of natural diuretics such as caffeine.
- *Nocturia* – lie in the left lateral recumbent position during the evening to encourage diuresis.
- *Risk of urinary tract infections* – screen urine culture at prenatal visits, encourage the use of the left lateral position to maximize renal output and urine flow.

Dependent Oedema

- Avoid the supine and upright positions for extended periods.
- Rest in the left lateral recumbent position with legs slightly elevated.
- Elevate the legs and feet at regular intervals and when sitting.
- Use support stockings, avoid tight clothing in the lower body and exercise regularly.
- Assess for signs of pre-eclampsia.
  Following birth: Alterations in bladder sensation can lead to overdistension with incomplete emptying and overflow incontinence. Promote adequate hydration and early ambulation, administer analgesia before attempting to void and place ice on the perineum to reduce swelling and soothe the discomfort.

---

renal blood flow and glomerular filtration rate (Blackburn, 2018). During the second trimester, the uterus is displaced upwards over the pelvic brim and the incidence of frequency is lower. Frequency becomes progressive until term, mainly because of pressure on the bladder by the growing uterus.

The increased reabsorption of sodium and water increases the need to pass urine through the night (**nocturia**). During the day, excess water is trapped in the lower extremities because of venous stasis. When the woman lies down at night, pressure on the large veins is reduced and there is increased cardiac return, cardiac output and renal blood flow with a subsequent increase in urinary output, particularly in the left lateral position. An increased risk of urinary tract infection occurs because of progesterone's effect on ureteric smooth muscle. This may cause **urinary reflux** or **stasis** (Blackburn, 2018). Clinical Application 30.5 provides guidance to address the common issues relating to the genitourinary system.

Leucorrhoea

An increase in white, non-irritant vaginal discharge is a normal feature of pregnancy. Some women still find this increase in vaginal discharge to be distressing or uncomfortable (NICE, 2021). Once the possibility of vaginal moniliasis or trichomonal infection has been excluded, simple personal hygiene will ensure comfort for the woman. Women need to be reassured and advised to wear cotton pants and avoid tights to increase comfort.

Risk Factors

The physiological adaptations occurring in the body systems during pregnancy are dramatic and profound. In addition, women also experience physical, psychological, emotional and social implications. In general, many women are resilient and cope with the changes and adaptations experienced and progress to have a positive pregnancy and birth outcome. This is not the case for all women, especially those who may be disadvantaged due to a range of risk factors that may negatively impact their health with potential adverse effects on pregnancy and birth outcomes. These risk factors need to be seriously considered during pregnancy, childbirth and the puerperium. The impact of death or serious health complications suffered because of maternity care cannot be underestimated. The impact on the lives of families and loved ones is profound and permanent (Kirkup, 2022; Ockenden, 2022).

Vigilance is crucial to ensure prompt action is taken with optimal teamworking as required (Kirkup, 2022; Ockenden, 2022). The worst-case scenario is maternal death and perinatal deaths for births. Box 30.1 summarizes the recent MBRRACE-UK report with key learning points and action points (Knight et al., 2022). Figs. 30.2 and 30.3 present the distribution of maternal deaths in risk categories from the MBRRACE-UK report and the key messages from the 2022 report, respectively. The key risk factors on maternal morbidity and deaths reported in previous surveillance reports are summarized in Table 30.1 (www.npeu.ox.ac.uk/ukoss/).

Risk factors are introduced at this point to set the context in relation to the subsequent medical, obstetric and mental health complications still to be discussed. Further details of the impact of risk factors in specific complications and emergency situations is provided as required. Table 30.1 summarizes key risk factors highlighted in previous surveillance reports on maternal morbidity and deaths.

Conclusion

Midwives play an essential role in the recognition and management of minor disorders of pregnancy. Women often discuss their discomforts with the midwife, who can reassure women that their problem is not health threatening and offer basic advice to minimize the problem. Occasionally with minor disorders, a more serious condition may be present, and midwives need to identify such cases and promptly seek medical advice.

• BOX 30.1　MBRRACE-UK Confidential Enquiry into Maternal Deaths During Pregnancy and One Year Following Pregnancy

MBRRACE-UK represents the gold standard around the world for rigorous investigations to drive improvements in maternity care. This recent ninth MBRRACE-UK annual report details the care of 536 maternal deaths between 2018 and 2020 and lessons learned to inform maternity care. Detailed chapters specifically focus on mental health and multiple adversity, cardiovascular care, hypertensive disorders, early pregnancy disorders, diabetic ketoacidosis in pregnancy and accidents.

The report recognizes the importance of learning from every woman's death during and after pregnancy and emphasizes the high level of vigilance required for all women, especially those women and their families who are disadvantaged due to existing or emerging risk factors during and following pregnancy.

Key messages for health professionals and those designing professional education programmes:

- Assess women with persistent and severe insomnia carefully for signs of underlying mental illness.
- Access services such as Psychiatric Liaison, Crisis and Street Triage Teams should alert specialist Perinatal Mental Health Teams to any referrals of self-harm in pregnant or postpartum women that they have received to allow triage regarding the need for specialist follow-up.
- Be alert to factors, such as cultural stigma or fear of child removal, which may influence the willingness of a woman or her family to disclose symptoms of mental illness, thoughts of self-harm or substance misuse.
- Wheeze can be due to pulmonary oedema; consider wheeze which does not respond to standard asthma management and exertional syncope as red-flag symptoms of cardiovascular disease in addition to orthopnoea and chest pain.
- Be aware of the common risk factors for heart disease and venous thromboembolism, such as extreme obesity, and consider on an individual basis whether women should be made aware of the symptoms and signs of heart disease as well as those of venous thromboembolism.
- Be aware that women using oral anticoagulation with warfarin may be more safely managed without transition to low-molecular-weight heparin treatment when having an early termination of pregnancy.
- Be aware of the added risk of fetal compromise when a woman's pregnancy is complicated by both hypertension and diabetes. It is not only babies predicted to be small for gestational age who may be at risk.
- Involve the critical care team in antenatal multidisciplinary treatment planning for women with serious morbidity who are anticipated to require admission to intensive care after giving birth.

For perinatal deaths for births in 2020, refer to Draper et al. (2022) and Knight et al. (2022).

For optimal care, it is essential for ongoing vigilance of women and new mothers to pick up early warning signs of the impact of risk factors and instigate immediate relevant action. Maternal risk factors need to be taken seriously to prevent and reduce adverse pregnancy, birth and maternal outcomes.

Missing Voices

Key messages from the report 2022

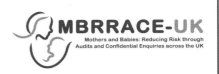

MBRRACE-UK
Mothers and Babies: Reducing Risk through
Audits and Confidential Enquiries across the UK

229 women died during
or up to six weeks after
the end of pregnancy
in 2018-20

10.9 women
per 100,000
giving birth
24% higher
than 2017-19

27 of their babies
died

**366 motherless
children** remain

A further **289 women**
died between six weeks
and a year after the
end of pregnancy
in 2018-20

13.8 women
per 100,000
giving birth

9 women
died from
covid-19

Excluding
their deaths,
10.5 women died
per 100,000
giving birth

19% higher
than 2017-19

**1 in 9 women
who died had
severe and multiple
disadvantage**

Most women died
in the postnatal
period **86%**

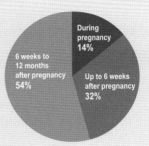

During
pregnancy
14%

6 weeks to
12 months
after pregnancy
54%

Up to 6 weeks
after pregnancy
32%

Black women were
3.7x more likely to die
than white women
(**34 women** per
100,000 giving birth)

Asian women
were **1.8x** more
likely to die than white
women (**16 women** per
100,000 giving birth)

More women from
deprived areas
are dying and this
continues to
increase

2009   **2020**

Number per 100,000 giving birth

20

10

0

2.5x

Most deprived

Least deprived

In 2020, women were
3x more likely to die
by suicide during or
up to six weeks
after the end
of pregnancy
compared
to 2017-19

1.5 women per
100,000 giving birth

• **Fig. 30.2** Missing Voices: key messages from the MBRRACE-UK report 2022.

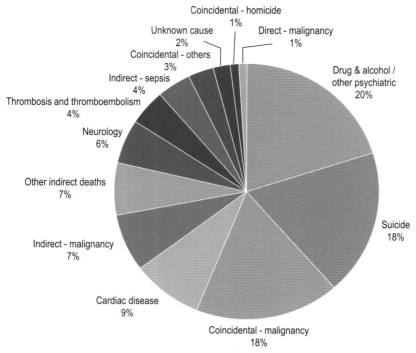

• **Fig. 30.3** Causes of death amongst women who died between 6 weeks and 1 year after the end of pregnancy, UK 2018–2020.

TABLE 30.1	Key Risk Factors Related to Maternal Deaths
Risk Factors	**Implications and Comments**
Mental health (see Chapter 56)	Mental ill health remains one of the leading causes of maternal death. When comparing 2020 rates with 2017–2019 rates, a statistically significant increase in the rate of suicide in the UK was reported. In 2020, women were three times more likely to die by suicide. Women dying through suicide had multiple adversities, substance misuse, homicide and accidental death. The increased rate of teenage maternal suicides remains a significant concern (all teenagers who died had Children's Social Services involvement with children and had complex problems involving mental health, substance misuse and domestic abuse).
Sleep and stigma	Sleep disturbance is very common in relation to mental illness. In women who died, the severity of insomnia was very marked.
Vulnerable and ethnic minority groups	Mortality rates remain high for babies born to Black or Black British and Asian or Asian British women. Compared to White women, there remains a more than three-fold difference in maternal mortality rates amongst women from Black ethnic backgrounds and an almost two-fold difference amongst women from Asian ethnic backgrounds.
Maternal socio-demographic profile	In the last decade, the rate of maternal mortality was higher amongst older women and those under 20, those living in the most deprived areas and amongst women from specific ethnic minority groups. Substance abuse, ethnicity and delayed access to antenatal care increases risk of adverse outcomes in women who do not use antenatal services (including obesity, teenagers, deprived and unemployed). Significant complex socio-demographic inequalities are associated with timing of access. Domestic abuse and obesity remain risk factors. Women with complex and multiple problems following discharge from hospital after birth are at risk.
Medical/obstetric complexity (see relevant Chapters 31–35, 47, 53 and 56)	Cardiac disease remains the leading cause of maternal death. Obesity is a risk factor in heart disease and venous thromboembolism. Medical conditions such as epilepsy, diabetes, high blood pressure, hyperthyroidism or infections present a potential risk to the baby. Admission to intensive care units is more likely for women of advanced maternal age, Black ethnicity, body mass index >35kg/m^2 and parity ≥3.

Refer to full report for further detail (Knight et al., 2022).

Main Points

- The corpus luteum of pregnancy is maintained due to the production of hCG by the cells of the syncytiotrophoblast as they invade the endometrium.
- Pregnancy is maintained by the corpus luteum secreting steroid hormones, mainly progesterone, until the placenta takes over this major role.
- Relaxin is a hormone produced by the luteal cells of the corpus luteum, with the levels peaking between 8–12 weeks and reducing by 20% as pregnancy progresses.
- Minor disorders of pregnancy refer to the range of inconvenient but not life-threatening symptoms commonly experienced by pregnant women. They can still impact negatively on daily functioning and quality of life.
- Minor disorders occur due to the maternal physiological adaptations to pregnancy. These are attributed to the effect of progesterone and other hormones on maternal smooth muscle and connective tissue.
- On occasion, a minor disorder can suddenly worsen to become a serious maternal condition.
- Whilst the aetiology of nausea and vomiting is not fully understood, it is likely to result from a combination of metabolic and endocrine factors, with many being placental in origin.
- Severe vomiting can persist to become the serious maternal condition known as hyperemesis gravidarum.
- Reflux oesophagitis with retrosternal burning is referred to as heartburn. It is caused by reflux of gastric acids into the lower oesophagus and is due to the relaxing effect of progesterone on the sphincter between the stomach and the lower oesophagus.
- Ptyalism refers to the excess salivation caused by the difficulty in swallowing saliva due to nausea and vomiting.
- Pica refers to the ingestion of non-nutritive substances such as coal and soap.
- Constipation primarily occurs from alterations to water transport and reabsorption from the large intestine.

- Melanocyte-stimulating hormone level increase results in increased skin pigmentation in pregnancy leading to a maternal condition called chloasma.
- Pruritus becomes a problem when the liver enzymes are raised and cholestasis of pregnancy is suspected.
- Supine hypotension is caused by the gravid uterus pressing on the inferior vena cava, preventing venous return to the heart and thus reducing cardiac output.
- PGP refers to the signs and symptoms of discomfort and pain in the pelvis and lower back (lumbopelvic) area, including musculoskeletal pain radiating to the upper thighs and perineum.
- CTS is due to fluid retention and swelling of connective tissue which compresses the median nerve running through the carpal tunnel in the wrist.
- Urinary tract infection risk is increased because of progesterone's effect on ureteric smooth muscle, which may cause urinary reflux or stasis.
- Midwives play a crucial role in the management of minor disorders of pregnancy. In cases where the minor disorder suddenly becomes serious and possibly life-threatening, midwives must be vigilant in seeking medical advice.
- Key risk factors identified from MBRRACE-UK report 2022 focused on mental health and multiple adversity, cardiovascular care, hypertensive disorders, early pregnancy disorders, diabetic ketoacidosis in pregnancy and accidents.
- Mental ill health remains one of the leading causes of maternal death.
- In 2020, women were three times more likely to die by suicide during or up to 6 weeks after the end of pregnancy compared to 2017–2019.
- Together, psychiatric disorders and cardiovascular disorders represent 30% of maternal deaths in the UK.
- There remains a more than three-fold difference in maternal mortality rates amongst women from Black ethnic backgrounds and an almost two-fold difference amongst women from Asian ethnic backgrounds compared to White women.

References

Blackburn, S.T., 2018. Maternal, Fetal and Neonatal Physiology: A Clinical Perspective, fifth ed. Elsevier, Philadelphia.

Bossuah, K.A., 2017. Fatigue in pregnancy. Int. J. Childbirth Educ. 32 (1), 10–20.

Brook, G., Brooks, T., Coldron, R., Hawkes, R., Lee, J., Vits, K., et al., 2017. Physiotherapy in women's health. Musculoskeletal Key. Available at: https://musculoskeletalkey.com/physiotherapy-in-womens-health/.

Coad, J., Pedley, K., Dunstall, M., 2019. Anatomy and Physiology for Midwives, fourth ed. Elsevier, London.

Crafter, H., Gordon, J., 2020. Problems associated with early and advanced pregnancy. In: Marshall, J., Raynor, M. (Eds.), Myles' Textbook for Midwives, seventeenth ed. Elsevier, London.

Draper, E.S., Gallimore, I.D., Smith, L.K., Matthews, R.J., Fenton, A.C., Kurinczuk, J.J., et al., (on behalf of the MBRRACE-UK collaboration), 2022. MBRRACE-UK Perinatal Mortality Surveillance Report UK Perinatal Deaths for Births from January to December 2020. Department of Health Sciences, University of Leicester, Leicester.

Fawcett, E.J., Fawcett, J.M., Mazmanian, D., 2016. A meta-analysis of the worldwide prevalence of pica during pregnancy and the postpartum period. Int. J. Gynecol. Obstet. 133 (3), 277–283.

Haufe, A., Leeners, B., 2023. Sleep disturbances across a woman's lifespan: what is the role of reproductive hormones? J. Endocr. Soc. 7 (5), bvad036.

Johnson, M.H., 2018. Essential Reproduction, eighth ed. Wiley-Blackwell, Oxford.

Kirkup, B., 2022. Reading the Signals: Maternity and Neonatal Services in East Kent – the Report of the Independent Investigation. Department of Health and Social Care, London. Available at: https://www.gov.uk/government/publications/maternity-and-neonatal-services-in-east-kent-reading-the-signals-report.

Knight, M., Bunch, K., Patel, R., Shakespeare, J., Kotnis, R., Kenyon, S., et al., (on behalf of MBRRACE-UK), 2022. Saving Lives, Improving Mothers' Care Core Report - Lessons Learned to Inform Maternity Care from the UK and Ireland Confidential Enquiries into Maternal Deaths and Morbidity 2018-20. National Perinatal Epidemiology Unit, University of Oxford, Oxford.

Matthews, A., Dowswell, T., Haas, D.M., Doyle, M., O'Mathúna, D.P., 2015. Interventions for nausea and vomiting in early pregnancy. Cochrane Database Syst. Rev. 9 (2015), CD007575.

Murray, I., Hendley, J., 2020. Change and adaptation in pregnancy. In: Marshall, J., Raynor, M. (Eds.), Myles' Textbook for Midwives, seventeenth ed. Elsevier, London.

National Institute of Health and Care Excellence (NICE), 2019. Gastro-oesophageal Reflux Disease and Dyspepsia in Adults: Investigation and Management. Available at: https://www.nice.org.uk/guidance/cg184.

National Institute of Health and Care Excellence (NICE), 2021. Antenatal Care. Available at: https://www.nice.org.uk/guidance/ng201.

Ockenden, D., 2022. Findings, Conclusions and Essential Actions from the Independent Review of Maternity Services at the Shrewsbury and Telford Hospital NHS Trust. Department of Health and Social Care, London. Available at: https://www.gov.uk/government/publications/final-report-of-the-ockenden-review.

Patil, C.L., Abrams, E.T., Steinmetz, A.R., Young, S.L., 2012. Appetite sensations and nausea and vomiting in pregnancy: an overview of the explanations. Ecol. Food Nutr. 51 (5), 394–417.

Pelvic Obstetric & Gynaecology Physiotherapy (POGP), 2015. Pregnancy Related Pelvic Girdle Pain and Low Back Pain during Pregnancy and after Having a Baby. Available at: https://thepogp.co.uk/patient_information/womens_health/pregnancy_pgp_lbp.aspx.

Royal College of Obstetricians and Gynaecologists (RCOG), 2022. Pelvic Girdle Pain and Pregnancy. Available at: https://www.rcog.org.uk/for-the-public/browse-all-patient-information-leaflets/pelvic-girdle-pain-and-pregnancy/.

Sedov, I.D., Cameron, E.E., Madigan, S., Tomfohr-Madsen, L.M., 2018. Sleep quality during pregnancy: a meta-analysis. Sleep Med. Rev. 38, 168–176.

Annotated recommended reading

Blackburn, S.T., 2018. Maternal, Fetal and Neonatal Physiology: A Clinical Perspective, fifth ed. Elsevier, Philadelphia.

This textbook provides a detailed description of the minor disorders of pregnancy. This includes up-to-date evidence to support the aetiology, underpinning physiological basis and management.

Kirkup, B., 2022. Reading the Signals: Maternity and Neonatal Services in East Kent – the Report of the Independent Investigation. Department of Health and Social Care, London. Available at: https://www.gov.uk/government/publications/maternity-and-neonatal-services-in-east-kent-reading-the-signals-report.

Knight M, Bunch K, Felker A, Patel R, Kotnis R, Kenyon S, Kurinczuk JJ (Eds.) on behalf of MBRRACE-UK. Saving Lives, Improving Mothers' Care Core Report - Lessons learned to inform maternity care from the UK and Ireland Confidential Enquiries into Maternal Deaths and Morbidity 2019-21. Oxford: National Perinatal Epidemiology Unit, University of Oxford 2023

This latest MBRRACE has reported a significant 33% increase in maternal death rates from direct causes between 2016-18 and 2019-21. COVID-19 was a leading cause of maternal death. Ethnicity and demography points remain unchanged.

Ockenden, D., 2022. Findings, Conclusions and Essential Actions from the Independent Review of Maternity Services at the Shrewsbury and Telford Hospital NHS Trust. Department of Health and Social Care, London. Available at: https://www.gov.uk/government/publications/final-report-of-the-ockenden-review.

These two reports are essential reading for students and midwives.

UK Obstetric Surveillance System (UKOSS). Current Surveillance. Available at: https://www.npeu.ox.ac.uk/ukoss/current-surveillance.

Students and midwives are strongly recommended to access UKOSS's excellent website for up-to-date information on obstetrics and maternity care. Information updates on the following UKOSS studies can be found on the website:

- *Amniotic Fluid Embolism.*
- *Pregnancy following Bone Marrow Transplant.*
- *New Therapies for Influenza.*
- *Pregnancy in Women with Known Cardiomyopathy.*
- *Thrombotic Microangiopathy Associated Pregnancy Acute Kidney Injury.*
- *Severe Respiratory Virus Infection in Pregnancy and Participating in the RECOVERY Trial.*
- *Biological Agents in Pregnancy.*
- *Severe Pyelonephritis in Pregnancy.*

Useful websites

National Institute of Health and Care Excellence (NICE), 2021. Antenatal Care. Available at: https://www.nice.org.uk/guidance/ng201.

NICE Guidance NG201 provides evidence evidence-based information and recommendations relating to the minor disorders of pregnancy.

www.pregnancysicknesssupport.org.uk.

Pregnancy Sickness Support is a charitable website offering information and support on nausea and vomiting in pregnancy to both women and professionals. Guidance is offered on hyperemesis gravidarum.

www.pelvicpartnership.org.uk.

Pelvic Partnership is a volunteer website offering personal experience of PGP for pregnant women. The information provides additional knowledge and guidance for student midwives.

www.rcog.org.uk.

The RCOG website provides invaluable information and guidance on best practice relating to gynaecological and obstetric-related situations. This includes PGP in pregnancy.

https://www.npeu.ox.ac.uk/ukoss/.

This site provides an excellent resource for ongoing surveillance in obstetrics.

www.npeu.ox.ac.uk/mbrrace-uk/reports.

All published MBBRACE-UK reports can be accessed on this site.

31

Bleeding in Pregnancy

THOMAS McEWAN AND JEAN RANKIN

Bleeding in pregnancy has the potential to be a life-threatening situation for the woman and baby. This chapter provides details of common conditions related to bleeding in early pregnancy and antepartum haemorrhage in later pregnancy. It is essential for students and midwives to have sound knowledge of these conditions due to the association with adverse pregnancy and birth outcomes.

Bleeding in Early Pregnancy

Bleeding from the genital tract during pregnancy is abnormal: sometimes it may lead to life-threatening situations and can adversely impact pregnancy at other times. Therefore all women reporting bleeding, irrespective of the amount, need to be assessed by a medical practitioner (Ekechi & Stalder, 2018). Bleeding before the 24th week of pregnancy may be caused by implantation bleeding, miscarriage (abortion), ectopic pregnancy, trophoblastic disease and lesions of the cervix or vagina.

Implantation Bleeding

Normal implantation involves three distinct processes (Blackburn, 2018) (see Chapter 12):

- Loss of the zona pellucida (hatching of the blastocyst) 5 days after fertilization, followed by rapid proliferation of the trophectoderm to form the trophoblast cell mass.
- Adherence of the blastocyst to the endometrial surface, which leads to the decidual reaction.
- Erosion of epithelium of the with burrowing beneath the surface (invasion).

Because the syncytiotrophoblast cells erode the endometrium during embedding, a small amount of bleeding may occur at about 5–7 days (Blackburn, 2018). By 10 days, the blastocyst is completely covered by the decidua. Because this is just before the menstrual period is due, women often think this is a normal but short menstruation. Implantation is a complex interaction between the blastocyst and the endometrium and 'various adhesion molecules'. At this early stage, women often do not know they are pregnant. If the blastocyst does not implant, then menstruation begins, although a little late, and the conceptus is lost with menstrual debris.

Miscarriage

Sensitive terminology needs to be used relating to the nature of pregnancy loss. Women find the term 'miscarriage' more acceptable for the spontaneous loss of a pregnancy than the medical term 'abortion'. Spontaneous miscarriage is the complete loss of the products of conception before the 24th week of pregnancy. Approximately 10–15% of diagnosed pregnancies are lost before 20 weeks. The aetiologies of miscarriage are shown in Table 31.1 and the classifications are presented in Fig. 31.1.

Many ova never implant, and it is estimated that only 50% of blastocysts that implant survive until the second week (Blackburn, 2018). Only 25% of implanted blastocysts will become clinically recognized later as miscarriages. About 80% of all miscarriages will occur before 12 weeks' gestation; the rest will occur between 13–24 weeks and are referred to as *late miscarriage*. Most early miscarriages are due to anembryonic pregnancies or blighted ova suggestive of genetic faults, whereas those with a formed fetus suggest many possible causes and occur after 13 weeks (Blackburn, 2018). Of the miscarriages, 65–90% are recognized as chromosomally abnormal. This may be linked to older age and pregnancy loss. The incidence of loss is higher in in vitro fertilization (IVF) pregnancies, probably due to the underlying causes of infertility.

TABLE 31.1	Aetiologies of Miscarriage	
Cause		**Percentage of Total**
Genetic abnormalities: mainly chromosomal abnormalities arising during meiosis of ovum or sperm		50–60
Endocrine abnormalities: progesterone deficiency, thyroid deficiency, diabetes, increased androgens, elevated luteinizing hormone as in polycystic ovary		10–15
Chorioamniotic separations: there may be bleeding beneath the chorion or between the amnion and chorion		5–10
Incompetent cervix: usually the result of cervical trauma		8–15
Infections: usually ascending, but occasionally due to systemic microbial infections such as rubella, listeria, toxoplasmosis or chlamydia		3–5
Abnormal placentation: failure of the trophoblastic invasion of the spiral arteries, linked to raised blood pressure		5–15
Immunological abnormalities: may be the cause of repeated spontaneous abortions and have recognizable serum antibodies		3–5
Uterine anatomic abnormalities: caused mainly by failure of the Müllerian ducts to unite in the embryonic stage, resulting in septate uterus; a fibroid uterus may also miscarriage (abortion)		1–3
Unknown reasons		<5

Classification of Miscarriage

Table 31.2 provides definitions of common terms relating to miscarriage (Ekechi & Stalder, 2018).

Gestational Trophoblastic Tumours

Chorionic tumours deriving from the placenta include **hydatidiform mole** (partial or complete), **placental site tumours** and **choriocarcinoma** with varying degrees of the diseased tissue spreading and causing malignancy (Ekechi & Stalder, 2018). Placental tumours are rare and generally treated with hysterectomy followed by chemotherapy.

Hydatidiform Mole

Hydatidiform mole is a benign neoplastic disease, an abnormal growth of the trophoblast where the chorionic villi proliferate, become avascular and are filled with fluid (Ekechi & Stalder, 2018). The mole looks like a bunch of grapes, often filling the uterus, which clinically palpates as being larger than expected for the gestational date (Fig. 31.2). Complete and partial moles have abnormal sets of chromosomes (Fig. 31.3); a complete mole will have a 46XX complement where all chromosomes are of paternal origin. The ovum has no nucleus but has been fertilized by one spermatozoon. A partial mole where a fetus may be present is usually triploid, either 69XXX or 69XXY, where two spermatozoa have fertilized one ovum (Blackburn, 2018).

Aetiology

Hydatidiform mole is a rare condition in the UK. However, there are wide worldwide variations in incidence: 2:1000 in Japan, 1:1000 in Europe and North America and 1:1945 in Ireland. It is suggested that diet and socioeconomic factors may play a role, particularly the lack of carotene and animal fats. There is an increased risk of a complete mole in women below 16 years and over 45 years with a history of a previous mole (Crafter & Gordon, 2020).

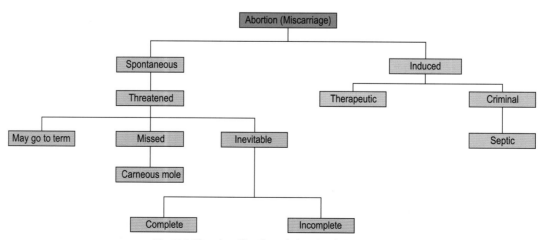

• **Fig. 31.1** The classification of abortion (miscarriage).

Signs and Symptoms

- Intermittent vaginal bleeding with increasing bleeding as the mole is aborted.
- Early onset of pre-eclampsia.
- The uterus is large for dates and no fetal parts will be palpated in a complete mole.
- There may be mild signs of thyrotoxicosis and hyperemesis gravidarum due to the action of human chorionic gonadotropin (hCG), which is similar to thyroid-stimulating hormone.
- Diagnosis is confirmed by ultrasound, which will show a snowstorm effect of multiple vesicles.
- Urinary or serum hCG is very high, exceeding that of a multiple pregnancy.

Management

Complete emptying of the uterus by suction and then curettage to eliminate all diseased tissue is essential. The molar tissue always expresses the RhD factor; therefore Rh-negative women require rhesus immunoglobulin after evacuation. As this condition has a high risk of carcinoma, follow-up is required. In the UK, hCG levels are monitored and if levels are within normal limits within 56 days of the end of the pregnancy, then follow-up continues for a further 6 months. If the hCG levels remain elevated, then follow-up will continue until these levels are normal.

Hormonal contraception should be avoided, as it increases the chance of developing malignant disease.

TABLE 31.2 Definitions of the Terms Relating to Miscarriage

Threatened miscarriage	Definition: Vaginal bleeding in the presence of a viable pregnancy. *In threatened miscarriage, painful or painless bleeding occurs, the cervical os is closed and ultrasound will define a live fetus when conservative treatment such as bed rest is advised. The outcome may be resolution and continuance of the pregnancy or an inevitable miscarriage.*
Inevitable miscarriage	Definition: Vaginal bleeding in the presence of an open cervical os and pregnancy-associated tissue still present. *Ultrasound will define if the fetus is alive. Blood loss may be heavy and cause maternal collapse with increasing abdominal pain. The uterus may spontaneously evacuate its contents, or medical removal with vaginal misoprostol may be necessary to remove retained products. Expectant management is sometimes an alternative for removing retained products of conception. If left to nature, most women will lose the retained products naturally. This management requires regular follow-up as an outpatient and access to the clinic by phone.*
Incomplete miscarriage	Definition: Vaginal bleeding that is ongoing where pregnancy tissue has already been passed but ultrasound suggests the presence of further tissue within the uterine cavity. *Offer vaginal misoprostol for the medical treatment of incomplete miscarriage (NICE, 2021a).*
Complete miscarriage	Clinical definition: Cessation of bleeding and a closed cervix following miscarriage. Ultrasound definition: An empty uterus with falling human chorionic gonadotropin (hCG) where an intrauterine pregnancy was previously confirmed.
Missed miscarriage (Early fetal demise)	Definition: Empty sac – a gestation sac with absent or minimal structure. *Miscarriage occurring in the absence of symptoms or minimal symptoms, where the empty gestation sac or non-viable embryo is still visible within the uterus.* *A blood-stained or brown loss may be evident, the woman may or may not still feel pregnant and the signs of pregnancy may disappear. Low levels of hCG may be found. The uterus needs to be removed of any remaining products of conception. Offer vaginal misoprostol for the medical treatment of missed miscarriage. If the uterus is larger than 13 weeks, a combination of vaginal prostaglandins and intravenous oxytocin may be prescribed. Although the uterus would eventually expel the conceptus, there is a risk of disseminated intravascular coagulation (DIC) because of the toxins produced by a dead fetus.*
Recurrent miscarriage	Definition: Three or more consecutive early pregnancy losses Only 0.4% of women suffer in this way but they have a 55% increased risk of having a fourth miscarriage. In some women the cause is unknown, but there is a specific group of women who suffer from **antiphospholipid antibodies (Hughes syndrome)**, some 10–16% who will continually miscarry. In other words, the mother produces antibodies against the fetus. These antibodies also affect clotting factors, and the process of abortion is thought to involve the activation of clotting mechanisms on the endothelial decidual cell surface.
Induced abortion (therapeutic) Legal: UK since 1967 Illegal: some countries	If a woman is pregnant and the pregnancy is unwanted, then she may choose the route to abort the fetus. Other women abort because of fetal abnormality, and this in itself is difficult for the woman and her partner. Some women are treated as outpatients using mifepristone or prostaglandins followed by a suction evacuation under a general anaesthetic if deemed necessary.
Illegal abortions	In countries with no abortion law, women put themselves at risk by seeking illegal abortions often carried out in unfavourable conditions by unskilled practitioners. This can end in a septic abortion due to infection – **septicaemia, endotoxic shock** and **DIC** (see Chapter 47).

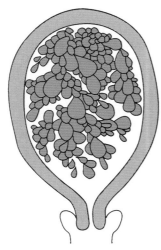

• **Fig. 31.2** A hydatidiform mole.

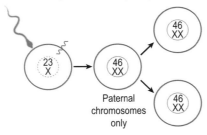

Paternal chromosomal origin of a complete hydatiform mole (46XX)

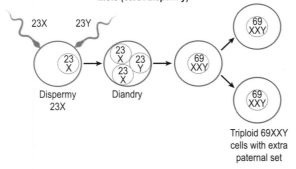

Triploid chromosomal origin of a partial mole (69XX dispermy)

• **Fig. 31.3** Genetic origins of complete and partial hydatidiform moles.

Choriocarcinoma and Placental Tumours

Choriocarcinoma, when untreated, is the most aggressive form of gestational trophoblastic neoplasia. Most cases occur following a complete hydatidiform mole (Goldblum et al., 2018). It is estimated that 1–2% of complete moles are followed by choriocarcinoma.

The diagnosis of a choriocarcinoma is the presence of a persistently raised level of hCG (>2000 IU/L). A tumour consisting of placental tissue and haemorrhage debris and spread to lung and brain is typical. In addition to raised levels of hCG, haemorrhage is another symptom to aid diagnosis. Treatment of this invasive tumour must be commenced immediately after diagnosis. Placental tumours can be difficult to diagnose, with hCG levels less elevated but not markedly as in choriocarcinoma; irregular bleeding may be a first sign.

Treatment

Choriocarcinoma in all its presentations responds very well to **chemotherapy** (Seckl, 2018). To assist in the treatment process, a scoring system is used: women scoring 0–8 are low risk and are administered methotrexate and folinic acid, while those scoring above 8 receive etoposide, methotrexate, cyclophosphamide and vincristine. Associated toxicities of these drugs include malaise, stomatitis, pharyngitis, diarrhoea, leucopoenia and alopecia occurring (Goldblum et al., 2018). Follow-up treatment will continue for life with some women opting for hysterectomy.

Ectopic Pregnancy

Maternal deaths from early pregnancy problems are almost all from ectopic pregnancy, especially in young women. In the recent MBRRACE-UK report, three women died from ruptured ectopic pregnancies after receiving thrombolysis (Knight et al., 2022). Causes may also be secondary to complications of termination of pregnancy, trophoblastic disease and miscarriage (Knight et al., 2022).

An ectopic pregnancy occurs when the fertilized ovum implants outside the uterine cavity, commonly diagnosed between 6–10 weeks (Blackburn, 2018). In 95% of cases, the site of implantation is the uterine tube. More rarely, the implantation site may be the ovary, the cervical canal or the abdominal cavity (Table 31.3). Ectopic pregnancy is a serious condition and is a major cause of maternal death. Primary reasons for death have been stated as missed diagnosis in primary care and accident and emergency. Offering a pregnancy test is recommended even when symptoms are non-specific to prevent missed diagnosis. Ultrasound will confirm diagnosis, with transvaginal scanning (TVS) confirming location of the pregnancy and whether there is a fetal pole and heartbeat (National Institute of Care and Health Excellence [NICE], 2021a). Diagnosis may prevent the drastic operative measures of salpingectomy.

Tubal Pregnancy

There is a rise in the incidence of tubal pregnancies due to the increase in sexually transmitted diseases, particularly by *Chlamydia trachomatis* (Greenhouse, 2018). Any condition that delays the transport of the zygote along the uterine tube may lead to a tubal pregnancy (Fig. 31.4). This may be due to malformation of the tubes but is more likely due to tubal scarring and the loss of cilia due to pelvic infection.

TABLE 31.3 Sites of Ectopic Implantation

Position	Percentage Occurrence
The fimbriated part of the tube	17
The ampulla	55
The isthmus	25
The ovary	0.5
The abdominal cavity	0.1

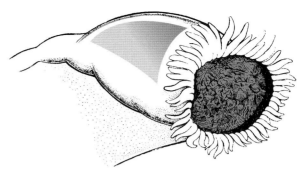

• **Fig. 31.5** Tubal abortion.

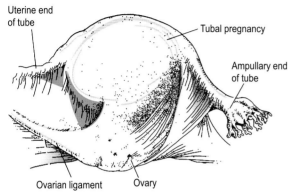

• **Fig. 31.4** Tubal pregnancy.

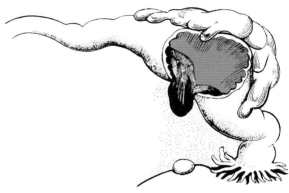

• **Fig. 31.6** Rupture of the uterine tube.

Risk Factors

Risk factors for tubal pregnancy include (Coudous, 2018):
- Increasing maternal age.
- Previous ectopic pregnancy.
- Previous pelvic/abdominal surgery (tubal ligation, appendectomy).
- Salpingitis.
- Pelvic inflammatory disease (PID).
- Chlamydia.
- Intrauterine contraceptive device.
- IVF and embryo transplantation.

Pathophysiology

Implantation may occur in various sites along the genital tract (Table 31.3). The outcome varies depending on where in the tube implantation occurs, the ability of the tube to distend and the size of blood vessels eroded. If the pregnancy occurs in the fimbriated end or the ampulla, the conceptus may continue to grow until 10 weeks. The gestation sac may be expelled into the abdominal cavity as a tubal abortion (Fig. 31.5). The blood clot may be organized around the separated sac to form a tubal mole, which may remain in the uterine tube or be expelled from the fimbriated end as a tubal abortion. Tubal rupture (Fig. 31.6) may lead to devastating haemorrhage. The most severe haemorrhage occurs if the zygote implants at the level of the isthmus where the mucosa is thinner and the blood vessels larger. Tubal rupture is likely to occur between the fifth and seventh weeks of pregnancy.

TABLE 31.4 Signs and Presenting History of Ectopic Pregnancy

Sign	Percentage Occurrence
Abdominal pain	97
Abdominal tenderness	91
Vaginal bleeding	79
Adnexal tenderness	54
History of infertility	15
Use of intrauterine device	14
Previous ectopic pregnancy	11

Diagnosis

The condition may be subacute or acute with signs of shock and collapse. The condition is serious and should always be suspected in women of childbearing age, especially if there is a history of amenorrhoea or previous salpingitis. The likely signs and presenting history of ectopic pregnancy are given in Table 31.4.

Delay in diagnosis may be fatal as the clinical picture is similar to PID or threatened abortion:
- The woman will give a history of early pregnancy signs.
- The uterus will have enlarged but feel soft.
- Abdominal pain may occur as the tube distends, and uterine bleeding may be present as the endometrium begins to degenerate.

- The abdomen is tender and may be distended.
- Shoulder tip pain may be due to referred pain.
- The woman may appear pale, complain of nausea and collapse.
- Severe pain may be felt during pelvic examination, especially if the cervix is moved.
- A mass may be felt in the adnexi on one or other side of the uterus.
- Hormonal assay will find progesterone levels to be low and hCG levels may be low or falling.
- Ultrasound may show fluid in the pelvic cavity, a mass in the pelvic cavity and absence of an intrauterine pregnancy.

Management

Although an acute emergency when rupture of the tube and bleeding occurs, surgery is indicated and salpingectomy is performed, ectopic pregnancy can be treated expectantly, particularly with early ultrasound diagnosis. Ectopic pregnancy resolves naturally in 88% of patients if the hCG titre is <1000 IU/L. The use of systemic methotrexate in women who have not ruptured and are haemodynamically stable has been beneficial; however it is not without side effects.

Prognosis

About 40% of women may never become pregnant after an ectopic pregnancy. About 75% of these women avoid pregnancy voluntarily, and 25% are infertile. The risk of a second ectopic pregnancy is 10% compared with only 0.4% in other women.

Bleeding from Associated Conditions

The following conditions may cause bleeding at any time in pregnancy but are not caused by the pregnancy.

Cervical Polyps

Cervical polyps are benign growths which are bright red, fleshy and attached by a pedicle. They usually originate in the cervical canal and can be seen on speculum examination. Polyps may have been present before the onset of pregnancy but bleed during pregnancy because of the increased blood supply.

Cervical Erosion

Cervical erosion (**eversion, ectropion**) forms when the columnar epithelium lining the cervical canal proliferates because of the influence of the pregnancy hormones. Columnar epithelium secretes mucin, and the woman may complain of profuse vaginal discharge. This may be bloodstained because of rupture of capillaries, especially after sexual intercourse. The epithelium should recede after delivery but, if it persists, treatment by diathermy or cryosurgery can be given.

Carcinoma of the Cervix

Carcinoma of the cervix, if diagnosed early, is a very treatable condition. Regular testing with the Papanicolaou test (Pap test) is effective. If diagnosed in pregnancy, treatment may depend on the stage of pregnancy and the severity of the findings. Prospective parents have a difficult choice to make and must be guided to make an informed decision. **Cellular dysplasia** (abnormal growth of cells) and **nuclear dyskaryosis** (abnormal chromosomes) are associated with human papillomavirus (HPV) infection types 6, 16 and 18, and between 10–30% of women have been affected by age 30. HPV is transmissible and is a cause of genital warts. About 60% of the partners of women with HPV infection of the cervix have penile infection. HPV acts with a co-agent to cause carcinoma of the cervix. Clinical findings may show **cervical intraepithelial neoplasia** (CIN; invasive carcinoma of the cervix).

Cervical Intraepithelial Neoplasia

Cervical cytology may show normal cells; mild, moderate or severe dysplasia; or carcinoma in situ. When carried out in the antenatal period, 1 in 200 mothers have abnormal cell changes. If these are consistent with CIN, a repeat Papanicolaou smear is taken and the cervix is assessed by **colposcopy.** A small cervical biopsy may be carried out. If the tissue is precancerous, treatment can be deferred until after delivery.

Invasive Carcinoma of the Cervix

Invasive carcinoma of the cervix occurs in about 1 in 5000 women of childbearing age. It is an aggressive cancer and may progress rapidly. The cervix feels hard and nodular and bleeds when touched. Decisions about treatment should be discussed with each woman and will depend on the degree of invasion and the duration of pregnancy.

Vaginitis

Occasionally the use of vaginal deodorants may lead to inflammation and bleeding from the vaginal epithelium. Infections by organisms such as *Candida albicans* or *Trichomonas vaginalis* are more likely causes of vaginitis, which may be accompanied by slight bleeding (Greenhouse, 2018). After culture of the organism, the correct antibiotic should be given.

Antepartum Haemorrhage

Antepartum haemorrhage is bleeding after the 24th week of pregnancy and before the birth of the baby and is always a serious complication. Bleeding from a placenta implanted wholly or partly in the lower uterine segment is termed **placenta praevia;** bleeding from a normally sited placenta is a **placental abruption. Intrapartum haemorrhage** occurs during labour and may be life-threatening for both mother and baby, necessitating emergency measures to deliver the baby.

Placenta Praevia

Normally, the chorionic villi surround the whole embryo but later degenerate under the decidua capsularis to form the chorion laeve. The fetus grows to fill the uterine cavity and the decidua capsularis fuses with the decidua vera by about 4 months. If the chorionic villi near the lower pole of the uterus fail to degenerate as the decidua capsularis fuses with the decidua vera, the area will become part of the placenta, encroaching on the lower uterine segment (Blackburn, 2018).

Placenta praevia is defined as a placenta developing within the lower uterine segment and graded according to the relationship and/or the distance between the lower placental edge and the internal os of the uterine cervix. The estimated incidence of placenta praevia at term is 1 in 200 pregnancies (Jauniaux, Alfirevic & Bhide, 2018). Risk factors include an association with the increased risk of placenta praevia in subsequent pregnancies, uterine surgery, the use of antiretroviral therapy and maternal smoking. Multifetal pregnancies are at risk of the placenta being large and covering a greater area of the uterus and thus covering the os.

Aetiology of Placenta Praevia

Evidence suggests that the placenta is low-lying because of defects in the uterine endometrium and musculature. The lower segment in later pregnancy appears to remove the placental site away from the internal os. As pregnancy advances, shearing stresses may detach the placenta from the uterine wall, resulting in haemorrhage.

Types of Placenta Praevia

Placenta praevia is defined as types I–IV as shown in Fig. 31.7 and described in Table 31.5.

Detection

Although a low-lying placenta may be detected on routine transabdominal scanning (TAS) in early pregnancy, it may be detected in as many as 20% of pregnancies in later trimesters (Hyett, 2018). TVS is safe and is superior for the diagnosis of placenta praevia or a low-lying placenta than TAS and transperineal approaches (Jauniaux, Alfirevic & Bhide, 2018). Determining the location of the placenta is one of the first aims of routine mid-pregnancy evaluation (18–21 weeks of gestation) (Jauniaux, Alfirevic & Bhide, 2018). If the placenta is low-lying at mid-pregnancy, then TVS ultrasound should define the exact position of the placenta. A follow-up ultrasound examination including TVS is recommended at 32 weeks of gestation to diagnose persistent low-lying placenta and/or placenta praevia. Defining the exact placental position enables subsequent management planning during pregnancy. Management decisions including plans for birth will depend on the amount of bleeding, the condition of the woman and fetus, location of the placenta and the stage of pregnancy. For example, the obstetrician may plan late preterm (34^{+0} to 36^{+6} weeks of gestation) delivery for women presenting with placenta praevia or a low-lying placenta and a history of vaginal bleeding or other associated risk factors for preterm delivery. Clinical Application 31.1 outlines the management of placenta praevia.

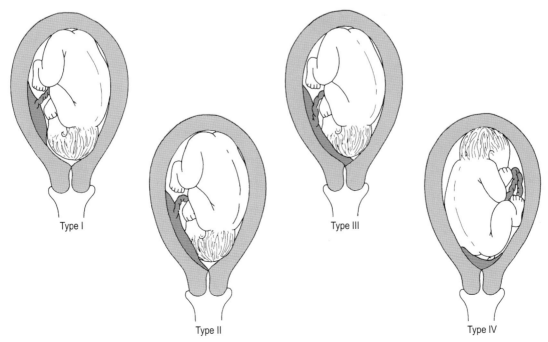

Type I   Type II   Type III   Type IV

• **Fig. 31.7** Placenta praevia types I–IV.

TABLE 31.5	Type of Placenta Praevia
Type	**Definition and Implications**
1. Grade I or *minor praevia*	Lower edge of placenta inside the lower uterine segment (LUS). *Blood loss is usually mild. Mother and fetus usually remain in good condition. Vaginal birth is possible.*
2. Grade II or *marginal praevia*	Lower edge of placenta reaching the internal os. *Blood loss is usually moderate. Condition of mother and fetus may vary. Fetal hypoxia is more likely than maternal shock. Vaginal birth is possible, especially if placenta is anterior.*
3. Grade III or *partial praevia* – major	Occurs when placenta partially covers the cervix. *Bleeding is more likely to be severe. As pregnancy progresses, the LUS stretches. Cervix begins to dilate in late pregnancy. As the placenta precedes the fetus, vaginal birth is not possible and inappropriate. Caesarean section is necessary.*
4. Grade IV or *complete praevia* – major	Occurs when placenta completely covers the cervix. *Torrential haemorrhage is very likely. Caesarean section is necessary to save mother and fetus.*

The Royal College of Obstetricians and Gynaecologists recommends the term 'placenta praevia' should be used when the placenta lies directly over the internal os (Jauniaux, Alfirevic & Bhide, 2018). For pregnancies greater than 16 weeks of gestation, the placenta should be reported as *'low-lying'* when the placental edge is less than 20 mm from the internal os, and as *'normal'* when the placental edge is 20 mm or more from the internal os on transabdominal or transvaginal scans (Jauniaux, Alfirevic & Bhide, 2018). This new recommendation better defines the risks of perinatal complications, such as antepartum haemorrhage and major postpartum haemorrhage.

Blood Loss

In 98% of cases painless, fresh, recurrent vaginal bleeding occurs after 24 weeks due to stretching of the lower uterine segment and detachment of the placenta, although it may occur earlier. Blood loss usually stops after a few hours and is rarely dangerous. Subsequent episodes of bleeding due to increased development of the lower uterine segment and further detachment of the placenta tend to become worse, and a blood transfusion may be required. Torrential maternal haemorrhage may occur at any time, especially if labour commences and the cervix begins to dilate. The fetus may be compromised if maternal bleeding is severe enough to reduce the uterine blood supply. The placenta may be torn,

and fetal bleeding occurs. Massive haemorrhage will require an emergency caesarean section (see Chapter 47).

Placental Abruption (Abruptio Placentae)

Placental abruption refers to premature separation of the normally situated placenta occurring after the 24th week of pregnancy (Blackburn, 2018; Fig. 31.8). It is also referred to as **abruptio placentae** and occurs in 0.49–1.8% of all pregnancies. Of this number, 65–80% are classified as revealed and 20–35% as concealed (Crafter & Gordon, 2020). This abruption can occur at any stage in pregnancy or labour with varying amounts of blood loss (Paterson-Brown & Draycott, 2018). Bleeding occurs into the decidua basalis beneath the placenta. A haematoma forms, separating the placenta from the maternal vascular system, and the fetus is deprived of oxygen and nutrients. If 50% of the placenta is involved, fetal loss is likely. Most maternal complications arise from hypovolaemia and collapse of the systems (Paterson-Brown & Draycott, 2018). The haemorrhage may be secondary to degenerative changes in the arteries supplying the intervillous spaces (Blackburn, 2018).

Risk Factors

In most cases, bleeding is slight and no cause may be found. The following risk factors are associated with this serious complication of pregnancy:

- **Hypertensive states**—chronic and/or gestational hypertension, or pre-eclampsia in 50% of severe cases.
- Sudden decompression of the uterus, as when membranes rupture in **polyhydramnios.**
- Preterm, pre-labour rupture of the membranes.
- Previous history of placental abruption, increasing parity.
- Trauma, as in a fall or road traffic accident, or domestic violence.
- Fetal growth restriction – non-vertex presentation, advanced maternal age, low body mass index, uterine infection.
- Smoking, illegal drug abuse such as cocaine.

Blood Loss

Blood loss comes from the maternal venous sinuses and may be revealed, partly revealed or concealed (Fig. 31.9; Table 31.6). The blood is darker than that seen in placenta praevia because of the time taken to appear out of the vagina. Some experts believe that the magnitude of placental separation is determined at the outset and that no further separation occurs. Others believe that abruption causes progressive placental separation. Table 31.7 summarizes the main features of bleeding in placental abruption (abruptio placentae).

Management of Placental Abruption (Abruptio Placenta)

The amount of bleeding per vagina does not give any indication to the degree of placental separation. Bleeding at home warrants immediate transfer to hospital. Table 31.8 outlines

• CLINICAL APPLICATION 31.1   Management of Placental Praevia

Possible findings on abdominal palpation:
- Malpresentation of the fetus.
- Non-engagement of the presenting part.
- The presence of a loud maternal pulse that originates in the placental bed below the umbilicus.

All women at home need to be aware that they must attend the hospital immediately if there is any bleeding, including spotting, contractions or pain (including vague suprapubic period-like aches) (Jauniaux, Alfirevic & Bhide, 2018). Antenatal care needs to be planned to meet the individual woman's needs and social circumstances, especially distance from the hospital (NICE, 2021b).

General Examination
- There may be a history of spotting or small blood loss.
- Observations of maternal pulse and blood pressure should correspond with the amount of blood loss and the degree of shock.
- Temperature should be normal.

Abdominal Examination
- The uterus should feel soft and should not be tender.
- The size will correspond to the period of gestation.
- There may be a malpresentation, an unstable lie and a high presenting part.
- Usually the fetus is in good condition with a normal heart rate and rhythm.
- Blood is taken for cross-matching and at least two units placed on standby. Blood loss is estimated. If bleeding, the woman remains on bedrest until the bleeding ceases.
- A speculum examination may exclude other reasons for bleeding.
- Management may be conservative or active.

Conservative Management

If bleeding is slight to moderate and occurs before the 38th week of pregnancy and both maternal and fetal conditions are satisfactory, conservative treatment is commenced. The aim is to maintain the pregnancy until 38 weeks to avoid preterm delivery of an immature fetus. The women will remain in hospital on bedrest until the bleeding has stopped and both woman and fetus are well. Maternal well-being and fetal growth will be monitored. Depending on the individual circumstances of the woman, the plan for delivery (timing and mode) will be made in advance with the obstetrician.

Delivery

If no serious haemorrhage occurs, the fetus is delivered at 38 weeks. A decision will be made in discussion with the woman about delivery including mode of birth. Placental localization

will be clarified. Vaginal birth is possible if the placental location allows. The potential hazards of vaginal delivery include:
- Profuse maternal haemorrhage (reduced number of oblique muscle fibres in the lower uterine segment (LUS) and reduced effects of the living ligatures).
- Malpresentation.
- Cord accidents.
- Placental separation.
- Fetal haemorrhage.
- Dystocia if the placenta is situated posteriorly.

Active and Immediate Management

This need for emergency management often occurs in the last 2 weeks of pregnancy. Therefore, severe vaginal bleeding or deterioration in the woman and fetus will require immediate delivery by emergency caesarean section in a unit with access to paediatricians. Stabilizing the woman's condition is crucial.

Blood must be cross-matched. Surgery can be complicated if the placenta underlies the site of normal surgical incision. Even if the fetus has died, caesarean section will be needed to stop the haemorrhage and stabilize the woman.

Third Stage

The lack of oblique fibres in the LUS may fail to control bleeding, and postpartum haemorrhage (PPH) may occur. **Placenta accreta** is a spectrum disorder ranging from abnormally adherent to deeply invasive placental tissue. It is often associated with placenta praevia as the thin decidua over the LUS increases the likelihood of myometrial invasion. The condition is difficult to diagnose and is associated with high maternal and neonatal morbidity and mortality. There is a wide variation in the incidence reported (i.e., 1 in 300 to 1 in 2000 pregnancies). There has been a 13-fold increase in placenta accreta rates correlated with increased caesarean section rates (Blackburn, 2018). Therefore, the incidence will continue to rise as caesarean section rates increase in addition to the increase in maternal age and use of antiretroviral therapy (Jauniaux, Alfirevic & Bhide, 2018). Hysterectomy may be required to control haemorrhage and to preserve life.

Complications:
- Moderate shock resulting from blood loss and hypovolaemia.
- Placenta accreta.
- Air embolism.
- Primary PPH.
- Anaesthetic/surgical complications.
- Maternal death.
- Fetal hypoxia/death
- (See Chapters 41–45 and 47 for obstetric complications and care of the acutely ill woman).

---

management of care. It is essential for clinicians to recognize the differences between placenta praevia and placental abruption (Table 31.9).

Complications

The serious complication of blood coagulation disorders may occur (Box 31.1). The complications of acute renal failure, Sheehan's syndrome, postpartum haemorrhage (PPH), infection, anaemia and mental disturbances are discussed in relevant chapters. Chapter 47 discusses the care of the

acutely ill woman. In addition, women with a history of placental abruption have a higher risk of complications such as spontaneous miscarriage or repeated abruption in later pregnancies.

Vasa Praevia

Vasa praevia is an unusual cause of bleeding in pregnancy where the blood lost is from the fetus. It occurs when the fetal vessels run through the free placental membranes

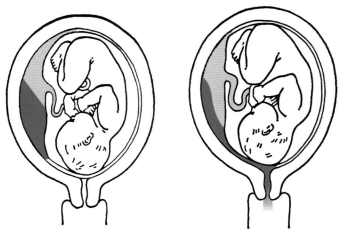

• **Fig. 31.8** Abruptio placentae.

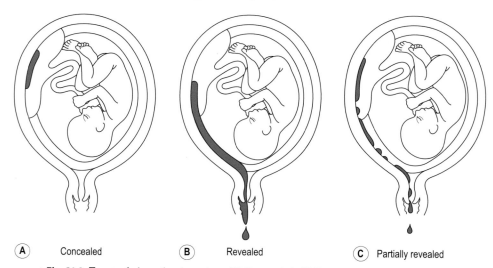

(A) Concealed (B) Revealed (C) Partially revealed

• **Fig. 31.9** Types of abruptio placentae. (A) Concealed. (B) Revealed. (C) Partially revealed.

TABLE 31.6 **Types of Placental Abruption (Abruptio Placentae)**

Type	Implication
Revealed bleeding	Occurs when the site of placental detachment is at the margin. Blood escapes between the membranes and decidua and is seen at the vulva. The woman's condition is directly related to the observed blood loss.
Partially revealed bleeding	Occurs when some of the blood remains in the uterus. The bleeding may exceed that which is visibly lost, and the degree of shock may be greater than expected.
Concealed bleeding	Occurs when the site of detachment is near to the centre of the site of placental attachment. Blood cannot escape and a large retroplacental clot forms. Extravasated blood may also infiltrate the full-thickness myometrium, a condition known as Couvelaire uterus. Under direct observation, the uterus would appear bruised and oedematous. No vaginal blood loss is noted but pain and shock are usually severe.

TABLE 31.7 **The Main Features of Bleeding in Placental Abruption (Abruptio Placentae)**

	Mild	Moderate	Severe
Blood loss	Slight	>1000 mL	>2000 mL
Uterus on abdominal examination	Soft, not tender	Firm and tender	Hard and tender (*if blood is trapped and concealed behind the placenta*); backache if the placenta is posterior
Pain	None or mild	Quite severe	Severe
Shock	No sign	Tachycardia, hypotension	Extreme shock
Fetus	Fetal heart normal	Signs of fetal distress	Fetal heart absent

TABLE 31.8 **Management of Placental Abruption (Abruptio Placentae)**

Placental Separation	Blood Loss and Presentation	Management
Mild	Includes episodes of bleeding where the mother and fetus are not compromised in any way. Uncertainty about diagnosis.	Ultrasound to define placental lie. Observe blood loss and fetal well-being. Stay in hospital until bleeding ceases.
Moderate Obstetric emergency	Moderate blood loss possibly ≥1000 mL and the fetus may be alive. The uterus may be tender and the woman in pain. Usually easy to diagnose.	Immediate caesarean section may be necessary if the fetus is distressed. • Woman may be hypovolaemic – commence intravenous (IV) therapy. Clotting screens should be undertaken. • If the fetus is dead, vaginal delivery is possible if woman is stable.
Severe separation of placenta Obstetric emergency	Life-threatening situation for the woman. Fetus nearly always dead. Usually easy to diagnose. Blood loss approximately ≥2000 mL (not all blood loss revealed). Uterus will be hard.	Maternal condition is poor with severe shock and pain. Resuscitation necessary. IV fluids to restore circulating volume. Analgesia to relieve pain.

Generic Management

- Possibly difficult to differentiate the cause of bleeding, especially if there is no sign of hypertension.
- Woman is initially treated as if placenta praevia is present until it is excluded by ultrasound.
- If the placenta is localized in the upper uterine segment, the bleeding usually ceases.
- With moderate and severe blood loss, the aim is to restore blood loss and deliver the baby as quickly as possible to empty the uterus to avoid complications.
- Bloods: grouping and cross-matching, full blood count, urea and electrolytes, clotting studies and fibrin degradation products.
- Monitoring of vital signs and urinary output is essential.
- Monitor cardiovascular and renal status closely to ensure a good maternal outcome.
- Postpartum haemorrhage is likely due to the poor ability of the uterine muscle to contract when it is infiltrated by blood; IV oxytocin infusion may be continued for some hours after delivery.
- Most maternal deaths occur in severe abruption of placenta.
- Potential complications: coagulation defects, kidney failure and Sheehan's syndrome.

TABLE 31.9 **Summary of Differences: Placental Praevia and Placental Abruption (Abruptio Placentae)**

Category	Placenta Praevia	Placental Abruption
Onset of bleeding	Usually unprovoked. Heavy. No clots present.	May follow a traumatic incident (e.g., road traffic accident). Usually unprovoked. May contain clots. Blood loss varies.
Signs and symptoms (for moderate to severe blood loss)	Painless. Fresh bleeding – bright red.	Generalized abdominal pain (mild to severe). After acute bleeding ceases, altered old brown-coloured blood will continue vaginally for some time.
	Temperature normal. Possible raised pulse and respiratory rate. Low blood pressure (BP).	Temperature may be raised (if infection present). Pulse and respiratory rate raised depending on level of blood loss and shock). BP may be low.
On abdominal palpation	Fetal malpresentation likely. Non-tender uterus. Fetal heart rate (FHR) may be normal, erratic or absent.	Uterus tense and painful if blood is getting concealed – palpation may not be possible. Fetal presentation or engagement is not affected by the abruption. FHR may be normal, erratic or absent.
On diagnostic ultrasound	Placenta is in the lower uterine segment.	Normally situated placenta. Blood clots may be seen in the cavity of the uterus.

• BOX 31.1   **Blood Coagulation Disorders**

Damage to tissue causes the release of **thromboplastins** from the cells. In normal circumstances, thromboplastin activates the clotting mechanism and **fibrinogen** is converted to **fibrin**, forming a clot to seal any broken blood vessels. This clot is later dispersed by **plasmin**, releasing **fibrin degradation products**. The tissue damage in placental abruption is so severe that there is a massive release of thromboplastin into the circulation. Widespread clotting occurs within the vascular tree, a condition called disseminated intravascular coagulation. At the same time, the anticlotting mechanisms are affected and shut down, preventing dissolution of the clots. The **microthrombi** produced occlude small blood vessels resulting in ischaemic damage in organs. The damaged tissue then releases more thromboplastins and a vicious circle commences:

- Damage to the kidney results in reduced urinary output and may result in **anuria**.
- The liver may be damaged, leading to **jaundice**.
- Damage to the lungs may result in **dyspnoea** and **cyanosis**.
- Brain involvement may result in **convulsions** or **coma**.
- The retina may be affected and cause **blindness**.
- If the pituitary gland is damaged, **Sheehan's syndrome** may occur.

Platelets and clotting factors are depleted and no further coagulation can occur. Spontaneous bleeding begins from puncture wound sites and mucous membranes, petechiae develop in the skin and there will be uncontrollable uterine bleeding. Transfusions of fresh frozen plasma, packed cells and platelets will be needed.

(Refer to Chapter 47 for care of the acutely ill woman).

between the presenting part of the fetus and the internal os of the uterus (Jauniaux, Alfirevic & Bhide, 2018). The two classifications of vasa praevia are:

- Type I: when the vessel is connected to a velamentous umbilical cord.

- Type II: when the vessel connects the placenta with a succenturiate or accessory lobe.

The vessels are unprotected by placental tissue or Wharton's jelly of the umbilical cord. Vasa praevia is likely to rupture in active labour, or when amniotomy is performed to induce or augment labour, particularly when located near or over the cervix, under the fetal presenting part. It is uncommon in the general population with a prevalence ranging between 1 in 1200 and 1 in 5000 pregnancies (possible under-reporting) (Jauniaux, Alfirevic & Bhide, 2018).

Fetal bleeding may be severe and there is a high incidence of perinatal mortality. The fetal mortality rate is at least 60% despite urgent caesarean delivery. However, improved survival rates of over 95% have been reported where the diagnosis has been made antenatally by ultrasound followed by planned caesarean section (Jauniaux, Alfirevic & Bhide, 2018).

Vasa praevia may be diagnosed during early labour by vaginal examination, detecting the pulsating fetal vessels inside the internal os, or by the presence of dark-red vaginal bleeding and acute fetal compromise after spontaneous or artificial rupture of the placental membranes (Hyett, 2018; Jauniaux, Alfirevic & Bhide, 2018).

If suspected during a vaginal examination, the membranes are left intact and the fetus delivered by emergency caesarean section. If the woman is in the second stage of labour, rapid delivery is made by forceps. Any sudden vaginal bleeding accompanied by fetal distress after rupture of the membranes should alert the practitioner and the blood should be tested for fetal cells. Although this sounds sensible, in reality there may be no time and the fetus should be immediately delivered. The baby may need a blood transfusion to restore blood volume.

Main Points

- Any bleeding from the genital tract during pregnancy is abnormal. All women should be medically reviewed.
- Causes of bleeding before the 24th week are implantation, miscarriage, ectopic pregnancy, cervical lesions, vaginitis and trophoblastic disease.
- Chorionic tumours deriving from the placenta include hydatidiform mole, placental tumours and choriocarcinoma with varying degrees of the diseased tissue and possible malignancy.
- Hydatidiform mole, a benign neoplastic disease, is an abnormal growth of the trophoblast where the chorionic villi proliferate and become avascular.
- An ectopic pregnancy occurs when the fertilized ovum implants outside the uterine cavity. In most cases, the implantation site is the uterine tube.
- Antepartum haemorrhage is bleeding after the 24th week of pregnancy and before the birth of the baby. Two main types are placenta praevia and placental abruption. These can quickly become obstetric emergencies with adverse pregnancy, birth and maternal outcomes.

- Placenta praevia causes bleeding from an abnormally sited placenta. It is defined as a placenta developing within the LUS and graded according to the relationship and/or the distance between the lower placental edge and the internal os of the uterine cervix.
- Placental abruption (abruptio placentae) refers to premature separation of the normally situated placenta occurring after the 24th week of pregnancy. The types are related to bleeding, being concealed, revealed or partially revealed.
- Risk factors for placental abruption include hypertensive states, sudden decompression of the uterus, preterm prelabour rupture of the membranes, previous history of placental abruption, trauma, smoking and abuse of cocaine.
- In moderate or severe placental abruption, blood needs to be restored and the baby delivered quickly to prevent complications such as renal failure and blood-clotting defects.
- Vasa praevia is associated with a velamentous insertion of the umbilical cord. The vessel may be torn when the membranes rupture and fetal bleeding may be severe.

References

Blackburn, S.T., 2018. Maternal, Fetal and Neonatal Physiology: A Clinical Perspective, fifth ed. Elsevier, Philadelphia.

Crafter, H., Gordon, J., 2020. Problems associated with early and advanced pregnancy. In: Marshall, J., Raynor, M. (Eds.), Myles Textbook for Midwives, seventeenth ed. Elsevier, London.

Coudous, G., 2018. Ectopic pregnancy. In: Edmonds, D.K., Lees, C., Bourne, T.H. (Eds.), Dewhurst's Textbook of Obstetrics and Gynaecology for Postgraduates, ninth ed. Wiley-Blackwell, Oxford.

Ekechi, C.I., Stalder, C.M., 2018. Spontaneous miscarriage. In: Edmonds, D.K., Lees, C., Bourne, T.H. (Eds.), Dewhurst's Textbook of Obstetrics and Gynaecology for Postgraduates, ninth ed. Wiley-Blackwell, Oxford.

Goldblum, J.R., Lamps, L.W., McKenney, J.K., Myers, J.L., 2018. Uterus: corpus. In: Rosai and Ackerman's Surgical Pathology, eleventh ed. Elsevier, New York.

Greenhouse, P., 2018. Sexually transmitted infection. In: Edmonds, D.K., Lees, C., Bourne, T.H. (Eds.), Dewhurst's Textbook of Obstetrics and Gynaecology for Postgraduates, ninth ed. Wiley-Blackwell, Oxford.

Hyett, J., 2018. Third trimester fetal assessment. In: Edmonds, D.K., Lees, C., Bourne, T.H. (Eds.), Dewhurst's Textbook of Obstetrics and Gynaecology for Postgraduates, ninth ed. Wiley-Blackwell, Oxford.

Jauniaux, E.R.M., Alfirevic, Z., Bhide, A.G., 2018. Placenta praevia and placenta accreta: diagnosis and management: Green-Top Guideline No. 27a. Br. J. Obstet. Gynaecol. 126 (1), e1–e48.

Knight, M., Bunch, K., Patel, R., Shakespeare, J., Kotnis, R., Kenyon, S., et al., (on behalf of MBRRACE-UK), 2022. Saving Lives, Improving Mothers Care Core Report–Lessons Learned to Inform Maternity Care from the UK and Ireland Confidential Enquiries into Maternal Deaths and Morbidity 2018–20. National Perinatal Epidemiology Unit, University of Oxford, Oxford.

National Institute of Health and Care Excellence (NICE), 2021a. Ectopic Pregnancy and Miscarriage: Diagnosis and Initial Management. Available at: https://www.nice.org.uk/guidance/ng126.

National Institute of Health and Care Excellence (NICE), 2021b. Antenatal Care. Available at: https://www.nice.org.uk/guidance/ng201.

Paterson-Brown, S., Draycott, T.J., 2018. Obstetric emergencies. In: Edmonds, D.K., Lees, C., Bourne, T.H. (Eds.), Dewhurst's Textbook of Obstetrics and Gynaecology for Postgraduates, ninth ed. Wiley-Blackwell, Oxford.

Seckl, M.J., 2018. Gestational trophoblast. In: Edmonds, D.K., Lees, C., Bourne, T.H. (Eds.), Dewhurst's Textbook of Obstetrics and Gynaecology for Postgraduates, ninth ed. Wiley-Blackwell, Oxford.

Annotated recommended reading

Blackburn, S.T., 2018. Maternal, Fetal and Neonatal Physiology: A Clinical Perspective, fifth ed. Elsevier, Philadelphia.

This textbook provides detailed and up-to-date evidence to support the aetiology and underpinning physiological basis for bleeding in early pregnancy.

www.nice.org.uk/guidance/.

The NICE website provides evidence-based information and recommendations relating to bleeding in early pregnancy.

https://www.hmole-chorio.org.uk/.

This excellent site is clearly set out and is full of very readable information on trophoblastic disease and hydatidiform mole.

Ockenden, D., 2022. Findings, Conclusions and Essential Actions from the Independent Review of Maternity Services at the Shrewsbury and Telford Hospital NHS Trust. Department of Health and Social Care, London. Available at: https://www.gov.uk/government/publications/final-report-of-the-ockenden-review.

Kirkup, B., 2022. Reading the Signals: Maternity and Neonatal Services in East Kent – the Report of the Independent Investigation. Department of Health and Social Care, London. Available at: https://www.gov.uk/government/publications/maternity-and-neonatal-services-in-east-kent-reading-the-signals-report

These two reports are essential reading for students and midwives.

Useful websites

www.nice.org.uk/guidance/.
https://www.npeu.ox.ac.uk/ukoss/current-surveillance.
https://www.hmole-chorio.org.uk/.

32
Cardiac and Hypertensive Disorders

THOMAS McEWAN AND JEAN RANKIN

CHAPTER CONTENTS

This chapter will focus on cardiac and hypertensive disorders. It is important for students and midwives to have fundamental knowledge of these key disorders and their associated management.

Introduction

In pregnancy, cardiac disease is a serious medical condition. Cardiac disease remains the largest single cause of indirect maternal deaths at 9% of reported deaths (Knight et al., 2022). Pre-existing cardiac conditions, increasing age and

---

> ### • BOX 32.1 Risk Factors for Maternal Deaths from Cardiovascular Disease
>
> - Existing cardiac problems were reported in 10% of maternal deaths.
> - Almost half of maternal deaths from cardiovascular disease were from socially deprived areas (i.e., twice as likely to die compared to women living in the least deprived areas) and tended to increase with age (i.e., women aged 40 were six times more likely to die than women aged 25–29 years).
>
> Chapter 30 provides further detail on risk factors related to MBRRACE-UK enquiry (Knight et al., 2022)

---

social deprivation are associated with maternal deaths (Box 32.1). This has implications within the maternity service for women of childbearing years. The most dangerous cardiac lesions are those that involve pulmonary hypertension, such as **primary pulmonary hypertension, Eisenmenger syndrome** and **Marfan syndrome,** an autosomal dominant disorder of connective tissue which may result in aortic dilatation and rupture late in pregnancy or in labour.

Rheumatic heart disease is still fairly common despite the reduction in rheumatic fever in the British population. The most commonly associated lesion, **rheumatic mitral stenosis,** may lead to **pulmonary oedema** late in pregnancy or immediately after delivery. Another cause for concern is the globally mobile population, with varied access to healthcare in their country of origin who have not been diagnosed with congenital and acquired heart disease.

Cardiac Disorders in Pregnancy

Maternal heart disease complicates up to 4% of pregnancies and up to 16% of pregnancies in women with previous cardiac conditions, with the associated risks depending on the underlying cardiac condition (Kotit & Yacoub, 2021). The incidence is increasing due to many factors including the association with co-existing medical conditions such as diabetes, hypertension in addition to obesity and substance misuse (Doughty, McLean & Coombes, 2020).

It is important to understand the physiological adaptation of the heart and circulation in pregnancy to understand the detrimental effects in pregnancy on the health of a woman with diagnosed heart disease (see Chapter 17). The changes in the cardiovascular system begin early, reach their maximum at about 30 weeks and are maintained until term. They include:

- An increase in cardiac output by up to 50%.
- An increase in blood volume up to 50%.
- A heart rate increase of 10–15 bpm.
- A decrease in total peripheral resistance.
- A lowering of blood pressure in the first and second trimesters with a rise at 34 weeks, myocardial hypertrophy and heart chamber enlargement in the third trimester.

The changes in cardiac output in normal pregnancy without pre-existing cardiac problems may produce signs and symptoms of cardiac disease: for example, dyspnoea, orthopnoea, breathlessness on exertion, altered heart sounds, oedema and occasional palpitations (Blackburn, 2018).

Risk Factors

In some women the adaptive changes may exceed the ability of the heart to function, and **congestive cardiac failure** with pulmonary oedema may occur (Adamson & Nelson-Piercy, 2018). More rarely, sudden death may be the outcome. There are times during pregnancy when **cardiac decompensation** is higher:

- At 12 and 32 weeks when the **haemodynamic changes** are increasing towards their maximum, with the most critical time between 28 and 32 weeks.
- The second dangerous period is during labour and delivery. During labour every uterine contraction injects blood from the uteroplacental circulation into the maternal bloodstream, which temporarily increases the cardiac output by 15–20%. This continuous demand on the heart may precipitate heart failure. Pushing during the second stage of labour also increases the risk further by reducing venous return.
- Finally, 4–5 days after delivery is a danger period, with thrombus formation and pulmonary embolism being a problem as blood constituents rapidly return to normal levels.

Main Types of Cardiac Disorders

Pregnancy is high risk for women with existing cardiac disorders and specialist care is essential (Adamson & Nelson-Piercy, 2018; Silverside & Warnes, 2021). Table 32.1 summarizes three key pre-existing cardiac disorders.

Assessment of Mothers with Heart Disease

Heart disease can present itself in pregnancy for the first time or as an ongoing existing problem. Assessment is made jointly by the cardiologist and obstetrician so that counselling and decision making can be considered. If a termination of pregnancy is suggested, this should take place in the first trimester. To assess client condition in heart diseases, the New York Heart Association classifications are commonly used to describe the severity of heart disease and how it affects daily activity (Caraballo et al., 2019). In practice this has little predictive value of the effect of pregnancy on the disease process.

- Class 1: no symptoms during ordinary physical activity.
- Class 2: ordinary physical activity, some fatigue, palpitations, dyspnoea.
- Class 3: symptoms during less than normal physical activity.
- Class 4: symptoms at rest, activity increases symptoms and discomfort.

If the woman is classified higher than class 2, it would indicate a poorer outcome in pregnancy. Increased risks to the fetus include maternal smoking, prescribed anticoagulants and maternal age under 20 and over 35.

TABLE 32.1	Key Cardiac Disorders
Disorder	**Aetiology and Implications**
Congenital heart disease	Categorization Septal defects: atrial septal defect, ventricular septal defect, atrioventricular septal defect. Obstruction defects: pulmonary stenosis, aortic stenosis, coarctation of the aorta (Otto & Bonow, 2021). Cyanotic defects: tetralogy of Fallot, transposition of great vessels (Valente et al., 2022). Some defects may not be problematic in pregnancy if the woman has been treated in childhood (Adamson & Nelson-Piercy, 2018). There is a need to prevent infective endocarditis; thus antibiotics in labour are necessary, and even though defects are repaired, some impairment may be present after the surgery. Uncorrected lesions may cause pulmonary hypertension and severe left ventricular failure. This will increase the risks of adverse pregnancy and birth outcomes. In women with aortic stenosis, hypertension must be avoided as it could cause increase the risk of left ventricular failure. Women with prosthetic valve replacement are at risk of **thromboembolism** and should be anticoagulated (Otto & Bonow, 2021).
Eisenmenger syndrome	Eisenmenger syndrome is an end-stage syndrome with pulmonary hypertension. The syndrome is a result of various congenital heart defects and causes systemic to pulmonary shunts (Lindman, Bonow & Otto, 2021). Women are advised not to become pregnant (Slaibi, Ibraheem & Nohanna, 2021) as this defect has a high risk of maternal mortality (between 30–50%). Pregnancy adaptation causes the right-to-left shunt to increase cyanosis and creates back-pressure on the pulmonary circulation. Intrauterine growth restriction is seen in 30% of cases because of poor cardiac output and thus low oxygen levels in the circulation (Edwards, 2021). Termination of pregnancy may be suggested. The woman is at the greatest risk of death during the third trimester, at birth and for 2 weeks postnatally and should be observed in hospital for at least 2 weeks post-delivery (Edwards, 2021).
Marfan syndrome	Marfan syndrome is an inherited condition (autosomal dominant chromosomal defect) involving connective tissue which causes skeletal, eye and heart abnormalities. High oestrogen levels present in pregnancy affect the structure of the aorta, where spontaneous rupture may take place (Adamson & Nelson-Piercy, 2018). This can happen in labour where pressures within the vascular system may be variable (Blackburn, 2018). However if there is no pre-existing heart disease, pregnancy should not pose a problem.

Management of Women with Heart Disease

The principles of management are to prevent or reduce the risk of major maternal complications. Care should be directed towards prevention of complications rather than treatment. The following treatments used would include:

- Endocarditis: routine antibiotics.
- Thromboemboli: anticoagulation.
- Cyanosis: rest, hospital admission.
- Arrhythmias: β-blockers, digoxin.
- Heart failure: hospital admission, dietary restriction of salt, diuretics.
- Respiratory and urinary tract infection: antibiotics.
- Hypertension.
- Anaemia.

It is important to be aware of the common risk factors for heart disease and venous thromboembolism, such as extreme obesity (Knight et al., 2022). Medical teams should be able to provide appropriate expertise and supervision for all women. All clinical teams caring for pregnant or postpartum women, irrespective of location, should be aware of 'red-flag' symptoms (RCP Acute Care Toolkit 15: Managing acute medical problems in pregnancy) (Engjom et al., 2022). Prior to pregnancy, any woman with a family history or genetic confirmation of aortopathy or channelopathy should be referred for cardiac assessment.

An assessment of risk can be made during pregnancy by using electrocardiography (ECG), echocardiography and maternal function in everyday circumstances (Adamson & Nelson-Piercy, 2018). Counselling is important, especially if the woman is at high risk. Assessment of the heart lesion by examining ventricular function, pulmonary pressure, persistence of shunts and valvular obstruction is crucial. Key messages from MBRRACE-UK reports are highlighted for information in Box 32.2. Specific aspects of care are presented in Clinical Application 32.1.

BOX 32.2 Key Messages Relating to Cardiac Disorders

Always investigate a persistent sinus tachycardia as a red flag, particularly when there is associated breathlessness.

Take a cardiac-specific history and heart failure suspected with the following symptoms (unless another cause is identified):

- Breathlessness when lying down (ruling out aortocaval compression) or at rest.
- Unexplained cough, particularly when lying down or which produces frothy pink sputum.
- Paroxysmal nocturnal dyspnoea – being woken from sleep by severe breathlessness and coughing (producing pink frothy sputum that is improved when upright).
- Palpitation (awareness of persistent fast heart rate at rest) (NICE, 2019).

(Engjom et al., 2022)

Action Points

Heart failure in cardiomyopathy can develop rapidly and guidelines for the management of acute heart failure and cardiogenic shock apply.

A raised respiratory rate, chest pain, persistent tachycardia and orthopnoea are important signs and symptoms of cardiac disease should always be fully investigated.

Wheeze can be due to pulmonary oedema. Consider wheeze (which does not respond to standard asthma management and exertional syncope) as red-flag symptoms of cardiovascular disease in addition to orthopnoea and chest pain.

For rapid diagnosis and decision-making, a pre-specified management algorithm and expert interdisciplinary team are crucial.

CLINICAL APPLICATION 32.1 Cardiac Disorders: Specific Aspects of Care

Intrapartum Care

Intrapartum care should be planned in a unit with full resuscitation facilities and an intensive care unit (Adamson & Nelson-Piercy, 2018). The cardiologist, obstetrician, anaesthetist and midwifery team should collaborate.

If possible, labour should be spontaneous in onset with a vaginal delivery desirable.

The use of intravenous fluids could increase circulating blood volume, which may result in pulmonary oedema, so accurate fluid balance is essential.

Blood should be cross-matched and oxygen and adult resuscitation equipment available.

The heart should be monitored by ECG and pulse oximetry with accurate blood pressure recording.

During active labour, the left lateral position is advantageous to assist venous return and prevent aortocaval compression.

Careful consideration should also be given to the woman's choice of pain relief.

Second Stage

This stage should be kept short and without exertion; if delay occurs, forceps or vacuum extraction should be considered.

Third Stage

To prevent blood loss, a continuous oxytocin infusion should be used for the third stage. When the uterus empties and contracts, approximately 500 mL of blood is returned to the central circulation.

Postnatal Care

The risk of cardiac failure with pulmonary oedema is greatest in the early puerperium (Adamson & Nelson-Piercy, 2018). Signs include tachycardia, cyanosis, oedema and distension of the liver. If pulmonary oedema occurs, acute dyspnoea with frothy sputum and haemoptysis may occur. In most units, the woman will be admitted to a high-dependency unit to stabilize her condition. Women with confirmed pre-eclampsia should be given an individual postpartum care plan on hospital discharge providing follow-up care, including medical review if needed (Knight et al., 2022).

Hypertension in Pregnancy

Hypertensive disorders during pregnancy can be associated with substantial complications for the woman and the baby. Women can have **hypertension** before pregnancy, in the first 20 weeks, in the second half of pregnancy or have new hypertension with features of multi-organ involvement (National Institute of Health and Care Excellence [NICE], 2019).

Terminology and Classifications

The terminology and classifications recommended by NICE (2019) are presented in Table 32.2.

Incidence

Hypertensive disorders during pregnancy affect around 8–10% of all pregnant women (NICE, 2019). Hypertensive disorders of pregnancy remain one of the leading causes of maternal death worldwide. In the UK, nine maternal deaths related to hypertensive disorders occurred in 2018–20, which is four times higher than the maternal deaths between 2012–14 (Knight et al., 2022). An increasing number of women are now entering pregnancy with risk factors for hypertensive pregnancy disorder, and multiple morbidities which add further complexity.

Pre-eclampsia is an idiopathic disorder with up to 5% of women developing pre-eclampsia in their first pregnancy (Waugh & Smith, 2018). However, blood pressure usually returns to normal within weeks of delivery. Proteinuria may persist for longer than the hypertension and may indicate underlying renal disease. Predisposing factors of pre-eclampsia are outlined in Table 32.3.

Pathogenesis

The cause of **gestational hypertension** is still not completely understood, and it has been described as a disease of theories (Waugh & Smith, 2018). Pre-eclampsia is associated with an increase in the inflammatory response, poor

---

TABLE 32.2 Terminology and Classification of Hypertensive Disorders

Terminology	Classification
Hypertension	Blood pressure of 140 mmHg systolic or higher, or 90 mmHg diastolic or higher.
Gestational hypertension	New hypertension presenting after 20 weeks of pregnancy without significant proteinuria.
Chronic hypertension	Hypertension that is present at the booking visit, or before 20 weeks, or if the woman is already taking antihypertensive medication when referred to maternity services. It can be primary or secondary in aetiology.
Hypertension	Diastolic blood pressure 90–109 mmHg, systolic blood pressure 140–159 mmHg (i.e., 140/90–159/109 mmHg).
Severe hypertension	Diastolic blood pressure 110 mmHg or more, systolic blood pressure 160 mmHg or more (i.e., 160/110mm Hg).

–	New onset of hypertension (over 140 mmHg systolic or over 90 mmHg diastolic) after 20 weeks of pregnancy and the co-existence of one or more of the following new-onset conditions:
	• **Proteinuria** (urine protein:creatinine ratio of 30 mg/mmol or more or albumin:creatinine ratio of 8 mg/mmol or more, or at least 1 g/L [2+] on dipstick testing) **or**
	• **Other maternal organ dysfunction:**
	  • *Renal insufficiency (creatinine ≥90 μM, ≥1.02 mg/100 mL)*
	  • *Liver involvement (elevated transaminases [alanine aminotransferase or aspartate aminotransferase ˃40 IU/L] with or without right upper quadrant or epigastric abdominal pain)*
	  • *Neurological complications (such as eclampsia, altered mental status, blindness, stroke, clonus, severe headaches or persistent visual scotomata)*
	  • *Haematological complications (such as thrombocytopenia (platelet count <150,000/μL), disseminated intravascular coagulation or haemolysis).*
	• **Uteroplacental dysfunction** (such as fetal growth restriction, abnormal umbilical artery Doppler waveform analysis or stillbirth).

Severe pre-eclampsia	Pre-eclampsia with severe hypertension that does not respond to treatment or is associated with ongoing or recurring severe headaches, visual scotomata, nausea or vomiting, epigastric pain, oliguria and severe hypertension, as well as progressive deterioration in laboratory blood tests (*such as rising creatinine or liver transaminases or falling platelet count, or failure of fetal growth or abnormal Doppler findings*).
HELLP syndrome	Haemolysis, elevated liver enzymes and low platelet count.
Eclampsia	A convulsive condition associated with pre-eclampsia.

(NICE, 2019)

TABLE 32.3	Predisposing Factors of Gestational Hypertension and Pre-eclampsia
Parity	Primigravida or a multiparous woman in her first pregnancy with a new partner.
Timing	A prolonged pregnancy interval (>10 years) or maternal age >40.
Genetic	Women more likely to develop disease if family history of gestational hypertension or pre-eclampsia (mother or sister).
Complex pregnancy	Multiple pregnancies and women who experience a hydatidiform mole may develop symptoms of hypertension before 20 weeks due to hyperplacentation.
Comorbidity	Underlying pre-existing vascular, kidney or medical problems, including hypertension, renal disease, diabetes, etc.
Raised body mass index	35 kg/m^2.

Refer to NICE (2019) for more detailed information.

placentation and poor placental blood flow to the fetus. Box 32.3 summarizes the pathogenesis of hypertensive disorders.

Eclampsia

The incidence of **eclampsia** is estimated to occur in 2.7 per 10,000 births. Symptoms often include headaches, visual disturbance, nausea, vomiting, convulsions and coma (Waugh & Smith, 2018). The underlying pathophysiology is a complicated process but is due to changes in pressure within the blood–brain barrier as a complication of the vascular changes within the circulatory system causing oedema in the brain.

It is difficult to predict the onset of eclampsia. Research into the increased numbers of endothelial cells is ongoing to try to identify a non-invasive test. Assessment of the risk for pre-eclampsia at the booking visit is essential, preferably before 10 weeks, and clinicians must be vigilant in detecting early signs and symptoms to prevent severe pre-eclampsia and eclampsia (NICE, 2019). Research has shown that women have a greater risk of cardiovascular disease if they have pre-eclampsia early in a first pregnancy,

• BOX 32.3 Pathogenesis of Hypertensive Disorders

In normal pregnancy, the spiral arterial walls are invaded by the trophoblast and are transformed into large tortuous channels that carry large amounts of blood to the intervillous space (see Chapter 12). This occurs by 22 weeks, leading to a fall in peripheral resistance. In gestational hypertension this does not occur, and the spiral arteries may only dilate to 40% of a normal pregnancy.

In women with pre-eclampsia, there is inadequate invasion of the spiral arterioles by trophoblastic cells so that a decreased uteroplacental perfusion occurs. Symptoms of gestational hypertension are a maternal response to poor placentation and an attempt to prevent poor oxygenation of the fetus. Maternal compensatory mechanisms may break down, causing the woman symptoms such as disseminated intravascular coagulation (DIC). This disruption of normal placentation may lead to altered endothelial cell function throughout the body, causing generalized vasoconstriction.

In normal pregnancy, the renin–angiotensin–aldosterone system increases in activity, maintaining salt and water balance. In gestational hypertension this system is depleted. Vasomotor tone depends on the relative influences of prostacyclin (a vasodilator) and thromboxane (a vasoconstrictor), which are substances from the prostaglandin family found in all tissues. In normal pregnancy, there is an increase in substances that cause vasodilatation, including nitric oxide, which is a potent relaxing factor within the endothelium.

The reduced trophoblast volume in the spiral arterioles leads to an underproduction of prostacyclin and a relative overproduction of thromboxane, which encourages vasospasm of the spiral arteries. The damaged endothelium of the spiral arteries undergoes acute atherosclerosis (thickening of the vessel walls), thus narrowing the lumen. This causes a rise in blood pressure to overcome the increased resistance.

Proteinuria is a serious sign in pre-eclampsia, resulting from a swelling of the kidney glomeruli partly due to the raised blood pressure causing leakage of protein through enlarged capillaries. Uric acid clearance is reduced and plasma urates rise, indicating kidney involvement showing impaired tubular function. The cardiac index (the ratio of cardiac output to body surface area)

is reduced by 22% in established pre-eclampsia and systemic vascular resistance is raised. This raised systemic resistance is not due to the action of the sympathetic nervous system. It is associated with vasoconstriction, a reduced plasma volume and haemoconcentration, and oedema usually develops. The reduced plasma volume is associated with intrauterine growth restriction.

Oxidative stress features as a component of pre-eclampsia, with excess free-radical generation initiating a cascade of events. This includes endothelial damage, reduced vasoconstriction ability and platelet aggregation, some of which may be mitigated by the use of the antioxidants vitamin C and E and low-dose aspirin prophylaxis.

Outcomes

This multisystem disorder eventually affects the kidneys, the liver and the placental bed. The kidney changes are only distinguishable from acute **glomerulonephritis** by electron microscopy. Narrowing of the capillary lumen by vasospasm is worsened by the deposition of **fibrinous material** between the endothelial cells and the basement membrane as the disease progresses. In glomerulonephritis the narrowing is caused by swelling of the basement membrane. The same fibrinous deposits have been found in the liver of patients with pre-eclampsia. **Intracapsular haemorrhages** and necrosis occur, and oedema of the liver cells may produce **epigastric pain** and impairment in liver function, showing diagnostically as raised liver enzymes.

The vessels supplying the placental bed may become constricted, and the reduction in uterine blood flow along with placental vascular lesions may result in **placental abruption**. The reduced maternal capillary blood flow in the placental villi may result in the placental tissue becoming ischaemic. These changes have grave implications for fetal growth and survival. The release of thromboplastin into the maternal circulation results in DIC. The brain becomes oedematous with the development of headache and visual disturbances. As blood pressure continues to rise, fitting may occur. Thrombosis and necrosis of the cerebral blood vessel walls may result in a **cerebrovascular accident** or **stroke**.

Refer to Huppertz & Kingdom (2018); Blackburn (2018).

showing symptoms of 'endothelial damage, abnormal lipids and insulin resistance' some years later (Chapter 47 includes care of the acutely ill woman).

HELLP Syndrome

HELLP syndrome is an acronym for **H**aemolytic anaemia, **E**levated **L**iver enzymes, **L**ow **P**latelet count. This is a serious multisystem disorder that can occur in up to 20% of women presenting with pre-eclampsia (Doughty, McLean & Coombes, 2020). Clinicians must be aware of the potential for HELLP syndrome to develop. There is uncertainty about whether **HELLP** syndrome is a severe form of pre-eclampsia or a process in itself. Women may present with malaise, nausea, vomiting, headache and epigastric pain in the second half of pregnancy (Martin, 2022). Typically this occurs just before term and less so immediately postpartum. They may have normal blood pressure and no proteinuria. As symptoms imitate gastric flu, women may be sent home to recover, but the practitioner should think again and take blood specimens for platelets and liver enzymes and await results before sending them home (Martin, 2022).

The resultant pathophysiology may be present alone or together with pre-eclampsia. The severe decrease in platelets alters clotting mechanisms, and the haemolysis damages the internal strata of the blood vessels. The multisystem involvement causes kidney failure, hepatic failure and neurological problems in the form of multiple emboli which block capillaries. The placenta is involved and abruptio placentae may occur with the death of the fetus. HELLP syndrome is a serious condition, and delivery is essential to prevent these complications. Criteria for diagnosis are perhaps a selection of abnormalities and not always all of them.

Management of Hypertensive Conditions

Vigilance is required in the observation and assessment of hypertensive disorders in antenatal women. Clinical Application 32.2 outlines the assessment.

Rest and Observation

Women with mild gestational hypertension can rest at home. However if the disease is moderate to severe or worsening with proteinuria, hospitalization is recommended as it allows greater surveillance of maternal and fetal conditions. Tables 32.4 and 32.5 summarize NICE (2019) recommendations for antenatal care management depending on the degree of hypertension.

A prime method of observing women antenatally is the assessment of blood pressure and urinalysis with estimation of maternal and fetal well-being. As the blood pressure rises, visual disturbances, headache and epigastric pain may be

---

• CLINICAL APPLICATION 32.2 **Antenatal Assessment for Hypertensive Disorders**

Assessment at the antenatal clinic: this needs to be conducted at each consultation by the midwife or another professional trained in the management of hypertensive disorder of pregnancy.

Concerns include:
- Sustained systolic blood pressure ≥160 mmHg.
- Any maternal biochemical or haematological investigations that cause concern. For example, a new and persistent:
  - Rise in creatinine (≥90 µM, or ≥1 mg/100 mL; **or**
  - Rise in alanine transaminase (>70 IU/L, or twice upper limit of normal range); **or**

- Fall in platelet count (<150,000/µL).
- Signs of impending eclampsia, pulmonary oedema or other signs of severe pre-eclampsia.
- Suspected fetal compromise.
- Any other clinical signs that cause concern.

Use a risk tool – consider using either the *fullPIERS* (use any time during pregnancy) or *PREP-S* (use up to 34 weeks of pregnancy) validated risk-prediction models to help guide decisions about the most appropriate place of care (such as in utero transfer) and thresholds for intervention (NICE, 2022).

TABLE 32.4 **Management of Pregnancy with Gestational Hypertension**

	Degree of Hypertension	
Recommendation	Hypertension (BP 140/90–159/109 mmHg)	Severe Hypertension (BP ≥160/110 mmHg)
Admission to hospital	Do not routinely admit to hospital	Admit If BP falls <160/110 mmHg then manage as hypertension
Antihypertensive pharmacological treatment	Offer pharmacological treatment if BP is >140/90 mmHg	All women – offer pharmacological treatment
Target BP once on antihypertensive treatment	Aim for BP ≤135/85 mmHg	Aim for BP ≤135/85 mmHg

TABLE 32.4   Management of Pregnancy with Gestational Hypertension—cont'd

Recommendation	Degree of Hypertension	
	Hypertension (BP 140/90–159/109 mmHg)	Severe Hypertension (BP ≥160/110 mmHg)
BP measurement	Once or twice a week (depending on BP) until BP is ≤135/85 mmHg	Every 15–30 min until BP <160/110 mmHg
Dipstick proteinuria testing	Once or twice a week (with BP measurement)	Daily while admitted
Blood tests	Measure FBC, liver function and renal function twice a week	Measure FBC, liver function and renal function three times a week
PlGF-based testing	Carry out (placental growth) PlGF-based testing on one occasion if there is suspicion of pre-eclampsia	Carry out PlGF-based testing on one occasion if there is suspicion of pre-eclampsia
Fetal assessment	Offer fetal heart auscultation at every antenatal appointment. Carry out ultrasound assessment of the fetus at diagnosis and, if normal, repeat every 2 to 4 weeks, if clinically indicated. Carry out a CTG only if clinically indicated.	Offer fetal heart auscultation at every antenatal appointment. Carry out ultrasound assessment of the fetus at diagnosis and, if normal, repeat every 2 weeks. If severe hypertension persists, carry out a CTG at diagnosis and only if clinically indicated.

BP, Blood pressure; CTG, cardiotocography; FBC, full blood count; PlGF, placental growth factor.

TABLE 34.5   Management of Pregnancy with Pre-eclampsia

Recommendation	Degree of Hypertension	
	Hypertension (BP 140/90–159/109 mmHg)	Severe Hypertension (BP ≥160/110 mmHg)
Admission to hospital	Admit if clinical concerns for woman and fetus or if deemed to be high risk of adverse events	Admit. If BP falls <160/110 mmHg then manage as hypertension
Antihypertensive pharmacological treatment	Offer pharmacological treatment if BP is >140/90 mmHg	All women – offer pharmacological treatment
Target BP once on antihypertensive treatment	Aim for BP ≤135/85 mmHg	Aim for BP ≤135/85 mmHg
BP measurement	At least every 48 h and more frequently if the woman is admitted to hospital	Every 15–30 min until BP <160/110 mmHg Thereafter, at least four times daily whilst the woman is an inpatient, depending on clinical circumstances
Dipstick proteinuria testing	Only repeat if clinically indicated (i.e., if new symptoms and signs develop or if there is uncertainty over diagnosis)	Only repeat if clinically indicated (i.e., if new symptoms and signs develop or if there is uncertainty over diagnosis)
Blood tests	Measure FBC, liver function and renal function twice a week	Measure FBC, liver function and renal function three times a week
Fetal heart auscultation	Offer fetal heart auscultation at every antenatal appointment	Offer fetal heart auscultation at every antenatal appointment
Fetal ultrasound	Carry out ultrasound assessment of the fetus at diagnosis. If normal, repeat every 2 weeks	Carry out ultrasound assessment of the fetus at diagnosis. If normal, repeat every 2 weeks
Cardiotocography	Carry out CTG at diagnosis, only if clinically indicated thereafter	Carry out CTG at diagnosis, only if clinically indicated thereafter

BP, Blood pressure; CTG, cardiotocography; FBC, full blood count.

experienced by the woman; these signs need investigated and acted on. Fetal observations are equally essential. Any signs of impending eclampsia may necessitate rapid delivery, regardless of the gestational period, to save the mother's life. Control of blood pressure using drug treatment is summarized in Table 32.6.

Control of Blood Pressure

Delivery

The only treatment for pre-eclampsia is delivery of the baby and placenta. A decision to deliver the baby will depend partly on the effectiveness of the treatment. The mode of delivery similarly depends on the risks to mother and baby, and delivery, whether by induction of labour depending on

TABLE 32.6	**Hypertension and Drug Treatment**
Degree of Hypertension	**Drug Treatment**
Gestational hypertension	Consider labetalol to treat gestational hypertension. Consider nifedipine for women in whom labetalol is not suitable, and methyldopa if labetalol or nifedipine are not suitable. Base choice on side-effect profiles, risk (including fetal effects) and the woman's preferences. *Labetalol is a β-adrenoreceptor antagonist. Effects can be seen in 2–5 min and it initiates a fall in blood pressure almost immediately. Labetalol does not pass through the placenta or decrease cardiac output.* *Nifedipine is a calcium-channel blocker that affects cell membranes and cardiac muscle. It is absorbed by the gut and is only used orally. It does not pass through the placenta but may have effects on labour as it is a tocholytic.* *Methyldopa, which affects noradrenaline (norepinephrine) synthesis, reduces systemic peripheral resistance without changing heart rate or cardiac output (Ritter et al., 2019).*
Treatment of chronic hypertension	Consider labetalol to treat chronic hypertension. Consider nifedipine for women in whom labetalol is not suitable, or methyldopa if both labetalol and nifedipine are not suitable. Base choice on any pre-existing treatment, side-effect profiles, risks (including fetal effects) and the woman's preference.
High risk of pre-eclampsia	Advise 75–150 mg of aspirin daily from 12 weeks until the birth of the baby. *(High risk: chronic kidney disease, autoimmune disease such as systemic lupus erythematosus or antiphospholipid syndrome, type 1 or type 2 diabetes, chronic hypertension)*
Moderate risk factor for pre-eclampsia	Advise pregnant women with more than one moderate risk factor for pre-eclampsia to take 75–150 mg of aspirin daily from 12 weeks until the birth of the baby. *(Moderate risks: nulliparity, age 40 years or older, pregnancy interval of more than 10 years, body mass index ≥35 kg/m² at first visit, family history of pre-eclampsia and multi-fetal pregnancy)*

Refer to NICE (2019) for further detail on drug treatment.

• BOX 32.4 Maternal Deaths (Cardiovascular and Hypertensive Disorders)

Cardiovascular

There has been an overall decrease in the rate of maternal cardiovascular deaths but it remained the leading cause of maternal death between 2018–2020 (Knight et al., 2022).

Reasons include acquired heart disease, older age and comorbid conditions such as obesity and hypertension.
Characteristics of maternal deaths:
- 61 women died from heart disease.
- Maternal mortality rates from cardiovascular disease increase with age.
- Almost half of women (29/61) were from some of the deprived quintiles of the UK.

Conclusions
- In almost one-third of instances (19/61), different care provision may have prevented women's deaths.
- There must be more awareness to consider cardiac causes as part of the differential diagnosis for women presenting with pain, wheeze and breathlessness.

- Only one in ten women were known to have cardiac disease prior to pregnancy.

Hypertensive Disorders

Characteristics of Maternal Deaths
- Eight women died from hypertensive disorders: two died following intracranial haemorrhage, two from acute fatty liver of pregnancy, two following eclamptic seizures and two women from pulmonary oedema at home.

Conclusions
- For three-quarters of these women (6/8), different care might have made a difference to the outcome.
- Fluid overload was seen in two women who subsequently died.
- Emphasis on prevention, early detection and optimal management of hypertensive disorders is paramount.
  See Chapter 30 for risk factors such as socio-demographic, ethnicity, mental health and combined adversities.

(Knight et al., 2022)

cervical ripeness or by caesarean section, depends on the condition of the mother and maturity of the fetus.

Main Points

- Patterns of heart disease are changing, with increasing numbers of women surviving congenital heart disease and an increase in coronary artery disease.
- For women with cardiac disorders, labour should be in a unit with full resuscitation facilities and an intensive care unit. Labour should be spontaneous in onset, with a vaginal delivery where possible. Intravenous fluids should be used cautiously. Antibiotic prophylaxis may be necessary in labour to prevent infective endocarditis. The second stage should be kept short and without exertion.
- Pre-eclampsia is associated with proteinuria and may lead to eclampsia. It is a multisystem disorder, which may result in maternal and fetal morbidity and mortality.
- In pre-eclampsia there is inadequate invasion of the spiral arterioles by trophoblastic cells, and decreased uteroplacental perfusion occurs. The common features of

Box 32.4 summarizes key outcomes from the MBRRACE-UK report relating to cardiovascular and hypertensive disorders.

pre-eclampsia, vasoconstriction and disseminated intravascular coagulation, can lead to changes in the kidney, liver and placental bed.

- The aim of care is to prolong the pregnancy until the fetus is mature enough to survive. Antihypertensive drugs are useful in protecting the woman's circulation against the risk of cerebrovascular accident but have no effect on the disease or on fetal growth.
- Plasma urate concentrations are useful biochemical indicators of kidney function, and severe disease is present if the platelet count falls.
- In a few women, severe pre-eclampsia may be complicated by HELLP syndrome. Immediate delivery will resolve the abnormal blood picture, but platelets or packed red cells may be used to lessen the risk of haemorrhage. The long-term prognosis is that the blood pressure returns to normal within weeks.

References

Adamson, D.L., Nelson-Piercy, C., 2018. Heart disease in pregnancy. In: Edmonds, D.K., Lees, C., Bourne, T.H. (Eds.), Dewhurst's Textbook of Obstetrics and Gynaecology, ninth ed. Wiley-Blackwell, Oxford.

Blackburn, S.T., 2018. Maternal, Fetal and Neonatal Physiology: A Clinical Perspective, fifth ed. Elsevier, Philadelphia.

Caraballo, C., Desai, N.R., Mulder, H., Alhanti, B., Wilson, F.P., Fiuzat, M., et al., 2019. Clinical implications of the New York Association classification. J. Am. Heart Assoc. 8 (23), e014240.

Doughty, R., McLean, M., Coombes, S., 2020. Medical conditions of significance in midwifery practice. In: Marshall, J., Raynor, M. (Eds.), Myles' Textbook for Midwives, seventeenth ed. Elsevier, London.

Edwards, C., 2021. Pregnancy plus atrial septal defect vs Eisenmenger syndrome. In: Libby, P., Bonow, R.O., Mann, D.L., Tomaselli, G.F., Bhatt, D.L. (Eds.), Solomon SD & Braunwald E 2021. Braunwald's Heart Disease: A Textbook of Cardiovascular Medicine, twelfth ed. Elsevier, Philadelphia.

Engjom, H., Clarke, B., Girling, J., Hillman, S., Holden, S., Lucas, S., et al., (on behalf of the MBRRACE-UK cardiac chapter writing group), 2022. Lessons on cardiovascular care. In: Knight, M., Bunch, K., Patel, R., Shakespeare, J., Kotnis, R., Kenyon, S., Kurinczuk, J.J. (Eds.), Saving Lives, Improving Mothers' Care – Lessons Learned to Inform Maternity Care from the UK and Ireland Confidential Enquiries into Maternal Deaths and Morbidity 2018–20. National Perinatal Epidemiology Unit, University of Oxford, Oxford.

Huppertz, B., Kingdom, J.C.P., 2018. The placenta and fetal membranes. In: Edmonds, D.K., Lees, C., Bourne, T.H. (Eds.), Dewhurst's Textbook of Obstetrics and Gynaecology, ninth ed. Wiley-Blackwell, Oxford.

Knight, M., Bunch, K., Patel, R., Shakespeare, J., Kotnis, R., Kenyon, S., Kurinczuk, J.J., (on behalf of MBRRACE-UK), 2022. Saving

Lives, Improving Mothers' Care – Lessons Learned to Inform Maternity Care from the UK and Ireland Confidential Enquiries into Maternal Deaths and Morbidity 2018–20. National Perinatal Epidemiology Unit, University of Oxford, Oxford.

Kotit, S., Yacoub, M., 2021. Cardiovascular adverse events in pregnancy: a global perspective. Glob. Cardiol. Sci. Pract. 2021 (1), e202105.

Lindman, B.R., Bonow, R.O., Otto, C.M., 2021. Aortic valves – diseases of the heart valves. In: Libby, P., Bonow, R.O., Mann, D.L., Tomaselli, G.F., Bhatt, D.L. (Eds.), Solomon SD & Braunwald E 2021. Braunwald's Heart Disease: A Textbook of Cardiovascular Medicine, twelfth ed. Elsevier, Philadelphia.

Martin Jr., J.N., 2022. HELLP syndrome. Br. Med. J. Best. Pract. Available at: https://bestpractice.bmj.com/topics/en-gb/1000.

National Institute of Health and Care Excellence (NICE), 2019. Hypertension in Pregnancy: Diagnosis and Management. Available at: https://www.nice.org.uk/guidance/ng133.

National Institute of Health and Care Excellence (NICE), 2021. Antenatal Care. Available at: https://www.nice.org.uk/guidance/ng201.

National Institute of Health and Care Excellence (NICE), 2022. Hypertension in Pregnancy: Scenario: Pre-eclampsia. Available at: https://www.nice.org.uk/.

Otto, C.M., Bonow, R.D., 2021. Approaches to the patient with valvular heart disease. In: Libby, P., Bonow, R.O., Mann, D.L., Tomaselli, G.F., Bhatt, D.L. (Eds.), Solomon SD & Braunwald E 2021. Braunwald's Heart Disease: A Textbook of Cardiovascular Medicine, twelfth ed. Elsevier, Philadelphia.

Ritter, J.M., Flower, R.S., Henderson, G., Loke, Y.K., MacEwan, D., Rang, H., 2019. Rang & Dale's Pharmacology, ninth ed. Elsevier, London.

Silverside, C.C., Warnes, C.A., 2021. Pregnancy and heart disease. In: Libby, P., Bonow, R.O., Mann, D.L., Tomaselli, G.F., Bhatt, D.L. (Eds.), Solomon SD & Braunwald E 2021. Braunwald's Heart Disease: A Textbook of Cardiovascular Medicine, twelfth ed. Elsevier, Philadelphia.

Slaibi, A., Ibraheem, B., Nohanna, F., 2021. Challenging management of a pregnancy complicated by Eisenmenger syndrome; a case report. Ann. Med. Surg. 69, 102721.

Waugh, J.S., Smith, M.C., 2018. Hypertensive disorders. In: Edmonds, D.K., Lees, C., Bourne, T.H. (Eds.), Dewhurst's Textbook of Obstetrics and Gynaecology, ninth ed. Wiley-Blackwell, Oxford.

Valente AM, Dorfman AL, Babu-Narayan SV, Kreiger E. 2021. Congenital heart disease in the adolescent and adult. In: Libby P, Bonow RO, Mann DL, Tomaselli GF, Bhatt DL, Solomon SD, eds. Braunwald's Heart Disease: A Textbook of Cardiovascular Medicine. 12th ed. Philadelphia, PA: Elsevier; 2021 chap 82.

Annotated recommended reading

Blackburn, S.T., 2018. Maternal, Fetal and Neonatal Physiology: A Clinical Perspective, fifth ed. Elsevier, Philadelphia.

This textbook provides a detailed description of the minor disorders of pregnancy. This includes up-to-date evidence to support the aetiology, underpinning physiological basis and management.

European Society of Cardiology, 2018. Cardiovascular Diseases during Pregnancy (Management of) Guidelines: ESC Clinical Practice Guidelines. Available at: https://www.escardio.org/Guidelines/Clinical-Practice-Guidelines/Cardiovascular-Diseases-during-Pregnancy-Management-of.

This international website provides standards and guidelines for cardiovascular diseases and the management during pregnancy. Other learning resources are also available.

https://www.npeu.ox.ac.uk/ukoss/current-surveillance.

Students and midwives are strongly recommended to access this excellent website for up-to-date information on obstetrics and maternity care. Current studies are ongoing in relation to key topic areas. The direct link for cardiac-related research is provided:

Pregnancy in women with known cardiomyopathy.

Libby, P., Bonow, R.O., Mann, D.L., Tomaselli, G.F., Bhatt, D.L., Solomon, S.D., Braunwald, E., 2021. Braunwald's Heart Disease: A Textbook of Cardiovascular Medicine, twelfth ed. Elsevier, Philadelphia.

This textbook (two volumes) provides current, comprehensive and evidence-based cardiology information for students and practitioners.

National Institute of Health and Care Excellence (NICE), 2019. Hypertension in Pregnancy: Diagnosis and Management. Available at: https://www.nice.org.uk/guidance/ng133.

A comprehensive guide to hypertension during pregnancy. Although providing a UK perspective, the information contained within this publication can be applied to any setting.

Useful websites

www.nice.org.uk/guidance/.
www.rcog.org.uk.
https://www.npeu.ox.ac.uk/ukoss/.

33
Anaemia and Clotting Disorders

THOMAS McEWAN AND JEAN RANKIN

CHAPTER CONTENTS

This chapter focuses on anaemia and clotting disorders. Iron deficiency anaemia, hyperglobinopathies, thromboembolism and consumptive coagulopathies during pregnancies are discussed.

Introduction

Worldwide, the effects of anaemia and clotting disorders on maternal and fetal morbidity and mortality are enormous. This remains an ongoing public health issue for women in reproductive years, especially during and following pregnancy (Stoltzfus, 2003). Box 33.1 summarizes the facts and key messages from the recent related maternal deaths in the UK (Knight et al., 2022).

Anaemia

Globally, almost 30% of the population are affected by anaemia (World Health Organization [WHO], 2020a). **Iron deficiency anaemia (IDA)** is the most common cause, especially in low-income populations (Stephen et al., 2018; WHO, 2020a). Women in childbearing years are compromised due to the loss of iron through pregnancy and menstruation (Stephen et al., 2018; WHO, 2020a). An estimated 75% of diagnosed anaemia arises from iron deficiency, with pregnant adolescents being at particular risk (Broughton Pipkin, 2018; WHO, 2022b). The reader is referred to Chapter 16, Box 16.1 for up-to-date information on the background and incidence of physiological anaemia of pregnancy, iron deficiency anaemia and evidence on interventions.

Anaemia is a condition in which the number of red blood cells (RBCs) or their oxygen-carrying capacity is insufficient to meet the physiological needs of the individual, which will vary by age, sex, altitude, smoking and pregnancy status. In its severe form, it is associated with fatigue, weakness and dizziness, and pregnant women and children are particularly vulnerable. There may be reduced resistance to infection, and life may be threatened by antepartum or postpartum haemorrhage. The fetus may suffer intrauterine hypoxia and growth restriction, although it is difficult to separate the effects of anaemia from other lifestyle factors.

Recognition and Types of Anaemia

The types of anaemia include:
- Iron deficiency anaemia (IDA).
- Folic acid deficiency.
- Hereditary haemoglobinopathies, sickle cell anaemias and the thalassaemias.
- Anaemia due to blood loss.

Anaemia is defined as a haemoglobin (Hb) level two standard deviations below the normal for age and sex (National Institute for Health and Care Excellence [NICE], 2021). Table 33.1 identifies the Hb levels for women, men and children.

Iron Deficiency Anaemia (IDA)

Pathology

Iron is essential for the bioavailability of oxygen to cells. Diminished iron levels are due to poor intake of available dietary iron. It is absorbed by the small intestine more readily in pregnancy. IDA is a common pathology of pregnancy but may be asymptomatic and difficult to diagnose (Davis & Pavord, 2018). The physiological changes of blood plasma volume expansion make it appear that Hb is lower.

Key Messages from the MBRRACE-UK Enquiry into Maternal Deaths

- Total number of maternal deaths: 229 women died from direct and indirect causes. (A statistically significant increase from direct causes was noted between 2015–17 and 2018–20).
  Related to anaemia and clotting disorders:
- Anaemia was directly associated with three maternal deaths.
- Thrombosis and venous thromboembolism (VTE) continue to be the leading cause of direct deaths occurring within 42 days of the end of pregnancy – i.e., 20 maternal deaths (4%) (1.4 in 100,000 maternities). This was a reduction from 32 deaths recorded in 2014–16.
- Of these maternal deaths, 11 (10%) died at less than 24 weeks.
- As maternal mortality rate from VTE remains a similar rate to 2015–17, this suggests that several of these deaths could be prevented with improvements to care.
  Raising awareness to:
- Common risk factors for heart disease and VTE, such as extreme obesity.
- Women with type 1 diabetes and nephropathy are at intermediate risk of VTE and antenatal thromboprophylaxis with low-molecular-weight heparin should be considered (RCOG, 2015b).
- Risk factors for ischaemic heart disease have significant overlap with those associated with VTE.
- In recent years, the diagnosis of pulmonary embolism has improved significantly but treatment should not be given until a focused assessment for trauma scan has excluded intra-abdominal pathology or bleeding.

(Knight et al., 2022)

TABLE 33.1 **Hb Levels for Women, Men and Children**

Category	Hb Levels
In pregnant women	Hb <110 g/L throughout pregnancy
	Hb ≥110 g/L appears adequate in the first trimester, and a level of 105 g/L appears adequate in the second and third trimesters. Postpartum — <100 g/L.
In non-pregnant women aged over 15 years	Hb <120 g/L
In men aged over 15 years	Hb <130 g/L
In children aged 12–14 years	Hb <120 g/L

Hb, Haemoglobin.
(NICE, 2021)

In pregnancy there is a greater demand for iron for Hb synthesis, which only increases during pregnancy (Broughton Pipkin, 2018). If Hb is low, there is a poor RBC uptake of oxygen and poor oxygen delivery to the placental bed and fetus. The fetus obtains its iron from transferrin in maternal blood across the placental–maternal interface, usually after 30 weeks of pregnancy. In the earlier weeks, maternal iron consumption increases and should meet the later demands, but if iron stores of ferritin are low, the demand may not be met.

IDA is a **microcytic anaemia** with a reduction in both mean cell volume (MCV) and **serum ferritin** (iron stores). This occurs before a reduction in Hb, which is a late sign when iron stores have already been depleted. Haemodilution should be considered when comparing pregnancy and non-pregnant reference values. Table 33.2 outlines the blood tests considered when making a diagnosis. Box 33.2 details the associated problems and complications. Clinical Application 33.1 outlines the signs, symptoms and assessment of IDA.

Treatment and Management

Oral iron should be the preferred first-line treatment for iron deficiency. Parenteral iron is indicated when oral iron is not tolerated or absorbed, if non-compliance is suspected or if the woman is approaching term with insufficient time for oral supplementation to be effective.

TABLE 33.2 **Blood Tests Used to Diagnose Iron Deficiency Anaemia**

Blood Test	Normal Reference Range	Validity in Diagnosis
Haemoglobin	11–15 g/dL (110 g/L) (pregnant)	Lacks specificity, affected by haemodilution and smoking
Mean cell volume	75–99 fL	Raised in pregnancy, decreased in IDA
Reticulocyte count	25–75 × 10^9/L	Increased by pregnancy, decreased by IDA
Serum ferritin	15–300 µg/L	Signifies iron stores, early indication of iron deficiency
Total iron-binding capacity	45–72 µmol/L	Non-specific in pregnancy, raised by pregnancy, false positive if infection present
Serum iron	13–27 µmol/L	Decreased by pregnancy and diurnal rhythm, non-specific in pregnancy

IDA, Iron deficiency anaemia.

Problems in Pregnancy and Generic Complications Associated with Iron Deficiency Anaemia

Pregnancy

- Maternal postpartum fatigue, altered cognition and depressive symptoms — this in turn may affect the woman's interactions with the infant and may negatively impact behaviour and development.
- Preterm delivery — increased risk of preterm delivery and perinatal mortality.
- Increased morbidity for the mother and infant and the possibility of lower birthweight.
- Infant iron deficiency in the first 3 months of life (by a variety of mechanisms).

Generic Complications

- Heart failure — high-output heart failure can occur in people with severe anaemia, especially in those with haemoglobin <50 g/L.
- Cognitive and behavioural impairment in children — especially attention deficits.
- Impaired muscular performance — endurance and exercise capacity are reduced.
- Adverse effects on immune status and morbidity from infection (for all age groups).

(Davis & Pavord, 2018; NICE, 2021)

Active management of the third stage is recommended to minimize blood loss. Women at high risk of haemorrhage should be advised to have their baby in hospital. Blood product specification in pregnancy and the puerperium: ABO-, rhesus D- (RhD-) and K- (Kell-) compatible red cell units should be transfused (NICE 2021; Royal College of Obstetricians and Gynaecologists [RCOG], 2015a).

Folic Acid Deficiency

During pregnancy, there is an increased demand for vitamins such as folic acid. With the high rate of unplanned pregnancy in the UK and increasingly obese pregnant populations, vitamin supplementation is an important public health issue, with potential significant impact on maternal and fetal morbidity and mortality (RCOG, 2022). Box 33.3 outlines folic acid deficiency and the role of folic acid.

Haemoglobinopathies

Haemoglobinopathies are one of the most common inherited disorders with abnormalities in Hb (Public Health England, 2018). In a multicultural society, the likelihood of **inherited haemoglobinopathies** should be considered, as well as the effects of nutrition and infection on iron status (RCOG, 2015b). Globally, at least 5% of adults are carriers for a Hb condition. Most countries have an uneven distribution of carriers because populations include different ethnic groups (with different carrier rates, types of haemoglobinopathy

and mutations) because of migration. Two of the most common diseases are the recessively inherited **sickle cell disease** (2.3%) and **thalassaemias** (2.9%) affecting Hb synthesis. In utero, the fetus is not affected as it carries fetal Hb (HbF) with a greater affinity to oxygen. Soon after birth, the switch between fetal and adult Hb (HbA) begins. The symptoms of inherited disease become evident as the ratio of HbF to HbA changes (Davis & Pavord, 2018).

The Globin Chains

The four protein chains in normal Hb take a particular shape which allows maximum uptake, delivery and release of oxygen into the tissues. All Hb variants have a tetrameric structure with four protein chains in association with four haem molecules. The gene for the α-globin chain family is located on chromosome 16 and for the β-globin chain family on chromosome 11. The α-globin chain is 141 amino acids long and the β-globin chain is 146 amino acids long.

Inherited genes produce abnormal proteins that cannot carry out their function efficiently, resulting in ill health with anaemia, hypoxia, tissue damage and haemolysis (Fig. 33.1). There are three forms of inherited haemoglobinopathies:

- Structural Hb variants, in which there is a fault in either the α-globin or β-globin chain.
- The thalassaemias, in which there is reduced production of either the α-globin or β-globin chain.
- Failure to switch from the production of HbF to HbA, which is clinically insignificant (and may help the sufferer as HbF absorbs oxygen easier).

Sickle Cell Disease

Sickle cell disease (SCD) is a disorder involving defects in the structure of Hb (Public Health England, 2018; Sickle Cell Society, 2018) (Table 33.3). A single amino-acid substitution of **valine** for **glutamic acid** results in a Hb molecule that is less soluble. When oxygen is low, the molecules form long, linear stacks that distort the RBCs into a sickle shape. The inheritance of one gene from each parent (homozygous genotype for HbSS) makes the individual sickle cell-positive. Those who inherit one gene (heterozygote) have the sickle cell trait (HbAS) and usually do not display signs of the disease. They do, however, have some protection against the organism *Plasmodium falciparum,* the cause of a severe form of malaria. The malarial parasite enters the RBC and causes sickling. This cell and its parasite are destroyed by the spleen, protecting the individual from malaria. Heterozygotic parents have a 50% chance of producing an infant affected by SCD (Sickle Cell Society, 2018).

The incidence of SCD varies from country to country and is about 1 in 4 in parts of Africa and 1 in 10 of the Black population of the United States and UK (Sickle Cell Society, 2018). Other variants of the disease are emerging and crossing racial and ethnic groups.

Common or very common signs include: Pallor, dry and rough skin, dry and damaged hair, diffuse and moderate alopecia, atrophic glossitis.

Other signs include: Ulceration of the corners of the mouth, nail changes such as ridging, worsening of pre-existing tachycardia, murmurs, cardiac enlargement and heart failure may occur if anaemia is severe (haemoglobin (Hb) <70 g/L). There may be an absence of signs, even if the person has severe anaemia.

Very common symptoms: Fatigue, dyspnoea, headache.

Common symptoms: Cognitive dysfunction, restless leg syndrome.

Rare symptoms: Syncope, haemodynamic instability, dysphagia (in association with gastrointestinal disorders).

Other symptoms: Dizziness or light-headedness, weakness, irritability, palpitations, pica, dysgeusia, pruritus, sore tongue, tinnitus, impairment of body temperature regulation (in pregnant women).

Serious symptoms such as worsening of pre-existing anginal pain, ankle oedema, or dyspnoea at rest are unlikely unless Hb <70g/L (indicates heart or lung pathology).

Angina may occur if there is pre-existing coronary artery disease.

Symptoms of iron deficiency may occur without anaemia. These symptoms include fatigue, lack of concentration and irritability.

Diagnosis is made through history, examination and investigations.

Assessment

Observe signs and explore if the woman has any symptoms.

A detailed history is essential and observational skills are crucial to pick up any signs.

- Personal history taking should be detailed enough to include general health and well-being, nutritional habits, weight loss, gastrointestinal upset, drugs, menstrual obstetric history, breastfeeding (as appropriate), demographics (to identify vulnerable groups) and any recent previous illness or conditions. Examples of chronic infections (low iron status affects immunity) include urinary tract infection (UTI), HIV, malaria and previous antepartum or postpartum haemorrhage.
- A family history of IDA or haematological disorders (e.g., thalassaemia).

Women should receive information on improvement of dietary iron intake and factors affecting absorption of dietary iron.

A urine sample will exclude UTI because ferritin levels may be artificially high when an infection is present.

Requirements for group and screen samples and cross-matching (in line with local protocols):

- Routine investigations at the initial antenatal booking include blood specimens for Hb concentration blood count. All women should also have their blood group and antibody status checked at booking and at 28 weeks of gestation.
- Borderline anaemia can be managed in the community setting and moderate to severe anaemia is referred to a consultant led unit.
- High-risk women should have precautionary blood tests and investigations in the event of emergency treatment and interventions and transfusion (e.g., placenta praevia).

Pathophysiology

Erythrocytes (RBCs) are fragile and have a significantly reduced life span (17 days) compared with healthy individuals (120 days). Deoxygenation is the most common cause of **sickling.** HbSS reacts by creating non-pliable intracellular fibres, pulling the cells into a banana shape or holly leaf shape. These block capillaries, creating the pain of a sickle cell crisis. Decreased plasma volume, hypothermia, infection and acidosis also precipitate sickling. This will occur with minor degrees of oxygen shortage with SCD, but lack of oxygen must be severe to cause sickling in people with sickle cell trait.

Vascular occlusion occurs anywhere, but especially in the kidney and brain. In pregnancy, the placental bed may be affected. Pain is severe, and death of tissues may occur within affected organs. Sickled cells are haemolyzed in the spleen, resulting in anaemia. Sickling is not permanent, and most RBCs regain their normal shape after reoxygenation and rehydration. The extent and clinical manifestations of sickling will depend on the percentage of Hb that is HbSS. Clinical Application 33.2 outlines the management of sickle cell anaemia in pregnancy.

Thalassaemia

More than 70,000 babies are born with **thalassaemia** worldwide each year, and there are 100 million individuals who are asymptomatic thalassaemia carriers. The basic defect in the thalassaemia syndromes is reduced globin-chain synthesis, with the resultant RBCs having inadequate Hb content. The pathophysiology of thalassaemia syndromes is characterized by extravascular haemolysis due to the release into the peripheral circulation of damaged RBCs and erythroid precursors because of a high degree of ineffective erythropoiesis (Davis & Pavord, 2018).

Thalassaemia is caused by a reduced rate of synthesis of either α-globin or β-globin chains. The heterozygote (**thalassaemia minor**) with one normal Hb gene is generally asymptomatic but with reduced Hb levels. The RBCs are thin, misshapen and short-lived. The homozygous condition (**thalassaemia major**) is life-threatening and, if untreated, leads to death in childhood. Homozygotes have severe anaemia which requires regular blood transfusions, but not replacement iron as stores are overloaded due to rapid breakdown of the short-lived RBCs.

β-Thalassaemia is much more common than α-thalassaemia and, in the carrier state, leads to mild **microcytic hypochromic anaemia** and hyperplasia of bone marrow due to increased haemopoiesis. Haemolysis of immature erythrocytes may cause a slight rise in serum iron. The spleen may be enlarged because of the increased haemolysis. Clinical Application 33.3 above outlines the management of thalassaemia.

Vitamins are essential for normal cell function, growth and development and should be an essential part of a healthy diet. This type of anaemia usually responds well to daily supplementation of folic acid. Certain vitamins taken around conception and in early pregnancy can reduce the likelihood of neural tube defects and other fetal anomalies.

Folic acid is necessary for RBC proliferation and DNA synthesis, and demands are high in pregnancy as the fetus develops and grows (Blackburn, 2018). Deficiency may occur in pregnancy in the undernourished, in multiple pregnancy, those on anticoagulants or anticonvulsants, or in heavy drinkers or smokers, causing megaloblastic anaemia (Davis & Pavord, 2018). Demands for folate (naturally occurring) and folic acid (synthesized) are high in pregnancy, and many women will have low reserves as the fetus grows. Synthesized folic acid is more readily acquired by body systems than folate; hence supplementation may be required and is more successful in raising levels in pregnancy.

In folic acid deficiency, RBCs are macrocytic (larger) and may be misshapen, fewer in number and the Hb level low. Plasma and RBC folate can be estimated. There may be a low platelet count and white cell count. Serum folic acid is lower than 4 μg/mL.

Management

Folic acid supplementation (400 μg/day) is recommended pre-conception and during the first trimester of pregnancy (NICE, 2023). Prevention of anaemia by administration of 300–500 μg prophylactic folic acid daily can be recommended for women:
- With malabsorption syndrome.
- With haemoglobinopathies (see later).
- With a multiple pregnancy.
- On anticonvulsant therapy.

Folate deficiency and the role in neural tube defects are detailed in Box 33.4. The role of vitamin supplements in pregnancy remains inconclusive. See Box 33.5 for current guidance (RCOG, 2022).

Glucose-6-Phosphate Dehydrogenase Deficiency

Glucose-6-phosphate dehydrogenase (G6PD) deficiency is a genetic metabolic abnormality. It is the most common X-linked enzyme deficiency found in people of African, Asian and Mediterranean origin. A gene frequency of 11% has been found in the American Black male population (Rogers, 2022). It is more common in males, only manifesting itself when both X chromosomes are affected. Neonates who inherit the gene may have prolonged jaundice.

It is caused by deficiency of the enzyme G6PD that is critical for the proper function of RBCs. If the level of this enzyme is too low, then RBCs can break down prematurely (haemolysis). When the body cannot compensate for accelerated loss, anaemia develops. Additional factors are required to *trigger* the onset of symptoms. Examples include certain infectious diseases and eating fava beans (this causes a potentially serious acute haemolytic anaemia known as favism). Symptoms can include fatigue, pale colour, jaundice or yellow skin colour, shortness of breath, rapid heartbeat, dark urine and enlarged spleen (splenomegaly).

Certain drugs also precipitate haemolytic crises and include antimalarial preparations, sulphonamides and some antibiotics (nitrofurantoin, nalidixic acid, chloramphenicol and hydralazine).

Thromboembolism and Pregnancy

Thrombosis in childbearing women is serious because of its association with deep vein thrombosis and pulmonary embolism (PE). Thrombosis and venous thromboembolism (VTE) continue to be the leading cause of direct maternal deaths (Box 33.1). The highest risk of thromboembolic diseases is the first 6 weeks after birth, with the risk increasing by 20-fold in the puerperium (Blackburn, 2018; RCOG, 2015b). Diuresis occurring in the first 24 hours after delivery changes the blood viscosity. The risk becomes even more significant with the increasing rate of operative deliveries. Thrombosis can be divided clinically into superficial **thrombophlebitis** and **deep vein thrombosis** (DVT).

Superficial Thrombophlebitis

The superficial veins of the legs are affected. The vein is tender and may be reddened and hard. It is usually a varicose vein that is affected, and there is no risk of PE unless there is a concomitant DVT. Women who are at risk tend to be older, overweight and of high parity. The use of supportive tights and thromboembolic-deterrent stockings assists in the treatment of this condition. The woman should elevate her legs when resting, but there is no need to restrict movement and anticoagulant therapy is not necessary.

Deep Venous Thrombosis (DVT)

The deep veins of the calf, thigh or pelvis are usually affected, particularly on the left side. If there is no accompanying inflammation (**phlebitis**) and the blood clot (thrombus) does not obstruct the blood vessel, there may be no clinical signs. If the clot is friable and pieces become detached from the vessel wall, they will travel around the circulation (**embolus**), through the heart and into the pulmonary circulation, leading to a **pulmonary embolus.** This may be fatal, but recovery could be complete.

Factors Associated with Pregnancy Predisposing to Thromboembolism

Risk factors include previous VTE or thrombophilia (a tendency to form blood clots); obesity; increased maternal age; immobility and long-distance travel; admission to hospital during pregnancy; and other comorbidities such as heart disease, inflammatory bowel disease and pre-eclampsia. Additional risk factors occurring during the first trimester of pregnancy include hyperemesis gravidarum, ovarian hyperstimulation and in vitro fertilization pregnancy. Caesarean section is a key risk factor.

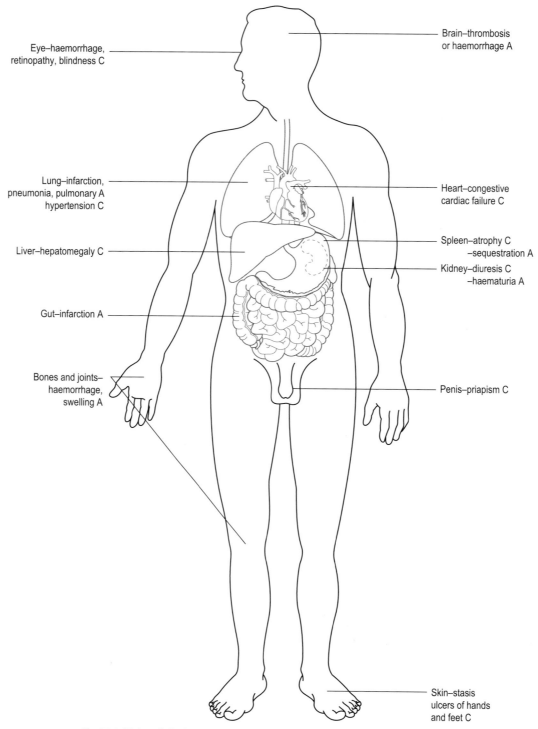

Eye–haemorrhage, retinopathy, blindness C

Brain–thrombosis or haemorrhage A

Lung–infarction, pneumonia, pulmonary A hypertension C

Heart–congestive cardiac failure C

Liver–hepatomegaly C

Spleen–atrophy C
–sequestration A

Kidney–diuresis C
–haematuria A

Gut–infarction A

Bones and joints–haemorrhage, swelling A

Penis–priapism C

Skin–stasis ulcers of hands and feet C

• **Fig. 33.1** Major clinical manifestations of sickle cell anaemia *A*, acute; *C*, chronic.

Pathogenesis

The hypercoagulable state of pregnancy is crucial in protecting the mother against excessive blood loss with delivery and placental separation (Blackburn, 2018). However, this can also be a disadvantage as it significantly increases the risk of thromboembolic disorders during pregnancy and postpartum. During pregnancy, some clotting factors are altered to prevent detrimental blood loss at delivery: von Willebrand factor; factors X, VIII and V; and fibrinogen are increased. There is impaired fibrinolysis, and the placenta produces plasminogen 1 and 2 activator inhibitors which prevent clotting at the placental bed. The three factors (**Virchow triad**) predisposing to thromboembolic disorders include venous stasis, altered coagulation and vascular damage. These are all present or potentially present during pregnancy (Blackburn, 2018).

TABLE 33.3	Common Variants of Haemoglobin in Sickle Cell Disease (SCD)

Haemoglobin	Disease
HbSS	Homozygous SCD (sickle cell anaemia)
HbSC	Heterozygous SCD (sickle cell C disease), mild anaemia and fewer crises; risk of retinal damage and thromboembolic problems in pregnancy
HbCC	Homozygous CC disease (not a sickling disorder)
HbS β-thalassaemia	Sickle β-thalassaemia, generally produces sickle haemoglobin
HbAS	Sickle cell trait, generally no problems

• CLINICAL APPLICATION 33.2 Management of Sickle Cell Anaemia in Pregnancy

Routine screening is recommended both antenatally and in the newborn. Diagnosis may be made in the first trimester of pregnancy by chorionic villus sampling. Molecular technology advances will soon be able to diagnose sickle cell disease (SCD) with a few fetal cells from maternal blood.

Principles of Treatment in Pregnancy

- Specialized care – haematologist, obstetrician and a sickle cell centre.
- Anaemia may be prevented by prophylactic use of folic acid and iron.
- Blood transfusion may be necessary if Hb is extremely low.
- Avoidance of infection, cold and stress.
- In labour, keep hydrated and prevent acidosis by intravenous therapy; use prophylactic antibiotics; oxygen may be necessary. Epidural for pain relief.
- If crisis occurs, give pain relief; this may be the first sign of sickling.
  In general, pregnancies are uncomplicated, whereas sickle cell-positive women may have complications. Women with SCD are more likely to have anaemia, proteinuric hypertension and low-birthweight babies (Sickle Cell Society, 2018).

• CLINICAL APPLICATION 33.3 Management of Thalassaemia

Routine Non-pregnant Treatment

The cornerstones of modern treatment in β-thalassaemia are blood transfusion and iron-chelation therapy.

Heterozygotes seldom need treatment. Treatment for homozygous β-thalassaemia is only partially successful. It involves:

- Blood transfusions to top up the haemoglobin (Hb) and haematocrit levels.
- Iron-chelation therapy with an agent such as desferrioxamine to allow the excess iron to be excreted from the body.
- Splenectomy to reduce the amount of haemolysis.
- Monitoring of hepatic iron and ferritin levels, which is essential.

Care in Pregnancy

Shared care with haematologist, specialist and obstetrician.

Full blood count will reveal low mean corpuscular Hb and low mean cell volume.

Bone marrow will reveal microcytic, hypochromic red blood cells (RBCs).

Hb analysis will reveal elevated HBA_2 levels.

Chorionic villi sampling and fetal blood sampling. Fetus has a 1:4 chance of inheriting a major condition if both parents are carriers.

Anaemia is common and similar to iron deficiency with microcytic cells. Avoid iron overload. Obstetricians sometimes treat this with folate supplementation. However, iron deficiency is not usually a problem as the reduced number of RBCs and mild haemolysis ensure that iron is available; folic acid supplementation is advised.

Genetic counselling is offered to couples, preferably before any pregnancies. Girls with homozygous β-thalassaemia die in childhood, but treatment increases the likelihood of them living long enough to become pregnant.

Optimizing care in childhood will prevent infertility, as the pituitary and hypothalamus are prone to damage because of high iron levels. There are maternal risks with an increase in cardiac disease and pre-existing diabetes. The fetus is more likely to inherit the condition with an increase in birth anomalies, preterm birth and growth restriction.

(Refer to UK Thalassaemia Society website (ukts.org/) for further detail on the four identified categories.).

DVT in pregnancy affects the left leg in 90% of cases (compared with 55% in non-pregnant women). This is due to compression of the left iliac vein by the right iliac and ovarian arteries; 70% are iliofemoral, as opposed to 10% in non-pregnant patients, and they carry a much higher chance of PE (Davis & Pavord, 2018).

Diagnosis and Treatment

DVT is most common in the first few days after delivery. The woman may complain of pain or discomfort in the leg, which is increased when the foot is dorsiflexed (**Homan's sign**). The affected leg (often the left leg) may be swollen and measures 2–3 cm more than the unaffected leg. There may be a slight rise in systemic temperature. Diagnosis on clinical signs alone is difficult, and there may be up to 50% error in diagnosing DVT of the lower extremity. Diagnosis is made by **Doppler** ultrasound. In 80% of pregnant women, the thrombosis starts in the iliac and femoral veins and can be diagnosed by non-invasive methods such as ultrasound. Blood estimation of **D-dimers** (fibrin degradation products (FDPs)) may be made, but results are inaccurate antenatally and of no value postnatally.

RCOG (2015b) guidance emphasizes that all women should undergo a thorough assessment for VTE in early pregnancy or pre-pregnancy and again intrapartum or immediately postpartum. Any woman with risk factors should be considered for prophylactic low-molecular-weight heparin, an injection administered to thin the blood. The duration of treatment depends on the number of risk factors a woman has. It may be offered both antenatally and after the baby is born.

Neural tube defects (NTDs), which comprise open **spina bifida,** anencephaly and encephalocele, complicate around 1000 pregnancies in the UK each year and represent the first congenital malformations to be preventable through public health measures (Throup & Prentis, 2022). In NTDs, the spinal cord is left unprotected by the spinal column. α-Fetoprotein (AFP) is a fetal protein found in small amounts in maternal serum in normal pregnancies. Any open fetal defect leads to the leaking of AFP into the amniotic fluid, with higher levels than usual entering maternal serum. Higher levels of AFP occur if the gestational age is over-assessed or if more than one fetus is present.

The routine use of ultrasound at booking, with later anomaly scan (~18–20 weeks), identifies most of these defects so prospective parents are informed to make a choice between continuing the pregnancy or termination. The cause may involve both genetic and environmental triggers. A dietary factor (like **folic acid**) was originally suspected as being an influencing factor from the 1960s. Folic acid is used in the metabolic chain to provide the chemical bases of three of the essential **DNA components:** guanine, adenine and thymine. Vitamin B_{12} is necessary to form an enzyme in the metabolic pathway of folate. Women suffering epilepsy are known to be at risk of congenital abnormalities, in part due to the antiepileptic medication altering the absorption of folate.

The effect of periconceptional folic acid on reducing the incidence of both occurrence and recurrence of NTDs has been confirmed in quality randomized controlled trials. Women are advised to take 400 μg folic acid daily before conceiving and up to the 12th week of pregnancy. The use of supplements requires a conscious effort on the part of women anticipating a pregnancy, as adequate folic acid is needed at the time of embryogenesis. Prophylaxis commenced after diagnosis of pregnancy is unlikely to prevent these serious handicapping malformations. Despite public health campaigns, only around one-third of women take folic-acid supplements preconceptionally. As many women do not plan a pregnancy, particularly those at nutritional risk because of poor dietary habits and/or socioeconomic status, the only reasonable approach to maintaining adequate periconceptional levels of folic acid would appear to be through food fortification.

The United States has fortified all cereal-based products since 1998. The UK has also added folic acid to foods made with flour, such as bread. This will actively help avoid around 200 NTDs (20% reduction) each year (Throup & Prentis, 2022).

Vitamin A and B supplementation are not required. There is currently no evidence to recommend additional vitamin E.

Vitamin C has important roles in collagen synthesis, wound healing, prevention of anaemia and as an antioxidant. Routine supplements of vitamin C are not specifically recommended when pregnant. However, this vitamin helps iron absorption and may be of benefit to prevent the risk of anaemia.

Vitamin D supplementation is recommended in women at risk of deficiency. Deficiency is often found in women of South Asian, African, Caribbean or Middle Eastern ethnic origin; women who have limited exposure to sunlight; and women with a pre-pregnancy body mass index of more than 30 kg/m². Vitamin D deficiency has been associated with infantile rickets (with severe deficiency), whereas supplementation has been linked with reduced childhood wheezing and reduced type I diabetes in children. Pregnant women at risk of vitamin D deficiency, particularly obese women, should be identified and encouraged to take supplements of 10 μg/day.

(RCOG, 2022)
Refer to Box 16.1 in Chapter 16 for iron deficiency anaemia.

Additionally, women with previous VTE must be offered pre-pregnancy counselling and a prospective management plan for VTE should be made, including appropriate treatment to be offered as early as possible with careful history documented.

Pulmonary Embolus (PE)

Diagnosis and Treatment

Chest pain, dyspnoea, cyanosis and hypotension are suggestive of PE and require action immediately. Oxygen may be given with intravenous (IV) heparin. The woman's physiological response depends on the size of the clot or clots. If she collapses and has a cardiac arrest, a major embolic event has taken place and is life-threatening. Resuscitation should continue as this may disperse the clot and IV heparin given.

Subsequent treatment should centre on positive diagnosis and immediate dissolution of the clot with streptokinase, urokinase or plasminogen activator. Anticoagulation over several months is necessary.

Consumptive Coagulopathies During Pregnancy

Disseminated Intravascular Coagulation

Disseminated intravascular coagulation (DIC) is a life-threatening situation that can arise from a variety of obstetrical and non-obstetrical causes (Blackburn, 2018). The condition is always secondary to some other occurrence. This may include (i) acute peripartum haemorrhage (uterine atony, cervical and vaginal lacerations and uterine rupture); (ii) placental abruption; (iii) pre-eclampsia/eclampsia/haemolysis, elevated liver enzymes and low platelet count syndrome; (iv) retained stillbirth; (v) septic abortion and intrauterine infection; (vi) amniotic fluid embolism; and (vii) acute fatty liver of pregnancy (Offer, Mastriola & Thachil, 2015).

DIC results from local activation of the clotting system, which releases thromboplastin into the circulation, leading to intravascular formation of fibrin. **Microthrombi** are released into the circulation, and these occlude blood vessels, which may lead to **multiple organ failure.** Consumption and reduction of clotting factors and platelets lead to severe bleeding. **Fibrinolysis** stimulated by DIC results in the formation of **FDPs**. These interfere with the formation of firm fibrin clots and a vicious circle is established, increasing the blood loss. FDPs are also thought to interfere with myometrial contraction and cardiac function. Clinical Application 33.4 outlines diagnosis and treatment of DIC.

• CLINICAL APPLICATION 33.4 Disseminated Intravascular Coagulation

Diagnosis

Swift diagnosis and understanding of the underlying mechanisms of disease leading to this complication are essential for a favourable outcome. Clinical obstetric and medical history and observations such blood loss (e.g., from intravenous site, nosebleed) or the presence of **haematuria** are key indicators. Laboratory tests will accurately diagnose disseminated intravascular coagulation (DIC), with the following values being abnormal:

- Platelet count.
- Clotting times (in series).
- Levels of antithrombin III.
- Fibrin degradation products.

Treatment

- *Priority:* The replacement of blood cells and clotting factors.
- Treating the underlying disorder may resolve DIC.
- Transfusion of fresh frozen plasma or plasma substitutes such as dextran and platelet concentrates.
- Whole blood is not usually given, but stored blood components are given separately.
- Teamwork and prompt treatment are essential.

(Refer to Chapter 47 – Care of the Acutely Ill Woman).

Idiopathic Thrombocytopaenia

Idiopathic thrombocytopaenia (ITP) is a disorder characterized by an autoimmune destruction of maternal and fetal platelets. Women aged between 18–40 years are typical sufferers. It is usually asymptomatic, although sufferers may report bruising easily and excessive bleeding. Platelet values are normal.

There is a low incidence in pregnancy (1:1000–1:10,000). This condition may be associated with preeclampsia or **HELLP syndrome** (**H**aemolysis, **E**levated **L**iver enzymes and **L**ow **P**latelet count) (see Chapter 32), and there is an increased rate of miscarriage. ITP is suspected in pregnancy when the platelet value is lower than normal for pregnancy, and the condition is confirmed with a full blood count.

In pregnancy, the aim is to maintain a platelet level $>100,000$ mm^3 by administering corticosteroids. It is important that the anaesthetist is happy with the level of platelets before epidural administration. IV γ-globulin may be used to suppress antiplatelet antibodies. Neonatal thrombocytopaenia is due to transplacental passage of antiplatelet antibodies, which may cause neonatal haemorrhage.

Main Points

- Anaemia occurs when the number of RBCs or their oxygen-carrying capacity is insufficient to meet the physiological needs of the individual.
- During pregnancy, anaemia occurs when Hb <110 g/L.
- If Hb is low, there is poor RBC uptake of oxygen and poor oxygen delivery to the placental bed and fetus.
- IDA, folic acid deficiency, hereditary haemoglobinopathies and anaemia due to blood loss are conditions associated with pregnancy.
- IDA is a microcytic anaemia with reduction in both MCV and serum ferritin (iron stores).
- Folic acid is necessary for RBC proliferation and DNA synthesis.
- Folic acid supplementation (400 μg/day) is recommended pre-conception and in early pregnancy.
- SCD (incidence 2.3%) and thalassaemias (incidence 2.9%) affect Hb synthesis.
- SCD is a structural Hb variant. A single amino-acid substitution of valine for glutamic acid results in an Hb molecule that is less soluble.
- In SCD, when oxygen availability is low, the RBCs are distorted into a sickle shape and cannot pass through the capillaries. Vascular occlusion occurs, especially in the kidney and brain.
- In haemoglobinopathies, chorionic villus sampling may also be used for DNA analysis.
- Thalassaemia is caused by a reduced rate of synthesis of either α-globin or β-globin chains. The heterozygote (thalassaemia minor) is generally asymptomatic but with reduced Hb levels. The RBCs are thin, misshapen and short-lived.

- The homozygous condition (thalassaemia major) is life-threatening and leads to death in childhood if untreated.
- Pregnant women with homozygous β-thalassaemia need specialized care. Treatment may include repeated blood transfusions.
- G6PD deficiency is a rare X-linked enzyme deficiency (affects people of African, Asian and Mediterranean origins). Certain drugs precipitate haemolytic crises. Neonates may have prolonged jaundice if they carry this gene.
- Thrombosis in childbearing women is serious because of its association with DVT and PE, which remains the most common cause of maternal death.
- The three factors (**Virchow triad**) predisposing to thromboembolic disorders include venous stasis, altered coagulation and vascular damage.
- In DVT, the deep veins of the calf, thigh or pelvis are affected. If the clot is friable and pieces become detached from the vessel wall, they will travel around the circulation (embolus), through the heart and into the pulmonary circulation, leading to a PE. Women with an inherited thrombophilia are at increased risk of developing a DVT in pregnancy.
- Women should be kept mobile because any treatment which immobilizes them will increase the risk of DVT.
- DIC results from local activation of the clotting system, which releases thromboplastin into the circulation, leading to intravascular formation of fibrin. Microthrombi are released into the circulation. These occlude blood vessels, leading to multiple organ failure.
- ITP is a disorder characterized by an autoimmune destruction of maternal and fetal platelets.

References

Blackburn, S.T., 2018. Maternal, Fetal and Neonatal Physiology: A Clinical Perspective, fifth ed. Elsevier, Philadelphia.

Davis, S., Pavord, S., 2018. Haematological problems in pregnancy. In: Edmonds, D.K., Lees, C., Bourne, T. (Eds.), Dewhurst's Textbook of Obstetrics and Gynaecology, ninth ed. Wiley-Blackwell, Oxford.

Knight, M., Bunch, K., Patel, R., Shakespeare, J., Kotnis, R., Kenyon, S., et al., (on behalf of MBRRACE-UK), 2022. Saving Lives, Improving Mothers' Care – Lessons Learned to Inform Maternity Care from the UK and Ireland Confidential Enquiries into Maternal Deaths and Morbidity 2018-20. National Perinatal Epidemiology Unit, University of Oxford, Oxford.

National Institute of Health and Care Excellence (NICE), 2021. Anaemia – Iron Deficiency: Scenario: Management of Iron Deficiency Anaemia. Available at: https://cks.nice.org.uk/topics/anaemia-iron-deficiency/management/management/.

National Institute for Health and Care Excellence (NICE), 2023. Pre-Conception – Advice and Management: Scenario: Pre-Conception Advice for all Women. Available at: https://cks.nice.org.uk/topics/pre-conception-advice-management/management/advice-for-all-women/.

Offer, E., Mastriola, S.A., Thachil, J., 2015. Disseminated intravascular coagulation in pregnancy: insights in pathophysiology, diagnosis and management. Am. J. Obstet. Gynecol. 213 (4), 452–463.

Pipkin, B.F., 2018. Maternal physiology. In: Edmonds, D.K., Lees, C., Bourne, T. (Eds.), Dewhurst's Textbook of Obstetrics and Gynaecology, ninth ed. Wiley-Blackwell, Oxford.

Public Health England, 2018. Guidance in Understanding Haemoglobinopathies. Available at: https://www.gov.uk/government/publications/handbook-for-sickle-cell-and-thalassaemia-screening/understanding-haemoglobinopathies.

Rogers, J.L., 2022. McCance and Huether's Pathophysiology: The Biologic Basis for Disease in Adults and Children, ninth ed. Elsevier, Philadelphia.

Royal College of Obstetricians and Gynaecologists (RCOG), 2015a. Blood Transfusion in Obstetrics. Green-top Guideline No. 47. Available at: https://www.rcog.org.uk/media/sdqcorsf/gtg-47.pdf.

Royal College of Obstetricians and Gynaecologists (RCOG), 2015b. Thrombosis and Embolism during Pregnancy and the Puerperium: Reducing the Risk. Green-top Guideline No. 37a. Available at: https://www.rcog.org.uk/media/qejfhcaj/gtg-37a.pdf.

Royal College of Obstetricians and Gynaecologists (RCOG), 2022. Vitamin Supplementation Could Have a Significant Impact on Maternal and Fetal Health. Available at: https://www.rcog.org.uk/for-the-public/browse-all-patient-information-leaflets/healthy-eating-and-vitamin-supplements-in-pregnancy-patient-information-leaflet/.

Sickle Cell Society, 2018. Standards for the Clinical Care of Adults with Sickle Cell Disease in the UK. Available at: https://www.sicklecellsociety.org/wp-content/uploads/2018/05/Standards-for-the-Clinical-Care-of-Adults-with-Sickle-Cell-in-the-UK-2018.pdf.

Stephen, G., Mgongo, M., Hussein Hashim, T., Katanga, J., Stray-Pedersen, B., Msuya, S.E., 2018. Anaemia in pregnancy: prevalence, risk factors, and adverse perinatal outcomes in northern Tanzania. Anemia 2018, 1846280.

Stoltzfus, R.J., 2003. Iron deficiency: global prevalence and consequences. Food Nutr. Bull. 24 (Suppl. 4), S99–S103.

Throup, M., Prentis, V., 2022. Folic Acid to Be Added to Non-wholemeal Flour across the UK to Help Prevent Life-Threatening Brain and Spinal Conditions in Fetuses. Department for Environment, Food & Rural Affairs, Department of Health and Social Care. Available at: https://www.gov.uk/government/news/folic-acid-added-to-flour-to-prevent-brain-and-spinal-conditions-in-fetuses.

UK Thalassaemia Society, 2018. Standards for the Clinical Care of Children and Adults with Thalassaemia in the UK. Available at https://www.stgeorges.nhs.uk/wp-content/uploads/2020/02/UKTS-adults-and-children-with-thalassaemia-guidelines-2016.pdf.

World Health Organization (WHO), 2020a. Worldwide Prevalence of Anaemia 1993–2005. WHO Press, Geneva.

World Health Organization (WHO), 2020b. WHO Guidance Helps Detect Iron Deficiency and Protect Brain Development. WHO Press, Geneva.

Annotated recommended reading

National Institute of Health and Care Excellence (NICE), 2021. Anaemia – Iron Deficiency: Scenario: Management of Iron Deficiency Anaemia. Available at: https://cks.nice.org.uk/topics/anaemia-iron-deficiency/management/management/.

This website provides up-to-date standards for the management of women with iron-deficiency anaemia during pregnancy.

Royal College of Obstetricians and Gynaecologists (RCOG), 2015a. Blood Transfusion in Obstetrics. Green-top Guideline No. 47. Available at: https://www.rcog.org.uk/media/sdqcorsf/gtg-47.pdf.

Royal College of Obstetricians and Gynaecologists (RCOG), 2015b. Thrombosis and Embolism during Pregnancy and the Puerperium: Reducing the Risk. Green-top Guideline No. 37a. Available at: https://www.rcog.org.uk/media/qejfhcaj/gtg-37a.pdf.

These two websites provide valuable up-to-date evidence-based information for obstetrics and maternity care relating to thrombosis and embolism during and following pregnancy.

Useful websites

Glucose-6-Phosphate Dehydrogenase Deficiency – National Organization for Rare Disorders (rarediseases.org).
nice.org.uk/guidance/.
npeu.ox.ac.uk/ukoss/current-surveillance.
rcog.org.uk/.
sicklecellsociety.org/coronavirus-and-scd/.
Thalassemia.com.
https://ukts.org/.

34

Respiratory, Renal, Gastrointestinal and Neurological Problems

SUSANNE CROZIER

CHAPTER CONTENTS

This chapter details common respiratory, renal, gastrointestinal and neurological problems that can impact on pregnancy. This includes pathophysiology, signs, symptoms and clinical management.

Respiratory Tract Problems

Asthma

Asthma is a serious health problem impacting over 300 million people worldwide with a rapid increase in prevalence during the late 20th century. More recent global data is variable and suggests there has been a plateauing of cases in some developed countries while numbers increase in low- to middle-income countries (Stern, Pier & Litonjua, 2020). It is the most common respiratory condition in the UK, affecting 6.5% of the population (Bloom et al., 2019). Asthma is an inflammatory clinical syndrome characterized by hyper-responsiveness of the airways with constriction of the smooth muscle in the bronchioles, hypersecretion of mucus and mucosal oedema. The work of breathing is increased, and excessive negative intrapleural pressures can increase the demands on the right ventricle. There is a rise in pulmonary arterial pressure and a decrease in arterial systolic pressure and pulse pressure.

Aetiology

Asthma is a complex disorder involving biochemical, autonomic nervous system, immunological, endocrine and psychological factors, which differ from person to person. Airway inflammation even when the person is symptom-free. There is a familial incidence, and environmental factors are recognized triggers that interact with inherited factors to cause **bronchospasm.** These include respiratory tract infections, dust mite allergens, pollens, foods, some drugs, smoking, cold air and exercise (National Institute of Health and Care Excellence [NICE], 2017). Asthma commonly develops in childhood (~50%) and before age 40 (~35%). Complete remission is common in children but less so in adults.

Pathophysiology

Respiratory rate is not changed by pregnancy; progesterone increases hyperventilation by term. The effects of the gravid uterus on the diaphragm cause a decrease in expiratory and residual volumes, and this may cause some problems for a woman who is pregnant and asthmatic (Blackburn, 2018). **Bronchoconstriction** occurs after exposure to an allergen and causes immunoglobulin E to bind to mast cell surface receptors. These release inflammatory substances such as **histamine, bradykinin, prostaglandins, thromboxane A_2** and **chemotactic factors** which attract eosinophils, neutrophils, T lymphocytes and platelets. Eosinophils produce a protein that stops epithelial cell cilia from beating, disrupts mucosal integrity and causes damage and sloughing of epithelial cells.

Asthma in Pregnancy

It is estimated that 10% of pregnant women have asthma, making it the most common chronic medical condition in

Ensure there is consideration of lifestyle factors or alternate diagnoses before starting or adjusting treatment and review within 4–6 weeks.

Establish that the person can use an inhaler correctly and develop a personalized asthma action plan.

It is safe to continue to take medicines prescribed for asthma during pregnancy, although reduced compliance has been noted amongst pregnant women.

The following is recommended usually in a stepwise approach with initial therapy based on the severity of the presentation.

- Bronchodilator (salbutamol) inhaler only.
- Bronchodilator (salbutamol) inhaler and corticosteroid inhaler (anti-inflammatory agent).
- Leukotriene antagonists (not as a new therapy).
- Steroid tablets if necessary to control severe asthma.

Labour: with **extreme caution** prostaglandin, ergometrine and syntometrine are used to reduce the risk of inducing bronchoconstriction.

(British Thoracic Society, 2019; Hindley, 2018; Murphy, 2015.)

pregnancy (Hindley, 2018; Murphy, 2015). Women with well-controlled asthma may have a healthy pregnancy and find that their asthma improves slightly due to endocrine changes (Baston, Hall & Samples, 2019). Poorly controlled asthma can be a cause of mortality and morbidity in women. However, for all women with asthma, there is an increased risk of complications such as preterm delivery, low birthweight, neonatal death, gestational diabetes and pre-eclampsia (Murphy, 2015). The risk is increased if the woman also smokes and this, along with respiratory susceptibility to infection, means that the influenza vaccination is an important part of protecting women's health during pregnancy (Hindley, 2018). Treatment considerations are outlined in Box 34.1.

A small number of women may develop **status asthmaticus,** a serious condition defined as recurrent asthmatic episodes resulting from spasm of the smooth muscle of the walls of the bronchi and bronchioles. This leads to atrial or complete obstruction of airways known as *bronchoconstriction.* This manifests with periods of coughing, wheezing and difficulty with exhalation. Air becomes trapped in the alveoli during exhalation with excessive secretions of mucus obstructing the airway. This is an emergency situation and needs hospitalization as the lives of the woman and fetus are at serious risk.

Tuberculosis

Worldwide, 10.6 million people are estimated to have fallen ill with tuberculosis (TB) in 2022. This includes 3.4 million women and 1.2 million children (World Health Organization [WHO], 2022) The incidence of TB has increased in the last 8 years and has overtaken HIV as a leading cause of morbidity due to infection, second only to COVID-19. In the UK, the incidence of TB has decreased following the implementation of a collaborative public strategy which has seen cases fall by 44% between 2011 and 2019 in England (Public Health England, 2019). Case numbers are also falling in Scotland, although it is noted that those with the disease are presenting with other complications that impact outcomes.

Aetiology

TB is an infectious bacterial disease which is both curable and preventable (WHO, 2022). It is caused by *Mycobacterium tuberculosis,* which most commonly affects the lungs. TB is transmitted from person to person via droplets from the throat and lungs of people with active respiratory disease and is associated with overcrowded living conditions and poor general health (Baston, Hall & Samples, 2019). Although the lungs are the most common site of infection, it can spread to other parts of the body including bone and the renal system. *M. tuberculosis* is a slow-growing bacterium with a waxy outer coat that protects it from immune system attack. The body responds by forming **fibrinous tubercles** to contain the microbe and these can then cause organ damage. It is estimated that 10% of people exposed to the infection will develop active TB within 2 years.

Signs and Symptoms

In healthy people, the infection often causes no symptoms because the person's immune system acts to 'wall off' the bacteria. It is not clear if pregnancy increases vulnerability either to TB infection or to progression to active disease; however pregnancy can make the diagnosis of TB more difficult (Miele, Morris & Tepper, 2020). Pregnancy increases the demands on the body's systems, so symptoms such as breathlessness and fatigue may be overlooked or classed as minor disorders until other factors emerge to alert health professionals. Equally, there may be a reluctance to perform investigations such as chest X-ray during pregnancy. Risk factors for TB include homelessness, poor housing, recent travel or residence in a country with high levels of TB and co-existing infections such as HIV. The woman's poor and deteriorating health may adversely affect fetal growth and perinatal loss is more likely (Miele, Morris & Tepper, 2020). The symptoms of active TB of the lung are coughing for more than 3 weeks, sometimes with sputum or blood, chest pains, weakness, weight loss, night sweats and fever (Baston, Hall & Samples, 2019; Miele, Morris & Tepper, 2020). The symptoms are often insidious with a feeling of general malaise. Box 34.2 describes TB management in pregnancy.

COVID-19

Coronavirus disease (COVID-19) is a new infectious disease. Infection is caused by a novel betacoronavirus known as severe acute respiratory syndrome coronavirus 2 (SARS-CoV-2). The associated disease is referred to as 'COVID-19'

• BOX 34.2 Tuberculosis Management in Pregnancy

Diagnosis

A tuberculin skin test (Mantoux test) will confirm tuberculosis (TB) infection but cannot differentiate between latent and active disease. Active infection is confirmed by *Mycobacterium tuberculosis* found in sputum and by chest X-ray.

Bacillus Calmette–Guérin (BCG) vaccination should not be performed in pregnancy as it is a live vaccine.

Specialist-shared care involves a respiratory physician, specialist nurses/health visitors, an obstetrician, a midwife, a general practitioner and possibly a social worker (as required by personal circumstances).

If infectious, the woman will need to be isolated from others (either in hospital or single room at home).

Treatment

In the general population, TB is treatable with a 6-month course of antibiotics (WHO, 2022).

TB drugs have side effects in pregnancy, although treatment is safe. Side effects include hepatitis, peripheral neuropathy and optic neuritis. Drugs safe for the fetus include rifampicin, isoniazid, pyrazinamide and ethambutol.

Treatment is usually over 6–9 months, with symptoms resolving and the patient becoming non-infectious within the first few weeks.

Mother and baby are not separated unless the disease is active.

Baby

Streptomycin is contraindicated due to the incidence of hearing loss in neonates exposed in utero.

No contraindications to breastfeeding.

BCG vaccination given and may be given syrup prophylactic isoniazid.

Vaccination: BCG

BCG, a live attenuated strain developed from bovine TB, is given by injection into the skin to stimulate an immune response. In babies, care must be taken to inject intradermally to prevent abscess formation. It can reduce the incidence of pulmonary tuberculosis by up to 80% and minimizes the risk of complications. The BCG vaccination is just one part of the public health effort to prevent the spread of TB in the community. It is recommended that all babies and young people be offered the BCG vaccination against TB if they are at risk (NICE, 2016).

(UK Health Security Agency [UKHSA] 2022; WHO 2023). The virus can spread from an infected person's mouth or nose in small liquid particles ranging from larger respiratory droplets to smaller aerosols. In 2020, the WHO declared a pandemic due to the rapid increase in cases observed worldwide (WHO, 2023). This unprecedented situation in modern times posed unique challenges to the medical community as the optimal treatment was uncertain and often at the discretion of emerging institutional guidelines.

Pregnancy is described as a high-risk state in the context of infectious diseases, given a particular susceptibility to pathogens and potential adverse outcomes. To date, studies have provided insight into the course of COVID-19 in the adult population. However, the implications of COVID-19 on pregnancy and pregnancy outcomes remain understudied. Guidelines continue to be updated based on emerging evidence (NICE, 2022; Royal College of Obstetricians and Gynaecologists [RCOG], 2022).

Current evidence suggests that pregnant women with no comorbidities have the same chance of having COVID-19 as other healthy adults and are more likely to have either mild or no symptoms (RCOG, 2022). However, a small number of pregnant women do become seriously ill with the risk possibly greater during the last 3 months of pregnancy. While the impact of COVID-19 infection on pregnant women remains relatively unknown, severe infection may result in complications like acute respiratory distress syndrome, acute myocardial or kidney injury, sepsis and venous thromboembolism (NICE, 2022). The physiological changes of pregnancy and hypercoagulability may further increase thrombotic risk (Crossette-Thambiah et al., 2021). Most women with severe COVID-19 were reported to be unvaccinated and vaccine coverage among pregnant women admitted to hospital with COVID-19 was low (Engjom et al., 2022). Black and Asian ethnic groups are particularly vulnerable to COVID-19 as they have increased risk factors for severe infection (NICE, 2022; (RCOG, 2022). Pregnant women are vulnerable and at increased risk of contracting COVID-19 if they have comorbidities such as pre-existing diabetes, body mass index (BMI) >25 kg/m^2 and gestational diabetes on insulin (RCOG, 2022.)

The management of pregnant women with COVID-19 is outlined in Clinical Application 34.1. Refer to (RCOG, 2022) for further detailed information.

Renal Disorders

Urinary Tract Infections (UTIs)

UTIs are a common problem affecting up to 50% of women. The infection usually occurs when bacteria from the gastrointestinal (GI) tract colonize the perineal area and migrate into the bladder via the urethra. Pregnant women are more susceptible to UTIs than non-pregnant women due to the anatomical and physiological changes that take place in the renal system and the increasing levels of oestrogen in the urine (Donaldson, 2019). The incidence of unsuspected asymptomatic infections is estimated at between 2–10% of pregnancies (NICE, 2019). If asymptomatic bacteriuria (ASB) is not diagnosed and treated during pregnancy, then up to 30% of women will go on to develop acute **pyelonephritis.** This complication occurs when the infection ascends and spreads into the renal system (Blackburn, 2018).

Women with a history of episodes of asymptomatic bacteriuria or UTI should have a midstream specimen of urine cultured. If the presence of a specific bacterium exceeds 100,000 organisms/mL of urine, then ASB is diagnosed. Appropriate antibiotics should be successful in treating the condition.

Clinical Implications of Acute Pyelonephritis

Fetus

- Risks associated with prematurity (e.g., respiratory distress, intraventricular haemorrhage).

Maternal Risks

- Anaemia.
- Sepsis.
- Renal compromise.

Signs and Symptoms

A small number of pregnant women (1–2%) will develop acute pyelonephritis, usually in the second and third trimesters (Grette et al., 2020). It begins with the onset of malaise, fatigue, chills and back pain located in the upper lumbar region, accompanied by muscle guarding. The pain follows the path of the ureters and may radiate round to the

suprapubic area. Some women complain of nausea, vomiting and uterine contractions. Affected women may have a temperature as high as 40°C with a corresponding increase in pulse rate. There may be dehydration and frequency of micturition with scalding on voiding. The urine appears cloudy and even bloodstained, and on urinalysis red blood cells, leucocytes and casts may be present, as well as bacteria. Clinical Application 34.2 provides clinical management.

Acute Kidney Injury (AKI)

AKI, formerly called *acute renal failure* (ARF), is commonly defined as an abrupt decline in renal function, clinically manifesting as a reversible acute increase in nitrogen waste products—measured by blood urea nitrogen and serum creatinine levels—over the course of hours to weeks. AKI usually results from a severe deficit in cortical renal

---

• CLINICAL APPLICATION 34.1   COVID-19: Management of Pregnant Women (RCOG, 2022).

Signs and Symptoms

Mild: Fever or chills, a new continuous cough, breathlessness, loss or change to sense of smell or taste, fatigue, muscle aches and pains, headache, sore throat, blocked or runny nose, loss of appetite, diarrhoea, nausea and/or vomiting.
Severe: Severe breathlessness, haemoptysis, hypoxia, cyanosis, feeling cold and clammy, pale or mottled skin, collapse or syncope, new confusion, drowsiness, reduced urine output.

Management

- Pregnant and postpartum women presenting with COVID-19 should be investigated and treated the same as non-pregnant women unless there is a clear reason not to do so.
- Decision for admission or for self-directed care at home depends on the overall clinical picture.
- Women with a fever should be cared for in line with RCOG (2012) Green-top Guideline No. 64a Bacterial Sepsis in Pregnancy.
- Bacterial (rather than viral) infection should be considered if the white blood cell count is raised (lymphocytes are

usually low with COVID-19) and antibiotics should be commenced.
- Perform radiographic investigations as for a non-pregnant adult; this includes chest X-ray and computed tomography (CT) of the chest.
- Consider a diagnosis of pulmonary embolism or heart failure for women presenting with chest pain, worsening hypoxia or a respiratory rate >20 bpm, or in women whose breathlessness persists or worsens after expected recovery from COVID-19. Further tests to investigate include electrocardiogram, echocardiogram, CT pulmonary angiogram and ventilation-perfusion lung scan.
- Disseminated intravascular coagulation can also occur, with low platelets and low fibrinogen levels, and sometimes prolonged prothrombin time and/or activated partial thromboplastin time.
    Nine maternal deaths (pregnant or within 6 weeks of the end of pregnancy) were directly attributable to COVID-19 in 2020 and many were from ethnic minority groups (Knight et al., 2022). See Chapter 47 for care of the acutely ill woman.

(Refer to UKHSA (2023) guidance on breastfeeding.)

• CLINICAL APPLICATION 34.2   Acute Pyelonephritis in Pregnancy: Clinical Management

Prompt diagnosis and immediate treatment are essential to avoid serious side effects. Hospital admission may be required.

Investigations and Management

- A midstream specimen of urine for culture and sensitivity tests.
- A blood specimen (for full blood count and electrolytes) if very ill.
- Intravenous fluids to correct any dehydration (as required).
- Commence antibiotic therapy intravenously if women are nauseated. Oral medication may be commenced after 48 h. *Escherichia coli* is becoming increasingly resistant to **ampicillin,** and a combination of antibiotics may be prescribed until sensitivity results are available.

- Pain relief and antiemetic to counteract nausea may be necessary.
- Renal function assessment during the acute illness and follow-up.
- Maternal observations: temperature, pulse and blood pressure (at least every 4 hours).
- Tachycardia and hypotension may indicate the development of sepsis.
- Maternal and fetal assessment and observations.
- Early onset of labour should be recognized.
    Most women respond to the combination of rehydration and antibiotics. In persistent problems, refer appropriately to assess for abnormality of renal tract.

blood flow that results in ischaemia. AKI is a rare disorder in developed countries and in pregnancy is usually linked to conditions such as pre-eclampsia and eclampsia, **HELLP** syndrome (**H**aemolysis, **E**levated **L**iver enzymes and **L**ow **P**latelet count), acute fatty liver of pregnancy and thrombotic microangiopathies (Jim & Garovic, 2017) (see Chapter 32).

If cortical hypoperfusion is allowed to persist, **acute tubular necrosis** or **cortical necrosis** may follow. Renal cortical necrosis is a severe form of AKI that usually results from large, sudden blood loss or vascular collapse such as in severe pre-eclampsia or haemorrhage. There is sudden onset of oliguria (<400 mL in 24 hours) or anuria and a rise in serum creatinine. Immediate treatment of AKI prevents necrosis. Clinical signs and symptoms include digital ischaemia, skin rash, slight jaundice and cardiovascular system irregularities including raised blood pressure (BP). Clinical Application 34.3 presents clinical management. This woman will be ill and requires shared care involving a renal physician, obstetrician, intensive care nurses, anaesthetists, haematologists and biochemists (Taber-Hight & Shah, 2020).

Chronic Renal Disease

The degree of success for a pregnant woman with chronic renal disease depends on the severity of renal impairment. As the reduction in renal function increases then the ability to conceive and sustain a pregnancy also decreases (Webster et al., 2017). Physiologically the kidney glomerular filtration rate and renal plasma flow increase in pregnancy by approximately 50%; if this does not occur, the woman's future health may be jeopardized even with a successful pregnancy. Normotensive women with mild renal disease before pregnancy do well, although there is a risk of pre-eclampsia, preterm birth and fetal growth restriction, and their renal prognosis is not significantly impaired (Blackburn, 2018). Women with moderate-to-severe disease have a greater risk of worsening renal function and greater risk of adverse maternal and fetal outcomes. Women with chronic renal impairment with poorly controlled hypertension, proteinuria, oedema and poor kidney function may not have successful pregnancies. These women should be offered pre-conception counselling to discuss the risks involved (Blackburn, 2018; Webster et al., 2017; Wiles et al., 2019).

Pathophysiologically oedema is present because of loss of protein in the urine, and electrolytes become imbalanced because kidney excretion of urine is low. Blood acid–base balance is compromised. Erythropoietin and red cell production are decreased and anaemia occurs. Renal tissue damage causes decreased blood supply, which results in the production of excess renin, which in turn increases BP.

Management and Care

Women with chronic renal disease will require specialist management involving a renal physician, obstetrician, specialist nurses, midwife, haematologist and biochemist. There may or may not be a history of prior kidney problems including:

- Glomerulonephritis.
- Chronic pyelonephritis.
- Renal calculi.
- Polycystic kidney disease.
- Nephrotic syndrome >3 g/day, a serum albumin of <3 g/dL plus oedema.
- Diabetic nephropathy.
- Systemic lupus erythematosus.

Maternal care includes early recognition of UTI, which is essential. The outcome is dependent on the degree of hypertension and kidney function, and optimum care should prevent deterioration in the mother and the delivery of a healthy infant. Regular antenatal assessment for maternal and fetal progress and well-being is essential. This is to monitor for fetal distress which occurs both antenatally and in labour in those pregnancies complicated by intrauterine growth restriction. Fetal mortality may also occur because of poor placental blood flow, abruptio placentae or hypoxia.

Pregnancy After Renal Transplant

Although pregnancy after kidney transplantation is feasible, the potential complications of pregnancy and impact on

---

• CLINICAL APPLICATION 34.3 Acute Kidney Injury in Pregnancy: Management

Aims: to re-establish urinary output and treat the underlying condition.
- **Investigations** include blood haematology and biochemistry, kidney function and urinalysis:
  - Blood: urea, electrolytes, plasma proteins, haematocrit and blood osmolality (to assess extent of dehydration) and blood culture.
  - Kidney function tests; urine investigation for culture and sensitivity of organisms, protein estimation, specific gravity and osmolality.
- Vigilant maternal and fetal assessment.

Re-establishing Kidney Function: Principles of Treatment

Treatment is guided by laboratory tests and includes:
- Control of bleeding, stabilization of raised blood pressure or sepsis.
- Intravascular volume expansion is critical but must be administered with caution to avoid pulmonary oedema.
- Dialysis if there is cardiovascular overload, **hyperkalaemia**, electrolyte imbalances, metabolic acidosis or **uraemia**.

(Taber-Hight & Shah, 2020)

renal function need to be carefully considered through pre-pregnancy counselling and clinical decision-making. Renal transplantation restores fertility in a woman with kidney failure. Transplantation is only performed in women with good kidney function, controlled BP and general good health. The pregnancy rate in kidney transplant recipients is lower than in the general population (Blackburn, 2018; Webster et al., 2017).

Transplant recipients need to continue immunosuppressive medications during pregnancy to prevent graft rejection. These drugs carry risks for the fetus, but the risks of prednisone, azathioprine, cyclosporine and tacrolimus are surprisingly low. Mycophenolate is teratogenic, except for sirolimus and mycophenolate mofetil (MMF), which are contraindicated during pregnancy. Published reports suggest that transplant recipients should wait 3 years before becoming pregnant to minimize the risk of allograft rejection (Webster et al., 2017).

Pregnancy post-transplant increases the risk of prematurity, intrauterine growth restriction, pre-eclampsia and caesarean section compared with the general population. The incidence of birth defects in live-born babies is similar to the general population, except for those pregnancies exposed to MMF, which have a high incidence of birth defects. Pregnancy in renal transplant patients should be planned with combined care from surgeons, nephrologists, obstetricians, paediatricians and dietitians, which offers the best chance of a favourable outcome in the mother and the fetus (Wiles et al., 2019).

Gastrointestinal Problems

Vomiting in Pregnancy

Slight nausea and vomiting are common symptoms of pregnancy, affecting approximately 70% of women in the first trimester (see Chapter 30). Causes and management of moderate-to-severe vomiting are now discussed.

Causes of Vomiting

Pregnant women may suffer from diseases causing vomiting not associated with pregnancy. These disorders, such as gastric ulceration or infection, must be excluded before accepting that moderate to severe vomiting is due to the pregnancy alone. Vomiting is a reflex which occurs because of stimulation of two centres in the brain (Ritter et al., 2019). These are the **vomiting centre** (VC) in the medulla and the **chemoreceptor trigger zone** (CTZ).

The VC controls smooth muscle movements in the stomach wall and the related skeletal muscle of the respiratory and abdominal muscles. The CTZ lies outside the blood–brain barrier and responds to circulating chemical stimuli from ingested drugs and endogenous toxins produced in uraemia and radiation sickness. This centre also produces motion sickness. Stimuli arising in the CTZ are passed to the VC, which then activates the relevant respiratory and GI

TABLE 34.1	Causes of Vomiting in Pregnant Women	
Non-pregnancy Causes	**Causes Due to Pregnancy**
Stimulation of the sensory nerve endings in the stomach and duodenum and of the vagal sensory endings in the pharynx	High levels of pregnancy hormones, such as human chorionic gonadotropin (hCG) or oestrogen, with multiple pregnancy and hydatidiform mole (trophoblastic disease)
Some stimuli to the heart and viscera, such as distension or damage or infection of the uterus, renal pelvis or bladder	Physiological changes in the gastrointestinal tract in pregnancy, resulting in decreased motility and in increased gastric reflux
Drugs or endogenous toxins produced because of radiation damage, infection or disease	Transient hyperthyroidism causing high levels of hCG, stimulating thyroid secretion
Disturbance of the vestibular apparatus, as in motion sickness	Metabolic changes, including carbohydrate deficiency and alteration in lipid pathways
Raised intracranial pressure, migraine, cerebral tumour	Pre-eclampsia, HELLP syndrome (Haemolysis, Elevated Liver enzymes and Low Platelet count)
Nauseating smells, sights or thoughts	Renal tract infections
Endocrine factors such as increased oestrogen	Torsion of an ovarian cyst
A fall in blood pressure and reduced circulation to the brain (vasovagal events)	Genetic incompatibility between mother and fetus
Viral gastroenteritis	Psychological factors
Hepatitis, acute liver failure	
Gall bladder disease	

See Chapter 47 for care of the acutely ill woman.

muscles, resulting in vomiting. Vomiting can be triggered by the factors outlined in Table 34.1.

Hyperemesis Gravidarum (HG)

HG is a severe condition that results in excessive vomiting throughout the day and often continues until birth. HG usually begins in the first trimester and is continuous, severe and often associated with excessive salivation. The incidence is about 0.3–0.6% of women. It is associated with multiple pregnancies, Black and Asian ethnicity, younger women and type 1 diabetes (Austin, Wilson & Saha, 2019).

Despite numerous studies, the aetiology remains unclear. Possible causes may be due to high levels of human chorionic gonadotrophin (hCG), increasing levels of oestrogen and progesterone and the decrease in the rate of GI peristalsis, which increases gastric reflux. Hyperthyroidism may be caused by high levels of hCG; this is similar in structure to thyroid-stimulating hormone and increases thyroid function (Blackburn, 2018). When the two conditions occur together, women may present with vomiting, weight loss and increased thyroid activity, which requires treatment to prevent adverse pregnancy outcomes.

Signs and Symptoms

HG is defined as when vomiting occurs more than three times per day and there is associated weight loss and ketonuria (Austin, Wilson & Saha, 2019). There is marked **oliguria** with dark urine of high specific gravity which may contain **ketones,** bile, protein and glucose. Electrolyte disturbances include **hyponatraemia** and **hypochloraemia** as sodium and chloride ions are lost in the vomit. Clinical assessment reveals a rapid pulse, lowered BP and the woman is pale and lethargic. It is important to consider other causes of vomiting and a careful abdominal examination should be undertaken by a medical practitioner (Austin, Wilson & Saha, 2019). Anaemia may occur because of the disruption in vitamin B_{12}, folic acid and vitamin C absorption.

Complications

HG is associated with poorer maternal and fetal outcomes:
- Micronutrient deficiency (e.g., vitamin B_1 (thiamine)) resulting in neuropathy such as **polyneuritis.**
- Muscle weakness.
- Retinal haemorrhage.
- Rarely, **Wernicke's encephalopathy** may occur. This is signalled by confusion, ataxia and impairment of short-term memory, leading to coma.
- Low birthweight, premature and neonates small for gestational age.

Management

The woman needs to be admitted to hospital for investigations, rehydration and correction of any electrolyte imbalance. The cause of vomiting may not be found, although initial tests will be carried out to exclude other conditions such as UTI, disorders of the GI tract or molar pregnancy. Treatment may include **antiemetics,** antihistamines or corticosteroids. Fluids and electrolytes are replaced by intravenous infusion such as Hartmann's solution. Vitamin B_{12}, thiamine, vitamin C, folic acid and iron may be needed to address any nutrition concerns and if severe enteral or parenteral nutrition may be required (Austin, Wilson & Saha, 2019).

The overall aim is to improve symptoms and stabilize the condition, preventing further complications. General observation of the woman's condition should be monitored with strict fluid balance until rehydrated. There is usually a rapid response to treatment, and oral fluids may be recommended when vomiting has ceased for 24 hours. Solid food should be then introduced gradually. Women may be readmitted with a recurrence of the condition.

Appendicitis in Pregnancy

The appendix is gradually displaced upwards by the growing uterus so that typical signs of appendicitis may not be present. Fever and diarrhoea are less common, and pregnant women may experience symptoms not often seen in adults, including uterus contractions, urination that is painful or difficult and pain in the upper right abdomen (changing position of appendix). In early pregnancy, appendicitis may be difficult to differentiate from threatened miscarriage (abortion); however there will be no bleeding. Later in pregnancy, the pain may be mistaken for UTI, abruptio placentae or the onset of labour (Wylie & Bryce, 2016). An ultrasound scan confirms the diagnosis, and an appendectomy is required to save life and prevent peritonitis.

The appendix can be surgically removed by performing the traditional abdominal procedure or by laparoscopic surgery. Laparoscopic surgery is gaining favour and has been used in pregnancy to remove ovaries and the appendix (NICE, 2021). Evidence suggests that local anaesthetic is safe and feasible for the treatment of acute appendicitis in all trimesters of pregnancy. Close maternal and fetal monitoring is essential during and after the operation.

Pregnancy in Women with a Stoma

The most common reasons for undergoing an ileostomy or colostomy are inflammatory bowel disease (IBD) and colorectal cancer. IBD affects women of reproductive age and decisions about stoma formation can impact their fertility and pregnancy outcomes (PAPooSE Study Group, 2022). Women with a stoma may report increased symptoms of nausea and other intestinal disorders. Later in pregnancy, as the uterus grows, there may be issues with the passage of stool from the stoma and potential bowel obstruction (Whiteley & Gullick, 2018).

Emerging data indicate a significantly increased incidence of birth by caesarean section (73%) compared to the general population (29%) and stoma-related complications (24%). The reasons for the increased use of caesarean sections are not clear and there was a higher risk of bladder trauma also noted during the study (PAPooSE Study Group, 2022).

Problems that may need careful management include:
- Changes in shape and position of the stoma as the uterus enlarges.
- Leaking from the stoma as the opening changes shape.
- Hormonal changes that alter skin secretions, leading to reduced adhesiveness of the appliance.
- Reduced absorption of nutrients—for example, vitamin B_{12} and folic acid—which may lead to anaemia.

- Increased risk of GI obstruction; the consequent abdominal pain is difficult to distinguish from appendicitis (Takahashi et al., 2007).

Intrahepatic Cholestasis of Pregnancy

Intrahepatic cholestasis of pregnancy (ICP) is an idiopathic condition of unknown cause, although genetic, geographical and environmental factors may be involved. It affects about 0.7% of pregnancies across all ethnicities and between 1.2–1.5% of those with Asian ethnic backgrounds (Wylie & Bryce, 2016). It usually begins in the third trimester of pregnancy (can occur earlier) and resolves spontaneously after birth. It is thought that this condition is an autoimmune response to pregnancy and affects those susceptible to raised oestrogen levels. There may also be a familial link and it recurs during subsequent pregnancies.

Clinical presentations may include pruritus without a rash (particularly hands and feet) resulting in insomnia, fever, abdominal discomfort, nausea and vomiting, darker urine and paler stools.

Investigations should include tests to exclude liver disease and other liver disorders, blood investigations for levels of bile acids (abnormally elevated in women with no evidence of liver inflammation), serum alkaline phosphate, bilirubin and liver transaminases (abnormally high levels). Jaundice is rare, occurring in less than 1% of those with ICP (Girling, Knight & Chappell, 2022).

Treatment can include topical emollients and antihistamines, although the evidence to support their use is weak. A recent review concluded that vitamin K was only required if there was evidence of coagulation problems (Girling, Knight & Chappell, 2022). The woman will need reassurance, psychological support, maternal and fetal monitoring and possible elective birth depending upon the severity of the condition. The incidence of stillbirth in pregnancies affected by ICP is dependent upon the degree of abnormality in blood results and is no higher than the general population for women with mild disease (Girling, Knight & Chappell, 2022).

Neurological Disorders

Epilepsy

Epilepsy is a general term for abnormal cerebral function and a tendency to have recurrent unprovoked seizures (Smithson & Walker, 2012) It is one of the most common serious neurological conditions. Epilepsy is not a single condition and encompasses numerous different types of conditions and syndromes. The prevalence is approximately 1 in 100 people (Epilepsy Action, 2022).

A seizure consists of a brief alteration in brain function with a high-frequency discharge that can involve motor, sensory, autonomic or psychic clinical features accompanied by an alteration in the level of consciousness.

Seizures may be provoked by hypoglycaemia, lack of sleep, raised temperature, emotional or physical stress, drinking large amounts of water, constipation, drugs, hyperventilation, strobe lights, loud noises, some music and being startled.

Classification of Seizures

- **Generalized seizures** involve neurons bilaterally, often without a focal onset and usually originating from a subcortical or deeper brain focus. Consciousness is always impaired or lost. Other terms used to describe seizures are *absence, myoclonic, akinetic* and *clonic-tonic,* and is often termed *grand mal* or *petit mal epilepsy.*
- **Partial seizures (focal)** such as temporal lobe epilepsy and **Jacksonian epilepsy** often have a local onset and usually originate from cortical brain tissue. Consciousness is maintained if the seizure is limited to one cerebral hemisphere, but voluntary loss of muscular control occurs in the affected part of the body. **Temporal lobe epilepsy** is often characterized by continuous inappropriate rubbing of hands or combing the hair.
- In **status epilepticus,** more seizures follow the first before consciousness is fully regained and the person is in the **postictal state** (a state after a seizure) when the next seizure begins. Cerebral hypoxia means that this state is a medical emergency, and failure to treat adequately may result in deterioration in mental health and death. Impairment of the conscious state may lead to the aspiration of the stomach contents.

Pathophysiology of Seizures

The abnormal discharge of electricity rapidly spreads throughout the brain to involve the cortex, basal ganglia, thalamus and brainstem, leading to a tonic phase with generalized muscle contraction and increased muscle tone. Respiration may stop, and involuntary urination or defecation may occur. This is followed by a clonic phase as inhibitory neurons begin to interrupt the seizure discharge, leading to an intermittent contraction/relaxation pattern of muscle action. The clonic bursts gradually become more infrequent and the seizure ends. Immediately before the onset of a seizure, there may be an aura involving a visual disturbance or sensing a peculiar smell (Ritter et al., 2019).

Treatment of Epilepsy

Investigation of seizures should be established to offer treatment. If no cause is found, which is common, antiepileptic medication, either as monotherapy or combination therapy, will be commenced. Epilepsy may be controlled but not cured. Drugs used in treatment are known to interact adversely, thus affecting the efficiency of the drug if used in combination therapy. Some drugs in use are:
- Valproate (Epilim).
- Phenytoin (Epanutin).
- Phenobarbital.
- Carbamazepine, oxcarbazepine and others.

Epilepsy in Pregnancy

It is estimated that 1 in 100 pregnancies involve a woman with active epilepsy (Morley, 2018). For most pregnancies, women can expect to be well and have normal outcomes. However there is a slight increase in the risk of major congenital malformations associated with antiepileptic drugs and increasing evidence of developmental problems in children exposed to some antiepileptic drugs during pregnancy (Bagshaw, Ferrie & Kerr, 2012; Morley, 2018).

Many pregnancies are unplanned, and antiepileptic drugs may increase the breakdown of oestrogens, rendering contraceptives less efficient. Pre-conception advice is, therefore, an important aspect of care for women with epilepsy. Women with epilepsy who are planning a pregnancy should be medically advised to take a higher dose of folic acid pre-pregnancy and in the first trimester (Stephen et al., 2019). The changing metabolism of pregnancy alters the effect of epilepsy medication, and there will be a need for careful medical management of both the type of drug used and the dose required to control seizures (NICE, 2022).

Specific abnormalities have been linked to specific drugs:

- Sodium valproate: neural tube and skeletal defects, particularly in higher doses.
- Carbamazepine: neural tube and cardiac anomalies.
- Phenytoin: orofacial clefts, cardiac anomalies and digital defects.

Seizures occurring during pregnancy may cause fetal hypoxia and therefore are a risk to fetal well-being—even more so if status epilepticus occurs. Many women are reluctant to take their medication during pregnancy as they are aware of the risks of congenital malformations. Physiological changes during pregnancy also mean that a higher dose may be required to prevent seizures. As a result, women may find their epilepsy less well-controlled and different in nature, resulting in more frequent seizures. Uncontrolled epilepsy can increase the risk of sudden unexpected death in epilepsy. Women with epilepsy should be managed by a multidisciplinary team including specialist nurses or midwives and be supported to continue their daily drug regimen (Bagshaw, Ferrie & Kerr, 2012).

Anticonvulsant drugs cross the placenta and decrease the production of vitamin K, which may lead to **haemorrhagic disease of the newborn.** Vitamin K should be administered to mothers from 36 weeks' gestation and to all babies after delivery (Nucera et al., 2022). If the baby is formula-fed, it may have withdrawal symptoms from maternal medication at approximately 1 week in the form of irritability, excessive crying and continuous hunger. Some babies may remain sleepy and difficult to feed. All drugs are excreted in breastmilk, and unless high levels of drugs are prescribed then there is no contraindication to breastfeeding.

Main Points

- Asthma is an inflammatory disease with hyper-responsiveness of the airways characterized by constriction of the smooth muscle in the bronchioles, hypersecretion of mucus and mucosal oedema.
- Pregnant women with asthma are susceptible to respiratory infections and should be encouraged to accept the influenza vaccination.
- Status asthmaticus is recurrent asthmatic episodes resulting from spasm of the smooth muscle of the walls of the bronchi and bronchioles.
- TB is second only to COVID-19 as a cause of death from infectious disease worldwide.
- TB is an infectious bacterial disease caused by M. tuberculosis, which most commonly affects the lungs. The symptoms of active TB of the lung are coughing, sometimes with sputum or blood, chest pains, weakness, weight loss, fever and night sweats.
- Pregnant women vulnerable and at higher risk of COVID-19 include Black and Asian ethnic groups and those with comorbidities such as pre-existing diabetes, BMI >25 kg/m² and gestational diabetes on insulin.
- Pregnant women are more susceptible to renal tract infections than other women. If UTIs are not diagnosed and treated then the infection can ascend to the kidneys, with 30% of women developing pyelonephritis.

- Signs and symptoms of acute pyelonephritis are malaise, fatigue, chills and back pain located in the upper lumbar region, accompanied by muscle guarding.
- AKI, formerly called *ARF,* is commonly defined as an abrupt decline in renal function.
- Women with chronic renal impairment with poorly controlled hypertension, proteinuria, oedema and poor kidney function may not have successful pregnancies.
- After kidney transplantation, fertility returns and pregnancy is likely. If kidney function is adequate and there is no hypertension, women with renal transplants tolerate pregnancy well. Common complications are preterm labour and pre-eclampsia.
- Transplant recipients are advised to wait 3 years before becoming pregnant to reduce the risk of rejection of the transplanted kidney.
- HG is a severe condition that results in excessive vomiting. It causes dehydration and metabolic imbalance and may lead to maternal death if not treated actively. Clinical investigations reveal dehydration, marked oliguria with dark urine of high specific gravity containing ketones, bile, protein and glucose. Electrolyte disturbances include hyponatraemia and hypochloraemia as sodium and chloride ions are lost in the vomit.
- In early pregnancy, appendicitis may be difficult to differentiate from threatened miscarriage (abortion), although there is no bleeding. Later in pregnancy, the pain may

be mistaken for UTI, abruptio placentae or the onset of labour.

- Women with a stoma may report increased symptoms of nausea and other intestinal disorders. Later in pregnancy, there may be stoma-related issues and there is a higher risk of birth via caesarean section.
- Cholestasis is a last-trimester problem with the development of pruritus (particularly of the hands and feet), abnormal liver enzymes and jaundice.
- An estimated 0.2–0.5% of pregnancies involve a woman with active epilepsy. Many pregnancies are unplanned,

and antiepileptic drugs may increase the breakdown of oestrogens, rendering contraceptives less efficient.

- Uncontrolled epilepsy will have a greater effect on pregnancy outcomes.
- Anticonvulsant drugs cross the placenta and decrease the production of vitamin K, which may lead to haemorrhagic disease of the newborn. Vitamin K should be administered to mothers from 36 weeks' gestation and to all babies after delivery.

References

Austin, K., Wilson, K., Saha, S., 2019. Hyperemesis gravidarum. Nutr. Clin. Pract. 34 (2), 226–241.

Bagshaw, J., Ferrie, C.D., Kerr, M.P., 2012. Special groups – women, children, learning disability and the elderly. In: Smithson, W.H. (Ed.), ABC of Epilepsy. Wiley-Blackwell, Oxford.

Baston, H., Hall, J., Samples, J., 2019. Respiratory disorders of childbearing. In: Baston, H., Hall, J., Samples, J. (Eds.), Midwifery Essentials: Medical Conditions. Elsevier, London.

Blackburn, S., 2018. Maternal, Fetal & Neonatal Physiology: A Clinical Perspective, fifth ed. Elsevier, Philadelphia.

Bloom, C.I., Saglani, S., Feary, J., Jarvis, D., Quint, J.K., 2019. Changing prevalence of current asthma and inhaled corticosteroid treatment in the UK: population-based cohort 2006–2016. Eur. Respir. J. 53 (4), 1802130.

British Thoracic Society, 2019. SIGN 158: British Guideline on the Management of Asthma: A National Clinical Guideline. Available at: https://www.sign.ac.uk/media/1773/sign158-updated.pdf.

Crossette-Thambiah, C., Nicolson, P., Rajakaruna, I., Langridge, A., Sayar, Z., Perelta, M.R., et al., 2021. The clinical course of COVID-19 in pregnant versus non-pregnant women requiring hospitalisation: results from the multicentre UK CA-COVID-19 study. Br. J. Haematol. 195 (1), 85–89.

Donaldson, C., 2019. Challenges in pregnancy. In: Pairman, S., Tracy, S., Dahlen, H.G., Dixon, L. (Eds.), Midwifery Preparation for Practice, fourth ed. Elsevier Australia, Chatswood.

Engjom, H.M., Ramakrishnan, R., Vousden, N., Bunch, K., Morris, E., Simpson, N., et al., 2022. Severity of maternal SARS-CoV-2 infection and perinatal outcomes of women admitted to hospital during the omicron variant dominant period using UK Obstetric Surveillance System data: prospective, national cohort study. BMJ Med. 1 (1), e000190.

Epilepsy Action, 2022. What Is Epilepsy? Available at: https://www.epilepsy.org.uk/info/what-is-epilepsy.

Girling, J., Knight, C.L., Chappell, L., 2022. Intrahepatic cholestasis of pregnancy. Br. J. Obstet. Gynaecol. 129 (13), 95–114.

Grette, K., Cassity, S., Holliday, N., Rimawi, B.H., 2020. Acute pyelonephritis during pregnancy: a systematic review of the aetiology, timing, and reported adverse perinatal risks during pregnancy. J. Obstet. Gynaecol. 40 (6), 739–748.

Hindley, C., 2018. Asthma in pregnancy: physiology, management and recommendations for midwives. Br. J. Midwifery 26 (7), 446–450.

Jim, B., Garovic, V.D., 2017. Acute kidney injury in pregnancy. Semin. Nephrol. 37 (4), 378–385.

Knight, M., Bunch, K., Patel, R., Shakespeare, J., Kotnis, R., Kenyon, S., et al., (on behalf of MBRRACE-UK), 2022. Saving Lives, Improving Mothers' Care – Lessons Learned to Inform Maternity Care from the UK and Ireland Confidential Enquiries into Maternal Deaths and Morbidity 2018–20. National Perinatal Epidemiology Unit, University of Oxford, Oxford.

Miele, K., Morris, B.S., Tepper, N.K., 2020. Tuberculosis in pregnancy. Obstet. Gynecol. 135 (6), 1444–1453.

Morley, K., 2018. Epilepsy in pregnancy: the role of the midwife in risk management. Br. J. Midwifery 26 (9), 564–573.

Murphy, V.E., 2015. Managing asthma in pregnancy. Breathe 11 (4), 258–267.

National Institute of Health and Care Excellence (NICE), 2016. Tuberculosis. Available at: https://www.nice.org.uk/guidance/ng33/chapter/Recommendations#latent-tb.

National Institute of Health and Care Excellence (NICE), 2017. Asthma: Diagnosis, Monitoring and Chronic Asthma Management. Available at: https://www.nice.org.uk/guidance/ng80.

National Institute of Health and Care Excellence (NICE), 2019. Urinary Tract Infection (Lower) – Women: Clinical Knowledge Summary. Available at: https://cks.nice.org.uk/topics/urinary-tract-infection-lower-women/.

National Institute of Health and Care Excellence (NICE), 2021. Managing Suspected Appendicitis: Clinical Knowledge Summary. Available at: https://cks.nice.org.uk/topics/appendicitis/management/managing-suspected-appendicitis/.

National Institute of Health and Care Excellence (NICE), 2022. Epilepsies in Children, Young People and Adults. Available at: https://www.nice.org.uk/guidance/ng217.

Nucera, B., Brigo, F., Trinka, E., Kalss, G., 2022. Treatment and care of women with epilepsy before, during, and after pregnancy: a practical guide. Ther. Adv. Neurol. Disord. 15, 1–31.

PAPooSE Study Group, 2022. Pregnancy outcomes after stoma surgery for inflammatory bowel disease: the results of a retrospective multicentre audit. Colorectal Dis. 24 (7), 838–844.

Public Health England, 2019. Tuberculosis Cases in England Hit Lowest Ever Levels. Available at: https://www.gov.uk/government/news/tuberculosis-cases-in-england-hit-lowest-ever-levels.

Ritter, J.M., Flower, R.S., Henderson, G., Loke, Y.K., MacEwan, D., Rang, H., 2019. Rang & Dale's Pharmacology, ninth ed. Elsevier, London.

Royal College of Obstetricians and Gynaecologists (RCOG), 2012. Green-top Guideline No. 64a. Bacterial Sepsis in Pregnancy. Available at: https://www.rcog.org.uk/media/ea1p1r4h/gtg_64a.pdf.

Royal College of Obstetricians and Gynaecologist. (RCOG), 2022. Coronavirus (COVID-19), pregnancy and women's health.

https://www.rcog.org.uk/guidance/coronavirus-covid-19-pregnancy-and-women-s-health/

Smithson, W.H., Walker, M.C., 2012. What is epilepsy? Incidence, prevalence and aetiology. In: Smithson, W.H., Walker, M.C. (Eds.), ABC of Epilepsy. Wiley-Blackwell, Oxford.

Stephen, L.J., Harden, C., Tomson, T., Brodie, M.J., 2019. Management of epilepsy in women. Lancet Neurol., 18(5), 481–491.

Stern, J., Pier, J., Litonjua, A.A., 2020. Asthma epidemiology and risk factors. Semin. Immunopathol. 42 (1), 5–15.

Taber-Hight, E., Shah, S., 2020. Acute kidney injury in pregnancy. Adv. Chron. Kidney Dis. 27 (6), 455–460.

Takahashi, K., Funayama, Y., Fukushima, K., Shibata, C., Ogawa, H., Kumagai, E., et al., 2007. Pregnancy and delivery in patients with enterostomy due to anorectal complications from Crohn's disease. Int. J. Colorectal Dis. 22 (3), 313–318.

UK Health Security Agency (HSA), 2023. A guide on the COVID-19 vaccine for women who are pregnant or breastfeeding. Available at: https://www.gov.uk/government/publications/covid-19-vaccination-women-of-childbearing-age-currently-pregnant-planning-a-pregnancy-or-breastfeeding

Webster, P., Lightstone, L., McKay, D.B., Josephson, M.A., 2017. Pregnancy in chronic kidney disease and kidney transplantation. Kidney Int. 91 (5), 1047–1056.

Whiteley, I., Gullick, J., 2018. The embodied experience of pregnancy with an ileostomy. J. Clin. Nurs. 27 (21–22), 3931–3944.

Wiles, K., Chappell, L., Clark, K., Elman, L., Hall, M., Lightstone, L., et al., 2019. Clinical practice guideline on pregnancy and renal disease. BMC Nephrol. 20 (1), 401.

World Health Organization (WHO), 2022. Tuberculosis. Fact Sheet. Available at: https://www.who.int/news-room/fact-sheets/detail/tuberculosis.

World Health Organization (WHO), 2023. Coronavirus disease (COVID-19) pandemic. Available at: https://www.who.int/europe/emergencies/situations/covid-19

Wylie, L., Bryce, H., 2016. The gastrointestinal system. In: Wylie, L., Bryce, H. (Eds.), The Midwives' Guide to Key Medical Conditions, second ed. Churchill Livingstone, London.

Annotated recommended reading

Useful websites

https://www.sign.ac.uk/media/1140/pat158_pregnancy.pdf.
https://www.asthma.org.uk/.
https://www.npeu.ox.ac.uk/ukoss/completed-surveillance/covid-19-in-pregnancy.
https://epilepsyresearch.org.uk/.
https://www.nice.org.uk/guidance/.
https://www.gov.uk/government/organisations/uk-health-security-agency.

These websites are excellent, up-to-date evidence-based resources for specific conditions including asthma, COVID-19 and epilepsy.

https://www.npeu.ox.ac.uk/ukoss/current-surveillance.

Students and midwives are strongly recommended to access this excellent website for up-to-date information on obstetrics and maternity care. Information updates on the following UKOSS studies can be found on the website:

- *New Therapies for Influenza*

- *Thrombotic Microangiopathy Associated Pregnancy Acute Kidney Injury*

- *Severe Respiratory Virus Infection in Pregnancy and Participating in the RECOVERY Trial*

- *Severe Pyelonephritis In pregnancy*

https://www.rcog.org.uk/guidance/coronavirus-covid-19-pregnancy-and-women-s-health/

This site provides information on Coronavirus (COVID-19), pregnancy and women's health. This includes: COVID-19, infection in pregnancy; vaccination; COVID-19 infection and abortion care.

35

Diabetes Mellitus and Other Metabolic Disorders in Pregnancy

DAWN CAMERON

This chapter discusses common metabolic disorders in pregnancy. Diabetes mellitus is detailed including the pathophysiology and general pathological effects. Other endocrine disorders impacting thyroid function are outlined.

Introduction

Midwives need to have a sound understanding of endocrine disorders, in the context of pregnancy and the postnatal period, to support and manage these conditions appropriately. If well controlled, most pre-existing endocrine conditions may have little impact on maternal or fetal morbidity. Uncontrolled endocrine conditions in pregnancy, whether poorly controlled pre-conception or newly diagnosed, are associated with adverse fetal outcomes and maternal morbidity (Calina et al., 2019). Three-quarters of maternal deaths are in women with co-existing medical complications (Knight et al., 2022). It remains a challenge to differentiate symptoms of normal pregnancy from pathological symptomatology (Neubergera & Nelson-Piercy, 2015).

Diabetes mellitus is by far the most common of these diseases, and much progress has been made in its management

(Ali & Dornhorst, 2018). Normal metabolism, including carbohydrate utilization, is discussed in Chapter 23.

Diabetes Mellitus

Diabetes mellitus is characterized by impaired carbohydrate utilization caused by an absolute or relative deficiency of insulin production by the endocrine pancreas. It is estimated that about 422 million people worldwide have diabetes, increasing from 108 million in 1980, and its prevalence continues to rise more rapidly in low- and middle-income countries than in high-income countries (World Health Organization [WHO], 2022). In 2019 it was estimated that diabetes was the direct cause of 2 million deaths (WHO, 2022). Type 2 diabetes now accounts for 95% of all diabetes worldwide including an increased incidence in children (WHO, 2016; WHO, 2022).

The changes in uncontrolled diabetes are a rise in blood plasma glucose (normal range 3–5 mmol/L), increases in glycogen breakdown (gluconeogenesis), fatty acid oxidation, ketone production and urea formation. There is reduced production of glycogen, lipid and protein in cells of tissue such as muscle and adipose that are normally dependent on insulin (Holt & Hanley, 2021).

Pathophysiology

Reduced uptake of glucose results in inhibition of **glycolytic enzymes** and activation of the enzymes involved in **gluconeogenesis**, resulting in in more blood glucose than can be utilized. Excessive glucose passes into the renal filtrate and **glycosuria** occurs. Glucose is osmotically active and pulls water after it, resulting in **polyuria** and **dehydration** (Holt & Hanley, 2021). **Thirst** increases to try to maintain adequate body fluids.

The body tries to mobilize energy from fats and proteins. Urea (a by-product of amino acid metabolism) is excreted in the urine. Fatty acid release always results in **ketogenesis,** but in people with diabetes, excess ketones are produced and excreted in the urine and on the breath. The ketones in the blood cause metabolic acidosis and lowering of pH (Holt & Hanley, 2021). Buffer systems become exhausted attempting to correct this, and other metabolic processes become disturbed, with all body systems affected. If untreated, acidosis leads to shock, coma and death.

Diabetes Mellitus in Pregnancy

Diabetes mellitus in pregnancy includes type 1 diabetes, type 2 diabetes and **gestational diabetes** (GDM). Recently, more pregnant women were found to have type 2 diabetes (WHO, 2014; Raets, Ingelbrecht & Benhalima, 2023). GDM is diagnosed if diabetes develops for the first time in pregnancy. Prevalence of GDM is increasing because of higher rates of obesity in the general population and more pregnancies in older women (Eades, Cameron & Evans, 2017; National Institute of Health and Care Excellence [NICE], 2020; WHO, 2014).

Aetiology

Type 1 Diabetes Mellitus

This condition results in almost a total lack of insulin production (rare before 9 months and peaks at 12 years of age). Hyperglycaemia, polyuria and ketosis are present at onset, and insulin treatment is necessary. Differences exist between populations both within and between countries. Type 1 diabetes accounts for about 10% of diabetes in developed countries. It is more prevalent amongst White people, with the highest incidence in Finland and the lowest in Japan.

Coxsackie virus B4 (CB4), causing childhood infection, may be implicated in the onset of type 1 diabetes (Holt & Hanley, 2021). The CB4 virus may destroy pancreatic islet cells and trigger an autoimmune response in genetically susceptible children. There is a long period of subclinical diabetes as β cells are progressively destroyed, and islet cell antibodies have been found years before the onset of clinical signs. There is impaired α-cell function, leading to excess **glucagon,** which exacerbates hyperglycaemia. Auto-antibodies have been found in most people with juvenile-onset diabetes.

Type 1 diabetes mellitus is subdivided into two distinct types:

- **Type 1A** develops in childhood (may be due to a genetic–environment interaction). There is a link with the human leucocyte antigen HLA-DR4, with the predisposing gene carried on chromosome 6. About 12% of people with newly diagnosed diabetes of this type have a first-degree relative with the disease.
- **Type 1B** tends to occur later in life, between 30–50 years, and is probably an autoimmune disorder linked to HLA-DR3.

Type 2 Diabetes Mellitus

More than 95% of people with diabetes have type 2 diabetes mellitus (WHO, 2022). The onset is usually in later life in people with obesity. Type 2 diabetes mellitus occurs more frequently in pregnancy and varies with ethnicity, suggesting a genetic–environment interaction (NICE, 2020). A form of diabetes called **maturity-onset diabetes of the young** is caused by an autosomal-dominant gene. Sufferers are usually of normal weight and under 25 years of age.

Amyloid deposits associated with islet cell destruction are seen in about 25% of cases, usually correlating with the person's age and severity of disease. The ratio of α to β cells is normal with no reduction of insulin in the blood, but insulin has a decreased ability to influence cellular uptake of glucose in people with obesity. This is probably due to increased circulating free fatty acids, although reactions with other substances have also been proposed (Holt & Hanley, 2021). There is increased **insulin resistance** because of decreased numbers of **cellular insulin receptors.**

Pregnant women with type 2 diabetes are likely to be obese and to suffer hypertension and hyperlipidaemia (overproduction of fatty acids).

Approximately 87.5% of women with diabetes during pregnancy have GDM (which may or may not resolve after pregnancy), 7.5% have type 1 diabetes and the remaining 5% have type 2 diabetes (NICE, 2020). Clinical Application 35.1 details the recommended plasma glucose levels in pregnancy for women with all forms of diabetes (NICE, 2020).

CLINICAL APPLICATION 35.1 Recommended Plasma Glucose Levels in Pregnancy

Women with Previously Diagnosed Diabetes

Women planning pregnancy should be advised to aim for the same capillary plasma glucose target ranges as recommended for all people with type 1 diabetes:

- Fasting plasma glucose level of 5–7 mmol/L on waking AND
- Plasma glucose level of 4–7 mmol/L before meals at other times of the day.

Antenatal Care with Any Form of Diabetes

Advise pregnant women to maintain their capillary plasma glucose below the following target levels (if achievable without causing problematic hypoglycaemia):

- Fasting: 5.3 mmol/L. AND
- 1 hour after meals: 7.8 mmol/L. OR
- 2 hours after meals: 6.4 mmol/L.

Diagnosis of Gestational Diabetes

If the woman has either:

- A fasting plasma glucose level of 5.6 mmol/L or above. OR
- A 2-hour plasma glucose level of 7.8 mmol/L or above.

Pre-pregnancy screening (or early in the first trimester) might help to differentiate between women with type 2 diabetes and those with GDM. Refer to the NICE (2020) guidelines.

Gestational Diabetes Mellitus

GDM develops in pregnancy and may be due to the diabetogenic effect of pregnancy, familial disposition to diabetes or impaired glucose tolerance in stressful situations.

These women have an increased risk of developing type 2 diabetes in later life, particularly if obese (Vounzoulaki et al., 2020). A previous diagnosis of GDM carries a lifetime risk of progression to type 2 diabetes of up to 60% (Noctor & Dunne, 2015).

The overall prevalence of GDM is 5.4% (Eades, Cameron & Evans, 2017) and is mostly in the third trimester. Clinical Application 35.2 details the maternal risk factors and recommended testing protocol for GDM. If women have not been screened before pregnancy or during the early part of the first trimester, it is difficult to differentiate this from pre-pregnancy-onset type 2 diabetes. GDM is associated with an increased risk of perinatal morbidity and mortality.

General Pathological Effects of Diabetes Mellitus

The metabolic changes and physiological effects of diabetes mellitus are extensive (Fig. 35.1). Deaths from **cardiovascular disease** and **renal disease** are much more common than in the general population. Acute complications include

• CLINICAL APPLICATION 35.2 Risk Factors and Recommended Testing Protocol for Gestational Diabetes Mellitus

Previous gestational diabetes (GDM) is a key risk factor.

Risk Factors (Assessed at Booking Visit)

- Body mass index above 30 kg/m².
- Previous macrosomic baby weighing ≥4.5 kg.
- Family history of diabetes (first-degree relative).
- Minority ethnic family origin with a high diabetic prevalence.
Glycosuria of ≥2+ on one occasion or ≥1+ or above on two or more occasions (detected by reagent strip testing during routine antenatal care) may indicate undiagnosed GDM and warrants further testing to exclude GDM.

Testing Protocol

The 2-hour, 75-g oral glucose tolerance test (OGTT) is used to test for GDM in women with risk factors (see earlier).
- Offer women who have had GDM in a previous pregnancy:
  - Early self-monitoring of blood glucose **or** a 75-g, 2-hour OGTT as soon as possible after booking (whether in first or second trimester) **and** a further 75-g, 2-hour OGTT at 24–28 weeks (if the first OGTT results are normal).
  - Offer women with any of the other risk factors for GDM a 75-g, 2-hour OGTT at 24–28 weeks.
  Refer to the NICE (2020) guidelines. See Clinical Application 35.1 for recommended plasma glucose levels in pregnancy.

hypoglycaemia and **diabetic ketoacidosis.** Pregnant women with insulin-treated diabetes for more than 10 years have increased risks of associated cardiovascular, ophthalmic, renal and neuropathic problems. In general, women with diabetes are at risk of poor pregnancy outcomes, particularly if their condition is poorly controlled.

Hypoglycaemia

Hypoglycaemia occurs in 90% of individuals with diabetes and is also known as **insulin shock** or **insulin reaction.** The balance of insulin versus available glucose becomes unbalanced and blood levels of glucose fall, brain cells are depleted of nutrients and loss of consciousness results in coma. Hypoglycaemia can be controlled by diet and insulin administration.

Symptoms

Hypoglycaemia causes secretion of glucagon, adrenaline (epinephrine) and growth hormone, which in turn causes tachycardia, palpitations, tremors, pallor and anxiety. Other symptoms include headaches, dizziness, irritability, confusion, visual disturbances, hunger and convulsions. Coma will occur if not treated with oral or intravenous glucose (White & Porterfield, 2018).

Diabetic Ketoacidosis

The body breaks down fatty acids, causing **ketoacidosis,** as glucose is not available for cell metabolism because of the deficit of insulin. This is a serious condition because as fatty particles are mobilized around the transport system, fatty deposits are left behind in the blood vessels, causing atherosclerosis with consequent cardiovascular problems. An increase in hormones such as catecholamines, glucagon, cortisol and growth hormone antagonize the effect of insulin. Liver glucose production increases and peripheral glucose usage decreases. Precipitating causes are likely to be the interruption of insulin administration, infection and trauma (White & Porterfield, 2018).

Symptoms and Treatment

Polyuria, polydipsia and dehydration will occur because of **osmotic diuresis.** Sodium, magnesium and phosphorus deficits may occur, but the most severe electrolyte disturbance is potassium deficiency. Hyperventilation may occur to compensate for the acidosis with postural dizziness, anorexia, nausea and abdominal pain. Both glucose and ketones will be present in the urine. There may be a smell of acetone on the breath. Treatment aims to decrease blood glucose levels by continuous administration of low-dose insulin and stabilizing electrolyte levels.

Box 35.1 outlines the long-term complications of diabetes mellitus.

Effects of Diabetes on Pregnancy

Pregnancy changes glucose metabolism, creating a **diabetogenic effect,** and women with carbohydrate intolerance

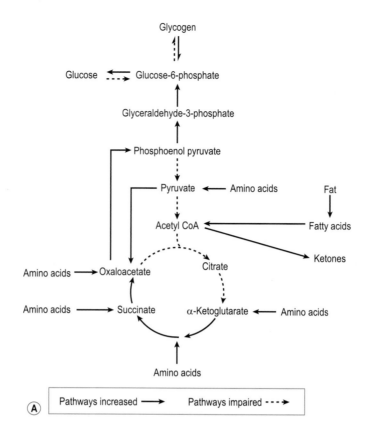

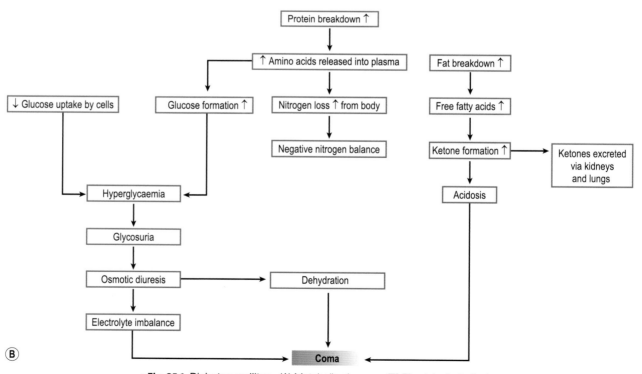

• **Fig. 35.1** Diabetes mellitus. (A) Metabolic changes. (B) Physiological effects.

• BOX 35.1 Long-term Complications of Diabetes Mellitus

- Diabetic neuropathy with sensory deficits.
- Microvascular disease appears to be directly linked to the duration of the disease and blood glucose levels. Retinopathy causes blood vessel changes, leading to loss of sight. Nephropathy may result in end-stage renal disease.
- Atherosclerosis appears at a younger age in people with diabetes and progresses more rapidly, leading to hypertension, coronary artery disease and stroke. This is unrelated to the severity of diabetes. Peripheral vascular disease, leading to gangrene and amputation, may result due to the abnormal level of glucose in the tissues.
- Infection is more common as pathogens utilize the increased tissue glucose to multiply and phagocytic white cell function is impaired.

• CLINICAL APPLICATION 35.3 Effects of Diabetes on the Pregnancy and Fetus

Diabetes in pregnancy is associated with risks to the woman and developing fetus , resulting in a significant increase in fetal and maternal morbidity.

Miscarriage, pre-eclampsia and preterm labour are more common in women with pre-existing diabetes. Maternal diabetic retinopathy can worsen rapidly during pregnancy.

Fetal Problems
- Higher incidence of fetal malformations with poor maternal diabetic control.
- Congenital malformations.
- **Fetal macrosomia** (i.e., birthweight >4500 g or >95th centile).
- Birth injury.
- Stillbirth.
- Neonatal asphyxia and respiratory distress syndrome.
- Perinatal mortality.
- Postnatal adaptation problems (such as hypoglycaemia) more common in babies born to women with pre-existing diabetes.
  Refer to the NICE (2020) guidelines (section 1.5.5) for admission of babies to neonatal unit.

may not show signs or symptoms of diabetes. Diabetes becomes more difficult to control in pregnancy, although after delivery women should return to their pre-pregnancy state. Clinical Application 35.3 outlines the effects on pregnancy and the fetus .

Effect of Pregnancy on Diabetes

Pregnancy places large demands on maternal metabolism, particularly in the last trimester, to allow more efficient storage of nutrients while minimizing catabolism of protein stores. In later pregnancy, there is progressive insulin resistance caused by the placental hormones (e.g., oestrogen and human placental lactogen), which decrease insulin efficiency. Normally, β cells increase the amount of insulin they release in the presence of insulin resistance, but glucose metabolism in pregnant women with diabetes becomes unstable and more insulin will be needed to achieve metabolic control (White & Porterfield, 2018).

Diabetic Nephropathy

Diabetic nephropathy (DN) complicates approximately 5% of pregnancies in women with pre-existing diabetes (Singh, 2012). Congenital malformation, pre-eclampsia, macrosomia, preterm birth and fetal growth restriction are the major obstetric complications. Therefore, in women of reproductive age with diabetes, a major concern is whether pregnancy increases the risk for DN and/or accelerates the progression of DN. Although risk factors are still concerning, pregnancy outcomes are good with vigilant management and assessment with close teamwork and specialist care (Singh, 2012; Spotti, 2019).

Diabetic Retinopathy

A significant proportion of women with diabetes continue to experience deterioration in retinopathy during pregnancy (Egan et al., 2015). It has been associated with poor control of blood glucose, blood pressure, albuminuria and poor perinatal outcome (Egan et al., 2015). Pre-pregnancy care has a key role to fully inform women of the need for more

frequent retinal assessments during pregnancy and allow preconceptual optimization of glycaemic control and blood pressure (Egan et al., 2015). NICE (2020) recommends a protocol for retinal assessment by digital imaging (with mydriasis using tropicamide) after the first antenatal clinic appointment.

Care in Pregnancy

Pre-Conception Advice

Pregnancy should be discussed with women with diabetes before conception. Further high-quality evidence is required to determine appropriate pre-conception care for women with diabetes for improving maternal and infant health (Tieu et al., 2017). Adequate blood glucose control before conception does help reduce congenital abnormalities, fetal macrosomia, polyhydramnios and stillbirth. Women with well-controlled diabetes before conception and during pregnancy have outcomes approaching the incidence of the non-diabetic population (Wahabi et al., 2010). Women should be offered a renal assessment, including a measure of albuminuria, before discontinuing contraception. Depending on the results, women may be referred to a nephrologist. These women should take folic acid (5 mg/day) until 12 weeks of gestation to reduce the risk of having a baby with a neural tube defect (NICE, 2020).

Management During Pregnancy

It is essential that women with diabetes are cared for during pregnancy by the midwife and obstetrician in collaboration with the specialist diabetic team. Antenatal care follows a particular protocol (NICE, 2020), and delivery should take place in a consultant unit with neonatal facilities.

Diabetic Control

Management before and during pregnancy requires control of blood glucose and prevention of ketosis. Hypoglycaemia may be problematic in the first trimester where excessive vomiting occurs. Dietary intake and insulin dosage should be monitored with blood glucose levels by self-assessment. Blood ketone testing is advised for women with type 1 diabetes who are planning a pregnancy and if a woman with any type of diabetes is hyperglycaemic or unwell. Ketoacidosis may present in pregnancy with normal glucose levels and is an emergency situation as the fetus has a greatly increased mortality rate (NICE, 2020).

Monitoring Blood Glucose

Advice to women during pregnancy:
* Type 1 diabetes: test fasting, pre-meal, 1-hour post-meal and bedtime blood glucose levels daily (NICE, 2020).
* Type 2 diabetes or GDM: women taking multiple daily insulin injections should be advised to test their fasting, pre-meal, 1-hour post-meal and bedtime blood glucose levels daily.

Type 2 diabetes or GDM: should be advised to test their fasting and 1-hour post-meal blood glucose levels daily during pregnancy if they are on diet and exercise therapy, taking oral therapy (with or without diet and exercise therapy) or single-dose intermediate-acting or long-acting insulin (NICE, 2020). Refer to Clinical Application 35.1 for plasma glucose levels.

The risk of *nausea and vomiting* occurring in the first trimester should be discussed, as well as how glucose metabolism is changed by the presence of the fetus . Reporting abnormalities should be emphasized and positive lifestyle factors discussed.

Insulin

This is necessary for all women with type 1 diabetes and occasionally those with type 2 diabetes. Glycaemic control can be obtained by tailoring the insulin regimen to the individual woman. After birth, women with pre-existing insulin-treated diabetes should reduce their insulin with careful monitoring of blood glucose levels.

Oral Blood Glucose–lowering Agents

Metformin may be offered to pregnant women with pre-existing type 2 diabetes and GDM (NICE, 2020).

Diet

Dietary advice should be offered, highlighting optimum nutrition for both the mother and fetus . Foods with a low glycaemic index and small frequent meals are recommended. It is an ideal time to educate the woman about a good diet in accordance with ethnic background.

Monitoring the Fetus

Ongoing fetal well-being should be monitored closely using the methods discussed in Chapter 13. Although fetal macrosomia is a risk, the babies of women with renal disease or superimposed pre-eclampsia may suffer from intrauterine growth restriction. Clinical Application 35.4 provides an overview of the baby of a mother with diabetes and Clinical Application 35.5 details the management of GDM.

Delivery and Birth

Care is under a consultant endocrinologist and obstetrician.
* Pregnant women with uncomplicated GDM are advised antenatally to give birth no later than 40+6 weeks and offer elective birth (by induction of labour or by caesarean section (CS) if indicated) to women who have not given birth by this time (NICE, 2020).
* Pregnant women with type 1 or type 2 diabetes and no other complications are offered to have an elective birth by induction of labour or by elective CS if indicated between 37+0 weeks and 38+6 weeks of pregnancy.

Care in the Puerperium

Control of Diabetes

Insulin requirements fall and re-stabilization is necessary. Women with type 2 diabetes or GDM can usually cease taking insulin and commence oral blood glucose-lowering therapy if needed, which is safe for breastfeeding (NICE, 2020).

• CLINICAL APPLICATION 35.4 **The Baby of a Mother with Diabetes**

* Baby may be large, weighing >90th centile and plethoric, especially with poor maternal control of diabetes mellitus.
* Despite being ≥4000 g (4 kg), these babies may be physiologically immature and have problems similar to those of a preterm baby, including respiratory distress syndrome (see Chapter 51).
* With good maternal glycaemic control, the baby is more likely to be of a weight appropriate for gestational age.
* Congenital defects are also related to the control of diabetes around the time of conception.
* Birth injuries such as Erb's palsy may occur if the baby is large (see Chapter 53). High maternal blood glucose levels in utero encourage the fetal pancreas to produce more insulin (hyperinsulinaemia). This state continues after birth, creating neonatal hypoglycaemia (which may need intravenous glucose to stabilize). Careful monitoring of neonatal blood glucose and early feeding prevent severe side effects. The baby will have high-fat deposits created by the hyperinsulinaemia which affects growth hormone.
* **Polycythaemia** with **hyperbilirubinaemia** may result from inadequate transfer of nutrients via the placenta. Polycythaemia results from the fetal needs to increase oxygen levels. This leads to hyperbilirubinaemia postnatally. Although lethargic at first, the baby has normal development (Blackburn, 2018; Coad, Pedley & Dunstall, 2019).
  Refer to NICE (2020) guidelines (section 1.5.5) for admission of babies to the neonatal unit.

Infection Prevention

Women with diabetes are at increased risk of infection, particularly breast infection. Therefore, care must be taken to control the blood glucose level and to inspect the breasts for early signs.

Breastfeeding

Breastfeeding is possible, but lactating women have a higher energy turnover, and this means diet and insulin dosage need to be monitored carefully. Women with diabetes gain the same benefits as all mothers who breastfeed.

In breastfeeding women with existing type 2 diabetes, metformin can be resumed but other glucose-lowering drugs should be avoided. Women with pre-existing diabetes can continue with breastfeeding. However, they still need to avoid any medication for diabetic complications discontinued for safety reasons before conception.

Contraceptive Advice

The oral contraceptive pill can be taken but may mimic pregnancy, increasing the need for insulin. Intrauterine contraceptive devices are not recommended as they may lead to infection. A barrier method is advised, and this is an ideal time to discuss future pregnancy and preconceptual care.

Box 35.2 summarizes the key messages from the MBR-RACE report for the care of women with diabetes during and following pregnancy.

Abnormalities of Thyroid Function

Overactivity and underactivity of the thyroid gland can produce serious illness. Women with a thyroid disorder who are planning pregnancy need to be given up-to-date guidance and care before conception, during pregnancy and in the postpartum period (NICE, 2021a).

Hyperthyroidism (Thyrotoxicosis) in Pregnancy

Hyperthyroidism is a biochemical diagnosis. It is confirmed when there is pathologically increased thyroid hormone production and secretion by the thyroid gland (NICE, 2019; NICE 2021b). **Thyrotoxicosis** is the clinical manifestation of excess circulating thyroid hormones due to any cause, including hyperthyroidism. Primary hyperthyroidism occurs when thyrotoxicosis is caused by an abnormality of the thyroid gland, such as Graves' disease or a nodular goitre (Labadzhyan et al., 2014; NICE, 2019, 2021b). Thyrotoxicosis occurs in about 0.2% of pregnancies, and **Graves' disease** accounts for 95% of cases.

• CLINICAL APPLICATION 35.5 **Management of Gestational Diabetes**

Treatment of gestational diabetes (GDM) is effective in reducing macrosomia, babies large for gestational age, shoulder dystocia and pre-eclampsia/hypertensive disorders in pregnancy. After delivery, glucose metabolism may return to normal. There are usually no symptoms, and diagnosis depends on abnormal blood plasma glucose results (see Clinical Application 35.1).

Complications of GDM

Macrosomia is more frequent, leading to a greater incidence of forceps delivery, caesarean section and shoulder dystocia (resulting in injury to mother or baby). Women should be reminded to maintain normal bodyweight, exercise regularly, have annual blood glucose tests and receive early care if they become pregnant again (NICE, 2020).

Management of GDM

Once diagnosed, treatment should aim to control blood glucose, establish additional fetal surveillance and decrease the risk of macrosomia. *NICE (2020) does **NOT** recommend fasting plasma glucose, random blood glucose, HbA1c, glucose challenge test or urinalysis for glucose to assess risk of developing GDM.*

Intervention Offered

- Initially dietary control is advised (diet and exercise are always encouraged for control).
- Metformin if blood glucose targets are not met within 1–2 weeks of diet and exercise.
- Insulin instead of metformin (if contraindicated or unacceptable).
- Addition of insulin to diet and exercise and metformin if blood glucose targets are not met.

(NICE, 2020)

- Immediate treatment with insulin, with or without metformin, with a fasting plasma glucose level of 7.0 mmol/L or above at diagnosis.
- Consider immediate treatment with insulin, with or without metformin (plus diet and exercise changes) where fasting plasma glucose level is between 6.0–6.9 mmol/L if there are complications (e.g., macrosomia or hydramnios).

Postnatal Care

In women diagnosed with GDM, blood glucose–lowering therapy is discontinued.

For women diagnosed with GDM and whose blood glucose levels return to normal after birth:
- Offer lifestyle advice (including weight control, diet and exercise).
- Offer a fasting plasma glucose test 6–13 weeks after the birth to exclude diabetes (at the 6-week postnatal check would be practical).
- If a fasting plasma glucose test has not been performed by 13 weeks, offer a fasting plasma glucose test or an HbA1c test if a fasting plasma glucose test is not possible >13 weeks.
- Do not routinely offer a 75-g, 2-hour OGTT.
- Offer an annual HbA1c test to women who were diagnosed with GDM who have a negative postnatal test for diabetes.

Raise awareness of risk of developing type 2 diabetes in later life and offer a referral onto a diabetes prevention programme if eligible based on the results of the fasting plasma glucose test or HbA1c test.

Thyroid-stimulating immunoglobulins (TSIgs) (antibodies) activate **follicular cell thyroid-stimulating hormone (TSH) receptors,** leading to increased production of **thyroid hormones.** It usually manifests with signs and symptoms including raised basal metabolic rate (BMR), heat intolerance and excessive perspiration, weight loss or lack of weight gain despite good calorific intake, tachycardia (bounding), palpitations, hypertension, anxiety and hyperreflexia (Labadzhyan et al., 2014). **Exophthalmos** (protrusion of the eyeballs) may occur (Cooper & Laurberg, 2013). Treatment before pregnancy may have included surgical removal of the thyroid gland or radioactive iodine to destroy the most active thyroid cells.

Rarer conditions causing hyperthyroidism include **autonomous thyroid nodules. Biochemical thyrotoxicosis** may occur in women who develop hyperemesis gravidarum because of the similarity between TSH and human chorionic gonadotrophin. In pregnancy, the thyroid increases in size without increased hormone levels; it may also become more nodular, making diagnosis of thyroid problems difficult. However the signs and symptoms and a rapid sleeping pulse and lid lag are suspicious. Thyroxine (T_4) assays will be higher than normally expected in pregnancy (Labadzhyan et al., 2014).

Severe hyperthyroidism is associated with infertility, but conception may occur if treatment has been successful or if the disease is mild. In mild hyperthyroidism, improvements may occur in pregnancy due to increased thyroxine-binding globulin, which can offset the excess of thyroid hormones. Thyrotoxicosis with the presence of goitre, ophthalmopathy and persistence of disease can be suggestive of Graves' disease (Labadzhyan et al., 2014). Women with Graves' disease may also experience improvement due to altered immune system functioning, and drug dosages can often be reduced.

Management

Clinical Application 35.6 summarizes the management of childbearing/pregnant women with thyroid disorders (NICE, 2021a).

Inadequately managed thyrotoxicosis is associated with severe pre-eclampsia and maternal heart failure. Pregnant women with hyperthyroidism also need more calories to compensate for the higher metabolic rate. Fluid loss may occur if there is diarrhoea. If antithyroid drugs are used, close monitoring of the effects is necessary to avoid too high levels of drug. The drugs commonly used to normalize thyroid function are **propylthiouracil** (PTU) or **carbimazole** (CBZ). PTU is the usual drug of choice in pregnancy and the puerperium. A **partial thyroidectomy** may be required if the disease is difficult to control or the woman has a large goitre.

Clinical Application 35.7 outlines the effects of maternal thyroid treatment on the fetus .

• BOX 35.2 Key Messages from the MBRRACE-UK Report

Maternal deaths of women with diabetes also had multiple, complex and interacting medical and social conditions. This level of complexity warrants a multidisciplinary (MTD) approach to care.

Care approaches should consider the multiple comorbidities and consider the following:

- Promote self-management of diabetes including both long-term physical and mental health conditions.
- Diabetes professionals need to have appropriate skills to support diabetes self-management in addition to the array of other complexities such as mental health.
- Antenatal thromboprophylaxis for women with type 1 diabetes and nephropathy due to the intermediate risk of venous thromboembolism.
- Professionals need to be alert to possible clinical or subclinical depression and/or anxiety, particularly if someone reports or appears to be having difficulties with self-management.
- Perinatal mental health services should involve face- to-face contact where necessary.
- Relevant skills and drills training on the management of diabetic ketoacidosis in pregnancy is essential to ensure that all maternity staff are aware of the symptoms and signs of diabetic ketoacidosis.
- Ensure the appropriate national Maternity Early Warning Score is used to monitor a pregnant woman wherever in the hospital she receives care in the hospital.
- Awareness of the added risk of fetal compromise when a woman's pregnancy is complicated by both hypertension and diabetes. It is not only babies predicted to be small for gestational age who may be at risk.

(Knight et al., 2022)

• CLINICAL APPLICATION 35.6 Management of Women with Thyroid Disorders

Pre-pregnancy

- Referral to an endocrinology specialist for all women with overt or subclinical hyperthyroidism for pre-pregnancy counselling.
- Baseline blood levels for serum thyroid-stimulating hormone (TSH) and free thyroxine (FT_4) levels and consider checking thyroid peroxidase antibody (TPOAb) status.
- Women with untreated hyperthyroidism are requested to delay pregnancy until the specialist assessment and thyroid function has normalized.

During Pregnancy

- Emergency admission and referral to specialist if the woman has a suspected serious complication (thyrotoxic crisis or hyperemesis gravidarum).
- Routine but urgent specialist referral (endocrinologist and obstetrician) for all other pregnant women with current or previous overt or subclinical hyperthyroidism.
- Monitor serum TSH, FT_4 and free triiodothyronine (FT_3) levels for all women.
- Monitor women taking antithyroid drug treatment.
- Postpartum – continue monitoring blood levels 6–8 weeks.
- Seek urgent advice from an endocrinologist if the woman experiences signs and symptoms of thyroid related complications.

Refer to NICE (2021a) for further details.

Thyroid Storm

The main complication of hyperthyroidism is the medical emergency of **thyroid crisis** (or **thyroid storm**), which is characterized by an extreme **hypermetabolic state.** It is a rare and potentially life-threatening complication, occurring in 1% of hyperthyroid pregnancies, usually due to a stressful delivery or infection (de Leo, Lee & Braverman, 2016; NICE, 2021b). The woman develops exaggerated features of thyrotoxicosis with hyperthermia (hyperpyrexia), tachycardia, cardiac dysrhythmias, congestive cardiac failure, altered mental states and ultimately coma. Goitre may also be present. This complication carries a high rate of maternal morbidity and mortality. The mortality rate is estimated at about 10% due to hyperthermia, cardiac arrhythmias, multi-organ failure and sepsis (Kahaly et al., 2018). Treatment in an intensive care unit is required and includes intravenous fluids, hydrocortisone and specific specialist drugs.

Hypothyroidism in Pregnancy

This underactivity of the thyroid gland may be due to autoimmune thyroiditis (Hashimoto's disease), viral thyroiditis or congenital absence of the thyroid gland (Gregory & Todd, 2013). This occurs due to a defect in the thyroid gland or in the control pathway of thyrotrophin-releasing hormone (TRH) or TSH release. The most common cause in pregnancy is autoimmune thyroiditis (goitre may or may not be present) (Gregory & Todd, 2013). Lack of dietary iodine can also cause goitre (enlarged thyroid tissue).

Hypothyroidism is familial and may be associated with other autoimmune diseases, like type 1 diabetes (Gregory & Todd, 2013). Other causes of hypothyroidism in pregnancy are those secondary to immune disorders or after destruction of thyroid tissue either surgically or with radioactive iodine.

Symptoms include a low BMR, weight gain, feeling cold, constipation, alopecia, dry skin, puffy eyes, oedema, hoarse voice, bradycardia, lethargy and cognitive impairment. Untreated hypothyroidism is often associated with infertility because TRH stimulation induces **hyperprolactinaemia,** which prevents ovulation. Confirmation is by measurement of triiodothyronine (T_3) and T_4 levels. Pregnancy complications include hypertension, low birthweight and psychomotor delay in the fetus . An endocrinologist is involved in early pregnancy to obtain baseline free T_4 and TSH levels (Lazarus et al., 2014). Treatment is by T_4 medication, and assessment of thyroid function once in each trimester is usually sufficient. As long as the fetus is not exposed to iodine deficiency or teratogenic drugs, development should be normal. Complications of increased fetal loss and prolonged pregnancy may occur.

Box 35.3 provides information on a range of adrenal disorders in pregnancy.

CLINICAL APPLICATION 35.7   Effect of Maternal Thyroid Treatments on the Fetus

Maternal pregnancy is high-risk and requires specialist care, which includes:
- Serial fetal growth ultrasound scans.
- Regular assessment of fetal heart rate to detect fetal tachycardia.
- Monthly measurements of scans and free thyroxine and thyroid-stimulating hormone levels (may require measurement by cordocentesis if poorly controlled) (Gregory & Todd, 2013).

Fetal risks include: thyrotoxicosis, intrauterine growth restriction, preterm labour and perinatal death. No teratogenic effects have been reported from drug therapy.

Fetal hyperthyroidism (uncontrolled) may develop in pregnancy (fetal heart rate >160 bpm). This results from placental transfer of **long-acting thyroid stimulator** from mother to fetus . Maternal drug therapy should include thyroxine (does not cross the placenta) to maintain normal thyroid function and thionamides to treat the fetus , using the fetal heart rate as a guide. The baby's thyroid function will return to normal within 3 months.

Fetal hypothyroidism may occur as maternal thionamide treatment of Graves' disease may cross the placenta and can block or suppress fetal and neonatal thyroid function.

Intrapartum care: meticulous monitoring of maternal and fetal vital signs is essential as labour can precipitate thyroid crisis/storm. Preterm labour should be treated with calcium-channel blockers such as nifedipine as β-agonists (e.g., salbutamol) are contraindicated due to risk of tachycardia.

BOX 35.3   Adrenal Disorders in Pregnancy

These conditions are uncommon in pregnancy. Disorders are usually diagnosed/treated before pregnancy.

Addison's Disease

Addison's disease is caused by inadequate secretion of the adrenal cortical hormones with deficiency of both glucocorticoids and mineralocorticoids. Symptoms include falling plasma sodium and glucose levels, rise in serum potassium levels, skin hyperpigmentation and weight loss. Severe dehydration and hypotension are common. The main cause is autoimmune destruction of the adrenal cortex (often combined with other autoimmune endocrine disorders; e.g., Graves' disease). Treatment in pregnancy is by replacement therapy with oral hydrocortisone (NICE, 2020). In an acute episode, intravenous hydrocortisone is necessary.

Cushing's Syndrome

Cushing's syndrome is excessive levels of **corticosteroids** often caused by pituitary or adrenal carcinoma. It is associated with amenorrhoea and anovulation (rare in pregnancy). Some

Continued

• BOX 35.3 Adrenal Disorders in Pregnancy—cont'd

normal pregnancy features mimic **Cushing's syndrome**. True Cushing's syndrome will also include moon face, hirsutism, acne and proximal myopathy. In the rare cases seen, there is an expected 25% chance of fetal loss and 50% chance of preterm birth.

Congenital Adrenal Hyperplasia

Congenital adrenal hyperplasia (CAH) is a group of inherited conditions with a block in the biosynthesis of **cortisol**. Undiagnosed women are often infertile (few pregnancies). Hormone treatment in childhood and adolescence may have clitoral and vaginal scarring, making vaginal delivery traumatic. Inappropriate masculinization of the pelvis causes **cephalopelvic disproportion**. Women with late-onset CAH usually have

polycystic ovary syndrome and require adrenal suppression with **glucocorticoids** to allow ovulation to occur (see Chapter 7). Caesarean section is usually performed to avoid a hypoadrenal crisis.

Phaeochromocytoma

A tumour of the **adrenal** medulla (rare in pregnancy) that can be misdiagnosed as pre-eclampsia or essential hypertension (blood pressure rises and proteinuria is present). Symptoms include intermittent or sustained hypertension, postural hypotension, sweating, palpitations and tachycardia, anxiety, nausea and vomiting. The tumour and symptoms are medically treated until the fetus is viable, when surgical removal of the tumour is carried out.

Main Points

- Diabetes mellitus is characterized by impaired carbohydrate metabolism and utilization caused by deficiency of insulin production.
- In pregnancy, abnormal carbohydrate metabolism occurs in women with type 1 diabetes, type 2 diabetes or GDM.
- GDM is likely to recur in subsequent pregnancies.
- CB4 virus may destroy pancreatic islet cells and trigger an autoimmune response in genetically susceptible children.
- Type 1 diabetes mellitus is subdivided into two types: type 1A begins in childhood and may be due to destruction of the β cells in the pancreas; type 1B occurs between 30–50 years and may be an autoimmune disorder.
- Type 2 diabetes occurs mainly in people with obesity.
- Long-term effects of diabetes mellitus include death from cardiovascular and renal disease. Chronic conditions include diabetic neuropathy, microvascular disease and atherosclerosis.
- Acute complications include hypoglycaemia and diabetic ketoacidosis.
- Fetal problems include first-trimester abortions, congenital abnormalities, macrosomia, polyhydramnios, traumatic delivery, stillbirth, neonatal asphyxia, respiratory distress syndrome and hyperviscosity syndrome.
- Diabetic management requires control of blood glucose and prevention of ketosis.
- Fetal complications include macrosomia with an increased incidence of shoulder dystocia, forceps delivery and CS. Women with unstable diabetes, complications or obstetric problems may be delivered earlier by CS to avoid intrauterine death.
- In the puerperium, insulin requirements fall and re-stabilization is necessary. Women who breastfeed may take oral glucose-lowering agents. Breast infection is higher in women with diabetes.
- The oral contraceptive pill may mimic pregnancy, increasing the need for insulin. Intrauterine contraceptive devices may lead to infection and are not recommended.

- With poor maternal diabetic control, the baby may be large and birth injuries may occur. The baby may be physiologically immature with problems similar to those of a preterm baby.
- High maternal blood glucose levels in utero encourage the fetal pancreas to produce more insulin. This hyperinsulinaemia continues after birth, creating neonatal hypoglycaemia which will require stabilizing, perhaps by intravenous glucose.
- Thyrotoxicosis occurs when TSIgs antibodies activate follicular cell TSH receptors, leading to increased production of thyroid hormones.
- Signs and symptoms of thyrotoxicosis include raised BMR, heat intolerance, excessive perspiration, weight loss, tachycardia, palpitations, hypertension, anxiety and hyper-reflexia. Exophthalmos (protrusion of eyeballs) may occur.
- The medical emergency of thyroid crisis (or thyroid storm) is characterized by an extreme hypermetabolic state.
- Fetal risks of hyperthyroidism include thyrotoxicosis, intrauterine growth restriction and preterm labour. Perinatal death may occur.
- Maternal hypothyroidism may be due to Hashimoto's disease, viral thyroiditis or congenital absence of the thyroid gland. Treatment is usually T_4 medication.
- Addison's disease is mainly caused by autoimmune destruction of the adrenal glands. In pregnancy, it is treated by oral hydrocortisone. In an acute episode, intravenous hydrocortisone is necessary.
- Women with congenital adrenal hyperplasia often have clitoral and vaginal scarring. Masculinization of the pelvis causes cephalopelvic disproportion.
- The symptoms of phaeochromocytoma are treated medically until the fetus is viable, when surgical removal of the tumour is carried out.

References

Ali, S.N., Dornhorst, A., 2018. Diabetes in pregnancy. In: Edmonds, D.K., Lees, C., Bourne, T.H. (Eds.), Dewhurst's Textbook of Obstetrics and Gynaecology, ninth ed. Wiley-Blackwell, Oxford.

Blackburn, S.T., 2018. Maternal, Fetal and Neonatal Physiology: A Clinical Perspective, fifth ed. Elsevier, Philadelphia.

Calina, D., Docea, A.O., Golokhvast, K.S., Sifakis, S., Tsatsakis, A., Makrigiannakis, A., 2019. Management of endocrinopathies in pregnancy: a review of current evidence. Int. J. Environ. Res. Publ. Health 16 (5), 781.

Coad, J., Pedley, K., Dunstall, M., 2019. Anatomy and Physiology for Midwives, fourth ed. Elsevier, London.

Cooper, D.S., Laurberg, P., 2013. Hyperthyroidism in pregnancy. Lancet Diabetes Endocrinol. 1 (3), 238–249.

De Leo, S., Lee, S.Y., Braverman, L.E., 2016. Hyperthyroidism. Lancet 388 (10047), 906–918.

Eades, C., Cameron, D., Evans, J., 2017. Prevalence of gestational diabetes mellitus in Europe: a meta-analysis. Diabetes Res. Clin. Pract. 129, 173–181.

Egan, A.M., McVicker, L., Heerey, A., Carmody, L., Harney, F., Dunne, F.P., 2015. Diabetic retinopathy in pregnancy: a population-based study of women with pregestational diabetes. J. Diabetes Res. 2015, 310239.

Gregory, R., Todd, D., 2013. Endocrine disorders. In: Robson, S.E., Waugh, J. (Eds.), Medical Disorders in Pregnancy, second ed. Wiley-Blackwell, Oxford.

Holt, R.I.G., Hanley, N.A., 2021. Essential Endocrinology and Diabetes, seventh ed. Wiley-Blackwell, Oxford.

Kahaly, G.J., Bartalena, L., Hegedüs, L., Leenhardt, L., Poppe, K., Pearce, S.H., 2018. 2018 European Thyroid Association Guideline for the Management of Graves' Hyperthyroidism. Eur. Thyroid J. 7 (4), 167–186.

Knight, M., Bunch, K., Patel, R., Shakespeare, J., Kotnis, R., Kenyon, S., et al., on behalf of MBRRACE-UK, 2022. Saving Lives, Improving Mothers' Care – Lessons Learned to Inform Maternity Care from the UK and Ireland Confidential Enquiries into Maternal Deaths and Morbidity 2018–20. National Perinatal Epidemiology Unit, University of Oxford, Oxford.

Labadzhyan, A., Brent, G.A., Hershman, J.M., Leung, A.M., 2014. Thyrotoxicosis of pregnancy. J. Clin. Transl. Endocrinol. 1 (4), 140–144.

Lazarus, J., Brown, R.S., Daumerie, C., Hubalewska-Dydejczyk, A., Negro, R., Vaidya, B., 2014. European Thyroid Association guidelines for the management of subclinical hypothyroidism in pregnancy and in children. Eur. Thyroid J. 3 (2), 76–94.

Neubergera, F., Nelson-Piercy, C., 2015. Acute presentation of the pregnant patient. Clin. Med. 15 (4), 372–376.

National Institute of Health and Care Excellence (NICE), 2019. Thyroid Disease: Assessment and Management Guideline. Available at: https://www.nice.org.uk/guidance/ng145.

National Institute of Health and Care Excellence (NICE), 2020. Diabetes in Pregnancy: Management from Preconception to the Postnatal Period. Available at: https://www.nice.org.uk/guidance/ng3.

National Institute for Health and Care Excellence (NICE), 2020. Addison's disease: Scenario: Management. Available at: https://cks.nice.org.uk/topics/addisons-disease/management/management/.

National Institute of Health and Care Excellence (NICE), 2021a. Hyperthyroidism: Scenario: Pre-conception, Pregnancy, and Postpartum. Available at: https://cks.nice.org.uk/topics/hyperthyroidism/management/pre-conception-pregnancy-postpartum/.

National Institute of Health and Care Excellence (NICE), 2021b. Hyperthyroidism: What Are the Complications? Available at: https://cks.nice.org.uk/topics/hyperthyroidism/background-information/complications/.

Noctor, E., Dunne, F.E., 2015. Type 2 diabetes after gestational diabetes: the influence of changing diagnostic criteria. World J. Diabetes 6 (2), 234–244.

Raets, L., Ingelbrecht, A., Benhalima, K., 2023. Management of type 2 diabetes in pregnancy: a narrative review. Front. Endocrinol. 14. DOI: 10.3389/fendo.2023.11.93271.

Singh, R., 2012. Pregnancy in women with diabetic nephropathy. J Nephrol 1 (2), 168–171.

Spotti, D., 2019. Pregnancy in women with diabetic nephropathy. J. Nephrol. 32 (3), 379–388.

Tieu, J., Middleton, P., Crowther, C.A., Shepherd, E., 2017. Preconception care for diabetic women for improving maternal and infant health. Cochrane Database Syst. Rev. 2017 (8), CD007776.

Vounzoulaki, E., Khunti, K., Abner, S.C., Tan, B.K., Davies, M.J., Gillies, C.L., 2020. Progression to type 2 diabetes in women with a known history of gestational diabetes: systematic review and meta-analysis. BMJ 13 (369), m1361.

Wahabi, H.A., Alzeidan, R.A., Bawazeer, G.A., Alansari, L.A., Esmaeil, S.A., 2010. Preconception care for diabetic women for improving maternal and fetal outcomes: a systematic review and meta-analysis. BMC Pregnancy Childbirth 10, 63.

White, B.A., Porterfield, S.P., 2018. Endocrine and Reproductive Physiology, fifth ed. Mosby, St. Louis.

World Health Organization (WHO), 2014. Diagnostic criteria and classification of hyperglycaemia first detected in pregnancy: a World Health Organization Guideline. Diabetes Res. Clin. Pract. 103 (3), 341–363.

World Health Organization (WHO), 2016. Global Facts and Figures about Diabetes. Available at: http://www.who.int/campaigns/world-health-day/.

World Health Organization (WHO), 2022. Diabetes. Available at: https://www.who.int/news-room/fact-sheets/detail/diabetes.

Annotated recommended reading

Imam, S.K., Ahmad, S.I., 2016. Thyroid Disorders: Basic Science and Clinical Practice, first ed. Springer International, London.

This book provides the reader with an excellent review of thyroid disease in pregnancy.

Lowe, L.P., Metzger, B.E., Dyer, A.R., Lowe, J., McCance, D.R., Lappin, T.R., et al., HAPO Study Cooperative Research Group, 2012. Hyperglycemia and Adverse Pregnancy Outcome (HAPO) Study: associations of maternal A1C and glucose with pregnancy outcomes. Diabetes Care 35 (3), 574–580.

Websites

https://www.diabetes.org.uk/

This is a useful website for providing information and data on diabetes in the UK.

https://www.nice.org.uk/guidance:

Type 2 Diabetes in Adults: Management, 2022, p. NG28.

Type 1 Diabetes in Adults: Diagnosis and Management, 2022, p. NG17.

Diabetes (Type 1 and Type 2) in Children and Young People: Diagnosis and Management, 2022, p. NG18.

Diabetic Foot Problems: Prevention and Management, 2019, p. NG19.

Intrapartum Care for Healthy Women and Babies, 2022, p. NG190.

Postnatal Care, 2021, p. NG37.

Obesity, 2022, p. NG189.

Thyroid Disease: Assessment and Management, 2019, p. NG145.

Fertility: Problems and Treatment, 2017, p. CG 156.

https://www.nice.org.uk/guidance/ng191/resources/covid19-rapid-guideline-managing-covid19-pdf-51035553326.

These NICE guidelines are evidence-based and provide clear and up-to-date guidelines for related management of care for individuals.

https://www.who.int/health-topics/diabetes#tab=tab_1.

In addition to providing facts and figures about diabetes, this WHO site provides an overview of various topics related to diabetes, including burden, prevention, risk factors, diagnosis, treatment, complications and economic costs.

https://www.btf-thyroid.org/thyroid-disorders-and-pregnancy.

This website provides excellent up-to-date evidence for pregnant women with thyroid disorders.

Labour—Normal

Birth is a challenging aspect of childbearing. Midwives are privileged to be the main carer during this meaningful life event for prospective parents. This section is dedicated to applied physiology in relation to uncomplicated labour and childbirth. The number of spontaneous vertex births is under threat due to the rising caesarean section rate. To preserve the skills in achieving normal physiological birth, it is imperative that midwives have fundamental knowledge and understanding of the physiological processes to facilitate labour and childbirth. In this context normal physiological birth is defined as the spontaneous onset of labour occurring between 37 and 42 weeks' gestation resulting in a vaginal birth. Labour is acknowledged to be a continuum. However, for educational purposes, the stages of labour will be subdivided into the recognized three stages. Firstly, the onset of labour is introduced and discussed in Chapter 36. The physiology and management of the first stage of labour is detailed in Chapter 37 with Chapter 38 dedicated to the physiology of pain and subsequent management. The second and third stages of labour are discussed in Chapters 39 & 40 respectively.

36

The Onset of Labour

LYZ HOWIE AND JEAN WATSON

CHAPTER CONTENTS

This chapter presents evidence to explore the physiology associated with normal uncomplicated labour. This process involves a complex interaction of many factors, with the origin and aetiology of labour not yet fully understood. The definitions of the stages of labour are provided and the possible reasons for the onset of labour are outlined. In addition, key areas are introduced including maternal physiological adaptations in labour and the clinical implications for midwives.

Introduction

The aetiology of labour is complex and is not fully understood (Blackburn, 2018). There are numerous hypotheses and theories, but the origin and process involve a complex interaction of many factors. Consequently, an outline of key areas is provided. If the onset of labour was fully understood, it would be easier to prevent preterm labour and the devastating fetal loss and morbidity resulting from extreme immaturity. The main issues in providing care for women in labour are to meet the social, psychological and spiritual needs and provide physiological safety for the woman and her baby.

The Onset of Labour

Spontaneous induction of labour at term is regulated by paracrine and autocrine systems.

- **Paracrine** signalling is a form of cell-to-cell communication where a cell produces a signal to induce changes in nearby cells, altering the behaviour or differentiation of those cells.
- **Autocrine** signalling is when a cell secretes a hormone or chemical messenger, called the *autocrine agent*, that binds to autocrine receptors on that same cell. This leads to changes in the cell and hormones acting on an integrated parturition cascade.

The factors responsible for maintaining uterine quiescence throughout pregnancy are shown in Fig. 36.1A. The factors responsible for the onset of spontaneous labour are shown in Fig. 36.1B. Factors include the withdrawal of the inhibition of progesterone on uterine contractility and the recruitment of cascades. These promote oestrogen (oestriol) production and lead to:

- upregulation of the contraction-associated protein in the uterus
- adrenocorticotrophic hormone (ACTH, corticotropin)
- contraction-associated proteins (CAPs)
- corticotrophin-releasing hormone (CRH)
- dehydroepiandrostenedione (DHEAS)
- 11β-hydroxysteroid dehydrogenase (11β-HSD)
- spontaneous rupture of membranes (SROM) (Blackburn, 2018).

In humans, the exact timing of the onset of labour is less precise. Normal labour occurs between 37–42 weeks (259–294 days) gestation (Coad, Pedley & Dunstall, 2019; Giussani, 2018). Major changes need to occur for the expulsion of the fetus. This is a cascade of fetal, placental/fetal membranes and maternal factors.

Fetal Factors Associated with the Onset of Labour

The timing may be related to fetal brain activity via ACTH and the pituitary–adrenal axis. Progesterone is metabolized to oestrogen. This gradually increases the sensitivity of the uterus to prostaglandins and oxytocin produced by both the fetoplacental unit and maternal tissues.

The Role of the Fetal Hypothalamus–Pituitary–Adrenal Axis

The fetus is largely responsible for triggering the onset of labour through the fetal hypothalamus–pituitary–adrenal axis

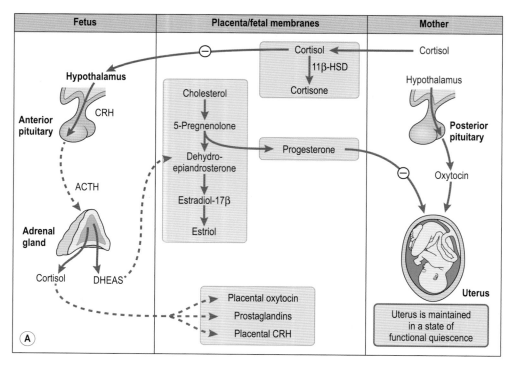

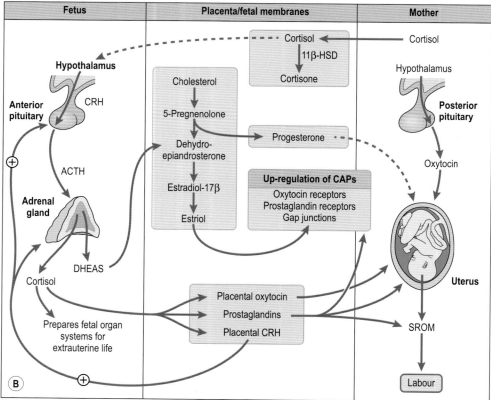

• **Fig. 36.1** Proposed parturition cascade for labour induction at term. The spontaneous induction of labour at term in the human is regulated by a series of paracrine and autocrine hormones acting in an integrated parturition cascade. (A) The factors responsible for maintaining uterine quiescence throughout pregnancy are shown. (B) The factors responsible for the onset of spontaneous labour are shown. They include the withdrawal of the inhibitory effects of progesterone on uterine contractility and the recruitment of cascades that promote oestrogen (oestriol) production and lead to upregulation of the contraction-associated protein in the uterus. *ACTH,* adrenocorticotropic hormone (corticotropin); *CAP,* contraction-associated protein; *CRH,* corticotropin-releasing hormone; *DHEAS,* dehydroepiandrostenedione; *11β-HSD,* 11β-Hydroxysteroid dehydrogenase; *SROM,* spontaneous rupture of membranes.

and uterine wall tension created from the growth of the fetus (Blackburn, 2018). The timing may be related to the fetus via ACTH and the pituitary–adrenal axis. The fetal hypothalamus stimulates the release of CRH from the anterior pituitary gland, which releases ACTH. This causes the fetal adrenal gland to produce cortisol and DHEAS. Alternatively, Coad, Pedley & Dunstall (2019) argue that the fetus has more of a supportive role in initiating labour rather than a direct one. Cortisol plays many roles such as helping mature fetal organ systems for extra-uterine life. It also acts on placental oxytocin, prostaglandins, placental CRH and the placental and fetal membranes (Blackburn, 2018) (Figs 36.2 & 36.3).

A change in steroid balance occurs, stimulating the release of prostaglandins from the placenta and myometrium. The

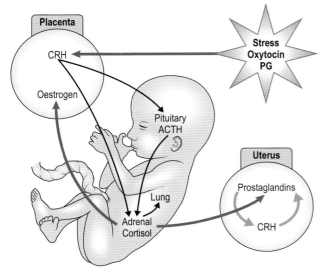

• **Fig. 36.2** The role of corticotrophin-releasing hormone (CRH) in human parturition. *ACTH*, Adrenocorticotrophic hormone; *PG*, prostaglandin.

myometrium forms oxytocin receptors, which are sensitive to the hormone oxytocin. During pregnancy, the hormone progesterone acts to decrease myometrial activity and irritability. Progesterone maintains uterine quiescence throughout pregnancy (Blackburn, 2018). The functional effects of progesterone decrease in late pregnancy resulting in increased levels of cortisol and uterine contractions (Blackburn, 2018). Near term, the effects of cortisol and oestrogen (from the fetoplacental unit) may override the effects of progesterone on the myometrium (Blackburn, 2018). Subsequently, uterine contractions are produced, which become powerful enough to expel the fetus.

Cortisol levels measured in the umbilical cord blood after delivery are difficult to assess (Coad, Pedley & Dunstall, 2019). They may increase because of the stress of labour rather than be responsible for initiating labour. Scalp blood cortisol measurements made in early labour showed no difference in spontaneous or induced labour, although there was a rise in fetal plasma cortisol as labour progressed. There is no dramatic rise in total cortisol level in fetal circulation before the onset of labour.

The administration of corticosteroids such as **beta-methasone** to women in late pregnancy results in a fall in maternal circulating oestrogen levels. However there is little effect on placental progesterone synthesis or the duration of pregnancy. In the human placenta, **glucocorticoids** do not induce the fall in progesterone and rise in oestrogen leading to labour. These are involved in fetal maturation (particularly the fetal lung), allowing survival of a fetus born 6 weeks early.

Dehydroepiandrosterone sulphate (DHEAS) is one hormone that may be implicated in fetal control of the onset of labour. This hormone is the major precursor of placental oestradiol and oestrone synthesis. The human fetal adrenal gland is relatively large at birth, with a fetal zone occupying 80% of the cortex and being responsible for the size. The

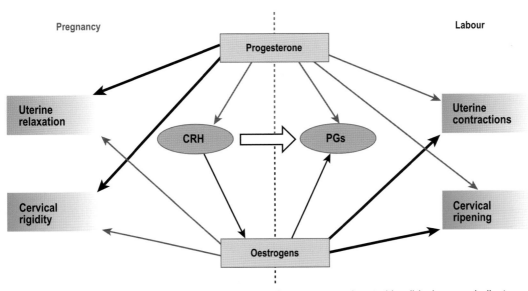

• **Fig. 36.3** Simplified scheme of hormonal control of pregnancy and parturition (*black arrows* indicate stimulatory effect and *green arrows* indicate inhibitory effect). *CRH*, Corticotropin-releasing hormone; *PG*, prostaglandin.

function of the adrenal cortex is different in the fetus from the adult, and the fetal zone atrophies after birth. Human chorionic gonadotrophin is a major stimulator of the fetal zone during pregnancy, and ACTH can also stimulate the production of DHEAS.

The Fetal Posterior Pituitary Gland

Higher concentrations of the posterior pituitary hormones vasopressin and oxytocin have been found in umbilical circulation than in maternal circulation. The source of this fetal oxytocin is not clear: the levels are higher in fetal arterial blood than venous blood, which suggests fetal origin. An argument against the fetal role is that labour almost always follows fetal death in utero (Coad, Pedley & Dunstall, 2019). This may depend on the gestational age of the fetus and possibly the release of prostaglandins is more important. The mechanism of hormone release differs when the fetus is dead, provoking the massive fall in progesterone level that accompanies fetal death.

The Role of the Placenta

Progesterone

The earlier hypothesis by Csapo, Pohanka & Kaihola (1974) expressed that labour is initiated by the withdrawal of the progesterone block on myometrial activity. High levels of progesterone during pregnancy inhibit the production of CRH and prostaglandins whilst preventing uterine activity and ripening of the cervix (Kamel, 2010). The use of progesterone could prolong the latency period in preterm labour and reduce rates of preterm birth less than 34 weeks (Dodd et al., 2013; Sirisangwon & Phupong, 2021). Therefore, progesterone's role is to suppress myometrial activity and aid uterine quiescence throughout pregnancy (Blackburn, 2018; Coad, Pedley & Dunstall, 2019). However, Blackburn (2018) proposes that it is the changing ratio of oestrogen to progesterone that may promote uterine contractions. This changing ratio may not be critical for labour onset.

Oestrogens

CRH has a stimulatory effect on fetal ACTH, which in turn stimulates the production of DHEAS and fetal glucocorticoids (Blackburn, 2018). Placental CRH seems to have an important role in the initiation of labour onset (Coad, Pedley & Dunstall, 2019). Placental production of **oestrogens** rises as pregnancy progresses (Blackburn, 2018). DHEAS of maternal and fetal origin contributes to the placental production of oestrogens, most importantly of oestradiol. Oestrogens stimulate uterine contractions and cervical ripening (Kamel, 2010). The contractions occur through the upregulation of CAPs and are oxytocin receptors, prostaglandin receptors and gap junctions (Blackburn, 2018).

Fetal Membranes

Fetal membranes have a relatively high concentration of progesterone. Both the chorion laeve and amnion contain enzymes that can reduce the level of progesterone, and both the chorion and amnion contain a protein which increases towards the end of pregnancy and can bind progesterone. These two mechanisms would produce a local progesterone withdrawal effect. However, the membranes are avascular, and any substance produced by them must travel by diffusion.

Prostaglandins

The amnion and chorion are both involved in the production of **prostaglandins** (Phillips, Fortier & López Bernal, 2014). Prostaglandins that are produced in fetal membranes and the decidua play a role in the initiation of labour by stimulating uterine muscle contraction (Blackburn, 2018). The fetal membranes contain significant amounts of **arachidonic acid**, and research indicates that the membranes are significantly involved in the synthesis of prostaglandins (Bitsanis et al., 2005; Okita, MacDonald & Johnston, 1982). Drugs such as non-steroidal anti-inflammatory drugs act as **prostaglandin inhibitors** (Blackburn, 2018; Loudon, Groom & Bennett, 2003), preventing the first step in the metabolism of arachidonic acid and prostaglandin production.

Labour may be promoted by brain neuromodulatory lipids and their receptors such as the endocannabinoids anandamide (*N*-arachidonoylethanolamide, AEA) and 2-arachidonoylglycerol (2-AG)), and the cannabinoid receptors (CB_1 and CB_2) (Chan et al., 2013). This occurs by anandamide converting to arachidonic acid within the presence of normal levels of fatty acid amide hydrolase, and with increased CB_1 receptor prostaglandin levels.

The endometrium decidua produces prostaglandins and is a major source of labour prostaglandins (Blackburn, 2018). Decidual cells have lysosomes containing **phospholipase A_2,** which is an enzyme necessary for the synthesis of prostaglandins. These lysosomes are fragile and degenerate under the influence of oestrogen in late pregnancy with falling progesterone and rising oestrogen levels (Giussani, 2018).

Early work showed that the primary prostaglandins present were PGE_2 and $PGF_{2\alpha}$. The precursor of the two prostaglandins is an essential fatty acid called *arachidonic acid*, which is derived from glycerophospholipids and involves several stages of conversion by enzymes. Prostaglandins are known to stimulate myometrial contractions (Blackburn, 2018).

Maternal Influences

The Endocrine System

The ovaries are not necessary for the initiation of labour (Coad, Pedley & Dunstall, 2019) and maternal oxytocin from the pituitary gland also plays little part. The maternal adrenal glands do not seem to be involved in any aspect of labour.

Neurohormonal Control

James Ferguson, a Canadian physiologist, discovered that if the cervix is stretched it increases the production of oxytocin

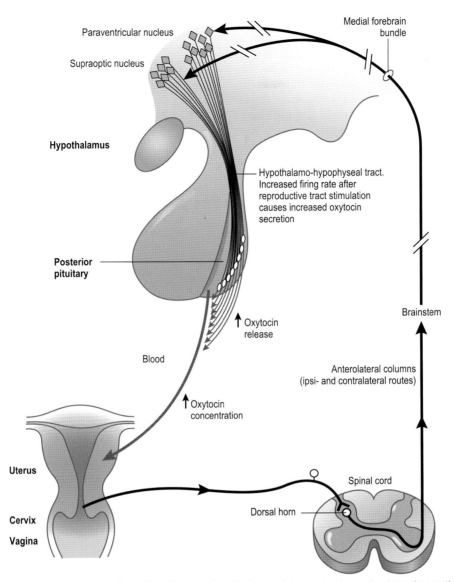

Paraventricular nucleus

Supraoptic nucleus

Medial forebrain bundle

Hypothalamus

Hypothalamo-hypophyseal tract. Increased firing rate after reproductive tract stimulation causes increased oxytocin secretion

Posterior pituitary

Brainstem

↑ Oxytocin release

Blood

Anterolateral columns (ipsi- and contralateral routes)

↑ Oxytocin concentration

Spinal cord

Uterus

Dorsal horn

Cervix

Vagina

• **Fig. 36.4** The neuroendocrine reflex (Ferguson's reflex) underlying oxytocin synthesis and secretion.

and subsequently increases uterine activity. **Ferguson's reflex** (Ferguson, 1941), a neurohormonal reflex (Fig. 36.4) arising from the genital tract, may be involved in the release of oxytocin and prostaglandin in labour (Giussani, 2018). The release of oxytocin could lead to increasing prostaglandin production as it does in some animal species. If this were so, then administration of epidural analgesia should block the spinal part of the reflex and oxytocin release, resulting in prolongation of the first stage of labour. As there is no evidence to suggest this happens, prostaglandin release in human labour probably does not involve oxytocin release.

Control of Cervical Changes in Labour

Two major physiological changes in cervical and myometrial tone are necessary for the expulsion of the fetus to proceed smoothly. Cervical change is called *softening* or **ripening** (Johnson & Taylor, 2023). Myometrial tone also changes to facilitate co-ordinated contractions of the myometrium (Giussani, 2018). The role of the cervix is now the outlet for birth rather than a protective barrier. Levels of **nitric oxide (NO)** play a key role during pregnancy and the onset of labour (Blackburn, 2018). During pregnancy, NO levels are elevated, relaxing the myometrium, but not raised within the cervix, maintaining cervical rigidity (Blackburn, 2018). This changes nearer term where NO levels increase in the cervix, which is believed to help cervical ripening. Simultaneously, the decrease in NO levels in the uterus is involved in the process of the onset of labour (Blackburn, 2018). Other factors considered to be involved in the initiation of labour are the hormone **relaxin** and **cytokines** (Blackburn, 2018). The role of relaxin along with progesterone is to maintain uterine quiescence and possibly suppress oxytocin (Coad, Pedley & Dunstall, 2019). Relaxin also has a role to play in cervical ripening and may help regulate the permeability of gap junctions (Blackburn, 2018). The secretion of proinflammatory cytokines promotes myometrial contractility for the onset of labour (Coad, Pedley & Dunstall, 2019).

It is essential that uterine contractions are co-ordinated with cervical dilatation (Li et al., 2022). The increasing pressure placed on the cervix by the presenting part during active labour is said to aid dilatation of the cervix by the mechanism of Ferguson's reflex (Coad, Pedley & Dunstall, 2019). Uterine contractions alone cannot bring about cervical softening and cervical dilatation. Changes in the collagen content of the cervix must occur, and there is evidence that these changes are brought about by the hormone oestradiol. Prostaglandins also play a part in the ripening of the cervix and are often used for induction of labour if the cervix is unfavourable (Bakker, Pierce & Myers, 2017).

Definitions of Labour

Labour progress must be achieved without compromising maternal or fetal safety. The key concepts associated with labour are defined in Clinical Application 36.1. Each stage of labour will be further explored in Chapters 37, 39 & 40.

The possible causes of the onset of labour have been discussed. The timing of onset is important as it allows decisions to be made about the progress and ongoing management of labour, yet it is difficult to establish with accuracy. The length of labour is variable and may be affected by parity, birth interval, psychological state, presentation and position, pelvic shape and size and the type of uterine contractions.

Maternal Physiological Adaptation in Labour

The physiological changes in labour are examined separately from the process of labour so that sufficient depth can be achieved.

Cardiovascular System

There are profound changes in the cardiovascular system due to the effect of uterine contractions (see Chapter 17). The woman's emotional response to labour may affect the cardiovascular system, especially in primigravidae. The first stage of labour is associated with a progressive rise in cardiac output as each contraction adds 300–500 mL of blood to the circulating blood volume (Adamson & Nelson-Piercy, 2018; Blackburn, 2018). During the first stage of labour, cardiac output rises 10–15% or up to 30% above pregnancy values and about 50% during the second stage of labour, with a peak just immediately after birth (Blackburn, 2018). These changes are limited by epidural analgesia or supine position and by alleviation of pain and anxiety.

Pain, anxiety and apprehension may add to this effect, causing an increase in systolic and diastolic blood pressure and heart rate by increasing sympathetic tone. Blood pressure begins to rise before the contraction begins and returns

• CLINICAL APPLICATION 36.1 Labour Definitions

- Labour is the process where the fetus, placenta and membranes are expelled through the birth canal.
- Normal labour is spontaneous in onset at term, with the fetus presenting by the vertex.
- First labours last on average 8 hours and are unlikely to last over 18 hours.
- Second and subsequent labours last on average 5 hours and are unlikely to last over 12 hours.
- Labour is a continual process subdivided into three stages (first, second and third).

First Stages of Labour

The first stage of labour is categorized into the latent and established phases:

The **latent phase** is a period which is not necessarily continuous, when:
- There are contractions **and** there is some cervical change, including cervical position, consistency, effacement and dilatation up to 4 cm.

The **established phase**:
- There are regular contractions **and** there is progressive cervical dilatation from 4 cm.

Second Stage of Labour

The **second stage** incorporates both passive and active phases of labour.

The **passive** second stage of labour is:
- When there is full dilatation of the cervix (determined by either vaginal examination or noting other external signs of full dilatation) before or in the absence of involuntary or active pushing.
- The passive second stage of labour may be up to 2 hours when a woman with an epidural in place has been advised to delay pushing (recommendations 1.9.7–1.9.10).

The **active** second stage of labour is:
- The baby is visible **or**
- There is involuntary or active pushing with full dilatation of the cervix.

Third Stage of Labour

This **stage** of labour is:
- The time from the birth of the baby to the expulsion of the placenta and membranes.

(From National Institute of Health and Care Excellence (NICE), 2023. Intrapartum Care.)

to its baseline after the contraction has ended. During the first stage of labour, there may be a rise in systolic blood pressure of 35 mmHg, and it may rise even higher in the second stage. The diastolic pressure can rise 25 mmHg in the first stage of labour (Blackburn, 2018).

After the delivery of the fetus, placenta and membranes, there may be cardiovascular instability because of dramatic haematological changes. The changes occur because of blood loss at delivery and compensatory mechanisms. Within 1–2 hours of delivery, cardiac parameters remain elevated above pre-labour levels and may take up to 6–8 weeks to return to pre-pregnancy levels (Blackburn, 2018).

Haematological System

There are changes in the haematological system and haemostasis to ensure that blood loss is kept to a minimum and tolerated (see Chapter 16). Haemoglobin levels tend to increase slightly in labour because of haemoconcentration from muscular activity and dehydration (Coad, Pedley & Dunstall, 2019). Erythropoiesis (formation of red blood cells) and white blood cell count increase due to stress in labour and postpartum (Coad, Pedley & Dunstall, 2019) and reach levels of 25,000–30,000/mm^3 (Blackburn, 2018).

The hypercoagulable state in pregnancy is further magnified in labour (Coad, Pedley & Dunstall, 2019). There is a transitory increase in the activity of the coagulation system during and immediately after placental separation so that clot formation in the torn blood vessels is maximized and blood loss from haemorrhage minimized. However, it also increases the risk of disseminated intravascular coagulation and thrombosis (Coad, Pedley & Dunstall, 2019). The placenta and decidua are rich in thromboplastin, and release of this factor during separation activates coagulation via the extrinsic system.

There is also a decrease in fibrinolytic activity, enhancing clot formation at the placental site. The placental site is rapidly covered by a fibrin mesh which utilizes about 5–10% of the circulating fibrinogen (Blackburn, 2018). Levels of fibrin/fibrinogen degradation products rise after delivery, increasing the risk of coagulation disorders in the immediate postpartum period.

Respiratory System
Maternal Acidosis

There is an increase in the work of the uterine and other muscles during labour and therefore a greater need for oxygen (see Chapter 18). Alterations in ventilation and acid–base status occur. If the contractions are occurring too frequently, there will be a decrease in the oxygenation of the myometrium with resulting metabolic acidosis. In the presence of strong, frequent uterine contractions, ischaemia and the resulting tissue hypoxia will occur with an increase in P_{CO2} because of the change to anaerobic metabolism leading to a fall in pH (maternal acidosis). The ischaemia will increase the pain experienced during contractions.

Respiratory rate and tidal volume are increased in labour due to pain (Coad, Pedley & Dunstall, 2019). Maternal P_{CO2} may rise during pushing and due to the use of voluntary muscles during bearing down. Fetal P_{CO2} will rise if the mother is acidotic because the build-up of maternal P_{CO2} will prevent placental transfer to the mother. This will lead to fetal acidosis and distress.

Maternal Alkalosis

In some women there is a tendency to hyperventilate, leading to respiratory alkalosis. This appears to be mainly caused by pain. Anxiety, drugs, breath-holding, panic and excessive use of breathing exercises learned in the antenatal period will also add to the likelihood of hyperventilation. The end result will be a fall in P_{CO2} and a level of 25 mmHg can commonly occur (Blackburn, 2018). The woman may complain of tingling of the fingers and toes and dizziness due to over-breathing. She should be encouraged to change her respiratory rate and slow it down by counting respirations and by taking slow, deep breaths between contractions to increase oxygenation.

Renal System

The renin–angiotensin systems of the mother and fetus are altered during labour and delivery (see Chapter 19). There is an increase in maternal and fetal renin and angiotensin, which may be important in reducing uteroplacental blood flow after delivery. The changes in pregnancy outlined in Section 2B affect fluid and electrolyte status so that administration of intravenous fluids and their electrolytic content must be carefully monitored to avoid water intoxication. Also, it is important to remember that oxytocin has an antidiuretic effect so that oxytocin infusion during labour reduces water excretion (Coad, Pedley & Dunstall, 2019).

Gastrointestinal System
Gastric Emptying

Evidence suggests that gastric motility is decreased and gastric emptying is mildly delayed during labour (Ditzenberger, 2018), with or without epidural analgesia. Factors dramatically increasing this delayed gastric emptying include:
- Fear and pain.
- Administration of opioid drugs.
- Intake of food during labour that contains high levels of fibre and fat.

There is also an increase in gastric acidity and relaxation of the lower oesophageal sphincter leading to reflux, thereby increasing the risk of aspiration if the woman requires a general anaesthetic (Ditzenberger, 2018). Aspiration pneumonitis is also known as **Mendelson's syndrome.** Nutrition and hydration in labour and the prevention of acid aspiration are discussed in the section on clinical implications later.

Metabolism

Generally, before labour, women have a degree of respiratory alkalosis and metabolic acidosis and a reduced ability to utilize glucose so that the main source of glucose for the fetus is met. Provision of glucose (gluconeogenesis) from the metabolism of body fat (lipolysis) occurs, causing an increase in plasma ketones throughout pregnancy. Labour influences maternal metabolism and plasma electrolytes, and these changes may affect the fetus.

The vigorous contractions of the uterus throughout labour require energy, and glucose is the main substrate for this. Most women have little reserve for aerobic metabolism and glucose stores are quickly used up, especially if there is restriction on oral intake in labour. The energy cost of active labour is estimated to be between 700–1100 calories

Recognition of the Onset of Labour

Women themselves usually recognize that labour has begun. The woman may notice a **show**, although this may occur after a vaginal examination in the antenatal clinic. A 'show' is when the operculum plug and blood from the shearing of the cervical vessels become dislodged when the cervix dilates (Coad, Pedley & Dunstall, 2019). **Contractions** which are regular, rhythmic and increase in **length**, **strength** and **frequency** occur, but the woman may only be aware of backache with hardening of her uterus. When the presenting part of the fetus is not well applied to the cervix, the membranes may rupture and the woman has a sudden gush of fluid per vagina. The woman should contact the midwife in this instance, as there is a small risk of cord prolapse. Sometimes women find it hard to distinguish the trickle of amniotic fluid from urine and this can be confirmed when seen by the midwife.

Initial Examination of the Woman

Whilst this is a physiology book, it is important to realize that the social and psychological background and approach to care may interfere with the process of labour. This interaction between the mind and body will be discussed in Chapter 57. The approach taken at this initial meeting of the woman and her midwife may influence not only her perception of labour, but also her physical progress towards delivery. Women need to have a meaningful experience and it is important that the physical safety of the mother and fetus are ensured. Good history-taking and risk assessment are crucial parts of the initial examination of the woman (NICE, 2023).

The History

When a woman contacts her midwife, information obtained will allow a decision either to visit at home, especially if there is to be a home birth, or admit to hospital. If there are no complications and the woman is in early labour, it will be beneficial for her to remain in her own surroundings. To assess the level of risk history of the woman's health, any previous pregnancies and this pregnancy up to the onset of labour should be carefully scrutinized (NICE, 2023).

General Examination

The general condition of the woman is important, and her appearance may indicate aspects of her well-being to the midwife. Her general stance and gait may indicate pain or even imminent delivery. The midwife should look for any abnormality in skin colour, which may indicate underlying problems. Behaviour may indicate how well the woman is coping with contractions and whether she is anxious or afraid. Observations of temperature, pulse rate, blood pressure, signs of oedema, urinalysis, contractions, vaginal loss and fetal well-being should be assessed and recorded (NICE, 2023).

Abnormal findings may indicate a problem with the general health of the woman or be associated with an abnormality of labour. If the temperature and pulse rate are elevated, it is necessary to find the cause, as infection may be present. A rise in blood pressure should be reported to the most relevant staff timeously. The presence of slight oedema of the feet and ankles may be normal, depending on the time of day, but pretibial oedema or puffiness of the fingers or face, especially if there is raised blood pressure, may indicate the presence of pregnancy-induced hypertension (PIH). Urine is tested for protein, which may indicate that the woman has had show or that the membranes have ruptured. Both are easily confirmed but may also indicate PIH or urinary tract infection. Glucose and ketones are also tested for and are considered in light of the woman's past medical history, when she last ate and how her labour is progressing. Assessment of fetal well-being is also conducted and is explored in more depth in Chapter 37.

Assessing Progress in Labour

As much detail as possible about the progress of labour pre-admission should be ascertained. On admission, the woman is examined to establish a baseline on which to judge further labour progress. An abdominal examination is conducted and may be followed by a **vaginal examination** (VE). A VE in low-risk women is not routine and only necessary if it adds further information to the decision-making relating to care (NICE, 2023). The health professional should use their clinical judgement along with fully informed consent from the woman before conducting a VE. Progress can be considered if there is descent of the presenting part through the pelvis and cervical dilatation. The presence of one in the absence of the other suggests lack of progress and is a cause for concern if this persists. These factors will be discussed in Chapter 37.

---

per hour (Coad, Pedley & Dunstall, 2019). Compensatory lipolysis occurs to meet the body's energy requirements, resulting in the production of ketones which, in excess, may depress fetal pH and interfere with myometrial activity (Coad, Pedley & Dunstall, 2019). Anaerobic metabolism causes the accumulation of lactate (see Krebs cycle, Chapter 23), and this produces a small drop in maternal plasma pH to about 7.34, a reduction in base excess to −5 mEq/L and a fall in P_{CO_2}.

An introduction to the clinical implications for labour is introduced in Clinical Application 36.2 (see Chapter 37 for further details).

Main Points

- In humans, the exact timing of the onset of labour is less precise than in many other species. Normal labour occurs between 37–42 weeks (259–294 days) gestation. A cascade of events occur, which are divided into fetal, placental/fetal membranes and the maternal factors.

- The thought is that the fetal hypothalamus stimulates the release of CRH from the anterior pituitary gland, which then releases ACTH. This causes the fetal adrenal gland to produce cortisol and DHEAS. Cortisol plays many roles such as helping to mature fetal organ systems for extra-uterine life and acting on placental oxytocin, prostaglandins, placental CRH and the placental and fetal membranes.

- Cortisol secreted by the fetal adrenal cortex acts on placental enzymes to convert progesterone to oestrogen.

The rapid change in steroid balance stimulates the release of prostaglandins from both the placenta and the myometrium.

- Increased sensitivity of the myometrium forms oxytocin receptors which are sensitive to the hormone oxytocin.
- During pregnancy, progesterone decreases myometrial activity and irritability.
- Progesterone has a role in maintaining uterine quiescence throughout pregnancy.
- Near term, the effects of cortisol and oestrogen override the effects of progesterone on the myometrium with the production of uterine contractions, which become powerful enough to expel the fetus.
- Uterine contractions are co-ordinated with cervical dilatation.
- Increasing pressure placed on the cervix by the presenting part during active labour aids dilatation of the cervix by the mechanism of Ferguson's reflex, which may be involved in the release of both oxytocin and prostaglandin in labour.
- Uterine contractions alone cannot bring about cervical softening and cervical dilatation. Change in the collagen content of the cervix must occur, and there is evidence that the hormone oestradiol brings about the change.
- Prostaglandins also play a part in the ripening of the cervix.
- Normal labour is spontaneous in onset at term, with the fetus presenting by the vertex, and with no complications arising.
- Labour is a continual process subdivided into three stages (i.e., first, second and third).
- First labours last on average 8 hours (unlikely to last over 18 hours) and second and subsequent labours last on average 5 hours (unlikely to last over 12 hours).
- Profound changes occur in the cardiovascular system because of uterine contractions. Pain, anxiety and uterine contractions may cause an increase in blood pressure and heart rate.
- Observations of temperature, pulse rate, blood pressure, signs of oedema, urinalysis, contractions, vaginal loss and fetal well-being should be assessed and recorded.
- Abnormal findings may indicate a problem with the general health of the woman or be associated with an abnormality of labour.

References

Adamson, D.L., Nelson-Piercy, C., 2018. Heart disease in pregnancy. In: Edmonds, D.K., Lees, C., Bourne, T.H. (Eds.), Dewhurst's Textbook of Obstetrics & Gynaecology, ninth ed. Wiley-Blackwell, Oxford.

Bakker, R., Pierce, S., Myers, D., 2017. The role of prostaglandins E1 and E2, dinoprostone, and misoprostol in cervical ripening and the induction of labor: a mechanistic approach. Arch. Gynecol. Obstet. 296 (2), 167–179.

Blackburn, S.T., 2018. Maternal, Fetal and Neonatal Physiology: A Clinical Perspective, fifth ed. Elsevier, Philadelphia.

Bitsanis, D., Crawford, M.A., Moodley, T., Holmsen, H., Ghebremeskel, K., Djahanbakhch, O., 2005. Arachidonic acid predominates in the membrane phosphoglycerides of the early and term human placenta. J. Nutr. 135 (1), 2566–2571.

Csapo, A.I., Pohanka, O., Kaihola, H.L., 1974. Progesterone deficiency and premature labour. Br. Med. J. 1 (5899), 137–140.

Chan, H.W., McKirdy, N.C., Peiris, H.N., Rice, G.E., Mitchell, M.D., 2013. The role of endocannabinoids in pregnancy. Reproduction 146 (3), R101–R109.

Coad, J., Pedley, K., Dunstall, M., 2019. Anatomy and Physiology for Midwives, fourth ed. Elsevier, London.

Ditzenberger, G.R., 2018. Gastrointestinal and hepatic systems and perinatal nutrition. In: Blackburn, S.T. (Ed.), Maternal, Fetal and Neonatal Physiology: A Clinical Perspective, fifth ed. Elsevier, Philadelphia.

Dodd, J.M., Jones, L., Flenady, V., Cincotta, R., Crowther, C.A., 2013. Prenatal administration of progesterone for preventing preterm birth in women considered to be at risk of preterm birth. Cochrane Database Syst. Rev. 2013 (7), CD004947.

Ferguson, J.K., 1941. A study of the motility of the intact uterus at term. Surg. Gynecol. Obstet. 73, 359–366.

Giussani, D., 2018. Giving birth. In: Johnson, M.H. (Ed.), Essential Reproduction, eighth ed. Wiley-Blackwell, Oxford.

Johnson, R., Taylor, W., 2023. Skills for Midwifery Practice, fifth ed. Elsevier, London.

Kamel, R.M., 2010. The onset of human parturition. Arch. Gynecol. Obstet. 281 (6), 975–982.

Li, P., Huang, Q., Wang, L., Garfield, R.E., Lui, H., 2022. Uterine electrical signals and cervical dilation during the first stage of labor. Arch. Gynecol. Obstet. 3 (1), 47–52.

Loudon, J.A., Groom, K.M., Bennett, P.R., 2003. Prostaglandin inhibitors in preterm labour. Best Pract. Res. Clin. Obstet. Gynaecol. 17 (5), 731–744.

National Institute of Health and Care Excellence (NICE), 2023. Intrapartum Care. https://www.nice.org.uk/guidance/ng235

Okita, J.R., MacDonald, P.C., Johnston, J.M., 1982. Mobilization of arachidonic acid from specific glycerophospholipids of human fetal membranes during early labor. J. Biol. Chem. 257 (23), 14029–14034.

Phillips, R.J., Fortier, M.A., López, B.A., 2014. Prostaglandin pathway gene expression in human placenta, amnion and choriodecidua is differentially affected by preterm and term labour and by uterine inflammation. BMC Pregnancy Childbirth 14, 241.

Sirisangwon, R., Phupong, V., 2021. Vaginal progesterone supplementation in the management of preterm labor: a randomized controlled trial. Matern. Child Health J. 25 (7), 1102–1109.

Annotated recommended reading

Blackburn, S.T., 2018. Maternal, Fetal and Neonatal Physiology: A Clinical Perspective, fifth ed. Elsevier, Philadelphia.

This book covers physiological changes that occur throughout the perinatal period, with the emphasis on the mother, fetus and the neonate and the relationship between them. The chapter on parturition and uterine physiology is a very useful resource to gain more depth on the onset of labour.

Johnson, M.H., 2018. Essential Reproduction, eighth ed. Wiley-Blackwell, Oxford.

This text provides a detailed account of parturition and the fetus and its preparation for birth.

37

The First Stage of Labour

LYZ HOWIE AND JEAN WATSON

CHAPTER CONTENTS

This chapter provides a detailed account of the first stage of labour. This includes the related physiology, assessment of progress and monitoring of the fetal condition. Other issues include maternal care in labour including positions, immersion in water, nutrition and hydration. It is essential for students and midwives to have sound knowledge and understanding of the fundamental issues to provide women with optimal care.

Physiology of the First Stage of Labour

Uterine Activity in Labour

In early labour, contractions may be fairly weak, lasting for approximately 30 s and 15–20 min apart. These may not be recognised as labour pains. In established labour, the uterus contracts three to four times every 10 min; in advanced labour each contraction may last 50–60 s. Contractions are measured in mmHg (millimetres of mercury) by the pressure they exert on the amniotic fluid. This is called the **intrauterine hydrostatic pressure** (Table 37.1).

The spread of each contraction across the myometrium begins in the fundus near the cornua, spreading outwards and downwards, remaining most intense in the fundus and being weakest in the lower uterine segment. This is known as **fundal dominance.** It takes up to 1 min for the spread of myometrial electrical activity to reach maximum intensity and the same time frame for the wave of contraction to subside. This allows progressive dilatation of the cervix and, as the upper segment thickens and shortens, the fetus is propelled down the birth canal. During contractions, the upper and lower poles of the uterus act in harmony, with contraction and retraction of the upper **pole** and dilatation of the lower pole to allow expulsion of the fetus. This is known as **polarity.**

Uterine muscle in labour has the unique property of **contraction** and **retraction** (Fig. 37.1). **Retraction** is where the muscle fibres do not completely relax between contractions but retain some of their shortening. This leads to progressive shortening and thickening of the upper uterine segment (UUS) and reduction of the uterine cavity to accommodate the descending fetus. A physiological ridge forms between the UUS and the lower uterine segment (LUS), known as a **retraction ring** (see Chapter 44 for the abnormal **Bandl's ring**, which is an exaggerated pathological retraction ring that develops in obstructed labour (Tinelli, Di Renzocand & Malvasib, 2015) and becomes visible above the symphysis pubis).

Effacement of the cervix is gradual merging of the cervix into the LUS. In primigravidae, this process is sometimes complete before the onset of labour and before dilation of the external cervical os occurs (Fig. 37.2A). In multigravidae, a cervical canal remains until labour is well established. During labour, there is **dilatation** of the external os until it is large enough for the widest diameter of the presenting part to pass through (Fig. 37.2B). In a fetus at term presenting by the vertex, the diameter of the cervix would normally have to reach 10 cm (Hassan et al., 2012). As the cervix begins to dilate, the operculum (mucous plug formed in pregnancy) will manifest as a mucoid discharge, which may be bloodstained. This is termed **'show'.** The blood stems from ruptured cervical capillaries on cervical stretching or where the chorion has become detached from the dilating cervix.

Mechanical Factors

There are also mechanical forces that aid cervical dilatation (Fig. 37.3).

TABLE 37.1	Levels of Intrauterine Hydrostatic Pressure	
Muscular Pressure		**Level of Hydrostatic Pressure**
Resting pressure of myometrium		5 mmHg
Uterine contraction pressure in pregnancy		30 mmHg
Uterine contraction pressure in labour		60–80 mmHg

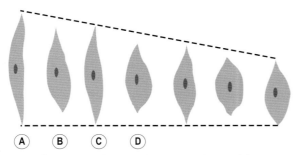

• **Fig. 37.1** Retraction of the uterine muscle fibres. (A) Relaxed. (B) Contracted. (C) Relaxed but retracted. (D) Contracted but shorter and thicker than those in (B).

When the membranes remain intact, the pressure of each contraction is exerted on the fluid and, as fluid is not compressible, pressure is equalized throughout the uterus. This is termed 'general fluid pressure' (Fig. 37.4A). If the membranes are ruptured and amniotic fluid is reduced, contraction pressure is applied directly to the fetus (Fig. 37.4B). The placenta is compressed between the uterine wall and the fetus, reducing the fetal oxygen supply. Therefore maintaining intact membranes reduces the risk of infection and a good oxygen supply to the fetus. The physiological moment for the membranes to rupture is when the cervix is fully dilated and no longer able to support the forewaters and the force of the uterine contractions reaches maximum. Smyth, Markham & Dowswell (2013) acknowledge that routine amniotomy during the first stage of labour is not justified, reporting no statistical difference in length of first stage of labour, caesarean section rates, Apgar score <7 at 5 min or maternal satisfaction of childbirth experience. The National Institute of Health & Care Excellence [NICE] (2023) concurs with not routinely performing amniotomy in normally progressing labour. If delay in the established first stage of labour is diagnosed, then NICE (2023) recommend considering amniotomy for all women with intact membranes, after explanation of the procedure and advice that it will shorten labour by about an hour and may increase the strength and pain of contractions.

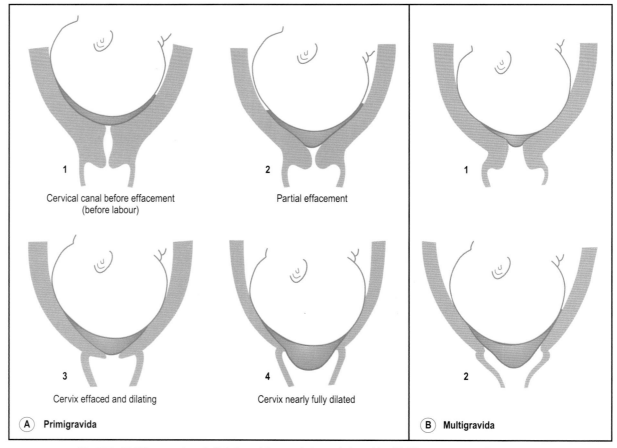

• **Fig. 37.2** (A) Effacement and dilatation of the cervix in a primigravida. (B) Effacement and dilatation of the cervix in a multigravida.

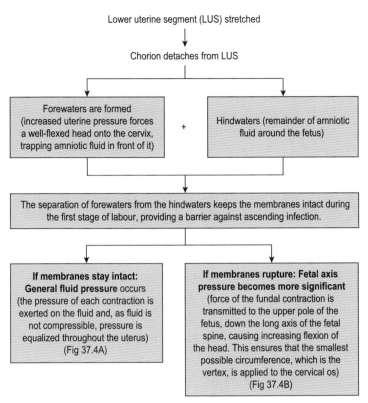

Lower uterine segment (LUS) stretched

↓

Chorion detaches from LUS

Forewaters are formed
(increased uterine pressure forces
a well-flexed head onto the cervix,
trapping amniotic fluid in front of it)

+

Hindwaters (remainder of amniotic
fluid around the fetus)

The separation of forewaters from the hindwaters keeps the membranes intact during
the first stage of labour, providing a barrier against ascending infection.

If membranes stay intact:
General fluid pressure occurs
(the pressure of each contraction is
exerted on the fluid and, as fluid is
not compressible, pressure is
equalized throughout the uterus)
(Fig 37.4A)

If membranes rupture: Fetal axis
pressure becomes more significant
(force of the fundal contraction is
transmitted to the upper pole of the
fetus, down the long axis of the fetal
spine, causing increasing flexion of
the head. This ensures that the smallest
possible circumference, which is the
vertex, is applied to the cervical os)
(Fig 37.4B)

• **Fig. 37.3** Mechanical factors of labour.

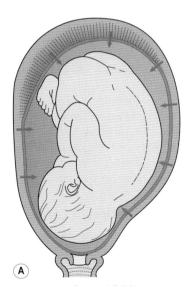

Ⓐ

• **Fig. 37.4a** General fluid pressure.

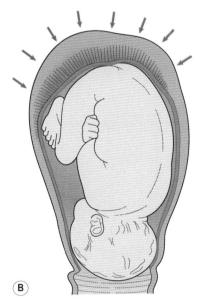

Ⓑ

• **Fig. 37.4b** Fetal axis pressure.

Phases of the First Stage of Labour

Freidman (1954) developed the graphic representation of labour by plotting cervical dilatation and descent of the presenting part against a time frame. Table 37.2 outlines the phases in the first stage of labour. Refer to Chapter 36, Clinical Application 36.1 for labour definitions including duration.

The length of established first stage of labour varies. First labours last on average 8 hours and are unlikely to last over 18 hours. Second and subsequent labours last on average 5 hours and are unlikely to last over 12 hours (NICE, 2023). Plotting the rate of cervical dilatation has been commonly carried out in labour (termed a **cervicograph**); an average duration is indicated in Fig. 37.5. Lundborg et al. (2020) question the exact timeframe for women as it can vary between different populations. They reported that dilatation accelerates after 5–6 cm. In the transitional stage of labour, a woman can display possible signs (see Clinical Application 37.1).

TABLE 37.2	**Phases of the First Stage of Labour**
Latent phase	This phase relates to a period of time, not necessarily continuous, when there are contractions **and** there is some cervical change, including cervical position, consistency, effacement and dilatation up to 4 cm (NICE, 2023). However the definition of the latent phase is still not clearly defined, and more research is required (Hundley et al., 2017).
Established/active phase	This established first stage of labour is when there are regular contractions **and** there is progressive cervical dilatation from 4 cm (NICE, 2023). During this phase, the cervix usually undergoes more rapid dilatation in the presence of rhythmic contractions (Jackson, Anderson & Marshall, 2020). Dilatation progresses to 10 cm or full dilatation. Duration of this phase remains a controversial issue where dilatation of the cervix can vary, for example by 1 cm/hour or less. More rapid dilatation occurs after 5–6 cm irrespective of parity (Lundborg et al., 2020).
Transitional phase (deceleration phase)	Where dilatation slows towards the second stage (Jackson, Anderson & Marshall, 2020).

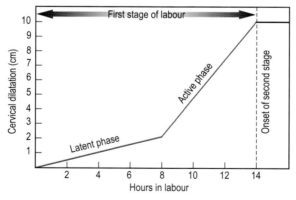

• **Fig. 37.5** A cervicograph.

Individualized Care

The childbearing experience for women encompasses a biological and a social event. When planning care with the labouring woman:

- Use a clear risk-assessment strategy.
- Plan care accordingly to specific needs and expectations.
- Carry out the plan of care.
- Evaluate the care given and modify if required.

• CLINICAL APPLICATION 37.1	Possible Signs of the Transitional Phase of Labour Displayed by Women

- Worried and anxious.
- Loss of control.
- Bewildered or confused.
- Feeling of not coping with labour and ability to carry on.
- Feeling of failure.
- Nausea and vomiting.
- Extreme shaking.
- Extreme pain and requesting further analgesia.
- Distress displayed vocally.
- Isolated and withdrawn.
- Heavy show.
- Extreme urge to bear down.
- Contractions reduce in frequency and strength.

(Downe, 2017)

The physiological aspects of care in labour also include assessing progress, positioning of the woman, nutrition and hydration and monitoring the condition of the woman and fetus.

Assessing Progress in the First Stage of Labour

The following is conducted when assessing progress in labour:

- Before admission, a clear and accurate history is taken from the woman to establish labour progress.
- On admission, a baseline assessment of maternal and fetal well-being is undertaken, comprising maternal observations and abdominal examination, and may be followed by a vaginal examination (VE).
- Labour progress is considered when there is descent of the presenting part and cervical dilatation. The presence of one in the absence of the other may suggest lack of progress and is a cause for concern.

Abdominal Examination in Labour

The aim of abdominal examination is to determine any deviations from normal by assessing:

- Fundal height.
- Fetal lie.
- Presentation.
- Position.
- Engagement.
- Fetal movements.
- Auscultation of fetal heart.

Abdominal examination should always be carried out before performing a VE and can be used to assess the descent of the presenting part. The procedure for undertaking abdominal examination is through inspection, palpation and auscultation (see Clinical Application 37.2). Terms used to describe fetal palpation are in Table 37.3.

• CLINICAL APPLICATION 37.2   Procedure for Abdominal Examination

Inspection

Uterus size and shape	Longitudinal-lie uterus: appearance is ovoid (primiparous), globular (parous). Transverse-lie uterus: may be low and broad. Occipitoposterior position: a saucer-shaped depression below the umbilicus may be visible.
Fetal movements	Important to assess fetal well-being. Can assist in fetal position.
Skin marks or changes	Linea nigra. Striae gravidarum. Operation scars.

Palpation (Fig. 37.6)

Fundal palpation	Overall size of uterus. Gestational age (Fig. 37.7). Fetal lie (Fig. 37.8). Length, strength and frequency of contractions.
Lateral palpation	Locate fetal back and limbs to determine position.
Pelvic palpation	Both hands used to identify the presenting part (Fig. 37.9). Amount of flexion (attitude) (Fig. 37.10) and engagement of head can be assessed by estimating the amount of head still present above pelvic brim. If head is engaged, then less than half of the fetal head will be felt above pelvic brim and head will not be mobile. Palpation to assess descent of the occiput of the head is not always possible if deeply engaged (Fig. 37.11). Engagement is a good sign and indicates that the bony pelvis is adequate for the passage of the fetus and a vaginal delivery should follow. Descent of head by abdominal assessment is described in fifths of the head felt above the pelvic brim.

Auscultation

Auscultation	Listening to the fetal heart is important to assess fetal well-being. Point of maximum intensity is located by considering position of the fetus (Fig. 37.12). As labour progresses and descent takes place, the point of maximum intensity will change. The position of the Pinard's stethoscope on the abdomen will also change to ensure clarity of the fetal heartbeat in assessing, rate, rhythm and frequency. Continuous fetal monitoring may be necessary where there is doubt about fetal well-being. The maternal pulse should be conducted at the same time to differentiate between fetal and maternal heart rate (Lewis & Downe, 2015).

TABLE 37.3   Terminology for Fetal Palpation

Lie	Relationship of long axis of the fetus and long axis of the uterus (longitudinal, oblique or transverse).
Presentation	Part of the fetus lies at pelvic brim or in lower pole of uterus (usually cephalic, but other presentations include breech, face, brow and shoulder).
Attitude	Relationship of fetal head and limbs to its body (fully flexed, deflexed or partially or completely extended).
Denominator	Name of the presenting part used when referring to fetal position in relation to pelvis. Each presentation has a different denominator: occiput (cephalic presentation), sacrum (breech presentation) and mentum (face presentation).
Position	Relationship of the denominator to key points on maternal pelvic brim: • Right and left anterior. • Right and left lateral. • Right and left posterior. • Direct anterior and direct posterior.
Engagement	Occurs when widest presenting transverse diameter has passed through brim of pelvis, i.e., biparietal diameter of 9.5 cm in cephalic presentation.

N.B. Presenting part refers to fetal part that lies over the cervical os during labour and where the caput succedaneum may form (e.g., in a cephalic presentation, the presenting part would be the posterior part of the anterior parietal bone).

Vaginal Examination (VE) in Labour

The rationale for a VE in a low-risk situation is still unclear (Moncrieff et al., 2022). NICE (2023) highlights that a VE is not always necessary and should not be considered as routine practice as it can be a painful and distressing experience (Moncrieff et al., 2022). It should be offered to the woman if there is uncertainty of established labour. With good physiological knowledge of labour, healthcare professionals can use their skills in deciphering progress rather than using intervention. The purple line, which is visualized at the 'natal cleft' (cleavage between the buttocks) (Byrne & Edmonds, 1990), may be a useful guide along with other techniques to measure descent of the fetal head (Moncrieff et al., 2022; Morvarid, Masoumeh & Habibollah, 2018). At the start of labour, the 'purple-red line' begins at the anal margin and gradually advances up the anal cleft as cervical dilatation occurs (Morvarid, Masoumeh & Habibollah, 2018). Health professionals should use their clinical judgement along with a fully informed decision from the woman before conducting a VE. Low-risk women with a strong history of pre-labour spontaneous rupture of membranes should not be offered a speculum examination routinely, but if there is any uncertainty then a speculum examination

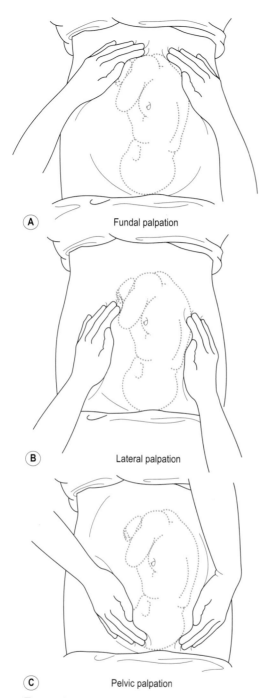

• **Fig. 37.6** Types of palpation per abdomen. (A) Fundal. (B) Lateral. (C) Pelvic.

should be offered (NICE, 2023). If no uterine contractions are present, then a digital VE should be avoided (NICE, 2023). It is acknowledged that VEs are not always required in labour but may be necessary. Clinical Application 37.3 identifies reasons to conduct a VE in labour.

Although VEs are not always necessary, when they are required, women accept the need for them. The woman should be treated with dignity and respect by the examiner and have the findings communicated to her (Lai & Levy, 2005; NICE, 2023).

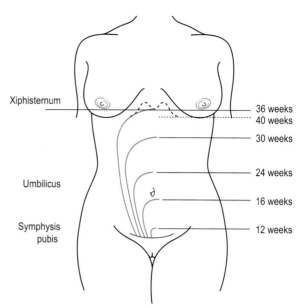

• **Fig. 37.7** The height of the fundus at different stages of pregnancy.

In any clinical examination, it is sensible to use the same order of findings each time (Table 37.4). This ensures there is less chance of missing an important feature. It is also important to continue with the examination until satisfied in all aspects, although it is essential to reduce the number of VEs to minimize the risk of infection (Gluck et al., 2020) and distress to the woman. The practitioner should adhere to local policies and procedures with regards to aseptic or non-aseptic technique. In some instances, if the woman has intact membranes it is a clean procedure; however if the membranes are ruptured, full aseptic technique should be used to prevent the risk of infection to both the woman and fetus. NICE (2023) specifies that tap water can be used prior to a VE as a cleansing agent but does not specify if this is for all VEs irrespective of membrane status.

The concept of a 'quick VE' is both futile and dangerous and should not be conducted! Contraindications to VEs are (Johnson & Taylor, 2023):

- Bleeding per vaginum.
- Placenta praevia.
- Preterm rupture of membranes, preterm labour.
- Pre-labour rupture of membranes.
- No consent from the woman.

Maternal Position in the First Stage of Labour

Low-risk labouring women should be encouraged to move about in labour and adopt the position they find to be most comfortable (Lawrence et al., 2013) (Fig. 37.13). This has shown to be a core attribute of physiological labour (Gould, 2000). Relating to the discussion on placental perfusion, it is proposed that there is better alignment between the descending presenting part and the pelvic brim. This facilitates engagement of the presenting part in the occipitoposterior presentation; rotation of the occiput to the anterior may be helped.

Labour normally begins with the fetal head in **asynclitism**. **Asynclitism** is a lateral flexion of the head

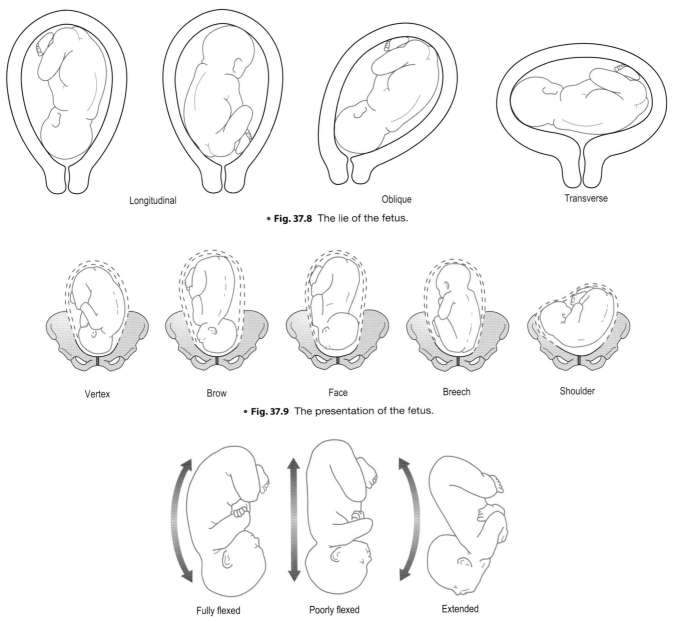

• **Fig. 37.8** The lie of the fetus.

Longitudinal   Oblique   Transverse

Vertex   Brow   Face   Breech   Shoulder

• **Fig. 37.9** The presentation of the fetus.

Fully flexed   Poorly flexed   Extended

• **Fig. 37.10** The attitude of the fetus.

(Dückelmann & Kalache, 2013). This means that the head is tilted so that one of the parietal bones enters the pelvis first. This tilting facilitates passage of the fetal head through the pelvic inlet. Once through the inlet, the head shifts to **synclitism** so that the vertex presents as the head descends farther through the pelvis. Encouraging women with firm abdominal muscles to adopt forward-leaning positions can promote the fetal head to adopt more favourable positions and increase the pelvic diameters (Simkin, Ancheta & Hanson, 2017). The forces of gravity may also lead to better application of the presenting part to the cervix, promoting Ferguson's reflex (Ferguson, 1941). The strength and length of uterine contractions are increased, leading to a more rapid dilatation of the cervix; the supine position should be avoided, as it can compromise uterine blood flow. Women who remain ambulant and adopt an upright posture during labour have a shorter labour, less risk of caesarean section, less epidural uptake and no reported negative impact on the well-being of the woman or the neonate (Lawrence et al., 2013). More evidence is required, however, due to the quality of the studies (Lawrence et al., 2013).

Immersion in Water

Immersion in water during labour has been shown to be effective for relaxation and pain relief.

Water immersion reduces the need for epidural/spinal analgesia and maternal pain, and there is no adverse effect on labour duration, operative delivery or neonatal outcome (Cluett, Burns & Cuthbert, 2018). However more research is needed to evaluate whether immersion in water affects

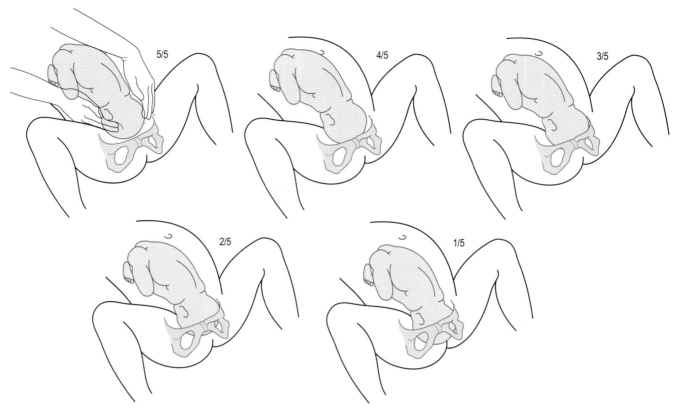

• **Fig. 37.11** Examination per abdomen to determine the descent of the fetal head in fifths.

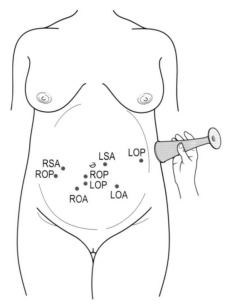

• **Fig. 37.12** The approximate points of the fetal heart sounds in vertex and breech presentations. *LOA,* left occipitoanterior; *LOP,* left occipitoposterior; *LSA,* left sacroanterior; *LSP,* left sacroposterior; *ROA,* right occipitoanterior; *ROP,* right occipitoposterior; *RSA,* right sacroanterior; *RSP,* right sacroposterior.

• CLINICAL APPLICATION 37.3	Reasons to Conduct a Vaginal Examination in Labour

- Make a positive identification of presentation.
- Determine whether the head is engaged.
- Ascertain if forewaters have ruptured or for artificial rupture.
- Exclude cord prolapse if forewaters rupture and presenting part is high.
- Assess progress/delay in labour.
- Following administration of oxytocin for delay in labour.
- Confirm full cervical dilatation.
- In multiple pregnancy, after the birth of the first baby, to confirm the lie and presentation of the second fetus and to rupture the second amniotic sac.

and enhances a state of mental relaxation. There may be a decrease in the release of stress hormones such as catecholamines, resulting in better uterine perfusion and more efficient contractions.

Nutrition and Hydration in Labour

Nutrition

The process of labour uses energy, and the body stores fat in pregnancy to use as fuel in longer labours. If insufficient carbohydrate is available, then body fat will be

neonatal or maternal morbidity (Cluett, Burns & Cuthbert, 2018). It may also increase maternal satisfaction, but more robust trial evidence is required (Cluett, Burns & Cuthbert, 2018). The warmth of the water may relax the muscles

TABLE 37.4   Order of Findings for Vaginal Examination (VE)

External genitalia	External genitalia inspected (e.g., genital herpes may influence the course and management of labour). Labia examined for any varicosities, warts or oedema. Perineum inspected for scarring, which indicates previous tear, episiotomy or female circumcision. Vaginal discharge or bleeding. If the membranes are ruptured, observe colour and quantity of liquor amnii. Any offensive odour identified might indicate infection.
Condition of vagina	The normal vagina in labour feels warm and moist. A hot and dry vagina could indicate prolonged or problematic labour. A cystocele and/or rectocele may be present in a multiparous woman. A loaded rectum can be easily felt through the posterior vaginal wall.
Condition of cervix	The cervix is palpated for length, consistency and dilatation (effacement). Position of the cervix is anterior, posterior or central. A long closed cervix indicates early stages of labour or that labour has not begun. Cervix in labour should feel soft and elastic. It will usually be applied closely to the presenting part. A primigravidae cervix has been described as the consistency of the nose. A parous cervix has been described as the consistency of the lips.
Assessing cervical os dilatation	Two examining fingers are gently inserted into the vagina and the cervical os is located. Fingers are then inserted into the cervical os and parted gently to assess the diameter of cervical dilatation in centimetres. A circular movement of the examining fingers in every direction ensures a complete circle or that no lip of cervix remains. Intact membranes can be felt through the dilating os; they feel smooth and will become tense during a contraction. If the membranes are absent, the slightly rougher fetal scalp can be felt.
Level or station of presenting part	Level of presenting part is judged in relation to the ischial spines so that descent of the fetus through the pelvis can be monitored. The distance above or below the ischial spines is estimated in centimetres (Fig. 37.14). If there is caput succedaneum, care must be taken to establish the true level of the skull under the swelling.
Presentation	96% will be a vertex presentation. Rarely will it be difficult to confirm presentation on VE; this usually indicates a very abnormal labour or a fetal anomaly (e.g., encephalocele).
Position	Landmarks such as sutures and fontanelles are used to confirm the position of the presenting part (Fig. 37.15). The most common landmark is the sagittal suture (i.e., vertex presentation) (Fig. 37.16). Identified by moulding that occurs with the leading anterior parietal bone overriding the posterior parietal bone and is usually in one or other of the oblique diameters. Posterior fontanelle can be identified by its small triangular size and its three sutures. Anterior fontanelle is larger, diamond-shaped and has four sutures.
Moulding of fetal skull	Moulding is described in Chapter 24. It is important to establish if the amount of moulding is normal or excessive. If excessive this suggests disproportion between the fetal skull and bony pelvis.
Pelvic capacity	Pelvic outlet estimation can be achieved by assessing the ischial spines and angle of the subpubic arch. Prominent ischial spines often accompany a pubic arch that is less than 90 degrees (these features suggest an android pelvis).
Fetal heart rate	An assessment of fetal heart rate should always be made after VE, especially if the membranes are ruptured, to ensure that the examination has had no adverse effect on the fetus.

utilized with the release of ketones and the development of ketoacidosis. Before admission, women can take normal diet and fluid intake. A problem with food intake in normal labour is the possible need for the administration of a general anaesthetic. Coupled with the delayed emptying of the stomach and the relative inefficiency of the cardiac sphincter brought about by the influence of progesterone is a risk of inhalation of acid gastric reflux,

resulting in **inhalational pneumonitis** (Mendelson's syndrome).

Practices for eating and drinking in labour vary considerably across the world and within the UK. Fasting in labour has been a feature of management since the relationship between anaesthesia and Mendelson's syndrome was established (Mendelson, 1946). In a review of the literature, Sleutal & Golden (1998) noted that anaesthetic research

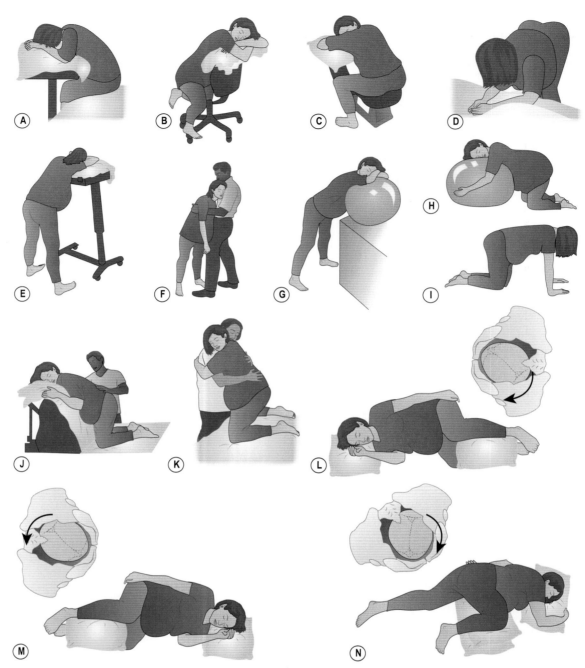

• **Fig. 37.13** Positions in labour.

has focused primarily on gastric emptying and that withholding of food does not necessarily ensure an empty stomach or reduce the acidity of stomach contents. Although death due to aspiration pneumonitis is rare, they concluded there was little difference in labour and birth outcomes between women who fasted or who did not fast in labour. There was no evidence that fasting improved the outcome for the woman and baby. Singata, Tranmer & Gyte (2013) suggest that there is no need to prevent low-risk women from eating and drinking in labour. A systematic review (Gyte & Richens, 2006) explored the use of the effects of antacids, H_2 receptor antagonists and dopamine antagonists

given routinely to labouring women to prevent gastric aspiration syndrome. They advocate that there is no evidence to support the routine use of these drugs in normal labour to prevent gastric aspiration syndrome. NICE (2023) also advocates no routine use of H_2 receptors or antacids to low-risk women on labour.

Policies for eating and drinking in labour may vary between maternity units.

A sensible protocol would be:
- Where there is no risk of general anaesthetic or instrumental delivery, women should be allowed to drink and eat a light diet as required.

- When narcotic analgesia has been given or general anaesthesia is anticipated due to risk factors, then food should be withheld, and sips of water given (NICE, 2023).

Hydration

Intravenous fluids are not routinely administered in labour. However there are some situations where it is required, such as:

1. During the administration of epidural analgesia (Hofmeyr, Cyna & Middleton, 2010).
2. For the administration of oxytocic drugs.
3. To correct dehydration (Dawood, Dowswell & Quemby, 2013).

There was no evidence in a systematic review by Toohill, Soong & Flenady (2008) to support the administration of intravenous fluids to correct ketonuria which has occurred because of metabolism of fat stores. The reviewers highlight that ketonuria can have some adverse effects and may be a normal physiological response to labour. More evidence is required on this issue.

Ehsanipoor et al. (2017) identified that labour was shortened and caesarean section rates were reduced when nulliparous low-risk women received normal saline or Ringer's lactate at a rate of 250 mL/hour compared with 125 mL/hour. They also stress that more evidence is required to discover the risk and benefits of hydration in labour. Monitoring of the maternal condition is outlined in Clinical Application 37.4.

Monitoring the Fetal Condition

The Fetus in the First Stage of Labour

Blood vessels in the myometrium, which supply the fetus with oxygen and nutrients, are compressed during each uterine contraction. Delivery of nutrients and oxygen is impeded when the strength of a contraction exceeds 40 mmHg. Therefore, increased myometrial tone or rapidly occurring contractions may cause fetal hypoxia and distress. When the membranes remain intact, the pressure of each contraction is exerted on the fluid and, as fluid is not compressible, pressure is equalized throughout the uterus. This is known as general fluid pressure (Fig. 37.4A).

If the membranes are ruptured and the amniotic fluid is reduced, the pressure of contractions is applied directly to the fetus and the placenta is compressed between the uterine wall and the fetus, further reducing the oxygen supply to

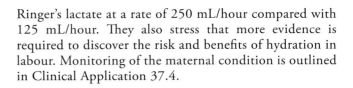

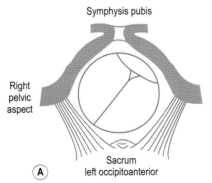

- **Fig. 37.14** The stations of the head. Descent in relation to the maternal ischial spines is expressed in centimetres.

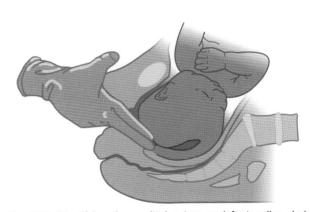

- **Fig. 37.16** Identifying the sagittal suture and fontanelles during vaginal examination.

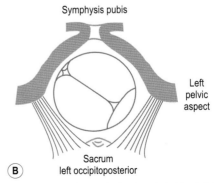

- **Fig. 37.15** Identifying the position of the fetus. (A) Left occipitoanterior: the sagittal suture is in the right oblique diameter of the pelvis. (B) Left occipitoposterior: the sagittal suture is in the left oblique diameter of the pelvis.

the fetus. Theoretically, oxygenation should improve by the avoidance of aortocaval compression. However, Mirzakhani et al. (2020) reported that there is no difference in outcomes for the mother or neonate from maternal position in labour. Additionally, Kibuka et al. (2021) acknowledge that there is limited evidence to support the benefit of upright position in labour and the authors advocate for more research to be undertaken on this topic.

In labour, the fetus is subjected to compression and hypoxic stress during uterine contractions and, if healthy, tolerates these conditions without a change in heart rate.

Distress in the fetus is indicated by alterations in heart rate, development of acidosis, passage of meconium, presence of excessive moulding and excessive movements. Information about fetal well-being is mainly obtained by recording fetal heart rate (FHR) and rhythm, either intermittently (Martis et al., 2017) or continuously (Alfirevic et al., 2017). Amniotic fluid is inspected for the presence of meconium and, where the FHR is abnormal, a fetal blood sample is taken to check the pH levels. A pH below 7.2 indicates fetal distress (NICE, 2022; Saling, 1965).

Heart Rate

Intermittent Monitoring

Intermittent monitoring of the FHR can be undertaken using Pinard's fetal stethoscope or a Doppler ultrasound apparatus such as Sonicaid. The **rate** is best counted over a full minute after each contraction and accelerations and decelerations recorded to allow for variations. The FHR should be between 110–160 bpm (NICE, 2022). It is recommended that maternal pulse should also be taken and documented to differentiate between the two heart rates (NICE, 2022). If there is bradycardia, hypoxia may be a problem. The **rhythm** of the fetal heart, as for any heart, is coupled and should remain steady. Any irregularity needs prompt action (NICE, 2022).

Continuous Fetal Heart Recording

Continuous recording of the fetal heart (**cardiography**) is a form of electronic fetal monitoring (Alfirevic et al., 2017) usually combined with continuous monitoring of maternal uterine activity (**tocography**) by using a **cardiotocograph (CTG) apparatus.** This allows a graphic response of the fetal heart to uterine activity to be recorded (Fig. 37.17). The midwife must also be able to use a Pinard's stethoscope to confirm the FHR, as the maternal heart rate can be mistaken for the FHR if solely electronic devices are used (Johnson & Taylor, 2023). Continuous monitoring is performed where there may be fetal compromise. It is important that an explanation is given to the woman if there is a need for continuous fetal heart monitoring. Fetal monitoring and the requirement for its use in emergency situations during labour should be discussed with the woman antenatally. NICE (2022) does not

---

• **CLINICAL APPLICATION 37.4** | **Monitoring the Maternal Condition**

Local protocols may vary, but observations for maternal monitoring established during the first stage of labour should include the following:

- A partogram or pictorial record of labour progress should be used adhering to the World Health Organization ((WHO 2021)) recommendations for actions.
- Half-hourly documentation of contractions.
- Pulse hourly, unless indicated more frequently.
- Temperature every 4 hours.
- Blood pressure every 4 hours.
- Monitor fluid and nutritional intake.
- Frequency of micturition.
- Urinalysis for protein, glucose and ketones. Small amounts of protein in the absence of known hypertensive or renal disease may indicate contamination by show or amniotic fluid. A small amount of ketosis is expected in normal labour and can be considered part of the physiological adaptation. Large amounts of ketones indicate exhaustion of the energy stores and may lead to uterine inertia if not corrected.
- Offer a VE every 4 hours or if there is concern about progress or in response to the woman's wishes (after abdominal palpation and assessment of vaginal loss).
- As psychological response to labour and to pain.
- Analgesia requirements (NICE, 2023).

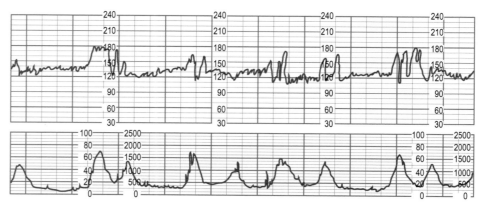

• **Fig. 37.17** Normal cardiotocograph (baseline 125–135 bpm; baseline variability 5–15 bpm; no decelerations; accelerations with some contractions).

recommend a continuous CTG for low-risk women when in established labour but they should be offered heart monitoring through intermittent auscultation.

External CTG involves strapping an ultrasound transducer to the abdominal wall over the point of maximum intensity of the fetal heart and the contraction transducer to the fundus of the uterus. The reading can be affected by maternal or fetal movement, the thickness of the abdominal wall and uterine contractions but is non-invasive. Internal cardiography (electrocardiogram) can be used by the application of an electrode to the fetal scalp (Ayres-de-Campos, Spong & Chandraharan, 2015). Membranes must be ruptured, and the cervix should be at least 2–3 cm dilated. Wiring attaches the electrode to the CTG.

Telemetry

If available, internal cardiography can be recorded by a portable battery-operated transmitter used to pick up the signal from the fetal heart and the woman can be ambulant (telemetry) (Ayres-de-Campos, Spong & Chandraharan, 2015). It is not possible to record uterine activity, however, and the woman is required to press a button at the onset of each contraction to mark the strip chart accordingly.

Findings

NICE (2022) categorizes CTG traces as normal, suspicious or pathological with reassuring, non-reassuring or abnormal features.

The CTG provides information about:
- Baseline FHR (NICE, 2022).
- Variability (NICE, 2022).
- Presence of accelerations (NICE, 2022).
- Presence or absence of decelerations (NICE, 2022).
- Contractions (NICE, 2022).

Each of these measurements are now discussed and graphs are used to demonstrate the points and to begin to develop the skills of reading and interpreting recordings.

Baseline FHR

The definition of the normal range of FHR is 110–160 bpm (NICE, 2022). The baseline FHR is the mean level of the FHR between contractions. If the heart rate is more than 160 bpm, it is termed **baseline tachycardia** (Fig. 37.18), whereas a baseline of less than 110 bpm is called **baseline bradycardia** (Fig. 37.19). These two features, with no other alteration, may indicate hypoxia, but tachycardia may be a response to maternal ketosis, infection or pyrexia. Continuous compression of the cord will cause prolonged severe bradycardia.

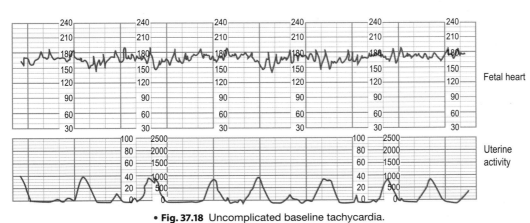

• **Fig. 37.18** Uncomplicated baseline tachycardia.

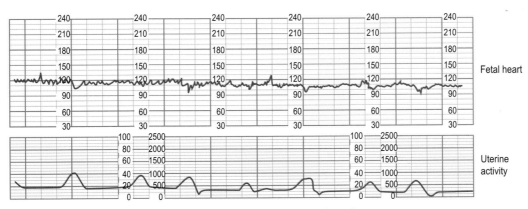

• **Fig. 37.19** Normal baseline bradycardia.

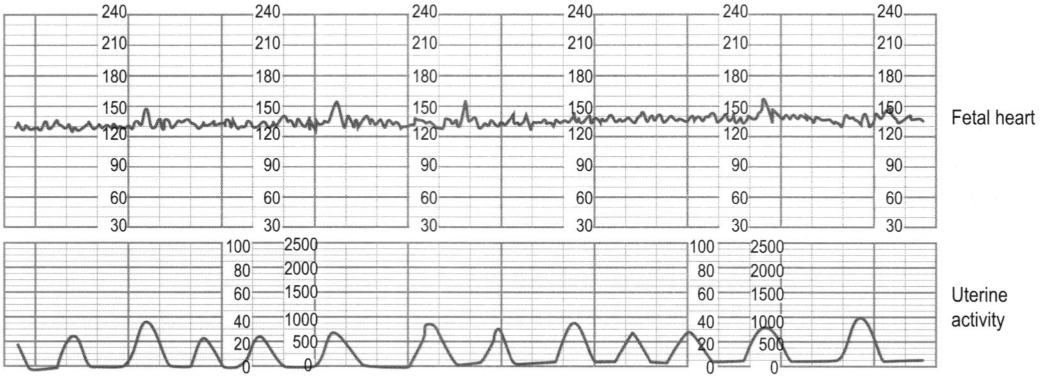

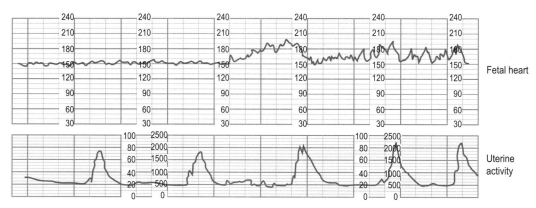

• **Fig. 37.20** Electrocardiogram trace showing variability in fetal heart rate.

• **Fig. 37.21** Physiological reduction of baseline variability in fetal heart rate (left). Normal baseline variability (right).

Baseline Variability

It is a normal function of the heart to have minute variations in the length of each beat. This is caused by electrical activity varying as a response to the environment and will produce a jagged rather than a smooth line on the graph called **baseline variability** (Fig. 37.20). The baseline rate should vary by at least 5–25 bpm (NICE, 2022). Loss of this (Fig. 37.21) may indicate fetal hypoxia (Gibb & Arulkumaran, 2017) or fetal sleep (intermittent short periods) (NICE, 2022), and has also been noted for a short time after the administration of opioid analgesia to the woman, which depresses the cardiac centre in the fetal brain. Where there is very poor baseline variability in the absence of accelerations, a VE and a fetal blood-sampling procedure may be performed to ascertain the fetal blood pH. An acceleration is an increase in the FHR of 15 bpm or more, lasting for at least 15 s and related to fetal movement (Ayres-de-Campos, Spong & Chandraharan, 2015). Fetal hypoxia may be indicated if no accelerations are present, there is a decrease of variability and/or an increase in heart rate (Gibb & Arulkumaran, 2017).

Response of the Fetal Heart to Uterine Contractions

It is normal for the FHR to remain steady or to accelerate during contractions (Fig. 37.22). The relationship of decelerations to the occurrence of uterine contractions must be considered closely to assess their significance. **Early decelerations** (Fig. 37.23) begin at or after the onset of a contraction, reach their lowest point at the peak of the contraction and return to the baseline rate by the time the contraction has finished (Gibb & Arulkumaran, 2017). They are commonly associated with compression of the fetal head (Gibb & Arulkumaran, 2017) but may be an early sign of hypoxia.

Variable decelerations are inconsistent in size, shape and in their relationship to uterine contractions (Gibb & Arulkumaran, 2017). They tend to have a rapid drop to nadir in less than 30 s (Ayres-de-Campos, Spong & Chandraharan, 2015) and accelerations often precede and follow the deceleration (termed *shouldering*) (Gibb & Arulkumaran, 2017). Variable decelerations are often mistakenly identified as early. These decelerations are related to cord compression (Gibb & Arulkumaran, 2017). The overall aim is to relieve the cord compression. Therefore management would be to change maternal position (avoid supine) (NICE, 2022), carry out a VE to exclude cord prolapse, stop oxytocic infusions, increase intravenous fluids and refer as appropriate. If variable decelerations continue, they can lead to fetal hypoxia and late decelerations.

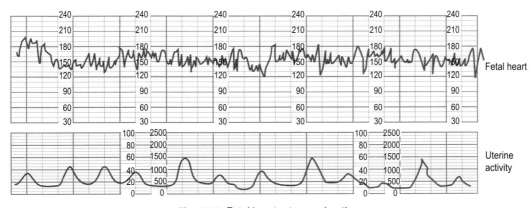

• **Fig. 37.22** Fetal heart rate accelerations.

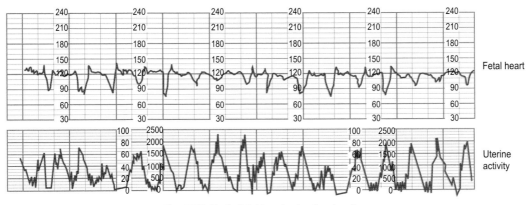

• **Fig. 37.23** Early fetal heart rate decelerations.

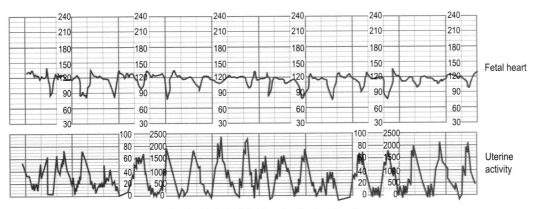

• **Fig. 37.24** Late fetal heart rate decelerations.

A **late deceleration** (Fig. 37.24) begins during or after a contraction, reaches its lowest point after the peak of the contraction and has not recovered by the time the contraction ends. These decelerations are related to uteroplacental insufficiency (Gibb & Arulkumaran, 2017). In severe deceleration, the heart rate may not have returned to normal by the onset of the next contraction. The **time lag** between the peak of the contraction and the low point of the deceleration is more significant than the actual fall in rate. This always indicates fetal hypoxia and should be treated as an emergency. The overall aim is to increase uterine blood flow and increase oxygen transfer. Management involves changing maternal position (avoid supine), increasing or commencing intravenous infusion (if the woman is hypotensive or has sepsis), stopping oxytocic infusions, considering a tocolytic (terbutaline),

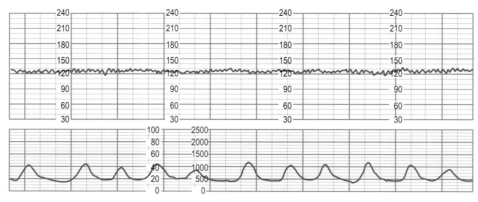

• **Fig. 37.25** A sinusoidal pattern.

expediating delivery (NICE, 2022) and obtaining fetal blood sampling.

A **sinusoidal** pattern is a regular, smooth, undulating signal resembling a sine wave, with an amplitude of 5–15 bpm and a frequency of 3–5 cycles per minute. This pattern lasts more than 30 min and coincides with absent accelerations (Ayres-de-Campos, Spong & Chandraharan, 2015). A sinusoidal pattern is considered abnormal and requires urgent attention (Fig. 37.25).

Fetal Blood Sampling

Hypoxia will lead to respiratory acidosis and a lowering of blood pH. Blood is taken by passing an amnioscope through the cervix and using a small blade to puncture the scalp skin (Fig. 37.26). A heparinized capillary tube is used to collect a blood sample for immediate analysis. The blood must not be allowed to clot or come into contact with atmospheric oxygen. East et al. (2015) highlight that serum lactate levels from fetal blood are more likely to be successful rather than pH estimation, although no differences were identified in neonatal outcomes in relation to low Apgar scores, low pH in their cord blood or admissions to the neonatal intensive care unit. There were no differences in caesarean sections, forceps or vacuum births (East et al., 2015).

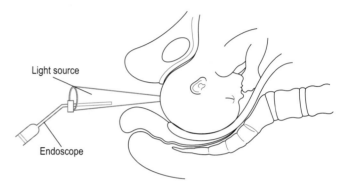

• **Fig. 37.26** Fetal blood sampling.

Amniotic Fluid

If the membranes have ruptured, clear or straw-coloured amniotic fluid will drain. The fluid should normally remain clear, but the fetus may pass meconium; this is common at term but may also be due to fetal hypoxia. Fresh meconium stains the amniotic fluid green and may indicate the fetus is hypoxic at that time; a muddy yellow colour indicates old meconium. Thick meconium may indicate breech presentation. A full discussion on fetal distress and neonatal asphyxia is presented in Chapter 46.

Main Points

- In early labour, contractions may be 15–20 min apart and inconsistent in strength, each lasting about 30 s. In established labour, the uterus contracts every 2–3 min, and in advanced labour each contraction may last 50–60 s, with contractions being powerful. Contractions are measured in mmHg by the pressure they exert on the amniotic fluid.
- Fundal dominance allows progressive dilatation of the cervix and, as the upper segment thickens and shortens, the fetus is propelled down the birth canal.
- Polarity during contractions allows the upper and lower poles of the uterus to act in harmony with contraction and retraction of the upper pole and dilatation of the lower pole.

- Contraction and retraction of the uterine muscle leads to the progressive shortening and thickening of the UUS and diminishing of the uterine cavity.
- A retraction ring forms between the UUS and the LUS. The external os dilates until it is large enough for the widest diameter of the presenting part to pass through.
- When the membranes remain intact, there is general fluid pressure. If the membranes are ruptured, the placenta is compressed between the uterine wall and the fetus, reducing fetal oxygen supply.
- During each contraction, fetal axis pressure causes increasing flexion of the head and is more significant during the second stage of labour.

- Upright postures facilitate engagement of the presenting part.
- Gravity may lead to better application of the presenting part to the cervix, promoting Ferguson's reflex and a rapid cervical dilatation.
- The process of labour uses energy. If insufficient carbohydrates are available, body fat will be utilized, with the release of ketones and the development of ketoacidosis.
- The main problem with food intake in labour is the possible need for a general anaesthetic and the subsequent risk of inhalation of gastric acid reflux, resulting in Mendelson's syndrome.
- Blood vessels in the myometrium are compressed during each uterine contraction, with impeded delivery of nutrients and oxygen when the strength of a contraction exceeds 40 mmHg. Fetal hypoxia may occur, especially if the membranes are ruptured.
- CTG allows recording of the response of the fetal heart rhythm and rate to uterine activity. Research findings do not support the value of CTG in normal labour. Serum lactate levels or fetal blood pH may be taken to assess fetal well-being.
- If the membranes have ruptured, there is continuous drainage of amniotic fluid, which should normally remain clear.
- During episodes of fetal distress in labour, hypoxia results and the fetus passes meconium, staining the fluid green. Presence of meconium requires closer vigilance on the fetal condition (paediatrician required at hospital birth).

References

Alfirevic, Z., Devane, D., Gyte, G.M., Cuthbert, A., 2017. Continuous cardiotocography (CTG) as a form of electronic fetal monitoring (EFM) for fetal assessment during labour. Cochrane Database Syst. Rev. 2017 (2), CD006066.

Ayres-de-Campos, D., Spong, C.Y., Chandraharan, E., 2015. FIGO consensus guidelines on intrapartum fetal monitoring: cardiotocography. Int. J. Gynaecol. Obstet. 131 (1), 13–24.

Byrne, D.L., Edmonds, D.K., 1990. Clinical method for evaluating the first stage of labour. Lancet 335 (8681), 122.

Cluett, E.R., Burns, E., Cuthbert, A., 2018. Immersion in water during labour and birth. Cochrane Database Syst. Rev. 2018 (5), CD000111.

Dawood, F., Dowswell, T., Quenby, S., 2013. Intravenous fluids for reducing the duration of labour in low risk nulliparous women. Cochrane Database Syst. Rev. 2013 (6), CD007715.

Downe, S., 2017. Care in the second stage of labour. In: Macdonald, S., Johnson, G. (Eds.), Mayes' Midwifery, fifteenth ed. Elsevier, Edinburgh.

Dückelmann, A.M., Kalache, K.D., 2013. Fetal progress in birth canal: state of the art. In: Malvasi, A. (Ed.), Intrapartum Ultrasonography for Labor Management. Springer, London.

East, C.E., Leader, L.R., Sheehan, P., Henshall, N.E., Colditz, P.B., Lau, R., 2015. Intrapartum fetal scalp lactate sampling for fetal assessment in the presence of a non-reassuring fetal heart rate trace. Cochrane Database Syst. Rev. 2015 (5), CD006174.

Ehsanipoor, R.M., Saccone, G., Seligman, N.S., Pierce-Williams, R.A.M., Ciardulli, A., Berghella, V., 2017. Intravenous fluid rate for reduction of caesarean delivery rate in nulliparous women: a systematic review and meta-analysis. Acta Obstet. Gynecol. Scand. 96 (7), 804–811.

Ferguson, J.K., 1941. A study of the motility of the intact uterus at term. Surg. Gynecol. Obstet. 73 (3), 359–366.

Freidman, E.A., 1954. The graphic analysis of labor. Am. J. Obstet. Gynecol. 68 (6), 1568–1574.

Gluck, O., Mizrachi, Y., Herman, H.G., Bar, J., Kovo, M., Weiner, E., 2020. The correlation between the number of vaginal examinations during active labor and febrile morbidity, a retrospective cohort study. BMC Pregnancy Childbirth 20 (1), 246.

Gould, D., 2000. Normal labour: a concept analysis. J. Adv. Nurs. 31 (2), 418–427.

Gyte, G.M.L., Richens, Y., 2006. Routine prophylactic drugs in normal labour for reducing gastric aspiration and its effects. Cochrane Database Syst. Rev. 2006 (3), CD005298.

Hassan, S.S., Romero, R., Gotsch, F., Nikita, L., Chaiworapongsa, T., 2012. Cervical insufficiency. In: Winn, H.N., Chervenak, F.A., Romero, R. (Eds.), Clinical Maternal-Fetal Medicine Online. CRC Press, London.

Hofmeyr, G.J., Cyna, A.M., Middleton, P., 2010. Prophylactic intravenous preloading for regional analgesia in labour. Cochrane Database Syst. Rev. 2010 (4), CD000175.

Hundley, V., Way, S., Cheyne, H., Janssen, P., Gross, M., Spiby, H., 2017. Defining the latent phase of labour: is it important? Evid. base Midwifery 15 (3), 89–94.

Jackson, K., Anderson, M., Marshall, J.E., 2020. Physiology and care during the first stage of labour. In Marshall, J., Raynor, M. (Eds.), Myles Textbook for Midwives, seventeenth ed, Elsevier, London.

Johnson, R., Taylor, W., 2023. Skills for Midwifery Practice, fifth ed. Elsevier, London.

Kibuka, M., Price, A., Onakpoya, I., Tierney, S., Clarke, M., 2021. Evaluating the effects of maternal positions in childbirth: an overview of Cochrane systematic reviews. Eur. J. Midwifery 5, 57.

Lai, C.Y., Levy, V., 2005. Hong Kong Chinese women's experiences of vaginal examinations in labour. In: Wickam, S. (Ed.), Midwifery Best Practice, vol. 3. Elsevier Butterworth-Heineman, Edinburgh.

Lawrence, A., Lewis, L., Hofmeyr, G.J., Styles, C., 2013. Maternal positions and mobility during first stage labour. Cochrane Database Syst. Rev. 2013 (10), CD003934.

Lewis, D., Downe, S., 2015. FIGO consensus guidelines on intrapartum fetal monitoring: intermittent auscultation. Int. J. Gynecol. Obstet. 131 (1), 9–12.

Lundborg, L., Åberg, K., Sandström, A., Discacciati, A., Tilden, E.L., Stephansson, O., et al., 2020. First stage progression in women with spontaneous onset of labor: a large population-based cohort study. PLOS ONE 15 (9):e0239724.

Martis, R., Emilia, O., Nurdiati, D.S., Brown, J., 2017. Intermittent auscultation (IA) of fetal heart rate in labour for fetal well-being. Cochrane Database Syst. Rev. 2017 (2), CD008680.

Mendelson, C.L., 1946. The aspiration of stomach contents into the lungs during obstetric anesthesia. Am. J. Obstet. Gynecol. 52 (2), 191–205.

Mirzakhani, K., Karimi, F.Z., Vatanchi, A.M., Zaidi, A., Najmabadi, M., 2020. The effect of maternal position on maternal, fetal and neonatal outcomes: a systematic review. J. Midwifery Reprod. Health 8 (1), 1988–2004.

Moncrieff, G., Gyte, G.M., Dahlen, H.G., Thomson, G., Singata-Madliki, M., Clegg, A., et al., 2022. Routine vaginal examinations compared to other methods for assessing progress of labour to improve outcomes for women and babies at term. Cochrane Database Syst. Rev. 2022 (3), CD010088.

Morvarid, I., Masoumeh, K., Habibollah, E., 2018. Relationship between length and width of the purple line and fetal head descent in active phase of labour. J. Obstet. Gynaecol. 38 (1), 10–15.

National Institute of Health and Care Excellence (NICE), 2022. Fetal Monitoring in Labour. Available at: https://www.nice-.org.uk/guidance/ng229/resources/fetal-monitoring-in-labour-pdf-66143844065221.

National Institute of Health and Care Excellence (NICE), 2023. Intrapartum Care. Available at: https://www.nice.org.uk/guidance/ng235.

Saling, D.E., 1965. A new method of safeguarding the life of the fetus before and during labour. J. Int. Fed. Gynaecol. Obstet. 3 (2), 100–110.

Simkin, P., Ancheta, R., Hanson, L., 2017. The Labor Progress Handbook: Early Intervention to Prevent and Treat Dystocia, fourth ed. Wiley-Blackwell, Oxford.

Singata, M., Tranmer, J., Gyte, G.M.L., 2013. Restricting oral fluid and food intake during labour. Cochrane Database Syst. Rev. 2013 (8), CD003930.

Sleutal, M., Golden, S., 1998. Fasting in labour: relic or requirement. J. Obstet. Gynecol. Neonatal Nurs. 28 (5), 507–512.

Smyth, R.M.D., Markham, C., Dowswell, T., 2013. Amniotomy for shortening spontaneous labour. Cochrane Database Syst. Rev. 2013 (6), CD006167.

Tinelli, A., Di Renzoc, G.C., Malvasib, A., 2015. The intrapartum ultrasonographic detection of the Bandl ring as a marker of dystocia. Int. J. Gynaecol. Obstet. 131 (3), 310–311.

Toohill, J., Soong, B., Flenady, V., 2008. Interventions for ketosis during labour. Cochrane Database Syst. Rev. 2008 (3), CD004230.

World Health Organization (WHO), 2021. Labour Care Guide User's Manual. Available at: https://www.who.int/publications/i/item/9789240017566.

Annotated recommended reading

Gibb, D., Arulkumaran, S., 2017. Fetal Monitoring in Practice, fourth ed. Elsevier, Edinburgh.

National Institute of Health and Care Excellence (NICE), 2023. Intrapartum Care. Available at: https://www.nice.org.uk/guidance/ng235.

The guideline agrees with the midwifery concept that childbirth is a normal physiological experience. It informs on caring for low-risk intrapartum women, but also highlights high-risk care.

Website

https://www.nice.org.uk/.

The NICE website provides the most up-to-date evidence-based guidance for all aspects of care during pregnancy, childbirth and following birth (intrapartum care). It offers a resource for evidence and best practice for mothers and babies.

38

Pain Relief in Labour

GAIL NORRIS

CHAPTER CONTENTS

This chapter focuses on pain in labour including perception of pain. Classification, physiological pathways and modulation of pain are detailed. The effects of pain and how pain is managed are described. It is essential for students and midwives to have sound knowledge and understanding of all aspects relating to the pain women experience.

Introduction

Pain is a complex process and is experienced differently by individuals depending on the physiological process, the context and their previous experience. The experience of pain can be discussed on three levels: pain transmission and perception; pain reception; and pain modulation.

Pain Perception

Pain is a complex, personal, subjective, multifactorial phenomenon which is influenced by psychological, physiological and sociocultural factors. Cognition and emotions such as fear and confidence affect how an individual cognition perceives pain (Boring et al., 2021; Jackson, Anderson & Marshall, 2020; Mander, 2011). The nature of pain depends on physiological parameters such as the part of the body affected, the extent of the injury and the psychological reaction to the pain. Pain is what the individual says it is, and pain exists when the individual says it does. It is not purely physical and can be modified by placebo drugs, emotions and other stimuli such as acupuncture (Birkett & Carlson, 2017). The translation of pain messages into unpleasant feelings ensures that an individual avoids repeating the experience if possible. These are all important factors to consider in the management of pain.

The physiological threshold for pain sensation appears to be similar in all people, whereas cognitive and emotive factors alter the individual's reaction to pain and the meaning attached to the experience. The anticipation of pain increases anxiety levels and the perceived intensity of pain. Facts known about pain can be applied to the pain in labour. When individuals have knowledge of events, this can reduce their anxiety and pain levels. In relation to the 'locus of control' theory, this suggests that pain is perceived as less threatening and with less intensity if women believe they are in control of events. Women should be placed at the centre of their care to facilitate labour and birth being less painful and less traumatic, even if problems such as occipitoposterior position occur.

Pain may also increase blood levels of catecholamines released, resulting in an increased heart and respiration rate with decreased blood flow to the internal organs such as the uterus. In labour, the uterus needs a good delivery of oxygen and nutrients to enable efficient contractions. As anxiety and fear increase pain and reduce uterine blood supply then this may prolong labour.

Pain Reception

The principle of pain reception is that several million bare sensory nerve endings weave their way through all tissues and organs of the body (except the brain) and respond to noxious stimuli (Marieb & Hoehn, 2022). **Bradykinin,** a chemical released from damaged tissue, seems to act as a universal pain stimulus. This in turn releases inflammatory chemicals such as **histamine** and **prostaglandin.** Bradykinin is thought to bind to receptor endings, resulting in an action potential. However, pain perception is much more than the simple sensation relayed by neurons.

Classification of Pain

Pain can be classified as somatic or visceral. **Somatic** pain arising from skin, muscles or joints can be deep or superficial. This is moderated by a range of somatic receptors, of which there are specific receptors for each sensation such as pressure, cold, hot and touch (Marieb & Hoehn, 2022). **Superficial pain** tends to be brief, highly localized and sharp or pricking in character. This pain is transmitted along large myelinated fibres – the Aδ fibres. **Deep somatic pain** is more likely to be described as burning or aching; it is more diffuse and longer lasting and always indicates tissue destruction. Impulses travel along small unmyelinated fibres called *C fibres*. The myelinated Aβ fibre is a third type of fibre which relays light touch. Refer to Chapters 26 and 27 for details of the central and peripheral nervous systems, respectively.

Pain Pathways

Visceral pain, resulting from the body's viscera or organs, is described as burning, gnawing or aching. **Visceral sensory neurons** (afferents) accompany autonomic sympathetic and parasympathetic fibres and send information about chemical changes, distension or irritation of the viscera. Both somatic and visceral pain stimuli pass along the **dendrites** of the **first-order neurons** to their cell bodies in the **dorsal root ganglia.** Their **axons** leave the dorsal root ganglia to enter the spinal cord and synapse with **second-order neurons** in the dorsal horns of the spinal cord. The pain impulse causes the release of the pain neurotransmitter, **substance P,** from the presynaptic membrane into the synaptic cleft.

The Anatomy of the Dorsal Horn

The cells in the spinal cord are arranged in **laminae** (layers) in a dorsal–ventral direction and running the full length of the spinal cord (Fig. 38.1). The **dorsal horn** contains six laminae numbered from the tip of the horn inwards. The **ventral horn** contains three other laminae, and another column of cells, lamina X, is clustered around the central canal. Laminae I and II are visible to the naked eye as a clear zone and are together called the **substantia gelatinosa.**

Ascending Pathways

Sensory fibres returning to the dorsal horns do so in an orderly fashion (Fig. 38.2). The rule is that the thicker the fibre, the deeper the fibre penetrates. The unmyelinated C fibres do not penetrate past lamina II; the small myelinated

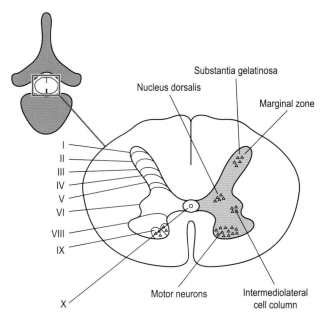

• **Fig. 38.1** Laminae (I–X) and named cell groups at midthoracic level.

Aδ fibres mainly terminate in laminae I and II, although a few make it to lamina V. The large myelinated fibres from the skin end mainly in laminae IV, V and VI. The specialized large-muscle stretch afferents reach level VI.

The axons of most of the second-order neurons cross the cord and enter the **anterolateral spinothalamic tracts** to ascend to the thalamus. There they synapse with **third-order neurons** to pass the pain message to the **sensory cortex** for interpretation. The second-order fibres may make abundant synapses in the brainstem, hypothalamus and limbic system before reaching the thalamus. This will add a state of arousal and emotion to the perception of pain. The limbic system is the affective (emotional) part of the brain, where emotions and thoughts are closely linked (Marieb & Hoehn, 2022).

Pain Modulation

Control Systems Descending from the Brain

Nerve fibres descending in the white matter penetrate the grey matter and innervate the nearest cells. The dorsolateral column is therefore able to send axons to the most dorsal laminae. Fibres from the **raphe,** from the **locus coeruleus** in the reticular formation and from the **hypothalamus,** as well as the **pyramidal tract** from the cortex, innervate the dorsal laminae III–VI. Descending fibres synapse in the dorsal horns and further modify the final ascending message by releasing endogenous opiates (opiate-like peptides) such as endorphins and encephalins into the synaptic cleft at the neural synapse. Endorphins are found in the limbic system, hypothalamus and reticular formation (Marieb & Hoehn, 2022). Endogenous opiates have been shown to inhibit prostaglandin production. Prostaglandin is thought to be a key chemical necessary for pain perception.

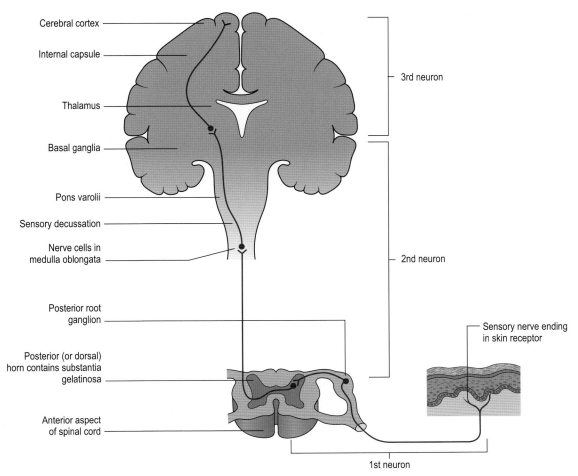

Cerebral cortex
Internal capsule
Thalamus
Basal ganglia
Pons varolii
Sensory decussation
Nerve cells in medulla oblongata
Posterior root ganglion
Posterior (or dorsal) horn contains substantia gelatinosa
Anterior aspect of spinal cord

3rd neuron
2nd neuron
Sensory nerve ending in skin receptor
1st neuron

• **Fig. 38.2** The sensory pathway showing the structures involved in the appreciation of pain.

The Gate Control Theory of Pain

The theories of pain include specificity patterns, affect and psychological/behavioural theory (Jackson, Anderson & Marshall, 2020; Mander, 2011). The following facts about pain perception must always be explained by any of the theories of pain:

- The high variability between injury and pain.
- The production of pain by innocuous stimuli.
- The perception of pain in areas seemingly removed from the area of damage.
- The persistence of pain in the absence of injury or after healing.
- The change in the location and nature of pain over time.
- The multidimensional nature of pain.
- The lack of treatment for some types of pain such as arthritic pain and migraines.

Many theories are not always applicable in the pain experienced in childbirth. The most widely used and accepted theory is the **gate control theory of pain** (McMahon et al., 2013). This theory was first proposed by Melzack and Wall in 1965 and modified in 1988. The theory involves:

- The ascending and descending tracts in the spinal cord.

- The relative conduction speeds of sensory nerve fibres returning to the spinal cord.
- The anatomy of the dorsal horns of the spinal cord.

Gating of the spinothalamic tract response to C-fibre activity can be achieved by stimulating large myelinated mechanoreceptor afferents by gentle stimulation (rubbing or tickling). These impulses inhibit the ascending pain impulse. Inputs from the large myelinated fibres conveying touch and smaller Aδ and C fibres conveying pain interact at the level of the spinal cord. The gate control theory declares that a neural or spinal gating mechanism occurs in the substantia gelatinosa of the dorsal horn of the spinal cord. The nerve impulses received by nociceptors, the receptors for pain in the skin and tissue of the body, are affected by the gating mechanism. It is the position of the gate that determines whether the nerve impulses travel freely to the medulla and the thalamus, thereby transmitting the sensory impulse or message to the sensory cortex. If the gate is closed, pain is blocked and does not become part of the conscious thought. If the gate is open, the impulses and messages pass through and are transmitted freely, resulting in pain being experienced.

Virtually the entire brain plays a part in pain perception; the thalamus, reticular system, limbic system and cortex add

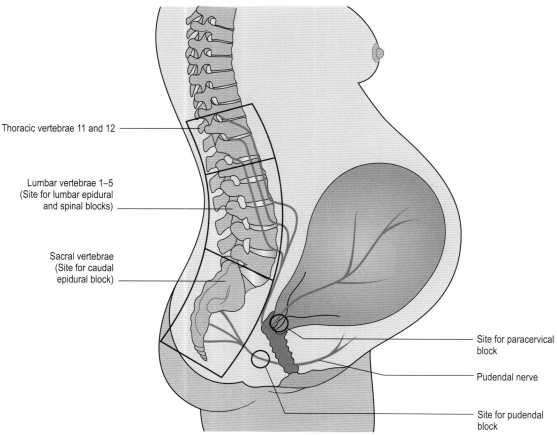

Thoracic vertebrae 11 and 12

Lumbar vertebrae 1–5
(Site for lumbar epidural
and spinal blocks)

Sacral vertebrae
(Site for caudal
epidural block)

Site for paracervical
block

Pudendal nerve

Site for pudendal
block

• **Fig. 38.3** Pain pathways in labour, showing the sites at which pain may be intercepted by local anaesthetic technique.

their effects to the physical, emotional and cognitive experience of pain. Knowledge of the multidimensional nature of pain perception allows the management of pain to be approached in an equally multidimensional manner. Techniques to inhibit the gate include stimulation of the large nerve fibres so that the pain impulses from the smaller fibres are blocked. Methods include heat, massage and pressure. Transcutaneous electrical nerve stimulation (TENS) works by applying a stimulating electrode to the skin at the level of the noxious C-fibre activity and delivering an electrical current sufficient to cause a buzzing sensation. **Descending-fibre impulses** also inhibit transmission of pain by release of natural opiates, and therefore concentration techniques may work in this way.

Visceral Sensory Neurons

Although the autonomic nervous system is considered to be a motor system, there are sensory neurons, mainly visceral pain afferents, in autonomic nerves. These visceral pain afferents travel along the same pathways as somatic pain fibres. Pain perception is referred to the somatic area of the specific dermatome of the surface of the body; for example, the pain of a heart attack is felt in the chest and along the medial aspect of the left arm.

Pain Pathways in Labour

Both visceral and somatic pain are perceived in labour. Visceral pain is caused by the uterine contractions, the dilatation of the cervix and, later, by the stretching of the vagina and the muscles and ligaments of the pelvic floor. The body of the uterus is served by autonomic nerves originating in thoracic 11 and 12 and lumbar 1 vertebrae (Fig. 38.3). Sensation from the body of the uterus is perceived as pain in response to stretch, infection and contraction and possibly ischaemia.

The cervix is innervated by the sacral plexus from sacral 2, 3 and 4 vertebrae nerves (Fig. 38.3), which then pass through the transcervical nerve plexi. Pain sensation from the cervix is in response to rapid dilatation. Somatic pain is caused by the pressure of the fetus as it distends the birth canal, vulva and perineum. Sensations from the pelvic floor are relayed from the pudendal nerve to the sacral plexus. Pain during the first stage of labour may be referred as nerve impulses from the uterus and cervix stimulate spinal cord neurons that innervate the abdominal wall. Pain may be felt between the umbilicus and the symphysis pubis, and around the iliac crests to the buttocks. Pain may radiate down the thighs and into the lumbar and sacral regions of the back.

The Effect of Pain

Besides the physical, emotional and cognitive factors affecting pain perception, abnormalities of labour may cause an increase in the pain perceived. Pain may be increased in labour complicated by prolongation, occipitoposterior position and borderline cephalopelvic disproportion.

Pain is a form of stress and may cause increased levels of catecholamine secretion, with these substances producing the normal physiological responses in the body. In labour, the physiological responses to pain are associated with the following:

- Increased cardiac output up to 20% increase in the first stage and 50% in the second stage of labour. The increase is brought about with the return of the uterine blood flow to the maternal circulation. Each contraction constitutes approximately 250–300 mL. The sympathetic response brought about by pain, fear and anxiety may also contribute to increased cardiac output.
- Increased heart rate and blood pressure (BP) associated with sympathetic response and increased cardiac output.
- Increased respiratory rate causes a decrease in $PaCO_2$ level with a corresponding increase in pH and a subsequent fall in fetal $PaCO_2$.
- Hyperventilation can alter the acid–base balance, resulting in maternal alkalosis. This alkalosis may affect the diffusion of oxygen across the placenta, leading to a degree of fetal hypoxia.
- Decreased cerebral and uterine blood flow due to vasoconstriction.
- Decreased uterine contractions.
- Delayed stomach emptying, leading to nausea and vomiting.
- Delayed bladder emptying.

Management of Pain

Understanding of pain pathways and perception leads to offering a range of pain-management strategies. These include non-pharmacological interventions (that aim to help women cope with pain in labour) and pharmacological interventions (that aim to relieve the pain of labour). In a Cochrane systematic review, Jones et al. (2012) reported on 18 conducted reviews of pain-management strategies in labour. The reviewers confirmed that there was insufficient evidence to make judgements on the effectiveness between non-pharmacological and pharmacological methods of pain relief (Jones et al., 2012). More evidence was available to support the efficacy of pharmacological methods, but these also have more adverse effects.

The range of strategies available includes:

- Non-pharmacological therapies and techniques for support.
- TENS.
- Systemic analgesia.
- Tranquilizers.
- Inhalational analgesia.
- Regional and local analgesia.
- Alternative methods.

'Working with Pain' Model

The relationship between the midwife and the woman and her partner has a crucial role to play in how the woman feels supported during pregnancy and childbirth and how she prepares for pain in labour. This relationship can affect how the woman perceives pain in labour. Midwifery care needs to be woman-centred and tailored to meet the specific wishes of women (Jones et al., 2012). This woman-centred approach includes the issue of pain in labour, which should not be medically oriented. The traditional goal of pain relief and the control of pain in labour need to be clearly differentiated. Midwives usually adopt one of two key paradigms: the *'working with pain' model* and the *pain relief model* (Leap & Anderson, 2008; Walsh, 2012). In the *'working with pain' model,* it is expected that some pain will usually be experienced in labour by women and that this is normal and fundamental to a physiological labour. The philosophy of the *'working with pain' model* encompasses women and midwives working together to plan and facilitate care, accepting that pain in normal labour is positive and has a purpose. In the *pain relief model,* midwives tend to present a list of pain-relieving options to the woman. This approach usually undermines the woman's confidence in herself and her body to give birth without the aid of medication. Table 38.1 presents the terminology and philosophy underpinning these two models of dealing with pain in labour.

Non-Pharmacological Support

An increasing number of women now wish to use other pain-relieving therapies and techniques (non-pharmacological methods) of relieving pain in labour and avoid pharmacological methods or the invasive technique of epidural analgesia. The midwife has a key role in working with the woman and her partner to support and facilitate the options for pain relief in labour. Clinical Application 38.1 provides information on the numerous ways that the midwife can support the woman to prepare during pregnancy and in labour. Clinical Application 38.2 details the list of therapies and techniques.

Mindfulness is a practice as well as a state of awareness. The practice consists of steering one's attention (commonly to the sensations of breathing) and aims at an awareness that makes it possible to have painful experiences without being reactive (Lönnberg, Nissen & Niemi, 2018). A current review of evidence examining relaxation therapies for pain management (including 19 studies) included relaxation, yoga, music and mindfulness found that relaxation, yoga and music may have a role with reducing pain and increasing satisfaction with pain relief, although the quality of evidence varies between low and very low. There is insufficient evidence for the role of mindfulness (Smith et al., 2018a).

TABLE 38.1	**Models of Labour Pain**	

Pain Relief Approach	'Working with pain' Approach
Language suggestive of pain as a problem	Language suggestive of pain as normative
Paternalistic – *'we can protect you from unnecessary stress'*	Egalitarian empowerment – *'we are alongside you'*
Techno/rationalism age, pain is preventable/treatable	Labour pain timeless component of *'rite-of-passage'* transitions
Neutral impact of environment	Seminal impact of environment
Clinical expertise of professional companions	Supportive role of birth companions
Special session/focus in antenatal education	Woven throughout labour preparation sessions
'Menu approach' to options for coping with pain	Supportive strategies for journey of labour
Pain as a *'management'* issue for assembly-line birth	Pain as one dimension of labour care in one-to-one, small-scale birth setting
Contributes to trend of rising epidural rates	Contributes to trend of less pharmacological analgesia
Risks of pharmacological agents outweighed by benefits	*'Cascade of intervention'* dynamic
First birth a special case for *'menu approach'*	First birth an optimal opportunity for 'working with pain'
Informed choice means all options must be presented	Informed choice within context of birthing plan and philosophy

Walsh, D., 2012.

- Antenatal discussions to explore attitudes to pain and expectations of women and birth partners.
- Everyday practice should support a *'working with pain'* philosophy and challenge a *'relief from pain'* approach.
- Encourage mobility, freedom of movement and upright positions, considering the woman's preferences (Simkin & Ancheta, 2017).
- Keep women informed of their progress and options. The woman and birth partner need to be involved in their decision making, which adds to their feeling of being in control.
- A range of non-pharmacological methods may be used:
  - During the latent phase of labour, women should be advised that breathing exercises, having a shower or bath, and massage may reduce pain. They should not be offered or advised to use aromatherapy, yoga or acupressure for pain relief.
  - In labour, women should be encouraged to use breathing to relax and TENS. They should be supported in their choices including, massage techniques, acupuncture, acupressure or hypnosis during labour.
  - Intracutaneous or subcutaneous sterile water injections may be a pain-relief option for women in labour with back pain (midwife needs to be trained). These are administered at four different injection points around the Rhombus of Michaelis, using doses of 0.1 mL intracutaneously or 0.5 mL subcutaneously at each injection point. (National Institute of Health and Care Excellence [NICE], 2023).
- Reduce the need for pharmacological agents by:
  - Providing one-to-one care and support in labour (especially the woman's choice of companion or a supportive midwife known to the woman) (Bohren et al., 2017).
  - Being particularly attentive in ensuring the birth environment is appropriate for physiological birth (friendly and welcoming staff and a relaxed atmosphere and comfortable physical surroundings) (Simkin & Ancheta, 2017).
- Provide women with clear information about the effectiveness, side effects and increased labour interventions with pharmacological agents, particularly epidurals.
- Be mindful that opioids and epidural agents are powerful drugs that are incompatible with physiological birth.
- Labouring and birthing in water or bathing may be soothing for some women, both as a direct reliever of pain and indirectly through relaxation and feeling fresher. Evidence from a systematic review (Cluett, Burns & Cuthbert, 2018) suggested that water immersion during the first stage of labour reduces the use of epidural/spinal analgesia. Other evidence from a systematic meta-thematic synthesis examining the views and experiences of women following water immersion during labour found that this offered effective analgesia (Feeley, Cooper & Burns, 2021). Limited information is available for other outcomes, with no evidence of increased adverse effects to the fetus/neonate or woman from labouring in water or waterbirth.

Current evidence examining the use of acupuncture or acupressure for pain management during labour (28 trials comparing acupuncture or acupressure with sham treatments as placebo, no treatment or usual care for pain management) found that most comparisons suggest a small benefit from acupressure, although supporting evidence is limited. Acupuncture may increase satisfaction with pain relief and reduce the use of pharmacological pain relief. More high-quality research is required (Smith et al., 2020). Evidence supporting the use of massage during labour reports that it may have a role in reducing pain, reducing the length of labour and improving women's sense of control and emotional experience of labour. However, the quality of the evidence varies from low to very low (Smith et al., 2018b).

Overall, based on the findings from numerous Cochrane systematic reviews, there is currently insufficient evidence to make judgements on the effectiveness of hypnosis, biofeedback, aromatherapy and TENS compared with placebos and pharmacological methods of pain relief. Whilst findings suggest there are benefits to women (i.e., promotes maternal relaxation and satisfaction, and reduces analgesia and rate of assisted

- Aromatherapy with oils placed in warm bath.
- Massage.
- Immersion in water.
- Hypnobirthing.
- Reflexology.
- Acupuncture or acupressure.
- Biofeedback.
- Nipple stimulation to increase oxytocin production.
- Music therapy.
- Mind–body and other calming techniques such as relaxation, meditation, visualization, breathing, yoga, hypnosis and herbal medicines or homoeopathy (these may not be readily accessible to women).
NICE (2023) recommend that women should be supported in their personal choice of method for pain relief.

vaginal births), there remains insufficient evidence (Jones et al., 2012). Further well-controlled trials in this area are required.

Health professionals need to support and facilitate these alternative therapies and non-pharmacological techniques within current evidence for safe practice if they are to embrace woman-centred care and respect women's choices. Midwives need to be appropriately trained in any of these alternative non-pharmacological therapies and techniques to relieve pain in labour before these are incorporated within their professional practice (Nursing & Midwifery Council, 2018).

Transcutaneous Electrical Nerve Stimulation (TENS)

TENS, a non-pharmacological method of pain relief, is based upon two hypotheses of pain physiology. First, is the gate control theory, according to which cells in the posterior horn of the spinal grey matter have a gate function. Electrical stimulation by TENS is thought to increase Aβ-fibre input to the central pain pathways, thus producing inhibitory neurotransmitters which cause presynaptic inhibition – the closing of the 'gate' (Melzack & Wall, 1988). Second, TENS may also stimulate the production of naturally occurring endogenous opiates, which act as neuromodulators. A TENS unit is an electronic stimulus generator emitting low-voltage electrical impulses which vary in frequency and intensity via electrodes attached to the skin. Four electrodes are placed over the areas of the skin on the woman's back which overlie the thoracic (T10) and lumbar (L1) nerve endings and over the sacral nerves (S2–S4) (Fig. 38.4).

Accurate positioning of electrodes is important for maximizing pain relief. TENS is self-administered, giving women a sense of *being in control,* and they should practice operating the equipment antenatally. Pressing a button causes a small electrical current to pass through the electrodes. The current can be controlled and may be pulsed – i.e., intermittent and

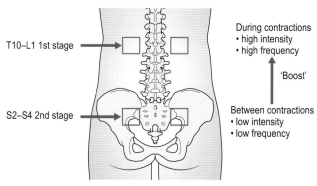

● **Fig. 38.4** Transcutaneous electrical nerve stimulation electrode positioning for use during labour.

low frequency – or it may be continuous and high frequency. Low-frequency TENS is thought to stimulate the release of endogenous opiates, whereas high-frequency TENS closes the pain gate. TENS is most effective when commenced early in labour (Jackson, Anderson & Marshall, 2020) but may not provide adequate analgesia for some women if used on its own. It is probably most useful in shorter multigravid labours, although many primigravidae find it useful. TENS equipment may interfere with electrical mechanisms within the heart if a woman has a cardiac pacemaker. This situation and immersion in water are really occasions when TENS cannot be used. TENS may also be used to stimulate acupuncture points or other parts of the body.

The use of TENS is within the midwives' sphere of practice. Therefore, practitioners should be responsible for keeping themselves updated in the use of TENS, the contraindications for its use and that equipment conforms to current safety standards.

Systemic Analgesia

An analgesic is a substance that reduces sensibility to pain without loss of consciousness and sense of touch. In labour, the substance should not compromise the safety of the mother or fetus, and it is advisable that there should be a specific antagonist. A strong analgesic drug is called a *narcotic,* and these include opioid drugs. The action lies in their ability to bind with receptor sites which are mainly found in the substantia gelatinosa of the dorsal horn of the spinal cord (Anderson, 2011). Others are in the hypothalamus, thalamus and midbrain. In the UK, three systemic opioids are commonly used: **pethidine, diamorphine** and **meptazinol.** See Clinical Application 38.3 for common opiates used in labour.

All of these opiate drugs have similar pain-relieving properties and there are numerous side effects. The extent to which the side effects are experienced is influenced by maternal metabolism of the drug used, the degree and speed of transfer of the drug and metabolites from maternal to fetal circulation, and the ability of the fetus to process and excrete both. Common side effects of opiate drugs include:

- Nausea and vomiting.
- Delayed emptying of the stomach.

Pethidine

- Also known as meperidine.
- Synthetic drug with powerful analgesic, sedative and antispasmodic effects.
- Administered intramuscularly (usual), intravenously (quicker effect) or by self-administered infusion (patient-controlled analgesia with built-in time limit to prevent overdose). Acts with rapid effect (within 20 min) and lasts up to 4 hours. Dose depends, depending on route of administration, maternal weight, labour progress and degree of pain.
- Maternal side effects include sedation, respiratory depression, delayed gastric emptying, nausea and vomiting. In addition, pethidine may cross the placenta and may cause complications such as respiratory depression and low Apgar scores in the newborn (Kadirogullari et al., 2021). This can depress the fetal respiratory centre. Preferably, it should not be given if birth is expected within 2–3 hours of administration. The effect on neonatal respiration is minimal if birth occurs within 1 hour of administration or more than 6 hours before birth. Pethidine administration can also result in a loss of baseline variability in the fetal heart rate pattern (may be observed within 40 min of administration).
- Avoid using pethidine for analgesia in women with sickle cell disease (Oteng-Ntim et al., 2021).
- There is insufficient evidence to assess which opioid drug provides the best pain relief (Smith, Burns & Cuthbert, 2018).

Diamorphine

- Provides effective analgesia for up to 4 hours and is an appropriate drug for pain in labour.
- Administered subcutaneously or intramuscularly. Dose will vary for increased maternal weight.
- More effectively metabolized and eliminated more readily from maternal and fetal plasma.
- Not suitable for long-term use, as repeated doses cause dependence and tolerance.
- Side effects of diamorphine include nausea and vomiting, constipation and drowsiness, and can cause respiratory depression and hypotension if used in large doses.

Meptazinol

- Fast acting and effective for up to 4 hours.
- Administered intramuscularly.
- Has little effect on cardiovascular and respiratory function.
- Little difference in the analgesic properties of pethidine and meptazinol, with both causing nausea and vomiting (local policies may apply).

Remifentanil patient-controlled analgesia (PCA)

- Intravenous remifentanil PCA (40 micrograms per bolus with a 2-minute lockout period) is an option for women who want ongoing pain relief during labour and birth (NICE 2023).

For analgesia and dosage refer to local protocols and follow NICE 2023 guidelines.

- Drowsiness or sedation in the woman (may impair decision-making).
- Reduction in fetal heart rate, variability and depression of the baby's respiratory centre at birth.

Entonox, 50% nitrous oxide (N_2O) and 50% oxygen (O_2), is:
- Colourless and odourless.
- Administered via the mouthpiece or face mask by maternal inspiratory efforts.
- Available by cylinder or by piped supply.
- N_2O is a heavier gas than O_2.
- Storage – cylinders should **always** be stored above 10°C and on their side until required.
- Gases may separate if stored at a temperature below −7°C.
- When required, the cylinder should be inverted several times to mix the contents.

- A sleepy baby, affecting the establishment of breastfeeding.
- If an intramuscular opioid is used, also administer an antiemetic (NICE 2023).

Inhalational Analgesia

The most commonly used inhalation analgesia in labour is **Entonox,** a pre-mixed gas made up of 50% nitrous oxide (N_2O) and 50% oxygen (O_2) administered via the Entonox apparatus. N_2O (also known as *laughing gas*) acts by limiting the neuronal and synaptic transmission within the central nervous system (CNS) and is known to induce opioid peptide release in the periaqueductal grey area of the midbrain. This leads to activation of the descending inhibitory pathways, resulting in modulation of the pain/nociceptive processing in the spinal cord.

The woman is instructed to begin to breathe the gas as soon as the uterus begins to contract and before the sensation of pain is felt. Entonox takes effect after about 20 s, with maximum effect after 50 s, which should coincide with the height of the contraction. It is excreted rapidly via the lungs as the mother exhales and therefore toxic levels do not build up to affect the fetus. Entonox does cross the placental barrier in both directions following a concentration gradient. This inhalation gas can be used in conjunction with narcotic drugs. Findings from a systematic review concluded that inhaled analgesia may help relieve labour pain without adversely increasing operative delivery rates (forceps or vacuum extraction, caesarean section), or affecting neonatal well-being (Nanji & Carvalho, 2020). Clinical Application 38.4 provides the practical implications involved.

Anaesthetics are used to make a patient unaware of and unresponsive to painful stimulation (Ritter et al., 2019). They are given systemically and exert their effect on the CNS. To be an effective anaesthetic, a drug must induce anaesthesia rapidly, be easily adjustable and be reversible. Inhalation anaesthetics include a wide variety of substances with no common chemical structure such as halothane, N_2O and xenon, and the mechanism for their action is not clear despite much research.

Stages of Anaesthesia

When inhalational anaesthetics are given on their own, four well-defined stages are passed through as the blood concentration increases:

- **Stage 1: analgesia.** The person is conscious but drowsy, and response to painful stimuli is reduced.
- **Stage II: excitement.** The subject loses consciousness and does not respond to non-painful stimuli but will respond in a reflex manner to painful stimuli. Cough and gag reflexes are also present. Irregular breathing may occur, and this is a dangerous state that modern procedures are designed to eliminate.
- **Stage III: surgical anaesthesia.** Spontaneous movement ceases and respiration becomes regular. If the anaesthesia is light, some reflexes are still present and muscle tone is still good. As the anaesthesia deepens, muscles become flaccid and reflexes disappear. Respirations become progressively shallower.
- **Stage IV: medullary paralysis.** Respiration and vasomotor control disappear and death would occur in a few minutes.

Obstetric Use of Inhalational Anaesthetics

An important characteristic of an inhalational anaesthetic is the rapidity with which the arterial blood concentration changes as the amount of drug inhaled changes. These drugs are generally used as obstetric anaesthetics in two ways: either as pain relief or as part of a combination of drugs to induce general anaesthesia during a caesarean section. Commonly, anaesthesia would be induced by an intravenous drug and then, to maintain the state, with an inhalational agent such as nitrous oxide or halothane. Muscle paralysis is obtained by the administration of a drug such as tubocurarine. Inhalation agents are time and dose dependent and may affect the fetus directly by being transported across the placenta or indirectly by altering uteroplacental blood flow.

Various factors, including the higher metabolic requirements and the presence of the fetus, make the pregnant woman more vulnerable to hypoxia should it occur during intubation. There is a rapid fall in PO_2, and hypoxia and respiratory acidosis may rapidly follow. Supine hypotensive syndrome may exaggerate the effect by reducing venous return and cardiac output so that the uteroplacental blood flow is poor; a left lateral tilt of the woman on the operating table will reduce the incidence of this problem. However, with safe techniques, light-to-moderate anaesthesia and adequate oxygen administration, women with normal health should not have problems.

Epidural Analgesia

Epidural analgesia is a central nerve block technique involving an injection of a local anaesthetic into the epidural space and close to the nerves that transmit pain. It is widely used as a form of pain relief in labour. A catheter is inserted so that further doses of local anaesthetic can be administered if

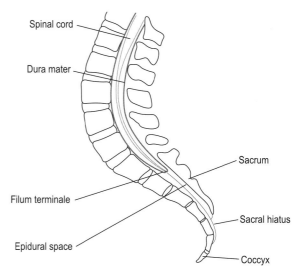

• **Fig. 38.5** The epidural space and sacral hiatus.

needed. Epidural analgesia provides adequate pain relief in about 90% of women who are given the technique.

Most women now choose epidural analgesia, especially primigravid women. Epidural and spinal analgesia are becoming more common as a method of pain relief for caesarean section.

Anatomy of the Epidural Space

The epidural space is a small space about 4 mm wide situated around the dura mater and contains blood vessels and fatty tissue (Figs. 38.5 and 38.6). The spinal nerves pass through it. Engorgement of the veins reduces the size of the space during pregnancy, and uterine contractions, which cause even more engorgement of the veins, further reduce the epidural space. The aim is to surround specific fibres of the spinal nerves to remove the sensation of pain. The procedure is similar to a lumbar puncture, but the meninges are not penetrated. Most commonly, the lumbar route is used, and the alternative of caudal anaesthesia is not popular in the UK. The anaesthetic is introduced between lumbar vertebrae 3 and 4 or 2 and 3 (Fig. 38.7). Clinical Application 38.5 details the procedure for administering epidural anaesthetic, and Box 38.1 provides the possible complications.

Indications for Epidural Analgesia

- The woman's choice of pain relief.
- Effective analgesia.
- Hypertensive conditions, to prevent the rise of BP (it may even cause a small reduction in BP).
- Preterm labour, to avoid the use of narcotic drugs.
- Prolonged labour, to allow rest and prevent exhaustion.
- Malpresentations such as breech, to prevent premature pushing and in case manipulations are required in the second stage of labour.
- Malposition of occipitoposterior, to reduce pain and early pushing. However there may be delay or no rotation of the head due to the reduced tone of the pelvic floor.

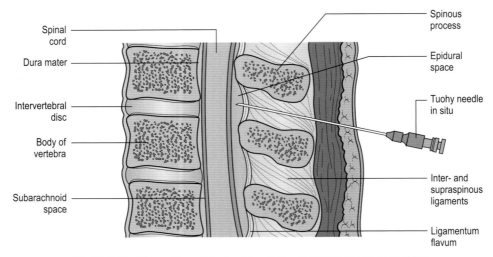

• **Fig. 38.6** Sagittal section of the lumbar spine with Tuohy needle in position.

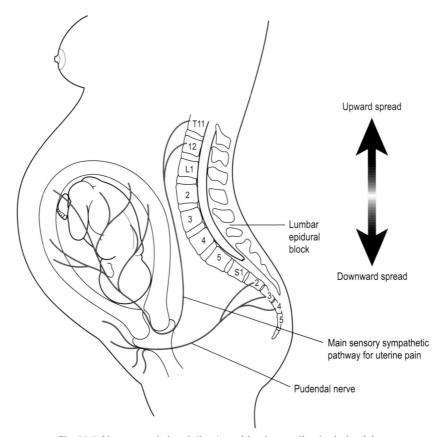

• **Fig. 38.7** Nerve supply in relation to epidural anaesthesia during labour.

- Multiple pregnancy, to prevent the administration of narcotic drugs and in case manipulations are needed in the second stage of labour.
- Cardiac and respiratory disease.
- Operative deliveries such as caesarean section.
- Possible difficulties with intubation during administration of a general anaesthetic.

Contraindications

- Maternal reluctance for this form of pain relief.
- Sepsis near the site of the injection or systemic sepsis.
- Haemorrhagic disease or clotting disorder.
- Neurological disease.
- Hypovolaemia or hypotension.
- Spinal deformity.
- Chronic back problems.

Continuous infusion of dilute bupivacaine and opioids (usually fentanyl) has resulted in significant reductions in the amount of local anaesthetic (LA) used whilst ensuring rapid analgesia. This regime has minimum motor block

• CLINICAL APPLICATION 38.5 Preparation and Procedure for Epidural

- Explain the procedure and risks to the woman and gain consent.
- Baseline recordings are essential, including temperature, pulse, blood pressure (BP) and fetal heart rate.
- Ensure the woman is encouraged to empty her bladder.
- Site an intravenous cannula for intravenous access. Preloading and maintenance fluid infusion need not be administered routinely before establishing low-dose epidural analgesia and combined epidural analgesia (NICE, 2023).
- Resuscitation equipment and drugs should always be available.
- When siting the epidural, the woman may be positioned on her left side or sitting up and asked to flex her back by drawing up her knees – positioning helps to separate the vertebrae and has better access to the epidural space.
- The technique is aseptic with the skin cleaned and sterile towels placed around the area of skin to be breached.
- A small amount of local anaesthetic is injected and a special epidural needle (Tuohy needle), a blunt needle with a stilette, is inserted.
- The needle is advanced carefully until resistance of the ligamentum flavum is reached, just before the epidural space (Fig. 38.6). The stilette is removed and a syringe containing air or normal saline is attached to the needle. Further needle advancement brings it into the epidural space. This is recognized by a sudden loss of resistance when the plunger of the syringe is depressed. Any leakage of cerebrospinal fluid (CSF) would indicate a dural tap has occurred.
- If no blood or CSF is seen, a fine catheter is introduced through the epidural needle until its tip is in the epidural space. This catheter is left in position to facilitate bolus injections or continuous infusion of the local anaesthetic. Epidural analgesia is established with a low-concentration local anaesthetic and fentanyl solution. The initial dose is essentially a test dose and is administered cautiously to ensure that inadvertent intrathecal or intravascular placement of the epidural catheter has not occurred (NICE, 2023). The infusion of local anaesthetic bathes the nerves of the corda equine, blocking the autonomic nerve pathways supplying the uterus. Once everything is satisfactory, the needle is removed and an antibacterial filter is attached to the end of the catheter, which is taped securely in place.
- Observations of maternal BP and pulse and fetal heart rate are recorded every 5 min for 20 min and then every 30 min. This is repeated with every epidural top-up.
- Assess the level of sensory block hourly (NICE, 2023).

effect, which enables the woman to move about freely and bear down more effectively in the second stage of labour (Anim-Somuah et al., 2018).

Other Drugs

Opiates have been injected into the epidural space, including diamorphine, morphine, pethidine and fentanyl. They do not produce a block so there is little risk of hypotension, but they may reduce the level of pain perceived, especially postoperative pain. The use of a dilute combination of opiate with LA may give a longer, more effective analgesia with less motor blockade. The LA blocks the Aδ fibres, whereas the opiates remove pain transmitted by the smaller C fibres. This allows careful mobilization of the woman, and she can be more active in the second stage of labour. The drugs commonly used are **bupivacaine** and **fentanyl,** given by epidural infusion or by bolus injection. Side effects include pruritus, urinary retention, postural hypotension, nausea, vomiting and respiratory depression.

Spinal Anaesthesia

Spinal anaesthesia is different from epidural anaesthesia in that the LA solution is injected into the subarachnoid space directly into the cerebrospinal fluid (CSF) rather than into the epidural space. It is quick, easy to perform and usually effective. It induces a total motor and sensory block below the anaesthetized area. There is more risk of profound hypotension occurring. It is useful for performing short procedures such as forceps delivery or manual removal of placenta. It can be used for performing a caesarean section, being cautious that its effects do not wear off before the end of the surgery.

Traditional epidural techniques are associated with prolonged labour, use of oxytocin augmentation and increased incidence of instrumental vaginal delivery. To reduce these adverse effects, the combined spinal-epidural (CSE) technique was introduced. A systematic review conducted revealed little basis for offering CSE over epidurals in labour, with no difference in overall maternal satisfaction despite a slightly faster onset with CSE and conversely less pruritus with low-dose epidurals (Simmons et al., 2012). They found no difference in ability to mobilize, maternal hypotension, rate of caesarean birth or neonatal outcome. However, the significantly higher incidence of urinary retention, rescue interventions and instrumental deliveries with traditional techniques would favour the use of low-dose epidurals. The review could not reach any meaningful conclusions regarding rare complications such as nerve injury and meningitis.

In a Cochrane review, Anim-Somuah et al. (2018) assessed the effectiveness and safety of all types of epidural analgesia, including CSE on mother and baby with non-epidural or no pain relief. They highlighted that women with epidurals reported this was more effective in reducing pain during labour. Women reported increased satisfaction with epidural as a form of pain relief in comparison to other non-epidural methods. Women with epidurals reportedly experienced more hypotension, motor blockade, fever and urinary retention. They also had a longer first and second stage of labour and were more likely to have augmentation using oxytocin. However, they were less likely to experience nausea and vomiting compared to women who used opioids for pain relief. Overall, epidural analgesia had no impact on the risk of caesarean section or long-term backache and did not appear to have an immediate effect on neonatal Apgar scores or admission into neonatal units (Anim-Somuah et al., 2018).

• BOX 38.1 Complications of Epidural Analgesia

Hypotensive Incident

This may occur as local anaesthetic (LA) blocks the transmission of both motor and sensory nerves. This affects the sympathetic nervous system by causing vasodilation and a possible fall in blood pressure (BP) (unless blood volume is increased by infusion (preload) prior to epidural block (effective in high-dose regional anaesthesia)) (Hofmeyr, Cyna & Middleton, 2004). There is probable fetal compromise.

The midwife should stop the epidural, assist the woman into the left lateral position and call for anaesthetic help. There should be rapid infusion of Hartmann's solution, with epinephrine (a vasopressor) to raise BP as required.

Dural Tap and Headache

This may occur if the dura mater is punctured with leakage of cerebrospinal fluid (CSF) causing stretching of brain tissue. Drops of CSF leak through the Tuohy needle. If more CSF leaks, the woman may develop a severe headache (up to 1 week). Lying flat will relieve headache. A blood patch of 10–20 mL of maternal blood into the epidural space may relieve headache.

Total Spinal Block

This is a rare complication occurring if the dura mater is punctured and LA is injected. There will be profound motor and sensory block with a dramatic fall in BP. The woman collapses and may have a respiratory arrest. The midwife should stop the epidural, and immediate resuscitation and ventilatory support are needed. Prevention of maternal hypoxia and restoration of normal BP may allow safe delivery of the baby where feasible.

Bloody Tap

This occurs if an epidural vein is punctured. Blood will be seen in the epidural cannula. Re-siting is necessary to avoid an intravenous injection of LA. The block may be patchy with a better effect on one side of the body occurring, usually the right side. A top-up by the anaesthetist with the woman lying on the affected side may work. Total analgesia may be impossible for a few women.

Local Anaesthetic Toxicity

This may be caused by overinfusion of LA or rapid administration and leads to cardiac arrest. There is probable fetal compromise. Stop the epidural with immediate resuscitation.

Neurological Sequelae (Damage)

This is rare but can be the result of any epidural complications. Serious damage is extremely rare. Weakness/sensory loss is uncommon and resolves quickly.

Other Related Complications

- Increased incidence in assisted vaginal births as confirmed by systematic review (Anim-Somuah et al., 2018). This is due to reduced muscle tone of the pelvic floor, resulting in difficulty in bearing down. A systematic review found insufficient evidence to support the discontinuation of epidural analgesia in late labour to reduce the rate of instrumental delivery (Torvaldsen et al., 2004).
- Loss of bladder sensation in labour often results in urinary bladder catheterization.
- Long-term backache is a common problem during childbirth due to pregnancy hormones softening ligaments. No evidence from systematic review to suggest epidurals have any impact (Anim-Somuah et al., 2018).

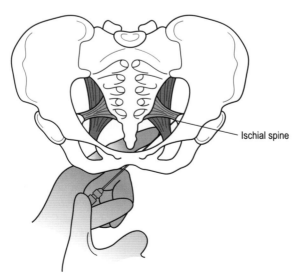

• **Fig. 38.8** Pudendal nerve block.

Ischial spine

Pudendal Block

This is the infiltration by the obstetrician of a LA agent via a transvaginal route into an area around the pudendal nerve (Fig. 38.8). The pudendal nerve originates from S2–S4 and passes across the ischial spine. A pudendal block needle is used, which is a special needle with a guide. Lidocaine (lignocaine) is introduced just below each ischial spine. Analgesia of the lower vagina and perineum results and is suitable for use in forceps or breech deliveries. Perineal repair may be carried out using the same analgesia, although perineal infiltration would be more usual.

Perineal Infiltration

This is the use of a LA to infiltrate the perineum for either performance of an episiotomy or suturing: 10 Lidocaine (lignocaine) 1% solution is distributed by fan-like injections (as per clinical guidelines). Precautions are taken to avoid the inadvertent intravascular injection of the drug.

Main Points

- The chemicals bradykinin, prostaglandin and histamine are involved in local production of inflammation and pain. Although the physiological threshold for pain sensation may be similar, cognitive and emotive factors alter the individual's reaction and experience of pain.

- Somatic pain is deep or superficial. Superficial pain tends to be brief, highly localized and sharp or pricking in character. Deep somatic pain is described as burning or aching, is more diffuse and lasts longer. Visceral pain results from organs of the body cavities and is described as burning, gnawing or aching. The brain plays a large part in pain modulation.

- Endorphins (opiate-like peptides) are found in the limbic system, hypothalamus and reticular formation. These inhibit prostaglandin production, a key chemical necessary for pain perception.

- The gate control theory of pain is one theory for childbirth pain. Inputs from large myelinated fibres conveying touch and fibres conveying pain interact at the spinal cord level. The large-diameter sensory nerve impulses come into the spinal cord more rapidly, inhibiting the slower pain impulses presynaptically. This constitutes the gate against small-diameter fibre impulses. If the gate is closed, pain is blocked (not part of conscious thought). If the gate is open, the impulses and messages pass through and are transmitted freely (pain is experienced).

- Besides physical, emotional and cognitive factors affecting pain perception, abnormalities of labour may cause an increase in perceived pain. Pain may be increased in labours complicated by prolongation, occipitoposterior position and cephalopelvic disproportion.

- Pain may cause increased levels of catecholamine secretion, leading to increased cardiac output, heart rate and BP; hyperventilation with maternal alkalosis, decreased cerebral and uterine blood flow due to vasoconstriction, decreased uterine contractions and delayed stomach and bladder emptying.

- Both pharmacological and non-pharmacological methods of pain relief are utilized in labour.

- TENS depends on the physiology of the gate in the spinal cord. It interrupts pain transmission and stimulates the release of endogenous opiates.

- The most common labour analgesics are diamorphine, pethidine and Entonox gas (50% O_2 and 50% N_2O). Entonox has no fetal side effects and can be used with other forms of analgesia.

- Epidural analgesia provides adequate pain relief. Indications for epidural analgesia include maternal choice, prolonged labour, malpresentations, malpositions, multiple pregnancy and hypertensive conditions.

- Contraindications for epidural analgesia include maternal reluctance, sepsis, haemorrhagic disease, clotting disorder and spinal deformity.

- Pudendal block results in analgesia of the lower vagina and perineum and is suitable for use in forceps or breech deliveries. Perineal infiltration is performed before an episiotomy or suturing.

- Alternative therapies and techniques (non-pharmacological methods) are accepted in labour. Midwives and others need to be appropriately trained in their use for professional practice.

References

Anderson, D., 2011. A review of systemic opioids commonly used for labor pain relief. J. Midwifery Wom. Health 56 (94), 222–239.

Anim-Somuah, M., Smyth, R.M., Cyna, A.M., Cuthbert, A., 2018. Epidural versus non-epidural or no analgesia for pain management in labour. Cochrane Database Syst. Rev. 5 (5), CD000331.

Birkett, A., Carlson, N.R., 2017. Physiology of Behavior. Pearson, Boston.

Bohren, M.A., Hofmeyr, G.J., Sakala, C., Fukuzawa, R.K., Cuthbert, A., 2017. Continuous support for women during childbirth. Cochrane Database Syst. Rev. 7 (7), CD003766.

Boring, B.L., Walsh, K.T., Nanavaty, N., Ng, B.W., Mathur, V.A., 2021. How and why patient concerns influence pain reporting: a qualitative analysis of personal accounts and perceptions of others' use of numerical pain scales. Front. Psychol. 12, 663890.

Cluett, E.R., Burns, E., Cuthbert, A., 2018. Immersion in water during labour and birth. Cochrane Database Syst. Rev. 5 (5), CD000111.

Feeley, C., Cooper, M., Burns, E., 2021. A systematic meta-thematic synthesis to examine the views and experiences of women following immersion during labour and waterbirth. J. Adv. Nurs. 77 (7) 2942–2942.

Hofmeyr, G.J., Cyna, A.M., Middleton, P., 2004. Prophylactic intravenous preloading for regional analgesia in labour. Cochrane Database Syst. Rev. 2004 (4), CD000175.

Jackson, K., Anderson, M., Marshall, J.E., 2020. Physiology and care during the first stage of labour. In: Marshall, J., Raynor, M. (Eds.), Myles' Textbook for Midwives, seventeenth ed. Elsevier, London.

Jones, L., Othman, M., Dowswell, T., Alfirevic, Z., Gates, S., Newburn, M., et al. 2012. Pain management for women in labour: an overview of systematic reviews. Cochrane Database Syst. Rev. 2012 (3), CD009234.

Kadirogullari, P., Yalcin Bahat, P., Sahin, B., Gonen, I., Seckin, K.D., 2021. The effect of pethidine analgesia on labor duration and maternal outcomes. Acta Biomed. 92 (2), e2021065.

Leap, N., Anderson, P., 2008. The role of pain in normal birth and empowerment of women. In: Downe, S. (Ed.), Normal Childbirth Evidence and Debate, second ed. Churchill Livingston, London.

Lönnberg, G., Nissen, E., Niemi, M., 2018. What is learned from mindfulness based childbirth and parenting education? – participants' experiences. BMC Pregnancy Childbirth 18 (1), 466.

Mander, R., 2011. Pain in Childbearing and its Control: Key Issues for Midwives and Women, second ed. Wiley-Blackwell, Oxford.

Marieb, E.N., Hoehn, K., 2022. Human Anatomy and Physiology, twelfth ed. Pearson, Harlow.

McMahon, S., Koltzenburg, M., Tracey, I., Dennis, C., 2013. Wall & Melzack's Textbook of Pain, sixth ed. Elsevier Saunders, Philadelphia.

Melzack, R., Wall, P., 1988. The Challenge of Pain. Penguin, Harmondswift.

Nanji, J.A., Carvalho, B., 2020. Pain management during labor and vaginal birth. Best Pract. Res. Clin. Obstet. Gynaecol. 67, 100–112.

National Institute of Health and Care Excellence (NICE), 2023. Intrapartum Care. Available at: https://www.nice.org.uk/guidance/ng235.

Nursing and Midwifery Council (NMC), 2018. The Code: Professional Standards of Practice and Behaviour for Nurses, Midwives and Nursing Associates. Available at: https://www.nmc.org.uk/standards/code/read-the-code-online/.

Oteng-Ntim, E., Pavord, S., Howard, R., Robinson, S., Oakley, L., Mackillop, L., Pancham, S., et al., 2021. Management of sickle cell disease in pregnancy. A British Society for Haematology Guideline. Br. J. Haematol. 194 (6), 980–985.

Ritter, J.M., Flower, R.S., Henderson, G., Loke, Y.K., MacEwan, D., Rang, H., 2019. Rang & Dale's Pharmacology, ninth ed. Elsevier, London.

Simkin, P., Ancheta, R., 2017. The Labor Progress Handbook: Early Interventions to Prevent and Treat Dystocia, fourth ed. Wiley-Blackwell, Oxford.

Simmons, S.W., Taghizadeh, N., Dennis, A.T., Hughes, D., Cyna, A.M., 2012. Combined spinal-epidural versus epidural analgesia in labour. Cochrane Database Syst. Rev. 10 (10), CD003401.

Smith, L.A., Burns, E., Cuthbert, A., 2018. Parenteral opioids for maternal pain management in labour. Cochrane Database Syst. Rev. 6 (6), CD007396.

Smith, C.A., Levett, K.M., Collins, C.T., Armour, M., Dahlen, H.G., Suganuma, M., 2018a. Relaxation techniques for pain management in labour. Cochrane Database Syst. Rev. 3 (3), CD009514.

Smith, C.A., Levett, K.M., Collins, C.T., Dahlen, H.G., Ee, C.C., Suganuma, M., 2018b. Massage, reflexology and other manual methods for pain management in labour. Cochrane Database Syst. Rev. 3 (3), CD009290.

Smith, C.A., Collins, C.T., Levett, K.M., Armour, M., Dahlen, H.G., Tan, A.L., et al. 2020. Acupuncture or acupressure for pain management during labour. Cochrane Database Syst. Rev. 2 (2), CD009232.

Torvaldsen, S., Roberts, C.L., Bell, J.C., Raynes-Greenow, C.H., 2004. Discontinuation of epidural analgesia late in labour for reducing the adverse delivery outcomes associated with epidural analgesia. Cochrane Database Syst. Rev. 2004 (4), CD004457.

Walsh, D., 2012. Evidence-based Care for normal Labour and Birth: A Guide for Midwives, second ed. Routledge, London.

Annotated recommended reading

McMahon, S., Koltzenburg, M., Tracey, I., Dennis, C., 2013. Wall & Melzack's Textbook of Pain, sixth ed. Elsevier Saunders, Philadelphia.

This textbook of pain remains current and provides a more in-depth and detailed explanation and illustration of the gate control theory.

Ritter, J.M., Flower, R.S., Henderson, G., Loke, Y.K., MacEwan, D., Rang, H., 2019. Rang & Dale's Pharmacology, ninth ed. Elsevier, London.

The approach of this comprehensive textbook emphasizes the mechanisms by which drugs act and relates these to the overall pharmacological effects and clinical issues.

Websites

https://www.cochranelibrary.com/cdsr/about-cdsr.

This website provides a series of systematic reviews on pain management as it relates to childbirth. The reader should visit this site to obtain evidence-based, informed specific strategies for pain in labour.

https://www.nice.org/uk/.

This website provides an excellent resource for evidence-based guidelines in a wide range of topics. These include care of the woman and fetus/baby during pregnancy, childbirth and the postnatal period. In particular refer to the guidelines on methods and doses of pain relief in the Intrapartum Care section.

39

The Second Stage of Labour

LYZ HOWIE AND JEAN WATSON

This chapter details the physiological processes involved in the second stage of labour. The mechanisms involved in labour and birth are described in depth with illustrations. Routine management of labour includes maternal position, maternal effort with details of the intervention of episiotomy and repair. It is essential for students and midwives to have robust knowledge and clear understanding of these processes and management to provide optimal care to the woman in labour.

Introduction

The physiological changes that occur in the second stage are a continuation of the forces that have been occurring in the first stage of labour. There is now no impediment to descent of the fetus through the birth canal and to its birth. The second stage of labour begins when the cervix is fully dilated (Fig. 39.1) and ends when the fetus is fully expelled from the birth canal (Coad, Pedley & Dunstall, 2019).

Physiology of the Second Stage of Labour

Contractions

There is often a brief lull in uterine activity at the end of the first stage before the contractions take on their expulsive nature. The character of the contractions changes from that of the first stage. They become longer and stronger but may be less frequent so that the woman and fetus can recover between each expulsive effort. There is continued contraction and retraction of the upper uterine segment as oxytocin receptors are more dominant in the fundal region (Coad, Pedley & Dunstall, 2019). The fetus descends the birth canal, and fetal axis pressure increases flexion and reduces the size of the presenting part.

The Secondary Powers

A reflex occurs when pressure is exerted on the rectum and pelvic floor, where the woman feels a compelling urge to push (the **active phase**). Ferguson's reflex (Ferguson, 1941) has been discussed in Chapter 36. Spontaneous bearing-down efforts made by a woman occur for about 5–6 s several times during the contraction. Compaction of the fetus occurs during the contraction, and pressure on the fetal head may evoke vagal stimuli, causing a transient fall in fetal heart rate with a rapid recovery. Reduction in oxygen supply due to compression of the placenta will add to this effect. A recent systematic review highlighted that there was no routine pushing style that was more effective when comparing indirect or direct pushing and more research is required (Lemos et al., 2017). Women in the expulsive phase of the second stage of labour should be encouraged and supported to follow their own urge to push (National Institute of Health and Care Excellence (NICE), 2023; World Health Organization (WHO), 2018).

Descent of the Fetus

As the fetus descends the birth canal, it displaces the soft tissues contained in the pelvis. Anteriorly, the bladder is pushed up into the abdominal cavity, which results in stretching and thinning of the urethra (Coad, Pedley & Dunstall, 2019). Posteriorly, the rectum becomes flattened in the sacral curve, and any faecal matter may be expelled. The muscles of the pelvic floor thin out and are displaced laterally (Coad, Pedley & Dunstall, 2019). The perineal body is stretched and thinned.

The fetal head now becomes visible at the vulva and advances with each contraction to recede slightly between contractions until crowning. The baby is born thereafter, accompanied by a gush of amniotic fluid. The second stage culminates as soon as the baby is completely born.

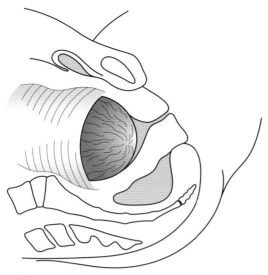

• **Fig. 39.1** The os uteri is fully dilated and the head enters the vagina.

Onset of the Second Stage

There is often no clear demarcation between the end of the first stage and the beginning of the second stage. Several signs can be taken as indicative that the second stage has begun. Downe & Marshall (2020) outline the **presumptive signs** of the onset of the second stage of labour and differential diagnoses (Table 39.1). The appearance of several of the signs together may indicate that the second stage of labour has begun, but the midwife must use her skills to confirm this. It is sometimes necessary to confirm the absence of the cervix by vaginal examination (VE).

Duration of the Second Stage

NICE (2023) defines the second stage of labour as passive and active. Passive is where the cervix is found to be fully dilated before or with no involuntary or expulsive contractions present. Active is where the fetus is now visible along with expulsive contractions and full dilatation of the cervix on VE or other signs of full dilatation of the cervix, or active maternal effort after confirmation of full dilatation of the cervix on VE without expulsive contractions (NICE, 2023).

The duration of the active second stage for primigravidae can be up to 3 hours (NICE, 2023; WHO, 2018). Consider inadequate progress after 1 hour of the active second stage (in terms of rotation and/or descent of the presenting part) and offer VE and amniotomy (if membranes are not ruptured) (NICE, 2023). Action and referral to medical staff should be undertaken after 2 hours if birth is not imminent (NICE, 2023). In multiparous women, it can be up to 2 hours (WHO, 2018). Consider inadequate progress after 30 min of the active second stage (in terms of rotation and/or descent of the presenting part) and offer VE and amniotomy (if membranes are not ruptured) (NICE, 2023). Action and referral should be after 1 hour if birth is not imminent (NICE, 2023). Women can be unpredictable and may have a second

TABLE 39.1	The Presumptive Signs of the Second Stage of Labour
Presumptive Sign	**Differential Diagnosis**
Expulsive uterine contractions	An urge to push before full cervical dilatation may occur if the rectum is full; more a physiological response in some woman than a pathological response.
Rupture of forewaters	May occur at any time in labour.
Dilatation and gaping of anus	Deep engagement of presenting part and premature maternal pushing may be the cause.
Anal cleft line	A purple-red line which is observed at buttock cleft and climbs up anal cleft as labour progresses. Positive correlation between purple line and station of the fetal head in Iranian woman and other research is required for other races (Irani, Kordi & Esmaily, 2018).
Rhomboid of Michaelis	A 'dome-shaped curve' is seen in the woman's lower back. This is displacement of sacrum and coccyx as the occiput progresses into sacral curve. The woman throws her buttocks forward, arches her back and throws her arms back to grasp onto something. This is thought to be a physiological response to optimize the process of the fetus through the birth canal by lengthening and straightening the curve of Carus.
Upper abdominal pressure and epidural analgesia	Women who have been epiduralized have reported upper abdominal pressure or discomfort under the ribs when the second stage occurs. More evidence is required to substantiate this finding.
Show	Bloodstained mucous from rapid dilatation of cervical os. Cause of this bleeding must be identified to exclude antepartum haemorrhage.
Appearance of presenting part	Usually, conclusive. However excessive moulding and caput succedaneum formation may protrude through the cervix before full dilatation, as may a breech presentation.

(Downe & Marshall, 2020)

stage that lasts only a few minutes. There have been challenges to the concept that the exact timing of the second stage of labour is possible, and rather than an estimated time limit, progress is a more useful indicator of normality. Therefore, base decisions on progress with evidence of adequate uterine contractions, descent and continuing good maternal and fetal well-being rather than timings.

As the fetal head descends due to the force of uterine contractions and stretches the tissues of the vagina and pelvic floor, it will become visible at the vaginal orifice. Once the fetal head is visible, pressure on the rectum will normally provide the reflex stimulus for maternal expulsive pushing and the active phase begins. Pressure of the fetus on the sacral nerves will result in the woman experiencing pain from trauma to the tissue and sometimes leg cramps (Coad, Pedley & Dunstall, 2019).

Mechanisms of Labour

The fetus is in effect a cylinder which must negotiate the curved birth canal formed of the bony pelvis and soft tissues of the perineal body. Moulding of the skull to reduce the presenting diameters is described elsewhere. This section will discuss the passive movements that the fetus makes in response to the forces exerted on it by the birth canal.

Collectively, these movements are called the **mechanisms of labour** and the fetus is turned slightly to take advantage of the widest part of each plane of the pelvis. The plane of the inlet is widest in the transverse, and the outlet is widest in the anteroposterior diameter. Knowledge of mechanisms enables the midwife to use skills to facilitate birth with least trauma to the mother and fetus. It may be lifesaving to understand what is occurring inside the woman's body so that external manoeuvres can be used to complete delivery.

Different mechanisms occur depending on the presentation and position of the fetus, and there are principles common to all:

- Descent of the fetus takes place.
- The part of the fetus that leads and meets the resistance of the pelvic floor will rotate forwards to come to lie anteriorly under the symphysis pubis.
- Whatever part of the fetus emerges will pivot around the pubic bone.

The Mechanism of a Normal Labour

There is a classical way of recalling the situation of a fetus at the commencement of the second stage of labour. The terms are described in Chapter 37. Box 39.1 provides an overview of the situation of the fetus for a normal labour.

The Movements

The movements of the fetus involved in the normal mechanisms of labour are:
- Descent.
- Flexion.
- Internal rotation of the head.
- Crowning and extension of the head.
- Restitution.
- Internal rotation of the shoulders and external rotation of the head.
- Lateral flexion.

For a further explanation see Box 39.2 and for illustrations of the movements see Figs. 39.2–39.8.

• BOX 39.1 Situation of a Fetus in Normal Labour

- The **lie** is longitudinal.
- The **attitude** is one of good flexion.
- The **presentation** is cephalic.
- The **position** is right or left occipitoanterior.
- The **denominator** is the occiput.
- The **presenting part** is the posterior part of the anterior parietal bone.

• BOX 39.2 Normal Mechanisms of Labour

Descent: Descent of fetal head into the pelvis may have occurred in the antenatal period so the woman, especially a primigravidae, begins labour with the head engaged. This may indicate that vaginal delivery is likely. The sagittal suture is in the transverse diameter of the pelvis. There is continued descent during the first stage of labour, and this is speeded up by maternal effort during the second stage of labour.

Flexion: The attitude determines which diameter will present in labour. The fetal head is in an attitude of natural flexion. Flexion of the fetal head on the trunk is increased during labour because the skull is attached to the fetal spine nearer the occiput than the sinciput. Pressure transmitted from the fundus of the uterus down the fetal spine will force the occiput lower than the sinciput, increasing flexion and resulting in the conversion of the suboccipitofrontal diameter of approximately 10 cm to the favourable suboccipitobregmatic diameter of approximately 9.5 cm.

Internal rotation of the head: As the leading part is driven onto the pelvic floor, the resistance of the muscular diaphragm and its gutter shape, sloping downwards anteriorly, cause the

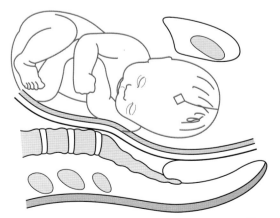

• Fig. 39.2 Descent of a well-flexed head into the pelvis. The sagittal suture is in the transverse diameter of the pelvis.

Continued

• **BOX 39.2** **Normal Mechanisms of Labour—cont'd**

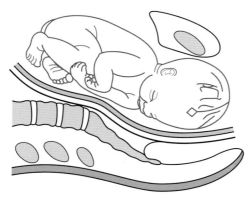

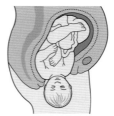

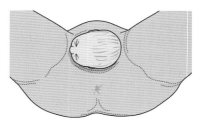

• **Fig. 39.6** Internal rotation of the shoulders and external rotation of the head.

• **Fig. 39.3** Internal rotation. The sagittal suture is normally in the oblique diameter of the pelvis and as further descent occurs rotates into the anteroposterior diameter of the pelvis.

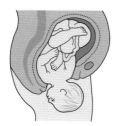

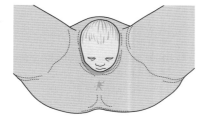

• **Fig. 39.4** Crowning and extension of the head.

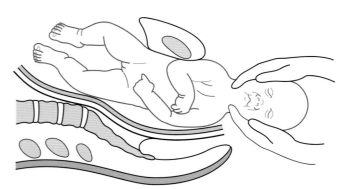

• **Fig. 39.7** Gentle downward traction is applied to deliver the anterior shoulder.

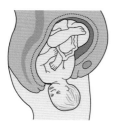

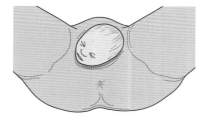

• **Fig. 39.5** Restitution of the head.

occiput to rotate forwards in the pelvis by one-eighth of a circle (45 degrees) to lie under the symphysis pubis; the anteroposterior diameter of the head now lies in the anteroposterior diameter of the pelvis, which is the largest diameter. This causes a slight twist on the fetal neck so that the head is misaligned to the shoulders.

Crowning and extension of the head: The occiput escapes from beneath the subpubic arch and the smallest possible diameters (suboccipitobregmatic approximately 9.5 cm and biparietal approximately 9.5 cm) distend the vaginal orifice. This is termed *crowning,* and the head no longer retracts in between contractions. The head is now born by extension as it pivots on the suboccipital region around the pubic bone. The sinciput, face and chin sweep the perineum. The widest diameter to distend the vagina is the suboccipitofrontal (approximately 10 cm) as the sinciput is born.

Restitution: Restitution is a movement made by the head after delivery which brings it into correct alignment with the shoulders. This will be one-eighth of a circle towards the side from which it started.

Internal rotation of the shoulders and external rotation of the head: The anterior shoulder is the first to reach the pelvic floor, and this now rotates forward to lie under the symphysis

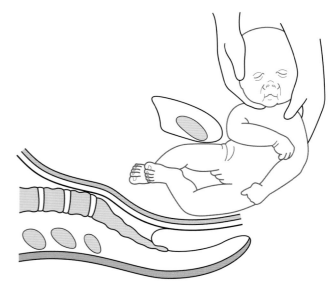

• **Fig. 39.8** The posterior shoulder is delivered and then the trunk by lateral flexion.

pubis. This movement is accompanied by external rotation of the head by one-eighth of a circle (45 degrees) more in the direction of restitution. The occiput now lies laterally, turned towards the woman's thigh.

Lateral flexion: Shoulders are born sequentially, where the anterior shoulder is usually born first and slips under the pubic arch and then the posterior shoulder passes over the perineum. The remainder of the body is born by lateral flexion as the spine bends laterally on its way through the curved birth canal.

Physiological Changes

Coad, Pedley & Dunstall (2019) outline some of the physiological principles which should underlie the management of the second stage of labour. These include:

- Hormonal influences and primitive physiological processes.
- Position of the mother.
- Passage of the fetus through pelvis.
- Condition of mother and baby.
- The bearing-down reflex.
- Thinning of the perineum.

The Length of the Second Stage of Labour

The definition at the beginning of this chapter states that the second stage begins with full cervical dilatation. At the time the woman's cervix has reached full dilatation, it may be 3 or 4 hours from a previous VE and it is not possible to know exactly when full dilatation occurred. Therefore this could introduce elements of bias in determining the actual overall length of the second stage of labour.

The second stage of labour begins when the cervix is fully dilated and ends when the fetus is fully expelled from the birth canal (Coad, Pedley & Dunstall, 2019; WHO, 2018). Midwives and medical colleagues have used this definition to base the management of the delivery of the baby according to a time regimen. This suggests that the exact timing of the second stage of labour is possible. This concept has been challenged. It is probable that careful monitoring of progress (NICE, 2023) rather than an estimated time limit is more useful as an indicator of normality.

Management

An important milestone for midwifery practice was a review of the management of women in the normal second stage of labour undertaken by Thomson (1988). She described with feeling and accuracy the control exerted over the labouring woman, including position, forced expulsive efforts and the concentration on the vulva. She concluded that the available literature on managing the second stage suggested an inter-relationship between three factors:

1. The position of the woman.
2. The means by which the woman exerts pressure to assist the uterus to expel the baby.
3. The length of the second stage of labour.

These three factors remain valid today and will be used as a plan for discussing the physiological management of labour.

Position of the Woman

In most other cultures in the world and in Europe until the 18th century, women used a variety of positions during the second stage of labour. Irrespective of the position used for delivery, women have tended to deliver with abducted thighs in an upright position. Upright positions include standing, kneeling, sitting on birthing chairs and squatting. The lying-down dorsal position may have originated in France because of the wish of Louis XIV to witness the delivery of the baby of his mistress but has been perpetuated for the ease of the medical profession. In Britain, the left lateral position may have originated as the 'London position' advocated by Smellie in 1752 (Thomson, 1988). The position a woman will adopt in labour is related to the context in which the birth is taking place (Walsh, 2012). Most standard labour ward rooms have a bed as the central feature. Walsh (2012) advocates that measures could be taken to position the bed against a wall or remove it altogether from the room to decrease the bed's status in childbirth!

Historically the recumbent position has been the most common position for delivery, where supine hypotension can occur, which may adversely affect fetal oxygenation. Adopting a more upright position might lead to a slight reduction in length of second stage (mainly primigravidae), reduction in episiotomy rates and reduction in assisted deliveries (Gupta et al., 2017). If the woman lies on her back, there will be a significant reduction in maternal cardiac output and circulation of oxygenated blood through the placental tissue due to compression of the inferior vena cava and descending aorta. This does not happen if the woman lies on her side or if the uterus is tilted to the left. The upright posture has many beneficial physiological effects on the progress of the second stage, which are identified in Box 39.3. It is worthy of consideration about a woman's preference for position in labour, especially if they have been subjected to abuse as some positions may act as a trigger (Simkin, Hanson & Ancheta, 2017).

Squatting

Squatting is probably the most common position for childbirth in the developing world. The mother may need the support of two people, or she may support herself with her back to a wall or firm surface. The flexion and abduction of the thighs brought about by squatting has several advantages (Simkin, Hanson & Ancheta, 2017) (Box 39.4). However, if the fetal head is at a relatively high station and asynclitic, squatting may impede correction of the angle of the head

---

> ### BOX 39.3 Physiological Effects of an Upright Position in Labour

- Allows gravity to play its part in the descent of the fetus.
- Increases the diameters of the pelvic outlet.
- Better alignment of the fetus through the birth canal.
- Increases the efficiency and strength of uterine contractions.
- Reduces the incidence of aortocaval compression, which ultimately improves the acid–base balance of the baby.

(See Chapter 24)
(Gupta et al., 2017; Simkin, Hanson & Ancheta, 2017)

- Provides the advantage of gravity.
- Enlarges the pelvic outlet by increasing the intertuberous diameter.
- Reduces bearing-down effort.
- Enhances fetal descent.
- Allows freedom to shift weight comfortably.
- Provides mechanical advantage: upper trunk presses on fundus more than any other position.
- Enhances the urge to push.
- Relieves backache.

(Gupta et al., 2012; Simkin, Hanson & Ancheta, 2017)

- Aids fetal rotation from the occipitoposterior or occipital transverse position.
- Aids in reduction of an anterior lip in late first stage.
- Allows the woman freedom to sway, crawl or rock the pelvis, which can promote rotation and increase comfort.
- Reduces back pain and relieves pressure on the anus (haemorrhoids).
- May resolve fetal heart problems that are mainly due to cord compression.

(Simkin, Hanson & Ancheta, 2017)

by reducing the space available for the fetus to move into synclitism (Simkin, Hanson & Ancheta, 2017). If squatting is continued for a prolonged period, the woman should lean back or rise after every contraction to prevent compression of the blood vessels and nerves located behind the knee joints (Simkin, Hanson & Ancheta, 2017).

Hands and Knees/All-Fours Positions

Women may often adopt a kneeling position themselves. This position also has advantages, which are outlined in Box 39.5. The position allows access for VE (Simkin, Hanson & Ancheta, 2017), provides an excellent view of the fetus and perineum and causes less perineal trauma, although there may be an increase in vulval trauma.

Birthing Chairs

Birthing chairs have been an alternative for supporting women in the squatting position, giving the midwife good vision and access to the fetus. However, problems are associated with their use, including a higher mean blood loss and an increase in postpartum haemorrhage (PPH). However, there is a lack of robust-quality evidence to determine the overall effect of their use on maternal and fetal outcomes (Gupta et al., 2017).

Review of Upright Positions

There has been controversy about whether being upright or lying down has advantages for women birthing their babies.

In a systematic review of research studies, Gupta et al. (2017) considered the benefits and risks associated with the upright positions in the second stage of labour. The reviewers concluded that upright positions were associated with a reduction in both assisted deliveries and episiotomies and a small reduction in duration of the second stage for primigravidae. They reported a small increase in second-degree tears and an increased risk of blood loss >500 mL, although the results were inconclusive (See Chapter 24). These are tentative findings, and further well-controlled studies are required. Women should be encouraged to give birth in the position they find most comfortable but avoiding supine or semi-supine positions (NICE, 2023).

Maternal Effort in the Second Stage of Labour

The second stage of labour begins with full dilatation of the cervix (Coad, Pedley & Dunstall, 2019), but the presenting part may not yet be visible at the pelvic outlet and the woman may not have an urge to bear down. As the fetal head descends due to the force of uterine contractions and stretches the tissues of the vagina and pelvic floor, it will become visible at the vaginal orifice. Once the fetal head is visible, pressure on the rectum will normally provide the reflex stimulus for maternal expulsive pushing and the active phase begins (NICE, 2023).

Before the 1990s, it was customary practice for birth attendants to give women formal instructions during the second stage of labour (Watson, 1994). The rationale for this was to reduce the length of the second stage of labour and reduce fetal stress. Women were often encouraged to take a big breath at the start of each contraction and bear down as long and as hard as they could. This is known as the *Valsalva manoeuvre* and uses forced expiration against a closed glottis (Pstras et al., 2016) to increase intra-abdominal pressure to aid the uterus to expel the fetus. This manoeuvre causes the blood pressure to drop and rise again, and women using the technique have shown alterations in heart rate and brain wave patterns. Forced pushing has been implicated as the cause of burst capillaries in the face and eyes, and rarely cerebrovascular accidents (strokes) may occur. Fetal outcome is also affected if this manoeuvre is utilized (Monteiro et al., 2021).

There is no evidence to suggest that any benefits are gained from routine directed pushing (Lemos et al., 2017). Current practice now recommends that directed pushing be abandoned and women should be encouraged to follow their instincts and preferences (Coad, Pedley & Dunstall, 2019; Lemos et al., 2017). The midwife's role should be to affirm physiology, not control it or deny it, and to encourage women-centred approaches, which promote normality.

Effect on Pelvic Soft Tissues

Beynon (1957) theorized that in the early part of a contraction, the vaginal muscles are drawn taut to prevent the bladder supports and transverse cervical ligaments being pushed down in front of the baby's head. Bearing down by the mother helps to overcome the resistance of the soft tissues of the vagina and the pelvic floor. Spontaneous pushing with its associated breaks is a natural process to help prevent perineal trauma (Coad, Pedley & Dunstall, 2019). Active pushing during the latent phase of the second stage of labour may strain the uterine supports and the vaginal and perineal muscle before these tissues have a chance to stretch gradually. Early expulsive effort may lead to incontinence and prolapsed uterus later in life.

Perineal Lacerations

During the second stage of labour, **perineal lacerations** may occur. Previously an episiotomy was conducted to control the extent of these lacerations. However, evidence does not support routine episiotomy being conducted (NICE, 2023; Jiang et al., 2017). NICE (2023) also advocates that routine episiotomy is not offered for previous third- and fourth-degree tears. Perineal lacerations are classified depending on the depth of tissue involved in the tear (Box 39.6).

An **episiotomy** is a surgical incision of the perineum made to increase the diameter of the vulval outlet during the last part of the second stage of labour or delivery (Carroli & Mignini, 2009). The tissues involved are the same as those in a second-degree tear, namely perineal skin or vaginal mucosa, perineum and perineal body (superficial bulbospongious (previously known as bulbocavernosus) and transversus perinei muscles, deep pelvic floor pubococcygeus muscle) (NICE, 2023; Royal College of Obstetricians and Gynaecologists [RCOG], 2015; Wilson, 2017).

Other tissues may be lacerated during delivery. **Labial lacerations** are not usually severe enough to require suturing but can be very painful, especially during micturition. However, if they are bilateral labial lacerations, suturing might be required to prevent abnormal fusion of these tissues. **Vaginal lacerations** may bleed severely and need immediate pressure to control bleeding followed by suturing.

The Episiotomy

An episiotomy is a deliberate surgical incision of the perineum, through the structures involved in a second-degree tear. A midwife's role is to perform an episiotomy and infiltrate the perineum with local anaesthetic when this procedure is required. The midwife must assess the need for this procedure and deliver evidence-based care to a high standard of practice (Nursing & Midwifery Council, 2018). The rationale for the incision is to enlarge the vulval outlet to facilitate delivery (Carroli & Mignini, 2009). Early studies demonstrated that the performance of an episiotomy was not a valid reason to prevent perineal trauma (Sleep, 1984a; Sleep, 1984b). Findings indicated that there was no reduction in trauma to the pelvic floor, nor did women suffer less pain or swelling; indeed many women felt more pain. The perineal wound, whether a tear or episiotomy, healed in a similar manner. RCOG (2015) guidelines acknowledge that the protective effect of episiotomy is conflicting but stipulate that the mediolateral episiotomy should be considered for instrumental deliveries.

• BOX 39.6 Classification of Perineal Laceration

- **First-degree** tear: a tear that only involves the perineal skin and/or vaginal mucosa.
- **Second-degree** tear: a tear that involves perineal skin, vaginal mucosa and perineal muscles (superficial bulbospongious (previously known as bulbocavernosus) and transversus perinei muscles, deep pelvic floor pubococcygeus muscle) but not the anal sphincter.
- **Third-degree** tear: a tear that involves perineal skin, vaginal mucosa and perineal muscles (superficial bulbospongious (previously known as bulbocavernosus) and transversus perinei muscles, deep pelvic floor pubococcygeus muscle) and the anal sphincter. This category is further divided depending on the degree of anal sphincter involvement:
  - **3a:** less than 50% of external anal sphincter torn.
  - **3b:** more than 50% of external anal sphincter torn.
  - **3c:** external and internal anal sphincters torn.
  N.B. If there is any doubt about third-degree classification, it is advisable to opt for the higher degree rather than the lower one.
- **Fourth-degree tear:** a tear that involves the perineal skin, vaginal mucosa and perineal muscles (superficial bulbospongious (previously known as bulbocavernosus) and transversus perinei muscles, deep pelvic floor iliococcygeus muscle), as well as the external and internal anal sphincters and anal mucosa (Hinshaw & Arulkumaran, 2018; NICE, 2023; RCOG, 2015; Wilson, 2017).

Recommendations for Performing an Episiotomy

During the antenatal period, women should be given a chance to discuss the possible need for the midwife to make an episiotomy to avoid confrontation situations in an emergency. The WHO, (2018) recommends that there should be no routine or liberal use of episiotomy for spontaneous vaginal birth. The woman's wishes should be recorded on her birth plan. Informed consent and adequate analgesia are essential when performing an episiotomy (WHO, 2018), unless in an emergency for acute fetal compromise (NICE, 2023).

Guidance on when to perform an episiotomy in current practice are in Box 39.7.

The Incision

There are two types of incisions: the mediolateral and the midline (Fig. 39.9). The mediolateral is the recommended incision because it avoids damage to Bartholin's gland and is less likely to extend in the midline and involve the anal sphincter. To perform the mediolateral episiotomy, the start of the episiotomy incision starts at the middle of the vaginal fourchette with the scissors directed to the maternal right (NICE, 2023). It is important that the angle to the vertical axis be between 45 and 60 degrees when making the episiotomy incision (NICE, 2023).

The perineum is infiltrated along the line of the intended episiotomy using 5–10 mL of lidocaine (lignocaine) 1% (Wilson, 2017) (Fig. 39.10). The practitioner should check carefully to avoid giving the injection intravenously and causing bradycardia or collapse. The anaesthetic takes effect very quickly, and the incision can then be made using episiotomy scissors. The incision is best made during a

- Performed for fetal compromise (NICE, 2023).
- Elective episiotomies for previous third- or fourth-degree tear are not routinely recommended (NICE, 2023).
- An episiotomy is performed for an instrumental birth (NICE, 2023; RCOG, 2015).
- Adequate analgesia is administered before episiotomy unless an emergency situation arises with fetal compromise (NICE, 2023).
- Informed consent should be obtained from the woman (WHO, 2018).

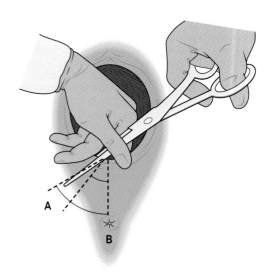

• **Fig. 39.9** Types of episiotomy incisions. (A) Mediolateral, (B) midline.

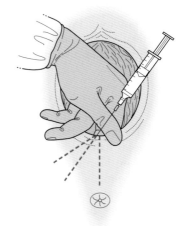

• **Fig. 39.10** Infiltration of the perineum.

contraction when the perineum is thinned out and should be approximately 4 cm long (Johnson & Taylor, 2023; Wilson, 2017). The practitioner should protect the fetal head during administration of the local anaesthetic and perform the episiotomy by inserting two fingers between the head and perineum (Figs. 39.9 and 39.10).

Suturing the Perineum

Many women who have a vaginal birth will have some degree of perineal trauma, with a large proportion of women requiring perineal suturing. Repair of the perineum is an integral part of the role of the midwife in intrapartum care. However, midwives must recognize situations where it is not appropriate for them to suture such as a third- or fourth-degree tear. The midwife should comply with the local policies for the use of suture materials, which should be based on up-to-date research. Aseptic technique is universal. The most important point is to explore the depth of the wound and ensure that the first suture is placed above its apex to prevent the development of a vaginal haematoma. A rectal examination should also be performed when identifying the degree of perineal trauma (NICE, 2023; RCOG, 2015)

Infiltration of the Perineum

Using an aseptic technique, infiltrate the perineum using 15–20 mL of lidocaine (lignocaine) 1% or equivalent (NICE, 2023) (the woman should be offered the use of Entonox inhalation analgesia if she has not had an effective epidural). Infiltration of the local anaesthetic can be inserted into the perineum using the following technique (Johnson & Taylor, 2023) (refer to Fig. 39.11 and to Clinical Application 39.1).

The perineum is then sutured in layers from the inside out (Fig. 39.12). A loose, continuous, non-locking subcuticular method of suturing is recommended (NICE, 2023) using synthetic suture material compared with catgut, as this results in less short-term pain with less requirement for analgesia and less requirement for re-suturing (Kettle, Dowswell & Ismail, 2010), although some women require removal of synthetic sutures due to lack of absorption (Kettle, Dowswell & Ismail, 2010). Women who had standard absorbable synthetic materials and more rapidly absorbing stitches experienced similar short- and long-term pain (Kettle, Dowswell & Ismail, 2010). After a systematic review, Kettle, Dowswell & Ismail (2012) stated that the continuous suturing techniques for perineal closure, compared with interrupted methods, are associated with less short-term pain, requirement for analgesia and removal of sutures. Another advantage is that using the continuous suture method involves less suture material being utilized (Kettle, Dowswell & Ismail, 2012).

Obstetric Anal Sphincter Injuries

Obstetric anal sphincter injuries (OASIS) are third- and fourth-degree perineal tears and are associated with maternal morbidity such as faecal incontinence, flatus, perineal pain and dyspareunia (Fernando et al., 2013). A midwife must be able to identify OASIS (Wilson, 2017) so that appropriate referral can be made, resulting in appropriate management and subsequent care. The structures that are involved in OASIS are specified in Box 39.6. All OASIS injuries should be repaired in theatre under regional or general anaesthetic by an appropriately trained medical practitioner (RCOG, 2015). Specific OASIS postoperative care includes antibiotic therapy, laxatives, physiotherapy input and follow-up review with clinicians specialized in OASIS (RCOG, 2015).

The Fetus in the Second Stage of Labour

The second stage of labour is a time of risk for the fetus, with distress related not only to hypoxia, but also to mechanical stress and trauma. The fetus in the second stage of labour will be discussed in Chapter 46.

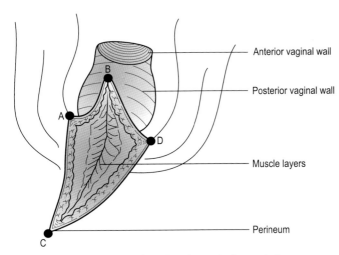

• **Fig. 39.11** Infiltration of perineum before suturing.

• CLINICAL APPLICATION 39.1 Infiltration of the Perineum

1. The tissue at point A is held with a pair of tissue forceps. The needle of the local anaesthetic syringe is injected into point A of the laceration with the tip of the needle going through the tissues and ending at point B.
2. The plunger of the syringe is then withdrawn, making sure that the needle is not in a blood vessel (the same method that is used before administering an intramuscular injection).
3. The local anaesthetic is then infiltrated into the perineal tissue using the withdrawal technique (i.e., infiltrating the local anaesthetic while withdrawing the needle backwards through the tissue from point B to point A).
4. Without removing the needle from point A, redirect the needle through the tissues so that the tip of the needle is at point C and continue to infiltrate the perineal tissue using the previously explained infiltration withdrawal technique.
5. Repeat these steps for the other side of the laceration by removing the needle completely and reinserting it into point D of the laceration.
6. Infiltrate this side of the tear by following the same principles so that you infiltrate from B to D and from C to D using the previously explained withdrawal technique.
7. Once adequate analgesia is effective, suturing may commence. If at any point the woman still feels discomfort stop and reassess for more analgesia.

(Johnson & Taylor, 2023)

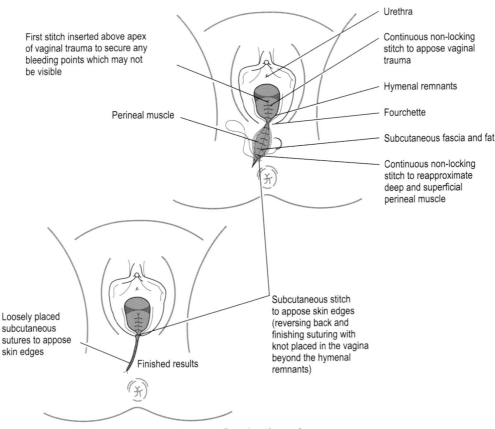

• **Fig. 39.12** Suturing the perineum.

Main Points

- At the end of the first stage of labour, there is often a brief lull in uterine activity before the contractions take on their expulsive nature, becoming longer and stronger but less frequent. The fetus descends the birth canal, and increasing flexion reduces the size of the presenting part.

- The second stage of labour begins with full dilatation of the cervix and ends when the fetus is fully expelled from the birth canal. Progress made during this stage rather than an estimated time limit is more useful as an indicator of normality.

- The duration of the second stage in multigravidae may be very short, whereas in primigravidae the process may take up to 3 hours. Two phases of the second stage of labour can be described: the passive and active phases. The passive phase begins at full dilatation of the cervix, but the woman may not have involuntary or expulsive contractions. The active phase is where the fetus is now visible, along with expulsive contractions and full dilatation of the cervix on VE or other signs of full dilatation of the cervix. Pressure on the rectum normally provides the stimulus for maternal expulsive pushing and the active phase begins.

- The upright posture allows gravity to aid descent of the fetus, increases uterine contraction efficiency and reduces the incidence of fetal distress and neonatal asphyxia. The squatting position for labour and delivery has several additional advantages: it enlarges the pelvic outlet, allows freedom to shift weight comfortably, may enhance the urge to push and hasten descent of the head and may relieve backache. The hands and knees position appears to relieve backache, aids rotation and descent and causes less perineal trauma.

- Current practice recommends that directed pushing should not be routine practice, with women encouraged to follow their instincts. The midwife's role should be to affirm physiology and to encourage women-centred approaches promoting normality.

- Perineal lacerations may occur during the second stage of labour. Labial lacerations may require suturing and can be painful during micturition. Vaginal and cervical lacerations may bleed severely and may need to be sutured immediately to control bleeding. OASIS injury requires specialist input and follow-up.

- The incision of an episiotomy aims to enlarge the vulval outlet immediately before delivery. Fetal compromise and clinical need are the justifications for performing an episiotomy. During the antenatal period, women should be given a chance to discuss the possible need for an episiotomy.

- Perineal repair is an integral part of the midwife's role. It is important to identify the degree of trauma sustained and ensure that the first suture is placed above its apex to prevent the development of a vaginal haematoma. The perineum is then sutured in layers from the inside tissues outwards with a continuous subcuticular method of suturing using synthetic suture material.

References

Beynon, C., 1957. The normal second stage of labour; a plea for reform in its conduct. J. Obstet. Gynaecol. Br. Emp. 64 (6), 815–820.

Carroli, G., Mignini, L., 2009. Episiotomy for vaginal birth. Cochrane Database Syst. Rev. 2009 (1), CD000081.

Coad, J., Pedley, K., Dunstall, M.J., 2019. Anatomy and Physiology for Midwives, fourth ed. Elsevier, London.

Downe, S., Marshall, J., 2020. Physiology and care during the transition and second stage phases of labour. In: Marshall, J., Raynor, M. (Eds.), Myles' Textbook for Midwives, seventeenth ed. Elsevier, Edinburgh.

Ferguson, J.K.W., 1941. A study of the motility of the intact uterus of the rabbit at term. Surg. Gynecol. Obstet. 73 (3), 359–366.

Fernando, R.J., Sultan, A.H., Kettle, C., Thakar, R., 2013. Methods of repair for obstetric anal sphincter injury. Cochrane Database Syst. Rev. 2013 (12), CD002866.

Gupta, J.K., Sood, A., Hofmeyr, G.J., Vogel, J.P., 2017. Position in the second stage of labour for women without epidural anaesthesia. Cochrane Database Syst. Rev. 2017 (5), CD002006.

Hinshaw, K., Arulkumaran, S., 2018. Malpresentation, malposition, cephalopelvic disproportion and obstetric procedures. In: Edmonds, D.K., Lees, C., Bourne, T.H. (Eds.), Dewhurst's Textbook of Obstetrics and Gynaecology, ninth ed. Wiley-Blackwell, Oxford.

Irani, M., Kordi, M., Esmaily, H., 2018. Relationship between length and width of the purple line and fetal head descent in active phase of labour. J. Obstet. Gynaecol. 38 (1), 10–15.

Jiang, H., Qian, X., Carroli, G., Garner, P., 2017. Selective versus routine use of episiotomy for vaginal birth. Cochrane Database Syst. Rev. 2017 (2), CD000081.

Johnson, R., Taylor, W., 2023. Skills for Midwifery Practice, fifth ed. Elsevier, London.

Kettle, C., Dowswell, T., Ismail, K.M.K., 2010. Absorbable suture materials for primary repair of episiotomy and second-degree tears. Cochrane Database Syst. Rev. 2010 (6), CD000006.

Kettle, C., Dowswell, T., Ismail, K.M.K., 2012. Continuous and interrupted suturing techniques for repair of episiotomy or second-degree tears. Cochrane Database Syst. Rev. 2012 (11), CD000947.

Lemos, A., Amorim, M.M., Dornelas de Andrade, A., de Souza, A.I., Cabral Filho, J.E., Correia, J.B., 2017. Pushing / bearing down methods for the second stage of labour. Cochrane Database Syst. Rev. 2017 (3), CD009124.

Monteiro, P.G., Coelho, T.S., de Lima, A.M., Ferreira, U.R., Monteiro, M.S.B., Esteche, C.M.G.C.E., et al., 2021. Neonatal outcomes associated with obstetric interventions performed during labor in nulliparous women. Rev. Rene. 22 (1), 1–8.

National Institute of Health and Care Excellence (NICE), 2023. Intrapartum Care. Available at: https://www.nice.org.uk/guidance/ng235.

Nursing & Midwifery Council (NMC), 2018. The Code. Available at: http://www.nmc-uk.org.

Pstras, L., Thomaseth, K., Waniewski, J., Balzani, I., Bellavere, F., 2016. The Valsalva manoeuvre: physiology and clinical examples. Acta Physiol. 217 (2), 103–119.

Royal College of Obstetricians and Gynaecologists (RCOG), 2015. The Management of Third- and Fourth-Degree Perineal Tears:

Guideline No. 29. RCOG, London. Available at: https://www.rcog .org.uk/guidance/browse-all-guidance/green-top-guidelines/third-and-fourth-degree-perineal-tears-management-green-top-guide-line-no-29.

Simkin, P., Hanson, L., Ancheta, R., 2017. The Labor Progress Handbook: Early Interventions to Prevent and Treat Dystocia, fourth ed. Wiley-Blackwell, Oxford.

Sleep, J., 1984a. Episiotomy in normal delivery 1. Nursing Times 80 (47), 29–30.

Sleep, J., 1984b. Episiotomy in normal delivery 2: the management of the perineum. Nursing Times 80 (48), 51–54.

Thomson, A.M., 1988. Management of the woman in normal second stage of labour: a review. Midwifery 4 (2), 77–85.

Walsh, D., 2012. Evidence and Skills for Normal Labour and Birth: A Guide for Midwives. Routledge, London.

Watson, V., 1994. Maternal position in the second stage of labour. Mod. Midwife 4 (7), 21–24.

World Health Organization (WHO), 2018. WHO Recommendations: Intrapartum Care for a Positive Childbirth Experience. WHO Press, Geneva. Available at: https://www.who.int/publications/i/item/9789241550215.

Wilson, A., 2017. The pelvic floor. In: MacDonald, S., Johnson, G. (Eds.), Mayes' Midwifery, fifteenth ed. Elsevier, Edinburgh.

Annotated recommended reading

Johnson, R., Taylor, W., 2023. Skills for Midwifery Practice, fifth ed. Elsevier, London.

This is a well-written book that covers the procedures related to perineal management.

Simkin, P., Hanson, L., Ancheta, R., 2017. The Labor Progress Handbook: Early Interventions to Prevent and Treat Dystocia, fourth ed. Wiley-Blackwell, Oxford.

This is an interesting book that explores labour and has in-depth information on positions for women.

Website

https://www.nice.org.uk/guidance/cg190/.

This site provides evidence-based guidelines for intrapartum care for healthy women and babies. The NICE site also offers good practice and evidence-based resources.

40

The Third Stage of Labour

LYZ HOWIE AND JEAN WATSON

This chapter focuses on the third stage of labour. The physiology of the separation of the placenta is described in detail along with the control of bleeding. Management of this stage is explained and examination of the placenta is described in detail. It is crucial that students and midwives have robust knowledge and clear understanding of the process of placenta separation and control of bleeding. This will prevent or minimize the risk of related obstetric emergencies.

Introduction

The third stage of labour is the period from the birth of the baby through to delivery of the placenta and membranes (National Institute of Health and Care Excellence [NICE], 2023) and ends with the control of bleeding. During this period vigilance is required, as emergency situations can occur and can lead to maternal morbidity and mortality. An understanding of the normal physiology allows choice between the physiological management and active management of the third stage. This will ultimately minimize the risk of complications by preventive management and rapid emergency treatment if necessary.

Physiology of the Third Stage of Labour

During the third stage, separation and expulsion of the placenta and membranes occur and bleeding from the placental site is minimized through normal haematological and physiological processes. This stage is most hazardous for the mother because of the risk of haemorrhage and other

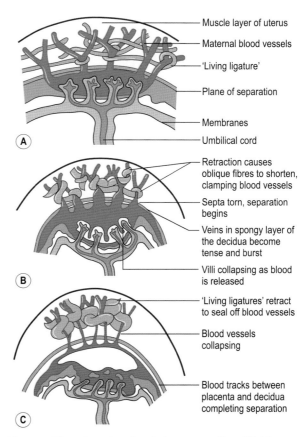

• **Fig. 40.1** The placenta site during separation. (A) Uterus and placenta before separation. (B) Separation begins. (C) Separation is almost complete.

complications (discussed in Chapter 45). The physiological third stage should be considered prolonged if it lasts for more than 30 min for active management or 60 min for physiological management (NICE, 2023).

Separation of the Placenta

Separation of the placenta usually begins with the contraction that delivers the baby (Figs 40.1 and 40.2). The sudden emptying of the uterus with the delivery of the baby rapidly reduces the surface area of the placental site to an area approximately 10 cm in diameter (Blackburn, 2018).

483

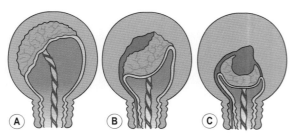

• **Fig. 40.2** The mechanism of placental separation. (A) Uterine wall is partially retracted, but not sufficiently to cause placental separation. (B) Further contraction and retraction thicken the uterine wall, reduce the placental site and aid placental separation. (C) Complete separation and formation of the retroplacental clot. Note: The thin lower segment has collapsed like a concertina after the birth of the baby.

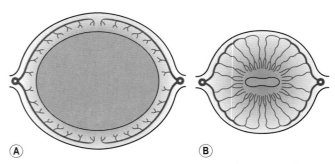

• **Fig. 40.3** Transverse sections of the uterus. (A) Relaxed before the third stage. (B) Contracted and retracted after the third stage; blood vessels are compressed and bleeding arrested.

This reduction in the support base for the placenta leads to compression and shearing of the placenta from the uterine wall. The placenta is compressed so that blood in the intervillous spaces is forced back into the spongy layer of the decidua. Retraction of the oblique muscle fibres constricts the blood vessels supplying the placenta so that the blood cannot drain into the maternal vascular tree. This causes the congested veins to rupture, the villi to shear off the spongy decidua basalis and the inelastic placenta to become wrinkled and peel away from the uterine wall. The weight of the placenta also increases due to congestion of blood, and this helps strip the membranes off the uterine wall (Coad, Pedley & Dunstall, 2019).

The placenta may separate from the central area to the borders with inversion so that the fetal surface presents first. This is known as the **Schultze** mechanism of placental delivery (named after the German anatomist who first described this method). Midwives have termed this process *shiny Schultze,* referring to the glistening appearance of the fetal surface of the placenta at the vulva.

Alternatively, the placenta may separate unevenly from the borders towards the centre with the side of the placenta appearing at the vulva (Duncan, 1871) like a button going through a buttonhole (Coad, Pedley & Dunstall, 2019). This process usually takes longer and there is more risk of incomplete expulsion of the membranes, often referred to as *ragged membranes.* This mechanism was first described by **Matthew Duncan,** an eminent Scottish gynaecologist (1826–1890), and has been called *dirty Duncan* due to the bulky blood ingested at the maternal surface appearing first.

Placentas implanted in the fundus of the uterus are more likely to separate via the Schultze mechanism; those implanted lower in the uterine wall usually separate by the Duncan mechanism, although these placentas may invert before expulsion (Blackburn, 2018).

Control of Bleeding

Once separation is complete, the uterus contracts strongly (Fig. 40.3) and the placenta and membranes fall

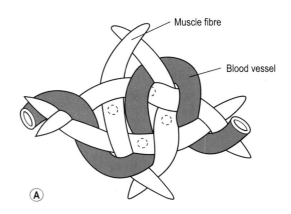

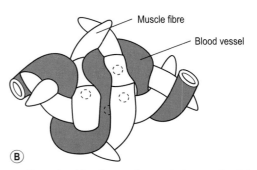

• **Fig. 40.4** How the blood vessels run between the interlacing muscle fibres of the uterus. (A) Muscle fibres are relaxed and blood vessels are not compressed. (B) Muscle fibres are contracted, blood vessels are compressed and bleeding is arrested.

into the lower uterine segment and then into the vagina. It is important to remember that 500–800 mL/min of blood flows to the uterus and placenta at term (Begley, 2020). This flow must be stopped in seconds to prevent serious haemorrhage. Three factors are involved in the process:

1. **Living ligatures**: The tortuous uterine blood vessels are surrounded by the oblique muscle fibres, which retract and act as 'living ligatures' (Fig. 40.4) and constrict the blood vessels.
2. **Pressure**: Once the placenta has left the upper segment, a vigorous contraction brings the walls of the uterus in opposition, applying pressure to the placental site.

1. **Active management** involves the following components:
- Routine use of uterotonic drugs.
- Deferred clamping and cutting of the cord (refer to NICE (2023) section 1.10.14 for specific guidance).
- Controlled cord traction after signs of separation of the placenta (Fig. 40.5) (Begley et al., 2019; Mavrides et al., 2016; NICE, 2023).

  Using this active method reduces the amount of bleeding. However some adverse effects are noted (Begley et al., 2019).

2. **Physiological management** involves:
- **No** routine use of uterotonic drugs.
- **No** clamping of the cord until pulsation has stopped or after delivery of the placenta.
- Delivery of the placenta spontaneously or by maternal effort.

  Physiological management involves letting nature take its course, using a 'hands-off approach'. The practitioner waits for signs of placental separation and allows the placenta to deliver spontaneously by maternal effort (Begley et al., 2019; NICE, 2023).

3. **Blood clotting**: There is a transitory increase in the activity of the coagulation system during and immediately after placental separation so that clot formation in the torn blood vessels is maximized. The placental site is rapidly covered by a fibrin mesh.

Attaching the baby on the breast may help with placental separation due to the stimulation of oxytocin. However a systematic review has reported there was no difference between third-stage blood loss and incidence of postpartum haemorrhage, but results should be viewed with caution (Abedi et al., 2016).

Management of the Third Stage of Labour

Management of the third stage of labour should be based on an understanding of the physiological process. Over recent decades, debate has surrounded the management of the third stage of labour in relation to the benefits of **active management** versus **physiological management** (expectant or conservative management) of the third stage. Box 40.1 details the components of active and physiological management.

The Use of Oxytocic Drugs

Active versus physiological management remains a controversial issue. In the first half of the last century, postpartum haemorrhage (PPH) was a major cause of maternal death (Begley, 1990). Today PPH still remains a key contributor to maternal mortality and morbidity (Escobar et al., 2022). Most maternal deaths occur within the first 24 hours post-delivery and a quarter of maternal deaths are caused by PPH (Oladapo et al., 2020). Box 40.2 provides the historical background related to active versus physiological management debate and the resulting series of key related research trials.

In a recent systematic review comparing active versus physiological (expectant) management of the third stage,

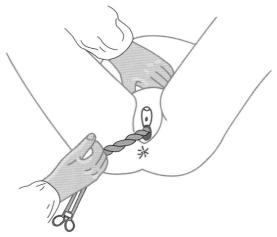

• **Fig. 40.5** Controlled cord traction.

Begley et al. (2019) concluded that routine active management of the third stage reduced the risk of primary PPH >1000 mL, although the quality of the evidence was poor. Active management was also reported to be associated with side effects such as increased blood pressure, pain and hospital readmission with vaginal bleeding. It was recommended that women should have an informed choice when opting for a method of the management of the third stage.

Syntometrine Versus Oxytocin

Research reviews comparing the effects of uterotonic drugs have reported that combined ergometrine–oxytocin may be effective in reducing blood loss and PPH. However side effects were reported such as elevated blood pressure, postpartum pain requiring analgesia, vomiting and nausea (Liabsuetrakul et al., 2018; McDonald, Abbott & Higgins, 2004; Salati et al., 2019). Therefore, side effects need to be considered when administering uterotonic drugs. Oladapo et al. (2020) compared intravenous (IV) with intramuscular (IM) administration of oxytocin and concluded that IM oxytocin was less effective in preventing PPH for vaginal birth compared with IV administration. For active management after vaginal birth, administer 10 units of oxytocin (by intramuscular injection), 5 units of oxytocin (by intravenous injection) or 5 units of oxytocin plus 500 micrograms of ergometrine (by intramuscular injection) immediately after the birth of the baby and before the cord is clamped and cut (NICE, 2023). Refer to Sections 1.10.9–1.10.13 for further details. NICE (2023) recommends the use oxytocin for active management as it is associated with fewer side effects than oxytocin plus ergometrine.

Examination of the Placenta

The placenta and membranes must be examined carefully after the birth (Fig. 40.7):
- To see whether the placenta and membranes have been completely expelled.
- To detect abnormalities which might provide information about any intrauterine problems.

• BOX 40.2 Background: Active Versus Physiological Management

An informative historical paper reporting on the use of ergot alkaloids in the management of the third stage of labour described ergometrine, which was first isolated in 1932 and synthesized in 1938 (Van Dongen & Groot, 1995). The first routine use of intramuscular (IM) ergometrine 0.5 mg was in 1951 (as the head crowned). This shortened the third stage and reduced blood loss in all deliveries. More significantly, it reduced the incidence of postpartum haemorrhage (PPH). Van Dongen & de Groot (1995) also indicated that oxytocin was safer and as efficient as ergometrine. The risks associated with ergometrine were severe hypertension, nausea and vomiting, and side effects due to vasoconstriction. Maternal deaths had occurred following administration.

Begley (1990) cited Embrey et al. (1963) and compared IM ergometrine with IM Syntometrine (ergometrine 0.5 mg and synthetic oxytocin 5 IU). Fig. 40.6 presents the speed of action of the drugs Syntocinon and ergometrine. Syntometrine rapidly became the drug of choice.

In the 1980s women were better nourished, younger, of less parity and less anaemic than their mothers and also better informed. There was a trend towards natural childbirth and many women requested oxytocic drugs be omitted in the third stage unless in an emergency. This was named *physiological management of the third stage of labour,* which led to a series of trials to ascertain the safety of this practice.

Clinical Trials

The *Bristol Third Stage Trial* was a major trial comparing routine obstetric procedures and their effects on the natural process of labour (Prendiville et al., 1988). Inch (1985) had suggested that routine management of the third stage led to a 'cascade of intervention', leading to controlled cord traction (CCT), because women delivered their placentas without the aid of gravity, the umbilical cord was clamped early and routinely and prophylactic oxytocic drug was administered. In particular, the use of an oxytocic, usually IM Syntometrine, was challenged. Comparisons were made on the effects on fetal and maternal morbidity of active and expectant (physiological) management and to determine if active management reduced the incidence of PPH. After 5 months, the researchers modified the protocol due to a high level of PPH in the physiological group (16.5% vs. 3.8%). The physiological group continued to show a high rate of PPH and the study was stopped after 1500 deliveries.

Prendiville et al. (1988) reanalysed the results to exclude the risk categories mentioned by Gilbert, Porter & Brown (1987). They found that active management was preferable, regardless of these first- and second-stage criteria. However, the effect of familiarity with management techniques suggests that midwives may find physiological management less acceptable because of the risks. The main conclusion was that active management of the third stage was justified.

After the Bristol Trial, the *Dublin Trial* involved a randomized controlled trial (1429 women) comparing active management using intravenous (IV) ergometrine 0.5 mg with physiological management of women (with low risk of PPH) (Begley, 1990). They reported an opposite viewpoint. Trial findings found the use of ergometrine was associated with complications such as a greater need for manual removal of placenta, nausea, vomiting and severe after-pains, hypertension and secondary PPH. Although the incidence of PPH and postnatal haemoglobin <10 g/dL was higher in the physiologically managed group, there was no difference in the need for blood transfusion. They stated there was no need to use IV ergometrine in women at low risk for PPH. In fact, administration resulted in more complications.

Thilaganathan et al. (1993) reported on another randomized controlled trial of active versus physiological management of the third stage, called the *Brighton Trial.* Randomization was achieved by consecutively numbered sealed envelopes and, like the other two trials, there were some post-randomization withdrawals due to circumstances such as retained placenta. The high-risk categories were grand multiparity, previous PPH, previous caesarean section, pregnancy-induced hypertension, antepartum haemorrhage and premature rupture of the membranes. Women who had previously consented and who presented in spontaneous labour between 37 and 42 weeks of gestation were admitted to the trial. Women who then required augmentation of labour, operative delivery, cervical laceration or third-degree tear during delivery were withdrawn from the trial. It was found that active management of the third stage of labour reduces the length of the third stage but may not reduce blood loss when compared with physiological management in women at low risk of PPH.

The Hinchingbrooke Randomized Controlled Trial compared active with physiological management of the third stage (Rogers et al., 1998). This trial was conducted to address the outcomes not answered by either the *Bristol* or *Dublin Trials.* Active management included IM Syntometrine (or Syntocinon for women with hypertension) within 2 min of birth, immediate cord clamping and cutting of the cord and delivery of the placenta by maternal effort or CCT. Physiological management involved no prophylactic drug, the cord was left intact until pulsation ceased and the placenta was delivered by maternal effort. Women (n = 1512) were recruited if deemed low risk for PPH, with information collected immediately after birth and up to 6 weeks postpartum. Midwives were experienced in both active and physiological management. Results indicated women who received physiological management had a PPH rate 2.5 times greater than women who were actively managed. There was more chance of these women requiring blood transfusion, and the average length of the third stage was 15 min compared with 8 min in the actively managed group (also noted to have a raised number of side effects). Women in the physiological group were three times more likely to make positive comments related to feelings of achievement. There were negative comments related to extra length of time.

This may be of help in planning neonatal care. See Clinical Application 40.1.

The midwife should remain with the mother for at least 1 hour after completion of the delivery, whether this is in the maternity unit or the home. The uterus should now be palpated gently to ensure that it remains well contracted, and the vaginal blood loss assessed. Maternal temperature, pulse, respirations and blood pressure should be recorded, and the woman is encouraged to pass urine, attend to personal hygiene and have fluids and nutrition. Any deviations from normal must be referred to appropriate medical staff.

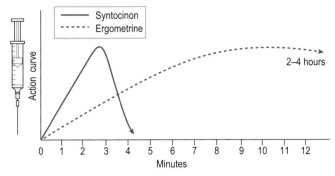

• **Fig. 40.6** Graph representing the relative speeds of action of the drugs Syntocinon and ergometrine.

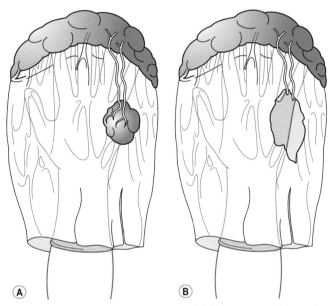

• **Fig. 40.7** (A) Succenturiate placenta. (B) The torn membrane; the missing lobe is in the uterus.

• **CLINICAL APPLICATION 40.1 Examination of the Placenta**

• Standard precautions should be taken (gloves, apron, goggles) to prevent the transmission of blood-borne diseases.
• The number of cord vessels (three: one vein and two arteries) should be ascertained. The absence of one of the umbilical arteries is sometimes associated with renal agenesis.
• The placenta (fetal surface) should be held up by the cord top to inspect the membranes for completeness. There should be a single hole through which the fetus was delivered.
• The amnion is stripped back from the chorion to the cord insertion to ensure that both membranes are present.
• The maternal surface of the placenta should be examined to make sure all the cotyledons are present. Any abnormalities such as calcification, infarctions or blood clots should be noted.
• Blood loss is measured and added to the estimated loss present in the bed linen and pads. Blood loss is documented and reported.
• Cord blood should be taken when the mother's blood group is rhesus-negative, where antibodies have been found in maternal blood and for haemoglobinopathy investigations.
• It is the midwife's responsibility to thoroughly examine the placenta and membranes and ensure that accurate contemporaneous documentation of the findings is executed.

Main Points

• In the third stage of labour, separation and expulsion of the placenta and membranes occur and bleeding from the placental site is minimal. This begins immediately after the birth of the baby. It should be considered prolonged if it lasts for more than 30 min for active management or 60 min for physiological management.

• The placental site rapidly diminishes in size, and the placenta is compressed so that blood in the intervillous spaces is forced back into the spongy layer of the decidua. Retraction of the oblique muscle fibres constricts the blood vessels supplying the placenta, preventing blood from draining into the maternal vascular tree.

• The Schultze mechanism describes separation occurring from the centre of the placenta and results in the fetal surface of the placenta first appearing at the vulva.

• The Duncan mechanism describes separation occurring from the borders and results in the side of the placenta/maternal surface of the placenta first appearing at the vulva.

• Three factors are involved in haemostasis: the action of the living ligatures, the walls of the uterus applying pressure to the placental site and a transitory increase in the activity of the coagulation system.

• Active management involves using a prophylactic oxytocic drug followed by controlled cord traction to control the length of the third stage and lessen the amount of bleeding. Physiological management involves a 'hands-off' approach, waiting for signs of placental separation and allowing the placenta to deliver spontaneously by maternal effort.

• Routine active management is better than physiological (expectant) management for some women. However depending on the drug administered, active management is associated with side effects such as nausea and vomiting. Women should have an informed choice when opting for a method of the management of the third stage of labour.

- The placenta and membranes must be examined after birth. This is required to identify complete or incomplete placenta and membrane tissue, and to detect abnormalities.

- The midwife should ensure that the uterus is well contracted and that vaginal blood loss is minimal. Blood pressure, pulse, respirations and temperature are taken and recorded. Any deviations from normal must be referred to appropriate medical staff.

References

Abedi, P., Jahanfar, S., Namvar, F., Lee, J., 2016. Breastfeeding or nipple stimulation for reducing postpartum haemorrhage in the third stage of labour. Cochrane Database Syst. Rev. 2016 (1), CD010845.

Begley, C.M., 1990. A comparison of 'active' and 'physiological' management of the third stage of labour. Midwifery 6 (1), 3–17.

Begley, C., 2020. 'Physiology and Care during the Third Stage of Labour'. In: Marshall, J., Raynor, M. (Eds.), Myles' Textbook for Midwives, seventeenth ed. Elsevier, Edinburgh.

Begley, C.M., Gyte, G.M., Devane, D., McGuire, W., Weeks, A., 2019. Active versus expectant management for women in the third stage of labour. Cochrane Database Syst. Rev. 2 (2), CD007412.

Blackburn, S.T., 2018. Maternal, Fetal and Neonatal Physiology: A Clinical Perspective, fifth ed. Elsevier, Philadelphia.

Coad, J., Pedley, K., Dunstall, M., 2019. Anatomy and Physiology for Midwives, fourth ed. Elsevier, Edinburgh.

Duncan, M.J., 1871. The mechanism of the expulsion of the placenta. Trans. Edinb. Obstet. Soc, 2, 331–339.

Escobar, M.F., Nassar, A.H., Theron, G., Barnea, E.R., Nicholson, W., Ramasauskaite, D., et al., FIGO Safe Motherhood and Newborn Health Committee, 2022. FIGO recommendations on the management of postpartum hemorrhage. Int. J. Gynecol. Obstet. 157 (1), 3–50.

Gilbert, L., Porter, W., Brown, V.A., 1987. Postpartum haemorrhage: a continuing problem. Br. J. Obstet. Gynaecol. 94 (1), 67–71.

Harding, J.E., Elbourne, D.R., Prendiville, W.J., 1989. Views of mothers and midwives participating in the Bristol randomized controlled trial of active management of the third stage of labor. Birth 16 (1), 1–6.

Inch, S., 1985. Management of the third stage of labour: another cascade of intervention? Midwifery 1 (2), 114–122.

Liabsuetrakul, T., Choobun, T., Peeyananjarassri, K., Islam, Q.M., 2018. Prophylactic use of ergot alkaloids in the third stage of labour. Cochrane Database Syst. Rev. 2018 (6), CD005456.

Mavrides, E., Allard, S., Chandraharan, E., Collins, P., Green, L., Hunt, B.J., et al., on behalf of the Royal College of Obstetricians and Gynaecologists, 2016. Prevention and management of postpartum haemorrhage. Br. J. Obstet. Gynaecol. 124, e106–e149.

McDonald, S.J., Abbott, J.M., Higgins, S.P., 2004. Prophylactic ergometrine-oxytocin versus oxytocin for the third stage of labour. Cochrane Database Syst. Rev. 2004 (1), CD000201.

National Institute for Health and Care Excellence (NICE), 2023. Intrapartum Care. Available at: https://www.nice.org.uk/guidance/ng235.

Oladapo, O.T., Okusanya, B.O., Abalos, E., Gallos, I.D., Papadopoulou, A., 2020. Intravenous versus intramuscular prophylactic oxytocin for reducing blood loss in the third stage of labour. Cochrane Database Syst. Rev. 11 (11), CD009332.

Prendiville, W.J., Harding, J.E., Elbourne, D.R., Stirrat, G.M., 1988. The Bristol Third Stage Trial: active versus physiological management of the third stage of labour. BMJ. 297 (6659), 1295–1300.

Rogers, J., Wood, J., McCandlish, R., Ayers, S., Truesdale, A., Elbourne, D., 1998. Active versus expectant management of the third stage of labour: the Hinchingbrooke Randomized Controlled Trial. Lancet 351 (9104), 693–699.

Salati, J.A., Leathersich, S.J., Williams, M.J., Cuthbert, A., Tolosa, J.E., 2019. Prophylactic oxytocin for the third stage of labour to prevent postpartum haemorrhage. Cochrane Database Syst. Rev. 4 (4), CD001808.

Soltani, H., Hutchon, D.R., Poulose, T.A., 2010. Timing of prophylactic uterotonics for the third stage of labour after vaginal birth. Cochrane Database Syst. Rev. 2010 (8), CD006173.

Soltani, H., Poulose, T.A., Hutchon, D.R., 2011. Placental cord drainage after vaginal delivery as part of the management of the third stage of labour. Cochrane Database Syst. Rev. 2011 (9), CD004665.

Thilaganathan, B., Cutner, A., Latimer, J., Beard, R., 1993. Management of the third stage of labour in women at low risk of postpartum haemorrhage. Eur. J. Obstet. Gynecol. Reprod. Biol. 48 (1), 19–22.

van Dongen, P.W.J., de Groot, A.N.J.A., 1995. History of ergot alkaloids from ergotism to ergometrine. Eur. J. Obstet. Gynecol. Reprod. Biol. 60 (2), 109–116.

Annotated recommended reading

Begley, C.M., Gyte, G.M., Devane, D., McGuire, W., Weeks, A., 2019. Active versus expectant management for women in the third stage of labour. Cochrane Database Syst. Rev. 2 (2), CD007412.

This is the latest updated review of active versus physiological management of the third stage of labour and is essential reading for evidence-based intrapartum care.

National Institute for Health and Care Excellence (NICE), 2023. Intrapartum Care. Available at: https://www.nice.org.uk/guidance/ng235.

This guideline explores the different managements of the third stage of labour to inform both practitioners' decision-making and maternal options.

Labour—Problems

Most labours progress normally. However problems may arise during labour that are life-threatening to both mother and fetus. The knowledge and experience necessary to recognize these problems is vital to the midwife who must immediately summon the obstetric team for assistance. This section is concerned with abnormal labour. Traditionally students have found it helpful for these problems to be grouped as the effects of the 'powers, passenger and passages' on the progress of labour. Chapter 41 examines the 'powers' and presents the problems of abnormal uterine action in detail. The next two chapters discuss problems with the fetus (i.e., passenger). Chapter 42 is concerned with breech presentation and Chapter 43 discusses all other abnormal positions and presentations. Except in extreme cases, it is artificial to discuss problems with the 'passages', as these almost always relate to the fetal size, position and presentation. Chapter 44 is concerned with cephalopelvic disproportion. The placenta and membranes are part of the 'passenger', and problems with their delivery are considered in Chapter 45. Perinatal fetal asphyxia connects labour and neonatal care and is considered in Chapter 46. Operative and assisted vaginal birth methods such forceps, vacuum extraction and caesarean section are detailed in Chapter 47. This final chapter also includes the critical situation when the woman becomes acutely unwell. Maternal collapse is life-threatening but can be reversible with prompt recognition and intervention. Therefore there is a clear focus on early recognition, assessment and resuscitation of the woman.

41

Abnormalities of Uterine Action and Onset of Labour

LYZ HOWIE AND JEAN WATSON

This chapter discusses the abnormalities of uterine action, onset of labour and active management of labour. Related problems include prolonged labour, prolonged second stage of labour and the timing of the onset of labour.

Introduction

The length of labour is variable and affected by different factors (Table 41.1). The abnormalities of uterine action are discussed. Each of these abnormalities are considered in turn, although in practice there may be some interaction. The association between the pattern of contractions and progress of labour is highly variable and the outcome difficult to predict. Abnormal uterine action may be inefficient, resulting in prolonged labour, or over-efficient, resulting in precipitate labour.

Normal labour begins spontaneously at term, i.e., after 37 completed weeks and before 42 completed weeks of pregnancy (Middleton, Shepher & Crowther, 2018; National Institute of Health and Care Excellence [NICE], 2023; Simkin, Ancheta & Hanson, 2017). Contractions increase in length, strength and frequency, resulting in progressive descent of the fetus and dilatation of the cervical os until the fetus, placenta and membranes are expelled from the uterus and bleeding is controlled. Normal labour is also characterized by harmonious interaction between the two uterine poles: the upper uterine segment contracts and retracts, the lower uterine segment thins out and the cervix dilates.

Abnormalities of Uterine Action

Prolonged Labour

The first stage of labour can be described as the **latent** and **established/active** phases and may be prolonged during any of these (see Chapter 36). During the latent phase, the uterus contracts and the cervix effaces and dilates (Simkin, Ancheta & Hanson, 2017). The latent phase lasts until cervical dilatation is about 4 cm (NICE, 2023). The established/active phase with normal dilatation of the cervix lasts approximately 12–14 hours for primigravidae but less for multigravidae (Coad, Pedley & Dunstall, 2019). Defining the term *prolonged labour* is problematic and related to a chosen length, mainly because of a belief that the longer labour lasts, the more danger there is for mother and fetus. Prolonged labour is common in primigravidae although it occurs less often in multigravidae. This may be due to obstruction of labour, where rupture of the uterus may follow the careless use of oxytocic drugs in a multigravid labour.

NICE (2023) acknowledges that the length of labour for a primigravida should be on average 8 hours and not last more than 18 hours, whereas a multigravida labour is shorter with an average of 5 hours and not lasting more than 12 hours. All aspects of labour progress should be assessed before diagnosing a delay in the first stage of labour. This includes cervical dilatation of less than 2 cm in 4 hours for both primigravida and multigravida or slowing down of labour in multigravida; a change in the frequency, duration and strength of uterine contractions; and descent and rotation of the fetal head (NICE, 2023). For labour to progress, six events must occur, which are detailed in Box 41.1.

TABLE 41.1	Factors Which Can Affect Labour	
Maternal	**Fetal**	
Type of uterine contractions	Presentation of fetus	
Pelvic shape	Position of fetus	
Parity	Size of the fetus	
Birth interval		
Psychological state		

• BOX 41.1 Six Events Needed for Labour to Progress

1. Posterior cervix changes to the anterior position.
2. Ripening and softening of the cervix.
3. Effacement of the cervix.
4. Dilatation of the cervix.
5. Flexion, rotation and moulding of fetal head.
6. Descent and further rotation of fetus and birth.

(Simkin, Ancheta & Hanson, 2017)

TABLE 41.2	Associated Maternal and Fetal Risks with Prolonged Labour	
Maternal Risks	**Fetal Risks**	
Maternal distress	Intrapartum hypoxia may cause acidosis, fetal distress, neonatal asphyxia and meconium aspiration, possibly leading to perinatal death	
Increased temperature, pulse and blood pressure		
Dehydration, oliguria and ketosis		
Vomiting	Cerebral trauma due to excessive pounding of the fetal head against the bony pelvis or excessive moulding	
Undetected cephalopelvic disproportion may cause uterine rupture		
Bladder trauma		
Operative interventions	Prolonged rupture of the membranes may result in neonatal infection (e.g., pneumonia)	
Postpartum haemorrhage		
Risk of intrauterine infection if prolonged rupture of membranes		
Haemorrhage is also associated with prolonged labour		

(Mavrides et al., 2016)

Timing of the Onset of Labour

Defining the onset of labour is difficult. The timing is important as it allows decisions to be made about the progress and ongoing management of labour (see Chapter 36). The onset is difficult to establish with accuracy. The concept of **pre-labour,** or preparation for labour, refers to the changes that occur in the last few weeks of pregnancy. It is often difficult to decide when the transition from the painless uterine contractions of pre-labour develops into true labour. Simkin, Ancheta & Hanson (2017) also suggest that slow labour may progress into normal labour patterns, and so it is difficult to accurately state that a labour is dysfunctional until the active phase.

Latent or Established/Active Phase?

There is lack of agreement about whether the onset of labour is from the start of the latent phase or the established/active phase of the first stage of labour (Chapman & Charles, 2018; Jackson, Anderson & Marshall, 2020). The most frequently used marker for the commencement of labour is the onset of regular rhythmic painful uterine contractions and advancing cervical dilatation (NICE, 2023; Simkin, Ancheta & Hanson, 2017). Vaginal examination of women at the time of admission suggests the decision to admit relies on various factors, including the advice the woman received about recognizing the onset of labour and her anxieties and expectations.

Inefficient Uterine Action

Uterine contractions are inefficient and do not result in dilatation of the cervix. Inefficient uterine action is the most common cause of abnormal labour in primigravidae and labour is prolonged. Inefficient uterine action caused delay in 65% of 9018 nulliparous women with prolonged labour (O'Driscoll, Meagher & Boylan, 1993). The remaining cases were caused by persistent occipitoposterior position (24%) and cephalopelvic disproportion (CPD) (11%). Therefore inefficiency may be due to weak contractions (**hypotonic uterine action**) or the loss of coordination between the upper and lower uterine segments (**incoordinate uterine action**). Prolonged labour increases maternal and fetal risks (Table 41.2).

Hypotonic Uterine Action

Hypotonic uterine action creates weak contractions of short duration, leading to slow or no dilatation of the cervix. If hypotonic contractions occur from the commencement of labour, they are said to be **primary.** Hypotonic uterine action occurs more commonly in primigravidae women. The cause is unknown. If hypotonic contractions begin after a period of normal uterine action, they are said to be **secondary** and there may be abnormalities of labour such as CPD, malposition of the occiput, a malpresentation, maternal dehydration or ketosis. The commencement of epidural analgesia sometimes causes hypotonic uterine action due to the relaxation of the pelvic floor, which interferes with the mechanisms of labour (Bartholomew, 2017).

Incoordinate Uterine Action

Incoordinate uterine action involves a loss of polarity and an increase in uterine resting tone. Contractions can be variable and painful, with the woman feeling the contraction before and after it is palpable abdominally. They often feel pain between contractions. The cervix dilates slowly or not at all. Placental blood flow is decreased, which might lead to fetal distress. This type of uterine action is associated with malpositions of the occiput. If there are no maternal problems or fetal distress, it is important to alleviate the woman's anxiety and try mobilization first. This might aid progress in labour before active management and the introduction of interventions (Lawrence et al., 2013).

Active Management of Labour

In the 1960s, O'Driscoll, Meagher & Boylan (1986) introduced the active management of labour for primigravidae. The active management care package includes routine amniotomy (artificial rupture of membranes), the use of oxytocin, diagnosis of slow progress in labour and appropriate one-to-one care. Whilst this management has demonstrated a small reduction in the caesarean section rate, it can lead to increase in medicalization, monitoring and interventions, where women have less control over their labour and reduced satisfaction (Brown et al., 2013). In some instances, amniotomy is carried out shortly after admission. Augmentation of labour with Syntocinon (oxytocin) may follow if there is inadequate progress after 1 hour (Wei et al., 2013).

Augmentation of Labour

Augmentation of labour is where a synthetic oxytocin (Syntocinon) is used to shorten labour and increase uterine contractions (Kenyon et al., 2013a). Once delay has been diagnosed and abnormalities of presentation or CPD ruled out, the membranes are ruptured and an intravenous infusion of Syntocinon is commenced. Any abnormality of fluid and electrolyte balance is corrected, and both mother and fetus are monitored carefully. Adequate pain relief and good psychological support of the woman should be provided, including explanations and reassurance (NICE, 2023). The progress of labour is recorded on a partogram to detect any deviations from normal (NICE, 2023) (Fig. 41.1). Lavender, Cuthbert & Smyth (2018) report that further evidence is required to support a specific type of partogram or routine use of partogram in practice.

Amniotomy

The benefits of intact membranes throughout labour include reduced risk of intrauterine infection and reduced risk of fetal hypoxia (due to less placental compression and less reduction in size of the placental site). Amniotomy is the artificial rupture of the fetal membranes resulting in drainage of liquor (Smyth, Markham & Dowswell, 2013). This procedure has been practiced for several decades and is performed to accelerate labour. Amniotomy may also be performed to examine the amniotic fluid for presence of meconium.

A clear indication of the need for amniotomy is required before the procedure is carried out. In a systematic review, Smyth, Markham & Dowswell (2013) studied the effects of amniotomy on the rate of caesarean sections and other indicators of maternal and neonatal morbidity. The reviewers found no difference in caesarean section risk, length of first stage of labour, maternal satisfaction or Apgar scores less than 7 at 5 min. They concluded that amniotomy in spontaneous labour should not be routinely practiced, but discussed with women before amniotomy is conducted in labour. NICE (2023) recommend against routine amniotomy in a normal progressing labour.

Oxytocin Infusion

Oxytocin is one of the most utilized drugs for augmenting labour and delivery. The administered dosage of oxytocin may vary. Further evidence is required to determine whether high-dose or low-dose oxytocin is the preferred regime for a term induction of labour (Budden, Chen & Henry, 2014). In their systematic review, Bugg, Siddiqui & Thornton (2013) reported that oxytocin infusion was associated with a shorter labour, no difference in caesarean section or instrumental delivery rate and no increase in vaginal delivery rate. Early use of oxytocin was associated with uterine hyperstimulation with no detectable adverse effects for mother or baby. Byrne et al. (1993) found no evidence that an oxytocic infusion generated excessive intrauterine pressures, although women could experience more painful contractions and restricted mobility.

Oxytocin infusion has its place in the management of women with prolonged labour. However other measures such as ambulation and intake of appropriate nutrition should first be considered prior to labelling a labour as abnormal and using medical intervention.

Prolonged Second Stage of Labour

A discussion on the acceptable length of the second stage of labour is presented in Chapter 39, and delayed progress may be due to the factors presented in Box 41.2.

Management

The condition of mother and fetus should be carefully assessed. More time may be given if progress is made, including slow progress. Actions to promote progress include adopting an asymmetrical upright, standing or kneeling position, closed-knee chest position, hands and knee position, side-lying or squatting position to enlarge the pelvic outlet (Simkin, Ancheta & Hanson, 2017). This directs the presenting part against the posterior vaginal wall, using Ferguson's reflex (Ferguson, 1941) for the release of oxytocin. If the maternal or fetal condition becomes worrying or there is no obvious progress, an assisted vaginal delivery or caesarean section may be needed.

Over-efficient Uterine Action
Precipitate Labour

A precipitate labour occurs when the uterine contractions occur frequently and are intense. There is rapid completion of

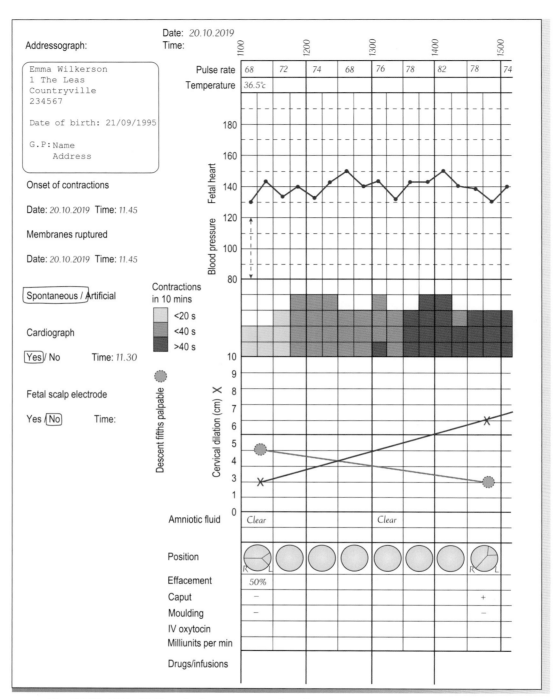

• **Fig. 41.1** World Health Organization partogram of cervimetric progress commencing at 4 cm dilatation. 'Alert' line outlines normal progress. 'Action' line indicates when augmentation should be instituted.

the first and second stages of labour, and birth normally occurs within less than 3 hours of commencement of contractions (Suzuki, 2015). This condition is more common in multigravidae and is usually caused by lack of resistance of the maternal soft tissues. Minimal pain might have been experienced in the first stage of labour, and the woman becomes aware of imminent delivery when the head is about to be born.

Dangers of Precipitate Labour

The woman may have lacerations to the cervix and perineum. Postpartum haemorrhage may follow (NICE, 2023). The baby may be hypoxic and may sustain intracranial injuries because of rapid descent through the birth canal. If the birth occurs in an inappropriate place, the baby may be injured. Any labouring woman with a history of a

Maternal:
- Inefficient uterine action (primary powers).
- Inefficient maternal effort (secondary powers).
- Uterine abnormalities.
- A full bladder or rectum, a rigid perineum.
- A contracted pelvic outlet.
- Maternal obesity.
- Psychological and or emotional sequelae.

Fetal:
- A large baby.
- A fetal abnormality such as hydrocephaly or abdominal enlargement.
- Persistent occipitoposterior position.
- Deep transverse arrest of the head.
- Malpresentation.

previous precipitate delivery should not be left alone and should be watched very closely when in labour. However NICE (2023) does not offer any recommendations regarding precipitate labour.

Tonic Contraction of the Uterus

This rare event, where the tone of the uterus is continuously high and there is no relaxation of the uterine muscle, is accompanied by intense pain. The fetus becomes distressed as the placental circulation is grossly restricted. Intrauterine death may occur. Causes may be obstructed labour or misuse of oxytocic drugs (Syntocinon and prostaglandins). This is an emergency, and immediate treatment may save the baby's life and prevent uterine rupture:

- If an oxytocic infusion is in progress, discontinue and consider tocolytics (NICE, 2023).
- Turn the mother onto her left side to enhance uteroplacental blood flow.
- Inform the obstetrician, who will review the woman about caesarean section.

Administration of maternal facial oxygen was common practice; however there is no evidence to support either prophylactic or short-term use of oxygen for fetal compromise (Fawole & Hofmeyr, 2012; NICE, 2023).

Cervical Dystocia

Cervical dystocia is where the cervix dilates slowly, if at all. This may be caused by scarring from procedures such as cautery, cryosurgery or other surgery, or congenital abnormalities (Simkin, Ancheta & Hanson, 2017). Failure to recognize the condition and prolonged pressure would result in ischaemia, and there would be annular detachment of the cervix.

If the anterior part of the cervix is trapped between the pelvic brim and fetal head, venous return is restricted, and the anterior lip may become swollen and oedematous. In this instance, it may feel as thick as a finger during vaginal examination. The first stage of labour will be prolonged, and occasionally the cervix may be seen blue and glistening

between the fetal head and the symphysis pubis. This is caused by the woman bearing down before full cervical dilatation, and it is commonly the result of a persistent occipitoposterior position (Simkin, Ancheta & Hanson, 2017). If the woman adopts other positions and uses inhalational analgesia, this may help avoid pushing. Epidural analgesia may occasionally be needed. It is sometimes possible to push an anterior lip of the cervix up behind the fetal head, but care must be taken not to tear the cervix. However, this would not be routine practice.

Problems: Timing of the Onset of Labour

Preterm Onset of Labour

Preterm labour begins before the end of the 37th week of pregnancy (World Health Organization [WHO], 2018). The WHO (2018) defines preterm birth as extremely preterm <28 weeks, very preterm from 28 to <32 weeks and moderate to late preterm from 32 to <37 weeks. This is a preterm baby, irrespective of birthweight. Not all preterm babies are of low birthweight (LBW), weighing less than 2500 g, but many babies are both preterm and LBW (Blencowe et al., 2019; UNICEF & WHO, 2004). Preterm babies have different problems and needs compared with LBW babies because of growth restriction (see Chapter 50).

The incidence of preterm birth affects approximately 15 million babies annually worldwide, indicating a global preterm birth rate of about 11% (Walani, 2020). Significant variations exist in preterm birth rates and mortality between countries. Particularly high rates are seen in low- and middle-income countries (especially Southeast Asia and sub-Saharan Africa) (Walani, 2020). Preterm birth is the single biggest cause of neonatal mortality and morbidity globally, and these babies also have a greater prevalence of disability and long-term health issues (WHO, 2019).

Woman may suffer feelings of inadequacy following a preterm birth (Henderson, Carson & Redshaw, 2016). However, maternal mortality and morbidity are rarely affected by preterm onset of labour.

Aetiology

Preterm births may follow a spontaneous onset of labour, or elective in instances of increased maternal or fetal risk (WHO, 2018). Table 41.3 highlights the risk factors associated with preterm labour (no known cause in ~40% of cases).

Although this list is comprehensive, it is difficult to predict which woman will begin labour before term. Even if the onset of preterm labour could be predicted, it is difficult to prevent the progress to delivery.

Because the risk factors are so wide, attempts at reducing some of the physical or social factors have had limited success. Risk-scoring systems using these factors are poor predictors, especially in primigravid women. Home monitoring of uterine activity has had no effect on the rate of

TABLE 41.3	A Summary of the Risk Factors Associated With Preterm Labour			
Biological/ Medical Factors	**Reproductive History**	**Current Pregnancy**	**Socioeconomic and Psychological**	**Cultural/Behavioural**
Age less than 16 or more than 35	History of previous preterm birth (two previous preterm births increases risk by 70%)	Poor nutrition and body mass index (BMI) less than 19.8	Poverty and social deprivation	Cigarette, alcohol or drug use
Low weight for height (low BMI)	Bleeding in previous pregnancy	Bleeding in this pregnancy	Psychological distress	Short interpregnancy interval
History of hypertension, renal disease or diabetes mellitus	Uterine abnormality (increases risk by 19%)	Retained intrauterine contraceptive device	Alcohol/substance abuse	Late antenatal booking and poor attendance for care
Generalized infections, especially viral	Poor obstetric history	Abdominal surgery Infections (e.g., pyelonephritis) Genital tract infection (e.g., bacterial vaginosis, chlamydia, group B haemolytic streptococcus) Fetal problems: multiple pregnancy, fetal malformation, rhesus disease, fetal death, polyhydramnios		
		Cervical incompetence		
		Congenital abnormality		
		Prolapsed cord		

(Hillier, Nugent & Eschenbach, 1995; Peacock, Bland & Anderson, 1995; Purisch & Gyamfi-Bannerman, 2017; Vogel et al., 2018)

preterm birth. Cervical effacement can be assessed, but it is not a good predictor of preterm birth and may also introduce infection.

Fetal Fibronectin

High levels of fetal fibronectin (fFN), a component of the extracellular matrix secreted by the anchoring trophoblastic villi, have been found in cervical and vaginal secretions before the onset of preterm labour (Berghella & Saccone, 2019). Separation of maternal and fetal tissue at the choriodecidual junction leads to a leakage of fibronectin. This can be detected using the fFN test. An fFN test taken within 7–10 days of testing has moderate accuracy in determining preterm labour for less than 37 weeks' gestation. NICE (2023) advocates the use of fFN testing. This test, as well as other clinical indicators, have recently been incorporated within a clinical tool (the QUIPP™ app) to aid decision making when

women present in threatened preterm labour (Carlisle, Watson & Shennan, 2021).

Preterm Rupture of the Membranes

Spontaneous preterm pre-labour rupture of the membranes is associated with genital tract infection (Kenyon, Boulvain & Neilson, 2013; NICE, 2023; RCOG, 2012) and cervical incompetence. Labour may begin soon after the event, but if delayed, bacteria may ascend the genital tract to colonize the uterus and fetus. The woman must be admitted to a hospital with a neonatal intensive care unit. No vaginal examination is performed in the absence of signs of labour, and a speculum examination is carried out to visualize the cervix (NICE, 2023). Although a high vaginal swab may be taken for culture and sensitivity testing, evidence is lacking to support this. Women should, however, be observed for signs of clinical chorioamnionitis (Thomson, 2019).

• BOX 41.3   The Use of Drugs in Preterm Onset of Labour and Preterm Rupture of the Membranes

Corticostroids

The risk of hyaline membrane disease for the neonate is high. Therefore the steroid dexamethasone is given to the mother to accelerate surfactant production in the lungs. Administration of corticosteroids to women expected to deliver preterm reduces mortality, respiratory distress syndrome and intraventricular haemorrhage in preterm infants (McGoldrick et al., 2020). A typical regimen is two doses of 12 mg given orally or by intramuscular injection 12 hours apart. The effects of the drug take 24 hours, and it is effective for up to 7 days. Research is ongoing to determine the optimal corticosteroids and regime for future clinical practice (Crowther et al., 2019; Williams, Ramson & Brownfoot, 2022).

Antibiotics

Chorioamnionitis is the cause of preterm labour in up to 30–40% of cases (Thomson, 2019). The cause is poorly understood. Intra-amniotic infection may exist without a rise in temperature, rise in white cell count, uterine tenderness or fetal tachycardia. The woman should still be regularly examined for such signs of intrauterine infection. Routine prophylactic use of antibiotics has resulted in the reduction of maternal and neonatal morbidity (Thomson, 2019). Overall there is insufficient evidence to recommend regular prophylactic use of antibiotics. More research is needed to evaluate any effects to the fetus (Thinkhamrop et al., 2015).

Tocolytic drugs

Tocolytic drugs for preterm premature rupture of membranes (PPROM) increases the risk of maternal chorioamnionitis (Mackeen et al., 2014). These drugs do not improve perinatal outcomes (Thomson, 2019). However when preterm membranes remain intact, tocolytic drugs may delay preterm birth (Wilson et al., 2022). Tocolytic drugs may have noticeable side effects for the mother and, as yet, undetermined effects on the neonate (Wilson et al., 2022). Examples of tocolytics include betamimetics, calcium channel blockers, magnesium sulphate,

oxytocin receptor antagonists and nitric oxide donors. They act by preventing contraction of smooth muscle. Some examples are outlined below:

β-adrenergic drugs, such as ritodrine hydrochloride, salbutamol and terbutaline, may be administered by intravenous infusion. They do, however, have maternal side effects, including tachycardia; cardiac dysrhythmias; palpitations; peripheral vasodilation, resulting in hypotension and flushing, decreased blood pressure, increased respiratory rate; nausea and vomiting; muscle tremors; increased blood glucose; fluid retention; and pulmonary oedema (Dodd, Crowther & Middleton, 2012; Ram et al., 2021; Ritter et al., 2019).

Magnesium maintenance therapy reduces uterine contractions by decreasing calcium uptake and depolarization of smooth muscle (Han, Crowther & Moore, 2013).

Cyclo-oxygenase (COX) inhibitors, such as indomethacin, may also be used; they block the production of the enzyme endoperoxide synthase, which is responsible for the conversion of arachidonic acid to prostaglandin. Reinebrant et al. (2015) identified that COX inhibitors might have some preventative measure for preterm labour and may have fewer maternal side effects than other tocolytics. Maternal side effects include nausea, vomiting, diarrhoea, dizziness and headaches. Fetal effects may be pulmonary hypertension, persistent patent ductus arteriosus, necrotizing enterocolitis and intraventricular haemorrhage (Reinebrant et al., 2015).

Calcium channel blockers (CCBs), such as nifedipine, inhibit muscle contraction. Although data suggests CCBs may prolong pregnancy by 48 hours, more robust evidence is needed (Flenady et al., 2014).

Other tocolytics have been explored, including oxytocin receptor antagonists (ORAs, e.g., atosiban), combinations of CCBs and ORAs, nitrous oxide donors (glyceryl trinitrate [GTN]) and progesterone. All these lack evidence of their effectiveness of delaying preterm birth (Dodd et al., 2013; Duckett et al., 2014; Flenady et al., 2014; Vogel et al., 2014).

Box 41.3 summarizes the evidence relating to the use of drugs in preterm onset of labour and preterm rupture of the membranes. The mother and fetus should be closely observed for signs of drug-related side effects. Delivery is probably inevitable if cervical dilatation progresses to 4 cm or if the membranes rupture.

Labour and Delivery

All tocolytic drugs are stopped and the condition of the woman and fetus is carefully observed. Analgesic drugs such as pethidine and morphine should be avoided. The preferred methods of pain relief are epidural anaesthesia or Entonox, neither of which adversely affects the fetus. An obstetrician and neonatal clinician should be present at the delivery, and an elective episiotomy considered to reduce pressure on the fetal head and minimize cerebral trauma. Forceps may offer better protection. Some preterm babies might be delivered by caesarean section, especially if in breech presentation. Limited data exists to support this practice for all preterm babies (Alfirevic, Milan & Livio, 2013). Stronger available data suggest caesarean section in extremely preterm babies (<28 weeks' gestation) results in reduced risk of fetal death

(Jarde et al., 2020). NICE (2023) highlights the difficulties associated with performing a caesarean birth for a preterm birth, especially the increased likelihood of a vertical uterine (classical) incision with the subsequent implications for future pregnancies.

Deferred cord clamping should be performed (NICE, 2023). Thereafter the cord should be clamped at least 10 cm away from its insertion into the abdominal wall – this facilitates care in the neonatal unit. Vitamin K 0.5–1.0 mg is usually given intramuscularly (with parental consent) to minimize the risk of haemorrhagic disease of the newborn.

Prolonged Pregnancy

A pregnancy is considered to be post-term if the gestational age is accurate, and it extends beyond 42 completed weeks (294 days) (Middleton et al., 2020). The risk of prolonged pregnancy is higher in primigravidae and obese women (30% vs. 20%) (Arrowsmith, Wray & Quenby, 2011). A prolonged pregnancy is high risk for the mother and neonate (Middleton et al., 2020; Walker, 2017).

Fetal maturity can be estimated if the first day of the last menstrual period is known (and the woman has a regular cycle). Abdominal examination is not an accurate way of measuring gestational age. An early ultrasound scan will provide good assessment of fetal age, and serial scans later in pregnancy can monitor ongoing fetal growth (Whitworth, Bricker & Mullan, 2015). Static maternal weight, abnormal fetal heart rate patterns and reduced fetal movements may indicate deterioration in fetal condition.

Risk Factors

A post-term pregnancy has associated problems for both the woman and the fetus. For the woman, this involves interventions such as induction of labour, possibly with an unfavourable cervix, caesarean section, prolonged labour, postpartum haemorrhage and traumatic birth (Middleton et al., 2020). Some outcomes may result from intervening when the uterus and cervix are not ready for labour. Post-term pregnancy also has a higher incidence of neonatal morbidity and mortality, and progressive placental insufficiency. Fetal stillbirth increases as pregnancies extend beyond 40 weeks (Muglu et al., 2018). The volume of amniotic fluid may diminish so that oxygen supply may be interrupted during contractions due to compression of the placenta. Meconium staining of the liquor is common, with the risk of meconium aspiration syndrome. Babies born after 42 weeks are more likely to weigh >4000 g. The increased size of the fetus may result in shoulder dystocia, accompanied by the typical trauma of brachial and facial palsy and fractured clavicle.

Management of Post-term Pregnancy

It is possible to monitor the well-being of the fetus by cardiotocography and ultrasound measurement of amniotic pool depth (Hofmeyr & Novikova, 2012; Middleton et al., 2020; NICE, 2021a). Irrespective of gestation, Doppler ultrasound of the umbilical artery in high-risk pregnancies may reduce the risk of fetal compromise (Alfirevic, Stampalija & Dowswell, 2017). However findings of the routine use in low-risk pregnancies having any benefit to mother or baby are inconclusive (Alfirevic, Stampalija & Medley, 2015). Biophysical profile is another surveillance method, where ultrasound assesses fetal movement, fetal tone, fetal breathing and amniotic fluid volume.

Omar et al. (2013) refute earlier claims that coitus during late pregnancy expedites labour. Unrestricted breast stimulation may reduce the need for induction, but more evidence is required (Kavanagh, Kelly & Thomas, 2005; Shahabuddin & Murphy, 2022). Digital separation of the membranes from the lower pole of the uterus (sweeping the membranes) may also help and should be discussed with and offered to women (NICE, 2021a).

Induction of labour is described below. Women who choose to wait for spontaneous labour should have regular fetal monitoring and should be advised to report any reduction in their pattern of fetal movements (NICE, 2021b).

Induction of Labour

Induction of labour is defined as 'the process of artificially stimulating the uterus to start labour' (WHO, 2018). It is associated with a lower risk of fetal death and caesarean section when compared with expectant management of labour (Middleton et al., 2020). The risks and benefits of expectant management versus induction of labour should be discussed with the woman, especially for women who go beyond 41 weeks' gestation, to help reach a decision on the timing of induction. NICE (2021a) reiterates this: although they do not specify an exact timing for induction of labour, they state that most labours will begin spontaneously before 42 weeks' gestation.

Induction of labour is usually performed by administering prostaglandins or oxytocin to the pregnant woman or by manually rupturing the amniotic membranes (WHO, 2018). Induction of labour is carried out for medical or obstetric reasons when it is thought that the health of the mother or fetus may be compromised by the continuation of pregnancy (Table 41.4). Box 41.4 highlights contraindications to induction of labour. Induction is more successful when the presence of favourable factors indicates readiness of the cervix (Coad, Pedley & Dunstall, 2019). This can be assessed by the Bishop scoring system (Table 41.5). For a score ≤6, the woman should be offered a form of mechanical or pharmacological induction; a score >6 indicates an induction using amniotomy and intravenous oxytocin infusion (NICE, 2021a).

TABLE 41.4	**Some Indications for Induction of Labour**	
Maternal Indications	**Fetal Indications**	**Joint Indications**
Prolonged pregnancy	Placental insufficiency	Pre-eclampsia
After spontaneous rupture of membranes	Rhesus isoimmunization with haemolysis	Placental abruption
Medical conditions such as diabetes mellitus	Intrauterine death	An unstable lie
Poor obstetric history such as a previous stillbirth	Severe congenital abnormalities	
Maternal request for social/psychological reasons		
Previous caesarean section		

Methods

Different methods are available for induction of labour. These include pharmacological vaginal prostaglandins in the form of gels, tablets or pessaries; surgical methods (amniotomy with or without intravenous oxytocin infusion); and mechanical methods such as balloon catheters and osmotic cervical dilator inserted into the cervical canal (NICE, 2021a).

Cervical Ripening

Prostaglandins

There are few oxytocin receptors in the cervix, making oxytocin inefficient at ripening the cervix. An unfavourable cervix at the commencement of induction is associated with a higher rate of failed induction, longer labour and an increased need for caesarean section. Some evidence supports the use of vaginal **prostaglandins** (PGE$_2$) for cervical ripening (Thomas et al., 2014), increasing the likelihood of a successful induction of labour with slightly reduced caesarean section rates. NICE (2021a) supports the use of vaginal PGE$_2$ for induction of labour, *unless* there are specific clinical reasons for not using it (i.e., a previous uterine scar). It can be administered as a gel, tablet or controlled-release pessary. In the event of hyperstimulation occurring following insertion of PGE$_2$, maternal and fetal monitoring is critical. There is no increase in operative deliveries with the use of PGE$_2$ (Denoual-Ziad et al., 2015; Thomas et al., 2014).

Mechanical Methods for Induction of Labour

Mechanical methods such as balloon catheters (Foley catheter) are inserted into the cervical canal to assist with cervical dilatation and stimulate uterine contractions (NICE, 2021a). When compared with PGE$_2$, there is less hyperstimulation (although rates of caesarean section remain similar). When compared with oxytocin, mechanical methods result in fewer caesarean sections (de Vaan et al., 2019). NICE (2021a) states that mechanical methods can be used for induction of labour in a woman *without* a previous caesarean section.

Sweeping the Membranes

Sweeping or stripping of the membranes is a relatively simple technique to perform during vaginal examination. The practitioner's finger is introduced into the cervical os, and the inferior pole of the membranes is detached from the lower uterine segment by a circular movement of the finger. This procedure has the potential to initiate labour by increasing local production of prostaglandins (Coad, Pedley & Dunstall, 2019). Findings from a systematic review confirmed that membrane sweep may reduce the need for induction of labour but did not reduce the rates of assisted vaginal births (Finucane et al., 2020). NICE (2021a) recommends that before formal induction of labour, women should be offered a vaginal examination for membrane sweeping. Only three studies reported on women's satisfaction with membrane sweeping, suggesting that although women reported it to be a painful procedure, they perceived the benefits to outweigh the risks.

Amniotomy With or Without Oxytocin

Rupturing the membranes is a point of no return in obstetric management of labour. Once performed, the risk of intrauterine infection increases. Amniotomy may be used on its own or alongside an oxytocic infusion (either immediately or if contractions have not commenced after a few hours) (Howarth & Botha, 2001). Syntocinon infusion must be carefully regulated to avoid hyperstimulation of uterine action and water retention. Amniotic fluid embolism is a rare complication that follows hyperstimulation of uterine action.

> • **BOX 41.4 Contraindications for Induction of Labour**
>
> - Placenta praevia.
> - Cephalopelvic disproportion (CPD).
> - Oblique or transverse lie.
> - Severe fetal compromise.
> - Lack of maternal consent.

TABLE 41.5 Bishop Scoring System

Bishop's Score	0	1	2
Length of cervix	3–4 cm	1–2 cm	<1 cm
Dilatation of the cervix (cm)	0	1–2 cm	>2 cm
Station of presenting part related	−3	−2	−1
Consistency of cervix	Firm	Soft	Very soft
Position of cervix	Posterior	Mid	Anterior
Total =	(Bishop's Score)		

(Coad, Pedley & Dunstall, 2019)

Systematic reviews highlight that evidence on this method of induction is sparse (Bricker & Luckas, 2000; Howarth & Botha, 2001; Mozurkewich et al., 2011).

Therefore decisions about induction of labour should use the best available evidence to inform practice, alongside discussions with women about the available options.

Main Points

- The length of labour is affected by the type of uterine contractions, parity, birth interval, psychological state, presentation and position, pelvic shape and size.
- The first stage of labour can be described as having latent and active phases. The term *prolonged labour* identifies that longer labours have increased risks for mother and fetus.
- Dangers of prolonged labour to the mother include physical effort, pain and anxiety, dehydration, ketosis and tiredness. Maternal distress could lead to maternal morbidity and mortality. Risks to the baby include intrapartum acidosis, fetal distress, neonatal asphyxia and meconium aspiration, perinatal death, cerebral trauma and ascending neonatal infections.
- Uterine contractions are inefficient if they do not result in dilatation of the cervix. The most common cause of abnormal labour in primigravidae is inefficient uterine action due to hypotonic uterine action or incoordinate uterine action. Progress is slow and labour is prolonged. The administration of oxytocin corrects inefficient uterine action and shortens labour.
- Delayed progress in the second stage of labour may be due to inefficient uterine action or inefficient maternal effort, a full bladder or rectum, cephalopelvic disproportion or obstructed labour. Adopting an upright position may enlarge the pelvic outlet and directs the presenting part against the posterior vaginal wall, bringing about increased uterine action.
- In precipitate labour, intense uterine contractions occur frequently, with delivery occurring within less than 3 hours. It is most common in multigravidae and is usually caused by lack of resistance of the maternal soft tissues. The woman may have lacerations to the cervix or perineum, and postpartum haemorrhage may follow. The baby may sustain intracranial injuries.

- Tonic uterine action is usually accompanied by intense pain. The fetus becomes distressed as the placental circulation is grossly restricted. Intrauterine death may occur. Causes may be obstructed labour or misuse of oxytocic drugs such as Syntocinon or prostaglandins. Immediate treatment will prevent uterine rupture and save the baby's life.
- Preterm labour begins before the end of the 37th week of pregnancy. Extremely preterm is defined as <28 weeks, very preterm from 28 to <32 weeks and moderate to late preterm from 32 to <37 weeks.
- If preterm labour is diagnosed and the membranes are intact, tocolytic drugs may be administered. Delaying the of onset of labour by 48 hours gives time for corticosteroids to be effective in maturing the fetal lungs. If delivery is inevitable, tocolytic drugs are discontinued. Prophylactic antibiotic therapy is recommended for use in preterm rupture of membranes, as it is associated with a delay in delivery and benefits for neonatal morbidity.
- A pregnancy is considered to be post-term beyond 42 completed weeks (294 days). The risk of prolonged pregnancy is higher in primigravidae and obese women (30% vs. 20%). A prolonged pregnancy is high risk for the mother and neonate.
- The introduction of vaginal or endocervical administration of PGE_2 for cervical ripening has increased the likelihood of a successful induction of labour. Stripping the membranes from the lower uterine segment possibly produces increased amounts of prostaglandin and may be a safe way of avoiding induction by promoting spontaneous onset of labour at term.
- Membrane sweep may reduce the need for induction of labour but rates of assisted vaginal births were not reduced (Finucane et al., 2020).

References

Alfirevic, Z., Milan, S.J., Livio, S., 2013. Caesarean section versus vaginal delivery for preterm birth in singletons. Cochrane Database Syst. Rev. 2013 (9), CD000078.

Alfirevic, Z., Stampalija, T., Medley, N., 2015. Fetal and umbilical Doppler ultrasound in normal pregnancy. Cochrane Database Syst. Rev. 2015 (4), CD001450.

Alfirevic, Z., Stampalija, T., Dowswell, T., 2017. Fetal and umbilical Doppler ultrasound in high-risk pregnancies. Cochrane Database Syst. Rev. 2017 (6), CD007529.

Arrowsmith, S., Wray, S., Quenby, S., 2011. Maternal obesity and labour complications following induction of labour in prolonged pregnancy. Br. J. Obstet. Gynaecol. 118 (5), 578–588.

Bartholomew, C.M., 2017. Supporting choices in reducing pain and fear in labour. In: Macdonald, S., Johnson, G. (Eds.), Mayes' Midwifery, fifteenth ed. Elsevier, Edinburgh.

Berghella, V., Saccone, G., 2019. Fetal fibronectin testing for reducing the risk of preterm birth. Cochrane Database Syst. Rev. 2019 (7), CD006843.

Blencowe, H., Krasevec, J., de Onis, M., Black, R.E., An, X., Stevens, G.A., et al., 2019. National, regional, and worldwide estimates of low birthweight in 2015, with trends from 2000: a systematic analysis. Lancet 7 (7), E849–E860.

Bricker, L., Luckas, M., 2000. Amniotomy alone for induction of labour. Cochrane Database Syst. Rev. 2000 (4), CD002862.

Brown, H.C., Paranjothy, S., Dowswell, T., Thomas, J., 2013. Package of care for active management in labour for reducing caesarean section rates in low-risk women. Cochrane Database Syst. Rev. 2013 (9), CD004907.

Budden, A., Chen, L.J.Y., Henry, A., 2014. High-dose versus low-dose oxytocin infusion regimens for induction of labour at term. Cochrane Database Syst. Rev. 2014 (10), CD009701.

Bugg, G.J., Siddiqui, F., Thornton, J.G., 2013. Oxytocin versus no treatment or delayed treatment for slow progress in the first stage of spontaneous labour. Cochrane Database Syst. Rev. 2013 (6), CD007123.

Byrne, M.B., Keane, D., Boylan, P., Stronge, J.M., 1993. Intrauterine pressure and the active management of labour. Journal of Obstetrics and Gynaecology 13 (6), 433–436.

Carlisle, N., Watson, H.A., Shennan, A.H., 2021. Development and rapid rollout of the QUiPP App Toolkit for women who arrive in threatened preterm labour. BMJ Open Quality 10 (2), e001272.

Chapman, V., Charles, C., 2018. The Midwife's Labour and Birth Handbook, fourth ed. Wiley, Oxford.

Coad, J., Pedley, K., Dunstall, M., 2019. Anatomy and Physiology for Midwives, fourth ed. Elsevier, London.

Crowther, C.A., Middleton, P.F., Voysey, M., Askie, L., Zhang, S., Martlow, T.K., et al., PRECISE Group, 2019. Effects of repeat prenatal corticosteroids given to women at risk of preterm birth: an individual participant data meta-analysis. PLoS Med. 16 (4), e1002771.

Denoual-Ziad, C., Aicardi-Nicolas, S., Creveuil, C., Gaillard, C., Dreyfus, M., Benoist, G., 2015. Impact of prolonged dinoprostone cervical ripening on the rate of artificial induction of labor: a prospective study of 330 patients. J. Obstet. Gynaecol. Res. 41 (3), 370–376.

de Vaan, M.D., Ten Eikelder, M.L., Jozwiak, M., Palmer, K.R., Davies-Tuck, M., Bloemenkamp, K.W., et al., 2019. Mechanical methods for induction of labour. Cochrane Database Syst. Rev. 2019 (10), CD001233.

Dodd, J.M., Crowther, C.A., Middleton, P., 2012. Oral betamimetics for maintenance therapy after threatened preterm labour. Cochrane Database Syst. Rev. 2012 (12), CD003927.

Dodd, J.M., Jones, L., Flenady, V., Cincotta, R., Crowther, C.A., 2013. Prenatal administration of progesterone for preventing preterm birth in women considered to be at risk of preterm birth. Cochrane Database Syst. Rev. 2013 (7), CD004947.

Duckitt, K., Thornton, S., O'Donovan, O.P., Dowswell, T., 2014. Nitric oxide donors for treating preterm labour. Cochrane Database Syst. Rev. 2014 (5), CD002860.

Fawole, B., Hofmeyr, G.J., 2012. Maternal oxygen administration for fetal distress. Cochrane Database Syst. Rev. 2012 (12), CD000136.

Ferguson, J.K., 1941. A study of the motility of the intact uterus at term. Surgical Gynaecology and Obstetrics 73 (3), 359–366.

Finucane, E.M., Murphy, D.J., Biesty, L.M., Gyte, G.M., Cotter, A.M., Ryan, E.M., et al., 2020. Membrane sweeping for induction of labour. Cochrane Database Syst. Rev. 2020 (2), CD000451.

Flenady, V., Wojcieszek, A.M., Papatsonis, D.N., Stock, O.M., Murray, L., Jardine, L.A., et al., 2014. Calcium channel blockers for inhibiting preterm labour and birth. Cochrane Database Syst. Rev. 2014 (6), CD002255.

Han, S., Crowther, C.A., Moore, V., 2013. Magnesium maintenance therapy for preventing preterm birth after threatened preterm labour. Cochrane Database Syst. Rev. 2013 (5), CD000940.

Henderson, J., Carson, C., Redshaw, M., 2016. Impact of preterm birth on maternal well-being and women's perceptions of their baby: a population-based survey. BMJ Open 6 (10), e012676.

Hillier, S.L., Nugent, R.P., Eschenbach, D.A., 1995. Association between a bacterial vaginosis and preterm delivery of a low birth-weight infant. N. Engl. J. Med. 333 (26), 1736–1742.

Hofmeyr, G.J., Novikova, N., 2012. Management of reported decreased fetal movements for improving pregnancy outcomes. Cochrane Database Syst. Rev. 2012 (4), CD009148.

Howarth, G., Botha, D.J., 2001. Amniotomy plus intravenous oxytocin for induction of labour. Cochrane Database Syst. Rev. 2001 (3), CD003250.

Jackson, K., Anderson, M., Marshall, J.E., 2020. Physiology and care during the first stage of labour. In: Marshall, J., Raynor, M. (Eds.), Myles' Textbook for Midwives, seventeenth ed. Elsevier, London.

Jarde, A., Feng, Y.Y., Viaje, K.A., Shah, P.S., McDonald, S.D., 2020. Vaginal birth vs caesarean section for extremely preterm vertex infants: a systematic review and meta-analyses. Arch. Gynecol. Obstet. 301 (2), 447–458.

Kavanagh, J., Kelly, A.J., Thomas, J., 2005. Breast stimulation for cervical ripening and induction of labour. Cochrane Database Syst. Rev. 2005 (3), CD003392.

Kenyon, S., Tokumasu, H., Dowswell, T., Pledge, D., Mori, R., 2013a. High-dose versus low-dose oxytocin for augmentation of delayed labour. Cochrane Database Syst. Rev. 2013 (7), CD007201.

Kenyon, S., Boulvain, M., Neilson, J.P., 2013. Antibiotics for preterm rupture of membranes. Cochrane Database Syst. Rev. 2013 (12), CD001058.

Lavender, T., Cuthbert, A., Smyth, R.M.D., 2018. Effect of partograph use on outcomes for women in spontaneous labour at term and their babies. Cochrane Database Syst. Rev. 2018 (8), CD005461.

Lawrence, A., Lewis, L., Hofmeyr, G.J., Styles, C., 2013. Maternal positions and mobility during first stage labour. Cochrane Database Syst. Rev. 2013 (10), CD003934.

Mackeen, A.D., Seibel-Seamon, J., Muhammad, J., Baxter, J.K., Berghella, V., et al., 2014. Tocolytics for preterm premature rupture of membranes. Cochrane Database Syst. Rev. 2014 (2), CD007062.

Mavrides, E., Allard, S., Chandraharan, E., Collins, P., Green, L., Hunt, B.J., et al., on behalf of the Royal College of Obstetricians and Gynaecologists, 2016. Prevention and management of postpartum haemorrhage. Br. J. Obstet. Gynaecol. 124 (5), e106–e149.

McGoldrick, E., Stewart, F., Parker, R., Dalziel, S.R., 2020. Antenatal corticosteroids for accelerating fetal lung maturation for women at risk of preterm birth. Cochrane Database Syst. Rev. 2020 (12), CD004454.

Middleton, P., Shepherd, E., Crowther, C.A., 2018. Induction of labour for improving birth outcomes for women at or beyond term. Cochrane Database Syst. Rev. 2018 (5), CD004945.

Middleton, P., Shepherd, E., Morris, J., Crowther, C.A., Gomersall, J.C., 2020. Induction of labour at or beyond 37 weeks' gestation. Cochrane Database Syst. Rev. 2020 (7), CD004945.

Mozurkewich, E.L., Chilimigras, J.L., Berman, D.R., Perni, U.C., Romero, V.C., King, V.J., et al., 2011. Methods of induction of labour: a systematic review. BMC Pregnancy Childbirth 11 (84), 84–103.

Muglu, J., Rather, H., Arroyo-Manzano, D., Bhattacharya, S., Balchin, I., Khalil, A., et al., 2018. Risks of stillbirth and neonatal death with advancing gestation at term: a systematic review and meta-analysis of cohort studies of 15 million pregnancies. PLoS Med. 16 (7), e1002838.

National Institute of Health and Care Excellence (NICE), 2021a. Inducing Labour. Available at: https://www.nice.org.uk/guidance/ng207.

National Institute of Health and Care Excellence (NICE), 2021b. Antenatal Care. Available at: https://www.nice.org.uk/guidance/ng201/resources/antenatal-care-pdf-66143709695941#page46.

National Institute of Health and Care Excellence (NICE), 2022. Preterm Labour and Birth. Available at: https://www.nice.org.uk/guidance/ng25/resources/preterm-labour-and-birth-pdf-1837333576645.

National Institute of Health and Care Excellence (NICE), 2023. Intrapartum Care. Available at: https://www.nice.org.uk/guidance/ng235.

O'Driscoll, K., Meagher, D., Boylan, P., 1986. Active Management of Labour, second ed. Mosby, London.

O'Driscoll, K., Meagher, D., Boylan, P., 1993. Active Management of Labour, third ed. Mosby, London.

Omar, N.S., Tan, P.C., Sabir, N., Yusop, E.S., Omar, S.Z., 2013. Coitus to expedite the onset of labour: a randomised trial. Br. J. Obstet. Gynaecol. 120 (3), 338–345.

Peacock, J.L., Bland, J.M., Anderson, H.R., 1995. Preterm delivery: effects of socio-economic factors, psychological stress, smoking, alcohol and caffeine. Br. Med. J. 311 (7004), 532–536.

Purisch, S.E., Gyamfi-Bannerman, C., 2017. Epidemiology of preterm birth. Semin. Perinatol. 41 (7), 387–391.

Ram, M., Anteby, M., Weiniger, C.F., Havakuk, O., Gilboa, I., Shenhav, M., et al., 2021. Acute pulmonary edema due to severe preeclampsia in maternal age women. Pregnancy Hypertension 25, 150–155.

Ritter, J.M., Flower, R.S., Henderson, G., Loke, Y.K., MacEwan, D., Rang, H., 2019. Rang & Dale's Pharmacology, ninth ed. Elsevier, London.

Reinebrant, H.E., Pileggi-Castro, C., Romero, C.L., Dos Santos, R.A., Kumar, S., Souza, J.P., et al., 2015. Cyclo-oxygenase (COX) inhibitors for treating preterm labour. Cochrane Database Syst. Rev. 2015 (6), CD001992.

Royal College of Obstetricians and Gynaecologists (RCOG), 2012. Sepsis in Pregnancy, Bacterial (Green-top Guideline No. 64a). Available at: https://www.rcog.org.uk/guidance/browse-all-guidance/green-top-guidelines/sepsis-in-pregnancy-bacterial-green-top-guideline-no-64a/.

Shahabuddin, Y., Murphy, D.J., 2022. Cervical ripening and labour induction: a critical review of available methods. Best Pract. Res. Clin. Obstet. Gynaecol. 79, 3–17.

Simkin, P., Ancheta, R., Hanson, L., 2017. The Labor Progress Handbook: Early Intervention to Prevent and Treat Dystocia, fourth ed. Wiley-Blackwell, Oxford.

Smyth, R.M.D., Markham, C., Dowswell, T., 2013. Amniotomy for shortening spontaneous labour. Cochrane Database Syst. Rev. 2013 (6), CD006167.

Suzuki, S., 2015. Clinical significance of precipitous labor. J. Clin. Med. Res. 7 (3), 150–153.

Thinkhamrop, J., Hofmeyr, G.J., Adetoro, O., Lumbiganon, P., Ota, E., 2015. Antibiotic prophylaxis during the second and third trimester to reduce adverse pregnancy outcomes and morbidity. Cochrane Database Syst. Rev. 2015 (6), CD002250.

Thomas, J., Fairclough, A., Kavanagh, J., et al., 2014. Vaginal prostaglandin (PGE2 and PGF2a) for induction of labour at term. Cochrane Database Syst. Rev. 2014 (6), CD003101.

Thomson, A.J., on behalf of the Royal College of Obstetricians and Gynaecologists, 2019. Care of women presenting with suspected preterm prelabour rupture of membranes from 24^{+0} weeks of gestation. Br. J. Obstet. Gynaecol. 126 (9), e152–e166.

United Nations Children's Fund (UNICEF), and World Health Organization (WHO), 2004. Low Birthweight: Country, Regional and Global Estimates. UNICEF, New York.

Vogel, J.P., Nardin, J.M., Dowswell, T., et al., 2014. Combination of tocolytic agents for inhibiting preterm labour. Cochrane Database Syst. Rev. 2014 (7), CD006169.

Vogel, J.P., Chawanpaiboon, S., Moller, A.-B., et al., 2018. The global epidemiology of preterm birth. Best Pract. Res. Clin. Obstet. Gynaecol. 52, 3–12.

Walani, S.R., 2020. Global burden of preterm birth. Int. J. Gynecol. Obstet. 150 (1), 31–33.

Walker, N., Gan, J.H., 2017. Prolonged pregnancy. Obstet. Gynaecol. Reprod. Med. 20 (10), 311–315.

Wei, S., Wo, B.L., Qi, H.-P., et al., 2013. Early amniotomy and early oxytocin for prevention of, or therapy for, delay in first stage spontaneous labour compared with routine care. Cochrane Database Syst. Rev. 2013 (8), CD006794.

Whitworth, M., Bricker, L., Mullan, C., 2015. Ultrasound for fetal assessment in early pregnancy. Cochrane Database Syst. Rev. 2015 (7), CD007058.

World Health Organization (WHO), 2007. Integrated Management of Pregnancy and Childbirth. Managing Complications in Pregnancy and Childbirth: A Guide for Midwives and Doctors. Available at: http://apps.who.int/iris/bitstream/10665/43972/1/9241545879_eng.pdf.

World Health Organization (WHO), 2018. WHO Recommendations: Induction of Labour at or beyond Term. Available at: https://srhr.org/rhl/article/who-recommendation-on-induction-of-labour-for-women-beyond-41-weeks-of-gestation.

World Health Organization (WHO), 2019. Survive and Thrive: Transforming Care for Every Small and Sick Newborn. Available at: https://www.who.int/publications/i/item/9789241515887.

Williams, M.J., Ramson, J.A., Brownfoot, F.C., 2022. Different corticosteroids and regimens for accelerating fetal lung maturation for babies at risk of preterm birth. Cochrane Database Syst. Rev. 2022 (8), CD006764.

Wilson, A., Hodgetts-Morton, V.A., Marson, E.J., Markland, A.D., Larkai, E., Papadopoulou, A., et al., 2022. Tocolytics for delaying preterm birth: a network meta-analysis (0924). Cochrane Database Syst. Rev. 2022 (8), CD014978.

Annotated recommended reading

National Institute of Health and Care Excellence (NICE), 2021. Inducing Labour. Available at: https://www.nice.org.uk/guidance/ng207.

This document sets out research-based guidelines for induction of labour. These provide an excellent resource for midwives and obstetricians.

National Institute of Health and Care Excellence (NICE), 2023. Intrapartum Care. Available at: https://www.nice.org.uk/guidance/ng235.

This document presents research-based guidelines for care in labour. It is essential reading for midwives and obstetricians. The overall responsibility for care remains with the lead professional caring for the woman.

Websites

https://www.nice.org.uk/.
https://www.rcog.org.uk/guidance/.
https://www.who.int/publications/.
https://www.cochranelibrary.com/.
https://www.npeu.ox.ac.uk/ukoss.

These websites provide evidence-based guidance and recommendations related to pregnancy and intrapartum care. The sites also provide excellent resources for good practice in high-quality care and related published evidence.

42

Breech Presentation

LYZ HOWIE AND JEAN WATSON

This chapter discusses breech presentation and management. This includes types of breech, aetiology, diagnosis and associated risk factors. For vaginal births, an understanding of fetal movements in response to the maternal pelvis will help prevent injury to the woman or her baby.

Introduction

Any presentation of the fetus other than a vertex is called a *malpresentation* (Yulia, Maksym & Lack, 2022). This includes breech, face, brow and shoulder. These presentations have an ill-fitting presenting part and may be associated with early rupture of membranes. There is also likelihood of poor uterine action, leading to prolongation of labour. Each malpresentation leads to a different mechanism for descent, and there may be difficulties in birth. Malpresentations increase the risk of morbidity and mortality for the fetus and may result in operative delivery. Other malpresentations are discussed in Chapter 43.

Breech Presentation

Breech presentation is where the lie is longitudinal but the fetal buttocks lie in the lower segment of the uterus. This presentation is found in 3–4% of all deliveries at term (Hofmeyr et al., 2015a; Impey et al., 2017a). Although one in five fetuses will present by breech at 28 weeks of pregnancy, spontaneous version to a vertex presentation is likely to occur, especially in multigravidae. Breech is more prevalent in nulliparous women and in preterm births (Impey et al., 2017a).

Aetiology

In many cases of breech there is no identifiable cause. Certain factors are, however, known to contribute to breech presentation. Many persistent breech presentations are associated with conditions which either restrict the movement or allow excessive movement of the fetus. Others involve the health of the fetus (Table 42.1).

Types of Breech Presentation

Four types of breech presentation can be described (depending on the relationship of the lower limb(s) to the fetal trunk): complete or flexed breech, extended or frank breech, footling presentation and knee presentation (see Clinical Application 42.1). The type can influence the diagnosis of breech presetation antenatally and the complications likely to occur at delivery.

In malpresentations, the fetus presenting by breech can take up different positions (Fig. 42.1).

Diagnosis of Breech Presentation

A history of a previous breech presentation could suggest a uterine anomaly and an increased risk of repeated breech. If the woman complains of discomfort under the ribs, it may be due to the presence of the hard fetal head in the fundus. The woman may also be aware of fetal kicking movements below the umbilicus.

On Abdominal Examination

Findings are:
- **Inspection:** usually reveals nothing unusual.
- **Palpation:** the presenting part feels firm but not hard or smooth. The head may be felt in the fundus as hard, round and ballotable. Clinical Application 42.2 presents possible findings on abdominal palpation of breech presentation.

TABLE 42.1	Possible Causes of Breech Presentation			
Restricted Space	**Excessive Space**	**Fetal Factors**	**Other Factors**
Primigravidae with firm uterine and abdominal muscles	Grand multiparity because of lax uterine and abdominal muscles	Fetal abnormalities	Use of anticonvulsant drugs
Uterine malformations such as bicornuate uterus	Polyhydramnios	Fetal death	Previous breech birth
Uterine fibroids		Decreased fetal activity	Preterm birth
Contracted pelvis preventing engagement of the presenting part		Impaired fetal growth	Nulliparity
Multiple pregnancy		Short umbilical cord	
Placenta praevia		Extended legs	
Oligohydramnios			

(Hofmeyr, Hannah & Lawrie, 2015; Hofmeyr, Kulier & West, 2015a; 2015b)

- **Auscultation:** fetal heart sounds may be heard above the umbilicus.

On Vaginal Examination

On vaginal examination (VE), either small parts or the breech itself may be detected. It is essential to distinguish between a hand and a foot (a hand might grasp the examiner's finger, whereas a foot will not). The breech itself is smooth and rounded and may feel like a vertex. Locating the anus may be mistaken for a mouth during VE and wrongly identified as a face presentation at term.

Ultrasound Scan

Diagnosis in a suspected breech presentation can be made by ultrasound to determine delivery options (National Institute of Health and Care Excellence [NICE], 2019; Yulia, Maksym & Lack, 2022). The fetus should also be examined for anomalies.

Associated Risk Factors

The increased risk of morbidity and mortality in breech deliveries may be four times that of cephalic presentation. It is unclear whether this is due to pre-existing problems or the effect of delivery. Associated factors include prematurity, congenital abnormalities, placenta praevia and placental abruption (Hofmeyr, Hannah & Lawrie, 2015). Prolapse of the umbilical cord may lead to anoxia and fetal death due to entrapment between the fetal breech and an incompletely dilated cervix. There are also increased risks for the woman due to possible delivery by caesarean section (CS).

Congenital Abnormality

The presence of a congenital abnormality occurs more frequently with breech presentation than with a cephalic

presentation (Mostello et al., 2014). The most common major abnormality is a defect of the neural tube such as meningomyelocele, hydrocephaly or anencephaly. Anomalies of the internal systems such as the gastrointestinal, respiratory, cardiovascular and urinary systems are also found. Developmental dysplasia of the hip is a common problem, occurring more frequently in girls.

Risks at Delivery

A breech birth is not without its risks. Risks to the fetus are outlined in Table 42.2.

Management of Pregnancy

Any woman found to have a breech presentation later in pregnancy or labour should have discussions regarding birth choices (e.g., benefits and risk of vaginal breech birth, CS and external cephalic version (ECV)) (Impey et al., 2017a & b; NICE, 2019). With her full involvement, a decision needs to be made about the safest option for delivery. Impey et al. (2017a) recommend that ECV should be offered at 36 weeks' gestation in a nulliparous singleton breech pregnancy, whereas in multiparous women this would be offered from 37 weeks' gestation. Women that may be excluded from ECV include labouring women, women with ruptured membranes, vaginal bleeding, uterine scar or abnormality, medical conditions and fetal compromise. There is, however, uncertainty about contraindications to ECV, and the risk is not deemed any greater for women who have had one previous CS (Impey et al., 2017a). If ECV is contraindicated or has been unsuccessful, then women with a singleton breech presentation should be offered choice of a vaginal or CS birth after being informed of all the risks, benefits and outcomes (NICE, 2019). Significant research continues on the optimization of care for women with breech presentation at term to support choice around planned vaginal breech birth (Walker et al., 2022).

• CLINICAL APPLICATION 42.1   The Four Types of Breech Presentation

Complete or flexed breech: The thighs and knees are flexed, and the feet are close to the buttocks (tailor sitting or squatting). This occurs in 10–15% of cases and is most common in multigravidae.

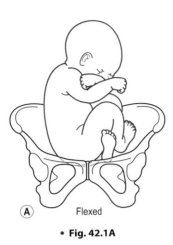

(A)   Flexed

• Fig. 42.1A

Extended or frank breech: The fetal thighs are flexed, and the legs are extended at the knees. The legs lie alongside the trunk with the feet near the head. This is the most common of the four types of breech presentation, occurring in 45–50%, most commonly in primigravidae near term. Firm uterine and abdominal muscles prevent fetal movement so that the fetus is unable to flex its knees. There is limited likelihood of a turn to cephalic presentation.

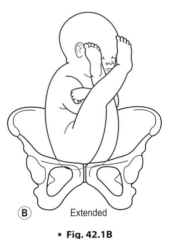

(B)   Extended

• Fig. 42.1B

Footling presentation: One or both hips and knees are extended, and the feet present below the buttocks. This rare complication is more common in preterm labour.

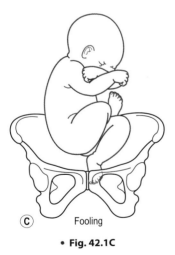

(C)   Footling

• Fig. 42.1C

Knee presentation: One or both hips are extended, and knees are flexed. The knee(s) present below the buttocks. This is the rarest of the four presentations.

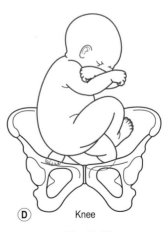

(D)   Knee

• Fig. 42.1D

• Fig. 42.1 The four types of breech presentation.

Cephalic Version
Promotion of Spontaneous Cephalic Version

Various exercises and maternal positions have been tried in an attempt to turn a fetus in breech presentation. As yet, there is no evidence to demonstrate their effectiveness (Hofmeyr & Kulier, 2012). However these exercises do not do any harm, and have no contraindications.

Moxibustion

Moxibustion (burning the herb *Artemisia vulgaris* close to the skin inducing a warming sensation) is a traditional Chinese method to help turn the fetus in a breech presentation (Coyle, Smith & Peat, 2012). Moxibustion and acupuncture have been increasingly combined. In this technique, a practitioner inserts heated acupuncture needles and then places small cones of moxa on the needle heads and ignites them. The acupuncture point Bladder 67 (BL67) is located at the tip of the fifth toe; its Chinese name is zhiyin (Coyle, Smith & Peat, 2012). It is a way of applying heat locally to regulate, tone and supplement the body's flow of qi (vital energy). This method is popular in China and Japan.

Although there are few high-quality trials available, there is enough evidence to conclude that moxibustion, combined with postural techniques and/or acupuncture, may reduce breech presentations at births and fewer CSs (Coyle, Smith & Peat, 2012). If using moxibustion, good ventilation should be available to prevent unpleasant odours and throat problems. More research is required to provide robust evidence on its use.

External Cephalic Version

During ECV, the fetus is manipulated with pressure through the abdominal wall to turn it from a breech to a cephalic presentation (Hofmeyr, Kulier & West, 2015b; Impey et al., 2017a) (Fig. 42.2). The timing for conducting this manual manoeuvre should be discussed and agreed upon with the woman (Hutton, Hofmeyr & Dowswell, 2015). Risks are attached to the procedure, including bleeding from the placental site, cord entanglement causing fetal distress,

converting the lie and presentation to an undeliverable one, and initiating preterm labour. Adhering to the contraindications in Box 42.1 will reduce these risks.

In a large multicentred randomized controlled trial, Hutton et al. (2011) concluded that ECV initiated at 34–35 weeks of gestation compared with 37 or more weeks increases the probability of cephalic presentation, does not reduce the rate of CS and may increase the rate of preterm birth. In a systematic review, Hofmeyr, Kulier and West (2015b) identified that there are reasons for the clinical use of ECV at term, with the appropriate precautions, in any woman in whom the value of an improved chance of a cephalic birth outweighs the risk of the procedure. The reviewers reported that breech births and CSs may be reduced by attempting ECV at or near term.

The interventions reviewed by Cluver et al. (2015) for ECV included routine tocolysis, fetal acoustic stimulation, regional analgesia, transabdominal amnioinfusion and systemic opioids. Tocolysis involves the use of drugs that act as relaxants to the uterine musculature, such as salbutamol and

---

• CLINICAL APPLICATION 42.2 Abdominal Palpation of Breech

Although abdominal examination is the main diagnostic tool, it may be difficult to recognize in the primigravid woman with an extended breech.
- Breech may be deep in pelvis and simulate an engaged head.
- Feet lie alongside head. Both prevent identification by palpation and movement of head on the neck elicited by ballottement.
- If breech is engaged, fetal heart may be heard in the expected position for a vertex presentation.

• BOX 42.1 Contraindications to External Cephalic Version

Strong Evidence to Support
- Placenta praevia or placental abruption.
- Severe pre-eclampsia.
- Abnormal fetal Doppler.
- No informed consent from woman.

Weaker Evidence to Support
- Rhesus isoimmunisation.
- Abnormal cardiotocograph.
- Current or recent vaginal bleeding (<1 week).
- Rupture of membranes.
- Multiple pregnancy (except after delivery of twin 1).
  Additional caution is required where there is oligohydramnios or hypertension.

(Impey et al., 2017a)

TABLE 42.2 Risks to Fetus from Breech Birth

Intrauterine and Extrauterine Asphyxia	Intracranial Haemorrhage	Skeletal Fractures and Dislocations	Genital Trauma
• Delay in delivery of head after birth of the thorax and arms. • Placental separation may occur before birth is complete. • Cord compression is inevitable. • Hypoxia may stimulate breathing with inhalation of blood, liquor and mucus.	• Previously thought to be due to rapid compression and decompression of the brain as the head descended through the pelvis, resulting in a torn tentorium cerebelli. • Now thought that the main cause of cerebral haemorrhage is anoxia and congestion of the cerebral vessels.	• Damage to muscles and nerves due to difficulties arising during delivery or to faulty delivery technique. • Rupture of abdominal organs due to difficulties arising during delivery or to faulty delivery technique.	• Bruising and swelling to male/female genitalia

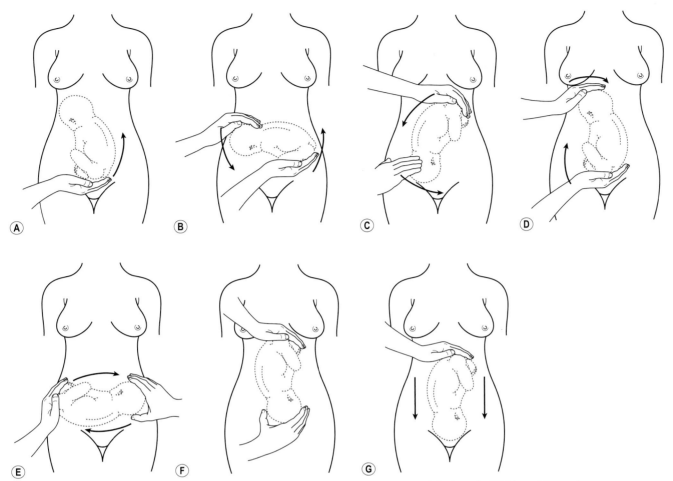

• **Fig. 42.2** External cephalic version. (A) Palpation and mobilization of the breech. (B) Manual forward rotation using both hands, one to push the breech and the other to guide the vertex. (C) Completion of forward roll. (D) Backward flip using both hands. (E) Quarter turn accomplished. Continue to push breech upwards and vertex downwards. (F) Completion of external version. (G) Gently push the breech downwards to direct vertex into pelvis.

ritodrine (beta stimulants), before carrying out ECV. Cluver et al. (2015) found that routine tocolysis appears to reduce the failure rate of ECV at term. Other types of tocolytic drugs such as calcium-channel blockers (CCBs) and nitric-acid donors and the use of systemic opioids are significantly negative (Bricker & Lavender, 2002).

Administering neuroaxial intravenous and inhalation anaesthetic techniques were reported to have a slightly higher success rate for ECV compared to the control group (Hao et al., 2020). As some findings appear promising, Cluver et al. (2015) suggest that further studies are warranted in fetal acoustic stimulation, combined regional anaesthesia with ECV and transabdominal amnioinfusion.

The Procedure for External Cephalic Version (ECV)

A skilled and experienced practitioner should carry out the procedure, where facilities for monitoring and immediate delivery are available (Impey et al., 2017a). A successful procedure not only depends on the practitioner, but also on the position and engagement of the fetus, volume of liquor and maternal parity. A cardiotocograph (CTG) and ultrasound

should be undertaken. The woman should give prior consent for the procedure. Some obstetricians prefer women to be fasted and prepared for theatre. Although this is usually not necessary, it is reasonable to have access to theatre close at hand. ECV is most likely to be successful when the presenting part is free, the head is easy to palpate and the uterus feels soft. The mother is asked to lie flat with a 30-degree lateral tilt. If the uterus is not soft, establish an intravenous tocolytic. Box 42.2 highlights the advantages and disadvantages of ECV at term.

Babies are more likely to turn headfirst during ECV and to remain headfirst for the start of labour if women receive beta stimulants (Cluver et al., 2015). Applying scanning gel to the abdomen allows easier manipulation and permits scanning during the procedure. If required, the obstetrician disimpacts the breech from the pelvis and applies pressure to both poles of the fetus to rotate it into a cephalic presentation (Fig. 42.2). It is safer to achieve this by making the fetus turn a forward somersault, or to 'follow its nose'! A backward somersault may sometimes achieve the version more easily, but there is a risk of extension of the neck, resulting in a brow presentation. Prior to the procedure and on completion of the manoeuvre, the fetal heart should be recorded for 30–40 min via CTG to ensure there is no fetal distress (Hinshaw & Arulkumaran, 2018). Uterine contractions, signs of rupture of the membranes and any vaginal bleeding are observed and reported to the obstetrician immediately. If the woman's blood group is Rh–, 500 IU of anti-D immunoglobulin is administered within 72 hours after ECV (Impey et al., 2017a).

The Role of Planned Caesarean Section at Term

Over recent decades it has become accepted that CS should be the mode of delivery for fetuses presenting by breech. Strong evidence demonstrates that CS is safer for term singleton breeches than planned vaginal deliveries; however there is an impact on maternal morbidity (Hannah et al., 2000; Hofmeyr, Hannah & Lawrie, 2015). These findings are not generalizable in areas where CS is not readily available or where women choose to give birth at home.

Although there are concerns that clinicians may become deskilled in vaginal breech delivery due to increased rates of elective CS, studies suggest that use of strict criteria before and during labour can result in a high level of safety for planned term vaginal breech births (Azria et al., 2012; Goffinet et al., 2006). More research is required to compare elective CS and planned vaginal delivery for breech presentations.

Vaginal Delivery

Women should be made aware of the risks of CS and vaginal breech birth so they are able to make informed decisions that best suit them and their babies (NICE, 2019). Although vaginal breech delivery remains controversial, the review by Berhan and Haileamlak (2016) has shown that vaginal breech birth has a low absolute risk. In the event of a persistent breech presentation, the following factors in Box 42.3 are considered before vaginal delivery.

There are fundamental differences in delivery between cephalic and breech presentations. With cephalic or vertex presentation, the largest part of the fetus, the head, delivers first. Moulding of the cranium can occur over several hours. In a breech delivery, the breech is first delivered followed by the shoulders and then the head. Each part of the fetus is larger and less compressible than the previous part. The after-coming head has not had time to mould because it enters the pelvis with the base of the skull leading. The biggest challenge, therefore, is that the head might not fit through the pelvis as it is the last and largest part to deliver. If women are selected carefully so that the pelvis is of adequate dimensions in relation to the fetus and there are no other adverse factors, they should be able to deliver safely per vagina.

It is essential to understand the mechanism of a breech delivery so that delivery can be completed without trauma. In ideal conditions, vaginal breech delivery should be performed by an experienced midwife or under the supervision of a senior obstetrician. A paediatrician or neonatal clinician should be present at delivery. The practice in normal spontaneous breech birth is to keep hands off and allow the breech to deliver spontaneously. However the practitioner must be able to intervene if necessary, and it is important to know the normal mechanisms of breech delivery.

Management
The Mechanism of a Breech Delivery

There are six possible positions for a breech delivery. These are right or left sacroanterior, right or left sacroposterior and right or left sacrolateral. The left sacroanterior position is outlined in Box 42.4.

The Movements

It is necessary to consider the birth of the fetus in three main stages: buttocks, shoulders and head.

- **Lie** is longitudinal.
- **Presentation** is breech.
- **Denominator** is the sacrum.
- **Attitude** is one of complete flexion.
- **Presenting part** is the anterior (left) buttock.
- **Bitrochanteric diameter**, 10 cm, enters the pelvis in the left oblique diameter of pelvic brim.

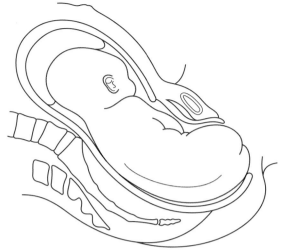

• **Fig. 42.3** Lateral flexion and birth of the buttocks.

Compaction and Flexion

Descent takes place with increasing compaction due to increased flexion of limbs on the trunk.

Internal Rotation of the Buttocks

The anterior buttock reaches the pelvic floor and rotates forwards in the pelvis by one-eighth of a circle to lie under the symphysis pubis. The bitrochanteric diameter now lies in the anteroposterior diameter of the pelvis.

Lateral Flexion of the Trunk

The anterior buttock escapes under the symphysis pubis, the posterior buttock sweeps the perineum and the buttocks are born by a movement of lateral flexion (Fig. 42.3).

Restitution

The anterior buttock turns slightly to the mother's right side.

Internal Rotation of the Shoulders

With the birth of the buttocks, the bisacromial diameter (~12 cm) of the shoulders enters the pelvis in the same diameter of the pelvis as the buttocks, the left oblique. The anterior (left) shoulder reaches the pelvic floor and rotates forwards by one-eighth of a circle to lie behind the symphysis pubis.

Birth of the Shoulders

The anterior shoulder and arm escape under the symphysis pubis, and the posterior shoulder and arm pass over the perineum.

Internal Rotation and Delivery of the Head

The flexed head engages with the suboccipitobregmatic diameter of 9.5 cm, or the suboccipitofrontal diameter of 10 cm, lying in the right oblique or transverse diameter of the pelvic brim. Internal rotation of the head carries the occiput behind the symphysis pubis. The face lies in the hollow of the sacrum. Internal rotation of the head is accompanied by external rotation of the trunk. The chin, face, vertex and occiput are born over the perineum by a movement of flexion.

The First Stage of Labour

The first stage does not differ from normal labour and may be allowed to continue spontaneously if there is progressive dilatation and descent with no fetal or maternal complications. In most resource-rich countries, the birth is advised to take place in a consultant unit (NICE, 2023) with an anaesthetist and neonatal clinician available (Impey et al., 2017b). This may not be the appropriate choice for all women, so informed decision-making outlining all the risks and benefits is paramount (Impey et al., 2017b; NICE, 2019). Induction of labour is not routinely recommended at term; if oxytocin is required for slow progress, then this should be administered alongside epidural analgesia. However it is noteworthy that epidural analgesia can increase intervention rates (Impey et al., 2017b). If the breech is flexed and not engaged, there may be early rupture of the membranes with the risk of umbilical cord prolapse. If the legs are extended, the breech is likely to be engaged and the risk of cord prolapse is lower. The woman may have a desire to push early when the buttocks slip through the incompletely dilated cervical os. This risks entrapment of the head. If this occurs, there is a possibility of delivery of the head by forceps.

Contractions in the first and second stages of labour may decrease in intensity after the commencement of epidural analgesia. If the woman has minimal analgesia, then she can labour standing up or on all fours, which facilitates the delivery of the breech. There is no evidence to support that routine epidural analgesia is essential (Impey et al., 2017b; Yulia, Maksym & Lack, 2022). Careful monitoring of the fetal heart is important as part of the continual assessment of the woman's progress in labour. Continuous electronic fetal monitoring by CTG should be offered to women throughout labour (Impey et al., 2017b).

The Second Stage of Labour

Once the breech is visible at the perineum, the woman can be encouraged to push. An experienced midwife or obstetrician will normally conduct the delivery. In hospital, with vaginal breech birth the woman's legs may be placed in the lithotomy position for the birth. There are other options, such as the use of upright postures, although there is currently no evidence to recommend these over the conventional postures (semi-recumbent and on all fours) with which most practitioners are familiar (Impey et al., 2017b). All midwives should be familiar with the manoeuvres necessary to deliver the baby in case of an emergency. Simulated practice is essential. An anaesthetist and paediatrician should be present at delivery in case of a sudden need for intervention.

Vaginal Breech Birth

The breech is engaged when the bitrochanteric diameter (10 cm) is at the pelvic brim, which is the diameter between the greater trochanters of the femora of the fetus.

Ideally the baby should be left alone to deliver itself ('hands off'), taking care to ensure the back remains uppermost when advancing. If there is undue delay or there are concerns about fetal well-being (e.g., movements stopping, baby becoming floppy, no response to stimuli), assisted delivery can be used to encourage a more rapid delivery. One key risk of breech delivery is that pulling may lead the head to extend and therefore become stuck at the pelvic brim. The importance of maternal effort at this stage, rather than traction from below, cannot be over emphasized – it allows the head to flex and minimizes the risk of it becoming stuck at the pelvic brim.

Breech extraction may be occasionally necessary where the fetus is extracted from the birth canal by manipulation rather than by assisting the normal mechanism. This is dangerous and is not often used in developed countries.

Assisted Breech Delivery

The woman's bladder is first emptied. Selective episiotomy is recommended to allow the practitioner to perform any required manipulations (Impey et al., 2017b).

The Buttocks

No handling is necessary, and delivery should proceed spontaneously until the fetal umbilicus appears at the introitus. Handling of the cord is not advised. The legs should normally deliver themselves. However, the knees can be flexed to deliver the legs by applying pressure to the popliteal fossa. Ensure that the buttocks remain sacroanterior. If the trunk appears to be rotating to a sacroanterior position, controlled rotation can be used with thumbs placed on the prominences of the sacroiliac crests.

Extended Legs

If the legs are extended, they may splint the body and prevent lateral flexion of the trunk. The legs of a frank breech may be delivered by inserting a finger behind the knee into the popliteal fossa to flex the knee and abduct the thigh (Pinard manoeuvre). However active efforts to deliver the legs are not mandatory, as the legs will deliver spontaneously and the feet will become free eventually.

The Body

Encourage spontaneous birth until the scapulae are visible. Traction of the baby can cause a nuchal arm and should be avoided. Handling or pulling of the cord should also be avoided.

The Arms

If the baby's arms cannot be found crossed over the chest or have not delivered spontaneously, they may be extended alongside the head, making the total diameter of the presenting part too large to descend into the pelvis. This often happens when the breech is pulled to deliver the legs and trunk.

Extended Arms

The arms must be brought down before the head can be delivered, and this is done by the Lövset manoeuvre (Fig. 42.4). The success of the manoeuvre arises from the relative positions of the two shoulders. The posterior shoulder is below the sacral promontory, and the anterior shoulder is above the symphysis pubis. Rotation by placing the thumbs on the iliac crest allows one arm to be freed, flexed and brought down, whereas rotation the other way allows the other arm to be similarly delivered. The practitioner gently holds the baby over the bony prominences of the hips and sacrum (avoiding pressure on the abdomen and abdominal organs) to keep the back uppermost to allow the fetal head to enter the pelvis with the occiput anterior. To release the uppermost arm, an index finger should be placed over the baby's shoulder and follow the baby's arm to the antecubital fossa; the arm is then flexed for delivery. The baby is rotated through 180 degrees to bring the posterior shoulder to the anterior position but beneath the symphysis pubis. The manoeuvre is repeated to release the second arm. After the arms are released, support the baby until the nape of the neck is visible.

The Head

If the hairline does not become visible after a few seconds of allowing the baby to hang by its weight, the head is probably extended. Forceps are usually used to deliver the head, but there are two alternative methods for delivering the head if the midwife is conducting the delivery: the Mauriceau–Smellie–Veit manoeuvre (Fig. 42.5) and the Burns–Marshall manoeuvre (Box 42.5; Fig. 42.6). Although both are discussed here, **the Mauriceau–Smellie–Veit manoeuvre is the recommended manoeuvre for breech delivery** (Impey et al., 2017b).

Mauriceau–Smellie–Veit (Modified) Manoeuvre

All movements in this manoeuvre promote head flexion. One of the practitioner's hands should be placed on the fetal back, with one finger inserted into the vagina and placed on the occiput and one finger on each of the fetal shoulders to promote flexion. The other hand is placed beneath the fetus; the modified manoeuvre involves placing two fingers on the maxillae whilst the practitioner's lower arm supports the body

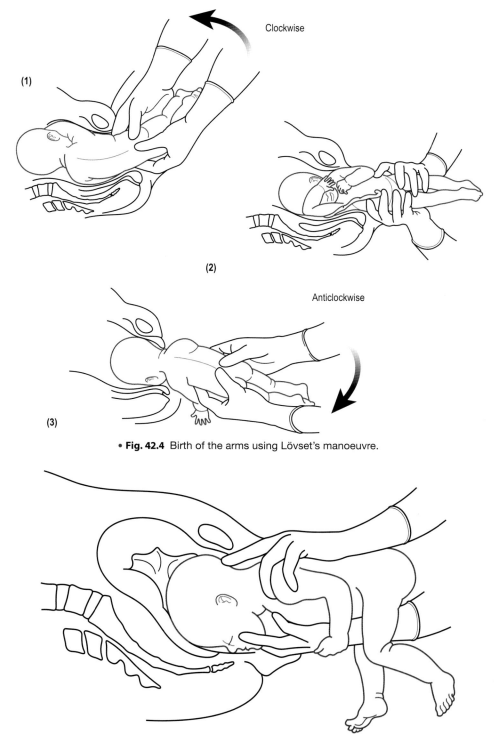

Clockwise

(1)

(2)

Anticlockwise

(3)

• **Fig. 42.4** Birth of the arms using Lövset's manoeuvre.

• **Fig. 42.5** The Mauriceau–Smellie–Veit manoeuvre.

(fetal legs straddle the practitioner's arm). An assistant should follow the head abdominally and be prepared to apply suprapubic pressure to flex the head through the pelvis.

Delivery of the head commences and is flexed through the pelvis by these separate mechanisms:
1. The occipital finger applies flexing pressure on the occiput.
2. The assistant applies suprapubic pressure on the occiput (if required).

3. The fingers on the maxillae apply pressure on the lower face, which tends to promote flexion.
4. Some traction is also required for the delivery by downward pressure of the fingers on the shoulders.

Oropharyngeal suction is not required as the mouth and nose appear over the perineum. The baby's head is carefully delivered following the curve of the birth canal (curve of Carus) slowly to prevent intracranial damage.

• BOX 42.5 Burns–Marshall Manoeuvre

This method of delivery for assisting birth of the head is not the preferred method and is no longer advised in the UK (Impey et al., 2017a). Concerns have been expressed in relation to the risk involved as it may lead to over extension of the baby's neck and cause injury (Winter et al., 2017, p.239). Included for background information only.

Method

The baby is allowed to hang by his own weight to encourage descent and flexion of the head, taking care not to allow

sudden delivery of the head (see Fig. 42.6 (1)). Once the nape of the neck and hairline can be seen, the baby's ankles are grasped (see Fig. 42.6 (2)) and, with slight traction, the trunk is carried in a wide arc up over the mother's abdomen (see Fig. 42.6 (3)). The other hand should support the perineum to prevent sudden delivery of the head. Once the mouth is clear, the baby can breathe, and time should be taken to complete the delivery of the head.

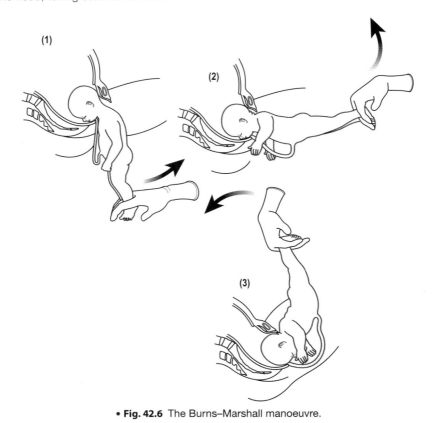

• Fig. 42.6 The Burns–Marshall manoeuvre.

Entrapment of the Fetal Head

This dangerous situation arises when the fetal body slips through an incompletely dilated cervix and the head is partially trapped behind the cervix. This is more likely in a preterm birth. The obstetrician will try to release the baby's head from the cervix, and one method that may help is the McRoberts manoeuvre, which is also useful in the delivery of a fetus with shoulder dystocia. The woman lies on her back, lifts her knees up to her chest and raises her buttocks off the bed. In the literature, several methods describe the management of head entrapment, with the most common being incising of the cervix at 10, 6 and 2 o'clock (to avoid the cervical neuromuscular bundles that run laterally in the cervix), thus releasing the head. There is a risk of extension into the lower segment of the uterus. To relax the cervix, tocolytics can be administered; for example an intravenous dose of terbutaline or intravenous nitroglycerin. Vaginal birth

can be possible in extremely preterm breech pregnancies with intact membranes by adopting the 'en caul' delivery method.

Undiagnosed Cephalopelvic Disproportion

In an unbooked woman or where there has been failure to diagnose a degree of hydrocephaly, this dire emergency may arise as the delivery proceeds. If the breech is delivered up to the head, there is usually difficulty in performing a CS. Symphysiotomy may save the baby's life.

Posterior Rotation of the Occiput

This is a rare complication. In this situation, the back of the baby is turned towards the mother's buttocks. To deliver the head, the chin and face are allowed to escape under the symphysis pubis as far as the root of the nose, and then the baby is lifted towards the mother's abdomen to allow the occiput to sweep the perineum.

Main Points

- One in five fetuses will present by breech at 28 weeks of pregnancy.
- Depending on the relationship of the lower limb(s) to the trunk of the fetus, breech presentation may be complete or flexed, extended or frank, footling or knee presentation.
- There is an increased risk of morbidity and mortality in breech deliveries. Associated factors include prematurity, congenital abnormalities, placenta praevia and placental abruption, prolapse of the umbilical cord and entrapment of the fetal head behind an incompletely dilated cervix.
- At delivery, the fetus is at risk from asphyxia, intracranial haemorrhage, skeletal fractures and dislocations, damage to muscles and nerves and rupture of abdominal organs, genital oedema and bruising.
- Any woman found to have a breech presentation later in pregnancy or labour should have discussions regarding birth choices (e.g., benefits and risk or vaginal breech birth, CS and ECV).

- Depending on parity, ECV would be offered at 36 weeks' gestation (primigravida) or 37 weeks' gestation (multigravida) to women with an uncomplicated singleton breech.
- The risks of a vaginal breech delivery mean that the birth should take place in a consultant unit.
- If the breech is flexed and not engaged, there may be early rupture of the membranes with the risk of umbilical cord prolapse.
- All midwives should be familiar with the manoeuvres necessary to deliver the baby presenting by breech in case of an emergency.
- The modified Mauriceau–Smellie–Veit manoeuvre is recommended for delivery of the head, as the movements promote flexion.
- An anaesthetist and paediatrician should be present at the delivery in case of a sudden need for intervention.
- Dangerous but rare complications such as entrapment of the fetal head, late diagnosis of cephalopelvic disproportion and posterior rotation of the occiput may lead to fetal morbidity and mortality.

References

Azria, E., Le Meaux, J.P., Khoshnood, B., Alexander, S., Subtil, D., Goffinet, F., PREMODA Study Group, 2012. Factors associated with adverse perinatal outcomes for term breech fetuses with planned vaginal delivery. Am. J. Obstet. Gynecol. 207 (4), 285.e1–285.e9.

Berhan, Y., Haileamlak, A., 2016. The risks of planned vaginal breech delivery versus planned caesarean section for term breech birth: a meta-analysis including observational studies. Br. J. Obstet. Gynaecol. 123 (1), 49–57.

Bricker, L., Lavender, T., 2002. Parenteral opioids for labor pain relief: a systematic review. Am. J. Obstet. Gynecol. 186 (5 Suppl. Nature), S94–S109.

Cluver, C., Gyte, G.M., Sinclair, M., Dowswell, T., Hofmeyr, G.J., 2015. Interventions for helping to turn term breech babies to headfirst presentation when using external cephalic version. Cochrane Database Syst. Rev. 2015 (2), CD000184.

Coyle, M.E., Smith, C.A., Peat, B., 2012. Cephalic version by moxibustion for breech presentation. Cochrane Database Syst. Rev. 2012 (5), CD003928.

Dasgupta, T., Hunter, S., Reid, S., Sandall, J., Shennan, A., Davies, S.M., Walker, S., 2022. Preparing for the OptiBreech Trial: a mixed methods implementation and feasibility study. Br. J. Obstet. Gynaecol. 129, 70.

Goffinet, F., Carayol, M., Foidart, J.M., Alexander, S., Uzan, S., Subtil, D., et al., PREMODA Study Group, 2006. Is planned vaginal delivery for breech presentation at term still an option? Results of an observational prospective survey in France and Belgium. Am. J. Obstet. Gynecol. 194 (4), 1002–1011.

Hannah, M.E., Hannah, W.J., Hewson, S.A., Hodnett, E.D., Saigal, S., Willan, A.R., 2000. Planned caesarean section versus planned vaginal birth for breech presentation at term: a randomised multicentre trial. Lancet 356 (9239), 1375–1383.

Hao, Q., Hu, Y., Zhang, L., Ross, J., Robishaw, S., Noble, C., et al., 2020. A systematic review and meta-analysis of clinical trials of neuraxial, intravenous, and inhalational anesthesia for external cephalic version. Anesth. Analg. 131 (6), 1800–1811.

Hinshaw, K., Arulkumaran, S., 2018. Malpresentation, malposition, cephalopelvic disproportion and obstetric procedures. In: Edmonds, K., Lees, C., Bourne, T. (Eds.), Dewhurst's Textbook of Obstetrics & Gynaecology, ninth ed. Wiley-Blackwell, Oxford.

Hofmeyr, G.J., Kulier, R., 2012. Cephalic version by postural management for breech presentation. Cochrane Database Syst. Rev. 2012 (10), CD000051.

Hofmeyr, G.J., Hannah, M., Lawrie, T.A., 2015. Planned caesarean section for term breech delivery. Cochrane Database Syst. Rev. 2015 (7), CD000166.

Hofmeyr, G.J., Kulier, R., West, H.M., 2015a. Expedited versus conservative approaches for vaginal delivery in breech presentation. Cochrane Database Syst. Rev. 2015 (7), CD000082.

Hofmeyr, G.J., Kulier, R., West, H.M., 2015b. External cephalic version for breech presentation at term. Cochrane Database Syst. Rev. 2015 (4), CD000083.

Hutton, E.K., Hannah, M.E., Ross, S.J., Delisle, M.F., Carson, G.D., Windrim, R., et al., 2011. The Early External Cephalic Version (ECV) 2 Trial: an international multicentre randomised controlled trial of timing of ECV for breech pregnancies. Br. J. Obstet. Gynaecol. 118 (5), 564–577.

Hutton, E.K., Hofmeyr, G.J., Dowswell, T., 2015. External cephalic version for breech presentation before term. Cochrane Database Syst. Rev. 2015 (7), CD000084.

Impey, L.W.M., Murphy, D.J., Griffiths, M., Eaton Bray, E., Penna, L.K., on behalf of the Royal College of Obstetricians and Gynaecologists, 2017a. External cephalic version and reducing the incidence of term breech presentation. Green-top Guideline No. 20a. Br. J. Obstet. Gynaecol. 124, e178–e192.

Impey, L.W.M., Murphy, D.J., Griffiths, M., Eaton Bray, E., Penna, L.K., on behalf of the Royal College of Obstetricians and Gynaecologists, 2017b. Management of breech presentation. Green-top Guideline No. 20b. Br. J. Obstet. Gynaecol. 124, e151–e177.

Mostello, D., Chang, J.J., Bai, F., Wang, J., Guild, C., Stamps, K., et al., 2014. Breech presentation at delivery: a marker for congenital anomaly? J. Perinatol. 34 (1), 11–15.

National Institute of Health and Care Excellence (NICE), 2019. Intrapartum Care for Women with Existing Medical Conditions or Obstetric Complications and Their Babies. Available at: https://www.nice.org.uk/guidance/ng121.

National Institute of Health and Care Excellence (NICE), 2023. Intrapartum Care. Available at: https://www.nice.org.uk/guidance/ng235.

Walker, S., Dasgupta, T., Shennan, A., Sandall, J., Bunce, C., Roberts, P., 2022. Development of a core outcome set for effectiveness studies of breech birth at term (Breech-COS) – an international multi-stakeholder Delphi study: study protocol. Trials 23, 249. https://doi.org/10.1186/s13063-022-06136-9

Winter, C., Crofts, J., Draycott, T., Crofts, J., Muchatuta, N., 2017. Practical Obstetric Multi-Professional Training (PROMPT). Cambridge University Press

Yulia, A., Maksym, K., Lack, N., 2022. Malpresentation. In: Fernando, R., Sultan, P., Phillips, S. (Eds.), Quick Hits in Obstetric Anesthesia. Springer, Cham.

Annotated recommended reading

Impey, L.W.M., Murphy, D.J., Griffiths, M., Eaton Bray, E., Penna, L.K., on behalf of the Royal College of Obstetricians and Gynaecologists, 2017a. External cephalic version and reducing the incidence of term breech presentation. Green-top Guideline No. 20a. Br. J. Obstet. Gynaecol. 124, e178–e192.

Impey, L.W.M., Murphy, D.J., Griffiths, M., Eaton Bray, E., Penna, L.K., on behalf of the Royal College of Obstetricians and Gynaecologists, 2017b. Management of breech presentation. Green-top Guideline No. 20b. Br. J. Obstet. Gynaecol. 124, e151–e177.

These two guidelines are recommended reading for practitioners working within obstetrics. They provide important information and guidance.

National Institute of Health and Care Excellence (NICE), 2023. Intrapartum Care. Available at: https://www.nice.org.uk/guidance/ng235.

This updated guideline provides evidence-based guidance for the provision and management of intrapartum care.

Winter, C., Crofts, J., Draycott, T., Crofts, J., Muchatuta, N., 2017. Practical Obstetric Multi-Professional Training (PROMPT). Cambridge University Press.

This PROMPT manual is an evidence-based training package that teaches healthcare professionals how to respond to obstetric emergencies. It is acknowledged by the Royal College of Obstetricians and Gynaecologists and the Royal College of Midwives.

Websites

https://www.nice.org.uk/.
https://www.rcog.org.uk/guidance/.
https://www.who.int/publications/.
https://www.npeu.ox.ac.uk/ukoss.

These websites provide evidence-based guidance and recommendations related to intrapartum care of the mother and baby. The sites also provide excellent resources for good practice in high-quality care and related published evidence.

43

Malposition and Cephalic Malpresentations

LYZ HOWIE AND JEAN WATSON

CHAPTER CONTENTS

This chapter discusses malposition and cephalic malpresentation in relation to diagnosis and management. The occipitoposterior position of the vertex is detailed first, followed by malpresentations (face, brow, shoulder and compound).

Introduction

In a cephalic presentation, if the vertex is the denominator the term *malpresentation* is not used. An occipitoposterior (OP) position of the vertex is a **malposition.** True cephalic malpresentations are face and brow. A shoulder presentation resulting from an oblique or transverse lie is a rare but dangerous event. Each of these situations may affect the length and outcome of labour and require vigilance to prevent maternal and fetal morbidity or mortality. OP position will be discussed first as it may lead to secondary brow or face presentation.

Occipitoposterior Position of the Vertex

In the OP position of the vertex, the occiput occupies one of the two posterior quadrants of the pelvis and the sinciput points towards the opposite anterior quadrant (Fig. 43.1). Malposition is common and affects about 15–33% of labours (Barrowclough et al., 2022). The outcome of such labour is generally a normal vertex delivery with rotation of the occiput to the anterior. There may be prolonged labour and mechanical difficulties associated with OP positions (Barrowclough et al., 2022).

Causes

There is no single cause for the OP position. However if the forepelvis is small (as found in android and anthropoid pelves), the head may take up a posterior position. Other possible causes include a pendulous abdomen, a flat sacrum, an anterior placenta, high body mass index (BMI), a sedentary lifestyle or epidural anaesthesia (Coates, 2017).

Attitude

Instead of the normal well-flexed attitude (with limbs and head flexed on the trunk and rounded back pointing towards the maternal abdominal wall), the fetal spine faces the forward curve of the maternal lumbar spine and good flexion is not possible. The fetal spine is straightened, the head is held in a deflexed position known as the *military position* and the anterior fontanelle is found directly over the internal os. This position of the head brings larger diameters

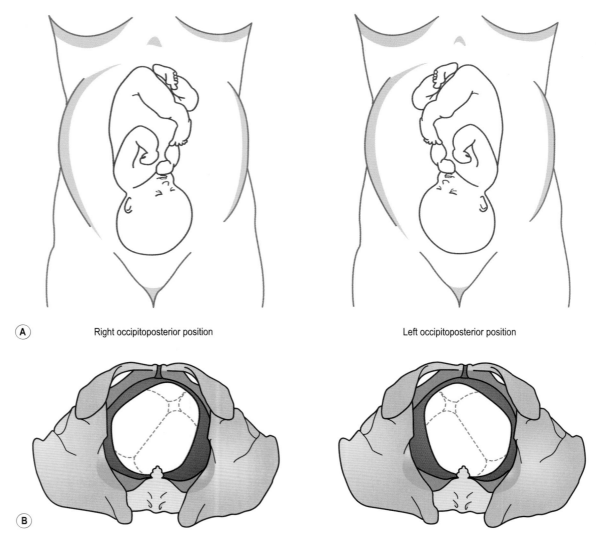

(A)   Right occipitoposterior position   Left occipitoposterior position

(B)

• **Fig. 43.1** Occipitoposterior positions. (A) Abdominal findings—the anterior shoulders are well out from the midline or the fetal limbs are easily palpable. This may cause a diagnosis of multiple pregnancy. (B) Vaginal findings—on vaginal examination, the anterior fontanelle is easily felt and recognized by its shape and size.

• BOX 43.1   Risks of Occipitoposterior Position

- Obstructed labour if either deep transverse arrest or brow presentation result.
- Maternal perineal trauma such as a third-degree tear and bruising.
- Cord prolapse if there is early spontaneous rupture of the membranes and ill-fitting presenting part.
- Neonatal cerebral haemorrhage due to upward moulding of the fetal skull. The falx cerebri may be pulled away from the tentorium cerebelli, resulting in a tear of the great vein of Galen.
- Chronic fetal hypoxia, if present, results in venous distension, which increases the likelihood of haemorrhage.

---

into relationship with the pelvic brim and engagement of the head may not occur. The risks of the OP position are presented in Box 43.1.

Diagnosis in Pregnancy

The OP position is the most common cause of a non-engaged head in late pregnancy in primigravidae. The woman may be aware of more fetal movement as the fetal limbs are anterior. Frequency of micturition might occur in the absence of infection. Abdominal examination to confirm the diagnosis is outlined in Clinical Application 43.1.

Diagnosis in Labour

Abdominal examination will indicate the presence of an OP position, although the head may be flexed and become engaged. On vaginal examination (VE), palpation of the anterior fontanelle is a diagnostic aid in determining the OP position (Leeman, 2020). If the head is reasonably well flexed, the anterior fontanelle will be felt anteriorly, and it may be possible to feel the posterior

Inspection: The abdomen appears flattened, with potentially a saucer-shaped depression below the umbilicus between the fetal head and limbs (Fig. 43.2).

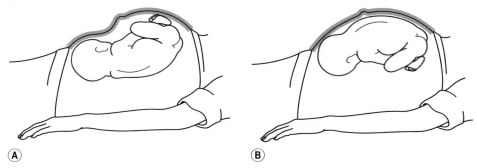

• **Fig. 43.2** (A) Abdominal contour with occipitoposterior position, showing depression at umbilicus. (B) Rounded abdominal contour with occipitoanterior position.[1]

Palpation: Fetal head is high and deflexed. May feel large if the occiput is more lateral, but small if the occiput is quite posterior and bitemporal diameter is palpated. Fetal limbs may be felt on both sides of the midline of the uterus, and the fetal back may be felt out in the flank (Fig. 43.3).

Auscultation: The fetal heart may be heard at or just above the umbilicus or out in the flank (Fig. 43.4).

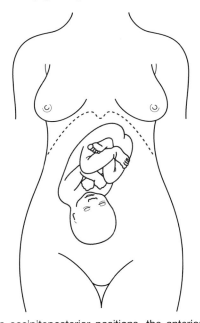

• **Fig. 43.3** In occipitoposterior positions, the anterior shoulder is well out from the midline and fetal limbs are readily palpable. This may cause a mistaken diagnosis of multiple pregnancy.[2]

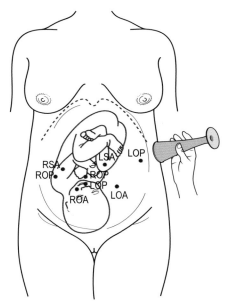

• **Fig. 43.4** The approximate points for fetal heart sounds in the occipitoposterior position.

1. From Henderson & Macdonald (2004), with permission of Elsevier; 2. From Beischer (1986), with permission of Elsevier.

fontanelle (Leeman, 2020). When the head is deflexed, the anterior fontanelle is almost central and easy to feel by its shape and size (Fig. 43.5).

First Stage of Labour

Fetal malposition of OP is associated with more painful, prolonged and obstructed labour and a difficult delivery (Phipps et al., 2014; Barrowclough et al., 2022). The course of labour partly depends on the degree of descent and flexion that occurs (Fig. 43.6). This, in turn, is influenced by the strength of uterine contractions. If the head flexes, it is likely that labour will proceed normally. The engaging diameter is the suboccipitofrontal (10 cm). When the occiput reaches the pelvic floor and rotates three-eighths of a circle, the baby is born with the occiput anterior.

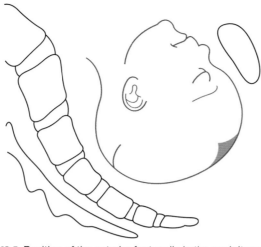

• **Fig. 43.5** Position of the anterior fontanelle in the occipitoposterior position.

Problems may arise if the head remains deflexed. The engaging diameter is occipitofrontal (11.5 cm). The head may be non-engaged at the commencement of labour, and early rupture of membranes may occur. If the presenting part is high and not well applied to the cervix, there is a risk of cord prolapse.

Labour is prolonged because of poor stimulation of the cervix, and dilatation is slow and uneven. Contractions may be excessive, uncoordinated and painful. The woman experiences severe backache. Encouraging the mother to take up a knee–chest position in the latter stages of pregnancy or labour does not necessarily rotate the vertex to an anterior position (Hunter, Hofmeyr & Kulier, 2007; Chapman & Charles, 2018). Augmentation of labour may be necessary (see Chapter 41). Care must be taken to prevent maternal loss of confidence, ketosis, dehydration and fetal distress. There may be difficulty in micturition with retention of urine. The woman should void urine frequently. Catheterization may be necessary.

The Role of Maternal Position

Hunter, Hofmeyr and Kulier (2007) discuss the benefits of upright and leaning-forward postures to encourage the fetal head to engage in the optimal occipitoanterior position. Taking up an all-fours posture may reduce the pressure of the fetus on the maternal spine and help reduce backache. All-fours does not, however, appear to reduce OP (Guittier et al., 2016) or transverse positions at delivery or reduce operative deliveries, and is not recommended as an intervention (Barrowclough et al., 2022; Guittier et al., 2016). The available evidence is inconclusive to support the suggestion that the incidence of the OP position of the fetal head at the commencement of labour can be reduced if the woman avoids the reclining position with knees higher than hips. However women should adopt positions they find comfortable, especially in labour, to reduce backache (Guittier et al., 2016).

Ambulation and forward-leaning positions have advantages in labour (Simkin, Ancheta & Hanson, 2017).

Freedom to move around in the first stage of labour and maintenance of an upright position can be achieved by sitting astride a chair and leaning forward onto its back. This may be beneficial in an OP position (Simkin, Ancheta & Hanson, 2017). Descent of the fetal head is encouraged, and good uterine contractions should follow. Progress is more likely to be normal, culminating in long internal rotation of the occiput (Fig. 43.6). In the second stage of labour, the squatting position increases the anteroposterior diameter of the outlet and may aid rotation, descent and delivery.

Warm packs are useful for pain management in labour (Smith et al., 2018), alongside massaging the woman's back in the lumbosacral region and immersion in a warm bath. Epidural analgesia is an effective method of relieving the pain in labour (Sng et al., 2014).

A difficult problem in the late first stage of labour is a strong urge to push before full cervical dilatation. Pushing presses the fetal head against the cervix; if oedema occurs this may lengthen the transitional stage of labour. Simkin, Ancheta & Hanson (2017) suggest that adoption of the knee–chest or hands and knees position may lessen pressure on the cervix and help reduce an anterior lip.

Second Stage of Labour

The five main possible outcomes of an OP position are (Stewart, 2017):

1. Long internal rotation of occiput and delivery as an occipitoanterior.
2. Deep transverse arrest of the head.
3. Short internal rotation of sinciput and delivery as 'face to pubes'.
4. Partial extension of head to a brow presentation.
5. Full extension of head to a face presentation.

For the mechanisms of long internal rotation of a right OP position, see Box 43.2; for the movements, see Table 43.1.

Deep Transverse Arrest of the Head

Deep transverse arrest is where the head remains in the occipitolateral position and is deep and low in the pelvis (Moir, 1938). If the head also remains deflexed, deep transverse arrest may occur. The fetal head begins long internal rotation but there is insufficient flexion to complete the process. The occipitofrontal diameter is caught above the ischial spines in the bispinous diameter. Labour becomes obstructed. Weak contractions or a straight sacrum with narrow outlet (android pelvis) may lead to this.

Diagnosis and Management

Diagnosis is made by finding the sagittal suture in the transverse diameter of the pelvis, with a fontanelle at each end of the suture. Caput succedaneum may obscure landmarks. It will be necessary to rotate the head to an OP position either manually or with Kielland's forceps before delivery. An alternative way of rotating and delivering the fetal head is by vacuum extraction. An instrumental

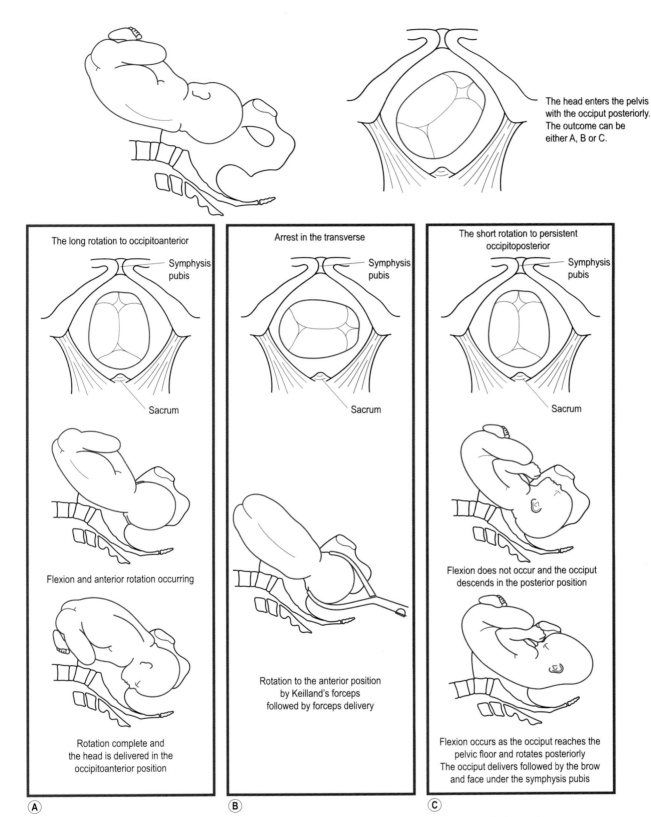

The head enters the pelvis with the occiput posteriorly. The outcome can be either A, B or C.

The long rotation to occipitoanterior

Symphysis pubis

Sacrum

Flexion and anterior rotation occurring

Rotation complete and the head is delivered in the occipitoanterior position

Arrest in the transverse

Symphysis pubis

Sacrum

Rotation to the anterior position by Keilland's forceps followed by forceps delivery

The short rotation to persistent occipitoposterior

Symphysis pubis

Sacrum

Flexion does not occur and the occiput descends in the posterior position

Flexion occurs as the occiput reaches the pelvic floor and rotates posteriorly
The occiput delivers followed by the brow and face under the symphysis pubis

Ⓐ   Ⓑ   Ⓒ

• **Fig. 43.6** Outcome of an occipitoposterior position. The head enters the pelvis with the occiput posteriorly. The outcome can be A, B or C.

• BOX 43.2 Mechanism of Long Internal Rotation of a Right Occipitoposterior Position

- **Lie** is longitudinal.
- **Attitude** of head is deflexed.
- **Presentation** is vertex.
- **Position** is right occipitoposterior.
- **Denominator** is occiput.
- **Presenting part** is the middle to anterior area of the left parietal bone.

TABLE 43.1   The Movements

Descent and flexion	There is continued descent with flexion during the first stage of labour. The presenting diameter of occipitofrontal (11.5 cm) is converted to suboccipitofrontal (10 cm).
Internal rotation of head	The occiput reaches the pelvic floor first and rotates forwards along the right side of the pelvis three-eighths of a circle to lie under the symphysis pubis. The anteroposterior diameter of the head now lies in the anteroposterior diameter of the pelvis. The shoulders follow and rotate two-eighths of a circle. The occiput escapes from beneath the subpubic arch.
Extension of head	The head is now born by extension as it pivots on the suboccipital region around the pubic bone. The sinciput, face and chin sweep the perineum.
Restitution	Restitution is a movement made by the head after delivery which brings it into correct alignment with the shoulders. This will be one-eighth of a circle towards the side of the occiput.
Internal rotation of the shoulders	The anterior shoulder is the first to reach the pelvic floor and rotates forwards to lie under the symphysis pubis. This movement is accompanied by external rotation of the head one-eighth of a circle more in the direction of restitution. The occiput now lies laterally turned towards the woman's thigh.
Lateral flexion	The anterior shoulder is usually born first and slips under the pubic arch and the posterior shoulder passes over the perineum. The remainder of the body is born by lateral flexion. Most common outcome, occurring for 65% of births.

delivery would not be performed if the head has not descended below the ischial spines (Hapangama, Navaratnam & Tempest, 2015).

When ventouse was used, Verma et al. (2021) highlighted that rigid vacuum cups were more successful than soft cups (although there was more injury to the baby). Handheld cups compared with other cups had similar success rates. This was from low-quality evidence. Forceps instruments were more successful, although they were associated with greater maternal morbidity, including perineal trauma, tears and increased pain (Verma et al., 2021). This was again from low-quality evidence. The use of either the vacuum extractor or forceps is based on clinical urgency of the situation and the skill of the practitioner. Both are associated with fetal or maternal risk (Verma et al., 2021).

Short Internal Rotation of Sinciput and 'Face to pubes' Delivery

In about 5% of labours, the occiput fails to rotate spontaneously to an anterior position (Vitner et al., 2015). This is known as *persistent occipitoposterior position* or POP. The head remains deflexed and the sinciput reaches the pelvic floor first and rotates forwards. The occiput comes to lie in the hollow of the sacrum and the head of the baby is born facing the pubic bone.

Diagnosis

- A delay may be present in the second stage of labour.
- Gaping of the vagina and dilatation of anus due to the presence of the large occiput.
- Confirmation is by finding the anterior fontanelle directly behind the symphysis pubis.

This may be masked by caput succedaneum. Feeling for the pinna of the ear will aid confirmation. In POP, the pinna will point towards the maternal sacrum.

Management of Spontaneous Delivery

The second stage is likely to be prolonged and even when the woman wishes to push, there may be incomplete cervical dilatation. Forward-leaning, side-lying and asymmetrical positions and movements may assist with a malpositioned fetus (Simkin, Ancheta & Hanson, 2017). Once the perineal phase of delivery is reached, to maintain the smallest possible diameters distending the perineum, the sinciput is allowed to emerge under the symphysis pubis as far as the root of the nose. Flexion is maintained and the occiput is allowed to sweep the perineum. The rest of the face is brought down from under the symphysis pubis. There is a high risk of perineal trauma, especially a 'buttonhole' tear in the centre of the perineum. An episiotomy may be required.

Face Presentation

The incidence of face presentation at term is about 1:500–800 (Hinshaw & Arulkumaran, 2018). The head and spine are fully extended and the limbs fully flexed. The fetal

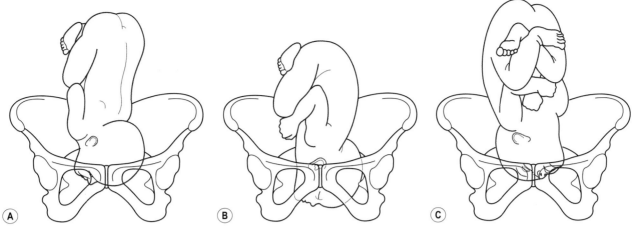

• **Fig. 43.7** Face presentations. (A) Right mentoposterior. (B) Right mentolateral. (C) Left mentoanterior.

occiput lies against its shoulder blades and the face is directly above the internal os (Fig. 43.7). Face presentation can lead to prolonged labour (Hinshaw & Arulkumaran, 2018).

Causes

Although face presentation may be present before the onset of labour, most face presentations are diagnosed during the second stage of labour (Hinshaw & Arulkumaran, 2018). Some OP positions may extend to a face or brow presentation (Stewart, 2017). The fetus is often abnormal and anencephaly, fetal goitre and neck tumours are present, which can cause head deflexion (Hinshaw & Arulkumaran, 2018). In a deflexed OP position, the biparietal diameter of the fetal head may be unable to pass through the sacrocotyloid diameter (9.5 cm) of the pelvic brim (the sacrocotyloid diameter is from the sacral promontory to the nearest point of the iliopectineal eminence). The bitemporal diameter descends more quickly and the head extends first to a brow presentation and ultimately to a face presentation. Other causes of face presentation include a flat pelvis, poor uterine muscle tone, prematurity, polyhydramnios or multiple pregnancy.

Risks

- Obstructed labour if either deep transverse arrest or brow presentation result.
- Maternal perineal trauma such as a third- or fourth-degree tear and bruising.
- Cord prolapse if there is early spontaneous rupture of membranes.
- Facial bruising as the caput forms over the face.
- Cerebral haemorrhage due to excessive moulding of the cranium.

Diagnosis
Per Abdomen

In pregnancy, the face presentation is rarely found, as most cases develop in labour (Coates, 2020). It may be difficult to diagnose face presentation. A deep groove may be palpated between the fetal head and back. The chest wall may be pressed up against the anterior wall of the uterus, and heart sounds are heard clearly on the side where the limbs are palpated. In mentoposterior positions where the chest faces posteriorly, heart sounds may be difficult to hear. In women who have a late ultrasound, a face presentation is sometimes found.

Per Vagina

In labour, the possibility of a face presentation should be suspected if the head remains high. On VE, feeling orbital ridges and a mouth with gum margins will confirm diagnosis. The fetus may suck the examining finger. The mouth feels very different from the soft anal orifice found in breech presentation. Care must be taken to avoid damage to fetal eyes (Stewart, 2017). It is important to determine whether the fetus is presenting in a mentoposterior or mentoanterior position. Unless a posterior face rotates to the anterior, there will be an obstructed labour. The position of the chin (mentum) is an important diagnostic tool.

Progress and Outcomes of Labour

There is an irregular high presenting part with possible early spontaneous rupture of the membranes and risk of cord prolapse. Contractions may be inefficient, leading to a prolonged labour. The face bones cannot mould and therefore large diameters must enter the pelvis.

Mentoanterior position

In the mentoanterior position, if contractions are good, descent and rotation of the head occur and labour progresses to a spontaneous delivery (Stewart, 2017). There are six possible positions: right mentoanterior, mentolateral and mentoposterior and left mentoanterior, mentolateral and mentoposterior. The mechanisms of the left mentoanterior position are shown in Table 43.2 and the movements in Box 43.3.

> **BOX 43.3 Mechanism of a Left Mentoanterior Position**
>
> - **Lie** is longitudinal.
> - **Attitude** of head and back is one of extension.
> - **Presentation** is face.
> - **Position** is left mentoanterior.
> - **Denominator** is mentum.
> - **Presenting part** is the left malar bone.

Mentoposterior Position

If the head is completely extended and the mentum reaches the pelvic floor first, the mentum rotates forwards into a mentoanterior position and delivery is possible. If the head is incompletely extended, there is a persistent mentoposterior position and the sinciput reaches the pelvic floor first. The chin comes to lie in the hollow of the pelvis and there can be no further progress. For further progress, the head and shoulders of the fetus would have to be in the pelvic cavity together. For birth to occur, the presenting fetal part must pivot around the subpubic arch either by flexion or extension. If the chin is posterior, vaginal birth cannot happen (Stewart, 2017), as the fully extended head cannot extend further and labour is obstructed.

Management

The **first stage** of labour is managed according to the risks. During VE, consideration should be taken of the descent of the mentum. If the head remains high or there is a suspicion of cephalopelvic disproportion, the fetus should normally be delivered by caesarean section (CS).

In the **second stage,** when the face appears at the vulva, the sinciput must be held back to permit extension. This allows the mentum to escape under the pubic arch before the occiput sweeps the perineum, thus ensuring the smallest possible diameter (submentovertical: 11.5 cm) distends the vaginal orifice rather than the mentovertical diameter (13.5 cm). An elective episiotomy would be required due to the large diameters distending the vaginal orifice. The chin escapes under the pubic arch and the head is born by flexion. If there is delay in descent or if the fetus remains in a persistent mentoposterior position, a forceps delivery, with rotation if necessary, may be successful. Otherwise, a CS is required (Collins et al., 2013) to reduce maternal and fetal morbidity and mortality.

Brow Presentation

The brow presentation occurs in about 1:1500–3000 deliveries (Hinshaw & Arulkumaran, 2018). Except for anencephaly, the causes are the same as for face presentation. The head is an attitude midway between full flexion and full extension (or face). The largest diameter of the head (mentovertical: 13.5 cm) cannot enter the widest possible diameter of the pelvic brim (transverse: 13 cm) (Fig. 43.8). Unless the brow presentation extends fully to a face presentation and the mentum comes anterior, labour is obstructed.

Diagnosis
Per Abdomen

The head is very high, and the presenting diameter is very wide. A groove may be felt between the occiput and the back.

Per Vagina

The presenting part may be so high it cannot be reached. If the brow is within reach, the orbital ridges are felt at one side and the anterior fontanelle on the other, with the frontal suture running between them (Fig. 43.9). The examination can be confusing due to oedema and unfamiliarity of presenting features (Leeman, 2020). Diagnosis can be confirmed by ultrasound.

Management

If brow presentation is diagnosed early in labour and both maternal and fetal conditions are satisfactory, time may be

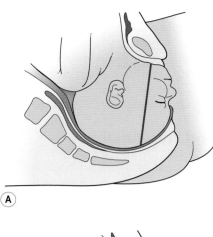

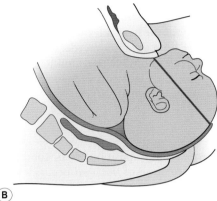

• **Fig. 43.8** Birth of the head in mentoanterior position. (A) The chin escapes under the symphysis pubis. Submentobregmatic diameter at the outlet. (B) The head is born by a movement of flexion.

allowed to see if the head will flex to a vertex or extend to a face presentation (Leeman, 2020). If brow presentation persists, a CS will be necessary (Hinshaw & Arulkumaran, 2018).

Shoulder Presentation

The shoulder presentation in labour results from an uncorrected abnormal lie in pregnancy. Instead of the normal longitudinal lie, the fetus lies across the uterus in either an oblique or a transverse lie (Fig. 43.10). The lie may be unstable. In a shoulder presentation where the fetus is in a transverse lie, the risk of cord prolapse is higher than in a vertex presentation (Coates, 2017). An uncorrected shoulder presentation leads to obstructed labour, and delivery should be by CS.

Causes

The most common cause is grand multiparity due to lax uterine and abdominal muscles. In this case, the fetus takes the transverse lie. Other causes include anything that prevents the fetus from adopting a longitudinal lie or fetal head from engaging. These include placenta praevia, multiple pregnancy, polyhydramnios, uterine abnormality, large

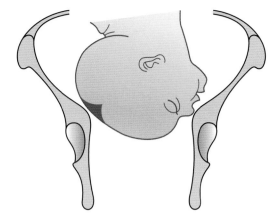

• **Fig. 43.9** Brow presentation.

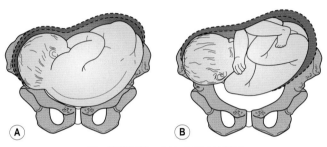

• **Fig. 43.10** Shoulder presentation.

uterine fibroid or contracted pelvis and over-extended bladder (Coates, 2017). If the fetus dies in utero, it may slump into an abnormal lie.

Diagnosis
Per Abdomen

A transverse lie is easy to diagnose in pregnancy because of the abnormal shape of the uterus. The uterus is broader and the fundal height lower than normal. There may be a discernible bulge at either side of the uterus. On palpation, the fetal head will be felt on one side of the uterus and breech on the other. The fetal back may be anterior (dorsoanterior) or posterior (dorsoposterior). There is no presenting part entering the pelvis (Fig. 43.10). In an oblique lie, the shape of the uterus may be indicative and one or other poles of the fetus is found in either iliac fossa. Ultrasound is useful to confirm diagnosis and detect the cause.

Per Vaginam

VE *should not* be performed if a transverse lie is suspected on abdominal examination in case there is a placenta praevia. Rarely, a woman will be admitted already in labour with the shoulder impacted at the pelvic brim. It may be mistaken for a breech presentation. The fetal cord and arm may prolapse into the vagina. On VE, the shoulder is recognized by feeling the fetal ribs and hand, which must be differentiated from a foot by length of the digits and presence of a heel.

The safest method of delivery is by CS, even if the fetus is dead.

Management

A full examination is made during pregnancy to exclude causes such as placenta praevia. If no major pregnancy abnormality is found, the obstetrician may attempt to correct the lie of the fetus to a longitudinal lie and cephalic presentation. Reversion to the original lie is common, and some doctors do not perform repeated external cephalic version (ECV) before the onset of labour, planned or otherwise. As pregnancy progresses, the lie of some fetuses will stabilize as longitudinal. However, at term 0.3% will be transverse or shoulder presentation (Leeman, 2020).

The woman may be admitted to hospital at 37–38 weeks, when the fetus is mature for ECV and induction of labour. There is a risk of labour commencing spontaneously with early rupture of the membranes and cord prolapse. When the contractions are established and the fetal head enters the pelvis, the membranes can be ruptured. If complications arise or if the woman has a poor obstetric history, a CS is performed.

In cases of twins, if the second twin takes up a transverse or oblique lie after the birth of the first twin, the fetus is turned by ECV. The second set of membranes is ruptured and delivery is completed.

Compound Presentation

This is where a hand or foot lies alongside the head. It is a rare complication, and the incidence is 1 in 377 to 1 in 1213 (Barth, 2021). Cord prolapse may occur if the fetus is small and the pelvis large (Leeman, 2020) or if there is any condition that prevents the descent of the head such as contracted pelvis, prematurity or multiple pregnancy. The limb may recede as the head advances and delivery proceeds normally. If the limb does not recede, it may be impossible for head and hand to be delivered simultaneously and a CS may be performed. If labour is progressing, then no intervention is required (Leeman, 2020).

Main Points

- There is no single cause for the OP position of the vertex, but if the forepelvis is small, as found in android and anthropoid pelves, the head may take up a posterior position.
- Antenatally, the OP position is the most common cause of a non-engaged head in late pregnancy in primigravidae.
- Possible outcomes of an OP position are occipitoanterior, deep transverse arrest of the head, 'face to pubes', brow or face presentation.
- If there is a deep transverse arrest, the head must be rotated to an occipitoanterior position either manually or with Kielland's forceps before delivery.

- In a mentoanterior position with good contractions, descent and rotation of the head occurs and labour progresses to a spontaneous delivery.
- In a mentoposterior position, a fully extended head cannot extend further and labour is obstructed.
- If brow presentation persists, CS is necessary.
- Shoulder presentation in labour is the result of an uncorrected abnormal lie in pregnancy.
- If the limb does not recede, it may be impossible for head and hand to be delivered simultaneously and a CS may be performed. If labour is progressing, then no intervention is required.

References

Barrowclough, J.A., Lin, L., Kool, B., Hofmeyr, G.J., Crowther, C.A., 2022. Maternal postures for fetal malposition in labour for improving the health of mothers and their infants. Cochrane Database Syst. Rev. 8 (8), CD014615.

Barth, W., 2021. Malpresentations and malposition. In: Landon, M., Galan, H., Jauniaux, E. (Eds.), Gabbe's Obstetrics: Normal and Problem Pregnancies, eighth ed. Elsevier, Philadelphia.

Beischer, N.A., Mackay, E.V., 1986. Obstetrics and the Newborn. Baillière Tindall, London.

Chapman, V., Charles, C., 2018. The Midwife's Labour and Birth Handbook, fourth ed. Wiley, Oxford.

Coate, T., 2020. Malpositions of the Occiput and malpresentations. In: Marshall, J., Raynor, M. (Eds.), Myles' Textbook for Midwives, seventeenth ed. Elsevier, Edinburgh.

Coates, T., 2017. Malpositions and malpresentations. In: Macdonald, S., Johnson, G. (Eds.), Mayes' Midwifery: A Textbook for Midwifery, fifteenth ed. Elsevier, Edinburgh.

Collins, S., Arulkumaran, S., Hayes, K., Jackson, S., Impey, L., 2013. Normal labour. In: Collins, S., Arulkumaran, S., Hayes, Jackson, S., Impey, L. (Eds.), Oxford Handbook of Obstetrics and Gynaecology, third ed. Oxford University Press, Oxford.

Guittier, M.J., Othenin-Girard, V., de Gasquet, B., Irion, O., Boulvain, M., 2016. Maternal positioning to correct occiput posterior fetal position during the first stage of labour: a randomised controlled trial. Br. J. Obstet. Gynaecol. 123 (13), 2199–2207.

Henderson, C., Macdonald, S., 2004. Mayes' Midwifery: A Textbook for Midwives. Elsevier, Edinburgh.

Hinshaw, K., Arulkumaran, S., 2018. Malpresentation, malposition, cephalopelvic disproportion and obstetric procedures. In: Edmonds, K., Lees, C., Bourne, T.H. (Eds.), Dewhurst's Textbook of Obstetrics & Gynaecology, ninth ed. Wiley Blackwell, Chichester.

Hunter, S., Hofmeyr, G.J., Kulier, R., 2007. Hands and knees posture in late pregnancy or labour for fetal malposition (lateral or posterior). Cochrane Database Syst. Rev. 2007 (4), CD001063.

Leeman, L., 2020. Malpresentations, malpositions, and multiple gestation. In: Leeman, L., Dresang, L., Quinlan, J.D., Magee, S.R. (Eds.), Advanced Life Support in Obstetrics (ALSO) Provider Mannual, ninth ed. AAFP, Kansas City.

Moir, C., 1938. The occipito-posterior positions of the vertex and their complications. Br. Med. J. 4053 (2), 555–557.

Phipps, H., de Vries, B., Hyett, J., Osborn, D.A., 2014. Prophylactic manual rotation for fetal malposition to reduce operative delivery. Cochrane Database Syst. Rev. 2014 (12), CD009298.

Simkin, P., Ancheta, R., Hanson, L., 2017. The Labor Progress Handbook: Early Intervention to Prevent and Treat Dystocia, fourth ed. Oxford, Wiley-Blackwell.

Smith, C.A., Levett, K.M., Collins, C.T., Dahlen, H.G., Ee, C.C., Suganuma, M., 2018. Massage, reflexology and other manual methods for pain management in labour. Cochrane Database Syst. Rev. 2018 (3),CD009290.

Sng, B.L., Leong, W.L., Zeng, Y., Siddiqui, F.J., Assam, P.N., Lim, Y., et al., 2014. Early versus late initiation of epidural analgesia for labour. Cochrane Database Syst. Rev. 2014 (10),CD007238.

Stewart, O., 2017. Malpresentations and malpositions. In: Boyle, M. (Ed.), Emergencies Around Childbirth, third ed. CRC Press, Boca Raton.

Tempest, N., Navaratnam, K., Hapangama, D.K., 2015. Management of delivery when malposition of the fetal head complicates the second stage of labour. Obstet. Gynaecol. 17 (4), 273–278.

Verma, G.L., Spalding, J.J., Wilkinson, M.D., Hofmeyr, G.J., Vannevel, V., O'Mahony, F., 2021. Instruments for assisted vaginal birth. Cochrane Database Syst. Rev. 2021 (9), CD005455.

Vitner, D., Paltieli, Y., Haberman, S., Gonen, R., Ville, Y., Nizard, J., 2015. Prospective multicenter study of ultrasound-based measurements of fetal head station and position throughout labor. Ultrasound Obstet. Gynecol. 46 (5), 611–615.

Walsh, D., 2012. Evidence and Skills for Normal Labour and Birth: A Guide for Midwives, second ed. Routledge, London.

Annotated Recommended Reading

Coates, T., 2020. Malpositions of the Occiput and Malpresentations. In: Marshall, J., Raynor, M. (Eds.), Myles' Textbook for Midwives, seventeenth ed. Elsevier, Edinburgh.

A chapter in an edited book in which Coates describes abnormal presentations and their management. It is an invaluable reference for those who provide intrapartum care.

Simkin, P., Ancheta, R., Hanson, L., 2017. The Labor Progress Handbook: Early Intervention to Prevent and Treat Dystocia, fourth ed. Oxford, Wiley-Blackwell.

A book based on aspects of care during pregnancy and childbirth. An interesting resource for intrapartum care.

44

Cephalopelvic Disproportion, Obstructed Labour and Other Obstetric Emergencies

LYZ HOWIE, JEAN WATSON AND JEAN RANKIN

CHAPTER CONTENTS

This chapter discusses diagnosis and management of cephalopelvic disproportion, obstructed labour and other obstetric emergencies. Uterine rupture, shoulder dystocia, cord presentation and prolapse are detailed.

Introduction

Evolutionary adaptations lead to problems between the female pelvis and fetal head due to the following:
- Anteroposterior diameter is reduced at brim, cavity and outlet.
- Widening of transverse diameters.

- Sacral promontory protrudes into the pelvic inlet.
- Sacrum makes an angle with the lumbar spine (**lumbosacral angle**).
- There is an inward protrusion of the ischial spines to support the strong pelvic floor.
- Sacrum is curved.
- Superior ramus is thinned and elongated with widening of the subpubic angle.

The fetal head can negotiate the pelvis successfully because of the following features (Coad, Pedley and Dunstall, 2019):
- Spheroid shape of the vertex.
- Mobility of the head on the neck, allowing flexion or extension.
- Moulding of the bones of the fetal skull.

Cephalopelvic Disproportion

Any condition leading to a misfit between the fetal head and maternal pelvis, with failure of descent of the head into the pelvis despite good contractions, results in **cephalopelvic disproportion** (CPD). Ultimately CPD interferes with the natural mechanisms of labour. The diameters of the fetal head are larger than the diameters of the pelvis (Heininen, Korhonen & Taipale 2015). The shape of the pelvis may be abnormal, but as long as the diameters allow passage of the fetal head, delivery should follow, as there should be no problem with the rest of the fetus. CPD is a cause of obstructed labour, and there is associated morbidity for both the woman and morbidity and mortality for the fetus (Cuthbert, Pattinson & Vannevel, 2017).

Diagnosis

In a primigravidae, it is expected that the fetal head should engage in the last 2–3 weeks of pregnancy. If the head does not engage, an attempt may be made to engage it and, if unsuccessful, CPD should be suspected. The most common cause for non-engagement of the head is the occipitoposterior, or

Maternal Indications of Possible CPD

- Bone conditions such as rickets or osteomalacia, resulting in alterations in the size and shape of the pelvis.
- Spinal deformities (e.g., scoliosis).
- Pelvic trauma and fractures, altering size and shape of the pelvis.
- Previous obstetric conditions (e.g., prolonged labour, difficult delivery or CS).
- Short stature of the woman. Height of women was a predictor of CPD (Fischer & Mitteroecker, 2015).

Fetal Conditions Leading to CPD

- Fetal abnormalities (e.g., hydrocephalus).
- Size of fetus in relation to the maternal pelvis. In a multigravida with deliveries of normal-sized babies, CPD is less likely, although there could be problems with larger fetuses.
- Abdominal palpation is an inaccurate method of judging fetal size.
- Estimation of fetal size is more accurate due to technological advances.
- Clinical or ultrasound examination is not a good estimator of fetal weight or diagnosing obstructed labour (Hofmeyr, 2004).

CPD, Cephalopelvic disproportion; CS, caesarean section.

OP position, with deflexed head and a presenting occipito-frontal diameter (11.5 cm). However in most of these cases, the head flexes and descent occurs in labour. Other causes of a non-engaged head include **pelvic tumours, placenta praevia** and **polyhydramnios.** A steep **angle of inclination** between the pelvic brim and the horizontal is found in some Afro-Caribbean women and may delay engagement until late in labour. Some reasons for maternal or fetal cephalopelvic disproportion are indicated in Box 44.1.

Assessing the Pelvis

A combination of careful history-taking and clinical expertise backed up by technology might enable the identification of women at risk. **Head fitting** or **pelvic assessment** examinations can be carried out to assess the woman's size of the pelvis through X-ray, CT or MRI (Cuthbert, Pattinson & Vannevel, 2017). Evidence is sparse surrounding this issue; interestingly, the National Institute of Health and Care Excellence (NICE, 2019; 2021; 2023) does not proffer any guidance surrounding pelvic examination as a method of determining CPD.

X-ray Pelvimetry

Erect lateral X-ray pelvimetry provides information about the size and shape of the pelvis and the relationship of the fetal head to the pelvic brim. There has previously been criticism of its use because of an association between prenatal irradiation and childhood leukaemia. Pattinson, Cuthbert

- Shape of the pelvis.
- Shape of the sacrum.
- Inclination between the sacrum and pelvic brim.
- Anteroposterior diameters of brim, cavity and outlet.
- Width of the sacrosciatic notch.
- Depth of pelvic cavity.

- Cephalopelvic disproportion is a cause that is unresolvable except by caesarean section (in remote areas of the world, symphysiotomy may prevent morbidity and mortality). More evidence is required to substantiate if this is an appropriate procedure (Hofmeyr & Shweni, 2012).
- Cephalic malpositions and malpresentations (Chapman, 2018).
- Fetal abnormalities such as hydrocephalus.
- Pelvic anomalies.
- Maternal tumours.
- Fibroids (Jackson, 2020).

& Vannevel (2017) stipulate that X-ray pelvimetry led to more caesarean sections (CSs) and the evidence does not support the use of pelvimetry in women with cephalic presentations. More studies are required to assess perinatal outcomes and the most effective method of pelvimetry using CT or MRI (Cuthbert, Pattinson & Vannevel, 2017). Box 44.2 outlines details that can be noted if X-ray pelvimetry is conducted.

There are three possible outcomes: disproportion is not present and vaginal delivery will be possible, there is a degree of CPD that may be overcome in labour or CPD is of such a degree that vaginal delivery is not possible (obstructed labour).

Obstructed Labour

Obstructed labour occurs when there is no advance of the presenting part with strong uterine contractions (Jackson, 2020). There is a large increase in maternal and fetal morbidity and mortality if labour is allowed to proceed with unrecognized obstructed labour. This situation is more common in remote areas of the world where women do not have access to trained personnel. However it can also occur in a developed country if a woman fails to disclose her pregnancy or to present herself for care in labour. Causes of obstructed labour are in Box 44.3 and signs and symptoms of obstructed labour are in Box 44.4.

Management

Prevention, by achieving a high standard of antenatal care and observations in early labour, would be the

Signs and Symptoms of Obstructed Labour

Early signs

- Little progress in labour.
- No descent of head despite efficient uterine action.
- High presenting part on VE.
- Cervix dilates slowly and is poorly applied to presenting part.
- Early rupture of membranes with risk of cord prolapse.
- In a primigravida, there may be active-phase arrest. The contractions stop for a while, finally restarting with increased strength. The woman may complain of severe and continuous pain.
- Multiparous woman may have tumultuous contractions that proceed rapidly to uterine rupture.

Late signs

- If presented late in labour and obstruction is not identified, the woman can develop a raised temperature, rapid pulse and dehydration.
- On abdominal inspection, the uterus would appear to be moulded around the fetus because of tonic contraction and loss of liquor amnii.
- A Bandl's pathological retraction ring may be seen as a ridge of tissue running obliquely across the abdomen. This denotes an extremely thinned lower uterine segment and imminent rupture of the uterus.
- Fetoplacental blood supply may be obstructed, causing lack of oxygenation leading to fetal morbidity and mortality.
- On VE, the vagina feels hot, dry and the presenting part is high. Excessive moulding and large caput succedaneum found obscuring the presenting part.
- Urinary output is reduced and a vesicovaginal fistula may occur due to tissue sloughing from prolonged fetal pressure.
- Abnormalities of fetal heart rate.

VE, Vaginal examination.
(Chapman, 2018; Jackson, 2020)

best management to allow early detection of likely difficulties and treatment before obstructed labour occurs. Removal of an ovarian cyst, correction of an abnormal lie or performing a planned CS are examples of actions that minimize the chances of obstructed labour occurring. There should also be caution in the use of amniotomy in obstructed labours. A systematic review (Dowswell, Markham & Smith 2013) explored amniotomy for

shortening spontaneous labour. The reviewers advocate that routine amniotomy is not recommended for normal labours, nor is it recommended for prolonged labours. If labour is advanced, an emergency CS is carried out regardless of whether the fetus is dead or alive. Rarely, especially in developing countries, if the fetus is dead and the cervix is fully dilated, destructive operations such as cleidotomy (division of the clavicles) or craniotomy (perforation of the skull) are performed. These allow for vaginal delivery, but there is a risk of perforation of the thin lower uterine segment (Sikka et al., 2011). However a systematic review and meta-analysis by Ayenew (2021) reported that CSs were more likely to be performed rather than destructive operations due to the lack of skilled operators in these procedures.

Uterine Rupture

Rupture of the uterus is an obstetric emergency, and the fetus and mother may die. Rupture may involve a previous scar, spontaneous rupture of an intact uterus or traumatic rupture. One MBRRACE report (Knight et al., 2014) highlighted four cases of uterine rupture. The incidence appears to be consistent in developed countries but may be rising in developing countries. Uterine rupture may occur due to vaginal delivery after a previous CS or due to inappropriate use of oxytocic infusions (Hinshaw & Arulkumaran, 2018). Ayenew (2021) attributed 30% of uterine ruptures in Ethiopia to obstructed labour.

Types of Uterine Rupture

Scar rupture is usually due to a previous CS in 0.5–0.9% of cases (Heinrichs, 2020). A longitudinal scar in the uterus (classical incision) is more likely to rupture than a transverse scar in the lower segment. Rupture of the classical scar occurs in about 2% of cases and is more likely to occur in late pregnancy when the upper segment is stretched to its limit. Performing a CS at 38 weeks may reduce this. Rupture of a transverse lower segment scar is more likely to happen in labour as the lower segment is thinned and extended. Uterine rupture after a lower-segment CS is less than 1%.

Traumatic rupture of the uterus may be caused using obstetric instruments such as forceps. These can cause tearing of the cervix which extends into the lower segment. Intrauterine manipulations such as the internal podalic version, where the foot of the fetus is grasped at delivery to convert a transverse lie (usually of the second twin) to breech or correction of a shoulder presentation in labour may lead to uterine rupture, as may the misuse of oxytocic drugs.

Spontaneous rupture of the uterus may follow strong spontaneous uterine action such as that occurring in obstructed labour. The rupture is found most often in the lower segment. Abruptio placentae, where there is extravasation of blood into the uterine muscle (Couvelaire uterus),

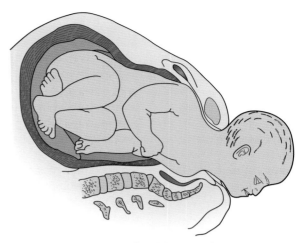

• **Fig. 44.1** Shoulder dystocia.

facilitates such a rupture. The signs and symptoms of uterine rupture are in Box 44.5.

Management

If a ruptured uterus is diagnosed, obstetric, anaesthetic and theatre emergency teams must be alerted, and the woman immediately transferred to the theatre. The anaesthetist will establish venous access and start resuscitative measures while the team prepares for an emergency CS. A blood transfusion will be necessary. The baby is delivered, and the uterus is repaired if possible. A hysterectomy may be necessary if the rupture is severe and bleeding difficult to control. Postoperative treatment should include observation of severe side effects of haemorrhage such as renal failure or, later, onset of Sheehan's syndrome (see Chapter 28). The psychological effect of the experience on the woman and her family should be anticipated and explanations and counselling made available.

Shoulder Dystocia

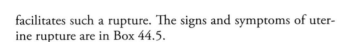

This arises when there is difficulty with delivering the shoulders after delivering the head (Ghermaine, Gonik & Ouzounian, 2021). Shoulder dystocia occurs when either the anterior or, less commonly, the posterior fetal shoulder impacts the maternal symphysis or sacral promontory (Fig. 44.1).

Definition

Shoulder dystocia is a condition requiring special manoeuvres to deliver the shoulders after an unsuccessful attempt

to apply routine axial traction. Shoulder dystocia is another obstetric emergency that may end in fetal and maternal morbidity and mortality. There is difficulty in delivering the anterior shoulder, and urgent manoeuvres are necessary. It is important to remember that this is a bony obstruction problem and NOT a soft tissue obstruction! There are two causes:
1. A large baby.
2. Failure of the shoulders to rotate into the anteroposterior diameter after delivery of the head.

The incidence of shoulder dystocia ranges from 0.58–0.70% (Royal College of Obstetricians and Gynaecologists [RCOG, 2012]; Bouthou, et al., 2021), and the risk rises as pregnancy becomes prolonged with increasing birthweight.

Recognition

The head fails to advance, and the fetus looks to be burying its chin in the perineum. This happens because the anterior shoulder is wedged firmly behind the symphysis pubis. Difficulty in delivering the face and chin is a warning sign (Coates, 2017; Coates & Green, 2020). The baby's head may fail to rotate or allow restitution to occur. This is sometimes referred to as a *'turtle sign'* (Gobbo, 2020).

Risk Factors

It is important to remember that shoulder dystocia can be an unpredictable event. However the following factors, most of them associated with a large fetus, should be taken into consideration so that the woman can be delivered in an appropriate setting. The risk factors are underlined in Box 44.6.

Management

Excessive force must not be applied to the fetal head or neck and fundal pressure must be avoided (Gobbo, 2020).

Risk Factors for Shoulder Dystocia

- Maternal age over 35 years may be associated with increased birthweight.
- Maternal body mass index of >30.
- Maternal diabetes mellitus (insulin dependent or gestational) and fetal macrosomia.
- Maternal high birthweight is associated with fetal high birthweight.
- In women with a platypelloid pelvis (anteroposterior diameter is reduced), shoulder dystocia can occur with a normal-sized infant.
- Previous shoulder dystocia.
- Induction of labour (oxytocin induction or augmentation).
- Prolonged first stage, secondary arrest, prolonged second stage.
- Assisted vaginal delivery.

These activities are unlikely to free the impaction and may cause maternal and fetal injury and may lead to uterine rupture (RCOG, 2012). Routine traction should be applied to the neck rather than a downwards traction to decrease the risk of fetal nerve injury (RCOG, 2012). There is little time to save the life of the baby, and the woman may be in her own home so the midwife must attempt to complete the delivery whilst summoning help (e.g., second midwife, paramedic or general practitioner). It may be necessary to try more than one manoeuvre, so it is necessary to keep calm and think clearly about what is happening inside the mother's pelvis. Shoulder dystocia should be treated as an obstetric emergency to prevent fetal morbidity, as 47% of babies die within 5 min of the head being delivered (RCOG, 2012).

Manoeuvres

Students and midwives need to have the skills required to relieve shoulder dystocia. The main focus should be concerned with comprehension, learning and regular opportunities to practice clinical judgment. Relevant and meaningful training needs to be in the form of mandatory multidisciplinary 'skills and drills' training. The mnemonic approach (such as HELPERR) is now considered limited and unhelpful (Coates & Green, 2020). In their study, Jan et al. (2014) reported a poor correlation between health practitioners' knowledge of manoeuvres and their eponyms. However different processes may be used depending on local policy and practice. Irrespective of the algorithm used, the current international guidance recommends four basic shoulder dystocia resolution manoeuvres (Winter et al., 2018). These include:

- McRoberts position / All-fours position
- Suprapubic pressure
- Delivery of the posterior arm
- Internal rotation

None of the manoeuvres/techniques described are superior, with the routine sequence of manoeuvres as identified. However in the situation with morbidly obese women where the McRoberts position or suprapubic pressure are difficult to perform, moving directly to delivery of the posterior arm may be more effective (Winter et al., 2018). Together the techniques are valuable for practitioners to effectively overcome this emergency situation. For the purpose of learning, each manoeuvre is detailed separately. The steps should be carried out efficiently and appropriately, as the time element is vital. The manoeuvres for managing shoulder dystocia are detailed in Clinical Application 44.1. An assistant should maintain relevant recordings of the events.

Manoeuvres have three main aims:
1. Increase the functional size of the bony pelvis.
2. Decrease the bisacromial diameter (~12 cm).
3. Change the relationship of the bisacromial diameter within the bony pelvis.

If possible, performing an episiotomy is recommended. This procedure will only make room for internal manoeuvres and prevent maternal trauma. Remember that the obstruction is bony. Delivery of the baby should be attempted after each manoeuvre through routine axial traction.

- Help must be summoned early with the obstetrician, neonatologist/neonatal specialist and anaesthetist in attendance.
- Explanation of the situation is given to the parents.
- Roles are allocated for those in attendance.

Time Available

No absolute time limit can be recommended for the management of shoulder dystocia. This is due to the head-to-body birth interval that each individual fetus can withstand without hypoxia occurring. This will vary depending on clinical circumstances and the vulnerability of the baby. At the eventual birth, the condition of the baby is dependent on the head-to-body interval and the condition of the fetus at the start of the dystocia. Box 44.8 summarizes findings from related cases of shoulder dystocia.

N.B. Shoulder dystocia should be managed effectively by using appropriate manoeuvres correctly and without using excessive and/or downward traction or fundal pressure. This will avoid unnecessary trauma. Manoeuvres need to be performed in a timely manner to avoid hypoxia.

Outcome for Mother and Fetus

Maternal death is rare but can happen. Maternal morbidity is more common. This can include lacerations (perineal, vaginal and cervical), uterine rupture, bladder problems, vaginal haematoma and haemorrhage. Primary postpartum haemorrhage (PPH) should be anticipated, and the genitalia carefully examined for trauma.

For the baby, birth asphyxia is a complication of shoulder dystocia. Birth injury is also commonly reported with brachial plexus injury.

• CLINICAL APPLICATION 44.1 **Manoeuvres to Manage Shoulder Dystocia (Winter et al., 2018)**

1. McRoberts Position / All-fours Position

The McRoberts manoeuvre is an effective intervention. However reports on success rates vary (<50% to as high as 90%) (Leung et al., 2011a; Hoffman et al., 2011). The McRoberts manoeuvre has a low rate of complication. It is usually employed first as it is one of the least invasive manoeuvres.

- Lie the mother flat and remove any pillows behind her back. With one assistant on either side, hyperflex the mother's legs against her abdomen so that her knees are up toward her ears (Fig. 44.2).
- If the mother is in the lithotomy position (for an operative vaginal birth), then remove her legs from the supports to reposition into the McRoberts position *(if the procedure is taking place in the maternity theatre, then the mother's legs may be secured using appropriate supports to achieve a comparable McRoberts position)*.

One feature of an effective McRoberts position is that the maternal buttocks are lifted off the bed during hyperflexion of the hips, thereby rotating the pelvis.

The McRoberts position increases the relative anteroposterior diameter of the pelvic inlet by rotating the maternal pelvis *(towards the mother's head)* and straightening the sacrum relative to the lumbar spine.

Routine Axial Traction

- The same degree of traction is applied as during normal birth and in an axial direction *(i.e., in line with the axis of the fetal spine, should then be applied to the baby's head)* to assess whether the shoulders have been released.
- If the anterior shoulder is not released with the McRoberts position, then move onto the next manoeuvre. Do not continue to apply traction to the baby's head.

Remember: shoulder dystocia is a bony problem where the baby's shoulder is obstructed by the mother's pelvis. If the entrapment is not released by the McRoberts position, another manoeuvre (not traction) is required to free the shoulder and achieve birth.

- It is **NOT** recommended to use a prophylactic McRoberts position before the birth of the baby's head. This is ineffective.
- If the McRoberts position is performed in anticipation of possible shoulder dystocia, then it would be unclear if there was truly a problem. This could have implications for the mother's birth choices in subsequent pregnancies.

All-fours Position

The all-fours position success rate of 83% was described in one small case series (Bruner et al., 1998).

- Positioning in an all-fours position with thighs against the abdomen has a similar effect on the maternal pelvis as the McRoberts position. In effect, the all-fours position is essentially the McRoberts position upside down.
- Individual circumstances should guide the accoucheur's *(i.e., one assisting at a birth)* decision on whether to use the McRoberts or all-fours positions. For slim mobile women with a lone midwifery birth attendant, the all-fours position is probably more appropriate, and clearly this may be a useful option in a homebirth setting.
- For women who are less mobile (e.g., regional anaesthesia in place), the traditional McRoberts position with the mother lying flat will be more appropriate.
- To achieve an all-fours position, ask the mother to roll over so that she is supporting herself on her upper arms and knees, with her hips and knees flexed.

- This simple of change of position may release the fetal shoulders.
- Routine axial traction should be applied to the fetal head to ascertain if the shoulder dystocia has been resolved. If dystocia remains, internal manoeuvres should be attempted.

Remember: when the woman is in an all-fours position, the maternal sacral hollow and the fetal posterior shoulder will both be uppermost.

2. Suprapubic Pressure

Suprapubic pressure aims to relieve shoulder dystocia by:
(1) reducing the fetal bisacromial (shoulder-to-shoulder) diameter, and
(2) rotating the anterior shoulders into the wider oblique diameter of the pelvis.

- The anterior shoulder is freed to slip under the symphysis pubis with the aid of routine axial traction.
- An assistant should apply suprapubic pressure from the side of the fetal back, which will reduce the diameter of the fetal shoulders by 'scrunching' (abducting) the shoulders in towards the fetal chest.
- Pressure should be applied just above the maternal symphysis pubis in a downward and lateral direction to push the posterior aspect of the anterior shoulder towards the fetal chest.
- If there is uncertainty regarding the fetal position, suprapubic pressure should be applied by the side where it is most likely that the fetal back will be, and, if this pressure is unsuccessful at relieving the dystocia, suprapubic pressure can be attempted from the other side.
- When applying suprapubic pressure, there is no evidence that rocking is better than continuous pressure, nor that pressure should be performed for 30 s for it to be effective.
- If this anterior shoulder is not released after attempting suprapubic pressure and routine axial traction, another manoeuvre should be attempted.

Evaluate the Need for an Episiotomy

- An episiotomy will not relieve the bony obstruction of shoulder dystocia but may be required to allow the accoucheur more space to facilitate internal vaginal manoeuvres (delivery of the posterior arm or internal rotation of the shoulders).
- A recent systematic review found no use of episiotomy in the prevention and management of shoulder dystocia (Sagi-Dain & Sagi, 2015).
- Often the perineum has already torn, or an episiotomy may have already been performed before the birth of the head. With the correct technique, there is almost always enough room to gain internal access without requiring an episiotomy (Johanson et al., 2002).

Internal Manoeuvres

Internal manoeuvres were originally described by Woods and Rubin (RCOG, 2012). There are two types of internal vaginal manoeuvre that can be performed if the McRoberts/all-fours position and/or suprapubic pressure are not effective:
i) Delivery of the posterior arm
ii) Internal rotational manoeuvres

There is no evidence demonstrating that either manoeuvre is superior or that one should be attempted before the other. The decision on which manoeuvre to attempt should depend on the clinical circumstances.

All internal manoeuvres start with the same action – inserting the whole hand posteriorly into the sacral hollow to locate the posterior arm or hand (Fig. 44.3A). Once access has been gained, a pragmatic decision can be made on the individual set of circumstances to determine the best manoeuvre to attempt first.

Gaining Internal Vaginal Access

When shoulder dystocia occurs, the problem is usually at the inlet of the pelvis, with the anterior shoulder trapped above the symphysis pubis.

When attempting to gain vaginal access for internal manoeuvres, the temptation is to introduce a hand anteriorly. However if the anterior fetal shoulder is trapped because there is not enough room, there will also be insufficient room to insert a hand anteriorly to perform any manoeuvre.

The most spacious part of the pelvis is in the sacral hollow, and therefore, vaginal access can be gained more easily posteriorly into the sacral hollow. If the accoucheur scrunches up his/her hand *(as if putting on a tight bracelet or reaching for a last Pringle crisp at the bottom of a container)*, internal rotation or delivery of the posterior arm can then be attempted using the whole hand.

3. Delivery of the Posterior Arm

- Delivering the posterior arm will reduce the diameter of the fetal shoulders by the width of the arm. This will usually provide enough room to resolve the shoulder dystocia.
- Babies will often lie with their arms flexed across their chest. Therefore, when the accoucheur inserts a hand into the vaginal posteriorly, it is often possible to feel the hand and forearm of the posterior arm (Fig. 44.3A).
- If this is the case, then the accoucheur can take hold of the fetal wrist (with fingers and thumb) and gently release the posterior arm in a straight line (Figs 44.3B, C & D). This involves a sweeping motion, taking the forearm over the anterior chest wall and face of the fetus – similar to putting your hand up in class.
- Once the posterior arm is delivered, gentle axial traction may be applied to the fetal head.
- If the shoulder dystocia is resolved, then the baby's body should be easily born.
- If the baby is lying with their posterior arm straight against their body *(in front of the fetal abdomen)*, it may be possible for the accoucheur to apply pressure with their thumb to the baby's antecubital fossa and flex the posterior arm, so that the wrist can be grasped and the arm delivered as previously described.

- However, this is much more difficult, and it may be easier to attempt internal rotation of the fetal shoulders instead.
- In addition if the accoucheur pulls on the upper arm rather than the wrist, then this is likely to result in a humeral fracture.

4. Internal Rotation Manoeuvres

The aims of internal rotation are to:
1. move the fetal shoulders (the bisacromial diameter) out of the narrowest diameter of the mother's pelvis (the anterior-posterior) and into a wider pelvic diameter (the oblique or transverse).
2. use the maternal pelvic anatomy to aid the descent of the shoulders: as the fetal shoulders are rotated within the mother's pelvis, the fetal shoulders descend through the pelvis owing to the bony architecture of the pelvis.
   - Internal rotation of the fetal shoulder should be easily achieved by pressing on the anterior aspect (*front*) or posterior aspect (*back*) of the posterior (*lowermost*) shoulder.
   - Pressure on the posterior aspect of the posterior shoulder has the added benefit of reducing the shoulder diameter by adducting the shoulders (*scrunching the shoulders together*).
   - Rotation should move the shoulders into the wider oblique diameter of the maternal pelvic, thereby resolving the shoulder dystocia and allowing release of the shoulders, aided by routine axial traction.
   - It is not necessary to attempt to place fingers from both hands in the vagina for internal rotation, nor is it necessary to rotate the shoulders more than 20 to 30 degrees.
   - A 180-degree rotation is anatomically very difficult to perform, if at all possible, and rotating the shoulders to such a degree is not usually necessary to achieve release of the shoulders.
   - If pressure in one direction has no effect, try to rotate the shoulders in the opposite direction by pressing on the other side of the fetal posterior shoulder (*that is, change from pressing on the back of the baby's shoulder to pressing on the front of the baby's shoulder or vice versa*).
   - If struggling, try to change the hand being used.
   - While attempting to rotate the fetal shoulders from the inside of the pelvis, a colleague can be instructed to apply suprapubic pressure. However ensure you are pushing with and not against each other.

Additional manoeuvres for shoulder dystocia are outlined in Box 44.7.

Cord Presentation and Prolapse

Births can be complicated by presentation of the umbilical cord when the cord lies in front of the presenting part with the fetal membranes still intact. If a loop of cord lies alongside the fetal presenting part, it is an **occult cord presentation.** If the membranes rupture, the cord is prolapsed. The incidence of cord prolapse is 0.1–0.6% (RCOG, 2014).

Causes of Cord Presentation and Prolapse

The characteristics of pregnancy that increase the risk of cord presentation and cord prolapse are not generally avoidable. Fetomaternal factors that lead to the maternal pelvis not being filled by the fetus and obstetric intervention are the two key risk factors. Common risk factors are in Box 44.9.

Diagnosis and Management

Cord presentation may be diagnosed in pregnancy by ultrasound scanning, but it is not a useful predictor of impending cord prolapse, and routine ultrasound scans to diagnose it are not recommended (RCOG, 2014). In early labour, vaginal examination (VE) may occasionally find the rope-like cord between the presenting part and membranes. It will be pulsating in time with the fetal heart rate. If cord presentation is suspected, it is essential to ensure that the membranes do not rupture. If there have been altered heart rate patterns after amniotomy or spontaneous rupture of

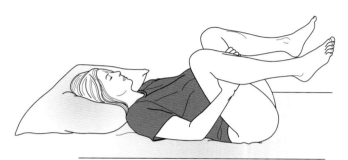

• **Fig. 44.2** McRoberts' position.

membranes, then cord prolapse should be suspected and a speculum examination or VE conducted (RCOG, 2014).

If cord presentation or prolapse is suspected or diagnosed, then the mother is best placed in one of the following positions depending on the environment and mode of transfer.

- A modified left lateral recumbent position (pelvis, hips and buttocks elevated to take pressure off the cord and membranes) (Fig. 44.4).
- Trendelenburg position (elevate the bottom of the bed with a maternal head down tilt) or knee–chest face-down position (Fig. 44.5).

This situation is an obstetric emergency and medical assistance should be obtained immediately. If cord presentation persists, an emergency CS will be needed. If the membranes have ruptured, the cord may have prolapsed through the cervix into the vagina or even outside of the vulva.

If the cord is prolapsed, it may be felt in the vagina or seen at the vulva. The cord may be compressed, especially if the presentation is cephalic, because of the hardness of the fetal head, and the fetal oxygen supply cut off. If the cord is external to the vagina, cooling, drying and handling may precipitate spasms in the umbilical vessels. If the woman is in hospital the prognosis can be good. However if the woman is at home the risk of fetal loss may be high.

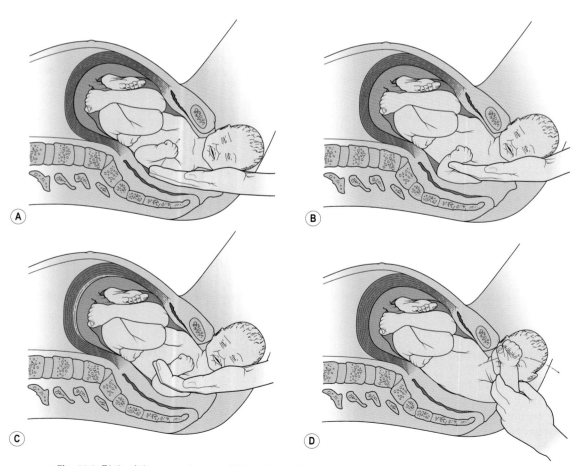

(A) (B) (C) (D)

• **Fig. 44.3** Birth of the posterior arm. (A) Location of the posterior arm. (B) Directing the arm into the hollow of the sacrum. (C) Grasping and splinting the wrist and forearm. (D) Sweeping the arm over the chest and delivering the hand.

• BOX 44.7 Additional Manoeuvres for Shoulder Dystocia

These last-resort or tertiary manoeuvres may be used in instances where key manoeuvres (as outlined in Clinical Application 44.1) have been unsuccessful. It is very rare that these are required if the manoeuvres described previously are performed correctly. In a recent series of more than 17,000 consecutive vaginal births with no permanent brachial plexus injuries, tertiary manoeuvres were not required (Crofts et al., 2016).

Vaginal replacement of the head (previously referred to as the *Zavanelli manoeuvre*) and subsequent birth by caesarean section has been described. This manoeuvre has variable success rates with a high fetal mortality rate (Vollebergh & van Dongen, 2000; Dharmasena et al., 2021). The long-term maternal consequences of this procedure are not reported. However a high proportion of fetuses have irreversible hypoxia-acidosis by the time this manoeuvre is attempted.

As the uterus will have retracted following the birth of the fetal head (i.e., the uterus is now smaller than when the fetal head was unborn), a tocolytic (e.g., terbutaline 0.25 mg subcutaneously or glyceryl trinitrate sublingually) should be given prior to any attempts to replace the fetal head inside the vagina to reduce the risk of uterine rupture.

Symphysiotomy (partial surgical division of the maternal symphysis pubis ligament) has also been suggested as a potentially useful procedure. However there is a high incidence of serious maternal morbidity and poor neonatal outcome (Goodwin et al., 2015).

Other techniques, including the use of a posterior axillary sling traction, have been reported but there is limited data to recommend their use (Cluver & Hofmeyr, 2015).

• BOX 44.8 Summary of Findings from Case Reviews of Shoulder Dystocia

In the UK, a review of fatal cases of shoulder dystocia reported that 47% of babies who died did so within 5 min of the head being born. Prior to shoulder dystocia, a high proportion of cases involved the fetus had a pathological cardiotocogram (Hope et al., 1998).

Two recent reviews reported low rates of hypoxic-ischaemic encephalopathy (HIE) if the head-to-body birth interval was less than 5 min (Lerner et al., 2011; Leung et al., 2011b). A Hong Kong study reported that the drop in cord arterial pH observed within increasing head-to-body birth interval was mostly related to the presence of an abdominal fetal heart rate prior to birth (Leung et al., 2011b). The prolonged interval of the head-to-body birth was associated with a clinically insignificant drop in cord arterial pH of 0.01 per minute. If a baby is in good condition before shoulder dystocia, the risk of HIE due to a prolonged head-to-body birth interval will be minimized.

Adequate assessment of fetal well-being in labour is crucial.

• BOX 44.9 Common Risk Factors

- A high presenting part, multiparous women, malposition of the occiput and malpresentations (brow, face, shoulder and breech).
- Transverse and oblique fetal lie.
- High assimilation pelvis found in Afro-Caribbean women.
- Preterm labour because of an increased ratio of liquor amnii to fetus and prevalence of malpresentations.
- Multiple births, especially after the birth of the first baby.
- Polyhydramnios.
- An unusually long cord.
- After obstetric manipulations such as external cephalic version or vaginal manipulations of the fetus with ruptured membranes.
- Fetal anomalies.
- Low-lying placenta.
- Induction of labour with large balloon catheter.

(RCOG, 2014; Leeman, 2020)

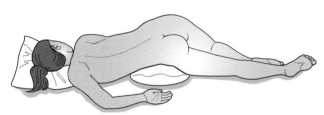

• **Fig. 44.4** Modified left lateral recumbent position. Pillows or wedges are used to elevate the woman's buttocks to relieve pressure on the umbilical cord

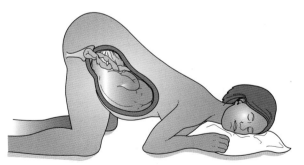

• **Fig. 44.5** Knee–chest position. Pressure on the umbilical cord is relieved as the fetus gravitates towards the fundus.

Factors to take into consideration are the stage of labour and whether the fetus is dead. If fetal death is confirmed, labour can be allowed to continue unless other conditions such as obstructed labour contraindicate vaginal delivery. If the fetus is thought to be alive, the treatment is immediate delivery by an emergency CS. In the meantime, pressure must be kept off the cord by positioning the woman in a knee–chest all-fours posture with buttocks raised (Fig. 44.5) or the modified left lateral recumbent position. (Fig. 44.4). Minimal handling of the cord is advocated to prevent vasoconstriction from spasm (RCOG, 2014). Evidence does not support the administration of maternal oxygen for use in fetal distress (Fawole & Hofmeyr, 2012).

In the early part of the second stage of labour with no CPD or malpresentation, a forceps delivery is performed. If the woman is multiparous and in late second stage, an episiotomy may allow early delivery.

Main Points

- Any condition leading to a misfit between the fetal head and maternal pelvis with failure of descent of the head into the pelvis despite good contractions results in CPD (obstructed labour dangerous for mother and fetus).
- Maternal indications of possible CPD include alterations in the size and shape of the pelvis, spinal deformities, pelvic trauma and fractures, tumours, previous difficulties with delivery and short stature.
- Fetal conditions include the size of fetus in relation to maternal pelvis and malpositions and malpresentations of the head, such as brow, posterior face or deep transverse arrest of the head, or fetal abnormalities.
- Rupture of the uterus may involve a previous scar, spontaneous rupture of an intact uterus or traumatic rupture.
- Rupture of the uterus may be complete or true, incomplete or silent.
- Shoulder dystocia is an obstetric emergency which may end in fetal and maternal morbidity and mortality. It may be due to a large baby or failure of the shoulders to deliver after delivery of the head.
- Causes of cord presentation and prolapse include high presenting part, breech presentation, CPD, placenta praevia, fibroids, preterm labour, multiple births, polyhydramnios, a long cord, external cephalic version, fetal anomalies, low lying placenta and induction of labour with a large balloon catheter.

References

Ayenew, A.A., 2021. Incidence, causes, and maternofetal outcomes of obstructed labor in Ethiopia: systematic review and meta-analysis. Reprod. Health 18, 61.

Bouthou, A., Apostolidi, D., Tsikouras, Iatrakis, G., Sarella, A., Iatrakis, D., et al., 2021. Overview of techniques to manage shoulder dustocia during vaginal birth. Eur. J. Midwifery 5, 48.

Bruner, J.P., Drummond, S.B., Meenan, A.L., Gaskin, I.M., 1998. All-fours maneuver for reducing shoulder dystocia during labour. J. Reprod. Med. 43 (5), 439–443.

Chapman, V., 2018. Malpositions and malpresentations in labour. In: Chapman, V., Charles, C. (Eds.), The Midwives' Labour and Birth Handbook, fourth ed. Wiley-Blackwell, Oxford.

Cluver, C.A., Hofmeyr, G.J., 2015. Posterior axilla sling traction for shoulder dystocia: case review and a new method of shoulder dystocia with the sling. Am. J. Obstet. Gynecol. 212 (6), 784.e1–787.e7.

Coad, J., Pedley, K., Dunstall, M., 2019. Anatomy and Physiology for Midwives, fourth ed. Elsevier, Edinburgh.

Coates, T., 2017. Shoulder dystocia. In: Macdonald, S., Johnson, G. (Eds.), Mayes' Midwifery, fifteenth ed. Elsevier, Edinburgh.

Coates, T., Green, K., 2020. Maternity emergencies. In: Marshall, J., Raynor, M. (Eds.), Myles' Textbook for Midwives, seventeenth ed. Elsevier, Edinburgh.

Crofts, J.F., Lenguerrand, E., Bentham, G.L., Tawfik, S., Claireaux, H.A., Odd, D., et al., 2016. Prevention of brachial plexus injury: 12 years of shoulder dystocia training: an interrupted time-series study. Br. J. Obstet. Gynaecol. 123 (1), 111–118.

Dharmasena, D., Berg, L., Hay, A., Yoong, W., 2021. The Zavanelli manoeuvre revisited: a review of the literature and a guide to performing cephalic replacement for severe shoulder dystocia. Eur. J. Obstet. Gynecol. Reprod. Biol. 266, 63–73.

Fawole, B., Hofmeyr, G.J., 2012. Maternal oxygen administration for fetal distress. Cochrane Database Syst. Rev. 2012 (12), CD000136.

Fischer, B., Mitteroecker, P., 2015. Covariation between human pelvis shape, stature, and head size alleviates the obstetric dilemma. Proc. Natl. Acad. Sci. U. S. A. 112 (18), 5655–5660.

Ghermaine, R., Gonik, B., Ouzounian, J., 2021. Shoulder dystocia. In: Landon, M., Galan, H., Jauniaux, E. (Eds.), Gabbe's Obstetrics: normal and Problem Pregnancies, eighth ed. Elsevier, Philadelphia.

Gobbo, R.W., 2020. Shoulder dystocia. In: Leeman, L., Dresang, L., Quinlan, J.D., Magee, S.R. (Eds.), Advanced Life Support in Obstetrics: Provider Mannual, American Academy of Family Physicians, Kansas City.

Goodwin, T.M., Banks, E., Millar, L.K., Phelan, J.P., 2015. Catastrophic shoulder dystocia and emergency symphysiotomy. Am. J. Obstet. Gynecol. 177 (2), 463–464.

Heinrichs, G., 2020. Late pregnancy bleeding. In: Leeman, L., Dresang, L., Quinlan, J.D., Magee, S.R. (Eds.), Advanced Life Support in Obstetrics: Provider Mannual, American Academy of Family Physicians: Kansas City.

Hinshaw, K., Arulkumaran, S., 2018. Malpresentation, malposition, cephalopelvic disproportion and obstetric procedures. In: Edmonds, K., Lees, C., Bourne, T. (Eds.), Dewhurst's Textbook of Obstetrics & Gynaecology, ninth ed. Wiley-Blackwell, Oxford.

Hoffman, M.K., Bailit, J.L., Branch, D.W., Burkman, R.T., Van Veldhusien, P., Lu, L., et al., 2011. A comparison of obstetric maneuvers for the acute management of shoulder dystocia. Obstet. Gynecol. 117 (6), 1272–1278.

Hofmeyr, G.J., 2004. Obstructed labour: using better technologies to reduce mortality. Int. J. Gynaecol. Obstet. 85 (1), S63–S72.

Hofmeyr, G.J., Shweni, P.M., 2012. Symphysiotomy for feto-pelvic disproportion. Cochrane Database Syst. Rev. 2012 (10), CD005299.

Hope, P., Breslin, S., Lamont, L., Lucas, A., Martin, D., Moore, I., et al., 1998. Fatal shoulder dystocia: a review of 56 cases reported to the confidential enquiry into stillbirths and deaths in infancy. Br. J. Obstet. Gynaecol. 105 (12), 1256–1261.

Jackson, K., 2020. Prolonged pregnancy and variations of uterine action. In: Marshall, J., Raynor, M. (Eds.), Myles' Textbook for Midwives, seventeenth ed. Elsevier, Edinburgh.

Jan, H., Guimicheva, B., Gosh, S., Hamid, R., Penna, L., Sarris, I., 2014. Evaluation of healthcare professionals' understanding of eponymous mnemonics and maneuvers in emergency care. Int. J. Gynaecol. Obstet. 125 (3), 228–231.

Johanson, R.B., Menon, V., Burns, E., Kargramanya, K., Osipov, V., Israelyan, M., et al., 2002. Managing Obstetric Emergencies and Trauma (MOET) structured skills training in America, utilising models and reality based scenarios. BMC Med. Educ. 2 (5).

Knight, M., Tuffnell, D., Kenyon, S., Bunch, K., Shakespeare, J., Kotnis, R., et al., 2014. Saving Lives, Improving Mothers' Care: Surveillance of Maternal Deaths in the UK 2011–13 and Lessons Learned to Inform Maternity Care from the UK and Ireland Confidential Enquiries into Maternal Deaths and Morbidity 2009–13. University of Oxford, Oxford.

Korhonen, U., Taipale, P., Heininen, S., 2015. Fetal pelvic index to predict cephalopelvic disproportion a retrospective clinical cohort study. Acta Obstet. Gynecol. Scand. 94 (6), 615–621.

Leeman, L.M., 2020. Malpresentations, malpositions, and multiple gestation. In: Leeman, L., Dresang, L., Quinlan, J.D., Magee, S.R. (Eds.), Advanced Life Support in Obstetrics: Provider Manual. American Academy of Family Physicians, Kansas City.

Lerner, H., Durlacher, K., Smith, S., Hamilton, E., 2011. Relationship between head-to-body delivery interval in shoulder dystocia and neonatal depression. Obstet. Gynecol. 118 (2), 318–322.

Lerner, H., Durlacher, K., Smith, S., Hamilton, E., 2011a. Comparison of perinatal outcomes of shoulder dystocia alleviated by different type and sequence of manoeuvres: a retrospective review. Br. J. Obstet. Gynaecol. 118 (8), 985–989 90.

Leung, T.Y., Stuart, O., Sahota, D.S., Suen, S.S., Lau, T.K., Lao, T.T., 2011b. Head-to-body delivery interval and risk of fetal acidosis and hypoxic ischaemic encephalopathy in shoulder dystocia: retrospective review. Br. J. Obstet. Gynaecol. 118 (4), 474–479.

National Institute of Health and Care Excellence (NICE), 2019. Intrapartum Care for Women with Existing Medical Conditions or Obstetric Complications and Their Babies. Available at: https://www.nice.org.uk/guidance/ng121.

National Institute of Health and Care Excellence (NICE), 2021. Antenatal Care. Available at: https://www.nice.org.uk/guidance/ng201.

National Institute of Health and Care Excellence (NICE), 2023. Intrapartum Care. Available at: https://www.nice.org.uk/guidance/ng235.

Pattinson, R.C., Cuthbert, A., Vannevel, V., 2017. Pelvimetry for fetal cephalic presentations at or near term for deciding on mode of delivery. Cochrane Database Syst. Rev. 2017 (3), CD000161.

Royal College of Obstetricians and Gynaecologists (RCOG), 2012. Shoulder Dystocia: green-top Guideline No. 42. Available at: https://www.rcog.org.uk/media/ewgpnmio/gtg_42.pdf.

Royal College of Obstetricians and Gynaecologists (RCOG), 2014. Umbilical Cord Prolapse: green-top Guideline No. 50. Available at: https://www.rcog.org.uk/media/3wykswng/gtg-50-umbilicalcordprolapse-2014.pdf.

Sagi-Dain, L., Sagi, S., 2015. The role of episiotomy in prevention and management of shoulder dystocia: a systematic review. Obstet. Gynecol. Surv. 70 (5), 354–362.

Sikka, P., Chopra, S., Kalpdev, A., Jain, V., Dhaliwal, L., 2011. Destructive operations—a vanishing art in modern obstetrics: 25 year experience at a tertiary care center in India. Arch. Gynecol. Obstet. 283 (5), 929–933.

Smyth, R.M.D., Markham, C., Dowswell, T., 2013. Amniotomy for shortening spontaneous labour. Cochrane Database Syst. Rev. 2013 (6), CD006167.

Vollebergh, J.H., van Dongen, P.W., 2000. The Zavanelli manoeuvre in shoulder dystocia: case report and review of published cases. Eur. J. Obstet. Gynecol. Reprod. Biol. 89 (1), 81–84.

Winter, C., Draycott, T., Muchatuta, N., Crofts, J., 2018. PROMPT (PRactical Obstetric Multi-Professional Training) Course Manual, third ed. RCOG Press, London.

Annotated recommended reading

Knight, M., Tuffnell, D., Kenyon, S., Bunch, K., Shakespeare, J., Kotnis, R., et al., 2014. Saving Lives, Improving Mothers' Care: Surveillance of Maternal Deaths in the UK 2011-13 and Lessons Learned to Inform Maternity Care from the UK and Ireland Confidential Enquiries into Maternal Deaths and Morbidity 2009-13. University of Oxford, Oxford.

This triennial report was produced for the Confidential Enquiries into Maternal Deaths in the UK. All health professionals providing care for women during pregnancy and childbirth are encouraged to read the full report.

Knight, M., Bunch, K., Felker, A., Patel, R., Kotnis, R., Kenyon, S., Kurinczuk, J.J., on behalf of MBRRACE-UK. Saving Lives, Improving Mothers' Care Core Report – Lessons learned to inform maternity care from the UK and Ireland Confidential Enquiries into Maternal Deaths and Morbidity 2019–21. Oxford: National Perinatal Epidemiology Unit, University of Oxford 2023

This report is the latest MBRRACE report on Maternal deaths in the UK 2019–2021.

Royal College of Obstetricians and Gynaecologists (RCOG), 2012. Shoulder Dystocia: green-top Guideline No. 42. Available at: https://www.rcog.org.uk/media/ewgpnmio/gtg_42.pdf.

Royal College of Obstetricians and Gynaecologists (RCOG), 2014. Umbilical Cord Prolapse: green-top Guideline No. 50. Available at: https://www.rcog.org.uk/media/3wykswng/gtg-50-umbilicalcordprolapse-2014.pdf.

These two RCOG guidelines are recommended reading for practitioners working within obstetrics.

Winter, C., Draycott, T., Muchatuta, N., Crofts, J., 2018. PROMPT (PRactical Obstetric Multi-Professional Training) Course Manual, third ed. RCOG Press, London.

This manual is an excellent and useful stand-alone resource for the management of a range of obstetric emergency situations. The manual provides evidence-based, up-to-date information for any health professionals in maternity care.

Websites

https://www.nice.org.uk/.
https://www.rcog.org.uk/guidance/.
https://www.who.int/publications/.

These websites provide evidence-based guidance and recommendations related to the management of emergencies in intrapartum care. The sites also provide excellent resources for good practice for high-quality care and related published evidence.

45

Postpartum Haemorrhage and Other Third-stage Problems

LYZ HOWIE AND JEAN WATSON

CHAPTER CONTENTS

This chapter discusses postpartum haemorrhage (PPH) including types, risk factors, causes, presentation and clinical management. Midwives need to have sound knowledge and understanding to recognize and effectively manage PPH in their everyday practice.

Introduction

The third stage of labour can be hazardous for the mother because of the risk of haemorrhage and other complications. The management of the third stage should be aimed at minimizing these possible serious complications but interfering as little as possible with the physiological process (discussed in Chapter 40) and the mother's enjoyment of her baby (National Institute of Health and Care Excellence [NICE], 2023). A role of the midwife is to explain the need for active interventions, such as the giving of an oxytocic drug or commencing an intravenous infusion, to the mother before labour so that women are enabled to make informed choices should the need suddenly arise.

Postpartum Haemorrhage

Definition

Postpartum haemorrhage (PPH) is defined as excessive bleeding from the genital tract after the birth of the baby and occurs in the period extending from the time of birth to the end of the puerperium. If bleeding occurs in the first 24 hours, it is called **primary PPH** (Mane et al., 2020; Mousa et al., 2014) and complicates about 6% of labours. If the bleeding occurs after the first 24 hours and before the end of the 12th week, it is called **secondary PPH**, a much less common occurrence that complicates less than 1% of labours (Gupta & Kakkar, 2020).

PPH is also classified according to the site of bleeding. Most commonly, the bleeding is from the placental site and there is poor tone of the uterine muscle. This is **atonic haemorrhage**. Bleeding may also be traumatic due to a laceration of the genital tract. In primary PPH, blood loss can be minor (500–1000 mL) or major (more than 1000 mL). Major blood loss can be further subdivided into moderate (1001–2000 mL) and severe (>2000 mL) and is sufficient to cause deterioration in the woman's condition, especially in women with lower body mass (Mavrides et al., 2016). Because of the diuresis and haemoconcentration that follow delivery, smaller amounts of blood loss are detrimental in secondary PPH.

Primary PPH is one of the most serious complications of labour. The incidence of mortality related to PPH is 0.76 per 1000 maternities (Knight et al., 2018). At term, maternal circulating blood flow to the uterus is 450–700 mL/min, where 80% is perfusion for the placenta and 20% for the myometrium. Blood loss may be rapid and devastating if the bleeding is not controlled. PPH is still a significant cause of maternal mortality after a caesarean section (CS) (Knight et al., 2014). Measuring blood loss at delivery can be difficult to estimate (Diaz, Abalos & Carroli, 2018). Importantly, blood soaks into sheets and towels and separates into clot and serum. Any clot placed in a jug and measured will

<table>
<tr><td colspan="4">**TABLE 45.1** **Risk Factors**</td></tr>
</table>

History	Current Pregnancy	Intrapartum
Grand multiparity	Anaemia	Prolonged labour
Multiple pregnancy	Antepartum haemorrhage	Precipitate labour
Obesity >35 kg	Overdistension of the uterus	Induction/oxytocin
Age >40	Uterine abnormalities/fibroids	Retained placenta
Previous postpartum haemorrhage	Pre-eclampsia	Placenta praevia
Bleeding disorder	Fetal macrosomia	Placenta accreta
		General anaesthetic
		Perineal trauma

(Mavrides et al., 2016; NICE, 2022; Trika & Singh, 2018)

• **BOX 45.1** **The Four T's**

Tone: Atonic uterus (most common).
Tissue: Retained placental tissue (important to check completeness of placenta and membranes).
Trauma: Trauma to the genital tract – tears to the perineum, uterus, clitoris, labia or cervix.
Thrombin: Abnormalities in clotting due to blood loss or clotting disorders.

---

only be 40% of the total loss, and so it is easy to underestimate the total loss by up to 50%.

Primary Postpartum Haemorrhage from the Placental Site

Causes

Uterine atony, which is failure of the uterine muscle fibres to contract and retract to compress the blood vessels, is the most common cause (Mousa et al., 2014). Despite the long list of risk factors outlined in Table 45.1, many cases of primary PPH occur in normal labours with no explanation. A useful way to assess for the cause of PPH is through the 4 T's outlined in Box 45.1.

Management of Postpartum Haemorrhage

In the antenatal period, prevention is the best form of management, and this begins with the booking interview and surveillance throughout pregnancy. Good history-taking and risk assessment is important (Mavrides et al., 2016). If any risk factors (Table 45.1) are present, the woman should deliver in hospital (Mavrides et al., 2016) so that if bleeding does occur then treatment is immediately available. As pregnancy progresses, detection and treatment of anaemia are important (Mavrides et al., 2016). NICE (2023) advocates that women who have a haemoglobin level <85 g/L at onset of labour should have a planned birth at an obstetric unit as anaemia is a risk factor for PPH. Haemoglobin of 85–105 g/L at onset of labour is not a reason for advising birth

within an obstetric unit, but indicates that further consideration of birth setting may be required (NICE, 2023).

In Labour

Women at risk of PPH must be managed carefully to minimize the likelihood of bleeding. When labour commences, an intravenous cannula (size 14 or 16 gauge) is inserted and blood is taken for a full blood count and confirmation of blood group. Serum is saved for 'cross-matching' blood should it become necessary to give the woman a blood transfusion. Prolonged labour, with its problems of dehydration and exhaustion, should be avoided. An oxytocin (Syntocinon) infusion should be started if labour progress is slow. The woman's bladder should be kept empty by encouraging micturition or by catheterization. A full bladder may inhibit uterine muscle activity and add to the risk of atony.

Management of the third stage should be discussed with the woman antenatally so that previous verbal consent can be given for any interventions. The benefits and risks associated with active and physiological management of the third stage should be discussed. The woman should be advised that the potential for PPH is greater with 'physiological management' of the third stage than it is with 'active management'. Advise the woman to have active management of the third stage because it is associated with a lower risk of PPH and/or blood transfusion (NICE, 2023). If a woman at low risk of PPH requests physiological management of the third stage, support her in her choice (NICE, 2023). In active management, an intramuscular injection of 10 IU oxytocin is usually given in preference to oxytocin plus ergometrine, as it is associated with fewer side effects than Syntometrine (refer to Chapter 40). The uterotonic is given immediately after the birth of the baby and before the cord is clamped and cut (NICE, 2023). Do not clamp the cord earlier than 1 min from the birth of the baby unless there is concern about the integrity of the cord or the baby has a heartbeat below 60 bpm. The placenta is delivered by controlled cord traction after signs of separation of the placenta for active management (NICE, 2023). If the woman starts to bleed, treatment needs to take into account the uterotonics already administered (NICE, 2023). This may include the administration of oxytocin intravenously or intramuscular ergometrine or oxytocin and ergometrine (NICE, 2023 section 1.10.34, Table 12).

One intervention is prophylactic radiology in the presence of a radiologist and appropriate equipment (Mavrides et al., 2016). This process involves inserting an arterial balloon into the blood vessels, causing occlusion and embolization, to prevent major blood loss. If this is procedure is unavailable, then uterine balloon tamponade might be a better treatment method (Mavrides et al., 2016). Radiological intervention may be used in the event of PPH if the cause is secondary to:

- Atonic uterus after normal or prolonged labour, with or without CS.
- Surgical complications or uterine tears at the time of CS.
- Bleeding continues on the postnatal ward or in the post-operative recovery area after a normal delivery or a CS.
- Bleeding after a hysterectomy.

Signs of Postpartum Haemorrhage

It would be difficult to miss the visible bleeding and maternal collapse that can occur. Other signs may be present if blood loss is not visible (e.g., clots retained in an atonic uterus (Box 45.2)). It is crucial that there is urgent management once PPH has been identified **after delivery of the placenta.** The algorithm for immediate management is outlined in Fig. 45.1.

After the placenta and membranes are expelled, they should be examined for completeness. If the placenta appears

> ### • BOX 45.2   Other Signs of Postpartum Haemorrhage if Blood Loss Not Visible
>
> - Pallor.
> - A rising pulse rate or paradoxical bradycardia.
> - Falling blood pressure (late sign).
> - Altered levels of consciousness.
> - Increased respiratory rate (air hunger).
> - An enlarged, 'boggy'-feeling uterus.

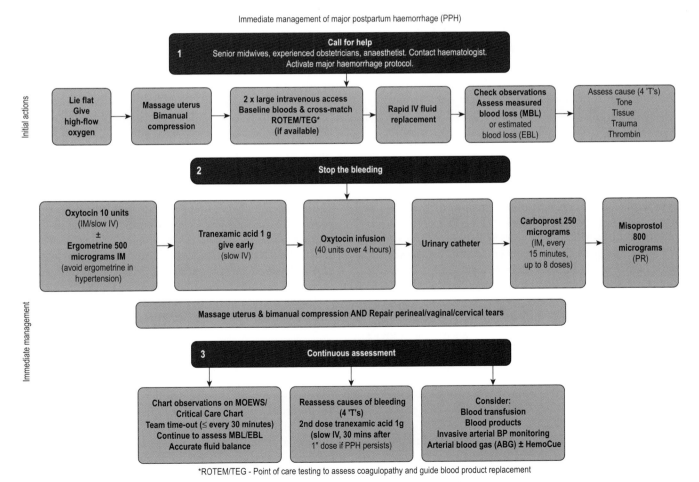

• **Fig. 45.1** Algorithm for initial management of major postpartum haemorrhage.
(Winter et al., 2018)

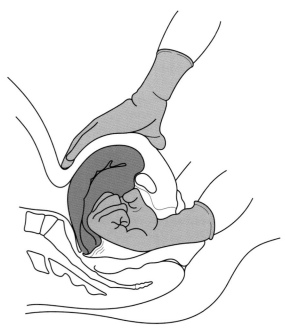

• **Fig. 45.2** Bimanual compression of the uterus.

incomplete, the doctor will carry out an exploration and evacuation of the uterus under spinal or epidural anaesthesia.

Bimanual Compression of the Uterus

This may be necessary where the woman is transferred into hospital by ambulance or transferred to the operating theatre. Bimanual compression is an excellent holding measure and should be continued until the haemorrhage is brought under control.

To perform **bimanual compression,** insert one gloved hand into the vagina like a cone. The hand is formed into a fist and placed into the anterior fornix of the vagina (Acosta & Aras-Payne, 2017; Begley, 2020). The other hand is placed behind the uterus abdominally with the fingers pointing towards the cervix (Fig. 45.2). The uterus is brought forward and compressed between the palm of the hand positioned abdominally and the fist in the vagina. To be effective, bimanual uterine compression must be maintained until the blood clots in the uterine vessels and the uterus may become firm. In several women, this is all that is needed. In others, it is a *temporary* measure in the management of PPH caused by uterine atony after vaginal delivery. If bleeding persists, a clotting disorder must be excluded before further exploration of the vagina and uterus under general anaesthetic (see Chapter 31). This procedure is extremely painful to the woman and is only undertaken without anaesthetic in cases of PPH if drugs are not available or if drug therapy fails.

Once bleeding is controlled, an intravenous infusion containing oxytocin is started to maintain uterine contraction. If blood loss is excessive or if the woman had a low haemoglobin level before delivery, a blood transfusion may be necessary. Therefore it is important not to underestimate the amount of blood lost. Knight et al. (2014) stress that it is not only the amount of blood loss that should be taken into consideration, but also the woman's stature, as smaller women will lose more of their total circulating volume than a larger woman.

In the case of serious PPH, the obstetrician and anaesthetist will agree on the management of fluid replacement. A total volume of 3.5 L of clear fluids (up to 2 L of warmed Hartmann's solution rapidly, followed by up to a further 1.5 L of warmed colloid if blood still not available) comprises the maximum that should be infused while awaiting compatible blood. However the evidence on colloid use is inconclusive for PPH (Mavrides et al., 2016). It is recommended that each obstetric unit should have a protocol on managing PPH that should be followed, and 'fire-drill' scenarios should be conducted to train and update practitioners on the protocol (Mavrides et al., 2016). Group O rhesus-negative blood should be available on the labour ward for use in emergencies. The importance of fluid administration for PPH is that it is infused rapidly and warmed (Mavrides et al., 2016). All maternity units should have access to rapid fluid warmers, which incorporate a blood-warming device (Knight et al., 2014). Appropriate personnel must be included, and there should be early involvement of a consultant obstetrician, anaesthetist, haematologist and blood bank.

If the uterus fails to contract even though oxytocic drugs have been used, a deep intramuscular injection of the prostanoid carboprost, which is 15-methyl-PGF$_{2\alpha}$ (Ritter et al., 2019), can be given and repeated as per regimen (maximum of eight doses administered 15 min apart). Carboprost can be administered to women who do not respond to ergometrine (Ritter et al., 2019). Carboprost is contraindicated in women with cardiac, renal, pulmonary and hepatic disease, as well as in acute pelvic inflammation. It should be used with care in women who have asthma, hypertension, diabetes, epilepsy, hypotension or hypertension (NICE, 2022). Different maternity units, according to their guidelines, may use different methods for controlling bleeding. In continuing haemorrhage, internal iliac artery ligation, uterine packing or intrauterine balloon tamponade and B-Lynch suture may be needed, or a hysterectomy performed. Knight et al. (2014) recommend early recourse to hysterectomy, especially where bleeding is associated with placenta accreta, or uterine rupture or when bleeding continues.

A systematic review by Mousa et al. (2014) compared misoprostol and oxytocin for PPH. They highlighted that oxytocin infusion is more effective and causes fewer side effects when used as first-line therapy for the treatment of primary PPH. When used after prophylactic uterotonics, misoprostol and oxytocin infusion worked similarly. The review suggests that among women who received oxytocin for the treatment of primary PPH, adjunctive use of misoprostol offers no added benefit.

Novikova, Hofmeyr and Cluver (2015) acknowledge that tranexamic acid along with uterotonics demonstrated some benefits for women at low risk for PPH, although more research is required for high-risk women following a vaginal or CS birth and the side effects of the use of tranexamic acid. However Escobar et al. (2022) recommend early use of intravenous tranexamic acid for PPH following a vaginal or CS birth as well as oxytocin for the early management of PPH. This recommendation is supported by the 2020 MBRRACE report (Tuffnell & Knight, 2020).

The evidence is contradictory regarding the effectiveness of mechanical and surgical interventions for PPH (Escobar et al., 2022; Kellie et al., 2020) and more high-quality research is required. Future studies should also focus on the best way to treat women who fail to respond to uterotonic therapy.

Observations

Once blood loss is controlled, the total loss is estimated, remembering how difficult this can be and that estimates become less accurate as blood loss increases. Knight et al. (2014) recommend that as well as accurate estimation of blood loss, a woman's stature should be taken into consideration. A woman of 70 kg who loses 1500 mL of blood will lose 20% of circulating volume, whilst a woman who weighs 55 kg would lose almost 30% (Paterson-Brown & Howell, 2014). Fluid intake is recorded, as is the hourly urine output. Central venous pressure measurement may be required depending on the blood loss and the severity of the woman's condition, which may require further fluid replacement. Respiratory rate, maternal pulse and blood pressure (BP) are recorded every 15 min to ensure her condition remains satisfactory. The uterine fundus is palpated frequently to ensure it remains contracted, and the vaginal blood loss is observed. All findings can be recorded using a Modified Early Obstetric Warning System (MEOWS) (Chu, Johnston & Geoghegan, 2020).

If the problem involves failure of blood coagulation, a haematologist should be involved (see Chapter 47 for maternal collapse). Fresh blood is usually the best treatment, as it contains both platelets and coagulation factors. Fresh frozen plasma, containing factors V and VIII and fibrinogen, cryoprecipitate and platelets may also be used along with recombinant factor VIIa therapy (Mavrides et al., 2016).

Traumatic Postpartum Haemorrhage

If the blood loss is from a laceration of the genital tract, bleeding should be stopped by direct pressure, if possible, and then sutured. Bleeding from a cervical or lower uterine tear should be suspected if the uterus is well contracted, no superficial bleeding can be seen and the blood loss is slow and steady. Tears of the upper part of the vagina, the cervix and lower uterine segment should be sutured under spinal or epidural anaesthesia. If severe bleeding is from the uterus and cannot be stopped, a hysterectomy may be necessary.

Secondary Postpartum Haemorrhage

Secondary PPH is any abnormal bleeding or excessive bleeding from the birth canal occurring between 24 hours and 12 weeks postnatally (Gupta & Kakkar, 2020). This is a complication of the puerperium and is most often seen between days 4 and 14. It is usually due to a retained piece of placenta, but other causes include the presence of a blood clot or a fibroid in the uterine wall or endometriosis. Secondary PPH is also commonly associated with infection. There may have been warning signs of heavy, red, offensive vaginal blood loss and subinvolution. If infection is present, pyrexia and tachycardia may be evident.

Management

If the uterus is palpable, it is massaged to make it contract. Any clots are expelled, and the bladder must be emptied. If bleeding is slight, it may be managed at home with antibiotics and oral ergometrine tablets.

If bleeding is severe, an intravenous injection of ergometrine or intramuscular oxytocin and ergometrine (adhere to local, regional or national guidance for dosage) is given. If the woman is at home, she should be transferred to hospital. A blood transfusion may be given, depending on the blood loss and the antenatal haemoglobin. The uterus is evacuated under spinal or epidural anaesthesia. Robust evidence from randomized controlled trials (RCTs) are needed to inform practice, and further robust RCTs are required to explore the different therapies for secondary PPH (Gupta & Kakkar, 2020).

Complications of Postpartum Haemorrhage

Unless adequately treated, the woman is likely to develop **iron-deficiency anaemia.** Infection is more common, and lactation may be poor. If shock develops, acute renal tubular necrosis may present with anuria. Anterior pituitary necrosis leading to Sheehan's syndrome may occur if the haemorrhage was severe (see Chapter 28). All women who have suffered PPH should be advised to book into hospital for any subsequent deliveries (NICE, 2023).

Haematoma Formation

PPH may be concealed if progressive haematoma formation occurs in the perineum or lower vagina. Bleeding into the broad ligament causing haematoma is more difficult to diagnose. Up to 1 L of blood may collect in the tissues, leading to increasing maternal pain due to pressure. The mother may collapse with signs of shock (see Chapter 47).

Management

The woman will have to be taken to theatre so that the haematoma can be drained and haemostasis achieved under spinal or general anaesthetic. Replacement of the lost blood may be necessary. Infection is a risk, and antibiotics are usually prescribed.

Prolonged Third Stage

Failure of the placenta to deliver spontaneously can cause PPH (Lewis, 2007; Mane et al., 2020). If labour is managed actively, the placenta and membranes should be delivered within 10 min. The third stage is considered prolonged if

- Uterine inertia.
- Full bladder.
- Mismanagement of third stage where 'fiddling' with the fundus causes irregular contractions and partial placental separation.
- The formation of a constriction ring or spasm between the upper and lower uterine segments.
- A uterine abnormality such as bicornuate uterus.
- Morbid adherence of placenta, more likely to occur in women who have had a previous caesarean section or placenta praevia.

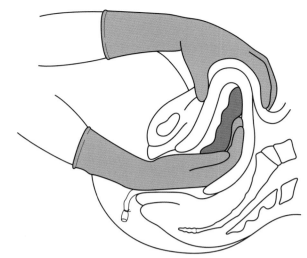

• **Fig. 45.3** Manual removal of the placenta.

the placenta is not delivered within 30 min of active management or within 60 min of physiological management (NICE, 2023). The placenta may be separated but be retained, trapped behind the reforming cervix, and bleeding is likely. Alternatively the placenta may be morbidly adherent to the uterine wall and, if there is no separation, bleeding will not occur. The causes of prolonged third stage are outlined in Box 45.3.

Types of Adherent Placenta

Placenta accreta where the decidua basalis is deficient, and the chorionic villi have attached to the myometrium.

Placenta increta where the villi penetrate deeply into the myometrium.

Placenta percreta where the villi have penetrated to the serous external coat of the uterus.

Management

As long as the placenta remains in the uterus, haemorrhage is a threat. Secure intravenous access is essential. If there is no success in delivering the placenta after emptying the bladder, manual removal of the placenta (under anaesthetic) is needed to avoid shock (Fig. 45.3).

An intravenous oxytocic injection is given after successful manual removal followed by an intravenous infusion of oxytocin. Different hospitals have different protocols for the dose of oxytocin to be used after manual removal of placenta. Prophylactic antibiotic therapy is commenced, as manual removal of the placenta may have introduced organisms into the uterus.

Acute Inversion of the Uterus

In this rare condition, which occurs in about 1 in 100,000 deliveries, the uterus is partly or completely turned inside out (Fig. 45.4). In partial inversion, the inner surface of the fundus is drawn down into the uterine cavity. In severe inversion, the inside of the fundus protrudes through the cervix into the vagina. If the uterus is fully turned inside out, it may appear outside the vulva. Profound neurogenic shock due to traction on the uterine supportive ligaments is

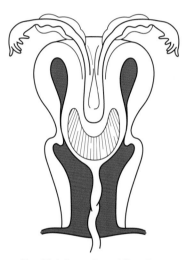

• **Fig. 45.4** Inversion of the uterus.

likely to occur. There will be pain and possibly haemorrhage if there is partial placental separation. Causes of inversion of the uterus are in Box 45.4.

Diagnosis and Management

The woman will complain of pain and may collapse. Cardiac arrest may occur. On palpation of the abdomen, it will be difficult to find the fundus of the uterus. A distinct hollow in the uterine fundus may be felt. The woman may complain of a feeling that something is in her vagina.

Methods of Replacement

Manual replacement: The rapid replacement of the uterus will prevent the development of shock. Replacement is easier if it is carried out immediately, before uterine congestion and oedema develop. Pressure is applied first to the part of the lower segment nearest the cervix, gently proceeding upwards towards the fundus. If replacement is not possible,

• BOX 45.4 Causes of Inversion of the Uterus

- Mismanagement of third stage by applying fundal pressure or cord traction with the uterus relaxed.
- A short cord, where the fundus descends with the fetus.
- Manual removal of placenta if the operator withdraws the hand in the uterus while still applying fundal pressure.
- Spontaneous inversion, possibly due to straining, which raises intra-abdominal pressure, such as a sudden cough or sneeze.

• CLINICAL APPLICATION 45.1 Diagnostic Criteria for Amniotic Fluid Embolism

In the absence of any other clear cause, a woman may present with the following:
1. Acute maternal collapse (see Chapter 47) with one or more of the following features:
   - Premonitory symptoms (e.g., restlessness, numbness, agitation, tingling).
   - Seizure.
   - Shortness of breath.
   - Cardiac arrest.
   - Cardiac rhythm problems.
   - Hypotension.
   - Disseminated intravascular coagulation (see Chapter 33).
   - Maternal haemorrhage.
   - Acute fetal compromise.
   (Excluding women with maternal haemorrhage as the first presenting feature in whom there was no evidence of early coagulopathy or cardiorespiratory compromise).
2. Women in whom the diagnosis was made at post-mortem examination with the finding of fetal squames or hair in the lungs (Knight et al., 2014).

the uterus should be replaced in the vagina and the foot of the bed elevated to reduce traction on the uterine ligaments, uterine tubes and ovaries. An injection of morphine will reduce pain. If the placenta is still attached to the uterine wall, it should not be removed.

O'Sullivan's hydrostatic method: This method can be performed in the labour ward without anaesthesia (Winter et al., 2018). First, exclude uterine rupture. Position the woman in lithotomy. Use two 1-L bags of warmed irrigation fluid (e.g., sodium chloride 0.9%) attached to a wide-bore giving set or cystoscopy irrigation set. The open end of the tubing may be inserted into the vagina and the introitus sealed by holding the vulva tightly around the forearm, using the other hand to prevent the warm fluid from leaking out (may require an assistant) *or* the open end of the tubing may be attached to a silastic ventouse cup, which is positioned in the lower vagina at the inner aspect of the introitus to create a seal. Copious amounts of warmed fluid are instilled through gravity or by pressure on the bag. Up to 4 L may be required. In most cases this will reduce the inversion, with rapid resolution of the shock. The placenta can then be removed under anaesthesia. Thereafter contraction of the uterus must be maintained by appropriate oxytocic treatment.

If there has been delay, the woman is anaesthetized and the uterus replaced manually, as previously described. This is by pressure in the fornices to replace the lower segment, which was last to invert, then finally inserting the fundus. If a retraction ring has developed between the upper and lower uterine segments, the replacement may be difficult. Uterine relaxants maybe useful to assist with the manual correction of the inversion. These include terbutaline (0.25 mg subcutaneously) or glycerol trinitrite spray (one metred dose sublingually). General anaesthesia might also promote uterine relaxation. However caution should be taken with the use of uterine relaxants as this may exacerbate atonic postpartum haemorrhage once the uterus is replaced.

Surgical intervention may be required if the previous methods have failed.

Amniotic Fluid Embolism

This obstetric emergency occurs when amniotic fluid is forced from the uterine venous sinuses of the placental bed into the maternal circulation. It usually follows uterine hyperactivity but may also occur near to term, before labour begins or in the third stage because of a tear in the lower uterine segment. The embolus travels around the systemic circulation, through the heart and into the pulmonary circulation to obstruct pulmonary arterioles or alveolar capillaries. This causes sudden maternal collapse and respiratory and cardiac arrest.

Risk Factors

Amniotic fluid embolism (AFE) is more likely to occur in women where intra-amniotic pressures are raised. Historically polyhydramnios, placenta praevia, abruptio placenta, cervical laceration, hyperstimulation and uterine rupture may all be risk factors leading to an increased risk of AFE, but there is a lack of evidence to support this (Tuffnell & Slemeck, 2017). However induction of labour, CS and older mothers from ethnic minorities are deemed risk factors (Knight et al., 2014). Diagnostic criteria for an AFE are outlined in Clinical Application 45.1.

Management

This is an obstetric emergency. The management of women with suspected AFE remains supportive rather than therapeutic, with emphasis on maintenance of oxygenation, circulatory support (cardiopulmonary resuscitation) and correcting coagulopathy. Because AFE has a multitude of presentations, management will depend on the clinical circumstances (see Chapter 47). The uterus must be emptied as quickly as possible and, if necessary, CS performed. Unfortunately, despite active management, this rare complication often results in maternal and fetal death. If the woman survives there may be renal failure, and dialysis may be necessary if the kidneys do not respond to diuretic drugs such as mannitol.

Shock in Obstetrics

Martin, Cheek and Morris (2018) define shock as being a condition in which the cardiovascular system (CVS) fails to perfuse the tissues adequately, resulting in widespread impairment of cellular metabolism and tissue function. Three functions of the CVS may be altered and result in shock. If the heart is thought of as a pump, these can be summarized as:

- **Heart function:** loss of the pump.
- **Blood volume:** nothing to pump.
- **Blood pressure:** no force in the pump.

Shock from any condition will inevitably cause progress to organ failure and death unless some compensatory mechanisms occur to reverse the situation or clinical treatments are successful (see Chapter 47). If shock remains untreated, the body's compensatory mechanisms are overwhelmed and a downward spiral towards death begins. Compensatory mechanisms function to maintain BP and blood flow to vital organs such as the brain and the heart.

Recognition of Shock

Because the body has many systems, all involving cells at the microscopic level, shock presents with many signs and symptoms. Tissue damage is diverse, and subjective symptoms can be vague. A person may report nausea, weakness, feeling cold or hot, dizziness, confusion, fear and anxiety, thirst and shortage of breath with air hunger. Clinical measurements will find pulse and respiration rate increased, BP and cardiac output decreased, diminished urinary output, cold and clammy skin, pallor (Martin, Cheek & Morris, 2018) and reduced core temperature.

Classification of Shock

There are various ways of classifying shock: for example, by pathophysiological processes, by clinical manifestations or by cause. Classification by cause is the most useful, as it will also indicate the likely pathophysiology underlying the shock and highlight the disorder that will need treating to reverse the shock (Tables 45.2 and 45.3). The three main cardiovascular functions that are impaired are obvious. All the following types of shock may occur in childbearing women and will be described in detail. Possible causes of obstetric shock will then be discussed. There is a danger that compensatory mechanisms may mask the signs of shock until maternal and fetal lives are at risk.

TABLE 45.2 **Types of Shock and their Immediate Cause**

Type	Cause
Cardiogenic	Heart failure
Hypovolaemic	Reduced blood volume
Neurogenic	Neural alterations of smooth muscle tone resulting in vasodilatation
Anaphylactic	Immune system pathology resulting in vasodilatation
Septic	Resulting in cardiac depression and dilatation with vasodilatation

TABLE 45.3 **Pathophysiological Causes of Shock in Childbearing**

Cardiogenic Shock	Hypovolaemic Shock	Neurogenic Shock	Anaphylactic Shock	Septic Shock
Pulmonary embolism	Haemorrhage associated with childbearing	Acute inversion of the uterus	Adverse drug reactions	Infection in septic abortion and puerperal infection Influenza
Severe anaemia	Ruptured ectopic pregnancy	Aspiration of acid gastric contents (Mendelson's syndrome)		
Cardiac disorders such as valvular or congenital problems	Ruptured uterus	Intrauterine manipulations without adequate anaesthesia		
Severe hypertension	Coagulopathy hypertension after amniotic fluid embolism or diabetic crisis			

Cardiogenic Shock

Heart failure or decreased cardiac output is the cause of cardiogenic shock (Martin, Cheek & Morris, 2018), and most cases are due to myocardial infarction. Shock may also occur in congestive cardiac failure, myocardial ischaemia and drug toxicity. It is not very responsive to treatment and often leads to death.

Compensatory Sequence of Events

- As cardiac output begins to decrease, renin produced by the kidneys stimulates aldosterone release so that sodium and water are retained.
- Hypothalamic responses cause catecholamine release from the adrenal glands, resulting in vasoconstriction to maintain BP.
- Cardiac performance is enhanced, but there is increased demand for oxygen and nutrients.
- Tissue perfusion begins to fall, and nutrient and oxygen delivery to the cells decreases.
- Cellular metabolism is impaired, and signs of shock appear.

Hypovolaemic Shock

Hypovolaemic shock is caused by loss of blood and fluid (Martin, Cheek & Morris, 2018) resulting in inadequate blood volume. Shock begins to develop when intravascular volume is decreased by 15%. The first sign is a thready pulse as intense vasoconstriction attempts to move blood from the periphery to supply the vital organs. A sharp decline in BP is a late and serious sign. It may occur because of:
- Loss of whole blood in haemorrhage.
- Loss of plasma as in burns.
- Loss of interstitial fluid.
- Diabetes mellitus.
- Excessive vomiting or diarrhoea.

Compensatory Sequence of Events

- Adrenals release catecholamines, which increase heart rate and systemic vascular resistance (SVR).
- Interstitial fluid moves into the vascular compartment.
- The liver and spleen disgorge stored red blood cells and plasma into the circulation.
- Renin produced by the kidneys stimulates aldosterone release, and sodium and water are retained.
- Tissue perfusion begins to fall, and nutrient and oxygen delivery to the cells decreases.
- Cellular metabolism is impaired, and signs of shock appear.

The management of shock is outlined in Clinical Application 45.2.

Neurogenic Shock

Another name for neurogenic shock is **vasogenic shock** (Martin, Cheek & Morris, 2018), referring to the massive vasodilatation that results because of a loss of balance between the sympathetic and parasympathetic stimulation of vascular smooth muscle. Although blood

CLINICAL APPLICATION 45.2 — Management of Hypovolaemic Shock

The crucial factor is to restore circulating blood volume. It is an emergency and requires immediate resuscitative measures (Lister, Hofland & Grafton, 2020).
1. Summon help, as time is of the essence. If hypovolaemic shock is not acted on promptly, it can lead to maternal death. Appropriate staff would be senior midwifery staff, obstetrician and anaesthetist.
2. Reassure the woman and her partner/birthing partner of what is happening.
3. Remember the important concepts of ABCDE: airway, breathing, circulation, disability and exposure (see Chapter 47).
4. Maintain or secure an airway. Intubation may be necessary if the woman is collapsed.
   - Oxygen via a non-rebreather, trauma mask (15 L/min).
   - Cannulate with two large-bore venflons (14 or 16 gauge) and commence an intravenous infusion using crystalloids (e.g., Hartmann's solution or normal saline).
   - Laboratory blood tests:
     - Blood type (group and crossmatch).
     - Full blood count.
     - Coagulation screen.
     - Urea and electrolytes.
     - Liver function tests.
     - Prepare for blood transfusion (non-cross-matched O negative or ABO cross-matched).
5. Assess maternal condition (when woman is stable, move to a high-dependency environment).
   - Observations taken and recorded: respiratory rate, blood pressure, pulse, oxygen saturation (every 5 min), temperature (every 15 min) and capillary refill (should be <2 s).
   - Accurate fluid balance (input/output including all blood loss)
   - Document findings on acute care and/or MEOWS chart.
   - Assess and stop cause of haemorrhage.

volume does not change, the vascular compartment is increased drastically, resulting in relative hypovolaemia with a decrease in SVR. Vascular resistance is normally maintained by the sympathetic stimulus, and if this is interrupted or inhibited for any length of time, neurogenic shock will follow. It may occur because of (Martin, Cheek & Morris, 2018):
- Trauma to the spinal cord.
- Cerebral hypoxia.
- Medullary hypoglycaemia.
- Anaesthetics and other depressive drugs.
- Pain and severe emotional distress.

Compensatory Sequence of Events

- An increase in sympathetic activity will correct the bradycardia and very low SVR.
- Fainting ensures that the person is prevented from maintaining an upright posture so that BP is equalized from head to toe and cerebral blood supply is maximized.

Anaphylactic Shock

Anaphylactic shock results from an allergic reaction resulting in anaphylaxis (Martin, Cheek & Morris, 2018). The pathophysiology is similar to that of neurogenic shock, with widespread vasodilatation and pooling of blood in the periphery and involves multiple body systems. It begins as an allergic reaction with an immune and inflammatory response to a proteinaceous substance such as insect venom, pollen, shellfish, drugs or foreign serum. The vascular component of this response includes vasodilatation and increased vascular permeability so that the relative hypovolaemia brought about by peripheral pooling is exacerbated by tissue oedema. There is bronchoconstriction so that the ability to provide oxygen to the tissues is severely compromised.

The onset of anaphylactic shock is rapid and can progress to death in minutes unless emergency treatment given. The signs are anxiety, difficulty in breathing, gastrointestinal cramps, oedema and urticaria with severe itching and burning sensations in the skin. A steep fall in BP follows with confusion and coma.

Emergency Management

There is little time for spontaneous compensatory mechanisms, and death occurs unless medical intervention is possible (see Chapter 47):

- Adrenaline (epinephrine) injection will reverse airway constriction and cause vasoconstriction.
- Volume expanders intravenously will reverse the relative hypovolaemia.
- Steroids will end the inflammatory process.

Septic Shock

Septic shock is caused by infection in the blood stream resulting in bacteraemia (Martin, Cheek & Morris, 2018). This is a vasodilatory or distributive form of shock and is defined as persisting hypotension despite adequate fluid resuscitation in the presence of sepsis. Gram-negative bacteria cause more than half of cases, and in the non-pregnant population the most common sources of infection are the respiratory and gastrointestinal tracts. Infections of the genital tract, in particular group A streptococcus, are of prime importance in the childbearing woman (Knight et al., 2014).

Septic shock is triggered by bacteraemia, and bacteria may be present in the blood for quite a long time before shock develops. It is most likely to be the elderly, critically ill or immunocompromised who develop bacteraemic shock. An example could be related to a woman becoming severely ill after insertion of an intrauterine contraceptive device. Uterine infection is followed by generalized infection and bacteraemia.

Four major body chemicals have been implicated in the development of bacteraemic shock:

1. **Interleukins** are cytokines produced by the white blood cells and cause vasodilatation and increase vascular permeability. They also influence the hypothalamus to cause fever, initiate the complement cascade and stimulate the release of **tumour necrosis factor (TNF).**

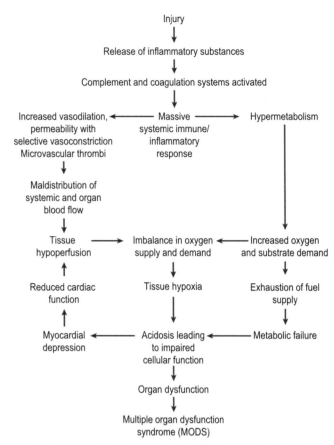

• **Fig. 45.5** The pathogenesis of multiple organ dysfunction.

2. **TNF** is a cytokine produced by macrophages, natural killer cells and mast cells. It activates both clotting and complement cascades. In addition, TNF causes vasodilatation and increases vascular permeability.

3. **Platelet-activating factor (PAF)** is released from mononuclear phagocytes, platelets and some endothelial cells in response to the presence of an endotoxin. It is directly toxic to multiple organs and causes vasodilatation and increased vascular permeability. PAF also mobilizes white cells, activates platelets and stimulates the release of TNF.

4. **Myocardial depressant substance (MDS)** is secreted by white blood cells in response to an endotoxin. The heart responds to MDS by becoming depressed and dilatated, which results in pump failure and hypotension.

As shock increases, carbohydrate metabolism is altered, with a serum increase in both insulin and glucagon. Serum glucose levels fluctuate and glucose usage by the tissues is enhanced. Glucose and glycogen stores become depleted. Depletion of glucose leads to heart failure and oxygen shortage, and **multiple organ dysfunction syndrome (MODS)** may develop. MODS is present if there is failure of two or more organ systems after severe illness or injury (Fig. 45.5).

Main Points

- In primary PPH, bleeding may be from the placental site, although occasionally from a genital tract laceration. Risk factors include previous PPH, high parity, over-distension of the uterus, fibroids, retained products of conception, inverted uterus, third-stage mismanagement and coagulation defects.
- Secondary PPH is usually due to a retained piece of placenta or membrane. Other causes include the presence of blood clots, a fibroid or infection.
- Failure of the placenta to deliver spontaneously is one of the main causes of PPH. Manual removal may be necessary in deeply adherent placentae.
- Causes of acute inversion of the uterus include mismanagement of the third stage, but spontaneous inversion does occur. Rapid replacement of the uterus will prevent shock.
- An AFE travels into the pulmonary circulation to obstruct pulmonary arterioles or capillaries. Mortality is high.
- Three functions of the CVS may be altered and result in shock: heart function, blood volume and BP. Shock progresses to organ failure and death unless compensatory mechanisms or clinical treatments can reverse the pathology.
- Types of shock are cardiogenic, hypovolaemic, neurogenic, anaphylactic and septic (see Chapter 47).
- It is important to diagnose the cause of shock so that effective treatment and management can occur.

References

Acosta, L., Aras-Payne, A., 2017. Complications related to the third stage of labour. In: Macdonald, S., Johnson, G. (Eds.), Mayes' Midwifery, fifteenth ed. Elsevier, Edinburgh.

Begley, C., 2020. Physiology and Care during the Third Stage of Labour. In: Marshall, J., Raynor, M. (Eds.), Myles' Textbook for Midwives, seventeenth ed. Elsevier, Edinburgh.

Chu, J., Johnston, T.A., Geoghegan, J., on behalf of the Royal College of Obstetricians and Gynaecologists, 2020. Maternal collapse in pregnancy and the puerperium. Br. J. Obstet. Gynaecol. 127 (5), e14–e52.

Diaz, V., Abalos, E., Carroli, G., 2018. Methods for blood loss estimation after vaginal birth. Cochrane Database Syst. Rev. 2018 (9), CD010980.

Escobar, M.F., Nassar, A.H., Theron, G., Barnea, E.R., Nicholson, W., Ramasauskaite, D., et al., FIGO Safe Motherhood and Newborn Health Committee, 2022. FIGO recommendations on the management of postpartum hemorrhage. Int. J. Gynecol. Obstet. 157 (1), 3–50.

Gupta, K.B., Kakkar, A., 2020. Secondary PPH. In: Sharma, A. (Eds.), Labour Room Emergencies. Springer, Singapore. Available at: https://doi.org/10.1007/978-981-10-4953-8_45.

Kellie, F.J., Wandabwa, J.N., Mousa, H.A., Weeks, A.D., 2020. Mechanical and surgical interventions for treating primary postpartum haemorrhage. Cochrane Database Syst. Rev. 2020 (7), CD013663.

Knight, M., Kenyon, S., Brocklehurst, P., Neilson, J., Shakespeare, J., Kurinczuk, J.J., on behalf of MBRRACE-UK, 2014. Saving Lives, Improving Mothers' Care: Surveillance of Maternal Deaths in the UK 2011-13 and Lessons Learned to Inform Maternity Care from the UK and Ireland Confidential Enquiries into Maternal Deaths and Morbidity 2009-13. University of Oxford, Oxford.

Knight, M., Bunch, K., Tuffnell, D., Shakespeare, J., Kotnis, R., Kenyon, S., et al., on behalf of MBRRACE-UK, 2018. Saving Lives, Improving Mothers' Care: Lessons Learned to Inform Maternity Care from the UK and Ireland Confidential Enquiries into Maternal Deaths and Morbidity 2014-16. National Perinatal Epidemiology Unit, University of Oxford, Oxford.

Lewis, G., 2007. Saving Mothers' Lives: The Seventh Report of the Confidential Enquiries into Maternal and Child Health Report. Royal College of Obstetricians and Gynaecologists, London.

Lister, S., Hofland, J., Grafton, H., 2020. The Royal Marsden Manual of Clinical Nursing Procedures, tenth ed. Wiley-Blackwell, Oxford.

Mane, S.V., Koravi, V.K., Kumar, P.D., Kandoria, M., 2020. Postpartum hemorrhage. In: Sharma, A. (Ed.), Labour Room Emergencies. Springer, Singapore. Available at: https://doi.org/10.1007/978-981-10-4953-8_36.

Martin, L.L., Cheek, D.J., Morris, S.E., 2018. Shock, multiple organ disfunction syndrome, and burns in adults. In: McCance, K.L., Huether, S.E. (Eds.), Pathophysiology: The Biologic Basis for Disease in Adults and Children, eighth ed. Elsevier, St. Louis.

Maternal & Critical Care Working Group, 2011. Providing Equity of Critical and Maternity Care for the Critically Ill Pregnant or Recently Pregnant Woman. Available at: https://www.oaa-anaes.ac.uk/assets/_managed/cms/files/Maternal_Critical_Care.pdf.

Mavrides, E., Allard, S., Chandraharan, E., Collins, P., Green, L., Hunt, B.J., et al., on behalf of the Royal College of Obstetricians and Gynaecologists, 2016. Prevention and management of postpartum haemorrhage. BJOG 124 (5), e106–e149.

Mousa, H.A., Blum, J., Abou El Senoun, G., Shakur, H., Alfirevic, Z., 2014. Treatment for primary postpartum haemorrhage. Cochrane Database Syst. Rev. 2014 (2), CD003249.

National Institute of Health and Care Excellence (NICE), 2022. Carboprost. British National Formulary. Available at: https://bnf.nice.org.uk/drugs/carboprost/.

National Institute of Health and Care Excellence (NICE), 2023. Intrapartum Care. Available at: https://www.nice.org.uk/guidance/ng235.

Novikova, N., Hofmeyr, G.J., Cluver, C., 2015. Tranexamic acid for preventing postpartum haemorrhage. Cochrane Database Syst. Rev. 2015 (6), CD007872.

Paterson-Brown, S., Howell, C., 2014. Managing Obstetric Emergencies and Trauma: The MOET Course Manual, third ed. Cambridge University Press, Cambridge.

Ritter, J.M., Flower, R.S., Henderson, G., Loke, Y.K., MacEwan, D., Rang, H., 2019. Rang & Dale's Pharmacology, ninth ed. Elsevier, London.

Royal College of Obstetricians and Gynaecologists (RCOG), 2015. Blood Transfusion in Obstetrics: green-top Guideline No. 47. Available at: https://www.rcog.org.uk/media/sdqcorsf/gtg-47.pdf.

Tuffnell, D., Knight, M., on behalf of MBRRACE-UK haemorrhage and AFE chapter-writing group, 2020. Lessons for care of women with haemorrhage or amniotic fluid embolism. on behalf of MBRRACE-UK. In: Knight M, M., Bunch, K., Tuffnell, D., Shakespeare, J., Kotnis, R., Kenyon, S., et al. (Eds.), Saving Lives, Improving Mothers' Care: Lessons Learned to Inform Maternity Care from the UK and Ireland Confidential Enquiries into Maternal Deaths and Morbidity 2016-18. National Perinatal Epidemiology Unit, University of Oxford, Oxford.

Tuffnell, D.J., Slemeck, E., 2017. Amniotic fluid embolism. Obstet. Gynaecol. Reprod. Med. 27 (3), 86–90.

Trikha, A., Singh, P.M., 2018. Management of major obstetric haemorrhage. Indian J. Anaesth. 62 (9), 698–703.

Winter, C., Crofts, J., Laxton, C., Crofts, J., Muchatuta, N., 2018. PROMPT (PRactical Obstetric Multi-Professional Training) Course Manual, third ed. RCOG Press, London.

Annotated recommended reading

Knight, M., Bunch, K., Felker, A., Patel, R., Kotnis, R., Kenyon, S., et al. (Eds.), on behalf of MBRRACE-UK, 2023. Saving Lives, Improving Mothers' Care Core Report – Lessons learned to inform maternity care from the UK and Ireland Confidential Enquiries into Maternal Deaths and Morbidity 2019-21. Oxford: National Perinatal Epidemiology Unit, University of Oxford..

Knight, M., Bunch, K., Patel, R., Shakespeare, J., Kotnis, R., Kenyon, S., Kurinczuk, J.J., on behalf of MBRRACE-UK, 2022. Saving Lives, Improving Mothers' Care – Lessons Learned to Inform Maternity Care from the UK and Ireland Confidential Enquiries into Maternal Deaths and Morbidity 2018-20. National Perinatal Epidemiology Unit, University of Oxford, Oxford.

These two triennial reports provide information on maternal deaths in the UK and Ireland between 2018 and 2021. Student midwives and midwives are encouraged to be familiar with the causes and current trends of maternal deaths in the UK.

McCance, K.L., Huether, S.E., 2018. Pathophysiology: The Biologic Basis for Disease in Adults and Children, eighth ed. Elsevier, St. Louis.

This is an excellence reference book, and the reader is encouraged to explore the pathophysiology and the fuller description of the management of MODS.

46

Perinatal Fetal Asphyxia

THOMAS McEWAN

CHAPTER CONTENTS

The risks of perinatal fetal asphyxia must be recognized by students and midwives to ensure this is managed appropriately during labour. This will optimize the fetal condition and reduce the likelihood of adverse outcomes for the baby.

Introduction

It has been known for centuries that labour, especially the second stage, is dangerous for the fetus. Compaction of the fetus occurs during the contraction, and pressure on the fetal head may evoke vagal stimuli, causing a transient fall in fetal heart rate (FHR) with a rapid recovery.

Reduction in oxygen supply caused by compression of the placenta will add to this effect. This may cause prolongation of the normal fall in FHR seen after contractions in the second stage of labour. Also, if the mother lies on her back there will be a significant reduction in cardiac output and circulation of oxygenated blood through the placental tissue due to aortocaval compression. This does not happen if the woman lies on her side or if the uterus is tilted to her left.

Uterine contractions interfere with umbilical and uteroplacental blood flow and affect fetal gas exchange. The result is a normal tendency to mild metabolic acidosis in the active phase of the first stage and in the early second stage of labour. Although healthy fetuses can withstand this as they have sufficient metabolic reserve, compromised fetuses might display fetal distress (da Silva, Moreira de Sá & de Oliveira, 2022). Terminology used for perinatal fetal asphyxia are in defined in Box 46.1.

Fetal Gas Exchange and pH Regulation

The bicarbonate buffer system regulating fetal acid–base balance is not as efficient in the neonate due to a decreased

• BOX 46.1 Perinatal Fetal Asphyxia Definitions

Fetal distress	General-purpose term indicating the fetus is in jeopardy, sometimes but not always because of hypoxia.
Acidosis	Increased concentration of hydrogen ions (H^+) in blood and at cellular level, resulting from an accumulation of acid or loss of base with a blood pH of <7.2.
Hypoxia	Decreased concentration of oxygen in blood (hypoxaemia) and at cellular level.
Hypercapnia (hypercarbia)	Increased concentration of carbon dioxide in blood and at cellular level.
Asphyxia	Greek word for 'pulseless'. A severe abnormality of gas exchange which results in hypoxia, hypercapnia and acidosis. Asphyxia is characterized by profound acidaemia (both metabolic and respiratory in nature) (Blackburn, 2018). The term *fetal asphyxia* is preferred to *fetal distress,* which refers to a state of fetal danger that may or may not be caused by asphyxia.

ability to eliminate carbon dioxide (CO_2). Because CO_2 cannot be expelled by the fetus into the air, it must be eliminated as molecular CO_2 via the placenta to be removed by the maternal respiratory system.

Respiratory Acidosis

In the placenta, there is a gradient between maternal and fetal circulations down which fetal CO_2 can diffuse. Fetal scalp blood Pco_2 is about 38–44 mmHg, and maternal blood Pco_2 is 18–24 mmHg. In most cases interference with fetal gas exchange involves a problem of elimination of CO_2, resulting in respiratory acidosis. An excessive rise in fetal Pco_2 causes fetal H^+ ions to be released from the unstable carbonic acid (H_2CO_3), which lowers fetal blood pH (acidosis). The buffering bicarbonate ions, which are also released, are insufficient to correct the acidosis. The full equation is:

$$\text{(Eqn. 46.1)}$$
$$CO_2 + H_2O \rightleftharpoons H_2CO_3 \rightleftharpoons H^+ + HCO_3^-$$

Metabolic Acidosis

Decreased oxygen transfer to the fetus will also cause acidosis. Oxygen deficiency causes cells to switch to anaerobic respiration, with the release of lactic acid and H^+ ions into the blood. If hypoxia persists, the excess H^+ ions cause CO_2 and water to be released from the buffer bicarbonate to add respiratory acidosis to the metabolic acidosis. Water is transferred across the placenta to the maternal circulation, but there is a delay in removing CO_2. Anaerobic respiration is inefficient and utilizes more energy, resulting in a decrease in glucose.

Intrauterine Hypoxia

Oxygenation of the fetus depends on maternal oxygenation, perfusion of the placental site, the fetoplacental circulation and adequate fetal haemoglobin (Blackburn, 2018). Disruption or impairment to the flow of oxygen from the air to the fetus will result in fetal hypoxia. Possible causes of intrauterine hypoxia are presented in Box 46.2.

Fetal Response to Hypoxia

The fetal response to hypoxia is an acceleration of heart rate to maintain oxygen supply to the brain and delivery of excess CO_2 to the placenta. As glycogen reserves become depleted, the increased supply of glucose demanded by the heart muscle because of the **tachycardia** cannot be met and the heart slows (**bradycardia**). The anal sphincter relaxes, and fresh meconium is passed into the amniotic fluid. Hypoxia may stimulate the fetus to make gasping movements, and meconium may be aspirated.

Physiological Control of the Fetal Heart

The cardiac regulatory centre is situated in the medulla oblongata. Baroreceptors found in the arch of the aorta and carotid sinus are responsive to changes in blood pressure, and chemoreceptors in the same blood vessels respond to changes in blood gas tensions (Blackburn, 2018). These receptors send messages to the cardiac regulatory centre, which in turn sends messages via the sympathetic and parasympathetic nervous systems to the heart. Sympathetic stimulation via the sinoatrial node will increase the heart rate, whereas parasympathetic stimulation via the vagus nerve will decrease the heart rate. The continuous interaction between these two branches of the autonomic system causes small fluctuations in heart rate, which lead to variability on cardiotocographs (CTGs).

Monitoring the Fetus in Labour

The fetal response to labour may be monitored clinically by observing the amniotic fluid and the rate and rhythm of the FHR. Monitoring is intermittent using a Pinard fetal stethoscope or Doppler ultrasound FHR detector, or by continuous CTG monitoring (see Chapter 37). Where it is difficult to monitor the FHR through the maternal abdomen (those with a high body mass index), the FHR can be monitored electronically using a fetal scalp electrode attached to the fetal head, which produces a direct **fetal electrocardiogram.** Contraction length, strength and frequency can also be monitored externally by a transducer.

Meconium-stained Liquor

The presence of meconium in amniotic fluid is only suggestive of intrapartum asphyxia in the fetus. Of all births, 14% of babies will pass meconium in utero with 3–12% of those going on to develop **meconium aspiration syndrome (MAS)** (Blackburn, 2018). Meconium is a non-specific finding that may be associated with fetal problems other than asphyxia. Meconium-stained amniotic fluid is associated with rhesus

---

• BOX 46.2 Possible Causes of Intrauterine Hypoxia

- Oxygenation of mother impaired by respiratory or cardiovascular disease.
- Perfusion of placental site may be reduced in:
  - Hypertension because of vasoconstriction.
  - Hypotension resulting from blood loss.
  - Aortocaval occlusion.
  - Shock.
  - Excessive uterine contractions.
- Prolapse, compression or a true knot in the umbilical cord may cause fetal hypoxia.
- Placental disease.
- Fetal haemolysis (reduced red cells).

isoimmunization, chorioamnionitis, cardiovascular malformations and pre-eclampsia (Blackburn, 2018). If the pregnancy is known to be high risk and the meconium is freshly passed (dark green or black, thick and tenacious), then the predictive value of asphyxia is high. Old or stale meconium giving rise to lightly stained yellowish or greenish amniotic fluid does not correlate well with fetal asphyxia.

Fetal Heart Monitoring

Intermittent Auscultation

The frequency of monitoring of the FHR by the midwife is decided by the frequency and strength of the uterine contractions and the effects on the fetus. Other risk factors likely to affect fetal oxygenation should be considered. In the first stage of labour for a woman with a low risk for complications, intermittent auscultation to listen to the heart rate and rhythm is usually carried out every 15 min immediately after a contraction for a duration of 1 min (National Institute of Health and Care Excellence [NICE], 2022) to assess whether decelerations are present. The maternal pulse should be palpated hourly to differentiate between these heartbeats. In the second stage, intermittent auscultation should be performed immediately after a contraction for at least 1 min and repeated every 5 min (NICE, 2022). The normal recommended reassuring FHR range is between 110 and 160 bpm (NICE, 2023). The faster rate is found in preterm babies and the lower in term and post-term babies. The rhythm is regular with a coupled beat.

Electronic Fetal Monitoring

Continuous electronic FHR monitoring (EFM), usually combined with continuous monitoring of maternal uterine activity (CTG), was introduced in the 1970s and adopted enthusiastically by obstetricians as 'a significant improvement in intrapartum fetal assessment'. The technique was introduced before evidence of its efficacy or safety had been sought and is explored further in Chapter 37. EFM can be used continuously or intermittently. The options for EFM are discussed in Box 46.3.

> ### • BOX 46.3 Implications for Practice–Options for Fetal Monitoring
>
> Options for fetal monitoring should be discussed with women and documented during their antenatal care. Furthermore, information on fetal monitoring should be provided during labour and the woman's decision supported (NICE, 2022). Fetal heart rate (FHR) monitoring provides only part of the information on fetal well-being and must be considered alongside the overall clinical picture (NICE, 2022).
>
> The main features to consider when interpreting cardiotocograph readings are baseline FHR, baseline variability, decelerations and accelerations. Variations in these measurements are categorized using a white, amber and red classification within the most recent UK guidance, which the reader should review (NICE, 2022).

Baseline FHR

The baseline rate of 110–160 bpm (NICE, 2022) is the rate present between periods of acceleration and deceleration. A rate >160 bpm is called **baseline tachycardia** (non-reassuring) and <110 bpm is **baseline bradycardia** (non-reassuring). Both tachycardia and bradycardia may be associated with fetal hypoxia. Tachycardia may be seen if the woman is ketotic or pyrexial. Some fetuses have a normal baseline of between 100 and 109 bpm. If there are no variable or late decelerations with a normal variability plus confirmation that it is not the maternal pulse, then continue usual care (NICE, 2022). A prolonged bradycardia occurs when there is continuous compression of the umbilical cord.

Baseline Variability

Continuous adjustments in the autonomic nervous stimulation of the heart caused by fetal response to the environment lead to minute variations in the length of each heartbeat. This leads to the CTG tracing having a jagged appearance, as the baseline rate is continuously adjusting, rather than being a straight line because each beat is the same length. There should be variance in the baseline rate of at least 5–25 bpm (NICE, 2022), estimated by examining the difference between the lowest and highest heart rate over a 1-min segment of trace between contractions. Loss of variance may be due to hypoxia. It is also seen after the administration of some opiate analgesics because of depression of the cardiac regulatory centre in the fetal brain. Fetal sleep lasting up to 30 min may also cause a reduction in variability.

Periodic Changes

The FHR normally remains steady or **accelerates** during a contraction. Accelerations of 15 bpm above the baseline lasting for 15 s are associated with fetal activity or contraction (Gauge, 2011). **Decelerations** are dips to below the baseline of varying degrees (see Box 46.4 and Figs 46.1–46.3).

> ### • BOX 46.4 Types of Decelerations
>
> - **Early deceleration** mirrors the pattern of the contraction. Commences at or after the onset of a contraction, reaches its lowest point at the peak of the contraction and then returns to normal by the end of the contraction. Associated with compression of the fetal head and vagal response (may indicate early fetal hypoxia).
> - **Late deceleration** begins during or just after a contraction. Reaches its lowest point after the peak of the contraction and may not recover until onset of the next contraction. The time lag between the peak of the contraction and low point of deceleration is more significant than the drop in fetal heart rate. Caused by a decrease in uterine blood flow during a contraction, reducing oxygen transfer. Indicates fetal hypoxia and inadequate fetal brain oxygenation.
> - **Variable decelerations**: Fetal heart rate decelerations vary in timing, frequency and amplitude in relation to contractions. Associated with cord compression where obstruction is to venous flow with a corresponding rise in fetal blood pressure. The pattern can be considered benign, although if decelerations are more atypical in characteristic, the fetus may be more compromised.

For interpretation of CTGs and subsequent management of abnormal CTGs, access the NICE (2022) guideline. Where concerns arise about fetal well-being, conservative measures related to possible causes may be useful and are outlined in Box 46.5.

Digital fetal scalp stimulation may be useful to determine the degree of fetal compromise. If an acceleration in the FHR results with a sustained improvement, then care may be continued with close monitoring. The absence of an acceleration in response to this stimulation is concerning and warrants urgent action (NICE, 2022).

Fetal Blood Sampling

CTG can suggest the presence of fetal hypoxia, although there can be false positives. Acidosis can be estimated by fetal blood sampling (FBS) for pH or lactate levels. The classifications for pH and lactate levels are presented in Table 46.1.

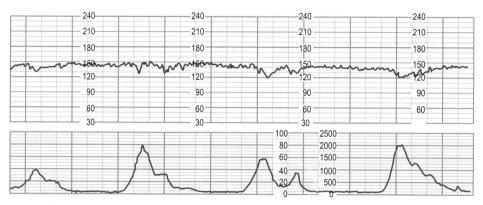

• **Fig. 46.1** Early deceleration.

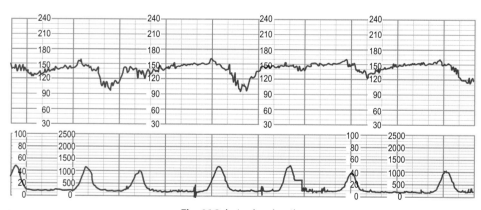

• **Fig. 46.2** Late deceleration.

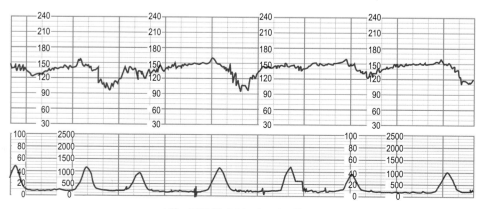

• **Fig. 46.3** Variable decelerations.

- **Maternal position:** Consider an alternative position or mobilization to alleviate any potential cord compression or reduced uterine blood flow.
- **Hypotension:** This may be secondary to an epidural top-up or maternal sepsis. Request an anaesthetic review as appropriate and consider a move to the left lateral position and intravenous fluids.
- **Excessive contraction frequency:** Consider reducing/ stopping oxytocin infusion. In severe cases, a tocolytic drug may be required.

(NICE, 2022)

Severe hypoxia may result in the baby being stillborn, asphyxiated at birth or suffering brain damage. If the condition of the fetus monitored by the earlier findings suggests a major problem, the obstetrician must be called to see the woman. If labour is being augmented by administration of oxytocin, it is sensible to reduce the force of the uterine contractions by discontinuing the infusion. The administration of oxygen to the woman for fetal distress is not advocated, unless for maternal hypoxia or preoxygenation before anaesthesia (NICE, 2022). Delivery will be either by caesarean section in the first stage of labour or by instrumental delivery in the second stage. If delivery is imminent, an episiotomy may only be required. A Resuscitaire should be present, and the neonatal team called to the delivery in all cases of fetal distress in preparation for resuscitation.

TABLE 46.1   Classification of Fetal Blood Samples

Lactate (mmol/L)	pH	Interpretation
≤4.1	≥7.25	Normal
4.2–4.8	7.21–7.24	Borderline
≥4.9	≤7.20	Abnormal

(Mukhopadhaya, Punder & Arora, 2020)

There is limited evidence to support the predictive value of FBS and its recommendation for use (NICE, 2022). A recent multicentre observational study found that FBS provided limited predictive value for neonatal acidaemia, low Apgar scores and admission to the neonatal intensive care unit (Watter et al., 2019). In addition, discordance between scalp pH and lactate levels has been noted by researchers, further complicating clinical decisions based on FBS results (Prouhèze et al., 2021). Despite this, it is commonly used as an adjunct to the overall assessment of fetal condition during labour where fetal compromise is suspected. The considerations for the management of confirmed fetal asphyxia are summarized in Box 46.6.

Neonatal Asphyxia and Resuscitation

Initiation of Respirations at Birth

From about 22 weeks, surfactant is produced in fetal lungs. The amount present increases until birth, and there is a surge of production at about 34 weeks' gestation. Surfactant has two main functions: to reduce surface tension in alveoli so that they can expand more easily and to help prevent alveoli collapsing at the end of each expiration. Fetal breathing movements have been identified as early as 10 weeks' gestation, and these increase in strength and frequency until they are present 30–40% in the last trimester (Blackburn, 2018). In the latent phase of labour, fetal respirations decrease to 10% of the time due to the effect of prostaglandins on the respiratory centre and are nearly absent towards the end of labour (Coad, Pedley & Dunstall, 2019). The rate varies between 30 and 70 bpm.

Establishing Respiration at Birth

This topic is summarized in this section and fully explored in Chapter 48.

- Where the fetal chest is compressed and squeezed during the process of birth, some lung and amniotic fluid are forced out of alveoli into the upper respiratory tract. Passive recoil of the chest after delivery helps draw air into the lungs and push the remaining fluid into the lymphatic system.
- Hypoxia during the late stage of delivery occurs with the birth of the head and the beginning of placental separation. Oxygen content of the blood falls and CO_2 content rises, stimulating chemoreceptors to send a message to the respiratory centre and cause onset of breathing.
- The respiratory centre is also bombarded with stimuli from handling of the baby and the temperature changes found in the nasopharynx and skin.
- Circulatory changes direct the blood away from the placental circulation to the pulmonary circulation and lungs for oxygenation.
- Effective oxygenation is achieved by respiratory exchange in alveoli and by adequate circulation. Most neonates establish respirations within 1 min of birth.

Birth Asphyxia

Lack of oxygenation to the cells, during birth or immediately after birth, where there is failure to initiate or

Sign	Score		
	0	1	2
Heart rate	Absent	Slow – below 100	Fast – above 100
Respiratory effort	Absent	Slow, irregular	Good, crying
Muscle tone	Limp	Some flexion of the extremities	Active
Reflex irritability	No response	Grimace	Crying, cough
Colour	Blue, pale	Body pink, extremities blue	Completely pink

• **Fig. 46.4** The Apgar scoring system based on points being awarded for five physiological signs.

sustain respirations can be termed **birth asphyxia, perinatal asphyxia** or **neonatal asphyxia.**

Causes

- Obstruction of airway by mucus, blood, meconium or amniotic fluid, especially if intrauterine anoxia has been present. Because of stimulation of the respiratory centre, the fetus may have gasped in utero, drawing the previously mentioned substances into the trachea and bronchi.
- Airways may not be patent due to congenital anomalies such as choanal atresia, hypoplastic lungs or diaphragmatic hernia.
- Lung function may be compromised by abnormalities in the cardiovascular system or central nervous system.
- Pain-relieving narcotic drugs or other drugs such as diazepam, as well as general anaesthetics, if given in large doses, may depress the fetal respiratory centre.
- Intracranial haemorrhage may cause pressure on the cerebellum and medulla, affecting the cardiovascular and respiratory centres.
- Severe intrauterine infections after prolonged rupture of the membranes, leading to pneumonia, meningitis and septicaemia, may inhibit the efficient establishment of respiration.
- Immaturity of the neonate may lead to mechanical dysfunction because of poor lung development, lack of surfactant and a soft rib cage.

Recognition

Birth asphyxia may be classified as mild, moderate or severe, depending on scoring systems such as that devised by Virginia Apgar in 1953. **Apgar scores** are well known to be poor predictors of hypoxia and acidosis; however they continue to be widely used in delivery suites. The principle of scoring systems such as the Apgar score (Fig. 46.4) is to assess the condition of the baby at birth, and the score may be affected by all the earlier causes of

neonatal asphyxia. It follows that babies may not always have shown pre-delivery signs of impending asphyxia, with many of the causes arising suddenly after delivery. Respiratory depression by fetal hypoxia is only one factor that may cause a baby to fail to breathe at birth (Fawke et al., 2021).

For each of the vital signs in Fig. 46.4, the neonate may be given a score of 0, 1 or 2 depending on the descriptors. The Apgar score at 1 min is recorded; the suggested parameters for asphyxia are:

- 7–10: no asphyxia (healthy baby).
- 4–6: mild-to-moderate asphyxia, response to treatment usually good (a less healthy baby).
- 3 or less: severe asphyxia, requires urgent resuscitation (an ill baby).

During this assessment, the impact of race and ethnicity must be carefully considered in relation to colour.

Management of Birth Asphyxia

Guidelines for resuscitation and support of transition of babies at birth provide a detailed step-by-step approach that all practitioners should be familiar with (Fawke et al., 2021). The approach is detailed in an algorithm from this guideline (see Fig. 46.5) and should be studied carefully. Some key points are summarized in Table 46.2.

Meconium

The practice of attempting to aspirate meconium from the nose and mouth of the unborn baby while the head is still on the perineum or delaying initial ventilation to routinely preform suction where a baby is born through thick meconium and is unresponsive (or not vigorous) at birth is not recommended (Fawke et al., 2021). These babies are at risk of requiring advanced resuscitation and, where possible, a competent practitioner in these skills or neonatal team should be available. The standard newborn life-support algorithm should be used (Fig. 46.5).

Newborn life support

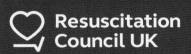

(Antenatal counselling)
Team briefing and equipment check

Birth
Delay cord clamping if possible

Start clock / note time
Dry / wrap, stimulate, keep warm

Assess
Colour, tone, breathing, heart rate

Ensure an open airway
Preterm: consider CPAP

If gasping / not breathing
- **Give 5 inflations (30 cm H$_2$O) – start in air**
- Apply PEEP 5–6 cm H$_2$O, if possible
- Apply SpO$_2$ +/– ECG

Reassess
If no increase in heart rate, look for chest movement

If the chest is not moving
- Check mask, head and jaw position
- 2 person support
- Consider suction, laryngeal mask/tracheal tube
- Repeat inflation breaths
- Consider increasing the inflation pressure

Reassess
If no increase in heart rate, look for chest movement

Once chest is moving continue ventilation breaths

**If heart rate is not detectable or < 60 min^{-1}
after 30 seconds of ventilation**
- Synchronise 3 chest compressions to 1 ventilation
- Increase oxygen to 100%
- Consider intubation if not already done or laryngeal mask if not possible

**Reassess heart rate and chest movement
every 30 seconds**

If the heart rate remains not detectable or < 60 min^{-1}
- **Vascular access and drugs**
- Consider other factors e.g. pneumothorax, hypovolaemia, congenital abormality

Update parents and debrief team
Complete records

**Preterm
< 32 weeks**

**Place undried in
plastic wrap +
radiant heat**

Inspired oxygen
28–31 weeks 21–30%
< 28 weeks 30%

If giving inflations,
start with 25 cm H$_2$O

Acceptable pre-ductal SpO$_2$	
2 min	65%
5 min	85%
10 min	90%

TITRATE OXYGEN TO ACHIEVE TARGET SATURATIONS

APPROX 60 SECONDS

MAINTAIN TEMPERATURE

AT ALL TIMES ASK "IS HELP NEEDED"

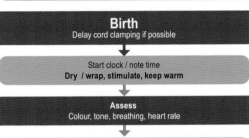

• **Fig. 46.5** Newborn life-support algorithm.

TABLE 46.2	Key Points for Newborn Resuscitation and Support of Transition at Birth

Clamping of the umbilical cord after at least 60 s is recommended. It should ideally take place after the lungs are aerated. This may not be practical or possible where immediate resuscitation is necessary. In these circumstances, cord milking should be considered for babies >28 weeks' gestation.

Keeping the baby warm is important, especially if preterm. Consider the environment and the use of polyethylene wrapping for those less than 32 weeks' gestation. Temperature should be maintained between 36.5°C and 37.5°C. Keep the baby warm and assess.

Whilst keeping the baby warm, an initial assessment should be performed. This includes **colour**, **tone**, **breathing** and **heart rate**. If the baby is not establishing adequate regular breathing or the heart rate is <100 bpm, then commence respiratory support.

To support breathing, ensure the airway is open by positioning the head in the neutral position. Provide five inflation breaths using an appropriate fitting face mask. Use an inflation pressure and % oxygen appropriate to gestation. Reassess **colour**, **tone**, **breathing** and **heart rate**. Where there is no heart rate response and the chest is not moving, repeat five inflation breaths ensuring mask size, position and seal are correct. If still no response, consider an airway manoeuvre or gradual increase in inflation pressure.

Following effective lung inflation where the baby is not breathing, commence ventilation breaths. Aim for 30 breaths per minute. Reassess **colour**, **tone**, **breathing** and **heart rate** after 30 s. If the heart rate remains slow (<60 bpm) or absent after 30 s of effective ventilation breaths, commence chest compressions. Request help if not already summoned.

The overall aim of chest compressions is to supply the heart with oxygenated blood. A two-handed technique is preferrable. Effective, synchronous ventilation must also continue at a rate of three compressions to one ventilation. The inspired oxygen should be increased to 100% when starting chest compressions.

Drugs are administered intravenously (usually via an umbilical venous catheter) or possibly through an intraosseous needle. The drugs associated with neonatal resuscitation are adrenaline, glucose and sodium bicarbonate. Volume replacement with blood or isotonic crystalloid is also recommended. The recommended doses and volumes are detailed in the Resuscitation Council guidelines (Fawke et al., 2021).

If chest rise is not seen after delivery of inflation breaths, then the airway should be inspected under direct vision. Only very rarely will tracheal intubation and suctioning be required. MAS is primarily the result of fetal aspiration of amniotic fluid containing meconium due to hypoxia (Monfredini et al., 2021).

Transfer to the Neonatal Unit

A baby who has suffered severe asphyxia should be transferred to the neonatal unit for further observation and post-resuscitation care. This should include monitoring of glucose levels and appropriate thermal care. Complications such as cerebral oedema, hypoglycaemia, hypothermia and electrolyte disturbance should be anticipated and treated, but where possible prevented. Where moderate or severe hypoxic-ischaemic encephalopathy is suspected, therapeutic hypothermia may be indicated. Neonatal follow-up is important to detect long-term problems such as developmental delay or cerebral palsy.

Correction of Acidosis

If only one of the two types of acidosis is present, the other system can be used to compensate. The lungs are central to the control of CO_2 level in respiratory acidosis, whereas the kidneys control the bicarbonate level in metabolic acidosis. Acidosis in neonates tends to be mixed, and the buffering systems may fail. The administration of sodium bicarbonate is controversial and should always follow blood gas analysis. The bicarbonate combines with hydrogen ions to form carbonic acid. This then dissociates into water and CO_2:

$$\text{(Eqn. 46.2)}$$
$$H^+ + HCO_3^- \rightleftharpoons H_2CO_3 \rightleftharpoons CO_2 + H_2O$$

If the CO_2 can leave the body by the lungs, there is no problem, but in respiratory difficulties it may accumulate in the body. It crosses cell membranes and the blood–brain barrier to cause intracellular acidosis, even if there seems to be a blood picture improvement in acidosis. This is because the bicarbonate buffer cannot cross cell membranes as readily as CO_2. The sodium content in sodium bicarbonate may result in an overloading of the baby's vascular system, resulting in cellular overhydration and damage.

Main Points

- Impairment of the distribution of oxygen to the fetus will result in fetal hypoxia with acceleration of FHR to maintain oxygen supply to the brain and deliver excess CO_2 to the placenta.
- Tachycardia and bradycardia may be associated with fetal hypoxia.

- Fetal acidosis can be estimated by FBS pH and lactate levels. Severe hypoxia may result in neonatal mortality and morbidity.
- A healthy baby will have good tone, a fast heart rate (>100 bpm) and will rapidly become pink. A less healthy baby will have less good tone, a slow heart rate (60–100 bpm)

and may not establish adequate breathing. A compromised baby will be born pale and floppy, not breathing and with a very slow/absent heart rate.

- The sequence of actions in neonatal resuscitation include appropriate cord management and keeping the baby warm; assess colour, tone, breathing and heart rate; support and open the airway using the neutral position; provide five inflation breaths to aerate the lungs (if required); 30 ventilation breaths per minute (if required); ratio of chest compression (if required) to inflations is 3:1; drugs may be required. Assess the baby every 30 s.
- A baby who has suffered severe asphyxia should be transferred to the neonatal unit for further observation.

References

Blackburn, S.T., 2018. Maternal, Fetal and Neonatal Physiology: A Clinical Perspective, fifth ed. Elsevier, St. Louis.

Coad, J., Pedley, K., Dunstall, M., 2019. Anatomy and Physiology for Midwives, fourth ed. Elsevier, Edinburgh.

da Silva, F.C., Moreira de Sá, R.A., de Oliveira, C.A., 2022. Perinatal asphyxia (acute fetal distress). In: Moreira de Sa, R.A., da Fonseca, E.B. (Eds.), Perinatology: Evidence-Based Best Practices in Perinatal Medicine. Springer, Cham.

Fawke, J., Wyllie, J., Madar, J., Ainsworth, S., Tinnion, R., Chittick, R., et al., 2021. Newborn Resuscitation and Support of Transition of Babies at Birth. Resuscitation Council (UK), London.

Gauge, S., 2011. CTG Made Easy, fourth ed. Elsevier, Edinburgh.

Monfredini, C., Cavallin, F., Villani, P.E., Paterlini, G., Allais, B., Trevisanuto, D., 2021. Meconium aspiration syndrome: a narrative review. Children 8 (3), 230.

Mukhopadhaya, N., Punder, J., Arora, M., 2020. Management of Labour. Part 1 MRCOG Revision Notes and Sample SBAs. Cambridge University Press, Cambridge.

National Institute of Health and Care Excellence (NICE), 2022. Fetal Monitoring in Labour. Available at: https://www.nice-.org.uk/guidance/ng229/resources/fetal-monitoring-in-labour-pdf-66143844065221.

National Institute of Health and Care Excellence (NICE), 2023. Intrapartum Care. Available at: https://www.nice.org.uk/guidance/ng235.

Prouhèze, A., Girault, A., Barrois, M., Lepercq, J., Goffinet, F., Le Ray, C., 2021. Fetal scalp blood sampling: do pH and lactates provide the same information? J. Gynecol. Obstet. Hum. Reprod. 50 (4), 101964.

Al Wattar, B.H., Lakhiani, A., Sacco, A., Siddharth, A., Bain, A., Calvia, A., et al., AB-FAB study group, 2019. Evaluating the value of intrapartum fetal scalp blood sampling to predict adverse neonatal outcomes: a UK multicentre observational study. Eur. J. Obstet. Gynecol. Reprod. Biol. 240, 62–67.

Annotated recommended reading

National Institute of Health and Care Excellence (NICE), 2022. Fetal monitoring in labour. Available at: https://www.nice-.org.uk/guidance/ng229/resources/fetal-monitoring-in-labour-pdf-66143844065221.

National Institute of Health and Care Excellence (NICE), 2023. Intrapartum care. Available at: https://www.nice.org.uk/guidance/ng235.

These publications set out evidence-based guidelines and recommendations for intrapartum care in all circumstances.

Resuscitation Council: Newborn resuscitation and support of transition of infants at birth. Available at: https://www.resus.org.uk/library/2021-resuscitation%20guidelines/newborn-resuscitation-and-support-transition-infants-birth.

This site provides clear guidelines for the management of the newborn at birth where resuscitation is required.

47

Operative Delivery and the Acutely Unwell Woman

LYZ HOWIE, JEAN WATSON AND JEAN RANKIN

CHAPTER CONTENTS

This chapter focusses on two key areas: operative delivery and the acutely unwell woman. The latter includes the recognition, assessment and resuscitation of maternal collapse and the management of sepsis.

Introduction

An operative delivery is performed if a spontaneous birth is judged to pose a greater risk to mother and baby. Operations are divided into assisted vaginal birth methods (forceps and vacuum extraction) and abdominal methods (caesarean section).

The operator must have the appropriate skill and knowledge to conduct the operative delivery and manage any complications, should they occur. Obstetricians should also have previous experience of vaginal deliveries before training in assisted vaginal birth methods (Murphy, Strachan & Bahl, 2020). Assisted vaginal births should be undertaken for the reasons outlined in Box 47.1.

Medical indications for caesarean section (CS) are cephalopelvic disproportion, major degrees of placenta praevia and HIV infection. CSs are also being performed for breech and previous CS more often upon maternal request (Lavender et al., 2012). The risks and benefits must be weighed before performing a CS (Murphy, Strachan & Bahl, 2020).

Forceps Delivery

Obstetric forceps have been utilized in difficult births since their invention by the Chamberlen family in the 17th century (Dunn, 1999). Since then, attempts to modify and improve their effectiveness and safety have led to a variety of instruments available for use in different obstetric situations (Fig. 47.1). Obstetric forceps consist of two blades, each with a handle and a shank. The blades are marked 'L' (left) or 'R' (right), according to the side of the mother's pelvis in which they lie when applied. There may be a locking device incorporated into the mechanism (Hayman & Raynor, 2020). Whatever the variation in shape, two considerations are important leading to the addition of **pelvic** and **cephalic curves**:
- The shape and size of the fetal head.
- The curve, shape and size of the bony pelvis.

The Use of Forceps

The shape and size of forceps depend on its use. Forceps may be applied in mid-cavity or at the pelvic outlet. They may be used to **rotate** the fetal head followed by **traction** in the direction of the curve of Carus (pelvic axis) to complete the delivery or to apply **traction** only (Bassett, 2017; Cunningham & Hinshaw, 2020). However rotation is rarely performed due to potential trauma to mother and baby (Bassett, 2017).
- For traction without rotation, nonrotational forceps such as those designed by **Wrigley** or **Simpson** are used for low-cavity delivery, or for delivery of the aftercoming head of the breech. **Neville–Barnes** or **Haig–Ferguson** forceps for mid-cavity delivery have a pelvic and cephalic curve, although these may be used for low-cavity nonrotational delivery, and the axis traction attachments are rarely used.

- It is important to understand that forceps deliveries are not undertaken when the fetal head is higher than station +2 cm because of the possibility of trauma. CS is more likely to be the method of choice in those cases.
- To correct malposition from occipitolateral or occipitoposterior to occipitoanterior before traction, rotational forceps such as **Kielland's forceps** are the design commonly used (Murphy, Strachan & Bahl, 2020; O'Brien, Siassakos & Hinshaw, 2020). These forceps have no pelvic curve (straight) so that they can be rotated in the confines of the birth canal. In malpositions there is often **asynclitism** (tilting of the fetal head). Kielland's forceps have a sliding lock so that asynclitism can be corrected before rotation and traction. There is a gap between the handles when the blades are applied, and there is a danger that too much pressure may be applied to the fetal head with the risk of cerebral trauma.

• BOX 47.1 Reasons for Operative Delivery

Fetal

- Suspected fetal compromise (cardiotocography pathological, abnormal fetal blood sampling result, thick meconium)

Maternal

- Nulliparous women – lack of continuing progress for 3 hours (total of active and passive second-stage labour) with regional analgesia or 2 hours without regional analgesia
- Parous women – lack of continuing progress for 2 hours (total of active and passive second-stage labour) with regional analgesia or 1 hour without regional analgesia
- Maternal exhaustion or distress
- Medical indications to avoid Valsalva manoeuvre

Combined (Fetal and Maternal)

- Indications for assisted vaginal birth often coexist

(Murphy, Strachan & Bahl, 2020)

Applying the Forceps
Positioning the Forceps

The blades are inserted separately on either side of the fetal head so that they are located alongside the head and over the ears (Fig. 47.2). They should be situated symmetrically between the eye orbits and the ears, reaching from the parietal eminences to the malar area and cheeks. They should come together and lock easily without the use of strength if they are applied correctly (Cunningham & Hinshaw, 2020). *'Ghosting'* is an important part of assembling the forceps. This is where the forceps are locked together in front of the perineum in the same position as they will lie in the pelvis. The line of application of the forceps blades is parallel to the fetal sagittal suture (Cunningham & Hinshaw, 2020).

The Skill of the Operator

The operator is a major determinant of the success or failure of instrumental delivery and should have appropriate training before conducting operative procedures (Murphy, Strachan & Bahl, 2020). Unfavourable results are almost always caused by the user's unfamiliarity with either the instrument or the rules governing its use (Murphy, Strachan & Bahl, 2020). It is important that the skills of using any instrument are acquired under supervision because of the devastating consequences that could arise if mother or baby is damaged during the operation.

Prerequisites for Forceps Delivery
No Obstruction to the Descent of the Fetus

- Engagement of the head (head one-fifth palpable abdominally).
- Vaginal examination performed to determine position and degree of caput and moulding for safe application of forceps.
- Vertex presentation.
- Cervix must be fully dilated; attempts to apply forceps blades with an undilatated cervix will lead to trauma without successful delivery.
- Ruptured membranes.
- No obvious contraindications such as cephalopelvic disproportion.

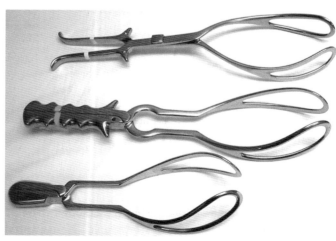

• **Fig. 47.1** Obstetric forceps.

Safeguarding the Mother

- Adequate anaesthesia must be available by epidural or pudendal block.
- A full explanation of the procedure should be given to the woman and her partner and informed consent obtained.
- An episiotomy may be performed (clinical judgement).
- The bladder must be empty to prevent trauma.

Verma et al. (2021) evaluated forceps and vacuum cup instruments for vaginal operative delivery. Forceps had a higher success rate, although there was more maternal morbidity such as perineal trauma and third- and fourth-degree tears. There were no differences between Apgar scores and umbilical cord pH. They concluded that the operator should choose the most appropriate method for a successful outcome whilst minimizing trauma to mother and baby. Although the use of episiotomy has been liberal in operative deliveries, it should not be done routinely but undertaken using clinical judgement (Murphy, Strachan & Bahl, 2020).

There should be as much safety, comfort and dignity for the woman as possible, although the lithotomy position is essential. The procedure is carried out aseptically using sterile instruments.

Safeguarding the Baby

- There should be careful and accurate identification of the presentation and position of the fetal head.
- Forceps blades must be applied correctly, and their position checked before rotation and/or traction is commenced.
- The paediatrician should be present at delivery.
- Neonatal resuscitation equipment should be available.
- Some obstetricians may manually rotate the head, as it is thought to be less traumatic than instrumental rotation. Rotational forceps delivery may cause a deterioration in fetal acid–base balance. Complications of forceps delivery for the mother and the neonate are in Box 47.2.

Vacuum Extraction (Ventouse Delivery)

Use of the Vacuum Extractor

Delivery using **vacuum extraction** has a history – as long as that of forceps delivery. The modern version was developed

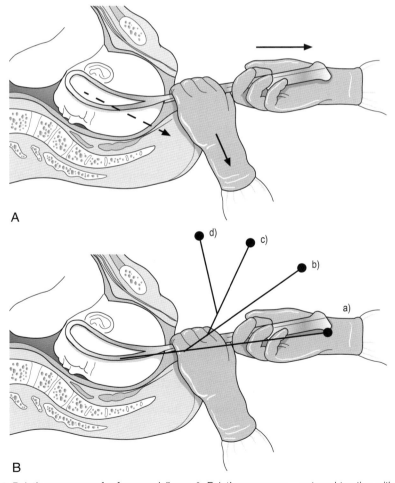

A

B

• **Fig. 47.2** Pajot's manoeuvre for forceps delivery. **A** Pajot's manoeuvre – outward traction with dominant hand, balanced by downward force using nondominant hand (solid arrows). Resultant force vector moves the head down the line of the pelvic axis, under the symphysis pubis (dashed arrow). **B** Lines indicating the angle of the handles as delivery progresses: (a) during Pajot's manoeuvre; (b) when the occiput passes under the pubic arch, elevate the handles after stopping Pajot's; (c) further elevation at the point of episiotomy; (d) handles over the symphysis pubis as head and chin finally deliver.

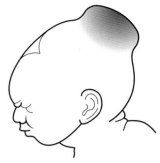

• **Fig. 47.3** Chignon.

• BOX 47.2 **Complications of Forceps Delivery**

Maternal

- Soft tissue damage to the lower uterine segment, cervix, vagina and perineum.
- Bleeding from tissue trauma leading to postpartum haemorrhage and shock.
- Retention of urine due to bruising and oedema of the urethra and neck of bladder.
- Perineal pain once anaesthesia has worn off.
- Dyspareunia in the long term.
- Psychological effects may lead to avoidance of future pregnancy.

Neonatal

- Cephalhaematoma due to friction between the fetal head and the blades or pelvic walls.
- Facial or scalp abrasions.
- Bruising of the scalp leading to neonatal jaundice. Intracranial haemorrhage (rare) but serious problem. May lead to convulsions.

in the 1950s and over the years has been modified. Originally, the vacuum extractor consisted of a rounded metal cup in three sizes: 40, 50 and 60 mm in diameter. The cup was attached to a **chain** and handle and a suction pump to extract air and create a vacuum. The largest cup size that can be passed through the cervix was chosen.

Cups are now made of silastic and plastic with cup sizes of 5 cm or 6 cm (van den Akker & Hinshaw, 2020). In a systematic review, Verma et al. (2021) compared soft versus rigid vacuum cups. They found that soft cups were significantly more likely to fail to achieve a vaginal delivery than rigid cups, although soft cups were associated with less fetal injury. Another form of cup for ventouse delivery is the Kiwi Omnicup (hand-held vacuum). The Omnicup is made of rigid plastic and can be used for malpresentations such as occipitoposterior and occipitoanterior positions. The Omnicup forms a chignon similar to that formed by metal/rigid cups. There was no difference found in delivery outcome between the hand-held compared with the standard vacuum (Verma et al., 2021).

Applying the Vacuum Extractor

Positioning

The cup is attached by suction to the fetal scalp as near to the occiput as possible and taking care to avoid the anterior fontanelle. A **vacuum** is created with negative pressure (Bassett, 2017) and may cause artificial caput (chignon) (Fig. 47.3) into the cup. The cup is checked for position to ensure that no maternal soft tissue such as the cervix has been included within the rim. The vacuum pressure is increased. This can either be done in stages or in one step. Evidence recommends that rapid versus stepwise negative pressure application for vacuum extraction-assisted vaginal delivery should be performed, as there is no difference in maternal or fetal morbidity and expedited delivery time (Suwannachat, Lumbiganon & Laopaiboon, 2012). Traction is then applied

following the curve of Carus (pelvic axis) to enhance the natural forces of uterine contractions and maternal expulsive effort for the vacuum birth (Fig. 47.4).

The Skill of the Operator

Used skilfully, the advantages of the **ventouse** are that there is no increase to the presenting diameters and the instrument can be used to flex and rotate the head and assist the mother to deliver her infant. However some operators may be too hasty or unskilled and apply traction before suction has been achieved, resulting in the cup coming away from the scalp. Some maternity units have trained midwives to perform ventouse deliveries. The technique is also useful where midwives work alone, without obstetric colleagues, in remote areas of the world. It is important that a midwife is properly trained and is confident in the use of this device and that their employing authority approves the use of ventouse equipment by midwives.

Prerequisites

- Same as for forceps delivery.
- Vacuum extractor not suitable for application in babies with suspected coagulability.
- Used with caution in preterm births of 32–36 weeks' gestation and avoided in infants below 32 weeks' gestation) (Murphy, Strachan & Bahl, 2020).
- Should not be used where contractions are weak or maternal effort is poor.

Although there are some maternal and neonatal complications from a vacuum extraction birth (see Clinical Application 47.1), there is less trauma to maternal tissues than with a forceps delivery (Verma et al., 2021).

Comparison of Forceps and Vacuum Extraction

Although **assisted vaginal delivery** is performed worldwide, there is a large variation in its application. In the UK, the rates for operative vaginal delivery have remained stable at between 10% and 15% (Murphy, Strachan & Bahl, 2020). In a systematic review, Verma et al. (2021) compared assisted vaginal delivery by obstetric forceps with ventouse extraction. The reviewers concluded that the use of the vacuum extractor appears to reduce maternal morbidity. The use of forceps delivery increased facial injury but reduced

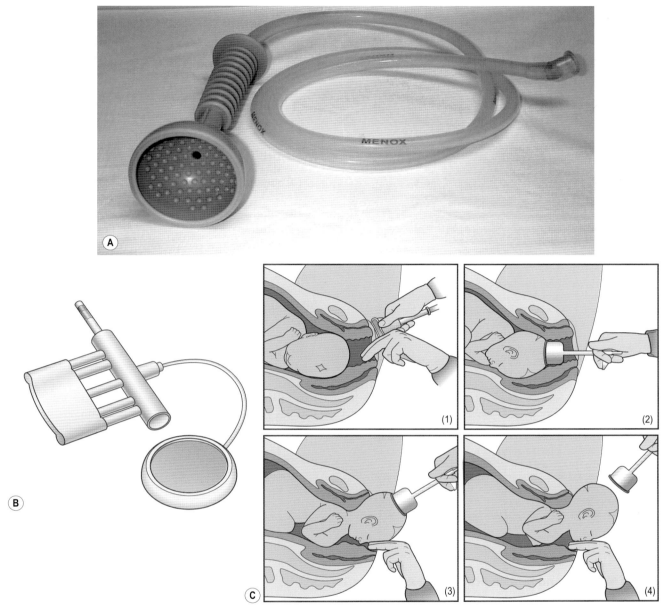

• **Fig. 47.4 A.** Example of Malmstrom vacuum extractor (rigid cup). **B.** Example of a Kiwi omnicup vacuum extractor (soft cup). **C.** Vacuum birth.

cephalohaematoma in the neonate. Therefore, the benefits and risks to the woman and fetus must be considered when choosing the method of operative delivery.

Caesarean Section (CS)

Overview

CS is a surgical procedure in which the abdomen and uterus are incised to facilitate the birth of the baby. There are records of this procedure being performed before the discovery of anaesthetic drugs, and usually for delivery of the fetus perimortem. CS may be carried out as an emergency in response to adverse conditions developing in late pregnancy or labour. Elective CS is a planned event where

the timing is chosen to maximize safety for the mother and fetus.

Current Rates

Rates of CS worldwide have increased steadily over the last few decades. According to the World Health Organization (WHO) (2021), CS rates are rising globally: in the 1990s, it was 7% compared to 21% today (1:5 women). The National Institute of Health and Care Excellence (NICE) (2023a) states that the current CS rate is 25–30% in the UK.

Within the UK, the figures for CS rates in relation to maternal mortalities is startling. In the last triennium report, 91 (64%) of the women who died had a CS birth, and 11% of these were perimortem as part of attempted resuscitation of the woman (Knight et al., 2022).

Indications

Countries in the UK compile statistics and offer explanations as to why CS rates continue to rise, such as higher rates in women aged 40 and over. One-to-one support in labour and women's choices also affect CS rates (WHO, 2018). Delivery of breech and preterm babies and increased maternal weight may also correlate to a rise in CS. The creation of

---

• CLINICAL APPLICATION 47.1 | **Complications of Vacuum Extraction Delivery**

Maternal

- Pelvic floor trauma.

Neonatal

- Trauma to the fetal scalp is the most common complication, although this is reduced if soft cups compared with rigid vacuum cups are used for assisted vaginal delivery (Verma et al., 2021).
- Some babies will have a chignon, which is a combination of oedema and bruising (Fig. 47.3).
- Abrasions of the scalp may be caused by the cup being pulled off during inexpert traction.
- Jaundice, usually mild and responding to phototherapy, may be due to the reabsorption of the red cells which have escaped the circulatory system during bruise formation.
- Neonatal cephalohaematoma, retinal haemorrhages and subgaleal haemorrhages are more common after vacuum extraction than forceps delivery.
- There is limited evidence to suggest that vacuum extraction may be associated with umbilical cord blood acid–base changes.
- Vacuum extraction can be used to deliver babies with fetal distress in the second stage of labour.

---

post-traumatic stress clinics for women who have had previous traumatic 'normal deliveries' may also have contributed to the rising numbers of CSs, as previously women may have opted for a CS for subsequent deliveries. However there are now vaginal birth after CS (VBAC) clinics to explore a woman's options around CS so that a fully informed choice is made for a subsequent delivery. Table 47.1 summarizes the indications for CS.

Method

The CS is an operative technique whereby the fetus is delivered via the abdominal route. It is important to be aware of the surgical techniques involved. Technically, there are two types of CS according to the incision in the uterus: the **lower segment** and the **classical.** There is no association with the type of abdominal wall incision, although a lower segment CS is most often performed through a transverse incision, also called the **Joel–Cohen** or **Pfannenstiel** or **bikini-line incision** (Bassett, 2017; Bergholt, 2020; Hayman & Raynor, 2020). The lower segment forms from about 32 weeks of pregnancy and is less muscular than the upper segment. A transverse incision into the lower uterine segment heals more rapidly than a vertical incision into the upper uterine segment and there is a reduced rate of rupture of the uterus in a subsequent pregnancy (Brennan & Palacios Jaraqemada, 2020). For this reason, classical CS is rarely performed unless the fetus is to be delivered before the 32nd week of pregnancy or there is an anterior placenta praevia. The anatomical layers incised and sutured for CS are in Box 47.3.

As the uterus is incised, the membranes are ruptured with the escape of amniotic fluid. There is likely to be substantial bleeding because of the increased blood supply to the uterus. The woman will wish to see and have contact

---

TABLE 47.1 Maternal and Fetal Indications for Caesarean Section

Maternal	Fetal	Maternal and Fetal
Severe pregnancy-induced hypertension	Severe rhesus isoimmunization	Cephalopelvic disproportion
Previous vaginal reconstructive surgery	Cord prolapse	Pelvic tumours
Previous third-degree tears	Multiple fetuses (three or more)	High-risk obstetric history
A large-for-date fetus (with previous shoulder dystocia)	Breech presentation	Antepartum haemorrhage
Eclampsia	Brow or shoulder presentation	Uterine rupture
Terminal illness of the mother	Severe intrauterine growth retardation (which may be complicated by maternal disease)	Failure to progress in labour
	Fetal distress in labour	Placenta praevia
	Fetal abnormality where damage may be increased by vaginal delivery	Fetal macrosomia
	Active genital herpes	Tumours

with her baby as soon as possible and to breastfeed if that is her intended method of feeding. Even though the woman has had a CS, the baby can still be placed skin to skin to initiate the first breastfeed if both the mother and baby's condition allow. Due to the proximity of the bladder to the lower uterine segment, urine output must be closely observed. A urinary catheter is inserted in the bladder until the woman is mobile but for no less than 12 hours after the last dose of the regional anaesthetic (NICE, 2023a), as there may be difficulty in micturition. Any presence of haematuria must be reported to the obstetrician. Immediate postoperative care is similar to any surgery.

Types of Anaesthesia Used for CS

Types of anaesthesia used for CS will depend on the reason why the CS is being performed. In the case of fetal distress, where a woman already has a working epidural, the epidural will be topped up with a stronger anaesthetic, with or without an opiate drug such as morphine or fentanyl. Spinal anaesthesia is used for an elective CS or when an epidural is ineffective. In the case of severe fetal bradycardia, where the fetus must be delivered quickly, a general anaesthetic might be administered. A general anaesthetic is also given when a woman who has had a spinal or epidural complains of pain during the operation. Women with clotting disorders will always have a general anaesthetic, as there is a high risk of bleeding. Patient-controlled analgesia (PCA) may be prescribed postoperatively if a woman has coagulation problems to avoid frequent intramuscular injections. Women who have had a general anaesthetic for an emergency CS may also have PCA. If the woman is having opioid analgesia, an antiemetic is usually given simultaneously. Postoperatively, analgesia and antiemetics are listed in Box 47.4.

> **• BOX 47.3 Anatomical Layers Incised and Sutured in a Caesarean Section**
>
> - Skin.
> - Fat.
> - Rectus sheath.
> - Muscle (rectus abdominis).
> - Abdominal peritoneum.
> - Pelvic (visceral peritoneum or perimetrium).
> - Uterine muscle (sutured in two layers).

> **• BOX 47.4 Postoperative Drugs**
>
> - Intramuscular or subcuticular analgesia (e.g., morphine sulphate).
> - Nonsteroidal anti-inflammatory drugs (e.g., diclofenac (Voltarol) per rectum or oral tablets (Brufen)) if maternal condition allows.
> - Oral analgesics (e.g., paracetamol or co-codamol).
> - Antiemetics (e.g., Stemetil (prochlorperazine) or Maxolon (metoclopramide)).
> - As per local protocol or clinical guidelines (NICE, 2023a).

Safety

Even with the benefit of modern surgical techniques, CS is still less safe for the woman than a vaginal delivery. **Pulmonary embolism**, **haemorrhage** and **infection,** as well as thromboembolic disorders, may occur. Long-term morbidity with **infertility,** voluntary or involuntary, may be a problem.

CSs can have an impact on the neonate, such as neonatal depression due to anaesthetics, fetal injury, respiratory distress syndrome and breastfeeding complications (Neu & Rushing, 2011). See Chapter 57 for the influence of drugs in labour on neonatal behaviour.

General Anaesthesia in Pregnancy and Childbirth

Reversible anaesthesia, which is a state of unconsciousness and muscle relaxation, is brought about by pharmacological preparations. There is a great difference in obstetric anaesthesia from general surgery, as two lives must be cared for: mother and fetus. The recent MBRRACE report continues to display a low rate of deaths due to anaesthetics in childbirth (1 woman) (Knight et al., 2023). However the need for vigilance in the care of the pregnant woman undergoing general anaesthesia and subsequent postoperative management is still crucial.

The altered physiology of the woman increases the danger and includes raised maternal intragastric pressure, acidity of gastric contents and delayed gastric emptying, leading to the risk of acid aspiration syndrome. Fetal monitoring is also required. Auscultation of the fetal heart is performed before the operation (Bassett, 2017).

General Anaesthetic Agents

For a drug to be used as an **anaesthetic agent,** it must affect the central nervous system appropriately and be controllable so that anaesthesia can be induced rapidly, be adjusted during the operation to provide the correct level of consciousness and the effects quickly reversed after the operation (NICE, 2023b). Humphrey Davy suggested the use of the gas **nitrous oxide** for relieving the pain of surgery in 1800. He tested its effects on himself and a few others, including the prime minister. It was found to cause euphoria, analgesia and loss of consciousness but became famous as 'laughing gas' until an American dentist, Horace Wells, had a tooth extracted under its influence.

Inhalational anaesthetics were used in surgery in 1846 when William Morton used ether to extract a tooth. He persuaded the chief surgeon at Massachusetts General Hospital to use it during a surgical procedure on 16 October 1846 and it was successful; subsequently, planned protracted surgical procedures could be carried out. The famous American Oliver Wendell Holmes invented the word 'anaesthesia'. In 1847 James Simpson, professor of obstetrics in Glasgow, used the agent **chloroform** to relieve pain in childbirth, but it only became popular after Queen Victoria gave birth to her seventh child under the influence of chloroform in 1853.

Modern Drugs

Although many CSs are now performed under spinal and/or epidural anaesthesia (see Chapter 38), general anaesthesia is still used. It is now common practice to administer antacid therapy, preoxygenate pregnant women, perform cricoid pressure and administer a rapid sequence induction of a general anaesthetic (NICE, 2023a). The woman is placed on a left lateral tilt of 15 degrees, which will help reduce supine hypotension (NICE, 2023a).

Problems

Failed Intubation

Failed intubation is an obstetric emergency requiring prompt and calm action. Most maternal deaths attributed directly to anaesthesia have been reported to be due to a misplaced endotracheal tube. It is important that there are regular training drills for airway management crisis (Knight et al., 2014). The anaesthetist may choose to maintain an airway with a laryngeal mask or another supraglottic airway device (Kinsella et al., 2015), with an assistant maintaining cricoid pressure throughout the anaesthetic, or **spinal anaesthesia** may be chosen. NICE (2023a) states that maternity units should have the necessary emergency drill procedure to be undertaken if failed intubation occurs. It is also pertinent that there are appropriately trained and skilled anaesthetists and anaesthetic assistants working within these facilities to deal with situations should they occur.

Aspiration Pneumonitis (Mendelson's Syndrome)

This life-threatening **aspiration pneumonitis** arises from the inhalation of acid gastric contents and was first described by Mendelson in 1946. The result of such aspiration is a chemical pneumonitis leading to **acute respiratory distress syndrome (ARDS)** with acute bronchospasm, dyspnoea, cyanosis, wheezing and tachycardia. The factors predisposing to this arise from the physiological effect of progesterone on the smooth muscle of the stomach, which causes delayed emptying; decreased lower oesophageal tone, which leads to reflux; and the altered position of the stomach due to the enlarged uterus. There is also gastric hypersecretion in labour. There is still controversy about oral intake during labour, with no firm evidence to support the policy of restricting food intake for all women in labour. Most maternity units now only restrict food intake in those women who have a higher risk of having an emergency CS.

Prevention of Acid Aspiration Syndrome

Prevention of this syndrome is essential. The administration of **antacid preparations** before anaesthetic induction of **histamine-2 (H$_2$) antagonists** or **proton pump antagonists** can be administered (NICE, 2023a). Paranjothy et al. (2014) argue that although the evidence quality was poor, they concluded that a combined approach of antacids plus H$_2$ antagonist was more effective than no intervention or antacid intervention alone for making the gastric pH less acidic. **Metoclopramide** acts centrally in the nervous system and locally in the gastrointestinal tract. These are antiemetic drugs and they act as stimulants to gastric motility, accelerating emptying without stimulating gastric juice production. Metoclopramide is a D$_2$ receptor antagonist which increases gastric motility and helps prevents gastro-oesophageal reflux (Ritter et al., 2019).

During induction of the general anaesthetic and intubation, **cricoid pressure (Sellick's manoeuvre)**, part of which is referred to as **crash induction**, along with the immediate passing of a cuffed endotracheal tube, is essential to prevent aspiration of acid stomach contents. The cricoid cartilage is compressed between the thumb and finger towards the cervical spine to occlude the oesophagus. Deaths have occurred due to inexperience of the practitioner, and it is recommended that an experienced anaesthetist be involved in obstetric anaesthesia (Knight et al., 2014). The Royal College of Anaesthetists (RCOA) (2022) stipulates that not only is it important to have the experienced obstetric anaesthetists, but there must also be the appropriate facilities for high-dependency monitoring and regular training updates for multidisciplinary staff on emergency drills.

Aortocaval Compression

The alternative name for **aortocaval compression** is *supine hypotensive syndrome*. A reduction in venous return and a fall in cardiac output are produced by the weight of the gravid uterus pressing on and partly occluding the inferior vena cava. It will occur whenever the woman lies supine in late pregnancy. If fetal distress is present, the interference with placental circulation will increase the severity of hypoxia.

Prevention of Aortocaval Compression

If the woman must lie supine, the sequence of events can be avoided by placing a rubber wedge under the mattress to tilt the woman's body about 15 degrees to the left. Modern operating tables and delivery beds have this function built into their design. Cluver et al. (2013) reviewed the use of maternal positions during CSs but there was limited evidence to prove or disprove the effects that positions had on fetal and maternal outcomes. Interestingly, they highlighted that there were no differences in Apgar scores, maternal pH, cord blood pH measurements or maternal diastolic blood pressure (BP). They concluded that a left lateral tilt might be better than a right lateral tilt and that manual displacement might be better than a left lateral tilt, but stress more evidence is required to confirm this.

The Acutely Unwell Woman

Maternal Collapse

Clinicians need to have the knowledge and skills to promptly recognize the signs and symptoms indicating deterioration and maternal collapse. **This is an urgent situation**. Maternal and fetal outcomes depend on swift action to summon assistance for effective resuscitation of the woman. The entire multidisciplinary team (MDT) will need to be involved. As students and midwives provide care to women in pregnancy, childbirth and the puerperium, it is more than likely they will have a key role in the recognition of maternal collapse and be involved in the resuscitation and subsequent care.

Midwives often deal with emergency situations that are resolved very quickly. These are termed 'near misses' and many have been discussed in Chapters 41–45. Whilst it is a rare occurrence, maternal collapse is a life-threatening event due to a wide variety of causes. This section emphasizes the essential skillset and tools needed by midwives to recognize and manage acute illness as part of the MDT providing maternity care for women (Chu, Johnston & Geoghegan, 2020).

Maternal collapse is defined as a sudden event involving the cardiorespiratory systems and/or brain, resulting in a reduced or absent conscious level (and potentially death) at any stage in pregnancy and up to 6 weeks after birth (Chu, Johnston & Geoghegan, 2020). Globally, maternal morbidity and mortality remains a major issue. In the MBRRACE-UK report, there was a total of 229 maternal deaths from direct and indirect causes (Knight et al., 2022). The MBRRACE-UK enquiry highlights that some maternal deaths occurred despite excellent care. Suboptimal care was also associated with maternal deaths – these may have been avoidable if optimal care had been provided. Examples included failing to recognize impending acute illness early enough to initiate prompt management (e.g., fluid replacement, antibiotics and oxygen therapy) and doing 'too little too late' or 'too much too soon' (Knight et al., 2022). Refer to Chapter 30 for a summary of the distribution of maternal deaths and the association with inequalities, vulnerable and ethnic minority groups, mental health and complex comorbidities.

Midwifery is a vital solution to the challenges of providing high-quality maternal and newborn care, in all countries (Renfrew et al., 2014). The increasing number of women now presenting in pregnancy with complex comorbidities, and their association with maternal deaths, is concerning. Therefore contemporary midwifery practice now must ensure midwives have the essential skills to deal with acute critical care situations. The common causes of maternal collapse are shown in Fig. 47.5. Many of the key predisposing obstetric and medical causes are previously covered in Chapters 31–35. The common obstetric emergencies arising during the intrapartum period are covered in Chapters 41–45. Sepsis will be discussed in this chapter and revisited

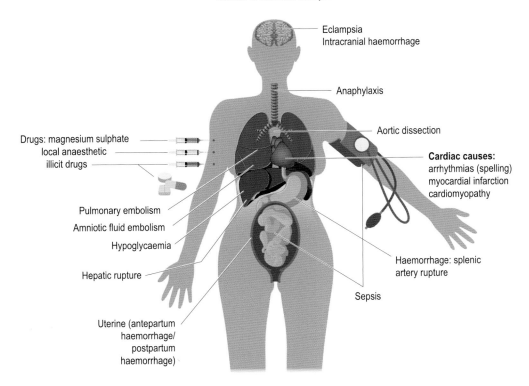

Causes of maternal collapse

Eclampsia
Intracranial haemorrhage

Anaphylaxis

Aortic dissection

Cardiac causes:
arrhythmias (spelling)
myocardial infarction
cardiomyopathy

Drugs: magnesium sulphate
local anaesthetic
illicit drugs

Pulmonary embolism
Amniotic fluid embolism
Hypoglycaemia
Hepatic rupture

Haemorrhage: splenic
artery rupture

Sepsis

Uterine (antepartum
haemorrhage/
postpartum
haemorrhage)

• **Fig. 47.5** Causes of maternal collapse.

in the puerperium Chapter 56. Disseminating intravascular coagulopathy is covered in several related chapters (e.g., Chapters 31 & 33).

This section will deal with the acutely ill woman who may rapidly deteriorate towards maternal collapse. The key areas to be addressed include:

- Recognition.
- Assessment.
- Resuscitation.
- Sepsis.

The physiology of shock and management are covered in Chapter 45. The types of shock include cardiogenic (heart failure), hypovolaemic (reduced blood volume), septic (infection), anaphylactic and neurogenic (see Boxes 45.2 & 45.3). In summary, failure of the cardiovascular system (CVS) to deliver oxygen to the body tissues may result in irreversible organ damage or death. However shock is reversible if detected early and prompt resuscitation measures put in place.

Recognition (Early)

A previous MBRRACE-UK report recommended a national obstetric early-warning scoring system should be introduced and used for all obstetric women, including those being cared for outside the obstetric setting (Chu, Johnston & Geoghegan, 2020; Knight et al., 2016). The Maternity Early-Warning Score (MEWS) or Modified Early Obstetric Warning Score (MEOWS) are tools designed to account for the normal physiological changes of pregnancy. The intention is to improve recognition of pregnant and postnatal women at risk of clinical deterioration and facilitate early intervention (Fig. 47.6). These tools do not replace clinical judgement but rather guide the clinician to make a clinical judgement based on the scores. MEWS (or MEOWS) uses a simple yellow and red colour code as a trigger. All triggers should be added up each time observations are recorded on the chart, documented at the bottom and acted upon accordingly.

All antenatal and postnatal women who enter an acute hospital setting should have their core observations recorded on the approved MEWS (or MEOWS) chart for their area. Core observations are:

- Respiratory rate.
- Oxygen saturations.
- Temperature.
- Maternal heart rate.
- Systolic BP.
- Diastolic BP.
- Neurological response.
- Urine output.
- Looks unwell.

The MEWS (or MEOWS) chart is an ideal recognition tool to clearly indicate the subtle changes that act as warning for physiological signs of shock. These include raised respiratory rate (tachypnoea) and raised heart rate (tachycardia).

In a pregnant woman the signs and symptoms of hypovolaemia could be delayed due to the normal physiological changes already present. Hypovolaemia may present with hypotension (low BP), pallor, reduced urine output or altered levels of consciousness. Respiratory rate is the first physiological parameter to be noticeably altered. Other maternal features such as tachycardia and hypotension are late signs. Therefore significant changes in respiration are a red flag. Action should be taken to prevent further deterioration in the woman's condition. Remember that deterioration is rapid, so prompt action is required to prevent a catastrophic situation. See Box 47.5 for key messages for midwives and the maternity services.

Assessment of Maternal Collapse

Assessment of the woman's physiological status must follow a systematic process by undertaking a detailed *A–E assessment approach* (Table 47.2). This process addresses all aspects of the woman's clinical status. The process also prescribes necessary interventions to address the abnormal features detected prior to moving onto the next level of assessment. Midwives must be familiar with this systematic assessment as it features in MDT training. The assessment process also references non-technical skills such as listening to the woman, assessing level of consciousness, and assessing any changes in skin colour.

Resuscitation

Box 47.6 summarizes the underlying principles and first steps in resuscitation. Box 47.7 outlines the key messages for adult resuscitation respectively (Resuscitation Council UK, 2021).

A key challenge in maternal resuscitation is airway obstruction, due to the increase of weight in pregnancy. **An anaesthetist must be alerted**. It is imperative to call immediately for an anaesthetist as early intubation is necessary for the unconscious woman. Cardiopulmonary resuscitation (CPR) is commenced if the woman is in cardiac arrest. The chain of survival describes the sequence of steps that together maximize the chance of survival following a cardiac arrest (Fig. 47.7).

- The first link in the chain is the immediate recognition of cardiac arrest and calling for help.
- The second is the prompt initiation of CPR.
- The third is performing defibrillation as soon as possible.
- The fourth is optimal post resuscitation care.

Like any chain, it is only as strong as its weakest link. If one stage is weak, the chances for successful resuscitation are compromised.

Sepsis

Globally, sepsis remains an acute critical illness that can cause maternal death if not identified and treated promptly. Sepsis is one of the most common direct causes of maternal death in the UK. There has been a steady increase from seven deaths in 2012–2014 to 17 deaths in 2018–2020 (Knight et al., 2022). Sepsis can occur at any time in pregnancy but is more common in the puerperium (see Chapter 56).

Sepsis (also known as blood poisoning) is the immune system's overreaction to an infection or injury, with the clinical presentation referred to as systematic inflammatory response syndrome. If not treated immediately, sepsis

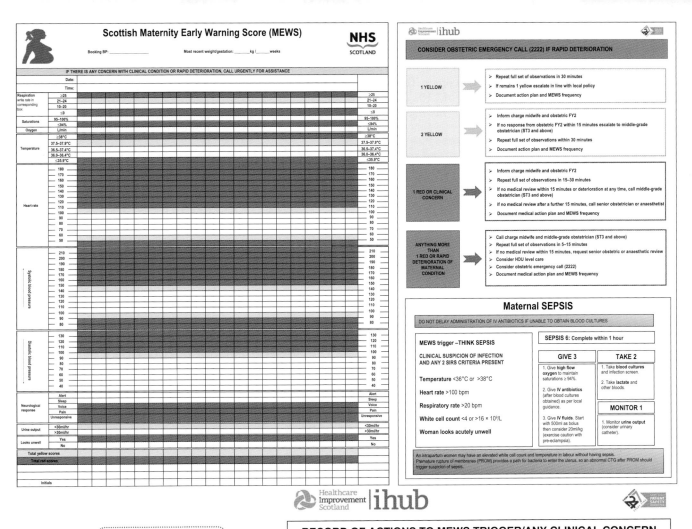

• **Fig. 47.6** Example of Maternity Early-Warning Score (MEWS). (https://ihub.scot/media/6721/fi nal-national-mews-chart_web.pdf)

can result in organ failure and death. Early recognition and management make a difference to the outcomes. The Sepsis Screening Tool for Acute Assessment (Fig. 47.10) is a critical tool identifying the physiological concerns that initiate the 'Sepsis 6' protocol. Clinical red flags are pyrexia, hypothermia, tachycardia, tachypnoea, hypoxia, hypotension, oliguria and reduced consciousness. All clinicians must *'think sepsis'* (Sepsis Trust, 2023).

• BOX 47.5 Key Messages on Early Recognition

For Midwives

- Do not presume normality.
- Be vigilant in using the MEWS (or MEOWS) chart.
- Escalate if any signs or symptoms of deterioration.
- Challenge assumptions – both your own and those of others to avoid a potential adverse maternal or fetal outcome.
- As part of the multidisciplinary team (MDT), share your concerns within the team – involve senior staff (midwives, obstetricians and anaesthetists)
- Use an SBAR (Situation, Background, Assessment, Recommendations) for effective communication. This is a straightforward structured tool used for communication between practitioners in the MDT. As part of the MDT, attend multiprofessional training including student midwives.
- Support student midwives to develop competency in using the MEWS (or MEOWS).

For Maternity Services

- A standardized tool for tracking changes in physiology is recommended, such as a MEWS or MEOWS.
- A physiological track-and-trigger system to monitor all antepartum and postpartum admissions in conjunction with the partogram in labour.
- The RCOA (2022) recommends that an early-warning score system modified for the maternity context acute services is needed by the acute services looking after women who are pregnant or within 42 days of having given birth.
- MDT teams need to train together and have the appropriate infrastructure and necessary resources in place to deliver high-quality service.
- An adult resuscitation team trained in resuscitation of the pregnant patient should be available immediately for related cases.
- RCOA (2022) recognizes the team must be able to work closely under stress in dynamic situations and should include obstetricians, anaesthetists, neonatologists, midwives, theatre staff, anaesthetic assistants and others.

For Pregnant Women and Mothers

Women need to 'Think Sepsis' and be aware of sepsis symptoms up to 6 weeks after birth.
Sepsis symptoms they need to be advised to look out for and seek advice:
- Slurred speech or confusion.
- Extreme shivering or muscle pain.
- Passing no urine (in a day).
- Severe breathlessness.
- It feels as though they are going to die.
- Skin mottled or discoloured.

(UK Sepsis Trust, 2023. Available at: https://www.sepsistrust.org.)

TABLE 47.2 Detailed Resuscitation Guidelines (Airway, Breathing, Circulation, Disability, Exposure [ABCDE] Approach)

Airway (A) Steps 1–3:	Airway obstruction is an emergency. Get expert help immediately. If untreated, airway obstruction causes hypoxia and risks damage to the brain, kidneys and heart, cardiac arrest and death.
1. Look for the signs of airway obstruction	Airway obstruction causes paradoxical chest and abdominal movements ('see-saw' respirations) and the use of the accessory muscles of respiration. Central cyanosis is a late sign of airway obstruction. In complete airway obstruction, there are no breath sounds at the mouth or nose. In partial obstruction, air entry is diminished and often noisy. In the critically ill patient, depressed consciousness often leads to airway obstruction.
2. Treat airway obstruction as a medical emergency	Obtain expert help immediately. Untreated, airway obstruction causes hypoxaemia (low PaO_2) with the risk of hypoxic injury to the brain, kidneys and heart, cardiac arrest and even death. In most cases, only simple methods of airway clearance are required (e.g., airway-opening manoeuvres, airways suction, insertion of an oropharyngeal or nasopharyngeal airway). Tracheal intubation may be required when these fail.
3. Give oxygen at high concentration	Provide high-concentration oxygen using a mask with an oxygen reservoir. Ensure that the oxygen flow is sufficient (usually 15 L/min) to prevent collapse of the reservoir during inspiration. If the patient's trachea is intubated, give high-concentration oxygen with a self-inflating bag. In acute respiratory failure, aim to maintain an oxygen saturation of 94–98%. In patients at risk of hypercapnic respiratory failure (see below), aim for an oxygen saturation of 88–92%.
Breathing (B)	During the immediate assessment of breathing, it is vital to diagnose and treat immediately life-threatening conditions (e.g., acute severe asthma, pulmonary oedema, tension pneumothorax and massive haemothorax).
	Look, listen and feel for the general signs of respiratory distress: sweating, central cyanosis, use of the accessory muscles of respiration and abdominal breathing.

TABLE 47.2 Detailed Resuscitation Guidelines (Airway, Breathing, Circulation, Disability, Exposure [ABCDE] Approach)—cont'd

	Count the respiratory rate. The normal rate is 12–20 breaths/min. A high (>25 breaths/min) or increasing respiratory rate is a marker of illness and a warning that the patient may deteriorate suddenly.
	Assess the depth of each breath, the pattern (rhythm) of respiration and whether chest expansion is equal on both sides.
	Note any chest deformity (this may increase the risk of deterioration in the ability to breathe normally); look for a raised jugular venous pulse (JVP) (e.g., in acute severe asthma or a tension pneumothorax); note the presence and patency of any chest drains; remember that abdominal distension may limit diaphragmatic movement, thereby worsening respiratory distress.
	Record the inspired oxygen concentration (%) and the SpO_2 reading of the pulse oximeter. The pulse oximeter does not detect hypercapnia. If the patient is receiving supplemental oxygen, the SpO_2 may be normal in the presence of a very high $PaCO_2$.
	Listen to the patient's breath sounds a short distance from their face: rattling airway noises indicate the presence of airway secretions, usually caused by the inability of the patient to cough sufficiently or to take a deep breath. Stridor or wheeze suggests partial, but significant, airway obstruction.
	Percuss the chest: hyper-resonance may suggest a pneumothorax; dullness usually indicates consolidation or pleural fluid.
	Auscultate the chest: bronchial breathing indicates lung consolidation with patent airways; absent or reduced sounds suggest a pneumothorax or pleural fluid or lung consolidation caused by complete obstruction.
	Check the position of the trachea in the suprasternal notch: deviation to one side indicates mediastinal shift (e.g., pneumothorax, lung fibrosis or pleural fluid).
	Feel the chest wall to detect surgical emphysema or crepitus (suggesting a pneumothorax until proven otherwise).
	The specific treatment of respiratory disorders depends upon the cause. Nevertheless, all critically ill patients should be given oxygen. In a subgroup of patients with chronic obstructive pulmonary disease (COPD), high concentrations of oxygen may depress breathing (i.e., they are at risk of hypercapnic respiratory failure – often referred to as type 2 respiratory failure). Nevertheless, these patients will also sustain end-organ damage or cardiac arrest if their blood oxygen tensions are allowed to decrease. In this group, aim for a lower-than-normal PaO_2 and oxygen saturation. Give oxygen via a Venturi 28% mask (4 L/min) or a 24% Venturi mask (4 L/min) initially and reassess. Aim for a target SpO_2 range of 88–92% in most patients with COPD but evaluate the target for each patient based on their arterial blood gas measurements during previous exacerbations (if available). Some patients with chronic lung disease carry an oxygen alert card (that documents their target saturation) and their own appropriate Venturi mask.
	If the patient's depth or rate of breathing is judged to be inadequate, or absent, use bag-mask or pocket-mask ventilation to improve oxygenation and ventilation, whilst calling immediately for expert help. In co-operative patients who do not have airway obstruction, consider the use of noninvasive ventilation (NIV). In patients with an acute exacerbation of COPD, the use of NIV is often helpful and prevents the need for tracheal intubation and invasive ventilation.
Circulation (C)	In almost all medical and surgical emergencies, consider hypovolaemia to be the primary cause of shock until proven otherwise.
	Unless there are obvious signs of a cardiac cause, give intravenous fluid to any patient with cool peripheries and a fast heart rate. In surgical patients, rapidly exclude haemorrhage (overt or hidden).
	Remember that breathing problems, such as a tension pneumothorax, can also compromise a patient's circulatory state. This should have been treated earlier on in the assessment.

Continued

TABLE 47.2	Detailed Resuscitation Guidelines (Airway, Breathing, Circulation, Disability, Exposure [ABCDE] Approach)—cont'd
	Look at the colour of the hands and digits: are they blue, pink, pale or mottled?
	Assess the limb temperature by feeling the patient's hands: are they cool or warm?
	Measure the capillary refill time (CRT). Apply cutaneous pressure for 5 s on a fingertip held at heart level (or just above) with enough pressure to cause blanching. Time how long it takes for the skin to return to the colour of the surrounding skin after releasing the pressure. The normal value for CRT is usually <2 s. A prolonged CRT suggests poor peripheral perfusion. Other factors (e.g., cold surroundings, poor lighting, old age) can prolong CRT.
	Assess the state of the veins: they may be underfilled or collapsed when hypovolaemia is present.
	Count the patient's pulse rate (or preferably heart rate by listening to the heart with a stethoscope).
	Palpate peripheral and central pulses, assessing for presence, rate, quality, regularity and equality. Barely palpable central pulses suggest a poor cardiac output, whilst a bounding pulse may indicate sepsis.
	Measure the patient's blood pressure (BP). Even in shock, the BP may be normal because compensatory mechanisms increase peripheral resistance in response to reduced cardiac output. A low diastolic BP suggests arterial vasodilation (as in anaphylaxis or sepsis). A narrowed pulse pressure (difference between systolic and diastolic pressures; normally 35–45 mmHg) suggests arterial vasoconstriction (cardiogenic shock or hypovolaemia) and may occur with rapid tachyarrhythmia.
	Auscultate the heart. Is there a murmur or pericardial rub? Are the heart sounds difficult to hear? Does the audible heart rate correspond to the pulse rate?
	Look for other signs of a poor cardiac output, such as reduced conscious level and, if the patient has a urinary catheter, oliguria (urine volume <0.5 mL/kg/h).
	Look thoroughly for external haemorrhage from wounds or drains or evidence of concealed haemorrhage (e.g., thoracic, intraperitoneal, retroperitoneal or into gut). Intrathoracic, intra-abdominal or pelvic blood loss may be significant, even if drains are empty.
	The specific treatment of cardiovascular collapse depends on the cause, but should be directed at fluid replacement, haemorrhage control and restoration of tissue perfusion. Seek the signs of conditions that are immediately life-threatening (e.g., cardiac tamponade, massive or continuing haemorrhage, septicaemic shock) and treat them urgently.
	Insert one or more large (14 or 16 G) intravenous cannulas. Use short, wide-bore cannulas because they enable the highest flow.
	Take blood from the cannula for routine haematological, biochemical, coagulation and microbiological investigations and cross-matching before infusing intravenous fluid.
	Give a bolus of 500 mL of warmed crystalloid solution (e.g., Hartmann's solution or 0.9% sodium chloride) over <15 min if the patient is hypotensive. Use smaller volumes (e.g., 250 mL) for patients with known cardiac failure or trauma and use closer monitoring (listen to the chest for crackles after each bolus).
	Reassess the heart rate and BP regularly (every 5 min), aiming for the patient's normal BP or, if this is unknown, a target >100 mmHg systolic.
	If the patient does not improve, repeat the fluid challenge. Seek expert help if there is a lack of response to repeated fluid boluses.
	If symptoms and signs of cardiac failure (dyspnoea, increased heart rate, raised JVP, a third heart sound and pulmonary crackles on auscultation) occur, decrease the fluid infusion rate or stop the fluids altogether. Seek alternative means of improving tissue perfusion (e.g., inotropes or vasopressors).
	If the patient has primary chest pain and suspected acute coronary artery syndrome (ACS), record a 12-lead electrocardiogram early.
	Immediate general treatment for ACS includes:
	• Aspirin 300 mg, orally, crushed or chewed, as soon as possible.
	• Nitroglycerine, as sublingual glyceryl trinitrate (tablet or spray).
	• Oxygen: only give oxygen if the patient's SpO_2 is less than 94% breathing air alone.
	• Morphine (or diamorphine) titrated intravenously to avoid sedation and respiratory depression.
Disability (D)	Common causes of unconsciousness include profound hypoxia, hypercapnia, cerebral hypoperfusion or the recent administration of sedatives or analgesic drugs.

TABLE 47.2 — Detailed Resuscitation Guidelines (Airway, Breathing, Circulation, Disability, Exposure [ABCDE] Approach)—cont'd

Review and treat the ABCs: exclude or treat hypoxia and hypotension.

Check the patient's drug chart for reversible drug-induced causes of depressed consciousness. Give an antagonist where appropriate (e.g., naloxone for opioid toxicity).

Examine the pupils (size, equality and reaction to light).

Make a rapid initial assessment of the patient's conscious level using the AVPU method: Alert, responds to Vocal stimuli, responds to Painful stimuli or Unresponsive to all stimuli. Alternatively, use the Glasgow Coma Scale score. A painful stimulus can be given by applying supraorbital pressure (at the supraorbital notch).

Measure the blood glucose to exclude hypoglycaemia using a rapid finger-prick bedside testing method. In a peri-arrest patient, use a venous or arterial blood sample for glucose measurement as finger-prick glucose measurements can be unreliable in sick patients. Follow local protocols for management of hypoglycaemia. For example, if the blood sugar is less than 4.0 mmol/L in an unconscious patient, give an initial dose of 50 mL of 10% glucose solution intravenously. If necessary, give further doses of intravenous 10% glucose every minute until the patient has fully regained consciousness, or a total of 250 mL of 10% glucose has been given. Repeat blood glucose measurements to monitor the effects of treatment. If there is no improvement, consider further doses of 10% glucose. Specific national guidance exists for the management of hypoglycaemia in adults with diabetes mellitus.

Nurse unconscious patients in the lateral position if their airway is not protected.

Exposure (E) — To examine the patient properly, full exposure of the body may be necessary. Respect the patient's dignity and minimize heat loss.

Additional Information

Take a full clinical history from the patient, any relatives or friends, and other staff.

Review the patient's notes and charts:
- Study both absolute and trended values of vital signs.
- Check that important routine medications are prescribed and being given.

Review the results of laboratory or radiological investigations.

Consider which level of care is required by the patient (e.g., ward, high-dependency unit, intensive care unit).

Make complete entries in the patient's notes of your findings, assessment and treatment. Where necessary, hand over the patient to your colleagues.

Record the patient's response to therapy.

Consider definitive treatment of the patient's underlying condition.

For further steps in resuscitation (i.e., steps F onwards) and equipment, refer to: Resuscitation Council UK 2021. The ABCDE approach, Available at: https://www.resus.org.uk/library/abcde-approach.
Reproduced with the kind permission of Resuscitation Council UK.

BOX 47.6 Summary: Underlying Principles and First Steps in Resuscitation (Airway, Breathing, Circulation, Disability, Exposure [ABCDE] Approach)

Underlying Principles

The approach to all deteriorating or critically ill patients is the same. The underlying principles are:
1. Use the ABCDE approach to assess and treat the patient.
2. Do a complete initial assessment and reassess regularly.
3. Treat life-threatening problems before moving to the next part of assessment.
4. Assess the effects of treatment.
5. Recognize when you will need extra help. Call for appropriate help early.
6. Use all members of the team. This enables interventions (e.g., assessment, attaching monitors, intravenous access) to be undertaken simultaneously.
7. Communicate effectively – use the Situation, Background, Assessment, Recommendation (SBAR) or Reason, Story, Vital signs, Plan approach.
8. The aim of the initial treatment is to keep the patient alive and achieve some clinical improvement. This will buy time for further treatment and making a diagnosis.
9. Remember – it can take a few minutes for treatments to work, so wait a short while before reassessing the patient after an intervention.

First Steps

1. Ensure personal safety. Wear an apron and gloves as appropriate.
2. First, look at the patient in general to see if the patient appears unwell.

Continued

• BOX 47.6 Summary: Underlying Principles and First Steps in Resuscitation (Airway, Breathing, Circulation, Disability, Exposure [ABCDE] Approach)—cont'd

3. If the patient is awake, ask 'How are you?' If the patient appears unconscious or has collapsed, shake her and ask 'Are you alright?' If she responds normally, she has a patent airway, is breathing and has brain perfusion. If she speaks only in short sentences, she may have breathing problems. Failure of the patient to respond is a clear marker of critical illness.

4. This first rapid 'Look, Listen and Feel' of the patient should take about 30 s and will often indicate a patient is critically ill and there is a need for urgent help. Ask a colleague to ensure appropriate help is coming.

5. If the patient is unconscious, unresponsive and is not breathing normally (occasional gasps are not normal), start cardiopulmonary resuscitation (CPR) according to the resuscitation guidelines. If you are confident and trained to do so, feel for a pulse to determine if the patient has a respiratory arrest. If there are any doubts about the presence of a pulse, start CPR.

- Current CPR guidelines are available from Resuscitation Council UK (www.resus.org.uk).
- The algorithm for *in-hospital* adult resuscitation is detailed in Fig. 47.8.
- The algorithm for *advanced life support* is detailed in Fig. 47.9 (Soar et al., 2021).

6. Monitor the vital signs early. Attach a pulse oximeter, electrocardiogram monitor and a noninvasive blood pressure monitor to all critically ill patients as soon as possible.

7. Insert an intravenous cannula as soon as possible. Take blood for investigation when inserting the intravenous cannula.

Reproduced with the kind permission of Resuscitation Council UK.

• BOX 47.7 Key Messages for Hospitals on Adult Resuscitation

For the prevention of in-hospital cardiac arrest, Resuscitation Council UK supports shared decision-making and advanced-care planning, which integrates resuscitation decisions with emergency care treatment plans to increase clarity of treatment goals and also prevent inadvertent deprivation of other indicated treatments, besides cardiopulmonary resuscitation.

Hospitals should:

- Use a track-and-trigger early-warning score system for the early identification of patients who are critically ill or at risk of clinical deterioration.
- Train staff in the recognition, monitoring and immediate care of the acutely ill patient.
- Empower all staff to call for help when they identify a patient at risk of physiological deterioration. This includes calls based on clinical concern rather than solely on vital signs.
- Have a clear policy for the clinical response to abnormal vital signs and critical illness. This may include a critical care outreach service and/or emergency team (e.g., medical emergency team, rapid response team).
- Use structured communication tools to ensure effective handover of information.
- Receive care in a clinical area that has the appropriate staffing, skills and facilities for their severity of illness.
- Review cardiac arrest events to identify opportunities for system improvement and share key learning points with hospital staff.

Reproduced with the kind permission of Resuscitation Council UK.

Chain of survival

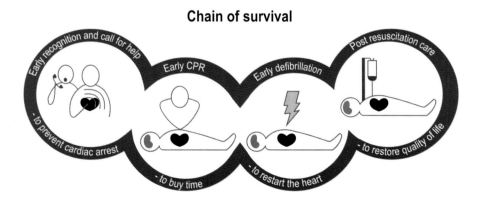

• Fig. 47.7 Chain of Survival.

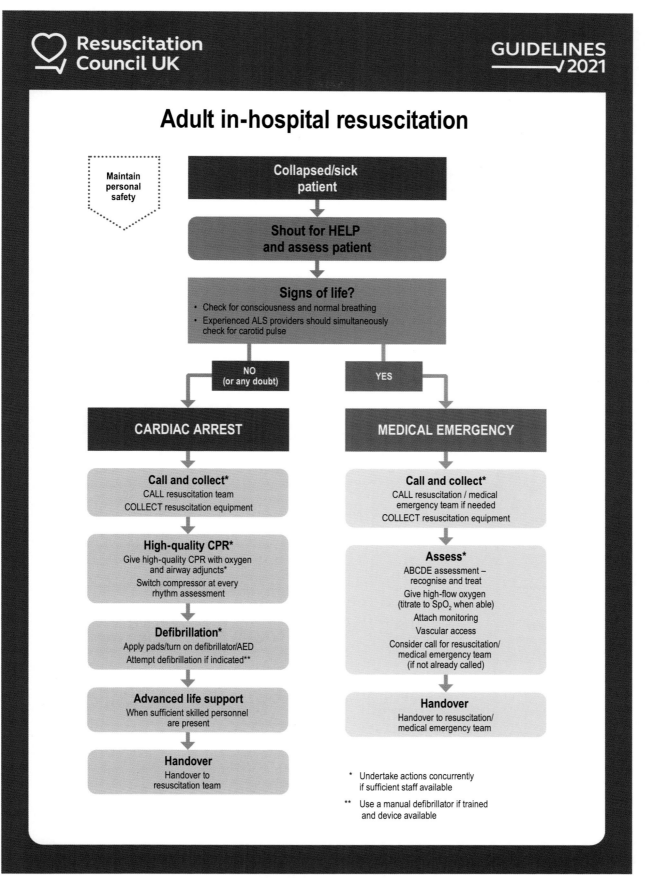

• **Fig. 47.8** Adult in-hospital resuscitation.

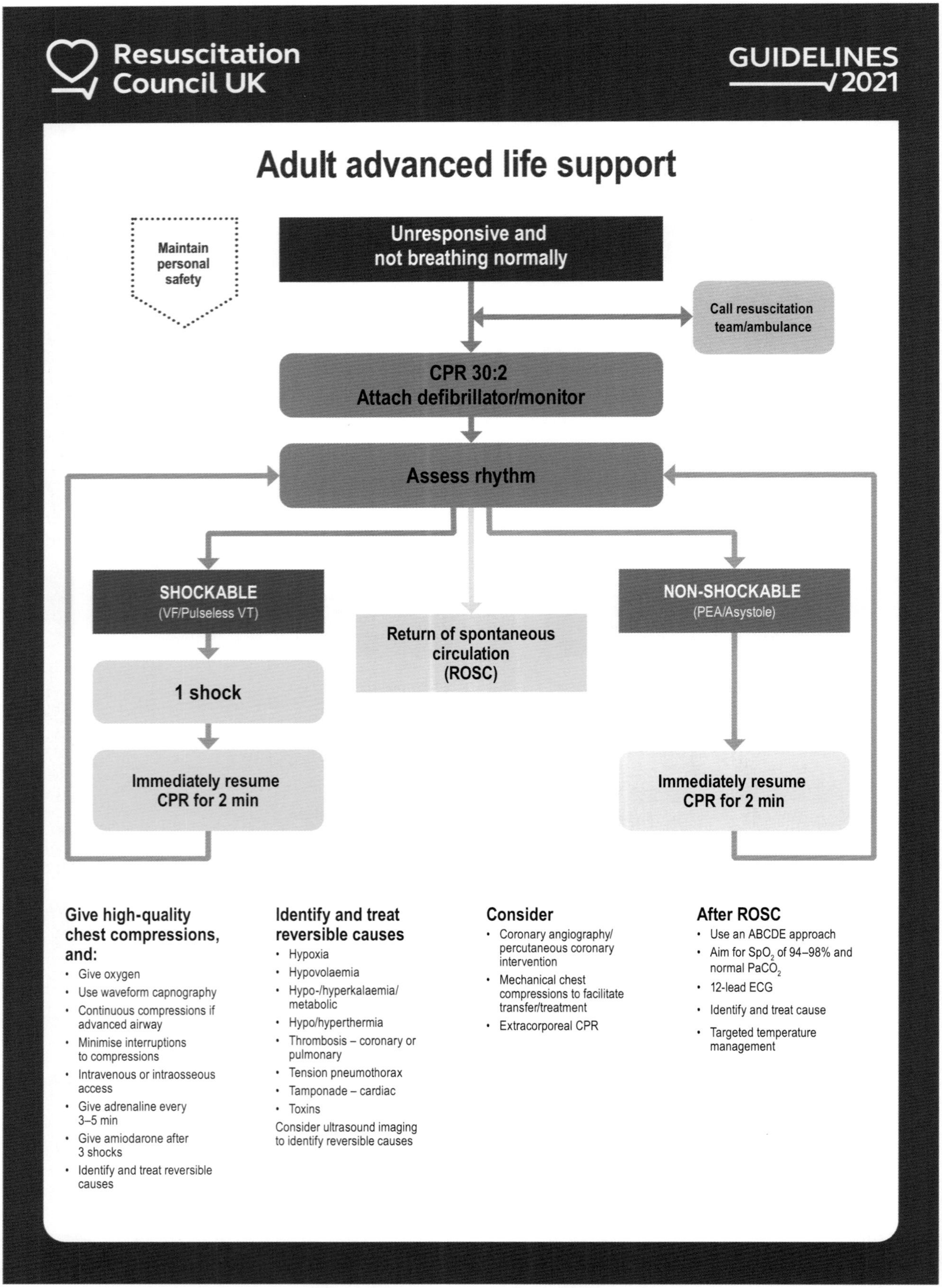

• **Fig. 47.9** Adult advanced life support (2021 guidelines).

SEPSIS SCREENING TOOL ACUTE ASSESSMENT

PREGNANT
OR UP TO 6 WEEKS POST-PREGNANCY

PATIENT DETAILS:

DATE: TIME:

NAME:

DESIGNATION:

SIGNATURE:

01 START THIS CHART IF THE PATIENT LOOKS UNWELL OR MEOWS HAS TRIGGERED

RISK FACTORS FOR SEPSIS INCLUDE:

☐ Impaired immunity (e.g. diabetes, steroids, chemotherapy)
☐ Recent trauma / surgery / invasive procedure

☐ Indwelling lines / IVDU / broken skin

02 COULD THIS BE DUE TO AN INFECTION?

YES

LIKELY SOURCE:

☐ Respiratory   ☐ Urine
☐ Breast abscess   ☐ Abdominal pain / distension

☐ Infected caesarean / perineal wound
☐ Chorioamnionitis / endometritis

NO → SEPSIS UNLIKELY, CONSIDER OTHER DIAGNOSIS

03 ANY RED FLAG PRESENT?

YES

☐ Objective evidence of new or altered mental state
☐ Systolic BP ≤ 90 mmHg (or drop of >40 from normal)
☐ Heart rate ≥ 130 per minute
☐ Respiratory rate ≥ 25 per minute
☐ Needs O_2 to keep SpO_2 ≥ 92%
☐ Non-blanching rash / mottled / ashen / cyanotic
☐ Lactate ≥ 2 mmol/l*
☐ Not passed urine in 18 hours (<0.5ml/kg/hr if catheterised)
   lactate may be raised in and immediately after normal delivery

YES →

RED FLAG SEPSIS

START

SEPSIS SIX

04 ANY AMBER FLAG PRESENT?

NO

☐ Acute deterioration in functional ability
☐ Respiratory rate 21–24
☐ Heart rate 100–129 or new dysrhythmia
☐ Systolic BP 91–100 mmHg
☐ Has had invasive procedure in last 6 weeks
   (e.g. CS, forceps delivery, ERPC, cerclage, CVs, miscarriage, termination)
☐ Temperature < 36°C
☐ Has diabetes or gestational diabetes
☐ Close contact with GAS
☐ Prolonged rupture of membranes
☐ Bleeding / wound infection
☐ Offensive vaginal discharge
☐ Non-reassuring CTG / fetal tachycardia >160
☐ Behavioural / mental status change

YES →

FURTHER REVIEW REQUIRED:

- SEND BLOODS AND REVIEW RESULTS
- ENSURE SENIOR CLINICAL REVIEW within 1HR

TIME OF REVIEW: ☐☐ : ☐☐
ANTIBIOTICS REQUIRED:
☐ Yes ☐ No

NO AMBER FLAGS = ROUTINE CARE /CONSIDER OTHER DIAGNOSIS

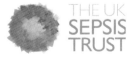

THE UK
SEPSIS
TRUST

UKST 2020 1.4 PAGE 1 OF 2

• **Fig. 47.10** Sepsis Screening Tool for Acute Assessment.

SEPSIS SCREENING TOOL - THE SEPSIS SIX

PREGNANT
OR UP TO 6 WEEKS POST-PREGNANCY

PATIENT DETAILS:

DATE:
NAME:
DESIGNATION:
SIGNATURE:

TIME:

COMPLETE ALL ACTIONS WITHIN ONE HOUR

01 ENSURE SENIOR CLINICIAN ATTENDS
NOT ALL PATIENTS WITH RED FLAGS WILL NEED THE 'SEPSIS 6' URGENTLY. A SENIOR DECISION
MAKER MAY SEEK ALTERNATIVE DIAGNOSES/ DE-ESCALATE CARE. RECORD DECISIONS BELOW
NAME: GRADE:

TIME
☐☐:☐☐

02 OXYGEN IF REQUIRED
START IF O_2 SATURATIONS LESS THAN 92% - AIM FOR O_2 SATURATIONS OF 94-98%
IF AT RISK OF HYPERCARBIA AIM FOR SATURATIONS OF 88-92%

TIME
☐☐:☐☐

03 OBTAIN IV ACCESS, TAKE BLOODS
BLOOD CULTURES, BLOOD GLUCOSE, LACTATE, FBC, U&Es, CRP AND CLOTTING
LUMBAR PUNCTURE IF INDICATED

TIME
☐☐:☐☐

04 GIVE IV ANTIBIOTICS
MAXIMUM DOSE BROAD SPECTRUM THERAPY
CONSIDER: LOCAL POLICY / ALLERGY STATUS / ANTIVIRALS

TIME
☐☐:☐☐

05 GIVE IV FLUIDS
GIVE FLUID BOLUS OF 20 ml/kg if age <16, 500ml if 16+
NICE RECOMMENDS USING LACTATE TO GUIDE FURTHER FLUID THERAPY

TIME
☐☐:☐☐

06 MONITOR
USE MEOWS. MEASURE URINARY OUTPUT: THIS MAY REQUIRE A URINARY CATHETER REPEAT LACTATE
AT LEAST ONCE PER HOUR IF INITIAL LACTATE ELEVATED OR IF CLINICAL CONDITION CHANGES

TIME
☐☐:☐☐

RED FLAGS AFTER ONE HOUR – ESCALATE TO CONSULTANT NOW

RECORD ADDITIONAL NOTES HERE:
e.g. allergy status, arrival of specialist teams, de-escalation of care, delayed antimicrobial decision making, variance

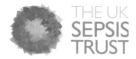

THE UK
SEPSIS
TRUST

UKST 2020 1.4 PAGE 2 OF 2

• **Fig. 47.10, cont'd**

A new MBRRACE report (Knight et al, 2023) was published at the time of this textbook going to print. There was a significant 33% increase in maternal death rates from direct causes between 2016–18 and 2019–21. COVID-19 was a leading cause of maternal death. Excluding the deaths due to COVID-19, the 2019–21 report showed morbidity and mortality rates are very similar to those reported in 2016 (Knight et al., 2016).

Of 2,066,997 women giving birth in the UK, **241** women died, giving a mortality rate of **11.7 women per** 100,000 during pregnancy or up to 6 weeks after childbirth or the end of pregnancy. Cardiovascular disorders and thrombosis and thromboembolism are now responsible for the same number of maternal deaths in the UK, followed by psychiatric disorders. Together, these three causes represent 38% of maternal deaths. Ethnicity and demography points remain unchanged. Chapter 30 summarizes the maternal deaths between 2018 and 2020 (Knight et al., 2022).

Main Points

- Forceps may be used to rotate the fetal head before traction is applied to complete the delivery or to apply traction only to complete delivery. It is necessary to confirm that there is no obstruction to the descent of the fetus before performing a forceps delivery.
- Maternal complications after forceps delivery include soft tissue damage to the lower uterine segment, cervix, vagina and perineum; bleeding from tissue trauma; retention of urine; post-delivery perineal pain; and dyspareunia.
- Neonatal complications can occur with operative delivery and include cephalhaematoma, abrasions, neonatal jaundice and intracranial haemorrhage.
- Equipment for vacuum extraction delivery has changed and cups are made of silastic and plastic with cup sizes of 5 cm or 6 cm.
- Midwives can be specially trained to perform this technique and can use the ventouse equipment for delivery if it is approved by their employing authority.
- Worldwide CS rates continue to rise. Even with modern surgical techniques it is still less safe for the woman than a vaginal delivery. During CS, the altered physiology of the woman increases the danger of acid aspiration syndrome but there are also other major hazards.
- Although many CSs are now performed under spinal or epidural anaesthesia, general anaesthesia is still used.

- Acid aspiration syndrome arises from the inhalation of acid gastric contents, resulting in chemical pneumonitis and ARDS. Prevention is essential, and antacid preparations and H_2 antagonists are recommended.
- Maternal collapse is defined as a sudden event involving the cardiorespiratory systems and/or brain, resulting in a reduced or absent conscious level (and potentially death) at any stage in pregnancy and up to 6 weeks after birth.
- Failure of the CVS to deliver oxygen to the body tissues may result in irreversible organ damage or death.
- Shock is reversible if detected early and prompt resuscitation measures put in place.
- The MEWS or MEOWS chart is a recognition tool to clearly indicate the subtle changes that act as warning for physiological signs of shock (i.e., tachypnoea and tachycardia).
- Significant changes in respiration are a red flag indicating urgent action is needed to prevent any further deterioration in the woman's condition.
- Sepsis is the immune system's overreaction to an infection or injury. If not treated immediately, sepsis can result in organ failure and death.
- Clinical red flags indicating sepsis include pyrexia, hypothermia, tachycardia, tachypnoea, hypoxia, hypotension, oliguria and reduced consciousness.

References

Bassett, S., 2017. Obstetric interventions. In: Macdonald, S., Johnson, G. (Eds.), Mayes' Midwifery: A Textbook for Midwifery, fifteenth ed. Elsevier, Edinburgh.

Bergholt, T., 2020. Caesarean section. In: Arulkumaran, S., Robson, M.S. (Eds.), Munro Kerr's Operative Obstetrics, thirteenth ed. Elsevier, Edinburgh.

Brennan, D.J., Jaraqemada, P.J.M., 2020. Uterine rupture. In: Arulkumaran, S., Robson, M.S. (Eds.), Munro Kerr's Operative Obstetrics, thirteenth ed. Elsevier, Edinburgh.

Chu, J., Johnston, T.A., Geoghegan, J., on behalf of the Royal College of Obstetricians and Gynaecologists, 2020. Maternal collapse in pregnancy and the puerperium. Br. J. Obstet. Gynaecol. 127 (5), e14–e52.

Cluver, C., Novikova, N., Hofmeyr, G.J., Hall, D.R., 2013. Maternal position during caesarean section for preventing maternal and neonatal complications. Cochrane Database Syst. Rev. 2013 (3), CD007623.

Cunningham, S., Hinshaw, K., 2020. Assisted vaginal delivery – non rotational forceps and manual rotation. In: Arulkumaran, S.,

Robson, M.S. (Eds.), Munro Kerr's Operative Obstetrics, thirteenth ed. Elsevier, Edinburgh.

Dunn, P.M., 1999. The Chamberlen family (1560–1728) and obstetric forceps. Arch. Dis. Child. Fetal Neonatal Ed. 81 (3), F232–F235.

Hayman, R., Raynor, M.D., 2020. Operative births. In: Marshall, J., Raynor, M. (Eds.), Myles' Textbook for Midwives, seventeenth ed. Elsevier, Edinburgh.

Kinsella, S.M., Winton, A.L., Mushambi, M.C., Ramaswamy, K., Swales, H., Quinn, A.C., et al., 2015. Failed tracheal intubation during obstetric general anaesthesia: a literature review. Int. J. Obstet. Anesth. 24 (4), 356–374.

Knight, M., Kenyon, S., Brocklehurst, P., Neilson, J., Shakespeare, J., Kurinczuk, J.J., on behalf of MBRRACE-UK, 2014. Saving Lives, Improving Mothers' Care: Surveillance of Maternal Deaths in the UK 2011–13 and Lessons Learned to Inform Maternity Care from the UK and Ireland Confidential Enquiries into Maternal Deaths and Morbidity 2009–13. University of Oxford, Oxford.

Knight, M., Noor, M., Tuffnell, D., Kenyon, S., Shakespeare, J., Brocklehurst, P., et al. 2016. Saving Lives, Improving Mothers' Care Surveillance of maternal deaths in the UK 2012–14 and lessons learned to inform maternity care from the UK and Ireland

Confidential Enquiries into Maternal Deaths and Morbidity 2009–14. Available at: https://www.npeu.ox.ac.uk/assets/downloads/mbrrace-uk/reports/MBRRACE-UK%20Maternal%20Report%202016%20-%20website.pdf.

Knight, M., Bunch, K., Tuffnell, D., Shakespeare, J., Kotnis, R., Kenyon, S., et al., on behalf of MBRRACE-UK, 2018. Saving Lives, Improving Mothers' Care: Lessons Learned to Inform Maternity Care from the UK and Ireland Confidential Enquiries into Maternal Deaths and Morbidity 2014–16. National Perinatal Epidemiology Unit, University of Oxford, Oxford.

Knight, M., Bunch, K., Patel, R., Shakespeare, J., Kotnis, R., Kenyon, S., et al., on behalf of MBRRACE-UK, 2022. Saving Lives, Improving Mothers' Care – Lessons Learned to Inform Maternity Care from the UK and Ireland Confidential Enquiries into Maternal Deaths and Morbidity 2018–20. National Perinatal Epidemiology Unit, University of Oxford, Oxford.

Knight, M., Bunch, K., Felker, A., Patel, R., Kotnis, R., Kenyon, S., et al. on behalf of MBRRACE-UK, 2023. Saving Lives, Improving Mothers' Care Core Report - Lessons learned to inform maternity care from the UK and Ireland Confidential Enquiries into Maternal Deaths and Morbidity 2019–21. Oxford: National Perinatal Epidemiology Unit, University of Oxford.

Lavender, T., Hofmeyr, G.J., Neilson, J.P., Kingdon, C., Gyte, G.M., 2012. Caesarean section for non-medical reasons at term. Cochrane Database Syst. Rev. 2012 (3), CD004660.

Maternity Early-Warning Score (MEWS). Available at: https://ihub.scot/media/6721/final-national-mews-chart_web.pdf

Murphy, D.J., Strachan, B.K., Bahl, R., on behalf of the Royal College of Obstetricians Gynaecologists, 2020. Assisted vaginal birth. Br. J. Obstet. Gynaecol. 127 (9), e70–e112.

National Institute for Health and Care Excellence (NICE), 2023a. Caesarean Birth. Available at: https://www.nice.org.uk/guidance/ng192/resources/caesarean-birth-pdf-66142078788805.

National Institute for Health and Care Excellence (NICE), 2023b. Anaesthesia (general). Available at: https://bnf.nice.org.uk/treatment-summaries/anaesthesia-general/

Neu, J., Rushing, J., 2011. Caesarean versus vaginal delivery: long term infant outcomes and the hygiene hypothesis. Clin. Perinatol. 38 (2), 321–331.

O'Brien, S., Siassakos, D., Hinshaw, K., 2020. Assisted vaginal delivery – an overview. In: Arulkumaran, S., Robson, M.S. (Eds.), Munro Kerr's Operative Obstetrics, thirteenth ed. Elsevier, Edinburgh.

Paranjothy, S., Griffiths, J.D., Broughton, H.K., Gyte, G.M., Brown, H.C., Thomas, J., 2014. Interventions at caesarean section for reducing the risk of aspiration pneumonitis. Cochrane Database Syst. Rev. 2014 (2), CD004943.

Renfrew, M.J., Homer, C.S.E., Downe, S., McFadden, A., 2014. Midwifery: An Executive Summary for the Lancet's Series. Available at: https://www.thelancet.com/pb/assets/raw/Lancet/stories/series/midwifery/midwifery_exec_summ.pdf.

Resuscitation Council UK, 2021. The ABCDE Approach. Available at: https://www.resus.org.uk/library/abcde-approach.

Ritter, J.M., Flower, R.S., Henderson, G., Loke, Y.K., MacEwan, D., Rang, H., 2019. Rang & Dale's Pharmacology, ninth ed. Elsevier, Edinburgh.

Royal College of Anaesthetists (RCOA), 2022. 2022 Edition of Guidelines for the Provision of Anaesthetic Services. Available at: https://rcoa.ac.uk/news/2022-edition-guidelines-provision-anaesthetic-services.

Soar, J., Böttiger, B.W., Carli, P., Couper, K., Deakin, C.D., Djärv, T., et al., 2021. Adult Advanced Life Support Guidelines. Available at: https://www.resus.org.uk/library/2021-resuscitation-guidelines/adult-advanced-life-support-guidelines.

Suwannachat, B., Lumbiganon, P., Laopaiboon, M., 2012. Rapid versus stepwise negative pressure application for vacuum extraction assisted vaginal delivery. Cochrane Database Syst. Rev. 2012 (8), CD006636.

UK Sepsis Trust, 2023. The UK Sepsis Trust. Available at: https://www.sepsistrust.org.

van den Akker, T., Hinshaw, K., 2020. Assisted vaginal delivery – vacuum. In: Arulkumaran, S., Robson, M.S. (Eds.), Munro Kerr's Operative Obstetrics, thirteenth ed. Elsevier, Edinburgh.

Verma, G.L., Spalding, J.J., Wilkinson, M.D., Hofmeyr, G.J., Vannevel, V., O'Mahony, F., 2021. Instruments for assisted vaginal birth. Cochrane Database Syst. Rev. 2021 (9), CD005455.

World Health Organization (WHO), 2018. WHO Recommendations: Non-clinical Interventions to Reduce Unnecessary Caesarean Sections. Available at: https://www.who.int/publications/i/item/9789241550338.

World Health Organization (WHO), 2021. Caesarean Section Rates Continue to Rise, amid Growing Inequalities in Access. Available at: https://www.who.int/news/item/16-06-2021-caesarean-section-rates-continue-to-rise-amid-growing-inequalities-in-access.

Annotated recommended reading

Murphy, D.J., Strachan, B.K., Bahl, R., on behalf of the Royal College of Obstetricians Gynaecologists, 2020. Assisted vaginal birth. Br. J. Obstet. Gynaecol. 127 (9), e70–e112.

National Institute for Health and Care Excellence (NICE), 2023. Caesarean Birth. Available at: https://www.nice.org.uk/guidance/ng192/resources/caesarean-birth-pdf-66142078788805.

These documents set out research-based guidelines for operative birth. They provide an excellent resource for midwives and obstetricians.

Arulkumaran, S., Robson, M.S., 2020. Munro Kerr's Operative Obstetrics, thirteenth ed. Elsevier, Edinburgh.

This book looks at operative delivery and is a useful resource to further explore these areas.

Royal College of Obstetricians and Gynaecologists (RCOG), 2019. Maternal Collapse in Pregnancy and the Puerperium (Green-top Guideline No. 56). Available at: https://www.rcog.org.uk/guidance/browse-all-guidance/green-top-guidelines/maternal-collapse-in-pregnancy-and-the-puerperium-green-top-guideline-no-56/.

This website provides access to the current guidelines for maternal collapse during and following pregnancy. The RCOG home webpage also provides a range of up-to-date related guidance on specific complications.

https://www.npeu.ox.ac.uk/mbrrace-uk/reports

This link provides access to previous and current MBRRACE reports.

Ockenden, D., 2022. Finding, Conclusions and Essential Actions from the Independent Review of Maternity Services at the Shrewsbury and Telford Hospital NHS Trust Final Report. UK Department of Health and Social Care. Available at: https://www.gov.uk/government/publications/final-report-of-the-ockenden-review.

Kirkup, B., 2022. Maternity and Neonatal Services in East Kent – the 'reading the Signals' Report. UK Department of Health and Social Care. Available at: https://www.gov.uk/government/publications/maternity-and-neonatal-services-in-east-kent-reading-the-signals-reports.

These two reports are essential reading for students and midwives.

Useful websites

https://www.resus.org.uk/library/abcde-approach.
www.sepsistrust.org.
https://www.npeu.ox.ac.uk/ukoss/current-surveillance.
https://www.rcog.org.uk/

Puerperium—The Baby as a Neonate

Section 4 considers the mother and her baby during the puerperium. In the postnatal period, midwives care for mothers/partners and their babies to support the transition to parenthood. It is essential that midwives are able to distinguish between normal appearances and behaviours of the mother and her baby and deal responsibly with any deviations present. Section 4A focuses on the baby. Chapters 48 and 49 provide a detailed account of the adaptation of the fetus to independent extrauterine life. The remaining chapters introduce some commonly encountered serious disorders that neonates can present with. Chapter 50 is about the care of the low-birthweight baby, Chapter 51 examines cardiac and respiratory problems, Chapter 52 is concerned with neonatal jaundice and some common metabolic disorders and Chapter 53 discusses problems arising from infection or trauma. These chapters provide fundamental information on the neonate at the level necessary for students and midwives to provide appropriate neonatal care. Specifically written neonatal textbooks provide more detailed and in-depth information. The interested reader is referred to one of the many excellent textbooks and papers within the chapter reference lists.

48

Adaptation to Extrauterine Life 1: Haematological, Cardiovascular, Respiratory and Genitourinary Considerations

THOMAS McEWAN

CHAPTER CONTENTS

Students and midwives should have a robust knowledge and understanding of the adaptation required by the newborn for successful extrauterine life. Within this chapter, those related to the haematological, cardiovascular, respiratory and genitourinary systems are considered.

Introduction

Understanding the complex anatomical features and physiological processes provides the practitioner with a foundation for the competent assessment of the neonate. For clarity, the masculine pronoun is used to distinguish the neonate from his mother.

This chapter considers many anatomical, physiological and biochemical adaptations that characterize the transition of a term fetus to an independent neonate. Throughout intrauterine life, fetal survival is dependent on the mother. However, at birth anatomical, physiological and biochemical changes contribute to independent extrauterine life. Every system contributes to the ever-changing homeostatic conditions crucial to independence. The respiratory and cardiovascular systems are amongst the first to respond. They initiate changes leading to a considerable rise in the partial pressure of carbon dioxide (PCO_2) in the neonate's blood. This initiates the respiratory drive that enables the neonate to take the first breath and maintain effective respiration. Blood oxygen content increases and favourable haemodynamic changes support and adjust cardiorespiratory functions, affecting oxygen perfusion of every organ and system. Oxygen supports cell metabolism and the production of energy while metabolic waste is efficiently eliminated. It is important that healthcare practitioners understand the complex changes that occur at this stage of life.

The Appearance of the Normal Neonate

The following information provides a general overview of the common findings within a general examination of the neonate. For those conducting the Newborn and Infant Physical Examination, the related chapter in *Myles Textbook for Midwives* "Recognising the healthy baby at term through examination of the newborn screening" may be of interest (Ransome & Marshall, 2020).

General Appearance and the Skin and Hair at Birth

At 40 weeks' gestation, the **neonate** weighs about 3500–4000 g and averages 50–55 cm in length. His occipitofrontal head circumference averages 35 cm, making his head almost 25% of total body mass; the brain weighs between

300 and 400 g (Collins, Hall & Brown, 2021). A healthy neonate appears plump with a rounded abdomen, largely due to deposition of subcutaneous fat and water. At birth, the upper and lower limbs are of a similar length, although primary ossification is present only in the upper limbs. All four limbs should have five separated digits with well-formed nails and well-defined palmar and sole features.

Fine hair usually covers the scalp. Some neonates appear fairly bald, but others have luxuriant straight or curly hair. Abnormally unruly hair on the forehead or the back of the head and neck, especially when accompanied by unusual facies, may imply underlying genetic or chromosomal problems (Boardman, Groves & Ramasethu, 2021). Remnants of **lanugo,** the fine hair that covers the entire body during the second and third trimesters of pregnancy, may be present if the neonate is premature. The degree of skin pigmentation is determined by the neonate's gestation and the ethnicity of his natural parents.

In healthy neonates, the skin, mucous membranes and nails should be a good colour, indicating favourable tissue perfusion and oxygenation. Generally, pigmentation of the nipples and genitalia is deeper in neonates with darker skin complexions. Some normal skin components are summarized in Table 48.1.

Posture and Crying

After birth, most neonates lie in a flexed position emulating the fetal position and resisting limb extension. Once their arms are extended, neonates show a tendency, possibly by reflex, to move both arms outwards. When placed on their back, there is a distinctive tendency to turn their heads spontaneously to one side. Conversely, when placed in the prone position, neonates tend to draw their knees under their abdomen, elevating their buttocks and turning their head to one side. At term, healthy neonates are active and should move all four limbs spontaneously. These postural phenomena may not be evident in premature neonates due to the structural immaturity of the neural and locomotor systems.

Crying is a physiological response to many different stimuli. The duration and type of crying vary with the severity of the distress (see Chapter 57), and attentive mothers quickly learn to discern between the different types of crying. Kline et al. (2018) suggest that a 2-week-old neonate may cry intermittently on average 2 hours per day, increasing to 3 hours per day by 6 weeks of age. Thereafter, crying reduces to about 1 hour per day as most healthy babies are physically more comfortable and secure.

Eyes

Competent examination of a neonate's eyes requires knowledge, skills and patience. The external appearance of the eyes can reflect ethnicity. **Epicanthic folds** (vertical pleats of skin that overlap the medial angles of the eyes) are common in neonates of Asian origin and are also noted in those born with Down syndrome. It is important to establish the

TABLE 48.1	Normal Skin Components
Linea nigra	A dark vertical line that may be present in the lower abdominal midline, especially in those with more pigmented skin.
Slate grey nevus	Depending on ethnic origin, a diffuse bluish-black skin colouration that may be present, usually over the sacrum. Previously referred to as a Mongolian blue spot.
Sebaceous glands	Humans are unique amongst primates in having large sebaceous glands that produce sebum over the scalp, face and upper back. These glands are very active in utero, producing waxy substances that mix with dead skin cells and form vernix caseosa, which initially covers the entire fetal skin. Term neonates show only residual vernix caseosa being present.
Milia	Distended sebaceous glands that may present over the nose, forehead and chin.
Eccrine glands (sweat glands)	Eccrine glands first appear in fetuses at 5 months of gestation on the palms and the soles of its feet. They are used for sweat cooling when the body temperature rises above a critical physiological point (Lakshminrusimha & Carlton, 2018). Although the eccrine glands are inactive for the first few days of life, most neonates experience a regional eccrine gland maturation in the craniocaudal direction, with the earliest perspiration occurring on the forehead followed by the chest, upper arms and then the rest of the body (Collins, Hall & Brown, 2021).
Apocrine glands (scent glands)	Apocrine glands develop throughout the body. By 7 months, the apocrine glands disappear except for in the armpits, pubic area and around the nipples and lips, while the eccrine glands continue to spread all over the body.

structural features of the eyes, and gentle attempts should be made to establish their presence, position, relative size and shape. Gross structural anomalies should be identified promptly. The colour of the neonate's eyes are generally dark blue-grey, although some dark-skinned neonates tend to have brown eyes at birth. Permanent colouring of the iris may take several years to develop.

Assessing a neonate's vision by an observed reaction to light is adequate unless significant structural anomalies warrant a fuller assessment. Assessment of vision is best achieved when the neonate is content but alert, although neonates startle in response to a bright light even if their eyelids are closed, indicating that the optic pathways are functioning (Boardman, Groves & Ramasethu, 2021).

Neonates cannot generally produce naturally lubricating and antiseptic tears. This contributes to a higher incidence of eye infections such as conjunctivitis, often further complicated by temporary blockage of the lacrimal ducts, which under normal conditions help to keep the conjunctiva moist and clean. Boardman, Groves and Ramasethu (2021) advocate that any symptoms of tearing or persistent discharge from the eyes appearing after the second day after birth should be investigated to exclude underlying pathology or acquired infection.

Ears

A considerable range of factors, including the amounts of cartilage and activity of the auricular muscles, determine the shape, position and resistance to deformation of the external ears. Both ears should be placed symmetrically on either side of head. The position of the ear lobes generally approximates with the vertical distance from the arch of the brow to the lower parts of the nose (Boardman, Groves & Ramasethu, 2021). Preauricular pits and skin appendages are fairly common (Lakshminrusimha & Carlton, 2018), but more significant malformations, low-set ears and other dysmorphic features may be associated with urogenital malformations, deafness and autosomal-dominant problems. Alert neonates with normal auditory capability are startled or cry in response to sudden, unaccustomed loud noise and turn spontaneously towards human speech. The absence of such behaviours requires more systematic audiometry assessments.

Nose

Most neonates are obligate nose-breathers, and their respiratory function depends on the patency of both nares. Nasal deformities and nasolacrimal duct obstructions should be excluded. Although unilateral or bilateral anatomical obstructions caused by choanal atresia are rare, these must be ruled out, especially in neonates who develop respiratory difficulties and cyanosis soon after birth or during feeding.

Mouth and Throat

The shape of the mouth and oral cavity is partly determined by neuromotor activity that occurs during fetal life. The tongue, buccal surfaces, palate, uvula and posterior aspects of the oral cavity should be inspected visually, but the gum and hard palate are best examined by gentle finger palpation. This careful visual and digital examination is required to exclude palate deformities. Healthy neonates should have a gag reflex and usually suckle vigorously on a finger. In some neonates, the tongue may be attached to a short central frenulum, but this anomaly rarely interferes with feeding or later speech development. The presence of facial asymmetries on feeding or crying may suggest facial nerve paresis.

Neck and Chest

Mature neonates have a full range of spontaneous neck movements despite the short neck and the weak muscles, incapable of supporting the weight of the head. The absence of or abnormalities in spontaneous movements may indicate cervical spine abnormalities or the presence of space-occupying lesions such as goitre or cystic hygromas which may compress and distort the trachea, causing inspiratory obstruction. In instances where the phrenic nerve(s) is damaged, the neonate will develop corresponding paralysis of the diaphragm with respiratory difficulties. The chest at term should be symmetrical, barrel-shaped with a prominent xiphoid sternum and compliant ribs. The chest circumference is generally 1–2 cm less than the head circumference. The neonate's lung sounds are more tubular than vesicular due to better sound transmission from the large airways across the small chest.

Major Systemic Characteristics of the Neonate

The Haematological System

Circulatory Volume

The separation of the fetus from the placental circulation after birth is a major physiological event. The **umbilical arteries** taking deoxygenated blood from the fetus to the placenta for oxygenation constrict while the umbilical vein remains dilated, limiting fetal blood loss. Fetoplacental blood volume varies from 110–120 mL/kg (Kline et al., 2018) throughout the latter parts of pregnancy, although approximately 80 mL/kg of this blood is probably in the neonate. Clamping of the umbilical cord after birth, which stops all blood flow, is an important haemodynamic step for the neonate.

Deferred Clamping of the Umbilical Cord

Although no consistent definition or guideline for the practice exists, deferred cord clamping (DCC) is accepted and supported by most international professional bodies (Peberdy et al., 2022). It improves haemodynamic parameters during the transition to extrauterine life, lowers the incidence of anaemia and improves neurodevelopment (Bruckner, Katheria & Schmölzer, 2021). As such, both the National Institute of Health and Care Excellence (NICE) and the Royal College of Obstetricians and Gynaecologists (RCOG) recommend routine DCC, subject to some clinical considerations (NICE, 2023; RCOG, 2015). The reader is referred to this literature for a more detailed account.

Adaptations in the Neonate's Haematological Parameters

Circulating blood volume at term averages 85–90 mL/kg of bodyweight (Sinha, Miall & Jardine, 2018). Haemopoiesis proceeds at a relatively steady pace and is highly responsive, with a unique capacity to upregulate or downregulate the

---

• BOX 48.1   **Genetic, Epigenetic and Physiological Variables**

Genetic, epigenetic and a range of physiological variables influence the differentiation of the red bone marrow's pluripotent stem cells into mature blood (Pocock, Richards & Richards, 2017). These include haematopoietic growth factors, such as granulocyte colony-stimulating factor (G-CSF), granulocyte–macrophage CSF (GM-CSF), interleukin 6 (IL-6) and IL-8 (see Chapter 29).

• BOX 48.2   **Primary Function of Haemoglobin**

A primary function of haemoglobin is to combine reversibly with oxygen and carbon dioxide, allowing the delivery of oxygen from the lungs to the tissues to support cellular metabolism (see Chapter 18). This function is best demonstrated by the oxygen dissociation curve, whereby the oxygen saturation of the blood is plotted against oxygen tension or partial pressure of the whole blood (Pocock, Richards & Richards, 2017). Due to the high concentration of fetal haemoglobin (HbF) in healthy neonates, the oxygen dissociation curve is placed firmly to the left, denoting its high oxygen affinity. This phenomenon is necessary for efficient extraction of oxygen from the maternal circulation during fetal life. After birth HbF, while capable of extracting large quantities of oxygen in the lungs, releases oxygen to the tissues only as needed.

---

production of any cell type on demand. This responsiveness is also crucial in ensuring that the transition in the composition of the neonate's blood is successful. Genetic, epigenetic and physiological variables are summarized in Box 48.1. Changes continue during the transitional period of the first week of life with fetal haemoglobin (HbF) being gradually replaced by adult haemoglobin (HbA), which is more suited to extrauterine life. The complex processes that regulate haemopoiesis lead to equilibrium between cell production, maturation, function and biodegradation. The neonate's blood cells gradually change from their fetal state to that of the child in whom mature **erythrocytes** function for 120 days, **platelets** for 10 days and **neutrophils** for 6–8 h.

The erythrocyte count at birth averages $5.1–5.3 \times 10^{-6}$ cells/mm^3 in term infants and $4.6–5.3 \ 10^{-6}$ cells/mm^3 for preterm infants (Boardman, Groves & Ramasethu, 2021). Because many of these erythrocytes are nucleated or contain HbF, they are rapidly degraded by the reticuloendothelial system, and it is unusual to find nucleated erythrocytes in circulation after the first week of extrauterine life. The earliest erythrocytes are **normoblasts,** which differentiate into **reticulocytes** and subsequently mature into erythrocytes containing predominantly HbA.

The maturation of precursor cells into competent erythrocytes is controlled by a vast range of factors, including **erythropoietin,** which is produced in the liver during fetal life and the kidneys after birth. Erythropoietin binds to specific receptor sites found in the membrane of myelocytic cells and erythroblasts, accelerating their differentiation and maturation, respectively, by mechanisms that are not fully understood (Pocock, Richards & Richards, 2017). Normal erythropoiesis also depends on the presence of iron, vitamin C and the vitamin B group.

The relative increase in erythrocytes due to **plasma reduction** and **haemoconcentration,** which occurs in the first few hours to days of life, is a transitional phenomenon, corrected by the rapid destruction of excess erythrocytes which occurs after birth. A more physiological erythrocyte count is achieved by 6 months (Andersen et al., 2018). Nucleated, immature erythrocytes are seen in large numbers during the first 24 hours after birth, possibly due to stressors associated with birth, but these usually disappear within 4 days. Significantly, the fetal blood erythropoietin values observed during intrauterine life fall within the first 24 hours, gradually returning to physiological values during the first 2–3

months after birth. This coincides with the steady resumption of erythropoiesis. Erythrocytes are more specialized in composition than most other cells because of the presence of haemoglobin, which accounts for 95% of total cellular protein content. The primary function of haemoglobin is summarized in Box 48.2.

In healthy term neonates, haemoglobin ranges from 15–23.5 g/dL (Sinha, Miall & Jardine, 2018). This may increase slightly over the first 24 hours due to a shift in fluid distribution, associated diuresis, reduction in circulating blood volume and haemoconcentration. There is a gradual reduction in HbF concentration back to umbilical cord blood values by the end of the first week of life. By 3 months, the haemoglobin level in healthy infants tends to fall to around 12 g/dL (Andersen et al., 2018). As new erythrocytes are produced, the rate of HbF production is reduced and the rate of HbA production increases so that at 4 months of age the average healthy child has less than 20% of HbF.

Affinity of HbF and HbA to oxygen is influenced by pH, Pco_2, 2,3-diphosphoglycerate (2,3-DPG) and blood temperature. After birth, the shift in the **oxygen dissociation curve** to the right is partly attributable to organic phosphates, which decrease the affinity of HbA to oxygen by competing for the same binding sites.

2,3-DPG is formed during anaerobic glycolysis (mature erythrocytes lack mitochondria and their glucose metabolism is anaerobic) and enhances the release of oxygen from haemoglobin. HbF has a lower affinity for 2,3-DPG than HbA and can bind oxygen more tenaciously. This accounts for the shift of the oxygen dissociation curve to the left in the fetus and neonate. Finally, the postnatal shift of the oxygen dissociation curve to the right is directly attributable to the gradual replacement of HbF by HbA, thus enhancing oxygen release to the tissues (Marieb & Hoehn, 2022).

White blood cells (WBCs) defend the body against genetically different antigens (see Chapter 29). At birth, most neonates show an initial increase in the number of circulating WBCs, possibly provoked by the stress of birth. However gradual reduction in these cells brings about normal WBC values by the fifth day after birth. The two main functions of WBCs are **phagocytosis** and **competent immune response** (see Chapter 29). In neonates, neutrophils make up approximately 50% and lymphocytes about 30% of the total WBCs. However the proportion of lymphocytes increases rapidly within the first few months to an average of 60%, and this value persists for the first 2 years of life. Monocytes are the most abundant cells in the first few weeks of extrauterine life but gradually decline to the much lower adult value.

A range of structural and biochemical differences exist in the immature neutrophils and lymphocytes, which may contribute to their less effective response to infection. For instance, cell immaturity may interfere with intracellular signal transduction or hinder cell mobility because of cytoskeletal rigidity and poor microfilament contraction. These factors could also affect neutrophil migration from capillary blood into the surrounding tissue, which may compromise tissue healing after injury.

Haemostasis (see Chapter 16) depends on the interaction between injured vessels, **platelets** and a group of **clot-promoting factors (coagulation system).** However neonates are most likely considered to be at risk of spontaneous bleeding between the third and sixth days of life due to the relative deficiency of **vitamin K,** which, amongst other functions, plays important roles in the synthesis of important clotting factors within the liver. Vitamin K is often administered to neonates at birth. However because a constant supply of vitamin K is required, milk feeding is the best means of colonizing the neonate's sterile gastrointestinal tract by bacteria capable of synthesizing it. It is worth noting that when the neonate requires treatment with broad-spectrum antimicrobials, the vitamin K–producing bacteria may be destroyed, leaving the neonate with low vitamin K and increased risk of bleeding. Vitamin K and haemorrhagic disease of the newborn (HDN) are outlined in Clinical Application 48.1.

The Cardiovascular System
The Fundamentals of Fetal Circulation

Successful transition from fetal to extrauterine life is dependent on gradual adaptation of the **fetal circulation** (Fig. 48.1) to the anatomical configuration that characterizes the adult cardiovascular system (Fig. 48.2). Under normal conditions, immediate changes take place within the first 60 s, although full cardiovascular transformation can take up to several weeks or months. The neonate's first breath followed by sustained spontaneous respiration contributes to the successful transition by ensuring that the lungs hold sufficient oxygenated air required to support pulmonary gas exchange. In addition, several anatomical modifications need to be made, closing specific cardiovascular structures and establishing a dual circulatory network capable of supporting the uniqueness of the pulmonary and systemic circulation.

The blood vessels and structures that transport blood between the fetus and placenta are described in Box 48.3.

> **• CLINICAL APPLICATION 48.1** **Vitamin K and Haemorrhagic Disease of the Newborn (HDN)**
>
> The reduction of vitamin K and clotting factors results from poor placental transfer of vitamin K to the fetus and the absence of appropriate fetal intestinal flora. There is a further decline in these factors over the first few days after birth, particularly in breastfed babies, because breastmilk contains lower levels of vitamin K. Breastfed babies may eventually develop prolonged prothrombin deficiency which could contribute to HDN or vitamin K-deficiency bleeding, which occurs in an estimated 35 per 100,000 live births, reducing to 8.8 per 100,000 live births in high-income countries (Sankar et al., 2016).
>
> The awareness of some of the benefits of vitamin K has resulted in its prophylactic administration (since the 1950s) to neonates at risk of spontaneous haemorrhage, especially within the gastrointestinal tract, resulting in **haematemesis** and the passage of **melaena stools**. Bleeding from the umbilical cord and the more serious risk of **intracranial haemorrhage** in susceptible premature and hypoxic neonates must also be guarded against.
>
> Although some past controversy regarding the intramuscular administration of vitamin K exists (see Golding et al., 1992, later refuted by Ekelund et al., 1993; Hull, 1992; Kline et al., 2018; Merenstein et al., 1993), current evidence recommends all babies should receive vitamin K prophylaxis (Jullien, 2021). This is preferably by intramuscular administration of a single dose of 1 mg phytomenadione (vitamin K). The oral route requires multiple doses in exclusively breastfed babies and is also dependent on the formulation used.
>
> Mature **platelets** (see Chapter 16) are complex fragments of megakaryocytes released into circulation when required to support normal coagulation. Platelets enjoy a lifespan of 10 days when structurally intact. The platelet surface properties, as well as their internal constituents, play crucial roles in haemostasis. Platelet counts in adults range from 150–400 $\times$ 10^9/L and, although term neonates show similar values, premature neonates frequently have lower values (Boardman, Groves & Ramasethu, 2021). Furthermore the release of stored substances enhancing the clotting cascade may be reduced, further compromising the neonate's ability to form insoluble clots in injured blood vessels. For instance, the lack of vitamin K reduces **prothrombin** values and clotting factors such as **factors VII, IX** and **X**. Neonatal fibrinogen levels are similar to those of adults, so it is important that an effective fibrinolytic system exists to limit blood clot formation either at any vessel injury or within intact blood vessels. To achieve a balance between clot formation and fibrinolysis, the fibrinolytic system is activated simultaneously with the coagulation system (Andersen et al., 2018).

The ductus venosus lies between the layers of the lesser omentum in a groove between the left and caudate lobes of the liver (Collins, Hall & Brown, 2021). It connects the umbilical vein to the left hepatic vein or the inferior vena cava. Obliteration of this vessel is gradual, initiated in the second week after birth at the portal vein end and moves gradually towards the vena cava. Its lumen tends to be completely closed by the second or third month. The hypogastric arteries branch off from the internal iliac arteries, enter the umbilical cord and become the umbilical arteries. The ductus arteriosus leads from the bifurcation of the pulmonary arteries to the

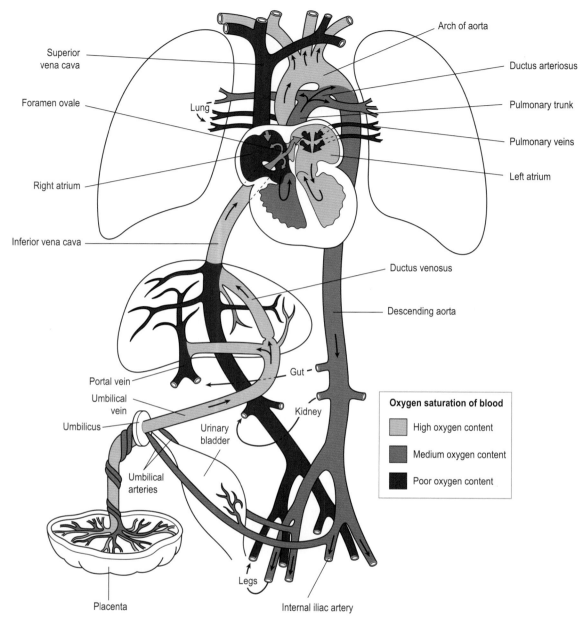

• **Fig. 48.1** Schematic illustration of the fetal circulation. The colours indicate the oxygen saturation of the blood, and the arrows show the course of the blood from the placenta to the heart. The organs are not drawn to scale. Observe that three shunts permit most of the blood to bypass the liver and lungs: ductus venosus, foramen ovale and ductus arteriosus. The poorly oxygenated blood returns to the placenta for oxygen and nutrients through the umbilical arteries.

aortic arch, entering it just after the exit of the subclavian and carotid arteries. The membranous foramen ovale is about 4–6 mm in length and 3–4 mm in width (Collins, Hall & Brown, 2021), located within the atrial septum and diverts blood away from the lungs during intrauterine life.

The path taken by the fetal blood flow, referred to as the *fetal circulation,* begins at the placenta. The sequence of events is best understood by reading the following résumé and referring to Fig. 48.1:

- Oxygenated blood flows from the placenta to the fetus via a single umbilical vein.
- Some of this blood enters the liver directly, reaching the inferior vena cava via the hepatic veins. A considerable

amount of blood circulates through the liver with the portal venous blood before also entering the hepatic veins.

- Blood from the ductus venosus and hepatic veins mixes in the inferior vena cava with the deoxygenated blood returning from the lower limbs and abdominal wall. This reduces the oxygen content of the blood contained in the upper parts of the inferior vena cava.
- As the inferior vena cava enters the heart, its position is aligned with the foramen ovale. The free edge of the atrial septum (the crista dividens) separates the blood flow into two streams. Most of this blood passes from the right atrium through the foramen ovale to the left atrium,

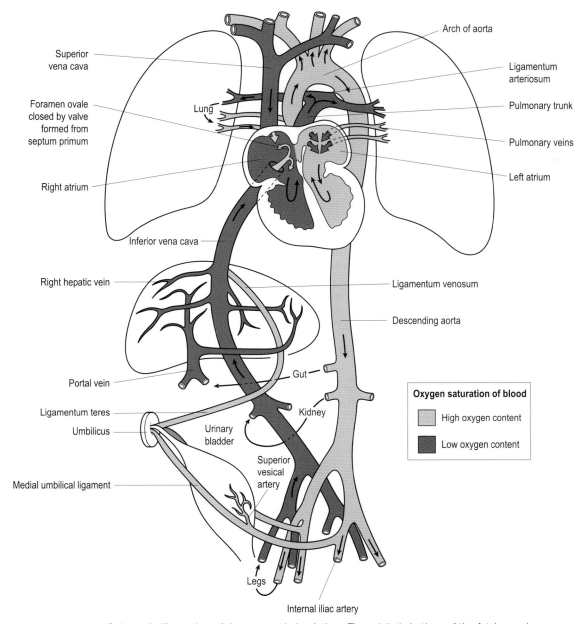

• **Fig. 48.2** Schematic illustration of the neonatal circulation. The adult derivatives of the fetal vessels and structures that become nonfunctional at birth are also shown. The arrows indicate the course of the blood in the infant. The organs are not drawn to scale. After birth, the three shunts that short-circuited the blood during fetal life cease to function and the pulmonary and systemic circulations become separated.

• BOX 48.3 Fetal Circulation Vessels and Structures

The **umbilical vein** carries blood to the fetus. fetus. This vein branches internally to connect with the **ductus venosus** and the **portal vein**.

The umbilical arteries return blood from the fetus to the placenta, connected to the internal iliac arteries (or hypogastrc arteries).

Right-to-left shunts that allow 90% of blood flow to bypass the lungs are created by two components of the fetal circulation. The **ductus arteriosus** is located between the pulmonary artery and aorta. The **foramen ovale** is located in the membranous septum and divides the right and left atria.

creating a right-to-left shunt. From the left atrium, the blood flows to the left ventricle and then to the aorta, which distributes the oxygenated blood to the head and upper body.

• Significant amounts of the right atrial blood pass through the tricuspid valve into the right ventricle. This engagement of the right ventricle contributes to the morphological development of the ventricle, the pulmonary artery and their respective valves and ensures that the pulmonary artery directs a small quantity (10%) of oxygenated blood to the lung tissue. The remaining 90% of this blood is directed into the aorta via the second right-to-left shunt, the ductus arteriosus found between the pulmonary artery and aorta. As oxygenated and deoxygenated blood mix along the different sections of the fetal circulation, the upper part of the descending aorta carries mixed oxygenated blood, which is distributed via the iliac arteries to the lower limbs and some abdominal and pelvic organs.

- Deoxygenated blood from the head and neck returns to the right atrium via the superior vena cava. Here, this stream of blood crosses the stream of blood coming from the inferior vena cava en route to the right ventricle, thus reducing the oxygen content of that blood even further. The two streams in the right atrium remain separate due to the atrial shape, although there is some mixing of about 25% of the blood, allowing oxygen and nutrients to be taken to the lungs.

- By the time the circulating blood enters the internal iliac arteries, its oxygen content is significantly reduced as it returns to the placenta via the two umbilical arteries for reoxygenation, uptake of nutrients and elimination of metabolic waste products. Fetal metabolic waste is removed via the placental circulation into the maternal circulation and then eliminated via the mother's kidneys.

Résumé of Cardiovascular and Haemodynamic Changes at Birth

Some of the unique features of the fetal circulation must adapt at birth, or shortly thereafter, if the neonate is to survive independently. This adaptation to extrauterine life depends largely on the interplay between the cardiovascular and respiratory systems:

- The separation of the neonate from the placental circulation results in the cessation of blood flow, which contributes to the collapse of the umbilical vein and arteries. The **ductus venosus** and the **hypogastric arteries** gradually fibrose, giving rise to supporting ligaments.

- The resulting reduction in blood flow to the right atrium causes a fall in the right atrial pressure. As blood flow through the hypogastric arteries ceases, a significant volume of blood is contained in smaller systemic compartments, which increases systemic vascular resistance and improves venous and arterial returns to the heart and lungs. As larger quantities of blood are returned from the lungs to the left atrium via the pulmonary veins, the left atrial pressure rises, closing the **foramen ovale.**

- The initial equalizing of pressures in the two atria holds the flap of the foramen ovale in position, stopping the shunting of blood from the right-to-left atrium. However the foramen ovale can reopen and remain patent for a few days or weeks, especially if left atrial pressure falls.

- As the baby takes his first breath, the lungs expand and oxygenated air is inspired. This displaces the pulmonary fluid further and triggers mechanisms essential to effective respiration and pulmonary gas exchange. Oxygen content of the blood increases, causing vasodilation in the pulmonary vascular bed. Consequently, the pulmonary vascular resistance falls by 80%, dramatically increasing pulmonary blood flow.

- At the same time, the amount of blood being shunted via the ductus arteriosus decreases and, as oxygen tension in the blood rises, the oxygen-sensitive fibromuscular tissue in this ductus constricts, eventually closing this short vessel. In some neonates, the patency of the **ductus arteriosus** may persist for a few days or weeks, especially in premature infants and those born with cardiovascular and respiratory anomalies.

The obsolete structures reform and serve as ligaments in the following manner:
- The umbilical vein becomes the ligamentum teres.
- The ductus venosus becomes the ligamentum venosum.
- The ductus arteriosus becomes the ligamentum arteriosum.
- The foramen ovale becomes the fossa ovalis.
- The hypogastric arteries are known as the *obliterated hypogastric arteries.*

A small number of infants with unresolved respiratory or cardiac disorders will experience various degrees of persistent fetal circulation (or persistent pulmonary hypertension of the newborn [PPHN]). This will require careful diagnostic and therapeutic interventions (see Chapter 51).

It is now appreciated that neonates should undergo thorough cardiovascular assessment in conjunction with the Apgar score. At birth, most neonates will manifest heart murmurs, although these may disappear within 12 hours. The heart rate varies from 110–160 bpm and blood pressure may average 80/40 mmHg (Kline et al., 2018). Most neonates experience a gradual reduction in heart rate and increase in blood pressure within the first few days after birth.

The Respiratory System

At term, the acinar portion of the fetal lung is well developed and more than 25% of **true alveoli** are present (Fig. 48.3). However because the pulmonary blood vessels are quite narrow, only a small amount of blood perfuses the lungs. This is adequate for meeting the metabolic needs of pulmonary tissue because the fetus obtains oxygen and excretes carbon dioxide via the placenta and maternal circulation; the fetal lungs are not required for gas exchange. At term, the lungs hold about 25 mL/kg of **pulmonary fluid,** which is partially expelled when the chest is compressed during vaginal delivery. The remaining fluid is absorbed by the lymphatic and pulmonary vessels and returned into the cardiovascular system. The fetus exercises its muscles of respiration, particularly the diaphragm, by making irregular fetal breathing movements. This activity may encourage muscle development to prepare for independent respiration.

Surfactant

From about 32 weeks' gestation, increasing amounts of **surfactant,** produced by alveolar type II pneumocytes, prepare the lungs for effective gas exchange after birth. Surfactant is composed of several **phospholipids** and specialized **protein molecules.** After the successful first breath, these jointly

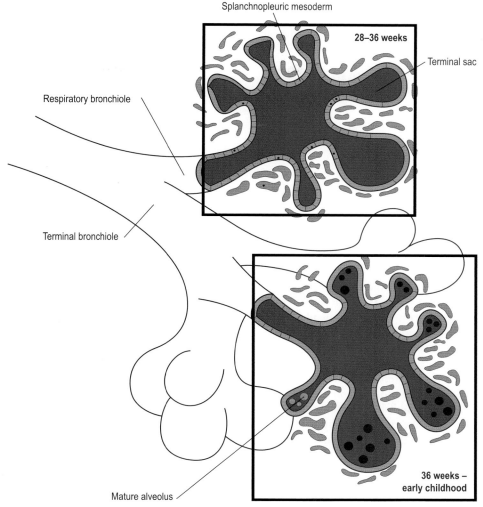

• **Fig. 48.3** Maturation of the lung tissue. Terminal sacs (primitive alveoli) begin to form between weeks 28 and 36 and begin to mature between 36 weeks and birth. Only 5–20% of all terminal sacs produced by the age of 8 years, however, are formed before birth.

reduce the **surface tension** of the alveolar fluid, thin out the alveolar membrane and increase the surface area for gas exchange. Glucocorticoids and thyroid hormones regulate the synthesis of surfactant in late fetal life (Sinha, Miall & Jardine, 2018). **Platelet-activating factor** stimulates the production of the phospholipids by triggering enzyme activities within the type II pneumocytes (Depicolzuane, Phelps & Floros, 2022; Whitsett, Wert & Weaver, 2015). At term, surfactant forms a monolayer lining within the alveoli, which acts as an air–liquid interface, reducing the surface tension within the terminal alveolar sacs (imagine blowing a soap bubble). This facilitates inspiration and prevents the alveoli from collapsing with each expiration.

Onset of Respirations

Most neonates gasp within the first few seconds of birth and establish regular respiration within minutes. It is important that this adaptation happens without delay to support the body's cellular metabolic needs by providing oxygen and removing carbon dioxide. The **respiratory centre** in the medulla oblongata matches respiratory effort to metabolic needs. **Chemoreceptors** and **stretch reflexes** influence the medulla oblongata's contribution to respiration, although the neonate's response to chemoreceptor stimuli is generally weak.

During birth, a reduction in blood oxygen values **(physiological hypoxia)** accompanied by a simultaneous accumulation of carbon dioxide **(physiological hypercarbia)** establishes a new respiratory drive within the medulla oblongata capable of sustaining successful pulmonary ventilation. Furthermore, the gradual elimination of the pulmonary fluid combined with the expansion of the pulmonary vascular bed and the elastic recoil of the respiratory muscles and the rib cage generates a negative pressure of up to 9.8 kPa, which assists in the taking of the first breath and subsequent sustained respiratory function (Ransome & Marshall, 2020). At the first inspiration, the diaphragm contracts strongly and the compliant ribs and sternum are pulled into

- Compression of the chest wall during vaginal delivery and the recoil of the chest wall immediately after birth.
- Chemoreceptor stimulation by the reduction in oxygen and increase in carbon dioxide in the blood.
- Sensory stimuli on the skin, such as touch, pressure and low environmental temperature.
- Stimulation of the senses by light, noise and touch.

a concave shape, but subsequent breaths require much less active work. The factors that initiate the first breath and lung expansion are summarized in Box 48.4.

The respiratory rate in a healthy neonate ranges from 30–60 breaths/min. However neonatal respiration is characteristically **irregular** with short periods of **apnoea** and involves the abdominal muscles. Although inspiration and expiration are initially energy-dependent, once established, the control of respiratory effort is thought to be like that in older children. However the inspiratory and expiratory time ratios in neonates and infants average 1:1 (i.e., the inspiration phase equals the expiratory phase).

Inflation of a normal lung in a term neonate is completed within the first few breaths, and most alveoli are expanded within the first few hours, establishing a lung volume of approximately 25 mL/kg bodyweight. The rhythmic inflation of the lungs encourages the **intra-alveolar fluid** to move into the peribronchial and perivascular spaces from which the pulmonary fluid is absorbed into the local blood and lymph vessels and sent to the heart. Delays in the removal of this fluid interfere with the efficiency of respiratory gas transfer, compromise lung compliance and functional residual capacity, and eventually cause significant cardiorespiratory distress, especially in immature neonates.

The Urinary System

Neonatal kidneys differ from that of the older child in both **glomerular** and **tubular function,** and its lobular appearance is different from the mature kidney. By 35 weeks' gestation, the fetal kidney has a full complement of **nephrons,** although these may be shorter and not as functionally mature. The **cortex** is morphologically more mature than the **medulla** by the end of the 36th week of gestation and **nephrogenesis** is believed to cease at this time, with each kidney having a complement of between 850,000 and 1,000,000 nephrons (Kline et al., 2018). In premature babies, nephrogenesis appears to continue for a variable period.

Postnatal Development of the Kidneys

At birth, the kidneys are lobulated and rounded in shape but capable of responding rapidly to haemodynamic changes and to endogenous and exogenous stressors. The clamping of the umbilical cord is one signal that increases renal function, and the kidneys take over the control of fluid, electrolyte, acid–base balance and the excretion of metabolic wastes. From a value of 10 mL/min/m^2 in term neonates, **glomerular filtration rate** (GFR) doubles during the neonate's first 2 weeks. The GFR is lower in very premature neonates but is gradually corrected as the glomeruli mature.

Although clamping of the umbilical cord is fundamental, the most likely factors enhancing renal maturation and function are the haemodynamic changes occurring at birth (Collins, Hall & Brown, 2021). These culminate in a decrease in **renal vascular resistance** and a corresponding increase in **systemic blood pressure,** thus improving filtration pressure. **Vasoactive substances** such as prostaglandins and prostacyclins also help mediate the renal haemodynamic changes and facilitate renal blood flow to enhance GFR.

Renal growth in early infancy depends on hypertrophy of existing microstructures within the pyramids. Kidney size correlates well with age and somatic growth, but the rate of glomerular growth varies and immature glomeruli may be present for months after birth, especially in premature neonates (Collins, Hall & Brown, 2021). Development of the lobulated kidneys proceeds from the corticomedullary junction out towards the periphery in a **centrifugal pattern** (Yu et al., 2020). This contributes to a process of budding from the ends of the collecting ducts to ensure that new nephrons are added to the outermost parts of the kidney. Recently formed nephrons are fitted into the developing cortical matrix, which eventually reshapes the external surface of the kidneys.

Neonatal Renal Physiology

Neonatal tubular functions are either effective at birth or mature rapidly to lower urinary osmolality and regulation of acid–base balance within acceptable values. Mechanisms involved in blood pressure control such as the **renin–angiotensin system** are very active at birth, possibly due to stimulation by excessive fetal **catecholamines** produced in response to the stress of birth. Because catecholamines enhance cardiac output and renal blood flow, it is likely that these enhance renal function. Another variable that may enhance renal function is the kidneys' capability to consume 7% of the total body oxygen.

Rapid renal growth ensures a functional relationship between the glomeruli and the nephrons. The average glomerular size of 100 μm, present at birth, increases to 300 μm. This is important for the transport and processing of vast amounts of solutes and water. In most neonates, tubular thresholds for the absorption of some solutes are lower, which can result in unwanted loss of sodium, glucose and other solutes in the urine. Although both full-term and premature neonates can excrete normal quantities of acid and bases via their kidneys, their reserve to cope with acidosis is limited. A lower corticomedullary gradient may contribute to limited excretion of urea and haphazard sodium chloride transport mechanisms in the **loop of Henle**. However neonates maintain a reasonable plasma sodium balance by the third day. The blunted response to sodium loading may be attributed to a high concentration of circulating aldosterone, which falls only gradually, in conjunction with similar decreases in renin and angiotensin, after the first week of life. Although the tubules are sensitive to **antidiuretic hormone,** which facilitates absorption of water thereby preventing life-threatening diuresis, the neonate's ability to dilute or concentrate urine is limited compared with that of older children, possibly due to the lower corticomedullary gradient and immature long loops of Henle. This may adversely affect the neonate's ability to excrete drugs such as gentamicin efficiently.

The Urinary Bladder and Micturition

The bladder in neonates is either fusiform (cigar-shaped) or egg-shaped (Collins, Hall & Brown, 2021) rather than pyramidal as in older children. It is situated almost entirely in the abdominal cavity and, when full, its apex extends to the umbilicus. The bladder descends gradually, locating in the pelvic cavity when the child is about 6 years old. This is accompanied by lengthening of the ureters, extending the distance to the kidneys. In neonates, the bladder empties by reflex action, and any distension will increase the intra-abdominal pressure and may exacerbate respiratory difficulties.

Most term neonates pass urine at or shortly after birth, although this may pass unobserved and unrecorded. The use of magnesium sulphate to control eclampsia or lidocaine (lignocaine) to induce epidural analgesia may delay the neonate's ability to void. Some delays may occur in premature neonates and those who experience perinatal asphyxia or severe stress. The neonate's overall haemodynamics, state of hydration/nutrition, cardiac output and renal perfusion must always be considered in evaluating urinary output. Term neonates excrete between 15 and 60 mL/kg of urine daily, increasing this four-fold by the end of the first week as fluid intake increases and the redundant pulmonary fluid is excreted. The urine is dilute, straw-coloured and odourless. It is important to observe the force and direction of the stream of urine and, in boys, whether the stream leaves the tip of the penis. In boys, effective voiding can be compromised by the presence of posterior urethral valves or a tight prepuce. The smallest quantity of urine that neonates should pass averages 0.5–1.0 mL/kg of bodyweight per hour.

Body Composition

For clinical convenience, **total body water** is divided into discrete compartments, which provides a basis for interpreting changes that occur in the distribution and composition of body fluids and electrolytes. **Intracellular fluid** is separated by cell membranes from **extracellular fluid,** which is divided into **intravascular** and **extravascular** components (see Chapter 2 & 20). Transcellular fluids formed by secretory activities of organs such as the biliary system are called **specialized (third space) fluids.**

The proportion and distribution of the body water varies with age, maturity, sex and white adipose tissue. The total water content of the normal neonate averages 77%, falling

TABLE 48.2	Total Body Water Content of Infants (3.0 kg Bodyweight)	
Body Fluid Compartment	**Body Fluid**	**Total Body Water (TBW)**
Intracellular	Fluid in body cells	38%
Extracellular	Fluid divided into interstitial fluid between cells (40%) and plasma (5%) (inside vascular system) Infants have larger interstitial lymph space	45%
Total	TBW ranges (73–83%) and is also due to lower bone mass and body fat	83%

TABLE 48.3	Total Body Water Content of Adults (70.0 kg Bodyweight)	
Body Fluid Compartment	**Body Fluid**	**Total Body Water (TBW)**
Intracellular	Fluid in body cells	70
Extracellular	Fluid divided into interstitial fluid between cells (16%) and plasma (4%) (inside vascular system)	30
Total		100%

to approximately 65% by 6 months (Kline et al., 2018). The distributions of body fluids in infants and adults are compared in Tables 48.2 & 48.3. In comparison to adults, neonates have more interstitial fluid. The gradual translocation of intracellular fluid into the interstitial compartment after birth may be attributed to withdrawal of maternal hormones. In any event, neonates are slightly oedematous, although a significant **diuresis** adjusts the distribution of water across the fluid compartments. In term neonates, a loss of 5–10% of bodyweight in the first week is attributed to this diuresis.

Maintenance of normal body water equilibrium also depends on a balanced fluid intake and output. During the first few days of extrauterine life, when neonates consume small volumes of liquid, a significant transfer of water from the intracellular fluid to the extracellular fluid compartment expands the already large extracellular fluid volume. This potentially protects neonates against dehydration during episodes of physiologically induced diuresis. Although healthy neonates seldom perspire, they are vulnerable to water loss because of their large body surface area, which enhances water evaporation.

Healthy neonates can exchange 50% of the total extracellular fluid volume over 24 hours in comparison to the 14–15% seen in adults. Midwives must remember that significant differences exist between the size of fluid compartments in neonates, pregnant mothers and newly delivered mothers and use this knowledge in caring for them. Fluid therapies and nutritional support must consider individual physiological differences to avoid iatrogenic problems that compromise cardiovascular and respiratory functions.

Sexual Characteristics

Both sexes have a small nodule of breast tissue averaging 1 cm in diameter surrounding the nipples. Initially, the breast tissue may be enlarged due to high plasma maternal oestrogens, and briefly a milky fluid, traditionally referred to as **witches' milk,** may be discharged. No attempt should be made to remove this milk because squeezing the nipple or breast tissue may lead to bruising and abscess formation.

In boys born at term, the testes are descended into the scrotum but can remain undescended in premature neonates. Although the foreskin adheres to the glans penis, this will not obstruct the voiding of urine unless there is obstruction caused by such anatomical problems as posterior urethral valves (often diagnosed antenatally). In girls, fat deposition in the genital area ensures that the labia majora covers and conceals the labia minora, a feature not present in premature neonates. Therefore the urethral and vaginal orifices can be seen when the labia minora are parted. Some female neonates also manifest a thick white vaginal discharge, which is probably a response to maternal oestrogens. Because the linings of the uterus and vagina consist of fairly mature epithelium, some girls may have a small **pseudomenstrual bleed,** although, as the maternal oestrogen levels in the neonate's blood fall, the genital tract returns to an infantile state.

Main Points

- Adaptation to an independent life after birth involves every body system establishing and maintaining new homeostatic values.
- Careful external examination of the newborn following birth is advised, including their general appearance and behaviour.
- Neonatal circulating blood volume varies from 85–90 mL/kg depending on blood flow in fetal life, the gestation of the infant and the time of clamping of the umbilical cord, with the average haemoglobin ranging from 15–23.5 g/dL.
- Prophylactic administration of vitamin K to prevent the risk of spontaneous haemorrhage between the third and sixth days of life is recommended.
- Fetal circulation differs from that of an adult as cardiovascular modifications bypass the lungs, transferring blood to and from the placenta for exchange of gases. Any respiratory or cardiac disorders accompanied by hypoxia and acidosis may lead to persistent fetal circulation.
- By 38–40 weeks' gestation, surfactant forms a monolayer lining for the alveoli, creating an air–liquid interface and reducing surface tension in the terminal sacs. This prevents the alveoli from collapsing at the end of expiration.
- Nephrogenesis is complete by 35 weeks of gestation, but in premature babies continues for a variable period. Improving renal function is most likely due to haemodynamic changes such as good cardiac output mediated by vasoactive substances such as prostaglandins.
- Neonates initially have more interstitial fluid than adults and may become slightly oedematous because of intracellular fluid shift after birth. Diuresis results in a loss of 5–10% of bodyweight in the first week. Renal perfusion, GFR and tubular filtration adjust to neonatal metabolic demands by the end of the second week.
- Tubular thresholds for solute reabsorption are lower in neonates, resulting in loss of sodium, glucose and other solutes in the urine. Infants are able to excrete normal quantities of acid via the kidneys but have little reserve to cope with increased levels that may occur in cardiorespiratory disturbances.
- The neonate's ability to dilute or concentrate urine is also limited. Most babies pass urine within 12 hours of birth. It is important to observe the force and direction of the stream of urine and, in boys, whether the stream leaves the tip of the penis.

References

Andersen, C., Keir, A., Hodyl, N., Stark, M., 2018. Hematologic abnormalities in the newborn. In: Kline, M., Blaney, S., Giardino, A., Orange, J.S., Penny, D.J., Schutze, G.E., Shekerdemian, L.S. (Eds.), Rudolph's Pediatrics, twenty-third ed. McGraw-Hill, London.

Boardman, J.P., Groves, A.M., Ramasethu, J., 2021. Avery's Neonatal: Pathophysiology and Management of the Newborn, eighth ed. Lippincott, Williams and Wilkins, Philadelphia.

Bruckner, M., Katheria, A.C., Schmölzer, G.M., 2021. Delayed cord clamping in healthy term infants: more harm or good? Semin. Fetal Neonatal Med. 26 (2), 101221.

Collins, P., Hall, M., Brown, K., 2021. Pre- and postnatal growth and the neonate. In: Standring, S. (Ed.), Gray's Anatomy: The Anatomical Basis of Clinical Practice, forty-second ed. Elsevier, London.

Depicolzuane, L., Phelps, D.S., Floros, J., 2022. Surfactant protein-A function: knowledge gained from SP-A knockout mice. Front. Pediatr. 9, 1542.

Ekelund, H., Finnström, O., Gunnarskog, J., Källén, B., Larsson, Y., 1993. Administration of vitamin K to newborn infants and childhood cancer. Br. Med. J. 301 (6896), 89–91.

Golding, J., Greenwood, R., Birmingham, K., Mott, M., 1992. Childhood cancer, intramuscular vitamin K, and pethidine given during labor. Br. Med. J. 305 (6849), 341–347.

Hull, D., 1992. Vitamin K and childhood cancer: the risk of haemorrhagic disease is certain; that of cancer is not. Br. Med. J. 305, 326–327.

Jullien, S., 2021. Vitamin K prophylaxis in newborns. BMC Pediatr. 21 (1), 1–7.

Kline, M., Blaney, S., Giardino, A., Orange, J.S., Penny, D.J., Schutze, G.E., et al., 2018. Rudolph's Pediatrics, twenty-third ed. McGraw-Hill, London.

Lakshminrusimha, S., Carlton, D., 2018. Transitional Changes in the Newborn Infant Around the Time of Birth. In: Kline M., Balney, S., Giardino, A., Orange, J.S., Penny, D.J., Schutze, G.E., et al. (Eds.), Rudolph's Pediatrics, twenty-third ed. McGraw-Hill, London.

Marieb, E.N., Hoehn, K.N., 2022. Human Anatomy and Physiology, twelfth ed. Pearson, Harlow.

Merenstein, G.B., Hathaway, W.E., Miller, R.W.S., Paulson, J.A., Rowley, D.L., 1993. Controversies concerning vitamin K and the newborn. Pediatrics. Available at: https://api.semanticscholar.org/CorpusID:70695904

Merenstein, K., Hathaway, W.E.S., Miller, R.W.S., Paulson, J.A., Rowley, D.L., 1993. Controversies concerning vitamin K and the newborn. Pediatrics 91 (5), 1001–1002.

National Institute for Health and Care Excellence (NICE), 2023. Intrapartum Care. Available at: https://www.nice.org.uk/guidance/ng235.

Peberdy, L., Young, J., Massey, D., Kearney, L., 2022. Integrated review of the knowledge, attitudes, and practices of maternity health care professionals concerning umbilical cord clamping. Birth 49 (4), 595–615.

Pocock, G., Richards, C., Richards, D., 2017. Human Physiology, fifth ed. Oxford University Press, Oxford.

Ransome, H., Marshall, J., 2020. Recognising the healthy baby at term through examination of the newborn screening. In: Marshall, J.E., Raynor, M.D. (Eds.), Myles' Textbook for Midwives, seventeenth ed. Elsevier, Edinburgh.

Royal College of Obstetricians and Gynaecologists (RCOG), 2015. Scientific Impact Paper no. 14: Clamping of the Umbilical Cord and Placental Transfusion. RCOG, London.

Sankar, M.J., Chandrasekaran, A., Kumar, P., Thukral, A., Agarwal, R., Paul, V.K., 2016. Vitamin K prophylaxis for prevention of vitamin K deficiency bleeding: a systematic review. J. Perinatol. 36 (1), S29–S35.

Sinha, S., Miall, L., Jardine, L., 2018. Essential Neonatal Medicine, sixth ed. Wiley-Blackwell, Sussex.

Yu, A.S.L., Chertow, G.M., Luyckx, V.A., Marsden, P.A., Skorecki, K., Taal, M.W., 2020. Brenner & Rector's the Kidney, eleventh ed. Elsevier Saunders, Philadelphia.

Whitsett, J.A., Wert, S.E., Weaver, T.E., 2015. Diseases of pulmonary surfactant homeostasis. Annu. Rev. Pathol. 10, 371–393.

Annotated recommended reading

Hockenberry, M.J., 2023. Wong's Nursing Care of Infants and Children, twelfth ed. Elsevier, Philadelphia.

This textbook offers detailed accounts of the relevant biophysical, psychosocial and nursing issues in managing the care of infants and children. It concludes with a range of helpful appendices, which include excellent developmental screening tools and biophysical nomograms and parameters invaluable in all aspects of childcare.

Sinha, S., Miall, L., Jardine, L., 2018. Essential Neonatal Medicine, sixth ed. Wiley-Blackwell, Sussex.

A compact but comprehensive textbook which provides an account of the myriad common problems and their management in neonatology. It provides a holistic focus for the care provided, including considerations of the multidisciplinary input and the involvement of parents within the neonatal unit. It includes an overview of practical procedures, an up-to-date neonatal pharmacopoeia and useful tables and charts for normal age-related ranges.

49

Adaptation to Extrauterine Life 2: Gastrointestinal, Metabolic, Neural and Immunological Considerations

THOMAS McEWAN

CHAPTER CONTENTS

Students and midwives should have a robust knowledge and understanding of the adaptation required by the newborn for successful extrauterine life. Within this chapter adaptations related to the gastrointestinal, metabolic, neural and immunological systems are considered.

Introduction

The human placenta is a discoid haemochorial organ that connects to a small part of the internal aspect of the uterus. It has many vital functions, including serving as a metabolic unit capable of exchanging nutrients and metabolic waste products between mother and embryo/fetus. At term, in a single pregnancy, a normal healthy placenta and its membranes weigh 470 g, which is directly proportional to the weight of the fetus (see Chapter 12). After birth, the neonatal systems support these physiological processes.

The Gastrointestinal Tract

Neonatal Characteristics

The embryological development of the gut described in Chapter 11 should be reviewed. Significant anatomical and physiological limitations exist in the neonatal gastrointestinal (GI) tract, many of which may be partly attributed to the requirement of the fetus to swallow amniotic fluid (Polin et al., 2022). The swallowing of small boluses of amniotic fluid may be fundamental to the patency of the GI tract. Although the fetal GI tract appears not to serve any nutritional purposes, it must process nutrients after birth.

The Oral Cavity

The walls of the oral cavity should be well formed with a central, short, broad but freely moveable tongue accommodated comfortably within it. The hard palate is slightly arched and gently corrugated by five or six irregular transverse folds which assist with suckling. Neonates have a high epiglottis that makes direct contact with the soft palate. As milk passes from the mouth to the pharynx, the larynx is elevated so that its opening is above the level of the oral cavity. The high position of the larynx, further elevated during suckling, directs its opening into the nasopharynx, enabling neonates to breathe when they suckle. Although neonates are thought to be obligate nose-breathers, oral breathing occurs in the presence of nasal occlusion (Sinha, Miall & Jardine, 2018).

The Stomach at Birth

The neonate's stomach has a small capacity, holding only 15–30 mL at birth, but increasing rapidly within the first few weeks. Neonatal swallowing may distend/enlarge the stomach capacity by four or five times and shift its position relative to other viscera. **Gastric emptying time** is initially slow, averaging 2–3 hours. This is influenced by nutrient digestibility: for example, carbohydrates increase emptying time, whereas fats decrease it. The presence of mucus in the stomach during the first 24–48 hours can delay gastric emptying, whereas weakness of the **cardiac sphincter** contributes to milk regurgitation.

Gastric acidity at birth equals that of an adult, but the pH rises gradually to alkaline values because of a fall in hydrochloric acid production. This rise in pH allows commensals essential to the production of vitamin K and vitamin B complex to colonize the large bowel. However it also allows pathogens to survive, making the baby vulnerable to infection (Ransome & Marshall, 2020). Furthermore, the intestinal mucosal barrier remains immature during the first 6 months, allowing the transport of **antigens** and other **macromolecules** across the epithelium into the systemic circulation. However maternal **colostrum** is rich in antibodies and helps the passage of **meconium** so that the risk of systemic infection is reduced. Postnatal maturation of the gut is stimulated by increases in peptide hormones such as **gastrin** and **motilin** (see Chapter 21), which are secreted after the commencement of feeding.

At term, the neonate's small intestine averages 300 cm in length and the large intestine averages 66 cm in length (Collins, Hall & Brown, 2021); both are about 1 cm in diameter. Both forms of intestine have many secretory glands and villi, but the muscular structures are weak and poorly developed. The villi increase the intestine's absorptive surface area. Because the haustra are not present for 6 months, the external surface of the large intestine appears smooth. Term neonates have a relatively long rectum that should connect to a patent anus. Digestive enzymes are synthesized and released as required. However the relative deficiency of **amylase** and **lipase** causes difficulties in digesting carbohydrates and fats. The entry of food into the stomach induces a **gastrocolic reflex,** resulting in **ileocaecal valve** opening. As the ileal contents enter the colon, they stimulate forceful **peristalsis** accompanied by a reflex emptying of the **rectum** (Ransome & Marshall, 2020).

Meconium

Meconium is a dark, rather sticky substance that collects in the intestines of the fetus from the 16th week and forms the first stools of the neonate. Its presence may ensure the patency of the intestine. Box 49.1 summarizes the characteristics of meconium.

Most neonates pass meconium within 24 hours of birth. Failure to do so could be an early indication of intestinal

---

• BOX 49.1 | Characteristics of Meconium

A viscid consistency and greenish-black colour are attributed to the accumulation of digestive enzymes, intestinal gland secretions, bile salts and components of amniotic fluid such as vernix, lanugo, fatty acids, epithelial cells, mucus and blood cells (Blackburn, 2018). Initially meconium is sterile but within 24 hours of birth it begins to be colonized with bacteria, largely in response to enteral feeding.

---

malformation, malfunction or obstruction such as an anorectal malformation or cystic fibrosis.

Milk feeding induces a change in the neonate's stools. As digested milk enters the colon, a gradual **transition** results in stools that are fairly liquid and yellow-brownish in appearance. After this, the consistency and frequency of the stools depend on the type of feeding. Breastfed babies pass loose, bright-yellow, inoffensive stools on average 6–10 times in 24 hours in the earlier days to once a day when feeding is established. By contrast, bottle-fed babies pass paler, more formed stools with a recognizable smell and generally less frequently with a tendency towards constipation.

The Liver

The fetal liver is a proportionally large organ, and the liver in mature neonates accounts for 4–5% of total bodyweight. Although immature, it is considered the central organ of homeostasis. The neonatal liver has less than 20% of the **hepatocytes** found in an adult liver, and ongoing mitosis is critical to the development of a functionally mature organ.

At birth, although physiologically immature, the liver produces small quantities of enzymes which metabolize substances by utilizing **oxidative** and **conjugation processes.** One major function the liver must be capable of is the synthesis of glucuronyl transferase, which is essential for bilirubin conjugation. Shortfalls in this enzyme lead to a rise in plasma values of **unconjugated bilirubin.** This situation is often exacerbated by the breakdown of superfluous erythrocytes during the first 6 weeks of postnatal life. Binding of unconjugated bilirubin to fatty tissue contributes to a transient neonatal jaundice on the third to fifth days. Feeding stimulates liver function and bacterial colonization of the gut, which in turn stimulates vitamin K production crucial to normal coagulation (see Chapter 52 for a fuller account of neonatal jaundice).

Metabolism

Fetal metabolic processes are mainly **anabolic,** required to support rapid growth. After birth, neonates must support their own metabolic needs by utilizing essential nutrients and gases as fuels. These adaptive changes are energy-demanding. The fetus prepares for independence by laying down a store of glycogen and lipids during the last few weeks of gestation; fetal blood glucose during the last trimester

The risk of a neonate developing hypoglycaemia is considerable. The relative excess water in neonates confers no protection against dehydration because the daily turnover of water equals 15–20%. Evaporative water loss is also costly in energy terms as the loss of 1 g of water causes a loss of 0.6 kcal of heat.

After birth, body heat production is attributed to brown adipose tissue and hepatic tri-iodothyronine synthesis, facilitating the transition from a net anabolic state to a catabolic state (Blackburn, 2018). These adaptations are influenced by factors such as maternal nutrition in late pregnancy, neonatal maturity, respiratory function and the ambient humidity and temperature.

averages 80% of maternal blood glucose concentration (Lakshminrusimha & Carlton, 2018). However nutrient reserves are fairly limited, and most neonates require an intake of glucose, protein, fat and water within the first few hours of birth. Box 49.2 provides further information on neonatal metabolism.

Glucose Metabolism

Glucose is the major substrate for carbohydrate metabolism in newborn babies (Sinha, Miall & Jardine, 2018). After birth, as the neonate loses the maternal glucose source, falling plasma insulin levels and slow production of insulin prevent cellular uptake of glucose. This is coupled with an increase in serum glucagon levels, which mobilize glucose from the intracellular glycogen stores.

Hepatic and muscle glycogen stores decrease rapidly after birth. Thereafter, gluconeogenesis is regulated by changes in the serum insulin: glucose ratio, catecholamine release, fatty acid oxidation and activation of liver gluconeogenic enzymes. The concentration of hepatic enzymes increases for the next 1–4 days. Lactose is the principal carbohydrate in human milk and many milk formulae, and term neonates consume 10–12 g/100 kcal/day.

Neonatal blood glucose falls rapidly after birth then stabilizes and equilibrates by the process of endogenous gluconeogenesis (Sinha, Miall & Jardine, 2018). The consensus for the lowest safe level for neonatal blood glucose is 2.6 mmol/L (McIntyre, 2020).

Fat Metabolism

Lipolysis increases rapidly after birth, reaching a maximum within a few hours of birth and adult levels by 24 hours, resulting in a rise in plasma free fatty acids. During this time, about two-thirds of neonatal energy is produced from fat oxidation, the major form of neonatal stored calories.

The major differences between human milk and formula milk (mainly derived from cows' milk) are the absence of long-chain unsaturated fatty acids in formula milk compared with high concentrations of long-chain unsaturated fatty acids and cholesterol in mature human milk (see

Chapter 54). The fat and protein content of colostrum is higher than in mature milk (McIntyre & Marshall, 2020). Mature human milk is optimal for neonates, with nutritional, digestive, immune, microbiotic and epigenetic properties unique to each mother and baby.

Alternative fat stores and ketone body release are stimulated by the release of catecholamines associated with the body cooling after birth. Ketone bodies are produced during fatty acid metabolism, and these form important metabolites. They also provide a major energy source for the developing brain and the myocardium (Polin et al., 2022).

Protein Metabolism

Whereas the basic fetal cellular building blocks are supplied by the placenta, the neonate must digest milk proteins into amino acids and oligopeptides, which requires proteolytic enzymes. The relatively high concentration of free amino acids and peptides in human milk probably enhances the release of gastrin and cholecystokinin, which promotes the release of proteolytic enzymes. The neonate's ability to synthesize protein is limited due to hepatic immaturity. Consequently, serum amino-acid levels are higher in the first few weeks, and there is significant urinary amino-acid excretion. Protein synthesis in mature fetuses and neonates is greater than later in life, likely attributable to the significant remodelling during a period of rapid cell differentiation and tissue growth (Kline et al., 2018).

Calcium, Phosphorus and Magnesium Balance

Compared with maternal blood values, most neonates manifest hypercalcaemia and hyperphosphataemia. Information on calcium, phosphorus and magnesium is presented in Table 49.1.

The Neonatal Nervous System

The mature central nervous system consists of approximately 100 billion neurons that interact to make consciousness, thought, learning, memory, vision and other nervous system properties possible. The nervous system and special sense organs originate from neural ectoderm, which forms the notochord and then the neural tube. This creates a range of specialized cells that form the nervous system. The term neonate is capable of processing incoming information from the environment and producing age-appropriate behaviours. The functions of the nervous system can be divided into three parts: the autonomic, sensory and motor state.

Autonomic Functions

At birth, the neonate's nervous system takes over control of functions such as hunger, thirst and satiety, which are balanced by hypothalamic centres. These are also thought to influence nutritive sucking and swallowing. Homeostasis

TABLE 49.1	Calcium, Phosphorus and Magnesium Levels and Function in the Neonate.
Calcium	Calcium is the most abundant mineral in the body. At term, most newborn babies have accumulated between 20 and 30 g, 80% of which is accrued in trimester three (Polin et al., 2022). Of this, 99% is in the neonate's developing skeleton. Serum calcium exists in three separate fractions: protein-bound, anion-bound and as the physiologically active free, ionized form. The ultimate balance in plasma calcium is partly determined by an ongoing exchange between the skeletal system, muscles, the intestine and the kidneys (Sherwood, 2016). This movement of calcium is controlled by parathyroid hormone, 1,25-dihydroxycholecalciferol and calcitonin. Calcium metabolism is also influenced by growth hormones, corticosteroids and some locally acting hormones and co-factors, including cytokines. In term infants, hypocalcaemia is defined as a total serum calcium concentration <2 mmol/L or ionized fraction <1.1 mmol/L. This level falls during the first 2 days of life, increasing back to normal once intestinal absorption of calcium matures. Renal excretion of calcium is efficient and continues to increase in conjunction with glomerular filtration rate (GFR). **Neonatal Aspects of Calcium Metabolism** As serum calcium levels decrease, parathyroid hormone (PTH) levels increase responsively by 3–4 days of age. Calcitonin levels are normal at birth, but this is followed by a surge in the next 24 hours, returning to normal values within the following 36 hours. Term neonates metabolize vitamin D in the liver and the kidneys, although absorption of exogenous vitamin D may be limited due to reduced fat absorption.
Phosphorus	Approximately 80% of the phosphorus in term neonates is accumulated by the fetus during trimester three. The total amounts of phosphorus are divided within the skeletal system (about 85% of the total), within body fluids and as inorganic phosphate. Although phosphorus levels decrease in the first 2 days after birth, they still remain higher than in the adult. This may be partly attributed to delayed renal excretion of phosphorus caused by an initial decrease in GFR and increase in tubular reabsorption rate. Furthermore increased cellular energy manufacture with conversion of adenosine triphosphate (ATP) to adenosine diphosphate (ADP) releases additional phosphate. If feeding is delayed, this catabolic process is increased even further.
Magnesium	Magnesium is the second most common **intracellular cation** in the body. Mature neonates contain about 20 mg of magnesium/100 g of fat-free weight (Polin et al., 2022). As usual, the total body magnesium is divided between three compartments: the skeletal system (about 60%), muscle tissue (about 29%) and the remainder can be found within soft and connective tissue. Only 1% of total body magnesium is in the extracellular space. The normal range for plasma magnesium is 0.7–1.0 mmol/L, with 60% existing as **free ions** and 20% bound to various **anions** such as phosphate and oxalate. Because no specific hormones have yet been identified as responsible for fine-tuning plasma magnesium, the kidneys are considered the primary regulators for reabsorption and loss of this ion.

is achieved by the regulation of respiration, heartbeat, body temperature and metabolic activity, and is adjusted to ensure the body generates sufficient heat to support important enzyme activity and off-loads redundant heat (see Thermoregulation).

Sensory Functions

The neonate can detect odour, differentiate between tastes, see and observe preferential stimuli and hear and discriminate sounds, all sensory modalities that are useful in the interaction with his carers (see Chapter 57). Many of these functions would have already been exercised in utero.

Motor Functions

Movements in neonates, as in adults, may be reflexive or volitional. Volitional movement is under the control of the motor cortex. At first, the neonate appears to make few volitional movements, but gradual motor control becomes evident as myelination of the major central and peripheral nerve tracts progresses. It is likely that environmental

stimulation encourages skeletal muscle movements, and these contribute to the generation of new dendrites (Fig. 49.1), motor neurons and interneuron connections. These ultimately contribute to the complexity of the many integrated functions of the central nervous system.

Ongoing Neural Development

The neonate's nervous system has a considerable complement of neurons, but many of these will be lost by **apoptosis,** and a new complement of neurons will be generated over the next 2 years (Derbyshire & Obeid, 2020). The significant increase in the size of the brain in the first year is attributed to the development of **neuroglia** and **myelin.** During infancy, the brain and spinal cord have a considerable degree of **plasticity** so that the developing nervous system can respond to environmental stimuli and balanced nutrition with ongoing modifications. Neonates learn by receiving, processing and responding to a vast range of sensory stimuli.

The characteristic neural development contributes significantly to the neonate's typical pattern of muscle tone, which causes ongoing neuromuscular growth and development.

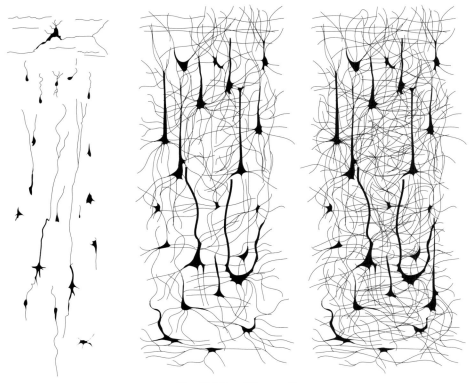

• **Fig. 49.1** Dendritic growth.

At first there is active **flexion** and **extension,** but these are replaced by purposeful movement allowing greater control and accuracy. Neuromuscular control proceeds in a **cephalocaudal** direction and amongst the first to develop are head and neck control, turning over, reaching, grasping and then crawling and walking.

Reflexes

Reflexes are autonomic, 'built-in' motor behaviours which generally occur in the spinal cord and are critical to safety and survival. These provide opportunities for assessing neonatal motor capabilities, responsiveness and needs. The absence, exaggerated state or persistence of many reflexes may signify brain damage. The key **neonatal reflexes** are described in Table 49.2.

Behavioural State Regulation

An excellent description of **behavioural states** is given by Prechtl and O'Brien (1982) in their seminal work. This term refers to the recognizable combination of behaviours repeated by the neonate over time. Such behavioural states have been investigated by observational studies, electroencephalography and polygraphy where physiological signals are studied. Prechtl & O'Brien (1982) defined five states using the four parameters of eyes open, respiration regular, gross movements and vocalization. This subject is further explored in preterm and term neonates (in relation to electroencephalography findings) by Dereymaeker et al. (2017)

and the assessment of pain (Eriksson & Campbell-Yeo, 2019).

Sleep States

Deep Sleep

The eyes are closed, respirations are regular, no eye movements are present and response to stimuli is delayed. Jerky movements may be present.

Light Sleep

Rapid eye movements occur. Respiration is irregular, nonnutritive sucking movements may occur, response to stimuli is rapid possibly resulting in an alteration of sleep state and random movements are noticed.

Awake States

Drowsy State

The eyes may be open or closed with some eyelid flutter and smiling may occur. Smooth limb movements interspersed with startle responses may be present and alteration of state occurs readily after stimulation.

Quiet but Alert State

Motor activity is minimal, but the baby is alert to visual and auditory stimuli.

Active Alert State

The baby is active and reactive to the environment. It is in this state that the baby will mimic facial expressions.

TABLE 49.2	**Neonatal Reflexes**
Moro (startle) reflex	This involves adduction and extension of the arms with the fingers fanned out, followed by abduction of the arms with flexed elbows in an 'embrace' position.
Palmar grasp and plantar grasp reflexes	These involve a neonate closing his fingers tightly around any object placed in his palm or cupping his toes and grasping the object when the sole of his foot is stimulated.
Rooting reflex	This is seen when the side of the mouth or cheek is gently stroked. The neonate will turn his head towards the source of the stimulus and open his mouth ready to suckle.
Sucking, swallowing and gag reflexes	These are well developed in the term neonate. Sucking and swallowing are coordinated with respiration, including gag, cough and sneeze reflexes.
Tonic neck (fencing) reflex	This is apparent when the neonate's head is turned to one side. He will extend the arm and leg on the side of body the head is turned to and flex the arm and leg on the other side. This helps stabilize the neonate and prevent him from rolling over.
Stepping reflex	The is seen when the neonate is held upright with his feet touching a solid surface, in response to which alternating stepping movements are made.
Traction response	This response is observed when the neonate is held by the wrists and pulled into a sitting position. The head lags at first, then rights itself, deploying neck muscles, before falling forward.

Active Crying State

The baby cries vigorously and may be difficult to console. There is considerable muscular activity. Neonates cry for different reasons such as hunger, thirst, pain, a need to change position or unsatisfactory room temperature. This is their only means of attracting attention to their needs. Although crying causes anxiety, mothers usually learn to recognize and respond to the different cries. Understanding these different behavioural states may lessen anxiety and allow greater parental enjoyment.

The Essence of Immunocompetence

Perhaps the most important components of the evolving **immune system** are the red bone marrow, the thymus gland and peripheral lymph nodes. The thymus gland weighs approximately 10 g and then grows steadily until puberty, when it weighs approximately 30 g. **Lymphopoiesis** (see Chapter 29) produces **immunocytes** capable of distinguishing between foreign and self-antigens, facilitating the elimination of foreign antigens and maintaining a memory of previous exposure to them. The development of lymphoid tissue proceeds along two classical pathways culminating in the formation of:

1. **Naïve B lymphocytes,** which on exposure to antigens become plasma cells capable of mounting **antibody-mediated immunity.**
2. **T lymphocytes,** which are predominantly responsible for coordinating **cell-mediated immunity.**

Both fetus and neonate are compromised by their immature immune systems. Also, lack of exposure to common pathogens and antigens contributes to significant delay in mounting an immune response. Because both pathways are functionally immature, the inflammatory response and complement cascade are limited. Immune system immaturity may also predispose to allergy formation and susceptibility to GI infections. Refer to Chapter 53 for a fuller account of the specific immune responses.

Gastrointestinal Perspectives

The initial mild acidity of the stomach secretions may afford some protection against ingested pathogens, and the colonization of meconium, which commences within a few hours of birth, rarely leads to infection. Breastfed babies develop a different pattern of bacterial colonization from that of neonates fed with formula milk. The acid environment in the gut in which protective organisms such as *Lactobacillus* can grow appears to prevent colonization by more harmful pathogenic organisms. Eventually the development of gut defence mechanisms such as 'gut closure', accompanied by the development of the mucosal barrier and other defences, renders the epithelium impermeable to pathogens. As further immune defence, the tonsils and peritoneal Peyer's patches develop.

Thermoregulation

Thermoregulation is the balance between the body's ability to produce heat and lose heat under physiologically appropriate conditions.

Adult Mechanisms

Humans are **homeotherms,** maintaining a constant body temperature independent of their environment. Skin receptors send signals to the **hypothalamus,** triggering autonomic nervous system responses. The transfer of these signals to the cerebral cortex triggers learned behavioural responses. Consequently, a rise in normal body temperature in humans is accompanied by an autonomically triggered **peripheral vasodilation,** sweating and a behavioural response of searching for a cooler environment and wearing appropriate clothing. If the body temperature falls, there is usually a reflex **peripheral vasoconstriction** and shivering and the person seeks a warmer environment and more suitable clothing (Hall & Hall, 2020).

Neonatal Mechanisms

At birth, the neonate passes from a thermoconstant intrauterine temperature of approximately 37.7°C to an environment where the room temperature averages between 21°C and 25°C. This contributes to rapid heat loss due to the wet, warm skin. Heat may be transferred down the internal gradient from the body core to the skin surface and to the environment at a speed dependent on capillary blood flow and the amount of subcutaneous fat present. In contrast, the loss of heat down the external gradient depends on the difference between the skin temperature and the external environment, which involves mechanisms of evaporation, convection, radiation and conduction. Table 49.3 shows the balance between heat gain and heat loss in the neonate.

Thermoregulation is a common physiological problem amongst neonates, largely due to immaturity and inefficiency of the control mechanisms observed in adults and their greater body surface ratio. The neonate has a much larger head surface area than an adult because the head makes up 25% of the **body mass.** Normally a neonate's core temperature may average 36.7–37.3°C (Sinha, Miall & Jardine, 2018).

Neonates are generally unable to shiver and are limited in their ability to generate heat from muscle action, so they are at a disadvantage. They can decrease their surface area exposed to the environment by flexing their limbs and taking up the fetal position. During the first 24 hours after birth, healthy term neonates will increase their heat production by 2.5 times as a physiological response to cold. This process appears to be activated by catecholamine release, which induces **lipolysis** in the brown adipose tissue (BAT), small amounts of which are also found in most human adults, other animal neonates and hibernating animals.

Heat Production and BAT

About 2–7% of the weight of a newborn infant probably consists of BAT which is mainly situated around the kidneys, in the mediastinum, around the nape of the neck and scapulae, along the spinal column and around the large blood vessels in the neck. **Brown adipocytes** (fat cells) begin to proliferate at 26–30 weeks' gestation and continue to increase in number for some months after birth. A small amount of BAT persists throughout life, with greater quantities being present in slender individuals.

BAT adipocytes differ from those in white adipose tissue by their scope for enhanced metabolic activity and heat production. The cells contain many small fat vacuoles, numerous mitochondria and other active organelles. BAT has extensive capillary perfusion, giving it a brownish colour. Activity of the sympathetic nerve fibres during cold stress causes the adrenal glands to release catecholamines, such as **noradrenaline** (norepinephrine), which stimulate the anterior pituitary gland to release **thyroid-stimulating hormone**. This causes the thyroid gland to increase production of **thyroxine** (T_4). **Adrenaline** (epinephrine) and thyroxine increase metabolic activity within BAT and heat is produced, providing adequate oxygen and glucose are available.

Thermal Care of the Neonate

It is important that parents and professionals caring for neonates are aware of the need to maximize their heat regulation after birth. This will involve careful consideration of the environment in which the birth will take place with many of the important elements of this identified in Clinical Application 49.1. Refer to Chapter 50 for additional information on the needs of small and sick neonates.

• CLINICAL APPLICATION 49.1	Thermal Care of the Neonate

Some of the actions that may support thermal care in the newborn include:

- **Skin-to-skin with the mother:** promotes conductive heat transfer from mother to baby.
- **Drying and wrapping of the baby after birth:** prevents evaporative heat loss from moisture and fluid on the baby's skin. The use of polyethylene wrapping applied before drying in the preterm infant (<32 weeks) with an external heat source is a standard approach to prevent transepidermal water and heat loss.
- **Closing windows/doors and switching off air conditioning in the birthing room:** prevents convective heat loss associated with cooler circulating air.
- **Warming of the weighing scales or the surface used for resuscitation:** reduces conductive heat loss when the baby is placed on a cold surface.
- **Ensuring the cot is not placed near to a cold wall or window with the baby dressed and covered appropriately:** minimizes heat transfer by radiation to the colder surroundings which are close to, but not directly touching, the baby.

TABLE 49.3	Sources of Heat Gain and Heat Loss in the Neonate
Heat Gain	**Heat Loss**
Metabolic processes such as oxidative metabolism of glucose, fats and proteins	Evaporation: water loss from the skin and respiratory tract, most common at birth Heat is also lost in urine and faeces
Physical activity such as crying, restlessness and hyperactivity Non-shivering thermogenesis generated through metabolism in brown adipose tissue	Convection: heat lost into the air around the baby Radiation: heat radiated to nearby cold solid surfaces, most common after the first week of life Conduction: heat lost by direct contact with cold surfaces touching the baby

Main Points

- The nutritional, excretory and metabolic needs of the fetus and its protection against pathogenic organisms and toxins are met by the placenta.
- The small stomach capacity increases rapidly within the first few weeks of life, allowing the infant to take larger feeds. The cardiac sphincter remains weak, and milk regurgitation is common.
- The intestinal mucosal barrier remains immature so that antigens and other macromolecules can be transported across the epithelium into the systemic circulation, especially from colostrum, which is rich in antibodies and helps the elimination of meconium.
- A gastrocolic reflex ensures that feeding is often accompanied by reflex emptying of the bowel.
- The immature liver has low production of enzymes such as glucuronyl transferase. Enteral feeding stimulates liver function and bacterial colonization of the gut, allowing vitamin K to be produced.
- The fetus lays down a fuel store of glycogen and lipids during the last few weeks of pregnancy for use after birth. Catecholamines released in response to body cooling stimulate the release of alternative fat stores and ketone bodies.
- Neonatal blood glucose levels fall to the lowest level between 2 and 6 hours after birth, become stable and then rise as the baby adapts to his extrauterine environment.
- Lipolysis increases rapidly after birth, reaching a maximum within a few hours. In the first 24 hours, two-thirds of the baby's energy is derived from fat oxidation. Protein synthesis remains limited due to immaturity of the liver enzyme systems.

- During the first 2 days of life, serum calcium levels fall, leading to physiological hypocalcaemia. This rises to normal values between 5 and 10 days as intestinal absorption of calcium increases.
- Only 1% of total body magnesium is in the extracellular space. The kidneys are the primary organs for serum magnesium regulation.
- Nervous system activity increases steadily throughout gestation. At term, the neonate processes incoming information from the environment and produces behaviour appropriate for its status. Plasticity of the brain ensures that new neural connections can be established and modified by environmental stimuli.
- The term neonate demonstrates a typical muscle tone which changes, giving rise to strong passive flexion and eventually to purposive movement. Reflexes are critical for the baby's safety and survival. The absence of such reflexes or unusual persistence may indicate brain damage.
- Neonatal behaviours include two sleep states (deep and light) and four awake states (drowsy, quiet alert, active alert and active crying). Helping parents to recognize these different behavioural states may contribute to better parenting skills.
- Breastfed babies develop a different pattern of bacterial colonization than artificially fed babies. The acid environment in the gut facilitates the growth of *Lactobacillus*, preventing colonization by pathogenic micro-organisms.
- Neonatal thermoregulation can be a problem because the large body surface area contributes to greater heat loss. Neonates can increase their heat production by 2.5 times in response to cold by BAT lipolysis.

References

Blackburn, S.T., 2018. Maternal, Fetal and Neonatal Physiology: A Clinical Perspective, fifth ed. Elsevier, St. Louis.

Collins, P., Hall, M., Brown, K., 2021. Pre- and postnatal growth and the neonate. In: Standring, S. (Ed.), Gray's Anatomy: The Anatomical Basis of Clinical Practice, forty-second ed. Elsevier, London.

Derbyshire, E., Obeid, R., 2020. Choline, neurological development and brain function: a systematic review focusing on the first 1000 days. Nutrients 12 (6), 1731.

Dereymaeker, A., Pillay, K., Vervisch, J., De Vos, M., Van Huffel, S., Jansen, K., et al., 2017. Review of sleep-EEG in preterm and term neonates. Early Hum. Dev. 113, 87–103.

Eriksson, M., Campbell-Yeo, M., 2019. Assessment of pain in newborn infants. Semin. Fetal Neonatal Med. 24 (4), 101003.

Hall, J., Hall, M., 2020. Guyton and Hall Textbook of Medical Physiology, fourteenth ed. Elsevier Saunders, Philadelphia.

Kline, M., Blaney, S., Giardino, A., Orange, J.S., Penny, D.J., Schutze, G.E., et al., 2018. Rudolph's Pediatrics, twenty-third ed. McGraw-Hill, London.

Lakshminrusimha, S., Carlton, D., 2018. Transitional changes in the newborn infant around the time of birth. In: Kline, M., Blaney, S., Giardino, A., et al. (Eds.), Rudolph's Pediatrics, twenty-third ed. McGraw-Hill, London.

McIntyre, J., 2020. Significant problems in the newborn baby. In: Marshall, J.E., Raynor, M.D. (Eds.), Myles' Textbook for Midwives, seventeenth ed. Elsevier, Edinburgh.

McIntyre, J., Marshall, J.E., 2020. Optimal infant feeding. In: Marshall, J.E., Raynor, M.D. (Eds.), Myles' Textbook for Midwives, seventeenth ed. Elsevier, Edinburgh.

Polin, R., Abman, S., Rowitch, D., Benitz, W.E., Fox, W.W., 2022. Fetal and Neonatal Physiology, sixth ed. Elsevier Saunders, Philadelphia.

Prechtl, H.F.R., O'Brien, M.J., 1982. Behavioural states of the full-term newborn. The emergence of concept. In: Stratton, P. (Ed.), Psychobiology of the Human Newborn. Wiley, Chichester.

Ransome, H., Marshall, J.E., 2020. Recognising the healthy baby at term through examination of the newborn screening. In: Marshall, J.E., Raynor, M.D. (Eds.), Myles' Textbook for Midwives, seventeenth ed. Elsevier, Edinburgh.

Sherwood, L., 2016. Human Physiology: From Cells to Systems, ninth ed. Cengage Learning, Boston.

Sinha, S., Miall, L., Jardine, L., 2018. Essential Neonatal Medicine, sixth ed. Wiley-Blackwell, Sussex.

Annotated recommended reading

Polin, R., Abman, S., Rowitch, D., Benitz, W.E., Fox, W.W., 2022. Fetal and Neonatal Physiology, sixth ed. Elsevier Saunders, Philadelphia.

This textbook offers detailed accounts of bioscientific concepts important in fetal and neonatal care. A résumé of genetics acts as a basis for a detailed exploration of normal embryonic development. The systematic exploration of biochemical, physiological, nutritional and pathophysiological principles makes a significant contribution to clinical practice and research.

50

Health Challenges and Problems in Neonates of Low Birthweight

THOMAS McEWAN

CHAPTER CONTENTS

Within this chapter, the health challenges for the low-birthweight neonate are considered. Students and midwives should have a comprehensive knowledge and understanding of these vulnerable neonates to ensure their needs, and those of their parents, are fully met.

Introduction

Initially this chapter provides information on the effect of deprivation and ethnicity on perinatal mortality and morbidity (see Box 50.1). It is crucial for health professionals to be aware of this background information if they are involved in supporting vulnerable groups during pregnancy and childbirth.

Thereafter, this chapter aims to define low birthweight (LBW), consider some of the common causes and address some of the most prevalent health challenges and problems that may occur in such neonates. These problems, which may be complex and diverse, highlight the need for all those providing care to have specialist knowledge and expertise.

This chapter also offers a résumé of relevant biological principles that may guide practice. This builds on some of the diagnostic accounts of congenital abnormalities in Chapter 15, giving due consideration to relevant aspects of physiology, pathophysiology and, where appropriate, therapeutic caring interventions.

Defining Low Birthweight (LBW)

The term LBW applies to all neonates, regardless of gestational age, whose bodyweight at birth is less than 2500 g. The improved survival of neonates weighing less than 1000 g required the introduction of the term **extremely** LBW (ELBW) to contextualize the challenges and outcomes related to these very small neonates. Given that about 70% of **perinatal mortality** (total of stillbirths and neonatal deaths) occurs in the 7% of babies whose birthweight is low or very low, this group of neonates clearly encounters complex problems. Regardless of the cause, these neonates are often grouped according to their birthweight in the following manner (Knight & Marshall, 2020):

1. LBW includes neonates weighing 2500 g or less at birth.
2. Very LBW includes neonates weighing 1500 g or less at birth.
3. ELBW includes neonates weighing under 1000 g at birth.

Causes of Low Birthweight

The two greatest reasons for LBW are **prematurity** and **intrauterine or fetal growth restriction** (IUGR/FGR) (Fig. 50.1). Premature neonates are born before 37 completed weeks of pregnancy, and the term *prematurity* is used regardless of birthweight. Neonates who are **small-for-gestational-age** (SGA) weigh less at birth than would be predicted for their gestational age. This group usually includes neonates born below the **10th centile.** Because these two groups of neonates are likely to present with a

• BOX 50.1 **Effect of Ethnicity and Deprivation on Perinatal Mortality**

Ethnicity and deprivation adversely impact on pregnancy, maternal and neonatal outcomes. Chapter 30 details risk factors during pregnancy. Draper et al. (2022) report the impact of ethnicity and deprivation on perinatal mortality.

1. Stillbirth and neonatal mortality rates increased with deprivation across all ethnic groups.
2. Stillbirth and neonatal mortality rates were lowest for babies of White ethnicity from the least deprived areas (2.78 stillbirths per 1000 total births and 1.26 neonatal deaths per 1000 live births).
3. The multiple impact of ethnicity and deprivation is highlighted by a stillbirth rate of 8.10 and 7.96 per 1000 total births for babies of Black African and Black Caribbean ethnicity, respectively, from the most deprived areas.
4. Neonatal mortality rates were over 3 per 1,000 live births for babies of Pakistani and Black African ethnicity from the most deprived areas.
5. Due to considerably higher proportions of babies of Black African, Black Caribbean, Pakistani and Bangladeshi ethnicity being from more deprived areas, they are disproportionately affected by the higher rates of stillbirth and neonatal death associated with deprivation.

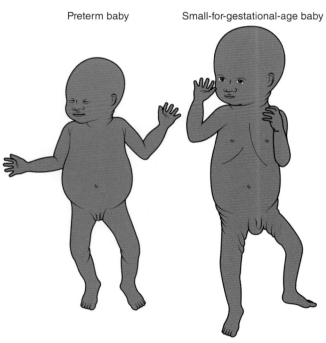

Preterm baby   Small-for-gestational-age baby

• **Fig. 50.1** Low-birthweight babies.

range of problems requiring specialist intervention, practitioners must be capable of assessing them at birth and identifying and managing problems which are present. Ongoing vigilance is needed to recognize new problems evolving in the first few days or even weeks of life. Specialist knowledge, clinical expertise and vigilance are crucial in providing optimal care.

Assessment of Gestational Age

One of the tools commonly used in the assessment of neonates is the **centile** chart (Fig. 50.2). Neonates suspected to be SGA can be confirmed by plotting their birthweight on an appropriate centile chart. This recording will invariably be more than two **standard deviations** below the mean or less than the 10th percentile of a population-specific birthweight for gestational age. It should be noted that within the World Health Organization (WHO) growth charts shown in Fig. 50.2 (now widely used within the UK), there is no **10th centile** line. Instead, a **9th centile** line is shown two standard deviations below the mean. This is the result of combining data collected by the WHO from healthy, exclusively breast-fed infants, showing optimal growth with the existing birth data from the UK 1990 growth reference, resulting in a more representative data set. Although variations in fetal growth exist, birthweight is frequently used to distinguish between neonates who are SGA from those who are small but normal for gestational age. Assessments of fetal growth, development and maturation must take into consideration variations in **genetic** and **environmental factors** which are known to affect the expectant mother's health and the growth of her fetus(es).

In most instances, assessment of fetal growth would be based on the length of gestation by considering the onset of the last menstrual period, the size and shape of the growing uterus and maternofetal hormone profile. **Ultrasonic studies** and, in some instances, **amniocentesis** provide additional information when required. Most fetuses fall into a **symmetric** or **asymmetric growth pattern.** Symmetric growth implies that both brain and body growths are limited, whereas asymmetric growth implies that body growth is restricted to a greater extent than head and brain growth. The mechanisms for such asynchronous growth are not understood, although Carducci et al. (2021) suggest that increased cerebral blood flow relative to the remainder of the systemic circulation may contribute. The birth of LBW neonates generally warrants the presence of experienced neonatal clinicians at the delivery.

In addition to establishing the birthweight, length, head circumference and gestational age, all small neonates must undergo a thorough physical assessment. This may include **scoring** of neurological and neuromuscular capabilities devised by Dubowitz, Dubowitz & Goldberg (1970) (Fig. 50.3). However because this scale awards points for neurological states and external criteria, it is not always suitable for assessing the gestational age of sick neonates. The Parkin score (Parkin, Hey & Clowes, 1976) and the New Ballard Maturational Score (Ballard et al., 1991), using physical and neurological criteria, are quicker to use. The Eregie score is another tool developed to estimate gestational age in African populations (Eregie & Muogbo, 1991). Raj et al. (2021) found that all these tools provided consistent scoring results.

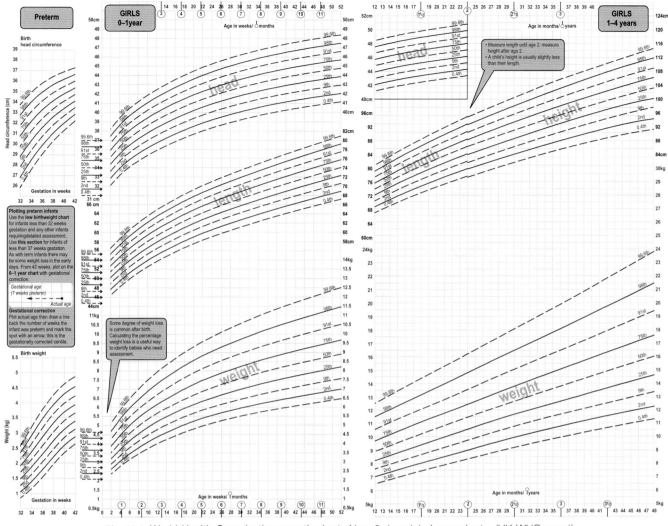

• **Fig. 50.2** World Health Organization growth chart. Now 0–1 and 1–4 year charts. (UK-WHO growth charts.)

The Preterm Neonate

Health challenges experienced by premature neonates can, to a large extent, be attributed to immaturity of body systems (Fig. 50.4). This means that some organs and systems have not reached the fully functional state required for adaptation to extrauterine life.

Characteristics of the Premature Neonate

- A large head and small face in proportion to the body.
- Soft skull bones with widely spaced sutures and large fontanelles.
- Neonates born before 24 weeks may present with fused eyelids.
- The skin is red and thin, subcutaneous fat is almost absent and surface veins are prominent.
- Lanugo is present, depending on the gestational age.
- A small narrow chest with little breast tissue.

- A large prominent abdomen with a low-set umbilicus.
- Thin limbs with soft nails not reaching the ends of the digits.
- Small genitalia: in girls, the labia majora do not cover the labia minora; in boys, the testes have not descended into the scrotum.
- Muscle tone is poor, and all four limbs may be held in the extended position.
- Normal reflexes, including sucking, gagging and coughing may be absent or feeble.

Causes of Preterm Birth

Although preterm births occur spontaneously, in many circumstances the sequence of events may be medically controlled for maternal or fetal safety. Whereas 40% of such births have no established causes, a range of contributing factors has been identified (Table 50.1). As illustrated, many suboptimal health problems appear to be the consequence of interplays between genetic and environmental factors (see Chapters 8 & 15).

Immediate Management

Proactive care of the premature neonate aims at supporting the physiological shortfalls which are apparent at birth. This care is often initiated before or during labour to ensure the neonate's survival. Ideally all premature neonates should be delivered in maternity units with specialist neonatal care facilities because the transfer of such small neonates is fraught with problems and increased risks.

Evidence-based considerations for care in labour and following birth are provided within the perinatal excellence to reduce injury in preterm birth (PERIPrem) care bundle (Williams et al., 2022). This builds upon earlier work in Scotland within the Preterm Perinatal Package (Maternity and Children Quality Improvement Collaborative, 2021) focused on births <34 weeks' gestation. The key elements of the PERIPrem care bundle are summarized in Table 50.2.

Ongoing Care of Premature Neonates
Potential Problems

Premature neonates may present with a potential for a range of problems. The main concerns are summarized in Box 50.2.

Any clinical evidence that some of these problems exist or could develop will require the premature neonate to receive specialist supportive care to prevent further escalation.

Maintenance of Temperature

Compared with term infants, premature infants have a narrower thermoneutral range where heat production cannot

External (superficial) criteria					
EXTERNAL SIGN	**SCORE** 0	1	2	3	4
OEDEMA	Obvious oedema hands and feet; pitting over tibia	No obvious oedema hands and feet; pitting over tibia	No oedema		
SKIN TEXTURE	Very thin, gelatinous	Thin and smooth	Smooth: medium thickness. Rash or superficial peeling	Slight thickening. Superficial cracking and peeling esp. hand and feet	Thick and parchment-like: superficial or deep cracking
SKIN COLOUR (infant not crying)	Dark red	Uniformly pink	Pale pink: variable over body	Pale. Only pink over ears, lips, palms or soles	
SKIN OPACITY (trunk)	Numerous veins and venules clearly seen, especially over abdomen	Veins and tributaries seen	A few large vessels clearly seen over abdomen	A few large vessels seen indistinctly over abdomen	No blood vessels seen
LANUGO (over back)	No lanugo	Abundant; long and thick over whole back	Hair thinning especially over lower back	Small amount of lanugo and bald areas	At least half of back devoid of lanugo
PLANTAR CREASES	No skin creases	Faint red marks over anterior half of sole	Definite red marks over more than anterior half; indentations over less than anterior third	Indentations over more than anterior third	Definite deep indentations over more than anterior third
NIPPLE FORMATION	Nipple barely visible; no areola	Nipple well defined; areola smooth and flat diameter <0.75 cm	Areola stippled, edge not raised; diameter <0.75 cm	Areola stippled, edge raised diameter >0.75 cm	
BREAST SIZE	No breast tissue palpable	Breast tissue on one or both sides <0.5 cm diameter	Breast tissue both sides; one or both 0.5–1.0 cm	Breast tissue both sides; one or both >1 cm	
EAR FORM	Pinna flat and shapeless, little or no incurving edge	Incurving of part of edge of pinna	Partial incurving whole of upper pinna	Well-defined incurving whole of upper pinna	
EAR FIRMNESS	Pinna soft, easily folded, no recoil	Pinna soft, easily folded, slow recoil	Cartilage to edge of pinna, but soft in places, ready recoil	Pinna firm, cartilage to edge, instant recoil	
GENITALIA MALE	Neither testis in scrotum	At least one testis high in scrotum	At least one testis right down		
FEMALE (with hips half abducted)	Labia majora widely separated, labia minora protruding	Labia majora almost cover labia minora	Labia majora completely cover labia minora		

(A)

• **Fig. 50.3 (A–C)** Dubowitz scoring system. **A** - External (superficial) criteria,

Neurological criteria						
NEURO-LOGICAL SIGN	**SCORE**					
	0	**1**	**2**	**3**	**4**	**5**
POSTURE						
SQUARE WINDOW	90°	60°	45°	30°	0°	
ANKLE DORSI-FLEXION	90°	75°	45°	20°	0°	
ARM RECOIL	180°	90–180°	90°			
LEG RECOIL	180°	90–180°	90°			
POPLITEAL ANGLE	180°	160°	130°	110°	90°	<90°
HEEL TO EAR						
SCARF SIGN						
HEAD LAG						
VENTRAL SUSPENSION						

Ⓑ

• **Fig. 50.3, cont'd** B - Neurological criteria,

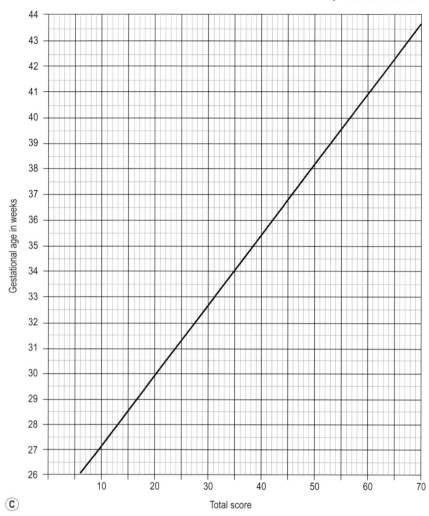

• **Fig. 50.3, cont'd** C - Total score (criteria A +B) to identify gestational age.

always match the rate of heat loss. This is further compromised by considerable heat loss due to a larger head-to-body ratio and the exaggerated body surface area that is characteristic of all premature and SGA neonates. The greater heat loss makes additional metabolic demands on the neonate, whose ability to assimilate nutrients and exchange gases can be compromised by multi-organ immaturity. Therefore although neonates are dependent on oxygen and glucose as energy, delivery of these substrates must not exceed the physiological norm.

To ensure that the neonate's body temperature is kept within the very narrow physiological range, ambient temperatures are held between 26°C and 28°C and the incubator temperature at about 36°C to maintain the neonate's body temperature at about 37°C. A temperature-monitoring skin probe (skin servocontrol) can be used to control the incubator temperature, allowing it to adjust automatically in response to changes in the neonate's temperature. Neonates born before 30 weeks of gestation have porous skin, allowing trans-epidermal water loss. Such neonates should be nursed in a humid atmosphere for the first week of their life.

Respiration

Premature neonates generally have a respiratory rate that averages closer to 60–80 breaths/min (Sinha, Miall & Jardine, 2018) with equal time for inspiration and expiration (ratio of 1:1). To ensure energy-efficient gas exchange, premature neonates use the apnoeic form of respiration: for instance, five short breaths are followed by a rest period. This physiological apnoea permits gas diffusion across the inflated alveolae and the pulmonary capillary interface. Ongoing observation and hourly monitoring should ensure that the neonate's respiratory functions are assessed, and distress is noted, including:

• The shape of the chest, assessing symmetry of inflation and expansion.
• The colour of the skin; evidence of central and peripheral cyanosis.
• The rate and rhythm and effort on respiration; evidence of sternal and subcostal recession.
• Breath sounds on chest auscultation; evidence of expiratory or inspiratory wheeze.

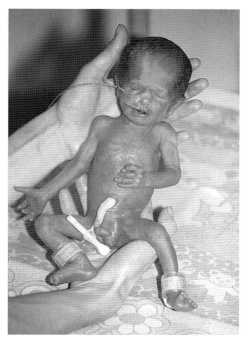

• **Fig. 50.4** A preterm infant.

TABLE 50.1 Causes of Preterm Birth

Fetal Causes	Maternal Causes
Multiple pregnancy	Pre-eclampsia
Polyhydramnios	Antepartum haemorrhage
Congenital abnormalities	Infection Rhesus incompatibility Systemic maternal disease such as diabetes mellitus Smoking, alcohol and drug abuse Maternal short stature Cervical incompetence Maternal age and parity Inappropriate maternal nutrition

TABLE 50.2 Key Elements of the PERIPrem Care Bundle

Birth in the right place	Delivery in a tertiary neonatal unit if <27 weeks, estimated fetal weight <800 g or multiple pregnancy <28 weeks.
Antenatal steroids	Administration of dexamethasone/betamethasone if <34 weeks. Aim for full course of two doses 12–24 hours apart.
Magnesium sulphate	For prevention of injury to neonatal brain. If <30 weeks optimally administer >4 hours and <24 hours from birth.
Early breastmilk (A)	Antenatal counselling of benefits and hand expression demonstrated. Assist mother to express <1 hour after birth.
Intrapartum antibiotic prophylaxis	If required, administered >4 hours pre-birth.
Optimal cord management	Aim for minimum of 60 s and lung aeration prior to cord clamping. Maintain thermal care throughout.
Thermoregulation	Aim for admission temperature of 36.5–37.5°C within 1 hour of admission to the neonatal unit.
Volume-targeted ventilation	If invasively ventilated, use this modality to minimize barotrauma.
Caffeine	If <30 weeks (but consider up to 32–34 weeks) and within 6 hours of admission.
Early breastmilk (B)	Early administration of colostrum/expressed breastmilk within 6 hours of birth.
Probiotics	Commence with non-nutritive feeds within first 24 hours.
Prophylactic hydrocortisone	If <28 weeks, commence 0.5 mg/kg dexamethasone/betamethasone started in the first 24 hours of life.

Oxygen Therapy

Oxygen therapy may be required in circumstances where respiratory distress and cyanosis develop (see Chapter 51). In such instances the temperature, humidity, flow rate and concentration of inspired oxygen must be monitored (Brown et al., 2021) to minimize the risks of oxygen toxicity. Oxygen-enriched air may be delivered to the neonate via head box, nasal cannula or, in more severe circumstances, by assisted mechanical ventilation. The amount of oxygen given must be adjusted to maintain arterial oxygen tension within a normal physiological range.

Too high concentrations of oxygen can have adverse effects, especially in premature neonates, contributing to the development of **retinopathy of prematurity** (Bhatt & Coats, 2018) and **bronchopulmonary damage.** Inadequate oxygenation or hypoxia can also be detrimental, particularly by contributing to episodes of profound bradycardia and cerebral hypoxia. Monitoring of oxygen administration by means of **pulse oxygen saturation (pulse oximetry)** and **arterial blood sampling** is therefore crucial, especially in very ill neonates. Because continuous pulse oximetry has many advantages over the intermittent sampling, it is the method of choice in most neonatal intensive care units. Non-invasive modes of respiratory support are now frequently used over **invasive assisted mechanical ventilation** for premature neonates (Boel et al., 2022). These include **heated humidified high-flow nasal cannula** and **nasal continuous positive airway pressure (nCPAP)**. These are effective means of life support where effective gas exchange cannot be sustained.

Potential Problems of the Premature Neonate

- Respiratory problems such as apnoea or respiratory distress syndrome.
- Metabolic problems such as hypoglycaemia and hypocalcaemia.
- Structural organic problems such as necrotizing enterocolitis and periventricular and intraventricular haemorrhage.
- Haematological problems such as jaundice and anaemia.
- Infection, either congenital or parentally acquired.

Nutrition

The neonate's specific nutritional requirements depend partly on his total body stores of fat, protein, glycogen, water and micronutrients. **Hypoglycaemia** is one of the most common problems of premature and LBW neonates, especially in the first 3 days of life (Hay, 2018). When planning a nutritional programme, intestinal uptake, assimilation of nutrients, energy expenditure and elimination must be taken into consideration in conjunction with the neonate's physical maturity and health.

For practical reasons, the neonate's energy requirements may be divided into two major roles: to support **physical growth** and **development** and to support metabolic activities and energy expenditure associated with **ill health.** In general, the energy requirements for metabolic activities take precedence over that required for growth. This becomes evident in circumstances where compromised nutrition and energy supply fail to meet the metabolic demands, resulting in poor growth.

Term neonates should be breastfed where circumstances allow. However the energy reserves and nutritional needs of premature and LBW neonates are more challenging. Milk expressed from the mothers of preterm infants has the correct whey:casein ratio and is preferable (Brown et al., 2021). Ideally appropriate nutritional support should commence within minutes of birth. However because the initial period tends to be complicated by a range of acute medical problems that require intervention, nutritional support is sometimes viewed as less important. Premature and SGA neonates should receive intravenous hydration and glucose within 30 min of their birth if homeostatic problems are to be avoided (Carducci et al., 2021). There is a need to be careful to prevent fluid overload, especially in infants whose mothers were given corticosteroids in labour (Nyp et al., 2021).

The nutritional considerations related to fat, protein and carbohydrate are summarized in Table 50.3.

Method of Feeding

The best method of feeding neonates depends on size, maturity and physical condition. Whenever possible, his inclination to suck should be used as an indication that breast or bottle feeding could be offered carefully. However premature neonates may have poor sucking and

TABLE 50.3   Nutritional Considerations Related to Fat, Protein and Carbohydrate

Fat	Fats are the main dietary source of energy in neonates, providing up to 50% of the total caloric needs. However all premature and low-birthweight (LBW) neonates have poor fat stores for energy production and for thermogenesis and lower plasma free fatty-acid levels in comparison to term neonates (Brown et al., 2021). Carducci et al. (2021) reported that these neonates appear to have deficient oxidation of free fatty acids and utilization of triglycerides, which could partly contribute to hypoglycaemia. Because fats are essential to the formation of cell membranes and contribute to the development of the nervous system, it seems logical that nutrition must contain the right kinds and quantities of fats to support the neonate's multifactorial needs.
Protein	Although dietary proteins supply less than 10–14% of the daily caloric needs, a daily intake of proteins is critical for growth, particularly in premature and LBW neonates whose muscle mass is deficient. Metabolic studies have shown that there is a need for higher protein intake in the preterm neonate than in the term infant, and protein supplementation is generally necessary. Protein loss may average 11–14% of the total body protein per day. Although neonates can synthesize some amino acids, some essential amino acids such as histidine, isoleucine, leucine, lysine, methionine, phenylalanine, threonine, tryptophan, taurine and valine must be given (Brown et al., 2021).
Carbohydrate	Enterally fed neonates use carbohydrates, and glucose in particular, as a major source of energy. The minimal 24-hour glucose utilization rate by the resting term neonate is estimated to be 4 mg/kg/min. An intake of glucose less than that rate may result in gluconeogenesis from non-carbohydrate sources such as amino acids. Conversely, excess glucose can be stored in the liver as glycogen and converted into glucose when required to support metabolic demands. However, in LBW neonates, glycogen stores are usually low in the early neonatal period, and this is a major contributing factor to the hypoglycaemia observed in these neonates. Other contributing factors may include deficient catecholamine release and decreased hepatic and muscle glycogen stores.

swallowing abilities so that **enteral tube feeding,** commonly **nasogastric,** may be necessary. Such feeding may be continuous or intermittent in circumstances where abdominal distension or severe regurgitation becomes apparent.

Neonates who require assisted mechanical ventilation may have the additional risk of milk aspiration, or the presence of milk in the stomach may impede respiratory function. In such instances **total parenteral nutrition** may be more suitable for providing nutritional support. If parenteral feeding is to be continued longer term, amino acids, lipids, vitamins and trace elements must be added. As the neonate's clinical condition improves, enteral feeding is introduced and gradually increased as the intravenous feeding regimen is reduced and discontinued.

Small and sick neonates will have additional nutritional requirements. Irrespective of whether enteral or parenteral feeding is chosen, the amount of fluid in which the nutrients are given must not exceed the kidney's ability to excrete metabolic waste products. Premature neonates grow more rapidly than term neonates and need, on average, 600 kJ/kg/day. To achieve this, 180–200 mL/kg/day of breastmilk or standard formula milk is necessary. Because this volume is excessive, the neonate's energy needs may be met by giving smaller amounts of LBW formula milk, fortifying breastmilk or adding calorific supplements to standard formula milk.

Supplements

Growing neonates require **nutritional supplements.** These include vitamins A and D from the age of 1 month to 2 years because premature babies have limited fat stores, which may have an impact on the neonate's ability to store and utilize fat-soluble vitamins. Vitamin C, a water-soluble vitamin, is also needed to support growth and healing and to aid iron absorption. Because there is a delay in the production of erythrocytes by the bone marrow, premature neonates can become very anaemic, sometimes requiring blood transfusion. In most instances, iron supplements are recommended from about the fourth week after birth until weaning.

The treatments themselves may contribute to problems. For instance, blood transfusion may suppress erythrocyte production, and iron supplementation can increase the risk of infection by inhibiting the anti-infective properties of lactoferrin, allowing *Escherichia coli* to multiply. Very small babies may also require folic acid supplements. Calcium and phosphate supplementation may be required to increase the rate of bone mineralization.

Excretion

As with all neonates, premature neonates should pass urine within 24 hours of birth and the amount should increase as fluid intake increases. All neonates cared for in a neonatal unit should have their urine output measured and the urine tested for glucose and **osmolality.** Glycosuria may indicate a lower renal threshold for glucose. This will require a review of the amount of glucose administered to avoid dehydration. The osmolality of the urine will indicate whether there is fluid retention or normal excretion, giving an indication of the amounts of fluids needing to be administered. Failure to produce urine, as well as failure to micturate, may be indicative of some haemodynamic problems such as hypotension, acute renal failure or urinary obstruction. Each of these problems is potentially life-threatening, and care must be taken to intervene in the earliest stages.

The passage of meconium may be delayed in small premature neonates, especially in those with moderately severe respiratory distress syndrome or suspected cystic fibrosis. Testing of the first meconium stool for the presence of abnormal constituents is important. The presence of blood and mucus in the stools may be indicative of a serious disorder such as necrotizing enterocolitis (Patel & Neu, 2018). Therefore this must be attended to immediately.

Pain

For many years, clinicians took little account of the pain suffered by neonates and small babies. Many believed neonates felt little pain (Gardner, Enzman-Hines & Agarwal, 2021). This view has now been largely dismissed by multiple studies showing that fetuses, neonates and small infants feel and respond to painful stimuli. From an evolutionary point of view, this would seem to be an essential adaptation to extrauterine life!

Balice-Bourgois et al. (2020) and Gardner, Enzman-Hines & Agarwal (2021) draw attention to the need for using adequate pain assessment tools and being proactive in the management of pain in neonates. Response to pain stimuli may be behavioural, such as crying, grimacing and startle or withdrawing limbs; physiological, such as tachycardia, bradycardia, hypertension and increased oxygen requirements; or metabolic, manifesting as increased metabolic rate in response to decreased insulin secretion and increased corticosteroid release, leading to hyperglycaemia and, in some instances, glycosuria, proteinuria, ketonuria and a raised urine pH.

The relief of pain includes caring for the environment. Staff should develop expertise in techniques such as heel prick and intravenous line siting, procedures known to induce pain. Comfort interventions such as stroking, non-nutritive sucking, positioning and cuddling can reduce pain. Non-pharmacological treatments such as **sucrose** and **skin-to-skin care** have been shown to reduce procedural pain (Nimbalkar et al., 2020). Analgesia, where required, must be used with caution, and anaesthesia should be used when invasive techniques and surgery are being carried out. Care must be taken not to suppress the neonate's respiratory drive and compromise respiratory function when postoperative analgesia is administered. Neonates whose respiratory function is supported by assisted mechanical ventilation may, if required, receive sedatives and, as an adjunct to analgesia, muscle-paralyzing agents.

Environmental Neonatology

The premature neonate is adapted to the intrauterine environment, and the effects of **noise, light, handling** and **positioning** may influence its well-being in the neonatal unit and beyond. Such neonates require a vast amount of sleep, yet neonatal units are not necessarily the most restful places for this. High noise levels, increased light levels and frequent handling disturbances are thought to contribute to apnoea and bradycardia and, in some instances, poor growth.

Noise

Noise levels are measured in logarithmic units called **decibels** (dB). The human ear is very sensitive and can hear sound over a wide range from a pin dropping to a shrieking steam whistle—a range from 0.1–120 dB. In adults, noise of 130 dB is invariably associated with inducing pain, with severe hearing dysfunction, and loss can occur with continuous exposure to sound over 90 dB.

Ongoing research into the effects of noise on these babies, such as the continuous noise levels inside an incubator, suggests that care should be taken to minimize all sounds. The mean recommended noise should not exceed 50 dB, and yet many incubator alarms can exceed 60 dB (Gardner & Goldson, 2021). Sudden loud noise can cause sleep disturbance, crying, tachycardia, hypoxaemia and raised intracranial pressure (Casey et al., 2020). This suggests that extra care must be taken when closing portholes and cupboard doors and moving incubators.

To observe neonates adequately, the level of light in neonatal intensive care units has increased 5- or 10-fold in the last two decades. Establishing a day/night pattern of lighting and dimming lights when not in use can reduce some of these harmful effects and is a key consideration in neonatal unit design (O'Callaghan, Dee & Philip, 2019).

Neonates undergoing **phototherapy** should have their eyes covered, and exposure to bright sunlight should be avoided. Phototherapy must be used vigilantly if the risks of encephalopathy caused by free or bound bilirubin are to be avoided.

Positioning

One significant problem in most neonatal units is the need to carry out invasive investigations whilst providing comforting care. Thoughtful planning to ensure that interventions are 'clustered' and carried out in a coordinated manner should ensure longer rest periods. Soothing and comforting interventions include massage and **'kangaroo mother care'** (Narciso, Beleza & Imoto, 2022) and **facilitated tucking** (containment of the infant's arms and legs in a flexed position close to his trunk) (Avcin & Kucukoglu, 2021; Balice-Bourgois et al., 2020).

Careful positioning that mimics the flexed position and extension normally adopted by the fetus during the last few weeks should be encouraged within the neonatal care setting (Sinha, Miall & Jardine, 2018). Premature neonates often develop flattened, elongated and asymmetrically shaped heads

which can be minimized by altering the resting position of the head and interspersing prone lying and lateral positioning with the hips and knees in optimal positions.

Infection

Exposure to pathogens is a major problem for premature neonates whose immune system cannot mount a full defence. Important considerations in the prevention of infection are detailed in Box 50.3.

Small for Gestational Age (SGA)

Neonates who are SGA are sometimes referred to as **'light for dates'** and can manifest symptoms of asymmetrical growth restriction or symmetrical growth restriction (see Chapter 13). Most of them are born after the 37th week of gestation and are frequently neurologically mature although lacking subcutaneous fat (Fig. 50.5). Their birthweight falls below the 10th percentile for gestational age (Hay, 2018). Because the fetal brain generally undergoes a growth spurt in the last trimester of pregnancy, there is sometimes a risk that this might have been compromised because of nutrient and oxygen deficiencies. Lack of energy stores can also compromise fetal ability to cope with the process of labour and birth. The risk of **hypoxia** during labour and **hypoglycaemia** after birth is high. Other health problems which may later be attributed to the condition of these fetuses in utero are **neurocognitive dysfunction, impaired renal** and **pulmonary function** and **metabolic syndromes** (Hwang, 2019).

Asymmetrical Growth Restriction

Asymmetrical growth restriction indicates that body growth is restricted to a much greater extent than growth of the head and the brain. In such cases, brain growth is considered **'spared'**. Maternal conditions such as pre-eclampsia

---

• BOX 50.3 Considerations for the Prevention of Infection

- Careful hand/forearm washing both before and after attending to each neonate.
- Regular use of appropriate liquid cleansing agents.
- Removal of jewellery and outdoor jackets.
- Use of personal protective equipment if body secretions are thought to be infectious.
- Each neonate must have a personal set of caring equipment stored in the vicinity of the incubator or cot.
- Allowance of sufficient space between cots or incubators to prevent cross-infection.
- Disposable items should be used where these are available, and continuous vigilance with cleaning of equipment is essential.
- Staff or visitors, including parents and siblings, with infections such as herpes simplex, upper respiratory tract infections, gastroenteritis or septic wounds should not enter a neonatal unit until their treatment is concluded and the infectious source eliminated.

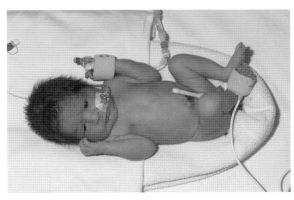

• **Fig. 50.5** A small-for-gestational-age (SGA) baby.

- The birthweight is low, but the head circumference and length of the baby are normal for gestational age.
- There is a lack of subcutaneous fat, and the body and limbs appear wasted.
- The ribs are visible, and the abdomen is flat or hollow due to the small size of the liver.
- The skin is dry, loose and peeling and may be stained with meconium.
- The umbilical cord is thin and may also be stained with meconium.
- The face often looks old and wizened with large eyes and an anxious and hungry expression.
- Muscle tone is generally good, and the neonate is active.
- The neonate is very hungry and sucks his fist.

may be a contributing factor, as it frequently affects placental function to the detriment of the fetus. Some features of fetal malnutrition are presented in Box 50.4.

Symmetrical Growth Restriction

Symmetrical growth restriction implies that the fetal brain and body growth are limited, a phenomenon which may be apparent throughout the pregnancy (Carducci et al., 2021). In this instance, the most common contributing factors could include intrauterine infections, maternal illness, fetal genetic or chromosomal abnormalities and maternal substance abuse. Characteristically, the neonate's head circumference is in proportion to body size and weight. These neonates may experience greater morbidity and mortality in comparison to neonates who present with asymmetrical growth restriction.

Immediate Management

SGA fetuses should be delivered in a maternity hospital with a suitably equipped neonatal unit capable of providing appropriate immediate care. Complications may include perinatal asphyxia (see Chapter 46), meconium aspiration syndrome, hypothermia, hypoglycaemia, **polycythaemia** and **pulmonary haemorrhage.** Most of these neonates also present with **immunological deficiencies** such as reduction in lymphocyte number and function. Many of these physical problems may extend beyond the neonatal period. Therefore early specialist intervention is invaluable in limiting undesirable outcomes. Some of these problems are discussed in Chapter 51.

Labour and Delivery

Recognition of fetal growth restriction in utero allows anticipation of poor energy reserves, including limited fat, muscle and glycogen stores. It is essential, therefore, particularly during labour, to monitor fetal well-being by continuously observing fetal heart rate patterns and noting the presence of fresh meconium in the liquor. A clinician skilled in resuscitation should be present at the delivery and initiate appropriate therapeutic and supportive intervention when required. Because these neonates lack subcutaneous fat, prompt drying and wrapping to prevent rapid heat loss is essential to minimize the risks of hypothermia developing.

Ongoing Care of SGA Babies

Many SGA neonates have different health-related problems from the premature neonate. However certain aspects of care such as the maintenance of body temperature, respiration, cardiac and renal function, nutrition and excretion require individual attention. Prevention of infection is a priority for both groups of babies. Because these babies are usually active, vigorous and alert and feed well, they may not require specialist care in a neonatal unit.

Transitional and Follow-up Care

Transitional care wards have been developed in many maternity units, situated near to the neonatal unit, allowing mothers to care for neonates with minor problems, supervised by experienced staff. Mothers and babies are not separated, and the mother is able to develop caring skills and, if breastfeeding, establish this effectively. Most of these neonates, regardless of their weight, are likely to be transferred home once they are well, providing that the home environment is suitable to their needs.

All neonates require **follow-up care** to ensure that their growth and **developmental milestones** are monitored, especially when growth has been symmetrically retarded. Because IUGR/FGR may be associated with ongoing and later health problems and complications, careful monitoring of these babies may be a considerable advantage.

Main Points

- About 70% of perinatal mortality occurs in the 7% of LBW babies. Such neonates may be small because of prematurity or because of being SGA.
- Care must be taken to minimize the neonate's excessive heat loss and body temperature should be maintained by creating a thermoneutral environment.
- Nutritional requirements will depend on total body stores of fat, protein, glycogen and ongoing energy expenditure.
- Premature neonates are poorly equipped in terms of maintenance of metabolic and nutritional homeostasis.
- In LBW, an infant's glycogen stores are usually lower in the early neonatal period, and this may contribute to hypoglycaemia.
- The method of feeding of neonates is determined by their maturity, size and state of health. Options include breastmilk, formula milk or total parenteral nutrition.
- All premature neonates should pass urine within 24 hours of delivery and the amount should increase as fluid intake increases.

- The passage of meconium may be delayed by several days in small premature neonates, especially if they experience respiratory difficulties. The presence of abdominal pain, blood and mucus in the stools may be indicative of the presence of necrotizing enterocolitis.
- The nervous system is sufficiently developed to allow neonates to feel and react to painful stimuli. Painful responses must be monitored and analgesia given if necessary. Comforting interventions such as stroking can sometimes reduce pain.
- The premature neonate gradually adapts to the extrauterine environment. Noise and light levels should be minimized to avoid any associated developmental problems.
- The immune system in all premature neonates is immature, contributing to an ongoing risk of infection; therefore high standards of infection control are essential.
- SGA neonates may present with asymmetrical or symmetrical growth restriction.
- SGA neonates may develop long-term problems as adults such as hypertension, cardiovascular disease and mature-onset diabetes mellitus.

References

Avcin, E., Kucukoglu, S., 2021. The effect of breastfeeding, kangaroo care, and facilitated tucking positioning in reducing the pain during heel stick in neonates. J. Pediatr. Nurs. 61, 410–416.

Balice-Bourgois, C., Zumstein-Shaha, M., Vanoni, F., Jaques, C., Newman, C.J., Simonetti, G.D., 2020. A systematic review of clinical practice guidelines for acute procedural pain on neonates. Clin. J. Pain 36 (5), 390–398.

Bhatt, A., Coats, D., 2018. Retinopathy of Prematurity. In: Kline, M., Blaney, S., Giardino, A., Orange, J.S., Penny, D.J., Schutze, G.E., et al. (Eds.), Rudolph's Pediatrics, twenty-third ed. McGraw-Hill, London.

Ballard, J.L., Khoury, J.C., Wedig, K., Wang, L., Eilers-Walsman, B.L., Lipp, R., 1991. New Ballard Score, expanded to include extremely premature infants. J. Pediatr. 119 (3), 417–423.

Boel, L., Hixson, T., Brown, L., Sage, J., Kotecha, S., 2022. Non-invasive respiratory support in preterm infants. Paediatr. Respir. Rev. 43, 53–59.

Brown, L., Hendrickson, K., Evans, R., et al., 2021. Enteral Nutrition. In: Gardner, S.L., Carter, B.S., Enzman-Hines, M., et al. (Eds.), Merenstein and Gardner's Handbook of Neonatal Intensive Care: An Interprofessional Approach, ninth ed. Elsevier, St. Louis.

Carducci, B., Campisi, S.C., Aleem, S., Bhutta, Z.A., 2021. The small-for-gestational age infant and IUGR. In: Boardman, J.P., Groves, A.M., Ramasethu, J. (Eds.), Avery & McDonald's Neonatology: Pathophysiology and Management of the Newborn, eighth ed. Lippincott, Williams & Wilkins, Philadelphia.

Casey, L., Fucile, S., Flavin, M., Dow, K., 2020. A two-pronged approach to reduce noise levels in the neonatal intensive care unit. Early Hum. Dev. 146, 105073.

Draper, E.S., Gallimore, I.D., Smith, L.K., Matthews, R.J., Fenton, A.C., Kurinczuk, J.J., et al., on behalf of the MBRRACE-UK Collaboration, 2022. MBRRACE-UK Perinatal Mortality Surveillance Report: UK Perinatal Deaths for Births from January to December 2020. The Infant Mortality and Morbidity Studies, Department of Health Sciences. University of Leicester, Leicester.

Dubowitz, L.M.S., Dubowitz, V., Goldberg, C., 1970. Clinical assessment of gestational age in the newborn infant. J. Pediatr. 77 (1), 1–10.

Eregie, C.O., Muogbo, D.C., 1991. A simplified method of estimating gestational age in an African population. Dev. Med. Child Neurol. 33 (2), 146–152.

Gardner, S.L., Goldson, E., 2021. The neonate and the environment: impact on development. In: Gardner, S.L., Carter, B.S., Enzman-Hines, M.I., Niermeyer, S. (Eds.), Merenstein and Gardner's Handbook of Neonatal Intensive Care: An Interprofessional Approach, ninth ed. Elsevier, St. Louis.

Gardner, S.L., Enzman-Hines, M., Agarwal, R., 2021. Pain and pain relief. In: Gardner, S.L., Carter, B.S., Enzman-Hines, M.I., Niermeyer, S. (Eds.), Merenstein and Gardner's Handbook of Neonatal Intensive Care: An Interprofessional Approach, ninth ed. Elsevier, St. Louis.

Hay, W., 2018. The small for gestational age infant. In: Kline, M., Blaney, S., Giardino, A., Orange, J.S., Penny, D.J., Schutze, G.E., et al. (Eds.), Rudolph's Pediatrics, twenty-third ed. McGraw-Hill, London.

Hwang, I.T., 2019. Long-term care, from neonatal period to adulthood, of children born small for gestational age. Clin. Pediatr. Endocrinol. 28 (4), 97–103.

Knight, M., Marshall, J.E., 2020. The healthy low birth weight baby. In: Marshall, J.E., Raynor, M.D. (Eds.), Myles' Textbook for Midwives, seventeenth ed. Elsevier, Edinburgh.

Maternity and Children Quality Improvement Collaborative (MCQIC), 2021. Preterm Perinatal Wellbeing Package (PPWP). Available at: https://ihub.scot/improvement-programmes/scottish-patient-safety-programme-spsp/spsp-programmes-of-work/maternity-and-children-quality-improvement-collaborative-mcqic/neonatal-care/preterm-perinatal-wellbeing-package/.

Narciso, L.M., Beleza, L.O., Imoto, A.M., 2022. The effectiveness of Kangaroo Mother Care in hospitalization period of preterm and low birth weight infants: systematic review and meta-analysis. J. Pediatr. 98 (2), 117–125.

Nimbalkar, S., Shukla, V.V., Chauhan, V., Phatak, A., Patel, D., Chapla, A., et al., 2020. Blinded randomized crossover trial: skin-to-skin care vs. sucrose for preterm neonatal pain. J. Perinatol. 40 (6), 896–901.

Nyp, M., Brunkhorst, J., Reavey, D., Pallotto, EK., 2021. Fluid and electrolyte management. In: Gardner, S.L., Carter, B.S., Enzman-Hines, M., Niermeyer, S. (Eds.), Merenstein and Gardner's Handbook of Neonatal Intensive Care: An Interprofessional Approach, ninth ed. Elsevier, St. Louis.

O'Callaghan, N., Dee, A., Philip, R.K., 2019. Evidence-based design for neonatal units: a systematic review. Matern Health Neonatol Perinatol 5 (1), 1–9.

Parkin, J.M., Hey, E.N., Clowes, J.S., 1976. Rapid assessment of gestational age at birth. Arch. Dis. Child. 51 (4), 259–263.

Patel, R.M., Neu, J., 2018. Necrotizing enterocolitis. In: Kline, M., Blaney, S., Giardino, A., Orange, J.S., Penny, D.J., Schutze, G.E., et al. (Eds.), Rudolph's Pediatrics, twenty-third ed. McGraw-Hill, London.

Raj, M., Kadirvel, K., Anandaraj, L., Palanisamy, S., 2021. Comparison of expanded new Ballard, Eregie and Parkin scores in predicting gestational age in newborns. J. Trop. Pediatr. 67 (4), fmab80.

Sinha, S., Miall, L., Jardine, L., 2018. Essential Neonatal Medicine, sixth ed. Wiley-Blackwell, Sussex.

UK-WHO growth charts - https://www.rcpch.ac.uk/sites/default/files/Girls_0-4_years_growth_chart.pdf.

Annotated recommended reading

Blackburn, S.T., 2018. Maternal, Fetal and Neonatal Physiology: A Clinical Perspective, fifth ed. Elsevier, St. Louis.

This textbook provides an invaluable account of the links between maternal, fetal and neonatal physiology. Written in an accessible yet detailed style, this is a valuable resource for any level of practitioner in maternity and neonatal care.

Draper, E.S., Gallimore, I.D., Smith, L.K., Matthews, R.J., Fenton, A.C., Kurinczuk, J.J., et al., on behalf of the MBRRACE-UK Collaboration, 2022. MBRRACE-UK Perinatal Mortality Surveillance Report: UK Perinatal Deaths for Births from January to December 2020. The Infant Mortality and Morbidity Studies, Department of Health Sciences. University of Leicester, Leicester.

This MBRRACE-UK report provides the latest information related to infant morbidity and mortality.

Gardner, S.L., Enzman-Hines, M., Agarwal, R., 2021. Pain and Pain Relief. In: Gardner, S.L., Carter, B.S., Enzman-Hines, M.I., Niermeyer, S. (Eds.), Merenstein and Gardner's Handbook of Neonatal Intensive Care: An Interprofessional Approach, ninth ed. Elsevier, St. Louis.

This textbook offers informative, highly readable systems-based accounts of common problems encountered by neonates and suggests a range of management and therapeutic interventions. The text is suitable for all students of nursing, midwifery and medicine when considering neonatal care.

51

Developmental Anatomy: Related Cardiovascular and Respiratory Disorders

THOMAS McEWAN

CHAPTER CONTENTS

Students and midwives should have a clear understanding of all the developmental anatomy relating to cardiovascular and respiratory disorders in the neonate..

Introduction

This chapter considers common neonatal **cardiovascular** and **respiratory problems.** Current research and specialist textbooks, such as those by Boardman, Groves & Ramasethu (2021) and Rogers (2022), give fuller accounts. Neonates can deteriorate and become ill very quickly. Therefore any neonate causing concern should be referred to a specialist clinician so that they are managed in a proactive manner. Prompt action will minimize short-term and long-term problems.

Aspects of Cardiovascular Development

The embryology of the anatomical structures of the heart is explained in Chapter 11, and the conducting system of the heart is detailed within Chapter 17. The student should refer to both sections for further information. Before the septation of the atria and the ventricles, specialized conducting cells form the sinoatrial ventriculobulbar and bulbotruncal junctions. This specialized conduction tissue is thought to originate from the cardiac myocytes, possibly in response to specialized signalling (Srivastava, 2018). The looping of the primitive heart allows the atrioventricular ring to invaginate so that it lies at the base of the atrial septum. This allows some of the specialized conduction cells to establish continuity between the atrioventricular node and the bundle of His. Failure in the various segments of these specialized conducting cells to contact each other causes congenital heart block.

Cardiovascular Problems

Cardiovascular Abnormalities

Cardiovascular malformations, or **congenital heart disease (CHD),** make up the largest group (approximately 30%) of congenital anomalies. This prevalence is around 6–11 per 1000 live births (Blundell, Jones & Crossland, 2021). Neonates may be born with **acyanotic** or **cyanotic cardiovascular anomalies** which will require expert intervention. Although the specific cause of cardiac anomalies is unknown, the occurrence of many of them is linked with chromosomal and genetic aberrations and poorly understood syndromes. For example, **atrioventricular canal** or **septal defects** are associated with trisomy 21, or Down syndrome. The affected chromosomes/genes in some syndromes have been identified as in trisomy 21. Other genetic mutations are discussed in Box 51.1. Because many of these anomalies are potentially life-threatening, parents will seek an explanation for these problems and any risks for recurrence in future pregnancies.

In general, cardiovascular anomalies are grouped according to the direction of blood flow. Therefore, defects that cause **'right-to-left shunts'** in the **heart** or **great vessels** almost always cause **central cyanosis.** In contrast, defects that cause **'left-to-right shunts'** in the **heart** or **great vessels** initially allow the neonate to be **acyanotic** (Table 51.1). Some cardiovascular anomalies cause obstruction, inhibiting either the right or the left ventricular outflow tract, as seen in neonates with pulmonary and aortic valve hypoplasia. Those neonates who develop **heart failure** eventually present with considerable peripheral and central cyanosis.

Risk Factors

Contributory factors thought to play a role in the development of some of the cardiovascular anomalies are presented in Box 51.2.

Presenting Features in a Neonate

Some of the following features may be present in neonates with cardiovascular anomalies, although some of these features may also be suggestive of respiratory problems:

- Tachypnoea/dyspnoea.
- Grunting.
- Pulmonary plethora.
- Peripheral/central cyanosis.
- Tachycardia.
- Heart murmurs.
- Poor feeding ability.
- Poor weight gain and growth retardation.
- Hepatomegaly.

An experienced neonatal clinician must examine all neonates presenting with any of these symptoms. However because some cardiovascular symptoms can be vague, the actual anomaly may not be diagnosed for several days or weeks and usually after extensive investigations in a specialist centre.

Investigations

Persistent tachypnoea may be the first indication of a cardiovascular or pulmonary anomaly. Generally, cardiovascular

anomalies that cause excessive pulmonary arterial blood flow and **pulmonary venous hypertension** enlarge the pulmonary vessels, causing **pulmonary oedema** and decreasing the neonate's lung compliance. The cumulative effects of all these events manifest in significant respiratory difficulties and cyanosis. In contrast, cardiovascular anomalies resulting in a decrease in pulmonary blood flow tend to contribute to intense cyanosis that elicits tachypnoea without significant respiratory distress. A persistent respiratory rate of 60 breaths/min or greater accompanied by increased respiratory depth commonly precedes clinical deterioration. Some standard investigations are discussed in Table 51.2.

Some Common Disorders: Acyanotic Lesions
Patent Ductus Arteriosus (PDA)

The incidence of isolated persistent **PDA** is about 0.1–0.2% of term infants and at least five-fold higher in premature infants (Anderson et al., 2021). In a term neonate, the ductus arteriosus usually closes within the first few hours of birth in response to increased blood oxygen saturation. This functional closure is then followed by an anatomical occlusion several days later. Premature neonates may take up to 3 months to achieve such spontaneous closures, which are attributed to the development of specialized contractile smooth muscle tissue and intimal thickening and fibrosis.

Where PDA persists, the fall in the neonate's pulmonary resistance reverses the direction of blood flow through

---

• BOX 51.2   Contributory Factors for the Development of Cardiovascular Anomalies

Maternal diabetes mellitus: ventricular septal defect (VSD), coarctation of the aorta and transposition of the great vessels.

Chromosomal abnormalities such as Down syndrome (40%): atrial septal defect, tetralogy of Fallot, VSDs and patent ductus arteriosus (PDA).

Genetic problems such as Williams syndrome.

Family history, where siblings or a parent has a cardiac defect.

Infectious agents such as those causing rubella or toxoplasmosis infection in pregnancy.

Nutritional/vitamin deficiencies such as folic acid deficiency (Obeid, Holzgreve & Pietrzik, 2019).

Environmental factors and maternal drug abuse (Kalisch-Smith, Ved & Sparrow, 2020).

• BOX 51.1   Genetic Mutations and Related Syndromes

Encoding for **extracellular matrix proteins**, with **fibrillin-1** being responsible for Marfan syndrome.

Deletion of material from chromosome 7 being responsible for Williams syndrome.

Genetic mutations on chromosome 22q11 may contribute to **aortic arch anomalies**, including **tetralogy of Fallot**.

TABLE 51.1   Cardiac Defects and their Relative Percentage Occurrence

Right-to-left Shunt	%	Left-to-right Shunt	%	Obstructive Disease	%
Transposition of the greater vessels	4	Ventricular septal defect	33	Aortic stenosis	6
Tricuspid atresia	1–2	Patent ductus arteriosus	10	Pulmonary stenosis	8
Total anomalous pulmonary venous drainage	1–2	Atrial septal defect	8	Coarctation of the aorta	6

the ductus from the aorta (left), shunting the oxygenated blood back into the pulmonary circulation (right). In some neonates, the ductus arteriosus remains open when cardiac anomalies such as pulmonary stenosis are present (Fig. 51.2). In such instances, the additional pulmonary blood flow is advantageous until the anomaly is surgically corrected. Failure of spontaneous closure of the PDA in premature neonates can contribute to persistence of respiratory distress syndrome (RDS). In term neonates, it may lead to congestive cardiac failure, pulmonary hypertension and subacute bacterial endocarditis.

Symptoms of PDA usually develop between the third and seventh days after birth. The neonate develops tachypnoea, dyspnoea and lethargy. Systolic and diastolic murmurs are almost always present. Therapeutic intervention includes avoidance of fluid overload, adequate oxygenation and, where necessary, diuretic therapy and correction of anaemia (Sinha, Miall & Jardine, 2018).

Indomethacin may be used to induce PDA closure in premature neonates, although term neonates are not as responsive to this drug, possibly due to its quicker clearance through the kidneys (Backes et al., 2018). As indomethacin binds to plasma albumin, its presence may displace bilirubin and contribute to jaundice. **Ibuprofen** can also induce ductal constriction (Surak, 2022). Alternatively, **paracetamol** has been shown to be efficacious to constrict the PDA (Gover et al., 2022). Where appropriate expertise is available, transcatheter device occlusion may be the method of choice for ductal closure; however more invasive methods of closure by means of a thoracotomy or thoracoscopy (Cabrera & Hoffman, 2018), which facilitate ligation, may be necessary if the earlier medical management fails.

TABLE 51.2	Standard Investigations for Cardiovascular Disorders
Pulse oximetry screening	A non-invasive and cost-effective investigation that can be useful in detecting critical congenital heart defects. False-positive results can arise, often indicating an underlying respiratory condition, but reduced if testing >24 hours. Site of testing (either postductal alone or pre- and postductal) has no significant effect on sensitivity or specificity (Jullien, 2021). Despite overwhelming evidence to support its use as a standard newborn screening tool and its current use for this purpose internationally, it is not currently supported by the UK National Screening Committee (Ewer et al., 2019).
Chest radiograph	A chest X-ray will establish the size and position of the heart in relation to the lungs and mediastinum because some cardiovascular defects and anomalies alter the normal size, shape and position of the heart. Any deviations from the normal appearance of the mediastinum, the heart, greater blood vessels and lungs contribute to the diagnosis.
Electrocardiography	Electrocardiography (ECG) is essential in cases of arrhythmia and may aid in the assessment of other conditions (Sinha, Miall & Jardine, 2018). ECG recordings often reflect the degree of neonatal adaptation to extrauterine life. Specialist practitioners should interpret the recorded evidence, distinguishing between the gradual transition in right ventricular dominance noticeable in the first 72 hours and electrophysiological anomalies that may help towards the overall diagnostic assessment.
Echocardiography	Exploration of the cardiovascular system by two-dimensional echocardiography involves ultrasound scanning (Fig. 51.1) and contributes to the analysis of cardiovascular and intracardiac structures (Swanson & Erikson, 2021). Neonates are good candidates for echocardiographic imaging because of their thin thoracic walls, with images of the heart chambers, valves and dimensions of the large vessels easily identifiable. Although many abnormalities can be identified in the fetus, new images are required after birth to confirm diagnosis. Colour images help to visualize the presence and direction of blood flow in neonates with persistent patent ductus arteriosus (PDA), septal defects, systemic venous anomalies and arteriovenous malformations. Pulsed and continuous-wave Doppler techniques can estimate pressure gradients across stenotic valves, septal defects and abnormal vessel structures such as the dimensions of PDA and coarctation of the aorta.
Magnetic resonance imaging	Magnetic resonance imaging detects intrathoracic abnormalities of the aortic arch, the peripheral pulmonary arteries and the systematic collateral vessels, which are not adequately evaluated by echocardiography.
	These are invasive procedures required in neonates with complex cardiovascular defects when explicit details are needed about the size of the defects and related haemodynamics. A fine catheter is inserted into the femoral vein, inferior vena cava, the right side of the heart, the pulmonary artery and its branches. In general, such procedures have diagnostic purposes, although occasionally cardiac catheterization can be used to provide emergency treatment for neonates born with transposition of the greater arteries or tricuspid atresia, whose life is dependent on interatrial blood flow. An intracardiac catheter can be used to carry out a balloon atrial septostomy, which enhances systemic and pulmonary blood flow. If a septal defect is present, it may be possible to pass the catheter into the left side of the heart. Abnormal tracts can be identified and blood pressure and oxygen saturation within the heart and great vessels can be measured (Qureshi & Justino, 2018).

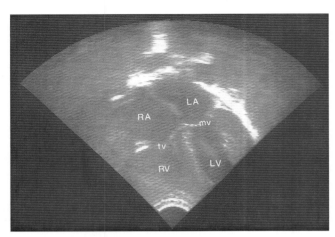

• **Fig. 51.1** A four-chamber ultrasound of the normal heart. *LA,* Left atrium; *LV,* left ventricle; *RA,* right atrium; *RV,* right ventricle; *tv,* tricuspid valve; *mv,* mitral valve.

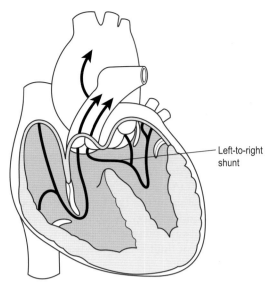

• **Fig. 51.3** Ventricular septal defect.

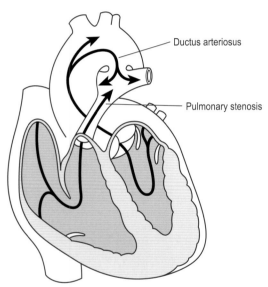

• **Fig. 51.2** Persistent ductus arteriosus in the presence of pulmonary stenosis.

Ventricular Septal Defects (VSDs)

VSDs are common and account for 40% of congenital heart malformations (Sinha, Miall & Jardine, 2018). A VSD can occur as an isolated intracardiac abnormality, or it can be an adjunct to other cardiovascular lesions, as is the case in about 50% of neonates born with congenital cardiovascular abnormalities. The defect usually occurs in the **membranous septum** but can present anywhere within the muscular part of the **interventricular septum** (Fig. 51.3).

The size and complexity of such defects vary from minute openings to almost complete absence of the interventricular septum. Knowledge of the precise size and position of the defect(s) is critical to successful therapeutic management. The incidence of spontaneous closure of a muscular defect is high, averaging 70%, although surgical repair is required where larger defects fail to close or membranous defects persist. Infants with small defects may be asymptomatic and eventually experience spontaneous closure, resulting in normal cardiac anatomy.

Larger defects are likely to lead to **congestive cardiac failure (CCF),** feeding problems and delays in growth. For this reason, VSDs are classified as acyanotic heart lesions with increased pulmonary blood flow caused by the increasing left ventricular pressure occurring after birth. The defect generates a left-to-right interventricular flow of blood. The presence of multiple VSDs or a large VSD allows the left-to-right shunt to equalize the pressure in both ventricles due to the shunting of oxygenated blood from the left ventricle into the right ventricle. This shunting will eventually lead to right ventricular volume overload, **pulmonary plethora** and CCF. Furthermore, the persistent increase in pulmonary blood volume increases pulmonary venous return to the left side of the heart. This eventually results in left ventricular volume overload, exacerbation of the left-to-right shunt and left ventricular hypertrophy.

For a time, the enlarged left ventricle pumps more efficiently, but eventually the heart fails, and pulmonary hypertension develops. If untreated, the persistent problems contribute to the development of **Eisenmenger syndrome** (Rogers, 2022). Pre-emptive therapeutic interventions are important if long-term problems are to be averted or minimized. Early diagnosis and proactive management of CCF as noted earlier should be considered until the defect is closed surgically. Where necessary, surgery is delayed until the infant is at least 12–18 months old, but all defects must ideally be closed, surgically if necessary, by the time the child enters school.

Atrial Septal Defects (ASDs)

ASDs are relatively common congenital cardiac malformations occurring in 1 in 1500 live births (Blundell, Jones & Crossland, 2021). Interference with sequential atrial septal development may cause a variety of ASDs (Bradley & Zaidi,

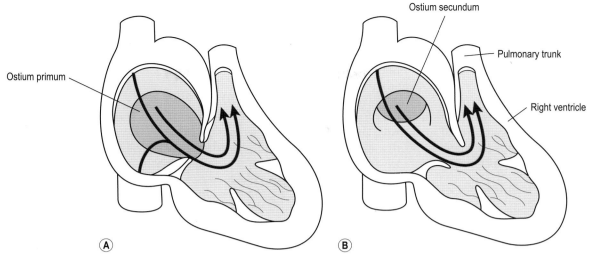

• **Fig. 51.4** (A) Ostium primum lesion. (B) Ostium secundum lesion.

2020; Srivastava, 2018). Some may be simple, involving only the foramen ovale, whereas others may be complex. Severe atrioventricular defects may extend to the ventricular septum and the **mitral** and **tricuspid** valves.

The most common of these defects are:

- **Ostium primum** with endocardial cushion defects. This defect is generally associated with abnormalities of the mitral valve and atrioventricular canals (Fig. 51.4A). Although this defect may occur in isolation in otherwise normal neonates, 30% of cases occur in neonates with Down syndrome in whom the involvement of the endocardial cushions may also contribute to the defective formation of the upper portion of the intraventricular septum.
- **Ostium secundum.** This defect is found in the central portion of the atrial septum. Because of its close anatomical association with the fossa ovalis, it is often referred to as the *fossa ovalis defect* (Fig. 51.4B).
- **Sinus venosus** defect. This defect is characteristically found in the superior portion of the atrial septum and generally extends into the superior vena cava.

Simple defects cause few problems and, if spontaneous closure does not occur, surgical repairs are carried out by about 2–5 years of age. However for neonates born with atrioventricular septal defect (AVSD), the management is more complex, as they may experience conduction problems. Complex ASDs may present in early life as these neonates develop tachypnoea, abnormal heart sounds, poor feeding and failure to gain weight (Kline et al., 2018).

Some Common Disorders: Cyanotic Lesions

Transposition of the Great Arteries (TGA)

Complete TGA is the most common cardiovascular cause of peripheral and central cyanosis in neonates; the aorta arises from the right ventricle and the pulmonary artery from the left ventricle. This complete switch of the great vessels (Fig. 51.5) leads to the formation of **two separate**

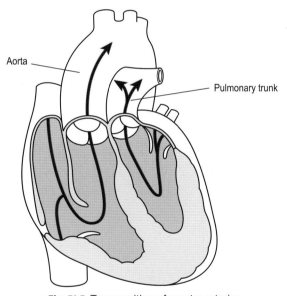

• **Fig. 51.5** Transposition of greater arteries.

closed circulatory systems, whereby the blood from the pulmonary circulation cannot enter the systemic circulation and vice versa. Survival of these neonates depends on the patency of the right-to-left shunts in the ductus arteriosus and/or the foramen ovale. The presence of a concurrent VSD also permits mixing of the oxygenated and deoxygenated blood at the interventricular level. Boys appear to be affected twice as often as girls (Blundell, Jones & Crossland, 2021).

A neonate with complete TGA and no accompanying ventricular defect will become increasingly cyanotic as the ductus arteriosus begins to close. This cyanosis is not relieved by administration of 100% oxygen, and urgent life-saving intervention is needed. This is likely to consist of **prostaglandin infusion** to maintain the PDA open until palliative or corrective **surgery** can be carried out.

The palliative intervention may consist of a balloon septostomy (e.g., **Rashkind's**), generally carried out as an emergency to enlarge the foramen ovale and increase the interatrial mixing of blood. When possible, corrective surgery will be carried out some weeks/months later (Fig. 51.6). This consists of switching the pulmonary artery and the aorta to the correct ventricles and closing any remaining cardiovascular defects. Care is taken to ensure that the **coronary arteries** can sustain **normal myocardial perfusion.** Most surgical corrections are successful, with a survival rate of up to 90% (Rogers, 2022).

Total Anomalous Pulmonary Venous Drainage

Total anomalous pulmonary venous connection occurs in 1 in 15,000 births and is characterized by the absence of any direct connection of the **pulmonary veins** to the left **atrium.** Instead, the pulmonary veins connect to the right atrium, various systemic veins or the liver. Central cyanosis,

dyspnoea, tachypnoea and CCF occur and urgent, life-saving surgical correction is necessary, with extracorporeal membrane oxygenation (ECMO) often used until surgery can be undertaken. Mortality can be between 5% and 25% (Swanson & Erikson, 2021).

Tetralogy of Fallot

Tetralogy of Fallot is the most common form of cyanotic congenital lesion in infants, affecting around 1 in 3600 births (Sinha, Miall & Jardine, 2018). Neonates can sometimes be asymptomatic. The four anatomic defects are (Fig. 51.7):
1. A high, large VSD.
2. An overriding aorta which straddles the VSD.
3. Pulmonary stenosis: a funnel-shaped opening at the entrance to the pulmonary artery. The pulmonary artery and valve may rarely be completely obliterated.
4. Right ventricular hypertrophy, developing because of the obstruction to blood flow.

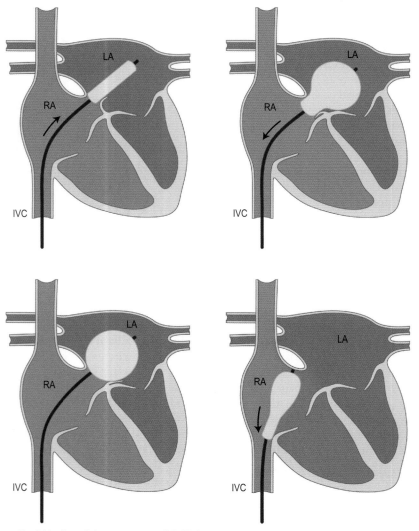

• **Fig. 51.6** Rashkind's atrial septostomy. *RA,* Right atrium; *LA,* Left atrium; *IVC,* Inferior vena cava.

These defects can be associated with Down syndrome, first-trimester rubella infection, Noonan's syndrome, Turner syndrome and other undefined genetic mutations (Bull, 2020; Huang, Olson and Maslen, 2021; Linglart & Gelb, 2020; Suryadevara, 2021). The clinical features of this defect relate to the neonate's pulmonary blood flow, which depends on:

1. The severity of the right ventricular outflow tract obstruction.
2. The relative resistance to ventricular outflow imposed by the systemic and pulmonary circulations.
3. The presence of systemic-to-pulmonary collateral blood flow through the bronchial arteries or, rarely, a PDA.

The symptoms vary depending on the degree of pulmonary stenosis, although the size of the VSD is important. Pulmonary stenosis decreases blood flow to the lungs, as well as the return of oxygenated blood to the left atrium. With a large VSD, blood may shunt from the right ventricle to the left ventricle, causing further reduction in systemic oxygen content and an increase in central and peripheral cyanosis. However, giving oxygen in this instance may result in the closure of the PDA, further increasing cyanosis. Hypoxia stimulates the kidneys to produce erythropoietin, so most children develop polycythaemia. Older children may have sudden spells of dyspnoea, cyanosis and restlessness and squat to alleviate these hypoxic spells.

Infants born with tetralogy of Fallot and pulmonary atresia usually require specialist surgical intervention of a corrective and/or palliative nature in the first few days or weeks of life. Because most such infants will have a history of CCF which might impair their growth and development, management in a specialist cardiac centre is advocated.

Some Common Disorders: Obstructive Lesions
Coarctation of the Aorta

Coarctation of the aorta occurs in 1 in 2500 births (Sinha, Miall & Jardine, 2018) and is characterized by an abnormal segmental narrowing of the aorta anywhere from the aortic arch to the bifurcation of the abdominal aorta at its lower end. However, 98% occur at the junction with the ductus arteriosus. The narrowing may occur **preductal** (Fig. 51.8) or **postductal**, appearing after the opening of the ductus arteriosus. Generally, coarctations of the aorta obstruct left ventricular outflow, leading to left ventricular failure, with many neonates presenting with life-threatening haemodynamic disturbances that lead to acute myocardial and renal failure.

In neonates presenting with postductal coarctation of the aorta, blood is delivered to the upper body from the ascending aorta via the subclavian arteries; this increases the blood pressure to the upper parts of the body. However as the aortic narrowing reduces blood flow to the descending aorta, the lower parts of the body are not so well perfused so that the blood pressure in the lower limbs is low and **femoral pulses** are weak and sometimes absent. If oxygen saturation monitoring is undertaken, the levels in the right arm (**preductal**) will be *higher* than that measured in the lower limbs (**postductal**).

CCF may be one of the first features manifested by such neonates and must be managed accordingly. However, *high oxygen levels must be avoided* and prostaglandin (PGE_1) may be given intravenously to maintain patency of the ductus arteriosus until the coarctation of the aorta is surgically corrected. Diuretics may be given to decrease fluid overload and correct pulmonary and systemic oedema. Surgery with correction and reconstruction of the defective segment of the aorta will be carried out as the neonate's clinical condition is stabilized.

Pulmonary Valve Stenosis and Aortic Valve Stenosis

Narrowing of the **pulmonary valve** occurs on its own in about 8% and **aortic stenosis** in about 6% of children born

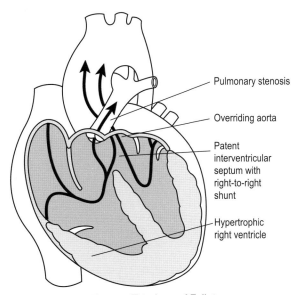

• **Fig. 51.7** Tetralogy of Fallot.

Pulmonary stenosis

Overriding aorta

Patent interventricular septum with right-to-right shunt

Hypertrophic right ventricle

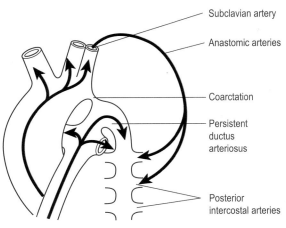

• **Fig. 51.8** Preductal coarctation of the aorta.

Subclavian artery

Anastomic arteries

Coarctation

Persistent ductus arteriosus

Posterior intercostal arteries

with congenital cardiac abnormalities. Mild valvular stenosis improves with age, although more severe narrowing produces symptoms in neonates, most commonly pulmonary oedema and CCF. Surgical correction or, less commonly, valve replacement may be necessary in early infancy or childhood if cardiorespiratory function is compromising the child's growth and exercise tolerance.

Hypoplastic Left Heart Syndrome

This syndrome is the consequence of specific cardiovascular malformations such as severe obstruction or atresia of the mitral valve, diminutive left ventricle, aortic atresia and malalignments of the **atrioventricular canals.** These neonates become symptomatic within the first few hours or days of life, developing CCF (see later). Cardiac enlargement, pulmonary plethora, hypotension and bradycardia require supportive intervention. Surviving neonates will require palliative surgery. Despite advances in paediatric cardiothoracic surgery, the mortality rate is high (Swanson & Erikson, 2021). **Cardiac transplantation** might be considered.

Congestive Cardiac Failure

CCF is a syndrome in which the failing heart cannot sustain a normal cardiac output or supply adequate oxygenated blood to the tissues. The major causes in neonates are **excessive volume overload, excessive pressure load** and **abnormal myocardial function.**

Excessive Volume Overload

Large valve incompetence or left-to-right shunts are the most common causes of volume overload, and in the neonate the cause is likely to be attributed to a PDA, large VSDs or endocardial cushion defects with gross valve incompetence. Less commonly, volume overload may be initiated by excessive placental transfusion at birth.

Excessive Pressure Load

Severe forms of aortic stenosis and coarctation of the aorta, commonly referred to as **left ventricular outflow tract obstruction,** lead to CCF in the first weeks of life. Infants with either of these lesions may present with very poor pulses and a large left-to-right shunt at the atrial level. The moderately severe pulmonary hypertension can be attributed to early CCF. Once the intra-atrial left-to-right shunt reverses or a large right-to-left shunt develops through the ductus arteriosus, neonates present with moderately severe peripheral and central cyanosis.

Arrhythmias in the Newborn

Often suspected after detection of a fetal arrhythmia, these are seen in 1% of neonates in the first week to 10 days of life (Joshi & Humagain, 2020). Causes include the physiological vulnerability of the myocardium, affected by trauma or birth asphyxia, and symptoms can range from mild to severe, may be transient or require significant treatment (Vlădăreanu, Vlădăreanu & Boţ, 2021). Dysrhythmias include:

- Supraventricular tachycardia (SVT), commonly narrow complex SVT in the newborn.
- Ventricular tachycardia and fibrillation.
- Congenital atrioventricular heart block.

Lower Respiratory Tract Problems in Neonates

Breathing difficulties are one of the most common clinical problems encountered in neonates, and it is often difficult to make a clear diagnosis, even after examining chest X-rays together with other diagnostic results. Lung infections are difficult to rule out, and many neonates are given antibiotics until microbiology results are available. Birth records detailing neonatal respiratory effort and the time of onset of respiratory difficulties are important in formulating a diagnosis. A major difficulty is to establish whether the neonate's cyanosis is caused by respiratory disorders or CHD (Blundell, Jones & Crossland, 2021), although a distinction must be made if treatment is to succeed. Neonates with significant respiratory dysfunction accompanied by cyanosis should be cared for in neonatal intensive care units.

Respiratory Distress Syndrome (RDS)

Most neonates initiate spontaneous respiration at birth. The inspired air gradually displaces the alveolar and interstitial fluid, allowing a greater pulmonary blood flow as the vascular tree expands. The 10-fold increase in pulmonary capillary blood facilitates an acceptable gas exchange across alveolar walls, providing the lungs are sufficiently mature and capable of synthesizing **surfactant** (further described in Box 51.3).

• BOX 51.3 **Surfactant**

Surfactant, a lipoprotein complex secreted by type II pneumocytes, consists of 90% **lipids**, including **lecithin**, **sphingomyelin** and **cholesterol**. The remainder is made up of substances such as specific proteins and some carbohydrates. Surfactant is extruded into the alveolar spaces where it unravels, forming complex lipid structures called **tubular myelin**. These form the **surface monolayer** at the alveolar air–liquid interface.

The fetal lungs secrete surfactant from about the 22nd week, with considerable surges at 33 weeks of gestation and at birth. Surfactant coats the inner aspect of the alveoli and reduces surface tension created by the alveolar fluid, ensuring that the alveoli do not collapse at the end of expiration. The ratio of lecithin to sphingomyelin (**L:S ratio**) is 1:1 at about 34 weeks of gestation, but the amount of lecithin increases until the ratio is 2:1, comparable to a mature lung. Amniotic fluid can be tested for these two substances to establish fetal lung maturity.

RDS occurs predominantly in premature neonates due to immature lung anatomy and physiology (Gardner, Enzman-Hines & Nyp, 2021). This severe lung disorder causes more neonatal deaths than any other condition. The incidence is inversely proportional to gestational age, occurring in >50% of neonates born at <28 weeks' gestation but declines sharply towards term (Gardner, Enzman-Hines & Nyp, 2021). The cause is multifactorial, but insufficient active pulmonary surfactant is the major contributing factor. Predisposing factors include:

- Immature lungs, especially in male neonates.
- Surfactant inactivation caused by endothelial damage.
- Birth by caesarean section before the onset of labour.
- Asphyxia neonatorum, as respiratory and metabolic acidosis interferes with surfactant synthesis.
- Second twin.
- Mother has a history of diabetes mellitus (this seems to delay lung maturity).
- Premature/prolonged rupture of membranes.

Pathophysiology

RDS is caused by the absence or immaturity of type II pneumocytes and their incapacity to produce enough functional surfactant. A greater inspiratory effort is needed to keep the alveoli open. Poor alveolar stability contributes to poor lung compliance, limited lung distensibility and reduced functional residual capacity. This directly affects **pulmonary perfusion,** and most neonates develop a right-to-left shunt, which contributes to significant hypoxia with a depressing effect on myocardial function. A moderate PDA may also add to the existing respiratory problems due to the additional pulmonary blood flow which compromises pulmonary function. Some neonates will eventually develop myocardial failure, hypotension and poor renal and peripheral perfusion.

Other problems such as **respiratory acidosis** and **atelectasis** (inadequate alveolar expansion and collapse of lung tissue) further compromise respiratory gas exchange. Atelectasis is generally attributed to unequal pressures and filling capacity in some alveoli. The normal alveoli become overdistended and the smaller alveoli collapse, reducing the functional residual capacity and creating a significant **dead space** within the lungs (Blackburn, 2018).

The resulting **hypoxia** and **hypercapnia** lead to pulmonary vasoconstriction and, sometimes, **persistent fetal circulation** with significant intracardiac right-to-left shunting of blood through the foramen ovale and ductus arteriosus. Lung ischaemia exacerbates the damage to the alveolar epithelial surfaces and capillaries. Metabolic and respiratory acidosis further suppresses the production of surfactant. Increased alveolar surface tension combined with the low plasma protein levels present in the premature neonates lead to a shift of interstitial fluid towards the alveolar space. Because the exudate is rich in **fibrinogen,** it is converted to **fibrin** as it lines the alveoli. Blood products and cellular debris present within the alveoli bind the fibrin, forming the **hyaline membrane,** which further reduces lung surface area (Blackburn, 2018) and makes the lungs less compliant.

Clinical Symptoms

Affected neonates gradually develop symptoms of RDS, typically about 4 hours after birth, with tachypnoea, increased respiratory effort and grunting on expiration. There is evidence of chest wall recession and peripheral and later central cyanosis (Fig. 51.9). A chest X-ray shows a 'ground-glass' appearance to the lungs (Fig. 51.10), whereas an air bronchogram shows air in the larger airways against the background opaqueness (Gardner, Enzman-Hines & Nyp, 2021).

Management of RDS

Prebirth Maternal Treatment with Corticosteroids

Management of RDS includes prevention and treatment. The production of surfactant in the fetal lung can be increased by treating the mother with a **corticosteroid** such as betamethasone for at least 24 hours before birth. Indications for commencing corticosteroid administration may be a low lecithin:sphingomyelin ratio or, if this invasive test is not possible, the anticipated premature birth. Roberts & Dalziel's (2006) review of the research concluded that this proactive management reduces the severity of RDS in susceptible premature neonates with significant reduction in morbidity and mortality, confirmed more recently by Uggioni et al. (2022).

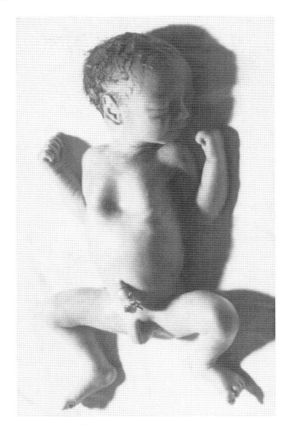

• **Fig. 51.9** A baby with respiratory distress syndrome. Note marked sternal recession.

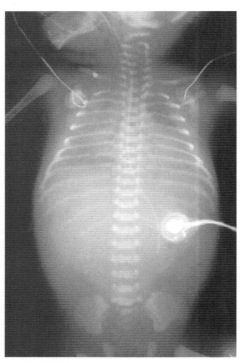

• **Fig. 51.10** Chest X-ray showing 'ground-glass' appearance of the lungs in hyaline membrane disease.

Surfactant Therapy

The use of natural and artificial surfactant postdelivery has been effective in the management of affected neonates. Reviews concerning **surfactant therapy,** comparing the benefits and drawbacks of natural versus synthetic surfactant, suggest both are effective in the treatment of established RDS, with naturally derived preparations the most desirable (Ardell, Pfister & Soll, 2015). There was earlier improvement in neonates who required assisted ventilatory support (Stevens et al., 2007), with fewer instances of **pneumothorax** occurring in neonates treated with natural surfactant extract (Hentschel et al., 2020).

Respiratory Support

Some neonates may require a **heated humidified high-flow nasal cannula** to support respiratory function, reducing nasopharyngeal dead space and decreasing CO_2 rebreathing whilst providing an oxygen reservoir. Alternatively **nasal continuous positive-airway pressure** (nCPAP) can reduce the work of breathing by maintaining a constant alveolar end-expiratory pressure or **non-invasive positive-pressure ventilation** (NIPPV), providing intermittent peak pressures (Mukerji et al., 2021). However, very small neonates and those with severe RDS may still require mechanical ventilation by **intermittent positive-pressure ventilation** (IPPV) (de Waal & van Kaam, 2018), and this group of neonates may also benefit from the use of surfactant therapies. See Box 51.4 for complications of oxygen therapy and IPPV.

• BOX 51.4   Complication of Oxygen Therapy and Intermittent Positive-Pressure Ventilation (IPPV)

Complications associated with excessive use of oxygen therapy and IPPV include:

- Pneumothorax, pulmonary interstitial fibrosis and later bronchopulmonary dysplasia.
- Periventricular haemorrhage when oxygen saturation is badly controlled or excessive.
- Infection and secondary pneumonia may follow endotracheal intubation and periodic lavage to keep the tube patent.
- Retinopathy (retrolental fibroplasia) most common in premature neonates exposed to high O_2 tension.
- Cellular damage due to the excessive production of oxygen-derived free radicals.

Bronchopulmonary Dysplasia

Bronchopulmonary dysplasia is a form of subacute or chronic **fibrosis of the lungs** associated with severe RDS, prolonged assisted mechanical ventilation and high oxygen requirement. This disorder affects infants weighing less than 1500 g at birth (Gardner, Enzman-Hines & Nyp, 2021; Jensen, Zhang & Kirpalani, 2018). Affected infants remain oxygen-dependent, have respiratory symptoms such as tachypnoea and intercostal recession and abnormal lung findings on radiography (Fig. 51.11) after 28 days (Rogers, 2022).

Scarring of the lung tissue, **emphysema,** failure of the alveoli to multiply and inflammatory destruction of the epithelial lining of the lungs and ciliated epithelial surfaces in the bronchi are characteristic features. In addition, mucous plugs and debris clog the small-diameter airways, contributing to recurrent pulmonary infection. The clinical picture may persist for some months or years and, whilst some infants recover with minimal residual lung damage, others die.

Meconium Aspiration Syndrome

When a fetus suffers from intrapartum asphyxia, meconium is passed into the amniotic fluid and inhaled as gasping movements are made. There is insufficient evidence to support routine nasal, oral or tracheal suctioning in the neonate when meconium is present. Following the birth of a non-breathing or ineffectively breathing neonate, the initiation of ventilation should not be delayed, regardless of the presence of meconium (Madar et al., 2021). Only if effective lung inflation is unsuccessful should the airway be inspected to exclude obstruction by meconium.

Meconium encourages growth of micro-organisms, and any neonate suspected of having inhaled meconium must be observed for the next 24–48 hours for signs of respiratory distress manifesting as tachypnoea and cyanosis. Oxygen therapy may be required, and a prophylactic course of antibiotics may be given to avert the onset of **pneumonia.** More severely affected neonates may show signs of persistent

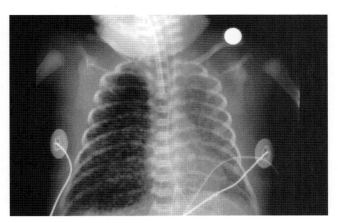

• **Fig. 51.11** Chest X-ray showing early stages of bronchopulmonary dysplasia.

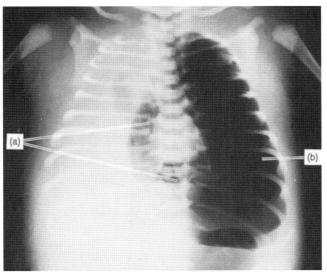

• **Fig. 51.12** Pneumopericardium (A) with a large left pneumothorax (B).

fetal circulation, resulting in cardiopulmonary problems such as pulmonary hypertension, systemic hypotension and hypoxia. Pneumothorax is a relatively common complication (Olicker, Raffay & Ryan, 2021).

The presence of meconium in the lung may inactivate surfactant, and short-term administration of surfactant, commenced within 6 hours of birth, improves oxygenation and reduced respiratory morbidity. However, where persistent fetal circulation and pulmonary hypertension are severe, more drastic measures involve assisted ventilatory support using high-frequency oscillatory ventilation and **inhaled nitric oxide (iNO).** However, the evidence to support surfactant therapy, either alone or in conjunction with nitric oxide or ventilation, remains inconsistent (Abdelaal, Abushanab & Al-Badriyeh, 2020; Soll & Dargaville, 2000). In severe cases, **ECMO** therapy may be required (Fichera et al., 2019).

Pneumothorax

A pneumothorax occurs because of injury to the pleural membranes, allowing air to leak into the pleural space. In neonates, the most likely cause is alveolar rupture and associated damage to the visceral layer of the **pleural membrane.** The affected lung collapses and may cause a mediastinal shift and displacement of the normal position of the heart and greater vessels. This in turn compromises cardiac function, initiating low cardiac output, hypotension and bradycardia. Recently, the selective use of surfactant therapy has contributed to a significant reduction in the number of neonates developing a pneumothorax and requiring additional supportive interventions.

A pneumothorax does not present with the classical symptoms seen in the adult and may be difficult to diagnose. The neonate collapses suddenly and becomes cyanotic with bradycardia. There may be cardiac displacement and **transillumination;** shining a cold light against the thorax may demonstrate air around the lung. Chest radiography will confirm the diagnosis (Fig. 51.12). If the neonate is otherwise in good health, draining the air may not be necessary, as it will be gradually reabsorbed. However, neonates who experience respiratory distress and haemodynamic changes will require the insertion of a pleural drain connected to underwater sealed drainage, which allows the air to escape and the lung to re-expand.

Transient Tachypnoea of the Newborn

Transient tachypnoea of the newborn is relatively common in term neonates who present with tachypnoea, intercostal retraction, expiratory grunting and possibly cyanosis. A chest X-ray shows enlarged lymph vessels and signs of **pulmonary interstitial oedema** (de Waal & van Kaam, 2018). This may persist from 2–5 days. Although the precise cause remains unknown, the most obvious factor is a mild immaturity in the surfactant system which may be responsible for surfactant deficiency or failure to absorb lung fluid after delivery. Most neonates require less than 40% oxygen to maintain systemic oxygenation.

Sudden Infant Death Syndrome

Sudden infant death syndrome (SIDS), regarded as a subset of all **sudden unexpected deaths in infancy,** is the unexplained death of an otherwise healthy infant. These deaths almost always occur during sleep, most commonly at night, during winter, and are usually unexplained by post-mortem examination (Dobson, Thompson & Hunt, 2021). The peak incidence of such deaths is between 2 and 4 months of age and 90% of cases occur before 6 months (Perrone et al., 2021). Boys are more likely to die than girls, and low-birthweight babies are at higher risk. Between 1 month and 1 year of age, SIDS remains the leading cause of death in infants (Horne, Hauck and Moon, 2015; Smith & Colpitts, 2020).

SIDS is a complex phenomenon, and key contributory factors include the infant's sleeping position, co-sleeping, overheating, sudden illness and cardiac arrhythmias such as prolonged Q-T syndrome (Dobson, Thompson & Hunt, 2021). Some evidence suggests bedsharing carries an inherent risk for SIDS (Tappin et al., 2023), whilst others suggest the risk with bedsharing is only increased where the parents smoke, drink alcohol or take drugs (Blair et al., 2022).

Main Points

- Cardiovascular anomalies are the most common forms of congenital malformations. Neonates may present with tachypnoea, dyspnoea, cyanosis, tachycardia, bradycardia, hypotension and hypertension, heart murmurs, poor feeding, grunting and systemic oedema.
- Closure of the ductus arteriosus in the preterm infant may take up to 3 months. Therapeutic interventions may be required to aid closure if neonatal compromise occurs.
- VSDs may be asymptomatic and close spontaneously. Large defects leading to haemodynamic problems and CCF must be treated before surgical closure.
- Simple ASDs cause few problems, with surgical closure advised before the child enters school. Those born with atrioventricular canal defects may experience conduction problems before and after surgical correction.
- Transposition of the great vessels leads to the formation of two separate circulatory systems preventing the transfer of oxygenated blood into the systemic circulation. Neonatal survival depends on the patency of the ductus arteriosus, the foramen ovale and the existence of a VSD, which must be preserved until corrective surgery is possible.
- The classical features of tetralogy of Fallot are a high, large VSD; an overriding aorta, which straddles the VSD; pulmonary stenosis; and right ventricular hypertrophy. Surgical correction is always necessary.
- Coarctation of the aorta commonly occurs at the junction with the ductus arteriosus.

- The major causes of neonatal CCF are excessive volume overload, excessive pressure load and abnormal myocardial function.
- In RDS, increasing inspiratory effort and expiratory difficulties may lead to respiratory failure and atelectasis. Hypoxia and hypercapnia lead to pulmonary vasoconstriction and persistent fetal circulation. Natural/synthetic surfactant administration to combat severe respiratory distress has significantly reduced neonatal morbidity and mortality.
- In bronchopulmonary dysplasia, neonates/infants may remain oxygen-dependent. Dexamethasone may reduce pulmonary inflammation, pulmonary scarring and ongoing respiratory problems.
- Inhalation of meconium can cause respiratory difficulties, with oxygen therapy and antibiotics required. Prognosis may be improved with administration of surfactant.
- A pneumothorax occasionally occurs because of other primary respiratory problems. Because this can influence haemodynamic stability, it will require invasive therapeutic intervention.
- Transient tachypnoea of the newborn may be caused by mild surfactant deficiency or failure to absorb lung fluid after birth. Oxygen therapy generally aids gradual recovery.
- SIDS almost always occurs during sleep, with a peak incidence in the winter. Low-birthweight babies are at higher risk. Causative factors include sleeping position, overheating, undetected illness and parental smoking. To date, no single common factor has been isolated.

References

Abdelaal, M.A., Abushanab, D., Al-Badriyeh, D., 2020. Surfactant therapy for meconium aspiration syndrome in neonates: a systematic overview of systematic reviews and recent clinical trials. J. Comp. Eff. Res. 9 (8), 527–536.

Anderson, J.E., Morray, B.H., Puia-Dumitrescu, M., Rothstein, D.H., 2021. Patent ductus arteriosus: from pharmacology to surgery. Semin. Pediatr. Surg. 30 (6), 151123.

Ardell, S., Pfister, R., Soll, R., 2015. Animal derived surfactant extract versus protein free synthetic surfactant for the prevention and treatment of respiratory distress syndrome (review). Cochrane Database Syst. Rev. 2015 (8), CD000144.

Backes, C., Kovalchin, C., Rivera, B., Smith, C.V., 2018. Patent ductus arteriosus: from bench to bedside. In: Kline, M., Blaney, S., Giardino, A., Orange, J.S., Penny, D.J., Schutze, G.E., et al. (Eds.), Rudolph's Pediatrics, twentythird ed. McGraw-Hill, London.

Blackburn, S.T., 2018. Maternal, Fetal and Neonatal Physiology: A Clinical Perspective, fifth ed. Elsevier, St. Louis.

Blair, P.S., Ball, H.L., Pease, A., Fleming, P.J., 2022. Bed-sharing and SIDS: an evidence-based approach. Arch. Dis. Child. 108 (4), e6.

Blundell, D., Jones, C., Crossland, D., 2021. Structural cardiac disease and cardiomyopathies. In: Boardman, J.P., Groves, A.M., Ramasethu, J. (Eds.), Avery & McDonald's Neonatology: Pathophysiology and Management of the Newborn, eighth ed. Lippincott, Williams and Wilkins, Philadelphia.

Boardman, J.P., Groves, A.M., Ramasethu, J., 2021. Avery & McDonald's Neonatology: Pathophysiology and Management of the Newborn, eighth ed. Lippincott, Williams and Wilkins, Philadelphia.

Bradley, E.A., Zaidi, A.N., 2020. Atrial septal defect. Cardiol. Clin. 38 (3), 317–324.

Bull, M.J., 2020. Down syndrome. N. Engl. J. Med. 382 (24), 2344–2352.

Cabrera, A., Hoffman, J., 2018. Congenital heart disease. In: Kline, M., Blaney, S., Giardino, A., Orange, J.S., Penny, D.J., Schutze, G.E., et al. (Eds.), Rudolph's Pediatrics, twentythird ed. McGraw-Hill, London.

de Waal, C.G., van Kaam, A.H., 2018. Respiratory distress syndrome. In: Kline, M., Blaney, S., Giardino, A., Orange, J.S., Penny, D.J., Schutze, G.E., et al. (Eds.), Rudolph's Pediatrics, twenty-third ed. McGraw-Hill, London.

Dobson, N., Thompson, M., Hunt, C., 2021. Control of breathing: maturation and associated clinical disorders. 2021. In: Boardman, J.P., Groves, A.M., Ramasethu, J. (Eds.), Avery & McDonald's Neonatology: Pathophysiology and Management of the Newborn, eighth ed. Lippincott, Williams and Wilkins, Philadelphia.

Ewer, A.K., Deshpande, S.A., Gale, C., Stenson, B.J., Upton, M., Evans, C., et al., 2019. Potential benefits and harms of universal newborn pulse oximetry screening: response to the UK National Screening Committee public consultation. Arch. Dis. Child. 105 (11), 1128–1129.

Fichera, D., Zanella, F., Fabozzo, A., Doglioni, N., Trevisanuto, D., Lolli, E., et al., 2019. H & S ECMO: preliminary experience with "hub and spoke" model in neonates with meconium aspiration syndrome. Artif. Organs 43 (1), 76–80.

Gardner, S., Enzman-Hines, M., Nyp, M., 2021. Respiratory diseases. In: Gardner, S.L., Carter, B.S., Enzman-Hines, M., Niermeyer, S. (Eds.), Merenstein and Gardner's Handbook of Neonatal Intensive Care: An Interprofessional Approach, ninth ed. Elsevier, St. Louis.

Gover, A., Levy, P.T., Rotschild, A., Golzman, M., Molad, M., Lavie-Nevo, K., et al., 2022. Oral versus intravenous paracetamol for patent ductus arteriosus closure in preterm infants. Pediatr. Res. 92 (4), 1146–1152.

Hentschel, R., Bohlin, K., van Kaam, A., Fuchs, H., Danhaive, O., 2020. Surfactant replacement therapy: from biological basis to current clinical practice. Pediatr. Res. 88 (2), 176–183.

Horne, R., Hauck, F., Moon, R., 2015. Sudden infant death syndrome and advice for safe sleeping. Br. Med. J. 350, 29–32.

Huang, A.C., Olson, S.B., Maslen, C.L., 2021. A review of recent developments in Turner syndrome research. J. Cardiovasc. Dev. Dis. 8 (11), 138.

Jensen, E., Zhang, H., Kirpalani, H., 2018. Bronchopulmonary dysplasia. In: Kline, M., Blaney, S., Giardino, A., Orange, J.S., Penny, D.J., Schutze, G.E., et al. (Eds.), Rudolph's Pediatrics, twenty-third ed. McGraw-Hill, London.

Joshi, A., Humagain, S., 2020. Neonatal arrhythmia. Kathmandu Univ. Med. J. 72 (4), 430–433.

Jullien, S., 2021. Newborn pulse oximetry screening for critical congenital heart defects. BMC Pediatr. 21 (1), 305.

Kalisch-Smith, J.I., Ved, N., Sparrow, D.B., 2020. Environmental risk factors for congenital heart disease. Cold Spring Harbor Perspect. Biol. 12 (3), a037234.

Kline, M., Blaney, S., Giardino, A., Orange J.S., Penny, D.J., Schutze. GE., & Shekerdemian, L.S., (Eds.), *Rudolph's Pediatrics*, twentythirdrd ed. McGraw-Hill, London.

Linglart, L., Gelb, B.D., 2020. Congenital heart defects in Noonan syndrome: diagnosis, management, and treatment. Am. J. Med. Genet. Part C: Semin. Med. Genet. 184 (1), 73–80.

Madar, J., Roehr, C.C., Ainsworth, S., Ersdal, H., Morley, C., Rüdiger, M., et al., 2021. European Resuscitation Council Guidelines 2021: newborn resuscitation and support of transition of infants at birth. Resuscitation 161, 291–326.

Mukerji, A., Abdul Wahab, M.G., Razak, A., Rempel, E., Patel, W., Mondal, T., et al., 2021. High CPAP vs. NIPPV in preterm neonates—a physiological cross-over study. J. Perinatol. 41 (7), 1690–1696.

Obeid, R., Holzgreve, W., Pietrzik, K., 2019. Folate supplementation for prevention of congenital heart defects and low birth weight: an update. Cardiovasc. Diagn. Ther. 9 (Suppl. 2), S424–S433.

Olicker, A.L., Raffay, T.M., Ryan, R.M., 2021. Neonatal respiratory distress secondary to meconium aspiration syndrome. Children 8 (3), 246.

Perrone, S., Lembo, C., Moretti, S., Prezioso, G., Buonocore, G., Toscani, G., et al., 2021. Sudden infant death syndrome: beyond risk factors. Life 11 (3), 184.

Qureshi, A., Justion, H., 2018. Cardiac catheterization and interventional cardiology. In: Kline, M., Blaney, S., Giardino, A., Orange, J.S., Penny, D.J., Schutze, G.E., et al. (Eds.), Rudolph's Pediatrics, twenty-third ed. McGraw-Hill, London.

Roberts, D., Dalziel, S., 2006. Antenatal corticosteroids for accelerating fetal lung maturation for women at risk of preterm birth (review). Cochrane Database Syst. Rev. 2006 (19), CD004454.

Rogers, J., 2022. McCance & Heuther's Pathophysiology: The Biologic Basis for Disease in Adults and Children, ninth ed. Elsevier, St. Louis.

Sinha, S., Miall, L., Jardine, L., 2018. Essential Neonatal Medicine, sixth ed. Wiley-Blackwell, Sussex.

Smith, R.W., Colpitts, M., 2020. Pacifiers and the reduced risk of sudden infant death syndrome. Paediatr. Child Health 25 (4), 205–206.

Soll, R.F., Dargaville, P., 2000. Surfactant for meconium aspiration syndrome in full term infants. Cochrane Database Syst. Rev. 2000 (2), CD002054.

Srivastava, D., 2018. Development of the cardiovascular system. In: Kline, M., Blaney, S., Giardino, A., Orange, J.S., Penny, D.J., Schutze, G.E., Shekerdemian, L.S. (Eds.), Rudolph's Pediatrics, twenty-third ed. McGraw-Hill, London.

Stevens, T.P., Harrington, E.W., Blennow, M., Soll, R.F., 2007. Early surfactant administration with brief ventilation vs. selective surfactant and continued mechanical ventilation for preterm infants with or at risk for respiratory distress syndrome. Cochrane Database Syst. Rev. 2007 (4), CD003063.

Surak, A., 2022. Pharmacological treatment of patent ductus arteriosus in preterm infants. In: Rao, P.S. (Ed.), Congenital Heart Defects: Recent Advances IntechOpen.

Suryadevara, M., 2021. Rubella. In: Domachowske, J., Suryadevara, M. (Eds.), Vaccines: A Clinical Overview and Practical Guide. Springer, Cham.

Swanson, Y., Erikson, L., 2021. Cardiovascular diseases and surgical interventions. In: Gardner, S.L., Carter, B.S., Enzman-Hines, M., Niermeyer, S. (Eds.), Merenstein and Gardner's Handbook of Neonatal Intensive Care: An Interprofessional Approach, ninth ed. Elsevier, St. Louis.

Tappin, D., Mitchell, E.A., Carpenter, J., Hauck, F., Allan, L., 2023. Bed-sharing is a risk for sudden unexpected death in infancy. Arch. Dis. Child. 108 (2), 79–80.

Uggioni, M.L.R., Colonetti, T., Grande, A.J., Cruz, M.V.B., da Rosa, M.I., 2022. Corticosteroids in pregnancy for preventing RDS: overview of systematic reviews. Reprod. Sci. 29 (1), 54–68.

Vlădăreanu, R., Vlădăreanu, S., Boţ, M., 2021. Fetal arrhythmia and related fetal and neonatal outcome. Donald Sch. J. Ultrasound Obstet. Gynecol. 15 (1), 87–96.

Annotated recommended reading

Rogers, J., 2022. McCance & Heuther's Pathophysiology: The Biologic Basis for Disease in Adults and Children, ninth ed. Elsevier, St. Louis.

Easy-to-read but in-depth descriptions of disease, disease aetiology and disease processes are included in this recent textbook. It includes full-colour illustrations and photographs providing unparalleled coverage of pathophysiology. An authoritative resource.

52

Jaundice and Common Metabolic Problems in Neonates

THOMAS McEWAN

CHAPTER CONTENTS

Students and midwives should have a clear understanding of all the adaptations for successful extrauterine life, including hepatic and metabolic changes. Within this chapter those related to hyperbilirubinemia (jaundice) and common metabolic disorders are considered.

Introduction

Transition to extrauterine life occurs normally when fetal organs are sufficiently mature to support neonatal survival. The liver plays a vital role in this transition. This chapter explores the developmental features of the liver, its contribution to the synthesis and excretion of bilirubin and draws attention to common metabolic problems that can occur in neonates.

Neonatal Jaundice

Morphological Factors

Details of the structure and function of the mature liver are provided in Chapter 22. Because hepatic immaturity and hyperbilirubinemia (jaundice) are common in neonates, it is important to understand the morphological features and functional scope of the liver and its biliary tract. The liver is one of the largest visceral organs in neonates and normally extends from the right hypochondrium, through the epigastrium into the left hypochondrium, descending just below the costal margin. As an outgrowth of the caudal part of the foregut, the liver retains its connection with the gastrointestinal system via the biliary tree. In mature livers the hepatocytes are arranged into plates which are usually one cell thick. These are separated by venous sinusoids which anastomose with each other, forming larger veins which join corresponding central veins. The hepatic parenchyma is supplied by nerves arising from the hepatic plexus and containing sympathetic and parasympathetic (vagal) fibres. Distension or disruption of the liver capsule may cause localized sharp pain (Rosen, 2021).

A complex network of systemic and portal vessels ensures that the liver benefits from a good blood supply and effective venous and lymphatic drainage. The portal venous system ensures that most of the blood from the gastrointestinal system is returned to the liver. In contrast, the hepatic venous system returns blood from the liver into the inferior vena cava. The protein-rich lymph is drained from the liver into the thoracic duct.

Synthesis and Metabolism of Bilirubin

Small amounts of **bilirubin** are detected in the amniotic fluid between the 13th and 37th weeks of gestation, possibly because of the limitations of the immature fetal liver. This implies that the major route for fetal bilirubin excretion is across the placenta. Because most of the fetal plasma bilirubin is unconjugated, it is easily transferred across the placenta into the maternal circulation and to the maternal liver for conjugation and excretion. Therefore, fetuses seldom manifest jaundice unless they suffer severe haemolytic disease.

In neonates, 75% of bilirubin is a by-product of haemoglobin of which 1 g yields 35 mg (600 µmol) of unconjugated bilirubin (Kamath-Rayne et al., 2021) (Fig. 52.1). About 25% is generated from other non-erythropoietic haem protein sources, principally in the liver, and from the destruction of immature erythrocytes in the bone marrow. Senescent (ageing) erythrocytes are removed and destroyed by the reticuloendothelial system where haemoglobin is catabolized and converted into bilirubin with the iron atoms at the centre of the haem skeleton reused. On leaving the reticuloendothelial system, unconjugated bilirubin is transported in the plasma

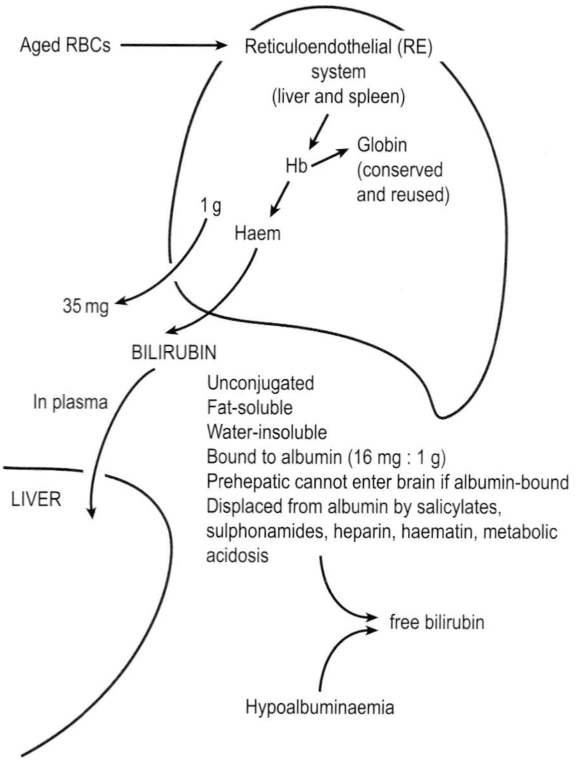

Aged RBCs → Reticuloendothelial (RE) system (liver and spleen)

Hb → Globin (conserved and reused)

1 g

Haem

35 mg

BILIRUBIN

In plasma

Unconjugated
Fat-soluble
Water-insoluble
Bound to albumin (16 mg : 1 g)
Prehepatic cannot enter brain if albumin-bound
Displaced from albumin by salicylates, sulphonamides, heparin, haematin, metabolic acidosis

LIVER

free bilirubin

Hypoalbuminaemia

• **Fig. 52.1** The formation of bilirubin.

• **BOX 52.1**   **Critical Processes for Bilirubin Conjugation**

Although hepatocytes easily take up the unbound lipid-soluble bilirubin, a carrier molecule is needed to take up any bound complexes. Once in the hepatocytes, bilirubin binds to ligandin and possibly other cytoplasmic-binding proteins. The unconjugated bilirubin is conjugated with a glucuronic acid by the enzyme glucuronyl transferase to form bilirubin monoglucuronide and diglucuronide pigments (Fig. 52.2). These are more water-soluble and can be excreted into the bile or through the kidneys into the urine. Bilirubin conjugation requires oxygen and glucose, and hypoxia or hypoglycaemia may slow down the conjugation process.

---

tightly bound to albumin. The critical processes that follow in bilirubin conjugation are summarized in Box 52.1.

Some of the conjugated bilirubin is carried in bile to the duodenum and metabolized in the terminal ileum and colon by bacterial enzymes to produce **urobilinogen** and **stercobilinogen.** The latter gives faeces the yellowish colour in infants and brown colour in adults. In its absence, faeces are greyish white. Small quantities of urobilinogen re-enter the circulation and are excreted by the liver and the kidneys as hydrophilic urobilinogen.

Bilirubin in the Neonate

After birth, the neonate's liver must take over bilirubin metabolism and clearance. Most of this bilirubin is diverted into the meconium; 200 g of meconium contains about 175 g

of bilirubin, 50% of which is conjugated. Delays in meconium excretion, which occur in premature neonates and neonates with **cystic fibrosis,** may contribute to the return of some unconjugated bilirubin into the systemic circulation via the **entero-hepatic circulation** (Fig. 52.2).

Term neonates hold about 137–171 μmol of bilirubin per litre of plasma (Bhutani & Wong, 2021). These high values compared with bilirubin values in adults are attributed to higher circulating erythrocytes at birth which are gradually biodegraded. The shorter erythrocyte life span of 80 days (as opposed to 120 days in adults) and a corresponding increase in immature or fragile erythrocytes means that more erythrocytes must be degraded (Bhutani & Wong, 2021). The less effective bilirubin binding to albumin, enhanced absorption of bilirubin through the enterohepatic circulation and the somewhat dormant hepatic conjugating system further complicate bilirubin conjugation and excretion. All neonates manifest a progressive rise in unconjugated bilirubin, which peaks at 180 μmol/L on the third or fourth day of life. This gives rise to **physiological jaundice.** The increase in unconjugated bilirubin, a relatively low liver uptake of bilirubin and the transient deficiency of the glucuronyl transferase enzyme culminate in reduced excretion of conjugated bilirubin. Higher levels of unconjugated bilirubin in neonates are explained in Box 52.2. Although healthy neonates produce almost twice as much bilirubin as adults, their plasma bilirubin values fall to physiological norms within 6 weeks of birth.

Kernicterus

Although bilirubin plays important physiological roles as an **antioxidant** and a **free-radical scavenger,** its tendency to aggregate increases the risks of neurotoxicity. Plasma pH significantly affects the solubility of bilirubin and its binding to tissue sites: solubility decreases as plasma pH falls. **Bilirubin-induced neurologic dysfunction,** as described by Brites & Fernandes (2015), may manifest with bilirubin accumulation, leading to deficits in cognitive processing and auditory function, with bilirubin preferentially deposited in the basal ganglia. Bhutani & Wong (2021) suggest this may be because bilirubin attaches first to nerve terminals with lower membrane potentials. This may decrease nerve conduction and allow a retrograde uptake of bilirubin into cell bodies where it binds with various cellular components, staining these and augmenting their function.

Delays in bilirubin conjugation are of concern as unbound, unconjugated fat-soluble bilirubin deposits in neural tissue and visceral organs. Although bilirubin flows constantly into and out of the brain under normal circumstances, under experimental conditions asphyxiated animals and those who have a defective blood–brain barrier experienced gross staining of the brain and electrophysiological changes (Bhutani & Wong, 2021). An intact blood–brain barrier probably excludes most water-soluble substances and protein but is permeable to lipid-soluble substances that are not protein-bound. Large proteins such as albumin are excluded from the brain but may cross the blood–brain barrier when it is compromised.

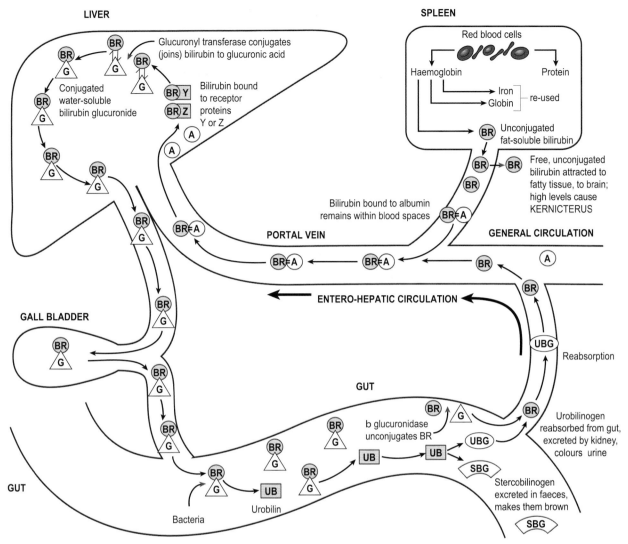

• **Fig. 52.2** Schematic diagram showing the conjugation of bilirubin. =, Bound to; *A*, albumin; *BR*, bilirubin; *G*, glucuronic acid; *SBG*, stercobilinogen; *UB*, urobilin; *UBG*, urobilinogen.

• BOX 52.2 Unconjugated Bilirubin in Neonates

Although the mechanisms involved in bilirubin conjugation are not fully understood, evidence shows that bilirubin is synthesized by and released from the reticuloendothelial system into the plasma and binds to plasma albumin. The higher levels of unconjugated bilirubin in neonates are attributed to lower plasma albumin values and lower albumin affinity for bilirubin. This is possibly due to the undeveloped molecular structure of the albumin (Blackburn, 2018) and that some albumin-binding sites may be occupied by other molecular substances such as drugs, including heparin and chloramphenicol (Bhutani & Wong, 2021).

However modest elevation of unconjugated serum bilirubin can produce reversible clinical and electrophysiological alterations in healthy full-term infants (Brites & Brito, 2012). Another mechanism for bilirubin entry into the brain occurs when there is a marked increase in unbound

bilirubin. Acidosis may facilitate the transfer of bilirubin across the blood–brain barrier and its subsequent deposition in the neural tissue of the brain (Bhutani & Wong, 2021). Although neural mitochondria contain the enzyme bilirubin oxidase, which converts bilirubin to biliverdin and other non-toxic products, the risk of irreversible brain damage caused by unconjugated bilirubin is high.

The risk of **bilirubin encephalopathy** (occurring in neonates with mild, reversible **hyperbilirubinemia**) is increased in low-birthweight neonates and those who experience hypoxic ischaemic insults. However autopsy reports on jaundiced neonates also reveal bilirubin staining of the aorta, pleural fluid and visceral organs (Bhutani & Wong, 2021). In the brain, unconjugated bilirubin leads to irreversible staining, especially in the basal ganglia and cerebellum, and causes **kernicterus** (yellow kernel; see Clinical Application 52.1). Deposition of larger quantities of unconjugated bilirubin may cause irreversible neural damage with long-term sequelae of **cerebral athetosis** and significant **developmental**

• CLINICAL APPLICATION 52.1   Kernicterus

Kernicterus is preventable in all but very small, sick neonates where the blood–brain barrier may be ineffective and quite low levels of bilirubin may damage the fragile tissues. Kernicterus is often exacerbated by bruising and trauma during birth. As such, prophylactic phototherapy is often commenced soon after admission for these vulnerable neonates (Okwundu et al., 2013; Sinha et al., 2018).

delay. Such events are most likely to occur when the neonate's serum bilirubin level rises above 350 μmol/L.

A Résumé of Common Causes of Neonatal Jaundice

Jaundice (yellow discoloration of the skin and sclera caused by deposits of conjugated and unconjugated bilirubin) becomes visible when the serum bilirubin rises above 90 μmol/L (Sinha et al., 2018). Bilirubin is a yellowish-green bile pigment which, before conjugation, is a weak acid. It is very soluble in lipids but only slightly soluble in water, making its excretion difficult. About 75% of bilirubin is released along with biliverdin when red blood cells are broken down in the liver and spleen, releasing haem and globin to the body stores. The remainder is derived from other haem products. Excessive bilirubin may enter the bloodstream in three ways (Rogers, 2022), all of which may affect the neonate:

1. During excessive haemolysis of red blood cells (prehepatic).
2. Where liver disease affects the metabolism and excretion of bile (hepatic).
3. Congenital obstruction of a component of the biliary system; e.g., congenital biliary atresia (posthepatic).

Because each of these problems requires different therapeutic interventions, an appropriate range of investigations is needed if:

- Jaundice appears within the first 24 hours after birth.
- Jaundice persists for longer than 2 weeks.
- Neonate's total bilirubin level is >250 μmol/L.
- Conjugated bilirubin portion is >20% of the total bilirubin level or a conjugated bilirubin level >25 μmol/L.
- Jaundice appears in an ill baby irrespective of its age and fails to respond to treatment.

It is important to distinguish between unconjugated and conjugated forms of bilirubin. The common causes of neonatal jaundice are shown in Table 52.1 and Figure 52.3 illustrates the sites of events leading to jaundice.

Prehepatic: Unconjugated Bilirubin

Physiological jaundice usually appears in otherwise healthy infants around the second to fifth day of life and fades gradually over the next 10 days. It is attributed to the increase in erythrocyte breakdown leading to greater bilirubin production and greater enteric reabsorption

and enterohepatic circulation of bilirubin. The immature liver cannot synthesize sufficient glucuronyl transferase to metabolize fat-soluble unconjugated bilirubin into water-soluble conjugated bilirubin. Because the unconjugated bilirubin cannot be excreted readily, it diffuses into body tissues. The less efficient binding of unconjugated bilirubin to plasma albumin increases diffusion, and the presence of meconium increases enteric reabsorption of unconjugated bilirubin. Deferred umbilical cord clamping may increase the **circulating blood volume** and **haematocrit,** both of which can exacerbate the rise in bilirubin. However the benefits of this intervention are outweighed by the risks. Neonates who present with physiological jaundice may be helped with periodic phototherapy and increased hydration.

Jaundice of prematurity is a more serious form of physiological jaundice. Due to a greater immaturity of the liver, premature neonates may manifest a more exaggerated form of jaundice which begins earlier, lasts longer and is more severe. Therapeutic interventions should be directed at minimizing the risks of bilirubin encephalopathy. If **phototherapy** only marginally improves bilirubin conjugation, **exchange blood transfusion** may be required.

Prominent non-physiological causes of jaundice are summarized in Table 52.2. Commonly these will result in visible neonatal jaundice in the first 24 hours of life, rapidly rising hyperbilirubinemia levels and warrant urgent investigation and management. These are often referred to as pathological causes of jaundice.

Breastfeeding-associated jaundice, also known as **breastfeeding jaundice,** may be noted in almost two-thirds of exclusively breastfed babies (Sinha et al., 2018), with bilirubin levels highest within the first week of life. The aetiology of this is uncertain but is most likely due to reduced fluid and calorie intake during this period whilst breastfeeding and maternal lactation are being established.

Hepatic: Unconjugated Bilirubin

Breastmilk jaundice occurs in 1–2% of breastfed babies who develop an unconjugated hyperbilirubinemia. It may occur from 3–4 days and persist for several weeks, after which there is a gradual decline in bilirubin levels. It causes no ill effects and *should not* lead to discontinuation of breastfeeding. However it often creates anxiety for parents, who see it as an illness. The cause of breastmilk jaundice has not been established although it may involve:

- Inhibition of glucuronyl transferase by substances found in breastmilk such as the maternal hormone pregnanediol and unsaturated fatty acids.
- The presence in breastmilk of lipase, which releases free fatty acids into the neonate's intestines.
- The presence in breastmilk of the enzyme β-glucuronidase, which splits conjugated bilirubin and increases shunting of unconjugated bilirubin from the intestine back to the liver.
- The delay in the passage of meconium seen in fully breastfed babies. Early breastfeeding with adequate colostrum

TABLE 52.1	Causes of Neonatal Jaundice				
Prehepatic: Unconjugated Bilirubin	**Hepatic: Unconjugated Bilirubin**	**Hepatic: Mixed Unconjugated and Conjugated Bilirubin**	**Posthepatic: Unconjugated Mixed and Conjugated Bilirubin**	**Posthepatic: Unconjugated Bilirubin**
Physiological jaundice/jaundice of prematurity Haemolytic jaundice Bruising and haematoma Polycythaemia Postnatal infections	Breastmilk jaundice	Congenital hypothyroidism Inborn errors of metabolism: galactosaemia Hepatitis, due to transplacental infections (TORCH organisms)	Congenital biliary atresia Bile plug syndrome	Paralytic ileus High intestinal obstruction such as duodenal atresia

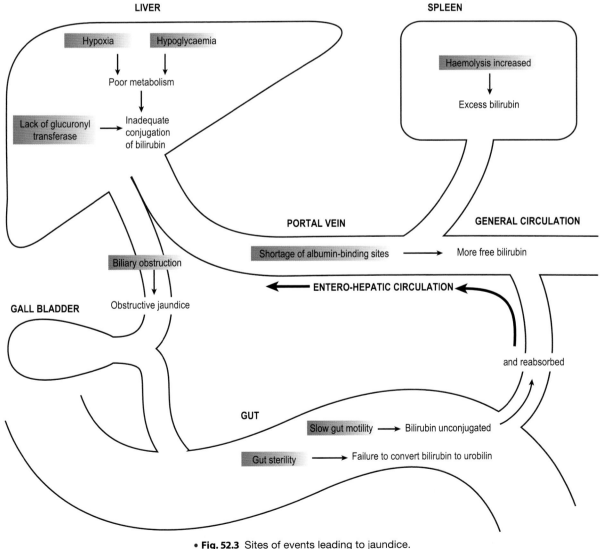

• **Fig. 52.3** Sites of events leading to jaundice.

TABLE 52.2	Non-physiological, or Pathological, Causes on Neonatal Jaundice

The two main causes of erythrocyte haemolysis are **rhesus isoimmunization,** a clinically serious problem, and **ABO incompatibility,** which is rarely severe (see Chapter 12). Both clinical problems cause **haemolytic jaundice** generally in the first 24 hours of life.

Bruising and haematomas such as cephalhematoma will lead to significant erythrocyte breakdown during the resolution of the bruise and cause jaundice which may last for several weeks.

Polycythaemia with excess erythrocytes that must be haemolyzed will increase bilirubin synthesis. This may occur in **twin transfusion syndrome,** delayed cord clamping and neonates of diabetic mothers.

Infections such as septicaemia, urinary tract infections, meningitis and ventriculitis may also cause significant haemolysis of erythrocytes which leads to jaundice.

Liver enzyme defects such as **Gilbert syndrome** and **Crigler–Najjar syndrome** can reduce bilirubin clearance significantly.

Neonates with **glucose-6-phosphate dehydrogenase (G6PD) deficiency** may be particularly susceptible to the haemolytic action of vitamin-K analogues. G6PD deficiency is a heterogeneous, sex-linked recessive trait whose occurrence has its greatest prevalence in Africa and Mediterranean and Asian countries. Because of this enzyme deficiency, erythrocytes cannot activate the pentose phosphate metabolic pathway and therefore are unable to defend adequately against oxidative stress. Haemolytic reactions and hyperbilirubinemia may occur in response to certain drugs and vitamin-K analogues, as well as other chemical and household products (Bhutani & Wong, 2021).

intake will act as a laxative and, at least in part, reduce the severity of breastmilk jaundice (Blackburn, 2018).

Hepatic: Mixed Unconjugated and Conjugated Bilirubin

Congenital hypothyroidism contributes to jaundice and the primary disorder must be treated, as well as the jaundice to avert neurological problems. Neonatal screening using the newborn blood-spot test should alert clinicians early to this major endocrine problem. Sometimes neonates present early with other features of hypothyroidism and jaundice, and these must be taken into consideration when using investigative procedures and planning treatment with levothyroxine (thyroxine) to avert developmental problems and intellectual disability.

Some **inborn errors of metabolism** such as cystic fibrosis and galactosaemia may cause severe jaundice due to adversely affected metabolic pathways releasing metabolites that alter or compromise liver function.

Hepatitis is often part of a syndrome accompanying transplacental infection by pathogens such as toxoplasmosis, cytomegalovirus and herpes simplex. The source and extent of the primary infection must be identified and treated in conjunction with any therapeutic interventions that may be required to minimize the severity of the jaundice.

Posthepatic: Mixed Unconjugated and Conjugated Bilirubin

Congenital structural anomalies of the biliary ducts interfere with normal bile flow and often lead to significant cholestasis, presenting as cholestatic jaundice in 1 in 2500 neonates (Feldman & Sokol, 2020). Some biliary malformations are extrahepatic biliary atresias, intrahepatic biliary hypoplasia, cystic dilatation of the major intrahepatic bile ducts and duodenal atresia. It is important to distinguish between these disorders because surgical correction of biliary malformations may be lifesaving. If cholestasis is caused by inflammatory response, infections or metabolic disorders, surgery is not needed.

Extrahepatic biliary atresia is the most common form of biliary malformation, with an incidence of 5–10 babies per 100,000 live births. It is more common in females. Associated histological features are proliferation of the hepatic interlobular bile ducts and periportal fibrosis. Such neonates develop a deep bronze jaundice in the second week of life, the stools are putty coloured and the urine contains bilirubin. The liver becomes firm and enlarged. Because the bilirubin is conjugated, the neonate is not at risk of developing kernicterus, although if the intrahepatic accumulation of bile is untreated the liver will be damaged, and such infants will go on to develop varying degrees of biliary cirrhosis, portal hypertension and liver failure.

Surgical intervention is usually required to reconstruct the defective biliary tree, but the prognosis is poor because only a few such neonates are suitable for early surgery before the liver is irreparably damaged. **Liver transplantation** is a long-term solution for some but is generally only carried out in older infants. When liver transplantation is not a realistic option, 80% of affected children die before the age of 3 years (Rogers, 2022).

Management of Jaundice

Investigations

Depending on the history, clinical evidence and gestational age, investigations may include serum conjugated and unconjugated bilirubin monitoring, blood group establishment, haemoglobin estimation, rhesus antibodies, screening for infection, monitoring of metabolic functions including thyroid function, digestive enzyme assays and enzyme deficiencies such as G6PD deficiency.

Phototherapy

If jaundice persists, the first line of treatment to prevent the development of kernicterus is phototherapy. When a light of wavelength 400–500 nm is shone on the skin, any unconjugated bilirubin is converted to a non-toxic water-soluble substance which is more easily excreted through the kidneys and gastrointestinal tract. Phototherapy may work by inducing **photo-oxidation, structural isomerization** and **configurational isomerization** (Itoh et al., 2017).

- Photo-oxidation is the reaction of bilirubin with singlet oxygen, leading to readily excreted, colourless, non-reactive products.
- Structural isomerization involves the molecule lumirubin, formed by intramolecular cyclization of the bilirubin molecule at the third carbon, leading to a polar compound.
- Configuration isomerization involves structural changes in the bilirubin molecules. The isomers are readily taken up by the liver and transported into the bile.

Phototherapy is not risk-free. Bilirubin is a **photosensitizer** and may sometimes induce skin blistering and bronze-baby syndrome. The phototherapy light may initiate retinal damage if the neonate's eyes are not protected, although the **photodecomposition products** have no known neurotoxic effects (Bhutani & Wong, 2021).

The National Institute of Health and Care Excellence (NICE, 2016) provides clear guidance on the investigation, management and treatment of neonatal jaundice, highlighting in particular:

- Visual inspection of the neonate is insufficient in the estimation of jaundice, advising the use of a **transcutaneous bilirubinometer** or serum sample.
- **Treatment threshold charts** should be used according to the gestation of the neonate.
- Expert advice should be followed in the management of **prolonged jaundice.**

Some recent studies have investigated new approaches to the management of neonatal jaundice. Due to the impact of the COVID-19 pandemic, the **use of telemedicine** for the evaluation of jaundiced babies, their ongoing management and provision of parental education was considered by Joshi et al. (2022). They identified that early assessment and management had the potential to greatly improve outcomes, but further research was required.

The **location of treatment,** either home or hospital, for non-haemolytic jaundice in the term neonate was found to have equivocal evidence following a review by Malwade & Jardine (2014). More recently, Anderson et al. (2022) conducted a systematic review of the efficacy of home phototherapy for physiological and non-physiological neonatal jaundice. They found it to be a safe and effective mode of treatment, conferring cost benefits and reducing parental anxiety, but further exploration of this intervention would be required.

Use of Immunoglobulin and Exchange Blood Transfusion

This treatment is mainly carried out in neonates with rhesus haemolytic disease where excess bilirubin and antibodies must be removed from the blood. Reducing the plasma bilirubin levels lowers the risk of kernicterus, and a reduction in antibodies lessens the severity of erythrocyte haemolysis.

Intravenous immunoglobulin (IVIG), when used in conjunction with phototherapy, has been shown to reduce the need for exchange transfusion in neonates with rhesus isoimmunization or ABO incompatibility (NICE, 2016; Sinha et al., 2018).

Exchange blood transfusion, a highly invasive therapy, carries a mortality risk of 0.7–2%. This is due to complications such as embolism, infection, electrolyte and glucose disturbances and bleeding but these can be minimized by careful technique during the procedure (Kamath-Rayne et al., 2021).

Common Metabolic Disorders

It is not within the scope of this book to explore the mainly recessively inherited **inborn errors of metabolism.** Detailed accounts of conditions such as **phenylketonuria, cystic fibrosis** and **galactosaemia** can be found in Rogers (2022). Preconception, antenatal and neonatal screening tests should be carried out where metabolic problems are anticipated. Disturbances in common substances such as glucose, calcium and sodium can alter cerebral tissue function and cause permanent neurological damage that could be avoided by proactive screening and prompt treatment.

Hypoglycaemia

Glucose homeostasis relies on the net balance in intake, production, storage and utilization of glucose. Because neonatal glucose homeostasis is less than optimal due to metabolic transitions around birth, problems occur when glucose utilization exceeds its availability or synthesis by the body. This leads to a fall in plasma glucose concentration. Conversely, glucose production can exceed utilization, resulting in an abnormal rise in plasma glucose. Regulation of hepatic glucose production is critical to homeostatic maintenance. Although the kidneys are capable of **gluconeogenesis,** their glucose contribution is insufficient to maintain homeostatic balance except in prolonged starvation and metabolic acidosis. Most neonates who develop hypoglycaemia in the first 24 hours have a history of:

- A mother who suffers from diabetes mellitus.
- A mother who developed pregnancy-induced hypertension.
- Stress related to neonatal asphyxia.
- Being large or small for gestational age.
- Hyperinsulinism.

Most hypoglycaemic infants make a gradual but spontaneous recovery. However recurrent or persistent hypoglycaemia may be caused by hepatic enzyme defects, endocrine deficiencies or hyperinsulinism. The consensus for the lowest safe level for neonatal blood glucose is not less than 2.6 mmol/L (McIntyre, 2020). A plasma glucose of <2.6 mmol/L in a symptomatic baby may lead to neurological dysfunction, manifesting as tremors and seizures (Hawdon & Boardman, 2021). The British Association of Perinatal Medicine (BAPM) provides a useful framework for the identification and management of hypoglycaemia in the full-term infant. This suggests an algorithmic approach based upon asymptomatic and symptomatic hypoglycaemia, with the acceptable safe level for blood glucose in this group as ≥2.0 mmol/L (BAPM, 2017).

Although hypoglycaemia is more common in low-birth-weight babies and in babies of diabetic mothers, it also occurs in neonates with a history of birth asphyxia, respiratory distress syndrome, hypothermia, cerebral damage, severe haemolytic disease or an inborn error of metabolism.

The Clinical Evidence

Hypoglycaemia may be asymptomatic or may be associated with other clinical problems such as lethargy, hypotonia, shallow respirations with periods of apnoea, cyanosis, muscle twitching, convulsions and coma. Prolonged hypoglycaemia may be associated with brain damage, and associated seizures may worsen the neonate's overall prognosis (Hawdon & Boardman, 2021; Kline et al., 2018). Management is outlined in Clinical Application 52.2.

Hypocalcaemia and Hypomagnesaemia

During the last trimester of pregnancy, free calcium diffuses from the mother to fetus, ensuring that by term his skeleton is mineralized. A manifestation of this positive calcium movement in favour of the fetus is reflected by calcium levels in the fetal blood, which are usually 10% higher than maternal values.

This **fetal hypercalcaemia** suppresses fetal **parathyroid secretion** and stimulates **calcitonin** release, favouring mineral deposition in the fetal skeletal system. This relative suppression of parathyroid function at birth contributes to the onset of a **transient hypoparathyroid state** with a fall in plasma calcium levels. The term neonate may show decreasing plasma calcium levels during the 24–48 hours after birth, reaching levels of <2.0 mmol/L. This physiologically induced **hypocalcaemia** may result in stimulation of the parathyroid glands and suppression of calcitonin secretion. See Clinical Application 52.3 for the management of hypocalcaemia.

Plasma calcium levels increase to acceptable levels within 5 days of birth. If the transition to normal calcium metabolism fails to happen, symptomatic hypocalcaemia develops. **Neonatal tetany** may occur when the plasma calcium level is low, with signs of this including irritability followed by muscle twitching, apnoea and hypocalcaemic convulsions (Vuralli, 2019). The neonate is generally conscious and alert between convulsions. Hypocalcaemia may occur in the first 3 days of life in premature neonates with a history of birth asphyxia, hypothermia or respiratory distress syndrome.

Late hypocalcaemia, 5–6 days after birth, is usually associated with feeding the neonate unmodified cow's milk and is rare in developed countries. Cow's milk is high in **phosphorus,** and the increase in serum phosphate causes the serum calcium to fall. Some immigrant mothers and mothers in lower socioeconomic groups may have **vitamin-D** and **calcium deficiencies** due to inadequate nutrition, leading to hypocalcaemia in pregnancy. Their babies may experience lower plasma calcium levels and higher risks of developing tetany.

Associated Hypomagnesaemia

Failure of plasma calcium concentration to respond to administration of intravenous calcium salts should raise the suspicion of coexisting **hypomagnesaemia.** In such circumstances, an intramuscular injection of 0.2 mmol/kg of **50% magnesium sulphate** is required to correct both metabolic conditions. Hypomagnesaemia is often associated with hypocalcaemia when the serum magnesium levels may be below 0.7 mmol/L (normal 0.7–1.0 mmol/L) (Polin et al., 2022). Its homeostasis is probably controlled by the kidneys and gastrointestinal tract. Long-term calcium and magnesium instabilities may contribute to hypoplasia of tooth enamel in the primary teeth.

Hypernatraemia

Neonatal hypernatraemia may result from excessive sodium intake, excessive fluid loss or insufficient fluid

---

• CLINICAL APPLICATION 52.2 | Management of Hypoglycaemia

- Prevention is the best form of management. Early feeding, preferably breastfeeding, and maintenance of normal body temperature are essential for those neonates at risk.
- Regular and accurate blood glucose monitoring for those at risk or when symptoms are noted.
- If a normal blood glucose level cannot be maintained despite adequate enteral feeding, an intravenous infusion of 10% glucose solution may be necessary. For full-term infants, administration of 40% buccal dextrose gel (200 µg/kg) may be considered as part of the feeding plan in asymptomatic hypoglycaemia when pre-feed blood glucose is 1.0–1.9 mmol/L (BAPM, 2017).
- If symptoms reappear, the neonate must have regular neurological and metabolic checks to identify or exclude more sinister problems.

• CLINICAL APPLICATION 52.3 | Management of Hypocalcaemia

- Advise expectant mothers at risk to increase their calcium intake.
- Encourage breastfeeding whenever possible, with modified cow's milk only given when breastfeeding is unachievable.
- If the neonate is asymptomatic, oral calcium supplements will usually be adequate (Kovacs, 2015).
- A slow intravenous infusion of **10% calcium gluconate** (1–2 mL/kg/dose) should be considered if a neonate experiences muscle twitching and convulsions (Vuralli, 2019).
- Oral calcium gluconate supplements may be continued when normal plasma calcium levels are restored. Because calcium has a direct impact on heart rate, rhythm and contractility, arrhythmias such as bradycardia may develop.

• BOX 52.3 Causes of Neonatal Hypernatraemia

- Excessive water loss—in those especially at risk from transepidermal water loss. This includes preterm infants with poorly keratinized skin, exacerbated by phototherapy and radiant heaters.
- Reduced renal excretion—more likely due to the immature newborn kidney unable to excrete excess salt, and more commonly losing excess water in the urine.

• CLINICAL APPLICATION 52.4 Management of Hypernatraemi

- Persistent hypernatraemia is associated with **cerebral haemorrhage** and **renal vein thrombosis** and must be managed carefully.
- Overaggressive correction may cause cellular overhydration, which can affect the structural integrity of the brain tissue. This may lead to convulsions.
- The neonate should be slowly rehydrated with either sufficient volume of enteral feeds or a slow intravenous infusion of a dextrose solution (Sinha et al., 2018).
- Any other electrolyte imbalance or hypoglycaemia must also be corrected.
- Ongoing care should observe for signs of potential neurological damage.

intake and is defined by a serum sodium level exceeding 150 mmol/L (Sinha et al., 2018). As such, any neonate receiving intensive care should have **plasma electrolytes** checked at least once a day. The main causes of this condition are outlined in Box 52.3.

Inappropriate infant feeding may lead to hypernatraemia. Where possible, breastfeeding should be encouraged. However to reduce the risk when formula milk is used, parents should be taught the principles of feed preparation and helped to understand the balanced hydration and nutrition that infants require.

Signs of Hypernatraemia

The infant may appear fretful and thirsty at first, followed by dehydration, pyrexia, hypertension and a bulging pulsatile fontanelle. If the condition remains untreated, convulsions occur (see Clinical Application 52.4). Sometimes the infant may present with encephalopathy and other neurological problems that could be life-threatening. There may also be failure to gain weight, irritability, hypertonicity and convulsions, especially when plasma sodium levels exceed 150 mmol/L (Sinha et al., 2018). Because the osmotic gradient favours maintenance of extracellular fluid at the expense of intracellular fluid, it may be difficult to establish the true diagnosis.

Main Points

- Neonates produce twice as much bilirubin as adults due to the excessive haemolysis of erythrocytes containing fetal haemoglobin. Excessive quantities of unconjugated bilirubin can be neurotoxic.
- Because the unconjugated fat-soluble bilirubin binds to tissue with high fat content, particularly the central nervous system, if left untreated it may cause kernicterus and related long-term neurological sequelae. Kernicterus is a preventable problem in all but very small, sick neonates.
- Prehepatic causes of neonatal jaundice with an excess of unconjugated bilirubin include physiological jaundice, jaundice of prematurity, haemolytic jaundice, bruising and haematoma, polycythaemia and some postnatal infections.
- Hepatic causes of jaundice include breastmilk feeding and congenital hypothyroidism. High values of mixed unconjugated and conjugated bilirubin may be attributed to such problems as inborn errors of metabolism and hepatitis caused by transplacental infections. Breastmilk jaundice should not be a reason to discontinue breastfeeding.
- Posthepatic jaundice owing to high mixed unconjugated and conjugated bilirubin values is generally caused by congenital biliary atresia and high intestinal obstruction such as duodenal atresia.
- Phototherapy and additional hydration are occasionally necessary in physiological jaundice, especially in premature infants. Immunoglobulin administration and exchange blood transfusion may have to be considered for neonates with significant haemolytic jaundice.
- Polycythaemia caused by twin transfusion syndrome may induce a non-physiological jaundice.
- Neonates with biliary atresia may present with deep bronze jaundice from the second week of life, often accompanied by light-coloured stools and dark urine containing bilirubin. Surgical intervention is necessary to prevent irreversible liver damage.
- Disturbances in glucose, calcium, magnesium and sodium homeostasis may lead to neurological changes and permanent neural tissue damage.
- Hypoglycaemia is more common in low-birthweight babies and in babies of diabetic mothers.
- Early symptoms of hypocalcaemia occur in premature neonates or those with a history of birth asphyxia, hypothermia or respiratory distress syndrome. Late hypocalcaemia is usually associated with feeding neonates unmodified cow's milk.
- Hypernatraemia may be caused by excessive fluid loss or excessive sodium intake as neonates cannot excrete high solute loads by concentrating urine; their urine is almost always dilute.

References

Anderson, C.M., Kandasamy, Y., Kilcullen, M., 2022. The efficacy of home phototherapy for physiological and non-physiological neonatal jaundice: a systematic review. J. Neonatal Nurs. 28 (5), 312–326.

Blackburn, S.T., 2018. Maternal, Fetal and Neonatal Physiology: A Clinical Perspective, fifth ed. Elsevier, St. Louis.

Bhutani, V., Wong, R., 2021. Neonatal hyperbilirubinemia. In: Boardman, J.P., Groves, A.M., Ramasethu, J. (Eds.), Avery & McDonald's Neonatology: Pathophysiology and Mof the Newborn, eighth ed. Lippincott, Williams and Wilkins, Philadelphia.

Brites, D., Brito, M.A., 2012. Bilirubin toxicity. In: Stevenson, D.K., Maisels, M.J., Watchko, J.F. (Eds.), Care of the Jaundiced Neonate. McGraw-Hill, New York.

Brites, D., Fernandes, A., 2015. Bilirubin-induced neural impairment: a special focus on myelination, age-related windows of susceptibility and associated co-morbidities. Semin. Fetal Neonatal Med. 20 (1), 14–19.

British Association of Perinatal Medicine (BAPM), 2017. Identification and Management of Neonatal Hypoglycaemia in the Full-Term Infant: A Framework for Practice. Available at: https://hubble-live-assets.s3.amazonaws.com/bapm/file_asset/file/37/Identification_and_Management_of_Neonatal_Hypoglycaemia_in_the__full_term_infant_-_A_Framework_for_Practice_revised_Oct_2017.pdf.

Feldman, A.G., Sokol, R.J., 2020. Recent developments in diagnostics and treatment of neonatal cholestasis. Semin. Pediatr. Surg. 29 (4), 150945.

Hawdon, J.M., Boardman, P., 2021. Homeostasis of carbohydrate and other fuels. In: Boardman, J.P., Groves, A.M., Ramasethu, J. (Eds.), Avery & McDonald's Neonatology: Pathophysiology and Mof the Newborn, eighth ed. Lippincott, Williams and Wilkins, Philadelphia.

Itoh, S., Okada, H., Kuboi, T., Kusaka, T., 2017. Phototherapy for neonatal hyperbilirubinemia. Pediatr. Int. 59 (9), 959–966.

Joshi, S.S., Benroy, B.R., Lawrence, I.N., Suresh, T.J., 2022. Telemedicine as progressive treatment approach for neonatal jaundice due to the coronavirus disease 2019 pandemic. Clin. Exp. Pediatr. 65 (5), 269–271.

Kamath-Rayne, B.D., Froese, P., Thilo, E., 2021. Neonatal hyperbilirubinemia. In: Gardner, S.L., Carter, B.S., Enzman-Hines, M., Niermeyer, S. (Eds.), Merenstein and Gardner's Handbook of Neonatal Intensive Care: An Interprofessional Approach, ninth ed. Elsevier, St. Louis.

Kovacs, C.S., 2015. Calcium, phosphorus, and bone metabolism in the fetus and newborn. Early Hum. Dev. 91 (11), 623–628.

Kline, M., Blaney, S., Giardino, A., Orange, J.S., Penny, D.J., Schutze, G.E., et al., 2018. Rudolph's Pediatrics, twenty-third ed. McGraw-Hill, London.

Malwade, U.S., Jardine, L.A., 2014. Home versus hospital-based phototherapy for the treatment of non-haemolytic jaundice in infants at more than 37 weeks' gestation. Cochrane Database Syst. Rev. 2014 (6), CD010212.

McIntyre, J., 2020. Significant problems in the newborn baby. In: Marshall, J.E., Raynor, M.D. (Eds.), Myles' Textbook for Midwives, seventeenth ed. Elsevier, London.

National Institute of Health and Care Excellence (NICE), 2016. Jaundice in Newborn Babies under 28 Days. Available at: https://www.nice.org.uk/guidance/cg98.

Okwundu, C.L., Okoromah, C.A., Shah, P.S., 2013. Cochrane review: prophylactic phototherapy for preventing jaundice in the preterm or low birth weight infants. Evid. Base Child Health 8 (1), 204–249.

Polin, R., Abman, S., Rowitch, D., Benitz, W., 2022. Fetal and Neonatal Physiology, sixth ed. Elsevier Saunders, Philadelphia.

Rogers, J., 2022. McCance & Heuther's Pathophysiology: The Biologic Basis for Disease in Adults and Children, ninth ed. Elsevier, St. Louis.

Rosen, C., 2021. Abdominal viscera: liver. In: Standring, S. (Ed.), Gray's Anatomy: The Anatomical Basis of Clinical Practice, forty-second ed. Elsevier, London.

Sinha, S., Miall, L., Jardine, L., 2018. Essential Neonatal Medicine, sixth ed. Wiley-Blackwell, Sussex.

Vuralli, D., 2019. Clinical approach to hypocalcaemia in newborn period and infancy: who should be treated? Int. J. Pediatr. 2019, 4318075.

Annotated recommended reading

Kline, M., Blaney, S., Giardino, A., Orange, J.S., Penny, D.J., Schutze, G.E., et al., 2018. Rudolph's Pediatrics, twenty-third ed McGraw-Hill, London.

A defining textbook within the paediatric field, it also provides comprehensive content related to neonatology. It offers an algorithmic approach to the body systems, as well as to diagnosis and treatment. Furthermore, most chapters include consideration of pathogenesis and epidemiology.

53

Risks of Infection and Trauma in Neonates

THOMAS McEWAN

Within this chapter infection and trauma are explored in relation to the fetus and newborn. The ability for the student and midwife to recognize the risks for these conditions, and their signs and symptoms, is imperative for timely and effective referral and clinical care.

Infections

Fetal and Neonatal Immunocompetence

Although not fully developed, the **neonatal immune system** is capable of mounting considerable defence against pathogens and is composed of **innate** and **adaptive** (specific) immunity. Innate immune mechanisms are generally well developed and responsive at birth. Components of innate immunity such as the neutrophils are responsible for immediate recognition, isolation and initiation of pathogen destruction. In contrast, the adaptive immune mechanisms are activated on exposure to specific pathogens (or vaccines) and can be further subdivided into **humoral** and **cellular** immunity (Kumar, Abbas & Aster, 2020). The most important component of the humoral immune system is the B lymphocyte and for the cellular immune system, the T lymphocyte. Both these naïve cell lineages must be exposed to and programmed by specific antigens. In response, the mature B lymphocytes are converted into antibody-producing plasma cells, whereas the activated T cells synthesize and release cytokines such as interferons.

In the fetus and neonate, the functional immaturity of the immune system is generally attributed to the limited exposure of the B and T lymphocytes to antigens and pathogens necessary for the generation of competent, specific immune responses. Those wishing to review the immune system should read Chapter 29. Although most neonates have some specific immunity obtained by passive means via transplacental transfer and from colostrum and breast milk (Albrecht & Arck, 2020), the relative immaturity of the acquired immune mechanisms can predispose some neonates to infection (Table 53.1). However this may also represent an active immunological strategy to allow for unimpeded intestinal colonization after birth (Bordon, 2014; Moore & Townsend, 2019).

Sources of neonatal infection can be divided into three categories (Pammi, Brand & Weisman, 2021):
1. Transplacental acquisition.
2. Perinatal acquisition.
3. Postnatal infection.

Specific pathogens related to these routes of infection are discussed in detail within Chapter 14.

Perinatal and Postnatal Infections

Neonates are colonized by **commensals** and **pathogens** during labour, as well as after birth when they are exposed to new environments. Some of these pathogens may cause systemic or localized neonatal infections. Neonatal infections are difficult to recognize because early signs may be nonspecific. These are presented in Box 53.1.

Because in some instances such neonates collapse suddenly, **differential diagnoses** such as metabolic disturbances, respiratory or cardiovascular problems or intracranial bleeding cannot be excluded. As such, healthy neonates who suddenly deteriorate must therefore be examined for evidence of infection.

The National Institute of Health and Care Excellence (NICE) guidance entitled 'Neonatal infection: antibiotics for prevention and treatment' (NICE, 2021) provides a risk-based strategy for the management of suspected infection. This includes the use of the *Kaiser Permanente neonatal sepsis calculator* for babies born >34 weeks receiving in-hospital care. Consideration of antibiotic therapy should only

<table>
<tr><td colspan="2">**TABLE 53.1**   Factors Predisposing to Neonatal Infection</td></tr>
</table>

Possible Barriers	Deficiencies in Host Defence Mechanisms
Anatomical barriers	Skin abrasions sustained during delivery
	Invasive procedures: airway lavage, endotracheal intubation, umbilical artery catheterization
Phagocytic cells	Small numbers of polymorphonuclear leucocytes
	Decreased polymorphonuclear cell activity
	Slow upregulation in neutrophil production
	Poor transmission of neutrophils into the tissue
Complement mechanisms	Decreased levels of complement proteins in the blood, possibly due to immaturity of the liver
Cellular immunity	Possible defects in T-cell immunoregulation
Humoral immunity	Low levels of immunoglobulins IgA and IgM
	Low levels of IgG in premature infants
	Impaired antibody function
	Low levels of cytokines, e.g., interferon and tumour necrosis factor

• BOX 53.1   Nonspecific Signs of Neonatal Infection

The neonate may be lethargic, reluctant to feed, fretful, develop jaundice and have unexplained vomiting and an unusual stool pattern with significant weight loss. Poor temperature control, manifesting as either pyrexia or more commonly hypothermia, accompanied by tachypnoea, apnoea, cyanosis and bradycardia, must be carefully monitored. A neonate's cold peripheries, mottled skin and grey or pale appearance are often late signs of systemic infection.

be commenced following appropriate risk assessment and clinical investigation. Thereafter, the duration of treatment will be guided by the results of the clinical investigations and condition of the baby, with the aim of stopping antibiotics at the earliest opportunity. The baby's parents and carers should be fully involved in all treatment decisions (NICE, 2021).

Skin and Surface Infections

All neonatal skin lesions must be considered potentially abnormal, particularly if they are associated with **staphylococcal infections** spread from the ear, nose, mouth and skin of a carer, another neonate or child. Due to the immaturity

<table>
<tr><td colspan="2">**TABLE 53.2**   Common Skin and Surface Infections</td></tr>
</table>

Pyoderma, the appearance of small spots or pustules on the skin, and **paronychia,** a localized staphylococcal nail-bed infection, may spread rapidly in premature and ill neonates causing systemic infections. Both infections may require early antimicrobial therapy to minimize the risk of systemic infection.

Staphylococcal scalded skin syndrome is a serious skin infection caused by staphylococci entering the superficial soft tissue through a broken skin surface such as a scratch. Such infections are highly contagious and may lead to epidemics that result in closure of maternity units. Therefore any blisters appearing on the neonate's skin should be notified early to neonatal clinicians because they may be caused by **exfoliative toxins** produced by staphylococci (Nusman, Blokhuis & Pajkrt, 2023). Generally, these lesions appear on the head and the trunk and, if unattended, fill with pus, break and leave raw skin surfaces open to further infection. Extensive blisters may coalesce, giving a 'scalded skin' appearance. Supportive interventions and care in isolation should be instituted. It is important to be aware of the prevalence of **methicillin-resistant** organisms that may not respond to the usual antibiotics.

Omphalitis (infection of the umbilicus) can be serious because of a possible spread of common staphylococcal pathogens through the umbilical vein to the liver and kidneys (Fig. 53.1). Widespread erythema around the umbilicus or discharge of fluid or pus indicates local infection and must be treated with appropriate antibiotics and meticulous hygiene.

Ophthalmia neonatorum means the presence of a purulent discharge from the neonate's eye(s). Such infections may develop within 21 days of birth. Both eyes must be treated with appropriate antimicrobial therapy to minimize the risks of blindness. In severe cases, systemic antimicrobials are required. Although such severe eye infections are now rarely seen, pathogens such as the penicillin-resistant strains of *Neisseria gonorrhoeae,* staphylococci species, *E. coli* and *Chlamydia trachomatis* can induce them.

of the neonate's immune system, simple lesions can rapidly lead to serious systemic infections. A selection of common infections is presented in Table 53.2.

Serious Infections

The most serious infections encountered in neonates are septicaemia, meningitis and pneumonia. In general, these infections present with nonspecific signs such as thermo-regulation problems, lethargy, apnoea, poor feeding and vomiting. Group B β-haemolytic *Streptococcus aureus* is frequently implicated in such neonatal sepsis (Walker, Kenny & Goel, 2019).

Septicaemia is a serious end result of localized infection which, in most instances, is confirmed by blood culture. Besides the nonspecific signs, abdominal distension, increased white blood cell count, hypotonia, unexplained metabolic acidosis and glycaemic variations may occur in premature and low-birthweight neonates. Occasionally

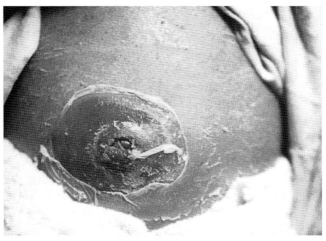

• **Fig. 53.1** Severe periumbilical infection.

the pathogens cause disseminated intravascular coagulopathy (DIC). In this case the septicaemia and coagulopathy require lifesaving supportive and therapeutic interventions.

Meningitis is most likely to occur in premature neonates or those born after difficult pregnancies and deliveries. Group B β-haemolytic streptococci and *Escherichia coli* are the most likely pathogens although *Listeria monocytogenes,* pneumococci, staphylococci and *Candida albicans* may be detected in cerebrospinal fluid cultures. The incidence of bacterial meningitis averages 0.4 per 1000 live births (Peros et al., 2020). Convulsions, bulging fontanelle, head retraction and hypothermia present in some neonates in the early stages of infection. Such symptoms must always be taken seriously and following investigative protocols managed proactively if mortality and the risks of long-term morbidity such as deafness, blindness and nerve palsies are to be minimized (Dhudasia, Flannery & Puopolo, 2021).

Neonatal pneumonia may follow the inhalation of infected amniotic fluid or meconium, causing respiratory distress within hours of birth. Conversely, **aspiration pneumonia** occurs in neonates who inhale milk, medicines or fluids given enterally. This is most likely to occur in premature neonates whose swallowing and coughing reflexes are absent or weak and may involve a range of pathogens.

Necrotizing Enterocolitis

Necrotizing enterocolitis (NEC) is an acute inflammatory change affecting the small and large bowel in predominantly premature neonates (Brown et al., 2021; Patel & Neu, 2018). Although the aetiology remains unclear (Patel & Neu, 2018), stress, infection, hypoxia, hypoglycaemia and inappropriate feeding may be contributing factors, with exclusive breastfeeding shown to reduce the incidence of NEC in preterm infants (Zhang et al., 2020). The prevention of pathogenic presence by the early colonization of the gut by **lactobacilli** may be crucial. If the neonate is not breastfed, factors such as **IgA** and **lymphocytes** from colostrum are absent, which allows invasion of the bowel wall,

portal system and bowel lymphatic glands by bacteria such as *Klebsiella, Clostridium* and *E. coli.*

Partial- or full-thickness intestinal **ischaemia** usually involves the terminal ileum. The sloughing of the ischaemic mucosal layer (Patel & Neu, 2018) contributes to gas formation within the muscular layers and the formation of **pneumatosis cystoides intestinalis,** detectable on abdominal X-ray films. Full-thickness **necrosis** leads to gut perforation and **peritonitis,** and the neonate becomes critically ill. **DIC**, septicaemia and peritonitis may develop. Hepatic portal venous gas collection usually implies that an extensive form of necrosis is present, and that the neonate requires surgery. Other clinical manifestations for NEC can include abdominal distension and tenderness; fresh blood in stools; feed intolerance; bilious vomiting; and haemodynamic, thermal and respiratory instability.

Predictive monitoring of low-birthweight infants using a heart rate characteristics index (HeRO) monitor has been shown to be effective in reducing mortality by detecting subtle clinical changes during developing neonatal shock, often from NEC (Sullivan & Fairchild, 2015). Furthermore, continuous vital sign analysis shows potential for predicting and preventing other neonatal diseases as a clinical analytic tool (Kumar et al., 2020).

Therapeutic Interventions

In mild forms of NEC, early **conservative treatment** consists of analgesia, cessation of gastric feeding, gastric decompression and intravenous antimicrobials. This may avert the severe form of gut necrosis and perforation. **Intravenous fluids** are used to maintain hydration, acceptable blood glucose and electrolyte values. Regular **analgesia** such as morphine or fentanyl is administered. It is often advantageous to establish **assisted mechanical ventilation,** particularly if respiratory distress and metabolic acidosis are evident. All affected neonates will require **antimicrobials** against Gram-negative and Gram-positive pathogens.

Surgical interventions are required if conservative medical interventions fail and the neonate shows signs of bowel perforation and peritonitis. Removal of the affected segments of the bowel with reanastomosis of the healthy segments of bowel later may have to be considered. If a functioning **ileostomy** is created, it is closed when the infant has recovered from the acute illness and surgery.

Gastroenteritis

Gastroenteritis is rare in breastfed babies, and outbreaks are commonly caused by **rotavirus,** which spreads rapidly and has a high risk of mortality (Sicard et al., 2020). Every effort must be taken to contain infection. *Salmonella* and certain strains of *E. coli* may also cause an outbreak. Most neonates deteriorate rapidly, as vomiting and frequent watery stools lead to severe dehydration. The gastrointestinal inflammatory changes may cause severe, spasmodic abdominal pain, requiring careful management. Segregation of the infected neonate is essential and, where more than one neonate is affected, the neonatal unit should be closed to new admissions. Affected neonates must be rehydrated and have their electrolyte imbalance and haemodynamic disturbances restored. Antimicrobial treatment is usually lifesaving. An affected neonatal unit may only reopen after treatment and discharge of all neonates, followed by disinfection of the clinical areas.

Birth Trauma

Uncomplicated labour rarely results in maternal or **neonatal trauma,** and severe birth traumas are therefore now rare and avoidable (Kline et al., 2018; Ojha, Tsilika & Mistry, 2020). However, minor injuries may occur during difficult deliveries such as rotational forceps, ventouse extraction, shoulder dystocia or breech presentation. Neonates who are large in relation to the mother's pelvis or of low birthweight, multiple fetuses and those born by precipitate birth are also at risk. **Neural tissue injuries** (Edwards, Counsell & Gressens, 2021; Whitelaw & Thoresen, 2021) and **fractures** of the long bones of the arm or leg may follow **shoulder dystocia** or **vaginal breech delivery.**

Head Injuries

Premature neonates are at great risk of sustaining head injuries, leading to **intracranial haemorrhage** from damage to the protective layers around the brain (Fig. 53.2). The most severe forms of intracranial bleeding are a major cause of perinatal death. A **tentorial tear** involving the great vein of Galen, a **subaponeurotic haemorrhage** or **subdural haemorrhage** (see later) may be fatal (Edwards, Counsell & Gressens, 2021; Kline et al., 2018).

Cephalhaematoma

A **cephalhaematoma** is a swelling on a baby's head caused by an effusion of blood under the periosteum of the affected skull bone (Fig. 53.3). Friction between the fetal head and the hard bone of the maternal pelvis or forceps may cause lacerations in the **periosteum,** leading to bleeding and haematoma formation. It may contribute to late onset of jaundice, as the excessive extravasated blood cells are reabsorbed. The cephalhaematoma is differentiated from the superficial oedema caused by **caput succedaneum** (see Chapter 24) by characteristic features (Table 53.3).

Subaponeurotic Haemorrhage

Subaponeurotic haemorrhage is a serious birth injury commonly associated with births assisted by vacuum extraction (Ojha, Tsilika & Mistry, 2020; Whitelaw & Thoresen, 2021). Bleeding occurs from beneath the **epicranial aponeurosis,** giving rise to a swelling which can cross suture lines. This problem must be differentiated from caput succedaneum. A subaponeurotic haematoma is present at birth and continues to increase in size. Haemorrhage is extensive and may extend into the subcutaneous tissues of the neck or eyelids, giving rise to painful swellings. The blood loss may cause anaemia, and a blood

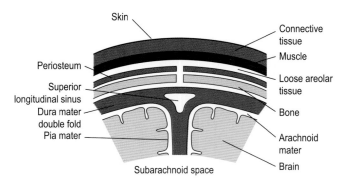
• **Fig. 53.2** A cross-section through the skull.

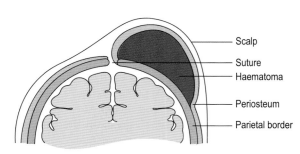
• **Fig. 53.3** Cross-section of a cephalhaematoma.

TABLE 53.3	Differentiation Between Cephalhaematoma and Caput Succedaneum	
Cephalhaematoma	**Caput Succedaneum**
It appears in the first 12 hours after birth	It is present at birth
It is clearly circumscribed and confined to one bone, never crossing a suture line	It may cross suture lines
It does not pit	Because it is oedematous, pitting can occur
It tends to grow larger rather than disappear	It resolves within the first few days of life
No treatment is needed, and the swelling usually disappears within 6–9 weeks, but may ossify	No treatment is necessary in normal circumstances

transfusion may be required. Clinical resolution is slow, extending over 2–3 weeks or longer, depending on extent and severity.

Intracranial Haemorrhage

Bleeding within the brain can occur in premature and low-birthweight neonates and is often detected when a cranial ultrasound is performed. The time of onset, duration and severity of bleeding are significant in planning a neonate's

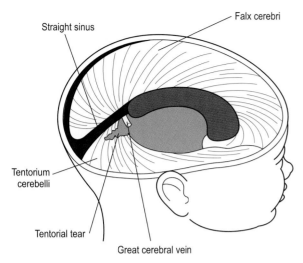

• **Fig. 53.4** A tentorial tear.

management. Intracranial haemorrhage is most likely to occur in premature neonates with a history of birth trauma, asphyxia or hypoxia. Poor autoregulation of cerebral blood flow may contribute. **Meningeal** and vessel tears occur in the **falx cerebri** or **tentorium cerebelli** (Fig. 53.4), although fragility of other cerebral blood vessels may be significant. The classical definitions of neonatal intracranial haemorrhage according to the site of bleeding are described in Table 53.4.

The site of bleeding is generally related to the gestation and developmental stage of the brain. The **subependymal germinal matrix** in the premature neonate is located adjacent to the lateral ventricles and contains actively dividing cells. From 24–32 weeks of gestation, a large capillary bed supplies these cells. The large cerebral blood flow contained in relatively fragile blood vessels is incapable of autoregulation, and the fragile capillary and related arteriovenous network is easily disrupted by hypoxia and hypercapnia, both capable of inducing cerebrovasodilatation. This matrix almost disappears in term neonates, and the risk of periventricular and intraventricular bleeding is reduced as the brain matures. In full-term neonates, intracranial haemorrhage is mainly from the **choroid plexus,** contrasting sharply with the predominantly **capillary bleeding** in the subependymal germinal matrix observed in premature neonates.

The neonate with a sudden, large periventricular or intraventricular haemorrhage presents with apnoea and circulatory collapse characterized by marked bradycardia. The **anterior fontanelle** may be enlarged and tense. Active resuscitation and respiratory support may be required (Ojha, Tsilika & Mistry, 2020). Balanced hydration and nutrition are administered intravenously, although fluids may have to be restricted if there is raised intracranial pressure. The prognosis for neonates with small haemorrhages is good, but neonates with massive haemorrhages may suffer from convulsions, localized **cerebral atrophy** and hydrocephalus (Edwards, Counsell & Gressens, 2021; Kline et al., 2018).

TABLE 53.4	Classical Definitions of Neonatal Intracranial Haemorrhage

Subdural haemorrhage is almost exclusively associated with trauma. A tear in the tentorium cerebelli at its junction with the falx cerebri causes rupture of the venous sinuses and the great vein of Galen. Initially the neonate may appear sleepy, but becomes irritable with a high-pitched cry, vomiting and a bulging anterior fontanelle. Convulsions may occur, requiring the use of anticonvulsant drugs and dexamethasone. A subdural tap may be performed to alleviate rising intracranial pressure and prevent the development of meningeal adhesions, which could contribute to later development of hydrocephalus (Kline et al., 2018; Whitelaw & Thoresen, 2021).

Subarachnoid haemorrhage occurs when there is bleeding from small vessels into the subarachnoid space after mild trauma or asphyxia. It may be asymptomatic and undetectable on ultrasound scan and is therefore more common than realized. There is blood-stained cerebrospinal fluid (CSF). The presence of blood may initiate local inflammatory changes, which may ultimately lead to **hydrocephalus.**

Intraparenchymal haemorrhage is bleeding into the cerebral tissue associated with birth asphyxia or with disseminated intravascular coagulopathy. The presence of blood within the cerebral tissue will cause local irritation, possibly leading to generalized or localized convulsions. Distortion and destruction of affected cerebral tissue leads eventually to the formation of **porencephalic cysts** (Edwards, Counsell & Gressens, 2021), although these are eventually reabsorbed. Many such neonates make a slow but full recovery.

Periventricular/intraventricular haemorrhage is the most common and most serious type of intracranial haemorrhage (Fig. 53.5) in premature neonates with a history of birth asphyxia, respiratory distress syndrome and stress. It is associated with direct trauma to neurons caused by accumulating blood, rising intracranial pressure and inflammatory changes. The accumulation of blood and inflammatory cells also interferes with normal production and circulation of CSF, which may lead to hydrocephalus. Long-term outcomes may include motor and sensory disabilities and cognitive developmental delay (Blackburn, 2018; Edwards, Counsell & Gressens, 2021; Kline et al., 2018). This form of haemorrhage is one of the most common causes of death in neonates born before 32 weeks.

In **periventricular leucomalacia** (PVL), cerebral tissue ischaemia leads to necrotic changes in the white matter surrounding the ventricles where blood flow may be interrupted due to hypotension. This area of the brain is vulnerable because it forms a boundary zone requiring blood supply from different arterial trees (Blackburn, 2018). PVL destroys neural tissue of the corticospinal motor pathways, resulting in **spastic cerebral palsy** (Fig. 53.6).

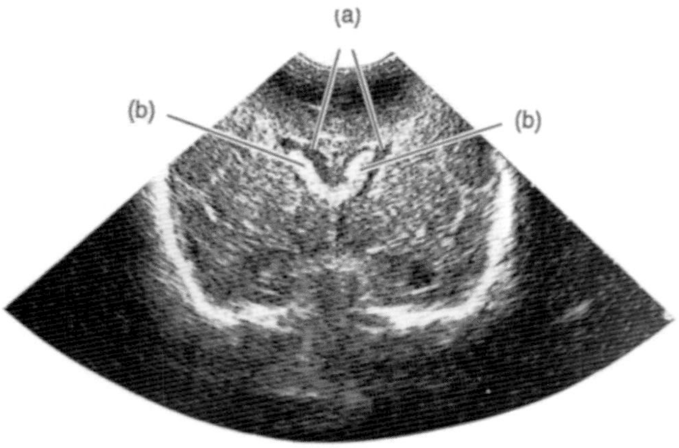

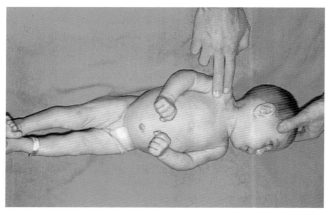

• **Fig. 53.5** Coronal cranial ultrasound scan showing intraventricular haemorrhages (B) in dilated lateral ventricles (A).

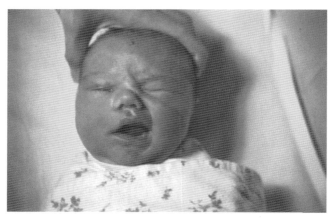

• **Fig. 53.7** Right-sided facial palsy.

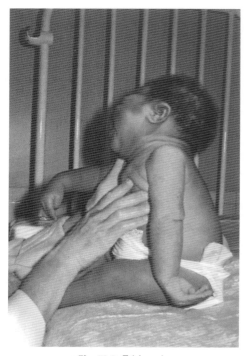

• **Fig. 53.6** Hypertonic baby with cerebral palsy.

• **Fig. 53.8** Erb's palsy.

Nerve Palsies

Facial Palsy

Facial palsy is commonly attributed to damage of the **seventh cranial nerve** by pressure applied to the facial nerve as it emerges near the angle of the jaw. The affected side of the face shows no spontaneous movement, the eye remains open and the corner of the mouth droops (Fig. 53.7). The neonate almost always recovers complete facial muscle movement.

Erb's Palsy

Erb's palsy results from damage to the **fifth** and **sixth cervical nerves** caused by **compression of the upper brachial plexus** by traction or rotation applied to the neck in a breech or difficult cephalic delivery. This results in paralysis of the arm, which is inwardly rotated and hangs limply at the side, and the half-closed hand is turned outwards in the characteristic 'waiter's tip position' (Fig. 53.8). Alternatively, the injury may present as flaccid upper extremities of one or both arms (Fig 53.9). As these nerves control the arm and some neck and chest muscles, any superficial or deep nerve injury will manifest in neuromuscular changes. Where spontaneous recovery does not occur, surgical treatment

with appropriate postoperative therapy may be necessary (Stutz, 2021).

Klumpke's Palsy

Klumpke's palsy is an uncommon problem caused by traction on the arm with damage to the **eighth cervical** and **first thoracic nerve roots** of the lower brachial plexus. The neonate presents with paralysis of the hand and 'wrist drop', although the upper arm generally has a normal range of movement. Physical assessment and radiographic screening rule out fractures to the humerus and clavicle and identify dislocated joints. Where fractures or joint problems are present, the neonate generally cannot move his affected arm. Most neonates make a slow recovery, which may take up to 2 years. **Analgesia** will limit pain and induce local muscle relaxation to aid healing. **Physiotherapy** encourages normal muscle movement

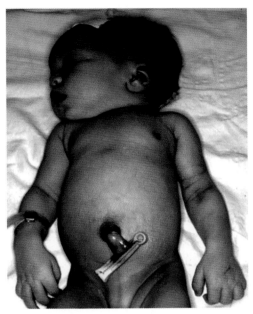

• **Fig. 53.9** Flaccid upper extremities due to bilateral brachial plexus injury.

and prevents contractures. As with Erb's palsy, **surgical intervention,** including nerve graft or repair, may be considered (Mutawakkil & King, 2023).

Soft Tissue Injuries

A common cause of soft tissue injuries is vaginal breech delivery (McKee-Garrett, 2019). Injuries include:

- Superficial bruising.
- Injury to liver and spleen.
- Injury to the kidneys and adrenal glands.
- Injury to the intestines.

Although painful superficial bruising is obvious, other more life-threatening complications may develop. This is particularly so where injury to the liver, spleen or adrenal glands results in bleeding and hypovolaemic circulatory collapse. Ultrasound scanning should establish the diagnosis. Where the neonate develops haemodynamic instability that could compromise vital organs, supportive interventions are necessary.

Main Points

- Fetal infection may be acquired transplacentally, perinatally or postnatally.
- Early signs of systemic infection in neonates are often nonspecific.
- Delays in diagnosing and treating local infections may contribute to the spread of the pathogens, causing severe systemic infection such as meningitis and septicaemia.
- Group B β-haemolytic streptococci and staphylococci are the most common pathogens in septicaemia. Meningitis is frequently caused by Group B β-haemolytic *S. aureus.*
- Gastroenteritis is rare in the breastfed baby. Outbreaks are commonly caused by rotavirus and are associated with a high mortality. Antibiotic therapy, rehydration and segregation of infectious neonates are necessary.
- Infectious neonates are isolated and, where appropriate, treated with antimicrobials. Omphalitis and ophthalmia neonatorum are potentially serious infections requiring antibiotic treatment and high standards of hygiene.
- Early diagnosis and swift medical intervention of NEC may reduce its severity. Neonates who develop bowel necrosis and perforation require specialist surgery.
- Normal labour rarely results in birth injuries, but minor soft tissue injuries may occur during a difficult labour.
- Friction between the fetal head and the maternal pelvis or forceps may cause a cephalhaematoma.
- Subaponeurotic haemorrhage is a serious birth injury commonly associated with vacuum extraction. Bleeding may extend into the subcutaneous tissues of the neck or eyelids.
- Intracranial haemorrhages are a major cause of perinatal death when prematurity is associated with hypoxia, asphyxia or trauma to the falx cerebri or tentorium cerebelli, resulting in subdural bleeding and subarachnoid bleeding, respectively.
- Intraparenchymal haemorrhage is frequently associated with birth asphyxia and may result in the formation of porencephalic cysts from the destruction of affected cerebral tissue.
- PVH/IVH haemorrhage is the most common and serious form of intracranial haemorrhage occurring in premature neonates. Some will develop a range of complications, including hydrocephalus; motor, sensory and cognitive disabilities; and leucomalacia leading to cerebral palsy.
- Nerve palsies include facial palsy, Erb's palsy and Klumpke's palsy.

References

Albrecht, M., Arck, P.C., 2020. Vertically transferred immunity in neonates: mothers, mechanisms and mediators. Front. Immunol. 11, 555.

Blackburn, S.T., 2018. Maternal, Fetal and Neonatal Physiology: A Clinical Perspective, fifth ed. Elsevier, St. Louis.

Bordon, Y., 2014. Neonatal immunity: hush-a by baby. Nat. Rev. Immunol. 14 (1), 4–5.

Brown, L., Hendrickson, K., Evans, R., Hay Jr, W.W., 2021. Enteral nutrition. In: Gardner, S.L., Carter, B.S., Enzman-Hines, M., Niermeyer, S. (Eds.), Merenstein and Gardner's Handbook of Neonatal Intensive Care: An Interprofessional Approach, ninth ed. Elsevier, St. Louis.

Dhudasia, M., Flannery, D., Puopolo, K., 2021. Evaluation and management of infection in the newborn. In: Boardman, J.P., Groves, A.M., Ramasethu, J. (Eds.), Avery & McDonald's Neonatology: Pathophysiology and Management of the Newborn, eighth ed. Lippincott, Williams and Wilkins, Philadelphia.

Edwards, D., Counsell, S., Gressens, P., 2021. Brain development and injury in preterm infants. In: Boardman, J.P., Groves, A.M., Ramasethu, J. (Eds.), Avery & McDonald's Neonatology: Pathophysiology and Management of the Newborn, eighth ed. Lippincott, Williams and Wilkins, Philadelphia.

Kline, M., Blaney, S., Giardino, A., Orange, J.S., Penny, D.J., Schutze, G.E., et al., 2018. Rudolph's Pediatrics, twenty-third ed. McGraw-Hill, London.

Kumar, V., Abbas, A., Aster, J., 2020a. Robbins and Cotran Pathologic Basis of Disease, tenth ed. Elsevier, Philadelphia.

Kumar, N., Akangire, G., Sullivan, B., Fairchild, K., Sampath, V., 2020. Continuous vital sign analysis for predicting and preventing neonatal diseases in the twenty-first century: big data to the forefront. Pediatr. Res. 87 (2), 210–220.

McKee-Garrett, T.M., 2019. Neonatal Birth Injuries. Available at: https://www.uptodate.com/contents/neonatal-birth-injuries.

Moore, R.E., Townsend, S.D., 2019. Temporal development of the infant gut microbiome. Open Biol. 9 (9):90128.

Mutawakkil, M.Y., King, E.C., 2023. Pediatric brachial plexus palsy. In: Sarwark, J.F., Carl, R.L. (Eds.), Orthopaedics for the Newborn and Young Child. Springer, Cham.

National Institute of Health and Care Excellence (NICE), 2021. Neonatal Infection: Antibiotics for Prevention and Treatment. Available at: https://www.nice.org.uk/guidance/ng195.

Nusman, C.M., Blokhuis, C., Pajkrt, D., 2023. Staphylococcal scalded skin syndrome in neonates: case series and overview of outbreaks. Antibiotics 12 (1), 38.

Ojha, S., Tsilika, L., Mistry, A., 2020. Trauma during birth, haemorrhages and convulsions. In: Marshall, J.E., Raynor, M.D. (Eds.), Myles' Textbook for Midwives, seventeenth ed. Elsevier, London.

Pammi, M., Brand, M.C., Weisman, L.E., 2021. Infection in the neonate. In: Gardner, S.L., Carter, B.S., Enzman-Hines, M., Niermeyer, S. (Eds.), Merenstein and Gardner's Handbook of Neonatal Intensive Care: An Interprofessional Approach, ninth ed. Elsevier, St. Louis.

Patel, R.M., Neu, J., 2018. Necrotizing enterocolitis. In: Kline, M., Blaney, S., Giardino, A., Orange, J.S., Penny, D.J., Schutze, G.E., et al. (Eds.), Rudolph's Pediatrics, twenty-third ed. McGraw-Hill, London.

Peros, T., van Schuppen, J., Bohte, A., Hodiamont, C., Aronica, E., de Haan, T., 2020. Neonatal bacterial meningitis versus ventriculitis:

a cohort-based overview of clinical characteristics, microbiology and imaging. Eur. J. Pediatr. 179 (12), 1969–1977.

Sicard, M., Bryant, K., Muller, M.L., Quach, C., 2020. Rotavirus vaccination in the neonatal intensive care units: where are we? A rapid review of recent evidence. Curr. Opin. Pediatr. 32 (1), 167–191.

Stutz, C., 2021. Management of brachial plexus birth injuries: Erbs and extended Erbs palsy. In: Shin, A.Y., Pulos, N. (Eds.), Operative Brachial Plexus Surgery: Clinical Evaluation and Management Strategies. Springer, Cham.

Sullivan, B.A., Fairchild, K.D., 2015. Predictive monitoring for sepsis and necrotizing enterocolitis to prevent shock. Semin. Fetal Neonatal Med. 20 (4), 255–261.

Walker, O., Kenny, C.B., Goel, N., 2019. Neonatal sepsis. Paediatr. Child Health 29 (6), 263–268.

Whitelaw, A., Thoresen, M., 2021. Brain injury at term. In: Boardman, J.P., Groves, A.M., Ramasethu, J. (Eds.), Avery & McDonald's Neonatology: Pathophysiology and Management of the Newborn, eighth ed. Lippincott, Williams and Wilkins, Philadelphia.

Zhang, B., Xiu, W., Dai, Y., Yang, C., 2020. Protective effects of different doses of human milk on neonatal necrotizing enterocolitis. Medicine 99 (37), e22166.

Annotated recommended reading

Volpe, J., Inder, T., Darras, B., de Vries, L.S., du Plessis, A.J., Neil, J., et al., 2017. Volpe's Neurology of the Newborn, sixth ed. Elsevier Saunders, Philadelphia.

This book offers a comprehensive account of neonatal neurophysiology and neuropathophysiology with the reader directed to the detailed chapters on perinatal trauma, intracranial haemorrhage and disorders of the motor system to further develop their understanding of the conditions identified within this chapter.

Wilson, C.B., Nizet, V., Maldonado, Y., Remington, J.S., Klein, J.O., 2015. Remington and Klein's Infectious Diseases of the Fetus and Newborn, eighth ed. Elsevier Saunders, Philadelphia.

This textbook is an authoritative reference, providing the most up-to-date and comprehensive guidance on infections found in the perinatal and neonatal period in both premature and term infants.

Puerperium—The Mother

This section focuses on the postpartum period. This involves the woman's return to normal physiology after childbirth, the onset and establishment of lactation and the physiological factors influencing the parent–baby relationship. Breast anatomy, lactation and related physiology are discussed in Chapter 54, and breastfeeding practices and problems are discussed in Chapter 55. Evidence-based practice and advances in technology provide further opportunity to revisit the lactating breast and lactation to facilitate understanding of the mechanisms of breastfeeding and practical advice given to lactating women. Chapter 56 addresses other physiolog ical changes occurring in the puerperium and the pathological conditions that may affect the woman. Some pathological conditions are discussed, including puerperal infection and mental health disorders. The final chapter of this book Chapter 57 considers the development of mother–baby relationships in terms of biological theories. This involves the role of midwives in using this information within their everyday practice to facilitate positive relationships with parents and their baby. However the student should not lose sight of the integration of biology, psychology and sociology which underpins all human behaviour.

54

The Breasts and Lactation

MARIA POLLARD

CHAPTER CONTENTS

This chapter details the anatomy and structure of the breasts. The development of the breasts through the stages from early life, puberty, pregnancy and lactation are discussed. The physiology of lactation and content of breastmilk are detailed.

Introduction

Lactation is the production of milk by specialized organs called **mammary glands,** named from the Latin word *mamma* for breast. Humans are classified as mammals and distinguished from other vertebrates because of their ability to produce milk for their young.

The Anatomy of the Breast

Situation, Shape and Size

The adult breasts are paired mammary glands situated on the anterior surface of the chest wall on either side of the midline and will vary in size depending on the amount of adipose tissue present. They possibly originate from modified apocrine sweat glands and subsequently form part of the skin. The shape of the breast varies, but it tends to be dome-shaped in adolescence, becoming more prominent, hemispheric and finally pendulous in parous females. The mature breast extends between the second rib and the sixth intercostal cartilage and lies over the pectoralis major muscle from sternum to axilla. Mammary glandular tissue projects somewhat into the axillary region blending with the anterior axillary fold, and this is known as the *tail of Spence.* The **nipple** is surrounded by areola and protrudes from the centre of each breast around the level of the fourth intercostal space depending on the size of the breast (Bazira, Ellis & Mahadevan, 2022).

Internal Structure

The mammary glands are modified exocrine glands comprising skin, subcutaneous tissue and the corpus mammae (body of the breast). The corpus mammae is the breast mass remaining after the breast is freed from the deep attachments and the skin, subcutaneous connective tissue and adipose tissue are removed.

The tissue of the mammary gland consists of two major divisions: the **parenchyma** and the **stroma.** The parenchyma or glandular (secretory) tissue is the functional component of the breast tissue. The stroma comprises adipose (fatty) tissue, blood and lymph vessels and nerve tissue, and is supported by a loose framework of fibrous connective tissue called *Cooper's ligaments.* The proportion of glandular and adipose tissue was found to be 2:1 in the lactating breast (Geddes et al., 2021). The parenchyma consists of epithelial glandular tissue with an extensive system of branching ducts (Fig. 54.1).

The Parenchyma

The basic glandular unit consists of alveoli. The alveoli (10–100) cluster to form lobules, which group into lobes (15–20) surrounded by a layer of fat. The alveolus is the site of milk synthesis and secretion, and consists of clusters of epithelial secretory cells (lactocytes) surrounded by myoepithelial cells to form smooth muscle contractile units responsible for ejecting milk into the lactiferous ducts from the lumen of the alveoli (Fig. 54.2). Milk is stored in the lumen of the alveolar until the 'let-down'

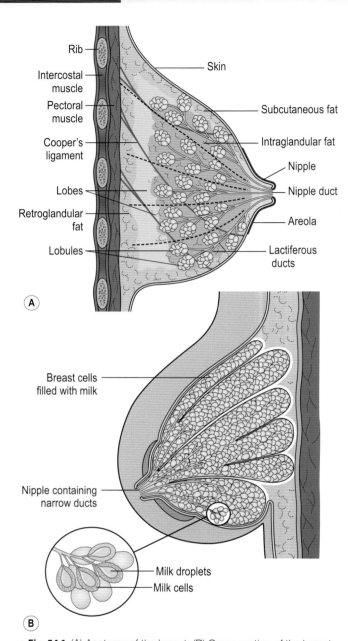

• **Fig. 54.1** (A) Anatomy of the breast. (B) Cross section of the breast.

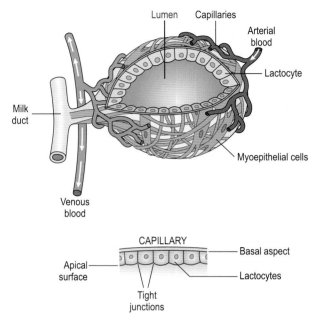

• **Fig. 54.2** The structure of the alveolus.

Women's breasts vary in size, but this is not an indicator of milk storage capacity. Milk storage capacity varies, but most mothers produce an average of 50–800 mL/day) (Geddes et al., 2021; Kent et al., 2006; Kent, Gardner & Geddes, 2016). Therefore women with lower milk storage capacity may feed more frequently than those with higher storage capacity. This supports the need for responsive feeding (Pollard, 2023).

reflex triggers the ejection of the milk into the ducts. Ramsay et al. (2005) found that each breast contains about nine milk ducts (range 4–18 ducts) arranged in a complex and erratic network and which converge at the nipple (Geddes et al., 2021). Contrary to previous understanding, Ramsay et al. (2005) found no evidence of lactiferous sinuses under the areola, which were previously thought to store breastmilk (Geddes et al., 2021). Clinical Application 54.1 highlights the role of breast size and storage capacity of milk.

Each alveolus is surrounded by a **basement membrane** (basal lamina). This provides a barrier between the epithelial and stromal components of breast tissue which cannot be crossed by cells other than leucocytes. Lymphocytes or monocytes are found wedged between the secretory cells of the alveoli and have migrated there. They play a role in local production of antibodies in the form of immunoglobulin A (IgA) for secretion into the breastmilk.

The Secretory Cells

The secretory cells, or lactocytes, lining the alveoli are cuboidal in shape if full and columnar if empty (van Veldhuizen-Staas, 2007) (Fig. 54.2). They are connected to each other and regulate milk synthesis. The basal surface of the cell has numerous infoldings for the uptake of substrate for milk production, whereas the apical surface facing the lumen is covered with microvilli for secretion of milk. Tight junctions connect these cells and are closed in the first few days after birth, stopping the passage of molecules into the milk. It is important to have knowledge of lactocytes when promoting effective breastfeeding. Clinical Application 54.2 outlines the implications for practice.

The Stroma

Connective and adipose tissue, which form the largest part of the mammary glands in the nonpregnant state, separate and support the glandular tissue. The breasts are held in position by the suspensory ligaments, or Cooper's ligaments, which form from the interlobar connective tissue. These fibrous bands of tissue attach the breast to the underlying muscle fascia and to the overlying dermis of the skin.

The Nipple and Areola

The skin of the breast includes the nipple and surrounding areola. The **nipple,** or papilla mammae, is a conic elevation located in the centre of the areola. The nipple contains about 4–18 milk (average 9) ducts (Geddes et al., 2021; Ramsay et al., 2005). The smooth muscle fibres in the nipple represent a closing mechanism for the milk ducts, and the nipple is richly innervated with sensory nerve endings. Nipple erection is induced by tactile, sensory or autonomic sympathetic stimuli. Local venostasis and hyperaemia occur to enhance the process of erection.

The **areola**, or areola mammae, is a circular pigmented area surrounding the nipple. Within the areola are about 18 sebaceous and lactiferous glands known as *Montgomery's tubercles.* These glands provide secretions to lubricate and protect the areola and nipple during pregnancy and lactation and a scent to attract the infant to the nipple (Zandro, 2018). Every woman's areola varies in size and colour but on average is 15 mm in diameter.

Blood and Lymphatic Supply

The internal mammary artery (also known as internal thoracic artery) and the lateral mammary branch of the lateral thoracic artery provide the major blood supply, with further sources of arterial blood from the superior thoracic, pectoral, lateral thoracic and subcapular. The venous supply parallels the arterial supply and have similar names. Veins end in the internal thoracic and axillary veins and create an anastomotic circle called the *circulus venosus* around the base of the papilla behind the nipple.

There is an extensive lymphatic drainage system forming a plexus beneath the areola and between the lobes of the breast with free communication between the two breasts. There are two main pathways by which lymph is drained from the breast and include the axillary nodes and the internal mammary nodes. Lymph from both the medial and lateral portions of the breast drains to the axillary nodes (75–80%), whereas the internal mammary nodes receive lymph from the deep portion of the breast (20–25%).

Nerve Supply

The breast skin is innervated primarily by the anterior cutaneous branches and lateral cutaneous branches of the second to sixth intercostal nerves and the nipple and areola by the third to fifth intercostal nerves (Smeele et al., 2022). The nerve supply to the corpus mammae is sparse and contains only sympathetic nerves accompanying blood vessels. The sensory innervation of the nipple and areola is extensive and consists of both sensory and sympathetic autonomic nerves:

- Somatic sensory nerves convey impulses from skin receptors to the central nervous system.
- Sympathetic (efferent) nerves innervate blood vessels and the contractile muscles of the nipple.

Development of the Breast

The mammary gland undergoes three major phases of growth and development before pregnancy and lactation: in utero, during the first 2 years of life and at puberty. **Embryogenesis** refers to the embryonic development of the organ in utero. **Mammogenesis** refers to the growth and development of the mammary glands. This stage occurs in two phases as the glands respond first to the hormones of puberty and then later to the hormones of pregnancy. **Lactogenesis** refers to the initiation and production of milk.

Early Development and Puberty

Mammogenesis or breast development commences around the fourth week of embryonic life, where a primitive milk streak develops from axilla to groin on the trunk of the embryo. This streak becomes the mammary ridge or milk line. Specialized cells differentiate into breast structures such as nipple, areola, glands, hair follicles and Montgomery's glands. Development is influenced by the placental sex hormones between 28 and 32 weeks to stimulate the formation of channels (canalization). From 32–40 weeks of gestation, lobular–alveolar structures containing colostrum develop. During this time, the fetal mammary glands increase four times, and the nipple and areola further develop and become pigmented. After birth, the neonate may secrete colostrum known as *witch's milk* due to the influence of the maternal hormones associated with breastmilk production.

Mammary gland development during childhood merely keeps pace with physical growth. At puberty, oestrogen becomes the major influence on female breast development but the increase in breast size is due to the deposition of adipose tissue (Geddes et al., 2021). Under the influence of oestrogen, primary and secondary ducts grow and divide and form terminal end buds, which develop into new branches and later become alveoli in the mature breast. During each menstrual cycle, proliferation and active growth of duct

GESTATION

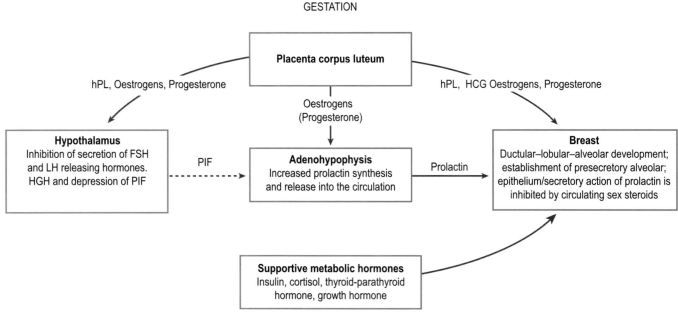

• **Fig. 54.3** Hormonal preparation of breast during pregnancy for lactation. *FSH*, Follicle-stimulating hormone; *LH*, luteinizing hormone; *HCG*, human chorionic gonadotropin; *HGH*, human growth hormone; *hPL*, human placental lactogen; *PIF*, prolactin-inhibiting factor.

tissue occurs during the follicular and ovulatory phases, reaching a maximum in the late luteal phase before regressing. Complete development of mammary function occurs only in pregnancy.

Development in Pregnancy

The breast reaches its full functional capacity at lactation and, as a result, several internal and external changes occur. Changes in levels of circulating hormones result in profound changes during pregnancy (Fig. 54.3). Breasts begin to exhibit changes at about the sixth week of pregnancy and may be useful in confirming pregnancy (Blackburn, 2018).

1. Early in pregnancy, the luteal and placental hormones are responsible for a marked increase in the development of the duct system and formation of lobes. Placental lactogen, prolactin and chorionic gonadotrophin contribute to the accelerated growth. Oestrogen is responsible for development in the duct system, and progesterone is responsible for lobular formation. This results in the breasts feeling nodular and lumpy, and the woman may feel the breasts tender and tingly. Growth continues throughout pregnancy, and the breasts increase in size.
2. By 12 weeks the nipples are now more prominent and the areola develops an increased fullness and brown pigmentation called the *primary areola of pregnancy*. Montgomery's tubercles further develop and become more prominent and appear as raised projections.
3. By approximately 16 weeks, colostrum is produced under the influence of prolactin, produced by the anterior lobe of the pituitary gland. During pregnancy, prolactin is

prevented from exerting its effect on milk excretion by the high circulating levels of progesterone.
4. Vascularity increases, and the appearance of a network of subcutaneous veins is visible beneath the skin. This network increases in size and complexity throughout pregnancy.
5. By the 24th week, there is further pigmentation around the primary areola known as the *secondary areola*.
6. By term the breasts usually enlarge by 5 cm overall and increase by 1400 g in weight.

Maternal Nutrition and Lactation

Lifestyle and dietary habits during pregnancy and breastfeeding will impact on the health of the mother and infant. The increased calorific requirements for breastfeeding, approximately 500 kcal/day for the first 6 months if exclusive breastfeeding, should be managed through a varied and balanced diet to ensure the adequate intake of nutrients such as iron, iodine, calcium, folic acid and vitamin D. Those at risk of not achieving sufficient intake of these nutrients include women on exclusion diets, women with underweight or overweight, smokers, adolescents and mothers who have had multiple pregnancies close together (Marangoni et al., 2016).

The Physiology of Lactation

Lactogenesis is the transition from pregnancy to lactation. There are three phases:
1. Lactogenesis I: the initiation of milk secretion, a neuroendocrine response commencing in pregnancy.

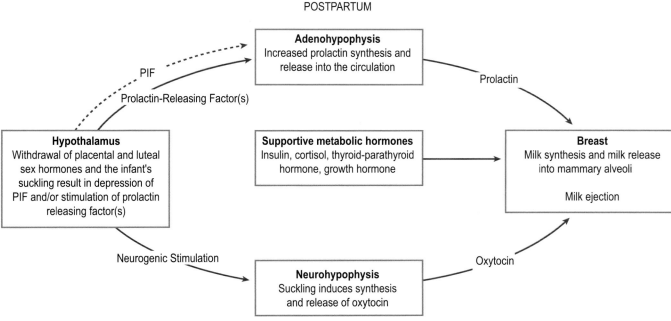

• **Fig. 54.4** Hormonal preparation of the breast postpartum for lactation. *PIF*, Prolactin-inhibiting factor.

TABLE 54.1	Stages of Lactogenesis
Stage	**Development**
Lactogenesis I	
Begins when milk components are first seen in breast tissue and colostrum can be expressed from the breast during pregnancy (normally from midpregnancy until day 2 after birth).	A specific milk protein called *α-lactalbumin* can be detected in maternal blood from midpregnancy. During this stage the physical changes in the breasts are accompanied by hormonal changes resulting from the interplay between the pituitary gland, the ovary and the placenta. Prolactin stimulates mammary secretory epithelial cells to produce milk. Developments culminate in the initiation of lactation after the birth of the infant.
Lactogenesis II	
Begins around days 2–3 after birth when 'milk comes in' and continues until about day 8.	Secretory activation is triggered by a rapid reduction in maternal plasma progesterone levels when the placenta is delivered. High levels of prolactin, which increase with suckling, stimulate copious milk production. There is a switch from endocrine to autocrine (local) control. Milk supply is regulated by removal of feedback inhibitor of lactation. There is fullness and warmth in the breast and major changes in milk continue until about day 8 after birth when mature milk is established.
Lactogenesis III (Galactopoiesis)	
Begins around days 8–9 after birth once the mature milk supply is established. It continues until involution of breastmilk tissues begins.	This involves the maintenance of established breastfeeding through milk production and removal of milk by the infant. Control by autocrine supply (supply and demand of milk).
Involution (Apoptosis)	
This stage begins once breastfeeding discontinues.	Apoptotic cell death and tissue remodelling happen when breastfeeding stops.

2. Lactogenesis II: the production of colostrum and transitional milk, a neuroendocrine response.
3. Lactogenesis III/galactopoiesis: the development of milk and the maintenance of established lactation. Control of milk production is by autocrine system – supply and demand.

Involution of the breast through apoptotic cell death and tissue remodelling happens when breastfeeding stops.

Fig. 54.4 summarizes the hormonal preparation of the breast postpartum for lactation and Table 54.1 details the stages of lactogenesis.

Neuroendocrine Control

Lactogenesis I commences around 16 weeks of pregnancy under **neuroendocrine control** leading to the production of colostrum. Although prolactin is present during pregnancy, it is inhibited by increased levels of oestrogen, progesterone, human placental lactogen (hPL) and prolactin-inhibiting factor (PIF), suppressing milk production.

Lactogenesis II, the onset of milk production, commences 30–40 hours after birth. After the delivery of the placenta and membranes, the pituitary gland produces low levels of follicle-stimulating hormone and luteinizing hormone, leading to low levels of oestrogen and progesterone enhancing the production of prolactin, releasing the lactocytes from their inhibitory state to respond to the circulating prolactin by producing milk. Mothers feel the milk 'coming in' about 2–3 days after birth.

Before lactogenesis II large gaps are evident between the alveolar cells, but after birth there is a decline in levels of chloride, sodium and protein, leading to closure of the tight junctions between the alveolar cells. In addition to this process, desmosome binds the cells, stopping the passage of substances between the alveolar cells (Garrod & Chidgey, 2008).

Prolactin

During pregnancy, prolactin increases breast mass and cell differentiation, and after birth is essential for the production and maintenance of milk. During pregnancy, concentrations of plasma prolactin rise steadily to term when they reach up to 20 times that of the nonpregnant woman. After delivery of the placenta, progesterone and oestrogen levels fall abruptly, and the anterior pituitary gland releases very large amounts of prolactin because it is no longer inhibited by these hormones. The decline in hPL removes any competition with prolactin for breast receptor sites, promoting the action of prolactin (Rassie et al., 2022). Prolactin is released via the anterior pituitary gland in pulses 7–20 times a day; it is at its highest rate 45 min after breastfeeding. The production of prolactin varies, but levels are higher at night than during the day (Freeman et al., 2000) (circadian rhythm) and therefore night feeds are important to promote milk production. Regular suckling (>8 feeds in 24 hours) during the early stages of lactation primes the prolactin receptor sites on the lactocytes to synthesize milk, resulting in an adequate milk supply. If not emptied and full of milk, the shape of alveoli becomes distorted, affecting the prolactin receptor sites. Prolactin is unable to enter the cells and the milk production rate decreases. When milk is emptied from the alveolus, its normal shape is returned and prolactin will bind to the receptor site, increasing milk production (van Veldhuizen-Staas, 2007). Where breastfeeding is not initiated, prolactin levels return to nonpregnant levels within 3 weeks postpartum (Rassie, 2022).

Oxytocin

Oxytocin is essential for the removal of milk from breast—neuroendocrine regulation. The effective removal of milk involves two closely related aspects of breastfeeding:

- The let-down (milk ejection) reflex and the role of the posterior pituitary hormone oxytocin.

- The important role the infant plays in suckling the breast to remove the milk.

Oxytocin is a peptide hormone produced in the hypothalamus and stored in the posterior pituitary gland. The nipple and areola have a rich supply of sensory nerves. The afferent fibres terminate in the dorsal horn of the spinal cord, where they synapse on ascending fibres which transmit the messages received from the suckling of the infant to the brainstem. The messages are then relayed to the midbrain and hypothalamus, resulting in the release of oxytocin (Fig. 54.5) from the posterior lobe of the pituitary gland. This hormone contracts the myoepithelial cells situated around the alveoli and dilates the ducts by acting on the smooth muscle cells lying in the duct wall propelling milk along the ducts. Smooth muscle contraction results in shortening and widening of the ducts to allow milk to flow. Some women may feel pressure and a tingling warm sensation during milk ejection. This is known as the *let-down* or *ejection reflex*.

Oxytocin levels in the blood often rise just before a feed, either due to the infant crying or becoming restless or the mother thinking about the infant (Uvnäs-Moberg et al., 2020). Oxytocin levels are raised within minutes of any breast stimulation. It is released in a pulsatile pattern and return to baseline levels within minutes after nipple stimulation has stopped (Uvnäs-Moberg et al., 2020).

The Effect of Higher Brain Centres

The **neuroendocrine regulation** of oxytocin release and the resulting milk ejection is a complex process that can be inhibited or stimulated by neural influences projected by nerves synapsing on the hypothalamus from higher centres of the brain. These include those parts of the brain involved in emotion, such as the limbic system, and the cognitive interpretation of all aspects of the activity from the prefrontal cortex. The control from higher centres can be more powerful than the nipple–hypothalamic pathway. The let-down reflex can be stimulated by other sensory pathways, such as visual, tactile, olfactory and auditory, or inhibited by emotional states. The mother can and will release milk by seeing, touching, hearing, smelling and/or just thinking about her infant. In addition, oxytocin can inhibit the release of cortisol and reduce stress levels, decrease anxiety and decrease blood pressure (Uvnäs-Moberg & Prime, 2013). Skin-to-skin contact at birth and early and regular breastfeeding have key roles to play in promoting effective breastfeeding. Clinical Application 54.3 summarizes the implications for practice.

> **• CLINICAL APPLICATION 54.3** Implications of Skin-to-Skin Contact at Birth and Early Breastfeeding
>
> Skin-to-skin contact at birth and beyond stimulates the production of prolactin and oxytocin.
> Early and regular breastfeeding inhibits the production of PIF and stimulates production of prolactin (Pollard, 2023).

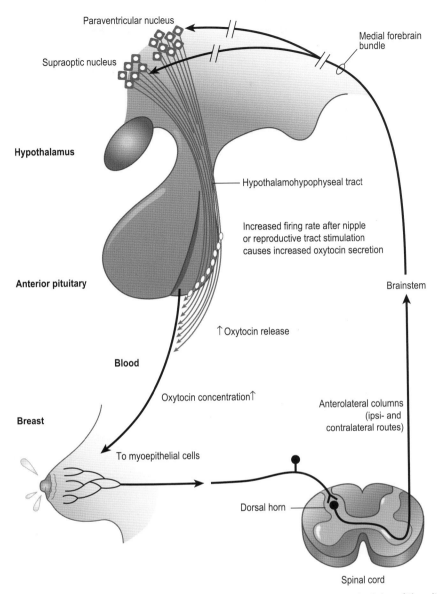

• **Fig. 54.5** Neuroendocrine reflex in the stimulation of oxytocin (from the posterior lobe of the pituitary gland) for milk ejection.

Autocrine Control

Lactogenesis III, or galactopoiesis, is where the supply and demand regulate milk production. An autocrine regulator of milk secretion has been identified called the **feedback inhibitor of lactation** (FIL). This factor – a whey protein present in secreted milk – can inhibit the synthesis of milk constituents (Wilde et al., 1995) and builds up in the breast as milk accumulates, exerting a negative control on the continued production of milk. Thus, milk production slows when milk accumulates in the breast (and more FIL is present) and speeds up when the breast is emptier of milk (and less FIL is present). Removing the milk removes the regulating protein, and milk then continues to be produced. This is a local mechanism and can occur in one or both breasts.

Suckling and Removal of Milk

The transition to extrauterine life is a critical period whereby the infants' survival instincts are developed or suppressed (Bergman et al., 2019). This innate behaviour is directed by the limbic system via the autonomic nervous system. Skin-to-skin contact encourages this neurobehavioural programme. Supporting early and frequent breastfeeding is a simple recommendation for the initiation and maintenance of breastfeeding. After birth, there is an early opportunity for the infant's suckling to stimulate prolactin receptors (Fig. 54.6), which in turn will enhance milk production. It is essential for newborn infants to be put to the breast as early as possible after birth, ideally in the first hour, and allow suckling as frequently as the infant demands. Some practices interfere with this process such as medication,

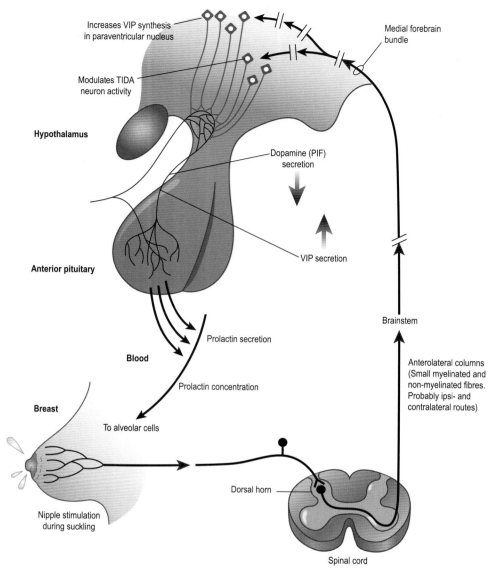

• **Fig. 54.6** Somatosensory pathways in the stimulation of prolactin (from the anterior lobe of the pituitary) for milk production. *PIF*, Prolactin-inhibiting factor; *TIDA*, tuberoinfundibular dopaminergic; *VIP*, vasoactive intestinal peptide.

particularly pethidine, or separation and may have negative effects on the ability of the newborn infant to respond with appropriate behaviour.

Widström et al. (2011) identify nine behavioural stages during the first hour following birth that facilitate and promote breastfeeding:

1. The birth cry – initial lung expansion.
2. Relaxation – no visible movements.
3. Awakening – eyes open, small mouth movement.
4. Activity – finger and limb movements, head lifting.
5. Resting between stages – with some activity.
6. Crawling – movement towards the breast and nipple.
7. Familiarization – touch, lick and taste the nipple.
8. Suckling – self-attachment to the nipple.
9. Sleeping.

The prone position of skin-to-skin allows the infant to move its head and lead with the chin to find the nipple.

This is called the **rooting reflex.** When the nipple brushes against the area between the nose and upper lip (philtrum), the infant will open its mouth wide enough to take in the nipple and surrounding breast tissue and start to suck. This is called the **gape response.**

The **sucking reflex** is complex in breastfeeding and different from sucking an artificial teat. Breast tissue is drawn into the infant's mouth by negative pressure at the anterior point of the junction between the hard and soft palate so that an elongated teat is formed. A vacuum occurs as the tongue and jaw move down drawing milk from the breast. The muscles of the cheeks create suction and a negative pressure within the mouth (Geddes et al., 2021). Clinical Application 54.4 summarizes the signs of good attachment to the breast.

The **swallowing reflex** is well developed in the term infant. Protection of the airway is important during

The mother is comfortable with no pain or nipple trauma.
The baby's mouth is wide open.
The cheeks are full and rounded.
There is more areola visible above the top lip.
There is audible rhythmic sucking and swallowing.

swallowing. The soft palate rises to close the nasal cavity, the vocal cords close the trachea and the hyoid bones rise to elevate the larynx. As the vacuum reduces and milk flow stops, the epiglottis moves backwards and downwards, closing the larynx as the milk is directed to the oesophagus.

Breathing is coordinated with swallowing by an **upper-airway reflex** to prevent aspiration. It is important that infants are free to move their heads to allow extension and stabilization of the airway.

Involution takes place during weaning or when milk is no longer removed from the breast. Prolactin is no longer produced, and there is a build-up of FIL inhibiting the production of milk. The epithelial cells die (apoptosis) and tissue remodelling occurs. However if there is further regular stimulation milk may be produced as a full return to the prepregnant state does not occur.

Breastmilk

The consistently identifiable stages of human milk are colostrum, transitional milk and mature milk, and their relative contents are significant to nourish newborns as they adapt to extrauterine life.

Colostrum, a thick yellow fluid, is synthesized in the breast from around the 16th week of pregnancy (lactogenesis I) and gradually changes into mature breastmilk between the 3rd and 14th day after birth. It is high in density and low in volume, containing more protein, minerals and fat-soluble vitamins (A and K) than mature milk but less lactose, fats and water-soluble vitamins. It also contains more anti-infective agents such as IgA, lactoferrin, lysozymes and leucocytes than mature milk. Colostrum facilitates the establishment of *Lactobacillus bifidus* in the digestive tract and has a purgative effect that facilitates the passage of meconium, reducing the possibility of jaundice.

Transitional milk is the milk produced between colostrum and mature milk (lactogenesis II). The content gradually changes from between 7–10 days and about 2 weeks after birth. The concentration of immunoglobulins and total protein decreases, and the lactose, fat and total caloric content increases. Water-soluble vitamins increase and fat-soluble vitamins decrease to the levels of mature milk.

Mature breastmilk is highly variable both within and between women. Its contents change from one feed to another, over the course of a specific feed and as the infant grows and develops. The milk obtained by the infant at the beginning of a feed is called the **foremilk** and differs from the **hindmilk** obtained towards the end of a feed when there is an increase in fat content. The highest volume of milk removal is in the morning and for infants up to 6 months old over a 24-hour period was 809 ± 171 mL, ranging from 549–1147 mL (Cregan, Mitoulas & Hartmann, 2002).

The Contents of Breastmilk

Breastmilk is sometimes referred to as a *living fluid*. Despite improvements in technologies, breastmilk cannot be replicated (Table 54.2). The properties include proteins, carbohydrates, fats, electrolytes, minerals, vitamins, enzymes, hormones and anti-infective substances and meet the infant's individual needs. Water makes up over 80% of the milk volume; therefore breastfed infants do not need supplementary drinks.

Protein

The main proteins of human milk are whey protein and casein. The composition changes depending on the stage of lactation changes depending on the stage of lactation from approximately 70/30 or 80/20 in early lactation to 50/50 or 60/40 in more mature breastmilk. These proteins form soft curds, which are easily digested by the infant. In addition to their nutritional function, milk proteins have immunological purposes. The chief fractions of whey protein are α-lactalbumin and lactoferrin. Lactoferrin is an iron-binding protein which is low in artificial milk. The total protein content and the balance of amino acids present are essential for the maximum functioning of enzyme systems. The amino acids phenylalanine and tyrosine are present in much lower amounts than in artificial milk. The important amino acids glutamic acid and taurine are abundant in human milk but low in artificial milk. Taurine is necessary for the conjugation of bile salts and fat absorption in the first week of life. It is also essential for the myelination of the central nervous system.

Carbohydrate

Lactose is the main carbohydrate in human milk (98%) and is formed from glucose or galactose in the Golgi apparatus under the influence of the enzyme lactose synthetase. The regulation of lactose is linked to the production of milk protein, in particular α-lactalbumin. Lactose in turn is linked to the water and mineral content of milk by exerting most osmotic pressure, drawing water from the cytoplasm into the Golgi apparatus. Water makes up more than 80% of milk volume.

Lactose is necessary for the promotion of the growth of the micro-organism *L. bifidus,* the presence of which leads to increased acidity of the stool.

Fats

The lipids found in human milk are mainly globules of triglycerides (98–99%) and are easy to digest and absorb.

TABLE 54.2 **Summary: Components of Human Breastmilk and Comparisons with Formula Milk**

Nutrient	Human Milk	Formula Milk	Comment
Carbohydrates	• Rich in lactose • Rich in oligosaccharides, which promote intestinal health	• No lactose in some formulae • Deficient in oligosaccharides	Lactose is an important carbohydrate for brain development.
Protein	• Soft, easily digestible whey • Increased absorption (higher in the milk of mothers who give birth to preterm babies) • Lactoferrin for intestinal health • Lysozyme, rich in brain and body-building protein components • Rich in growth factors • Contains sleep-inducing proteins	• Harder to digest nonhuman whey and casein curds • Not completely absorbed, more waste, harder on kidneys • No or only a trace of lactoferrin • No lysozyme • Deficient or low in some brain- and body-building proteins • Deficient in growth factors • Does not contain as many sleep-inducing proteins	Human infants are *not* allergic to human milk protein. The protein in human milk is ideal for the baby and is very different from formula milk.
Fats and fatty acids	• Rich in brain-building omega 3s, namely docosahexaenoic acid (DHA) and amino acids • Automatically adjusts to infant's needs • Levels decline as baby gets older • Rich in cholesterol • Nearly completely absorbed • Contains fat-digesting enzyme, lipase	• No DHA • Does not adjust to infant's needs • No cholesterol • Not completely absorbed • No lipase	Fat content in breastmilk provides about half of the calories. It is the most important nutrient in breastmilk. Absence of cholesterol/DHA (vital nutrients for growing brains/bodies), may predispose to adult cardiovascular and central nervous system diseases. Formula-fed babies: Unabsorbed fat and waste accounts for unpleasant-smelling stools.
Vitamins and minerals	• Improved absorption (e.g., iron, zinc and calcium) • 50–75% iron is absorbed • Contains more selenium (an antioxidant)	• Not absorbed as well • 5–10% iron is absorbed • Contains less selenium (an antioxidant)	A greater percentage of vitamins and minerals in breastmilk are absorbed, i.e., enjoy a higher bioavailability. Addition of vitamins to formula milk makes digestion more difficult for baby.
Anti-infective factors	*See Table 54.3* • Very rich in living white blood cells (leucocytes) • Rich in immunoglobulins • Contains lactoferrin and bifidus factor	• No live white blood cells – or any other cells • Less immunological benefit • Few immunoglobulins (bovine)	Antibodies made in response to maternal infection are transferred to the baby via breastmilk.
Enzymes and hormones	• Rich in digestive enzymes, such as lipase and amylase • Rich in many hormones, e.g., thyroid, prolactin, oxytocin • Epidermal growth factor and insulin-like growth factor increases maturity of baby's digestive system and reduces susceptibility to infection • Varies with mother's diet	• Processing destroys digestive enzymes • Processing destroys (bovine) hormones • Always tastes the same	Digestive enzymes promote intestinal health. Hormones contribute to the biochemical balance and wellbeing of the baby. Breastmilk shapes the tastes of the child to family foods.

Long-chain fatty acids are transported directly from maternal blood to the breast. Long-chain fatty acids make up most of the fat content of milk (95%).

Arachidonic acid and docosahexaenoic acid (DHA) are two long-chain fatty acids found in human milk that are essential for the development of the brain, nervous system and vascular tissue (Salem & Dael, 2020). The intake of biologically inappropriate fatty acids could have long-term effects on the growth of nervous tissue. The unavailability of some fatty acids with a corresponding alteration in body tissue composition may be a long-term problem for infants fed on artificial milk. In particular, the formation of the myelin sheaths may be affected permanently.

Arachidonic acid and another fatty acid, linoleic acid, are found in high quantities in human milk. These enable prostaglandin synthesis, which matures intestinal cells, aids digestion and adds to the anti-infective protective effect of human milk.

Variations in Fat Content of Milk

Fats are the most variable constituent of human milk, varying in concentration from breast to breast, over time and among individuals. The fat content of the hindmilk is significantly increased, especially in late morning and early afternoon (Ballard & Morrow, 2013; Kent, 2006). The fatty acid content varies according to dietary source, whereas the fat content varies with calorific intake. High quantities of free fatty acids and cholesterol are present in human milk and act as an important energy source for the infant, providing more than 50% of the calorific requirements.

Electrolytes

Lactose secretion is directly involved in the transfer of ions across the acinar cell membrane into the milk. The total content of mineral salts is less than one-third of that present in artificial milk, with only 0.2% of the sodium, potassium and chloride content. The kidney of the neonate does not cope well with an increased sodium load. Despite modification in artificial feeds, there is a risk of hypernatraemia with dehydration in formula-fed infants if the feed is reconstituted with too much milk powder over a period of time. High solute content leads to thirst and crying, which may be interpreted as hunger and offer more milk, which could predispose to long-term obesity. Although rare, severe hypernatraemia may result in irreversible brain damage. There may be a link between high solute loads and a predisposition to hypertension in later life.

Minerals

Calcium, phosphorus and magnesium are present in human milk at higher concentrations than in plasma, which suggests active transportation. Absorption in the gut of the neonate depends on the availability of fats and vitamin D. Calcium is more efficiently absorbed from human milk than from substitutes due to human milk's high calcium:phosphorus ratio.

Trace Elements

Trace elements in breastmilk are essential for growth and development in early life. The levels of iron, copper and zinc are higher in colostrum than in mature milk. Healthy term breastfed infants do not require iron supplements before the age of 6 months. Breastmilk has low levels of iron compared to artificial milk and is more bioavailable because it is bound by lactoferrin, preventing growth of bacteria in the intestine. Artificial milk has significantly more 'free iron', promoting growth of bacteria and the risk of infection. A small amount of zinc is necessary to ensure the infant's health. More zinc is present in artificial milk but is not as readily absorbed as that present in human milk. Other necessary trace elements such as copper, cobalt and selenium are present in optimal quantities. These elements are associated in small amounts with the protein casein, larger amounts with whey proteins and

moderate amounts with fats bound to specific carrier proteins (ligands).

Vitamins

The fat-soluble vitamins A, D, E and K are present in breastmilk. However vitamins D and K are not always at the desired level. Vitamin D is essential for bone development, but levels are dependent upon the mother's exposure to sunlight. Vitamin K is required for blood clotting. The need to give vitamin K to neonates is discussed in Chapter 48. All vitamin B-complex vitamins and vitamin C are also present in breastmilk.

Enzymes

The function of many of the enzymes present in breastmilk is unknown. The enzymes lipase, amylase and lysozyme are important. Lipase, the fat-digesting enzyme, is present in breastmilk in a form which becomes active in the infant's intestine, making fat digestion easier in breastfed infants. Also present is the carbohydrate-digesting enzyme amylase. The presence of amylase may compensate for low salivary and pancreatic amylase activity in neonates. Lysozyme is an important bacteriolytic enzyme that protects against bacteria such as *Escherichia coli* and *Salmonella*.

Hormones

Hormones present in breastmilk include prolactin, oxytocin, prostaglandins, insulin, thyroid-stimulating hormone, thyroxine and growth hormones, specifically epidermal growth factor, which is important for the development of the lining of the gut. Endocrine responses are different in breastfed infants from those who are artificially fed. Growth factor concentration is maximal in the colostrum produced on the first day of life.

Anti-infective Factors

The anti-infective factors present in breastmilk are outlined in Table 54. 3.

The Transmission of Viruses in Milk

In viral diseases, such as cytomegalovirus, rubella and hepatitis B, the virus may be present in breastmilk with no adverse effects on the infant. However human immunodeficiency virus (HIV) is transmitted through breastmilk (vertical transmission). The guiding practice statements of the World Health Organization (WHO) recommend that mothers living with HIV should breastfeed for at least 12 months and up to 2 years or longer (similar to the general population) while being supported for antiretroviral treatment (ART) adherence (WHO, 2016). Although exclusive breastfeeding is recommended, mixed feeding is not a reason to stop breastfeeding in the presence of ART and mothers living with HIV and healthcare workers can be reassured that shorter durations of breastfeeding of less than 12 months are better than never initiating breastfeeding at all.

TABLE 54.3	The Anti-infective Factors in Breastmilk

Factor	Effective
Leucocytes	A high level of leucocytes is present in breastmilk, especially in the first 10 days. These are mainly macrophages and neutrophils, whose purpose is to surround and destroy pathogenic bacteria.
Immunoglobulins	Immunoglobulins IgA, IgG, IgM and IgD are found in breastmilk. However the most important is IgA, which lines the intestinal mucosal surfaces to protect against: • Pathogenic bacteria such as *Escherichia coli, Salmonella* and *Shigella* spp., streptococci and staphylococci. • Pathogenic viruses such as poliovirus and the rotaviruses.
Lysozyme	This an important protein present in breastmilk in high concentrations. It is bacteriolytic and helps break down the cell walls of pathogenic organisms.
Lactoferrin	Lactoferrin, an iron-binding protein found in human milk, increases the absorption of enteric iron. It provides protection in breastfed infants by inhibiting the growth of certain iron-dependent bacteria such as *E. coli* in the gastrointestinal tract.
Bifidus factor	This factor present in human milk encourages the growth of the Gram-positive *Lactobacillus bifidus.* In turn, this discourages the growth of Gram-negative pathogenic organisms.
Human milk oligosaccharides	Although a carbohydrate, these are also potent antimicrobial factors. They act as antiadhesive antimicrobials which prevent viral, bacterial and protozoan pathogens adhering to mucosal surfaces, preventing colonization and subsequent infection. They also prevent and decrease inflammatory responses and support the maturation of the immune system (Quitadamo, Comegna and Cristalli, 2021).

Based on current evidence, mothers with COVID-19 should initiate and continue breastfeeding and should not be separated from their infant.

Antiallergic Properties

The newborn infant has an immature immune system and gut mucosa, and this allows the absorption of large foreign proteins. The IgA and other factors present in breastmilk encourage maturity of the gut mucosa to form a barrier against these large proteins. Oligosaccharides alter gene expression. These factors are different between individuals, and this has led to conflicting evidence in this area. However there is evidence of reduced risk of peanut sensitization in infants of mothers who eat peanuts (Dawod, Marshall & Azad, 2021).

Main Points

- *Embryogenesis* refers to the embryonic development of the organ in utero. *Mammogenesis* refers to the growth and development of the mammary glands during puberty and pregnancy. *Lactogenesis* refers to the initiation and production of milk (three stages).
- Mammary tissue is divided into parenchyma and stroma. The parenchyma (glandular tissue) is the functional component of the breast. The stroma comprises the other supportive tissues, including the skin.
- The glandular tissue contains secretory and ductal tissue within a lobuloalveolar system. Lobes are merged together within a complex network of alveoli, leading to an average of 9 (4–18) milk ducts converging at the nipple.
- Each alveolus contains lactocytes, which are milk-producing cells. Myoepithelial cells surround the alveoli and ducts.
- Developments of the breast in pregnancy include a marked increase in the ductal system and formation of lobes, the synthesis of colostrum, increased vascularity, development of Montgomery's tubercles, pigmentation of the areola and an increase in size.

- Montgomery's tubercles lubricate and protect the areola and nipple.
- The four hormones involved in the initiation and maintenance of lactation are oestrogen, progesterone, prolactin and oxytocin. During pregnancy, progesterone inhibits the effect of prolactin on breast tissue to produce milk. Prolactin is involved in milk production (galactopoiesis), and suckling is the main stimulus for its release.
- Stimulation of the areola and nipple initiates the release of oxytocin. This causes contraction of the myoepithelial cells surrounding the milk-secreting cells and propels milk along the duct. This is known as the *let-down reflex*. The let-down reflex can be also stimulated by sensory factors and inhibited by emotional states. Lactating women require an additional 500 kcal/day approximately.
- Mature milk is highly variable and changes from one feed to another.
- Reflexes in the newborn that influence breastfeeding include rooting, suckling, swallowing and breathing reflexes. Factors interfering with suckling will affect milk production.

- Build-up of FIL in milk inhibits the synthesis of milk. This is a local mechanism and can occur in one or both breasts.
- Some proteins in milk form soft curds in the stomach, providing a continuous flow of nutrients to the infant. Fats act as an important energy source for the infant, providing more than 50% of the calorific requirements. The fat-soluble vitamins A, D, E and K are present in breastmilk in addition to vitamin B complex and vitamin C.
- Immunity factors present in breastmilk include a high level of leucocytes and IgA. Other anti-infective agents include lysozyme, lactoferrin and the bifidus factor.
- Water makes up over 80% of the milk volume; therefore breastfed infants do not need supplementary drinks.
- Although HIV is transmitted through breastmilk, the WHO recommends that mothers living with HIV should breastfeed for at least 12 months and up to 2 years or longer while being supported for ART adherence.
- Based on current evidence, mothers with COVID-19 should initiate and continue breastfeeding and should not be separated from their infant.

References

Bazira, P.J., Ellis, H., Mahadevan, V., 2022. Anatomy and physiology of the breast. Surgery 40 (2), 79–83.

Ballard, O., Morrow, A., 2013. Human milk composition: nutrients and bioactive factors. Pediatr. Clin. North Am. 60 (1), 49–74.

Bergman, N.J., Ludwig, R.J., Westrup, B., Welch, M.G., 2019. Nurturescience versus neuroscience: a case for rethinking mother-infant behaviours and relationship. Birth Defects Research 111 (15), 1–18.

Blackburn, S.T., 2018. Maternal, Fetal and Neonatal Physiology: A Clinical Perspective, fifth ed. Elsevier, St. Louis.

Cregan, M., Mitoulas, L., Hartmann, P., 2002. Milk prolactin, feed volume and duration between feeds in women breastfeeding their full-term infants over a 24h period. Exp. Physiol. 87 (2), 207–214.

Dawod, B., Marshall, J., Azad, M., 2021. Breastfeeding and the developmental origins of mucosal immunity: how human milk shapes the innate adaptive mucosal immune systems. Gastroenterology 37 (6), 547–556.

Freeman, M.E., Kanyicska, B., Lerant, A., Nagy, G., 2000. Prolactin: structure, function and regulation of secretion. Physiol Rev 80 (4), 1523–1631.

Garrod, D., Chidgey, M., 2008. Desmosome structure, composition and function. Biochemica et Biophysica Acta 1778 (3), 572–587.

Geddes, D.T., Gridneva, Z., Perrella, S.L., Mitoulas, L.R., Kent, J.C., Stinson, L.F., et al., 2021. 25 years of research in human lactation: from discovery to translation. Nutrients 8 (12), 3071.

Kent, J.C., Mitoulas, L.R., Cregan, M.D., Ramsay, D.T., Doherty, D.A., Hartmann, P.E., 2006. Volume and frequency of breastfeeding and fat content of breastmilk throughout the day. Pediatrics 117 (3), 387–395.

Kent, J., Gardner, H., Geddes, D., 2016. Breastmilk production in the first 4 weeks after birth of term infants. Nutrients 8 (12), 756.

Marangoni, F., Cetin, I., Verduci, E., Canzone, G., Giovannini, M., Scollo, P., et al., 2016. Maternal diet and nutrient requirements in pregnancy and breastfeeding. An Italian consensus document. Nutrients 8 (10), 629.

Pollard, M., 2023. Evidence-Based Care for Breastfeeding Mothers: A Resource for Midwives and Allied Healthcare Professionals, third ed. Routledge, London (in press).

Quitadamo, P.A., Comegna, L., Cristalli, P., 2021. Anti-infective, anti-inflammatory, and immunomodulatory properties of breast milk factors for the protection of infants in the pandemic from COVID-19. Front. Public Health 8,589736.

Ramsay, D.T., Kent, J.C., Hartmann, R.A., Hartmann, P.E., 2005. Anatomy of the lactating human breast redefined with ultrasound imaging. J. Anat. 206 (6), 525–534.

Rassie, K.L., Giri, R., Melder, A., Joham, A., Mousa, A., Teede, H.J., 2022. Lactogenic hormones in relation to maternal metabolic health in pregnancy and postpartum: protocol for a systematic review. BMJ Open 12 (2):e055257.

Salem, N., van Dael, P., 2020. Arachidonic acid in human milk. Nutrients 12 (3), 626.

Smeele, H.P., Bijkerk, E., van Kuijk, S.M.J., Lataster, A., van der Hulst, R.R.W.J., Tuinder, S.M.H., 2022. Innervation of the female breast and nipple: a systematic review and meta-analysis of anatomical dissection studies. Plast. Reconstr. Surg. 150 (2), 243–255.

Uvnäs-Moberg, K., Prime, D., 2013. Oxytocin effects in mothers and infants during breastfeeding. Infant 9 (6), 201–206.

Uvnäs Moberg, K., Ekström-Bergström, A., Buckley, S., Massarotti, C., Pajalic, Z., Luegmair, K., et al., 2020. Maternal plasma levels of oxytocin during breastfeeding: a systematic review and meta-analysis of anatomical dissection studies. PLoS One 15 (8),e0235806.

van Veldhuizen-Staas, C., 2007. Overabundant milk supply: an alternative way to intervene by full drainage and block feeding. Int. Breastfeed. J. 2, 11.

World Health Organization (WHO), 2016. Guideline Updates on HIV and Breastfeeding: The Duration of Breastfeeding and Support from Health Services to Improve Feeding Practices Among Mothers Living with HIV. Available at: https://apps.who.int/iris/bitstream/handle/10665/246260/9789241549707-eng.pdf.

Widström, A.M., Lilja, G., Aaltomaa-Michalias, P., Dahllöf, A., Lintula, M., Nissen, E., 2011. Newborn behaviour to locate the breast when skin-to-skin: a possible method for enabling early self-regulation. Acta Paediatr. 100 (1), 79–85.

Wilde, C.J., Addey, C.V., Boddy, L.M., Peaker, M., 1995. Autocrine regulation of milk secretion by a protein in milk. Biochem. J. 305 (Pt 1), 51–58.

Zandro, V., 2018. Breast crawl: the attractive warmth of the mammary areola. Acta Paediatr. 107 (10), 1673–1674.

Annotated recommended reading

Lawrence, R.A., Lawrence, R.M., 2021. Breastfeeding: A Guide for the Medical Profession, ninth ed. Elsevier, Philadelphia.

This is a very good reference book for health professionals involved with breastfeeding issues. It provides in-depth information, well supported with evidence in the literature and is ideal as a reference book.

Pollard, M., 2023. Evidence-based Care for Breastfeeding Mothers: A Resource for Midwives and Allied Healthcare Professionals, third ed. Routledge, London (in press).

This book is designed for both undergraduate students and practitioners undertaking continuing professional development. Each chapter begins with specific learning outcomes linked to the UNICEF Baby Friendly outcomes.

Ramsay, D.T., Kent, J.C., Hartmann, R.A., Hartmann, P.E., 2005. Anatomy of the lactating human breast redefined with ultrasound imaging. J. Anat. 206 (6), 525–534.

This journal article details the original findings of a research study of the structure of the breasts that changed practice.

Watson Genna, C., 2022. Supporting Sucking Skills in Breastfeeding Infants, fourth ed. Jones and Bartlett Publishers, Burlington.

This book provides up-to-date evidence for health professionals supporting mothers and infants. It suggests clinical strategies and includes photographs to make recommendations easier to understand.

Useful Website:

http://www.unicef.org.uk/babyfriendly/.

This site provides updates on research findings and other interesting facts about breastfeeding, breastmilk and information available for health professionals and parents.

55

Breastfeeding Practice and Problems

ELIZABETH SMITH AND JEAN RANKIN

CHAPTER CONTENTS

This chapter provides information to enable students and midwives to share their knowledge of breastfeeding with mothers. This will help mothers develop and apply the practical skills necessary to successfully establish breastfeeding.

Introduction

Breastmilk contains all the essential nutrients to help babies to grow and develop. In addition, it also protects against infection and encourages development of a close and loving relationship between mother and child. Breastfeeding is an important public health intervention as it impacts on health inequalities through building on the potential of every child, optimizing physical, mental and social health. For these reasons, there are global efforts towards promoting, supporting and protecting breastfeeding and this is recognized in the United Nations Convention on the Rights of the Child (UNICEF, 2023).

Learning about breastfeeding is part of a lifelong process that begins at birth. Some of this is instinctive but a lot is social learning and involves seeing breastfeeding as being a normal and welcome sight, involving shared experiences within the family or community. However beliefs and attitudes about breastfeeding are very much dependent and influenced by culture, folklore and social context. For example, colostrum is accepted and encouraged as the first food for the baby in many cultures, whereas other cultures believe colostrum to be 'old' milk and unfit for the newborn.

Most women are physiologically capable of breastfeeding, and when this is not possible, commercial formula milk is available for the baby. Formula contains the nutrients for babies to grow but has none of the other benefits (see Chapter 54) and special measures are needed when making up feeds and sterilizing due to the inherent risks. Breastfeeding is seen as both an art and a science. The art of breastfeeding is a specialized aspect of the science of lactation and is at risk of being lost to future generations because mothers in developed countries may choose to formula-feed, and lay breastfeeding knowledge and skills are lost (Bergman, 2016). This is concerning and makes it even more necessary to promote, support and protect breastfeeding.

Although breastfeeding is partly instinctive behaviour, potential challenges when establishing breastfeeding mean that many mothers will need support to overcome these if they are to meet their breastfeeding goals. Breastfeeding is in part a learned behaviour and it is vital that midwives and other health professionals providing care and support have the necessary knowledge and skills to share with mothers.

Benefits of Breastfeeding

The benefits of breastfeeding for babies and mothers and society are well established. Evidence is continually emerging, and it is important that the strength of any research is critically analysed before it is accepted into practice (see Box 55.1). Refer to literature on the UNICEF Baby Friendly website (UNICEF Baby Friendly Initiative [BFI], 2022a; 2022b; 2022c).

Breastfeeding: the Climate—Smart Infant Feeding Choice

Breastfeeding is considered the most environmentally sustainable form of infant feeding. Despite this, it is largely absent from the global conversation on net-zero emissions and the circular economy, as well as climate and health policy generally. More discussion is needed to highlight how developing breastfeeding-friendly communities and services can help to protect both public health and the health of our planet. Midwives have an important role in sharing

• BOX 55.1   Overview from *The Lancet*
Breastfeeding Series

Victora et al. (2016) published findings from the largest and most detailed analysis to quantify levels, trends and benefits of breastfeeding around the world. The authors highlighted that while breastfeeding is one of the most effective preventive health measures for children, mothers and public health, there has been little recognition of this important issue. Increasing breastfeeding to near-universal levels for infants and young children has been estimated to save over 800,000 children's lives a year worldwide (equivalent to 13% of all deaths in children under two) and prevent an extra 20,000 deaths from breast cancer every year. It is often suggested that the benefits of breastfeeding are for poorer countries, but Victora et al. (2016) stated that *"our work for this series clearly shows that breastfeeding saves lives and money in all countries, rich and poor alike. Therefore, the importance of tackling the issue globally is greater than ever."*

The research shows that:
- In high-income countries, breastfeeding reduces the risk of sudden infant deaths by more than a third.
- In low- and middle-income countries, about half of all diarrhoea episodes and a third of respiratory infections could be avoided by breastfeeding.

Breastfeeding also increases intelligence and protects against obesity and diabetes in later life.

For mothers, longer duration breastfeeding reduces the risks of breast and ovarian cancer.

The authors suggest that political commitment and financial investment is needed to protect, promote and support breastfeeding at all levels—family, community, workplace and government.

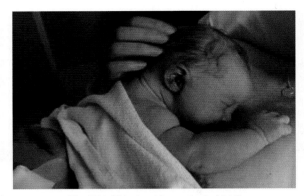

• **Fig. 55.1** Skin-to-skin contact at birth.

information on impact of breast and formula feeding on the environment. Nurses Climate Challenge (NCC) Europe provides a range of useful resources (NCC Europe, 2022a).

Breastfeeding Practices

In Western countries, many young women have had no direct experience of caring for a baby and live in a community where formula feeding is deeply embedded and breastfeeding is unseen. A first-time mother is faced with the need to rapidly acquire these skills of parenting and breastfeeding without the benefit of prior experience, and with a family and social circle who may have no breastfeeding knowledge and skills to share with her. Midwives must therefore take on this role as well as professional support. This requires that they are knowledgeable about the physiology of lactation and can apply this to practice; sharing this information with mothers and providing emotional support if they are to help mothers to continue breastfeeding. The mother must be enabled to develop self-efficacy and confidence that she has the necessary skills to feed her baby.

As practice has developed, several common breastfeeding practices have been shown to be unhelpful or even detrimental to breastfeeding success. It is important to ensure practices are evidence-based and up to date.

Antenatal Preparation

The decision to breastfeed by women in this society is often made before pregnancy or very early in pregnancy, whereas women tend to make the decision to formula-feed later in pregnancy. It is well established that the decision is influenced by culture, education and socioeconomic background. A couple's prenatal decision-making process is also important, although evidence suggests that the final decision most often lies with the mother (Henshaw et al., 2021).

It is crucial that midwives adopt a mother-centred, sensitive, nonjudgmental approach with women to help them make their own, and crucially fully informed, decision about infant feeding, as this can have an impact on the future relationships. The UNICEF Baby Friendly Initiative (BFI) emphasizes the importance of building relationships acknowledging that 'communication is at the heart of effective care and good communication skills are essential for maintaining relationships built on trust' (unicef.org.uk/babyfriendly/).

It is important to have meaningful conversations with parents to encourage them to connect with their baby, discuss the value of skin-to-skin contact and how to respond to the baby's needs with responsive feeding (UNICEF BFI, 2022a; 2022b; 2022c). The importance of loving relationships on brain development should also be discussed, as well as the value of breastfeeding and how to get breastfeeding off to a good start.

The First Feed

All mothers should have the opportunity to have unhurried skin-to-skin contact with their babies as soon as possible after birth. Immediate skin-to-skin contact helps regulate newborns' breathing and body temperature and exposes them to beneficial bacteria from their mother's skin (Fig. 55.1). These good bacteria protect babies from infectious diseases and help build their immune system. This experience is also important for preterm babies as it leads to improvements in cardiorespiratory stabilization (Linnér et al., 2022).

Skin-to-skin contact immediately after birth until the end of the first breastfeeding has many other benefits. It has been shown to increase the chances that babies are breastfed, to extend the length of breastfeeding and to improve rates of exclusive breastfeeding. Immediate skin-to-skin contact is important for babies who are delivered by caesarean section,

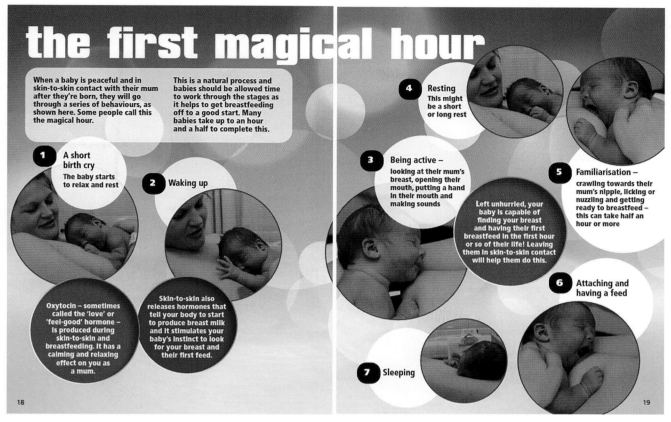

• **Fig. 55.2** Magical hour.

with research evidencing that it results in higher breastfeeding rates, improved bonding and reduced incidence of anxiety and depression for mothers (Sheedy, Stulz & Stevens, 2022).

When a mother holds her baby in skin-to-skin contact after birth, this initiates strong instinctive behaviours for both mother and baby. The increased mothering hormones mean that a mother will instinctually begin to touch, stroke, smell and gaze at her baby for long periods.

Babies' instincts after birth will result in an instinctive nine-stage process, which if left uninterrupted will result in them having a first breastfeed. This is often called the '*Magical Hour*'. Fig. 55.2 demonstrates these stages (Public Health Scotland, 2023). If the mother has taken drugs during labour, the baby may be a little sleepy and take a little longer, but most babies can be breastfeeding within 90 min. Babies will familiarize themselves with their mother's breasts and can self-attach. This first feed sets a pattern for feeding which babies will follow in subsequent feeds and can lead to fewer breastfeeding challenges (Table 55.1).

Communicating with Mothers

The role of health practitioners involved with mothers is to share information with mothers to allow them to come to an informed decision. The BFI believes it is important to communicate well and give key tips for achieving this:

- Explain the reasons for the information that is being given. If the mother understands why her baby is held nose-to-nipple, for example, she is more likely to remember and use the information.
- Use simple language and focus on key messages.
- Models, leaflets and other visual aids can support learning. They contribute to the mother's understanding and act as an aide memoire for the mother and those providing support.
- Use of visual resources such as links to films or other social media sites.

Positioning and Attachment

Positioning refers to how the mother holds her baby to help the baby attach effectively to the breast. There is a range of suitable positions the mother can choose to adopt to breastfeed her baby (unicef.org.uk/babyfriendly; UNICEF 2013). Irrespective of the position adopted, the mother needs to ensure the baby's body is turned towards her body so the angle is the same for both the baby approaching the breast and the breast coming towards the baby. Fig. 55.3 shows two common breastfeeding positions.

Attachment refers to how the baby takes the breast into their mouth to enable them to feed effectively; this is the most important aspect of breastfeeding (see Clinical Application 55.1). Therefore it is essential for the baby to be appropriately positioned to promote correct attachment of the baby to the

TABLE 55.1	Instinctive Stages of Initiating Breastfeeding	
Stage	**Description**	
Distinctive birth cry	Baby's lungs expand immediately after birth.	
Relaxation	Baby is relaxed. Skin-to-skin contact should be promoted with the mother. Baby should be covered with a warm, dry towel or blanket.	
Awakening	Baby begins to open their eyes and responds to the mother's voice. Initially moving their head and shoulders, the baby will begin to show some movements of the mouth.	
Activity	Baby begins to exhibit mouthing and sucking movements and the rooting reflex is seen. This stage usually begins soon after birth.	
Rest	Baby may have both periods of rest and activity.	
Crawling	Baby will begin to make crawling movement towards the breast.	
Familiarization	Baby begins to nuzzle, massage and lick the nipple.	
Sucking	Baby self–attaches to the breast and the first breastfeed begins. For a term baby, this is normally around an hour after birth if allowed to move through the instinctive stages.	
Sleeping	Baby falls asleep. The mother may also feel sleepy and fall asleep.	

(UNICEF BFI, 2022a; 2022b; 2022c).

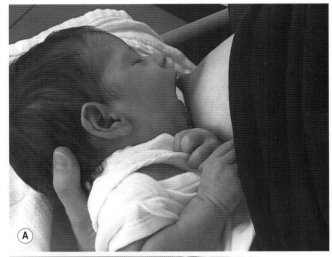

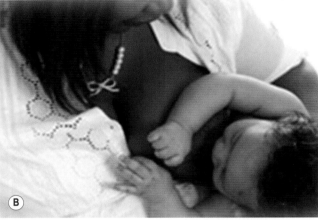

• **Fig. 55.3** Breastfeeding positions. A. Cradle hold. B. Underarm hold.

breast (Fig. 55.4). Ineffective attachment causes problems for both mother and baby. Fig. 55.5 shows effective and ineffective attachment to the breast. Appropriate information should be shared with the mother to help her attach her baby effectively (Box 55.2). This information will prevent any problems arising.

Positioning refers to how the mother holds her baby to help the baby attach effectively to the breast. There is a range of suitable positions the mother can choose to adopt to breastfeed her baby (unicef.org.uk/babyfriendly; UNICEF 2013). Irrespective of the position adopted, the mother needs to ensure the baby's body is turned towards her body so the angle is the same for both the baby approaching the breast and the breast coming towards the baby. Fig. 55.3 shows two common breastfeeding positions.

Attachment refers to how the baby takes the breast into their mouth to enable them to feed effectively; this is the most important aspect of breastfeeding (see Clinical Application 55.1). Therefore, it is essential for the baby to be appropriately positioned to promote correct attachment of the baby to the breast (Fig. 55.4). Ineffective attachment causes problems for both mother and baby. Fig. 55.5 shows effective and ineffective

attachment to the breast. Appropriate information should be shared with the mother to help her attach her baby effectively (Box 55.2). This information will prevent any problems arising.

Effective Milk Transfer

To maintain **milk production** (see Chapter 54), it is essential that there is effective removal of breast milk. The BFI recommends regular feeding assessments be carried out in the first week after birth and any time the mother is experiencing challenges with feeding.

Observation of a full feed is a crucial part of this assessment to ascertain signs of effective feeding.

Additional assessment includes:
- Assess breast for problems such as discomfort, nipple trauma or engorgement.
- Observe baby's appearance, colour, behaviour and tone.
- Number of feeds: can change day to day but new babies should be having 8–10 feeds in 24 hours.
- Length of feeds: Volume of milk transfer cannot be assessed by the amount of time spent feeding as this varies between individuals, but feeds routinely lasting less than 5 min or more than 40 min should lead to full feeding assessment and monitoring.

Positioning and Attachment (Figs. 55.4 & 55.5)

Effective Positioning

The acronym CHINS is a common way of remembering the key principles that enable the baby to access the breast using instinctive behaviour:

Close: baby is close to the mother.

Head free: the baby can tilt its head back to allow the chin to lead when attaching to the breast.

In line: the baby's head and neck are in alignment to avoid twisting.

Nose to nipple: will encourage rooting and the tilting of the head backwards to scoop the breast in the mouth.

Sustainable: make sure the mother is comfortable to sustain the position.

Key signs of good attachment:

- Feeding is pain-free.
- The baby's chin indents the breast.
- The baby's mouth is wide open.
- The cheeks are full and rounded.
- There is more areola visible above the top lip.
- There is rhythmic sucking and swallowing can be heard.

Impact of ineffective attachment:

Mother:
- Sore nipples.
- Engorgement.
- Mastitis.
- Decreased milk production.
- Loss of confidence.

Baby:
- Frequent feeding.
- Frustration.
- Poor weight gain.
- Jaundice.
- Hypernatraemia.

(UNICEF BFI, 2022a; 2022b; 2022c)

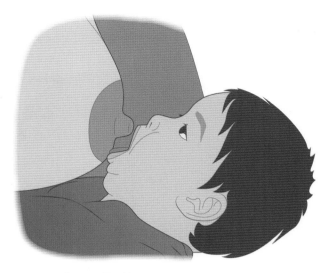

• **Fig. 55.4** Position of baby – pre-attachment.

- The sucking pattern: feeding begins with short rapid sucks to initiate milk flow. This changes for a period of active feeding with long, slow, rhythmical sucking and swallowing with pauses (1–2 sucks per swallow). The feed ends with flutter sucking and occasional swallowing as the baby reaches the fat-rich milk towards the end of the feed. After feeding, the baby should appear relaxed and often sleepy.
- Assessing urine and stool: this is a key indicator of effective feeding. If a baby does not pass a minimum of two soft stools per day, this suggests inadequate milk intake. Normally babies will pass at least two stools per day until 4–6 weeks (Table 55.2).
- Ask the mother about use of soothers or nipple shields or any supplementary feeds being given as they can interfere with responsive breastfeeding.
- Weight gain is a late indicator of effective feeding and is not a substitute for a quality breastfeeding assessment.

Responsive Feeding

Some mothers become anxious about lack of routines for breastfeeding; setting routines is common in formula-feeding cultures, and this can have a negative impact on breastfeeding (Brown & Arnott, 2014; Ventura, 2017). Responsive feeding is the best way to describe the unique relationship between mothers and babies responding to each other's needs and cues. Mothers should be assured that there is no need to know how much milk has been taken (one reason for wishing to formula-feed) and that sometimes babies, like adults, may just want a drink or snack rather than a full feed. Breastfeeding babies may also simply want the comfort of a cuddle and the interaction breastfeeding provides. A strong message to mothers should be that babies cannot be spoiled or overfed by frequent breastfeeds.

The baby will be getting sufficient nourishment if content after feeding and settling and sleeping well between feeds. Mothers need to understand that breastmilk is not designed to last for four full hours between each feed and that newborns do not differentiate night from day. At first, the mother may experience tiredness due to frequent feeding, but can be reassured this will settle down when breastfeeding is fully established.

Breastfeeding Challenges for Mother and Baby

Regular infant feeding surveys are conducted with the most common reasons for mothers stopping breastfeeding in the first 2 weeks cited as being:

- Breast refusal.
- Nipple trauma.
- Perception of insufficient milk supply.

Mothers tend to report they could have continued to breastfeed for longer if they had more support and guidance

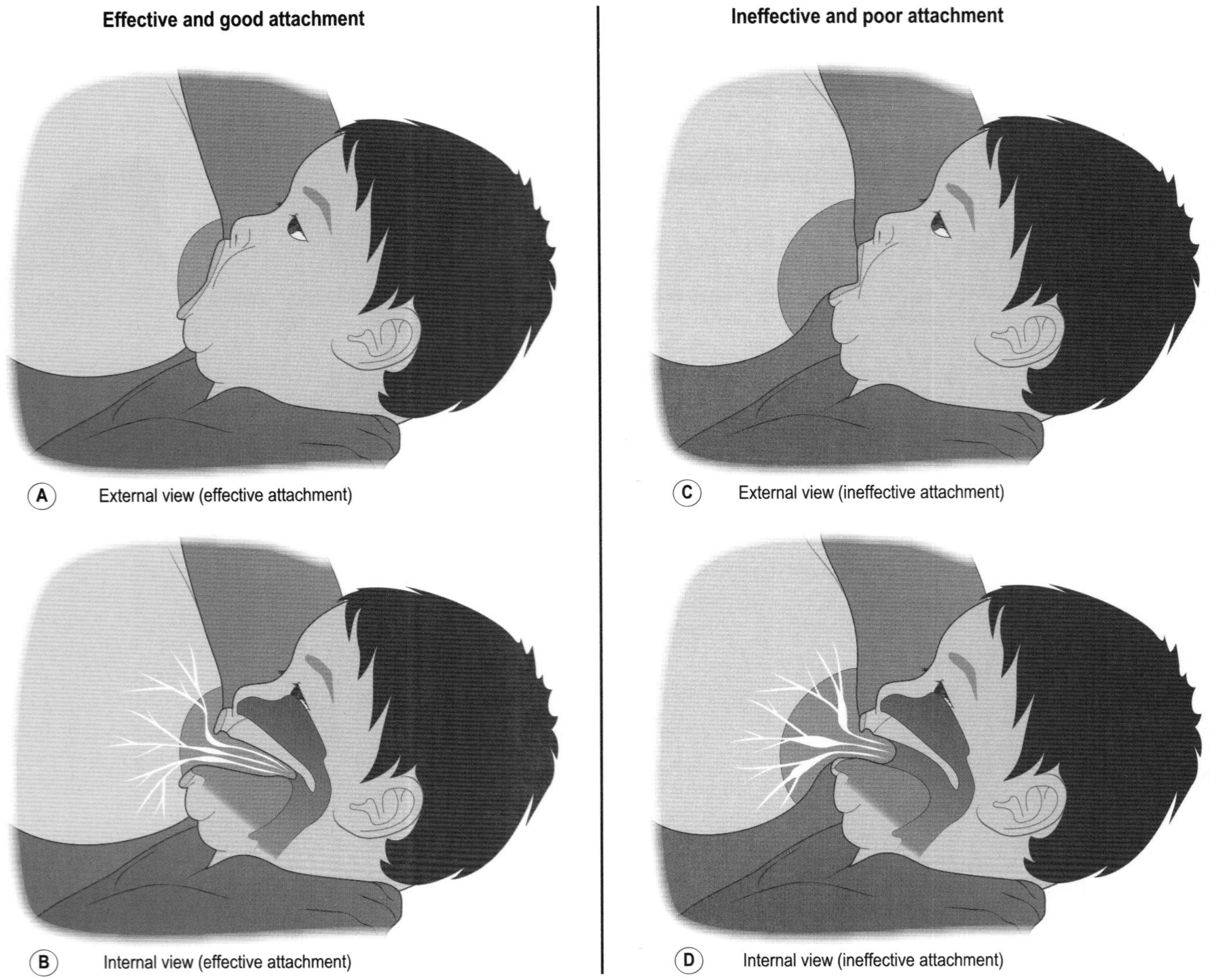

Effective and good attachment

Ineffective and poor attachment

(A) External view (effective attachment)

(C) External view (ineffective attachment)

(B) Internal view (effective attachment)

(D) Internal view (ineffective attachment)

• **Fig. 55.5** Effective and ineffective attachment. **(A and B) Effective and good attachment, external and internal views. (C and D) Ineffective and poor attachment, external and internal views.**

from healthcare professionals, were able to achieve better attachment to the breast or had pain-free breastfeeding.

Breast Refusal

In the first few days, babies may be slow to feed due to use of narcotics in labour, trauma, jaundice or separation. The mother may feel that the baby is refusing feeding, and this can be distressing. The baby may physically present with an arching back and stiffening when approaching the breast, crying and pushing away from the breast. Hands-off breastfeeding support is essential; hands-on support, where the helper takes hold of the baby's head and pushes it towards the nipple, is not only unhelpful and unpleasant for the mother, but can also lead to breast refusal from the baby and should never be practiced.

Nipple Trauma

Breastfeeding should be comfortable and pain-free. Some mothers may feel the nipples tender for the first few days with some discomfort on attachment, but this should quickly

resolve. The most common cause of nipple trauma is poor attachment to the breast, but thrush and other problems should be considered. Nipple pain can cause anxiety and stress, inhibit the let-down reflex and reduce the number of times the breast is offered, resulting in ineffective milk removal and a build-up of **feedback inhibitor of lactation** (FIL), resulting in reduced milk supply (Lawrence & Lawrence, 2021).

Treatment must address the cause of the problem first, with the most common being incorrect position and attachment. If the nipple is too painful for the mother to continue feeding, she can rest the affected breast, perform hand expression and offer the other breast. Moist wound healing, with use of an appropriate barrier cream, is advised. If there is a bacterial infection, this inhibits healing and may need treatment with antibiotics. Thrush infection will need treatment with an antifungal medication.

Perceived Insufficient Milk

A common reason for mothers introducing complementary feeding and stopping breastfeeding is the perception that they do not have enough milk, often due to a lack of confidence and a cultural need to measure the volume of milk.

Poor lactation can be categorized as follows:

- Primary inability to produce breastmilk. This may be due to a hormonal imbalance, such as hypothyroidism or diabetes; birth complications, such as retained placenta, preterm birth or caesarean section; or other factors such as postpartum haemorrhage (leading to Sheehan's syndrome, breast trauma and polycystic ovaries).
- Secondary due to poor techniques or management of problems such as lack of skin-to-skin contact, infrequent feeds, poor attachment, supplementary feeds and use of teats and pacifiers.
- Refer to the section on effective milk transfer.

The best means of preventing insufficient milk from occurring is recognizing the problem early by observing breastfeeds and taking a lactation history. The midwife should promote unrestricted feeding by encouraging skin-to-skin contact, a well-positioned baby and frequent and

---

BOX 55.2 Supporting the Mother with Effective Breastfeeding

The following information should be shared with new mothers:

- Skin-to-skin contact is not just for the period after birth; continued skin-to-skin contact promotes both instinctual feeding and mothering behaviours.
- The baby must be well positioned to feed effectively.
- Mother and baby should be calm – observe for baby's early feeding cues (Fig. 55.6) and act on these – avoid trying to feed a crying baby.
- Eliciting the rooting reflex from the baby and waiting until the baby's mouth is wide open.
- How to recognize when the baby is properly attached.
- How the mother can recognize signs of effective feeding. Sometimes there is a reluctance from the baby to feed. In these instances:
- If necessary, hand express colostrum/milk and cup feed or drip into the mouth. This stimulates her milk supply until the baby is ready for breastfeeding.
- Observe the baby for signs of illness.

Regular feeding in the early days is important, as colostrum has a purgative effect, clearing the bowel of meconium and reducing the possibility of jaundice.

TABLE 55.2 Assessing Urine and Stool

Day	Urine	Stool
1–2	2 or more wet nappies	1 (green/black and sticky meconium)
3–4	3 or more wet nappies (heavier)	3 or more (changing stool)
4–6	5 or more wet nappies (heavy)	2 or more soft yellow stools
4–6 weeks	6 or more wet nappies (heavy)	Individual pattern develops

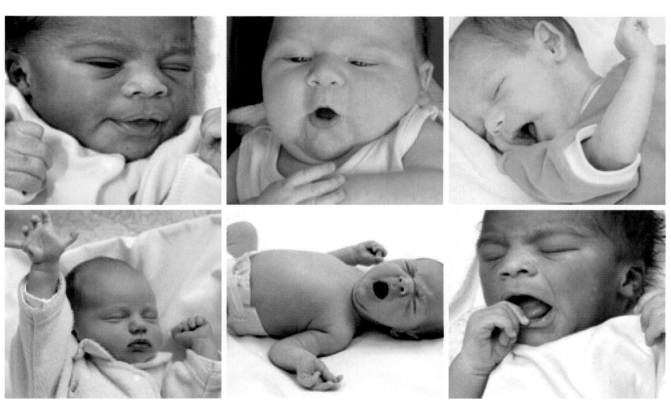

• **Fig. 55.6** Early and mid-feeding cues.

effective removal of breastmilk, while giving good practical and emotional support to the mother.

The following common situations and conditions can also cause difficulties with breastfeeding (see Table 55.3):

- Full and engorged breasts.
- Blocked ducts and mastitis.
- Breast abscess.
- Previous breast surgery.

Table 55.4 identifies problems with the baby (**cleft lip and palate, tongue-tie** and **prematurity**) and the support required for feeding. Drugs and substances in breastmilk with required feeding support are outlined in Table 55.5.

Suppression of Lactation

The suppression of lactation is necessary in a variety of situations such as when women choose not to breastfeed, when there are absolute contraindications to breastfeeding or after the loss of a baby. Because breastmilk is supplied on demand, there is no need for treatment, as lactation will cease spontaneously. Women are advised to wear a well-supporting bra, and although there may be discomfort for a day or two, it is rare to find extreme discomfort with engorgement.

TABLE 55.3   Common Breastfeeding Challenges

Full breasts and engorgement	Normal fullness of the breasts will occur a few days after delivery when the mother's milk is 'coming in'. The breasts may feel heavy and uncomfortable. The milk will be flowing well and can often be seen dripping from the breasts. The mother should be encouraged to breastfeed her baby frequently to remove the milk. The breasts will feel softer and more comfortable after the feed, and the breasts will adapt to suit the baby's needs within a few days. Importantly, the mother will feel well.
	Engorgement is not normal and means that the breasts are overfull, partly with milk and partly with increased tissue fluid and blood. The breasts appear flushed, shiny and hard. The mother may have a slight rise in pulse and temperature. The mother will report feeling unwell.
	Management of engorgement Engorgement will compress the arterial blood supply and the milk ducts, and build-up of FIL will further decrease milk production. Allowing the baby unrestricted access to the breast while properly positioned is the most effective method of treating and preventing breast engorgement. The removal of milk is essential to prevent further complications. Mothers should be encouraged to empty the breasts regularly, preferably by increasing the number of feeds or by hand expressing if the baby is unable to attach.
Mastitis	Mastitis is an area of inflammation that affects part of the breast, and usually one breast. The skin may appear red, although this may be more difficult to see on darker skin. Mastitis may follow a blocked duct and milk leaks into surrounding tissue, resulting in inflammation. Mastitis can be infective or noninfective; damage to the nipple may suggest infection has tracked into the breast, but both conditions can cause the same severe symptoms. Noninfective mastitis occurs in a substantial proportion of women. It is the result of poor drainage of the breast and this can be a result of ineffective feeding, pressure on the breast tissue from clothes or the mother holding her breast tightly.
	Signs and symptoms These are rarely seen before the eighth postpartum day. The affected wedge-shaped segment of breast tissue is swollen and painful, and the overlying skin is reddened. The woman complains of throbbing pain and tenderness, and it is common for her to develop a raised temperature and pulse rate. Aching flu-like symptoms are often accompanied by shivering attacks and rigour.
	Management of mastitis Effective breast drainage and includes assessment of positioning and attachment, and optimizing these when required. Mothers should be supported to continue breastfeeding with unlimited feeds and advising to feed from the affected side first, as milk stasis is an ideal culture for micro-organisms. Changing the position for feeding, with the baby's chin against the affected part of the breast, assists drainage. If unable to feed, she should be encouraged to express regularly. The mother should take anti-inflammatory medication unless contraindicated and pain relief if appropriate. Mothers should be advised to rest and increase fluid intake. Antibiotics may be commenced if there is no change in the mother's condition after a few hours of effective milk drainage and comfort measures. It is important to acknowledge that mastitis can lead to breast abscess and in some cases sepsis can develop. (Breastfeeding Network, 2016; NICE 2023).

TABLE 55.3 Common Breastfeeding Challenges—cont'd

Breast abscess	• Breast abscesses develop when a collection of pus forms in part of the breast as a result of untreated infection. • Diagnosis is by ultrasound examination and needle aspiration or surgical drainage may be required, as well as commencement of antibiotic therapy. • The baby will not be affected by the abscess and, if possible, should continue to feed from the breast. However if the abscess is too painful or the mother is unwilling to feed, she should be advised to express her milk until the incision has healed. (Breastfeeding Network, 2016; NICE, 2023).
Feeding after breast surgery	It is not uncommon for women to have undergone breast surgery before pregnancy and lactation. Surgery may be performed for pathological conditions and include biopsy and conservative surgery for cancer or for cosmetic reasons. The latter operations include the insertion of silicone breast implants and reduction mammoplasty. Several factors will influence the woman's ability to lactate after surgery, but success or failure will really depend on the degree to which surgery affected the internal structures involved in lactation.

UNICEF provides a range of useful leaflets for parents on breastfeeding challenges (UNICEF BFI, 2022c).

TABLE 55.4 Problems Arising with the Baby

Cleft lip and palate	Structural abnormalities of the lip and palate may make a mother feel she cannot breastfeed. In practice, there may be no difficulties if the cleft is only in the lip, especially if the cleft is small or narrow. Support may be needed with trying different positions and the cleft nurse specialist or infant feeding team should offer support. The cleft nurse specialist or infant feeding team should assess and develop a care plan together with the mother. This may include expressing breastmilk; a breast pump may be provided and responsive bottle feeding should be discussed. There are also alternative feeding methods that may be useful, including cup and spoon feeding and use of a supplemental nursing system. Some mothers have expressed their breastmilk until repair and then achieved successful breastfeeding.
Tongue-tie	Tongue-tie, or ankyloglossia, is when the frenulum, which holds the tongue to the floor of the mouth, is shorter than normal. This can lead to difficulties with attachment and lead to painful or damaged nipples and ineffective feeding. Some babies have no feeding difficulties and can attach and feel without any issues and so not every baby will need to have treatment. Some babies will exhibit feeding problems and this requires examination and a feeding assessment. If treatment is needed, a frenotomy is performed by a specialist practitioner and this usually does not require anaesthetic. The tongue-tie is snipped with sterile scissors and the mother asked to breastfeed as this can help to stop any bleeding, though this should be minimal. The baby should be reviewed to assess if the treatment has resulted in improvements with feeding.
Prematurity	Babies born preterm (<37 weeks) should be considered in the 'at risk' category for feeding and support; close monitoring will be required. For preterm babies, feeding can be challenging until the sucking and swallowing reflexes have fully developed. If the baby tires quickly at the breast, tube feeding with expressed milk may be needed. If volumes of expressed milk are low, donor breastmilk may be given with parental consent. Preterm babies require a good energy source, both for growth and development and to maintain an adequate body temperature. Unrestricted kangaroo care is recommended to regulate temperature, breathing, heart rate and access to the breast to facilitate instinctive behaviour (Moore et al., 2016).

The International Code of Marketing of Breast Milk Substitutes

The International Code of Marketing of Breast Milk Substitutes (World Health Organization, 1981) aims to protect and promote breastfeeding, to provide safe and adequate nutrition for infants, to ensure the correct use of breastmilk substitutes and to control marketing of formula milk products. The recommendations for manufacturers of infant formulae include:

TABLE 55.5	**Drugs and Substances in Breastmilk**
Medications	All women of childbearing age should be reminded that prescription and over-the-counter drugs may have adverse effects on the fetus or baby. Medical advice should always be taken in pregnancy or when breastfeeding. However any prescription medication should not be discontinued without consulting the prescriber. Many factors can influence the potential effects of the drug on the baby, such as the nature, characteristics and the route of administration. Individual assessment is needed. For health professionals working with pregnant or new mothers, a number of sources such as BNF/NICE (2023) guidelines should be consulted for guidance in the use of individual drugs.
Smoking	Smoking while breastfeeding is not recommended, but the benefits of breastmilk outweigh the risks from smoking. Mothers who smoke should be offered smoking cessation advice. Smoking during lactation results in a reduced milk supply and shorter duration of breastfeeding, and the baby may have colic. Nicotine replacement therapy reduces the amount of nicotine in the breastmilk. Mothers who choose to continue to smoke should be advised not to smoke before a feed, as levels of nicotine take approximately 95 min to clear, with levels peaking 30–60 min after smoking. Parents who smoke should be advised not to share a bed with their baby as parental smoking increases the risk of sudden infant death syndrome (SIDS).
Alcohol	Current NHS guidance recommends no alcohol intake. Alcohol may affect milk supply. If a mother chooses to drink alcohol while breastfeeding, she should be advised to avoid alcohol before breastfeeding. It takes up to 2 hours to clear 1 unit from breastmilk and peak levels appear 30–90 min after consumption. The level of alcohol in breastmilk will fall as the level of alcohol in the blood falls, so mothers do not need to 'pump and dump' their breastmilk before feeding the baby if sufficient time has passed. Excessive drinking when breastfeeding can lead to sleep, growth and developmental problems with the baby. Help is available for mothers who request support with alcohol-related issues. **A responsible adult should always be available to care for the baby if the mother is not able to.**
Recreational drugs	Mothers should be advised against taking all recreational drugs while breastfeeding. The benefits of breastfeeding can outweigh the negative effects of the drugs and lifestyle; individual assessment is needed and is dependent on drugs being consumed. These infants can be at greater risk of SIDS, poor nutrition and poor weight gain if drug taking results in a chaotic lifestyle.

(Breastfeeding Network, 2016. Mastitis and Breast Abscess. Available at: https://www.breastfeedingnetwork.org.uk/.)

- No advertising of breastmilk substitutes to the public.
- No free samples to pregnant women or mothers.
- No free or subsidized supplies to hospitals.
- No contact between marketing personnel and mothers.
- No free gifts such as discount coupons or special offers.
- No pictures of babies or idealizing images on formula labels.
- Materials for health workers should contain only factual and scientific evidence information.

UNICEF Baby Friendly accredited services must adhere to the code, but it is good practice for all services supporting pregnant and new mothers to do so. The UNICEF Baby Friendly standards UK provide a roadmap for improving care to support all mothers with feeding and to help parents build a close and loving relationship with their baby (UNICEF BFI, 2022b).

Main Points

- Breastfeeding provides the baby with nutrition, protection and comfort, and encourages development of close and loving relationships between mother and baby. Breastfeeding has benefits for mothers, babies, society and the planet.
- Beliefs and attitudes about breastfeeding are influenced by culture, folklore and social context.

- Learning to breastfeed is part of a lifelong process beginning at birth. Some parts of breastfeeding are instinctive, but a lot is about social learning.
- The baby should be placed in skin-to-skin contact and breastfed as soon as possible after birth. The position of the baby at the breast is important. Attachment to the breast is essential to the success of breastfeeding and in the prevention of problems.

- Breast refusal, nipple trauma and insufficient milk are the most common reason given by mothers for discontinuing breastfeeding. Prevention for all of these requires support for early and frequent effective feeding.
- Engorgement refers to breasts when they are overfull, partly with milk and partly with increased tissue fluid. Early and frequent feeding helps prevent its onset.
- Mastitis is an area of inflammation that affects part of the breast and occurs due to milk stasis. If untreated it may lead to abscess, and in some cases sepsis.

- Drugs may be passed from mother to baby in breastmilk. Mothers should avoid smoking, alcohol and recreational drugs and seek medical advice for prescription and over-the-counter drugs.
- The International Code of Marketing of Breast Milk Substitutes aims to promote and protect breastfeeding and health professionals should be aware if their responsibilities within the code.

References

Bergman, N., 2016. Breastfeeding and perinatal neuroscience. In: Genna, C.W. (Ed.), Supporting Suckling Skills in Breastfeeding Infants, third ed. Jones and Bartlett Learning, New York.

Breastfeeding Network, 2016. Mastitis and Breast Abscess. Available at: https://www.breastfeedingnetwork.org.uk/.

British National Formulary (BNF) and National Institute of Health and Care Excellence (NICE), 2023. British National Formulary. Available at: https://bnf.nice.org.uk/.

Brown, A., Arnott, B., 2014. Breastfeeding duration and early parenting behaviour: the importance of an infant-led, responsive style. PLoS One 9 (2):e83893.

Henshaw, E.J., Mayer, M., Balraj, S., Parmar, E., Durkin, K., Snell, R., 2021. Couples talk about breastfeeding: interviews with parents about decision-making, challenges, and the role of fathers and professional support. Health Psychol. Open 8 (2).

Lawrence, R.A., Lawrence, R.M., 2021. Breastfeeding: A Guide for the Medical Profession, ninth ed. Elsevier, Philadelphia.

Linnér, A., Lode Kolz, K., Klemming, S., Bergman, N., Lilliesköld, S., Markhus Pike, H., et al., 2022. Immediate skin-to-skin contact may have beneficial effects on the cardiorespiratory stabilisation in very preterm infants. Acta Paediatr. 111 (8), 1507–1514.

Moore, E.R., Bergman, N., Anderson, G.C., Medley, N., 2016. Early skin-to-skin contact for mothers and their healthy newborn infants. Cochrane Database Syst. Rev. 2016 (5):CD003519.

National Institute of Health and Care Excellence (NICE), 2023. Mastitis and Breast Abscess. Available at: https://cks.nice.org.uk/topics/mastitis-breast-abscess/.

Nurses Climate Challenge (NCC) Europe, 2022a. Climate-smart Infant Feeding Part 1: The Interconnection of Environment, Climate Change, and Infant Nutrition. Available at: https://www.qnis.org.uk/wp-content/uploads/2022/07/2022-05-03-NCCEurope-climate-smart-infantfeeding-part1.pdf.

Public Health Scotland, 2023. Off to a Good Start: All You Need to Know about Breastfeeding. Available at: https://publichealthscotland.scot/publications/off-to-a-good-start-all-you-need-to-know-about-breastfeeding/.

Sheedy, G.M., Stulz, V.M., Stevens, J., 2022. Exploring outcomes for women and neonates having skin-to-skin contact during caesarean birth: a quasi-experimental design and qualitative study. Women Birth 35 (6), e530–e538.

UNICEF Baby Friendly Initiative (BFI), 2022a. Guidance for Antenatal and Postnatal Conversations. Available at: https://www.unicef.org.uk/babyfriendly/baby-friendly-resources/implementing-standards-resources/guidance-for-antenatal-and-postnatal-conversations/.

UNICEF BFI, 2022b. Baby Friendly Standards. Available at: www.unicef.org.uk/babyfriendly/about/standards/.

UNICEF BFI, 2022c. Support for Parents. Available at: www.unicef.org.uk/babyfriendly/support-for-parents/.

UNICEF, 2023. How We Protect Children's Rights with the UN Convention on the Rights of the Child. Available at: https://www.unicef.org.uk/what-we-do/un-convention-child-rights/.

United Nations Children's Fund (UNICEF), 2013. Community Infant and Young Child Feeding Counselling Package. Available at: https://www.unicef.org/documents/community-iycf-package.

Ventura, A.K., 2017. Associations between breastfeeding and maternal responsiveness: a systematic review of the literature. Adv. Nutr. 8 (3), 495–510.

Victora, C.G., Bahl, R., Barros, A.J., França, G.V., Horton, S., Krasevec, J., et al., 2016. Breastfeeding in the 21st century: epidemiology, mechanisms, and lifelong effect. Lancet 387 (10017), 475–490.

World Health Organization (WHO), 1981. International Code of Marketing of Breast Milk Substitutes. WHO Press, Geneva.

Annotated recommended reading

Rosen-Carole, C., Blumoff Greenberg, K., 2021. Chestfeeding and lactation care for LGBTQ+ families (lesbian, gay, bisexual, transgender, queer, plus). In: Lawrence, R.A., Lawrence, R.M. (Eds.), Breastfeeding: A Guide for the Medical Profession, ninth ed. Elsevier, Philadelphia.

This interesting chapter was widely shared by Elsevier publishing to celebrate Pride Month. The chapter is informative and highlights the need for providers to both understand how to support and counsel families about their options with respect to lactation and to compassionately approach any constraints they may face. As with all families, lactation providers should be inclusive and offer bias-free care for everyone. This is an essential read for all providers including student midwives in preparation for practice.

Lawrence, R.A., Lawrence, R.M., 2021. Breastfeeding: A Guide for the Medical Profession, ninth ed. Elsevier, Philadelphia.

This is an excellent reference book for all aspects of breastfeeding.

Pollard, M., 2023. Evidence-Based Care for Breastfeeding Mothers: A Resource for Midwives and Allied Healthcare Professionals. Routledge, London (in press).

This is an up-to-date evidence-based textbook for students, midwives and all health professionals involved with breastfeeding parents.

NCC Europe, 2022a. Climate-Smart Infant Feeding Part 1: The Interconnection of Environment, Climate Change, and Infant Nutrition. Available at: https://www.qnis.org.uk/wp-content/uploads/2022/07/2022-05-03-NCCEurope-climate-smart-infantfeeding-part1.pdf.

NCC Europe, 2022b. Climate-Smart Infant Feeding Part 2: What Individual Nurses Can Do to Support Climate-Smart Infant Feeding. Available at: https://www.qnis.org.uk/wp-content/uploads/2022/07/2022-05-03-NCCEurope-climate-smart-infantfeeding-part2.pdf.

NCC Europe, 2022c. Climate-Smart Infant Feeding Part 3: Advocacy for Breastfeeding. Available at: https://www.qnis.org.uk/wp-content/uploads/2022/07/2022-05-16-NCCEurope-climate-smart-infantfeeding-part3.pdf.

These websites provide excellent training and information resources.

Public Health Scotland, 2023. Off to a Good Start: All You Need to Know about Breastfeeding. Available at: https://publichealthscotland.scot/publications/off-to-a-good-start-all-you-need-to-know-about-breastfeeding/.

This user-friendly document is informative and provides guidance for breastfeeding parents. It is useful for student midwives and other professionals involved in breastfeeding.

UNICEF sites:

www.unicef.org.uk/babyfriendly/news-and-research/baby-friendly-research/infant-health-research/infant-health-research-meta-analyses/the-impact-of-breastfeeding-on-maternal-and-child-health/.

www.unicef.org.uk.

www.unicef.org.uk/babyfriendly.

www.unicef.org/documents/community-iycf-package.

These websites provide excellent resources for students, midwives and other health professionals involved with breastfeeding parents. The site provides a range of related evidence-based documents and leaflets for health professionals and parents. In particular the IYCF-package provides a wide range of additional including:

- *Infant and Young Child Feeding Image Bank.*
- *Infant and young child feeding recommendations when COVID-19 is suspected or confirmed – Counselling package.*
- *Infant and young child feeding counselling: an integrated course | Global Breastfeeding Collective.*
- *Implementation guidance on counselling women to improve breastfeeding practices | Global Breastfeeding Collective.*
- *Operational Guidance on Breastfeeding Counselling in Emergencies | Global Breastfeeding Collective.*
- *First Foods for Young Children Video Series for Caregivers and Frontline Workers.*

Useful websites

https://www.breastfeedingnetwork.org.uk/.

https://bnf.nice.org.uk/.

https://www.unicef.org.uk.

https://www.unicef.org.uk/babyfriendly/.

56

The Puerperium

YVONNE GREIG AND JEAN RANKIN

The puerperium is a crucial time for the mother and baby. This chapter details the physiology of the puerperium and care and support of the mother. The influences on emotional reactions and perinatal mental health associated with childbirth are discussed.

Introduction

The postnatal period or **puerperium** is the time commencing after delivery of the placenta and membranes until 6–8 weeks following birth. It is described as a period of restoration (Blackburn, 2018). During this time, the pelvic organs return to their nonpregnant state, the maternal changes during pregnancy are reversed and lactation is established (Edmonds, 2018). The puerperium is deemed to be complete with the first ovulation and return to menstruation (Edmonds, 2018). Despite the lack of scientific agreement on the duration of the puerperium, the consensus appears to be 6–8 weeks (National Institute of Health and Care Excellence [NICE], 2021).

Globally, the postnatal period is steeped in customs and rituals (Edmonds, 2018; Weeks, 2017). This means that, in some cultures, medical recommendations have been developed because of social acceptability rather than from scientific evidence (Edmonds, 2018). In turn, this suggests some women may not be given appropriate care or treatment following the birth of their babies, leading to poor postnatal outcomes. The World Health Organization (WHO) now recognizes that many poor puerperal outcomes occur due to 'missed opportunities' for improvement and the subsequent omission of appropriate treatment or the delivery of suboptimal care (WHO, 2019). In the UK, midwives continue to provide care to new mothers for as long as they deem it to be clinically appropriate (Nursing and Midwifery Council (NMC), 2019). The midwife has autonomy in making the decisions for both the mother and baby rather than postnatal care being time limited.

The puerperium occurs during a time when the anticipation and excitement of the birth are over and with the expectation that both mother and baby will be well. It is now widely understood that a significant number of women suffer from mortality or morbidity postnatally (Knight, 2021; WHO, 2019). This means that midwives need to have a clear and thorough understanding of the physiological processes of the puerperium to accurately monitor the woman's recovery and identify any deviations from normal. In doing so, midwives will ensure any required referrals to specialists are made in a timely manner. Postpartum haemorrhage (PPH), maternal sepsis and blood pressure disorders are some of the most common causes of maternal morbidity and mortality in the puerperium (Knight et al., 2022; Knight et al., 2023). Pre-eclampsia and eclampsia can lead to venous thromboembolic disease and mental health disorders have resulted in an increase in maternal deaths by suicide (see Box 56.1).

Midwifery terminology related to the puerperium includes the descriptive term '**postpartum**' that is attributed to situations and conditions after birth (parturition) and the '**postnatal period**', which is a social concept involving mother and baby.

Chapter 45 provides more detailed information about PPH and Chapter 33 provides information on thromboembolic disorders, including thrombophlebitis, deep vein thrombosis and pulmonary embolism. Related aspects are considered in other chapters, including family planning (Chapter 6) and interactive aspects of parenting (Chapter 57). Details of remaining key disorders are provided in this chapter.

In total, 229 women died in the recent triennium from direct and indirect causes.

Of the total deaths:
- 42 (18%) women died on the day of birth.
- 123 (54%) died between days 1–41.

Place of deaths:
- Home: 5 women (4%).
- Hospital: 120 women (85%).
- Emergency unit: 17 women (12%)

Overview:
- Of all maternal deaths, 11% of women were at severe and multiple disadvantages such as mental health diagnosis, substance use and domestic abuse.
- Psychiatric disorders and cardiovascular disorders now represent 30% of maternal deaths.
- Deaths from mental health-related causes as a whole (suicide and substance abuse) account for nearly 40% of deaths occurring within a year after the end of pregnancy, with maternal suicide remaining the leading cause of direct deaths in this period.
- In the UK, the rate of suicide during pregnancy and up to 6 weeks after pregnancy from the previous triennium has significantly increased.

Refer to Chapter 30 for further details on the MBRRACE-UK enquiry into maternal deaths and the risk factors associated with maternal deaths.
(Knight et al., 2022)

Physiological Changes

During the puerperium, the physiological changes can be divided into:
- Involution of the uterus and genital tract.
- Secretion of breastmilk and establishment of lactation.
- Other physiological changes.

The major physiological event of the puerperium is lactation. Chapters 54 & 55 are devoted to lactation, including the anatomy of the breast, the initiation and maintenance of lactation and breastfeeding and complications.

Endocrine Changes in the Puerperium

Changes in hormone levels following delivery of the placenta initiates the rapid reversal of pregnancy-related changes in the woman's body (Blackburn, 2018). During pregnancy, it is the placenta that produces most of the steroid hormones (oestrogen and progesterone) (Coad, Pedley & Dunstall, 2019). Plasma levels of the placental protein hormones (human placental lactogen and human chorionic gonadotrophin hormone) fall more slowly due to their longer half-lives. Early in the puerperium, gonadotrophins suppressed during pregnancy are again produced.

Oestrogen levels return to prepregnant levels by the seventh day following birth. Progesterone levels return to those found in the luteal phase of the menstrual cycle by 24–48 hours postbirth and to the follicular phase by 7 days postbirth (Fig. 56.1) (Coad, Pedley & Dunstall, 2019). The mother's metabolic rate returns to normal, with the thyroid hormones returning to their nonpregnant levels at 4 weeks after birth and the thyroid gland (i.e., increased in size during pregnancy) returning to its normal size by 12 weeks postbirth (Edmonds, 2018).

Resumption of Menstruation and Ovulation

Most women are relatively infertile during the early postnatal period due to having low levels of gonadotrophins, whose production has been inhibited during pregnancy. In the absence of breastfeeding, the reproductive cycle may start again within a few weeks of birth. This varies from woman to woman. The return of ovulation is preceded by an increase in plasma progesterone. In most cases, the first menstrual cycle after delivery is anovulatory (Coad, Pedley & Dunstall, 2019). However ovulation may occur before menstruation in 25% of women, meaning conception could occur prior to the woman having had a menstrual period. It is understood that for most women, ovulation will recommence by 12 weeks postpartum irrespective of infant feeding choice (Edmonds, 2018). Menstruation usually resumes at approximately 6 weeks postpartum in nonlactating women, although this does vary (Blackburn, 2018; Coad, Pedley & Dunstall, 2019).

Prolactin and oxytocin are maternal hormones involved in the initiation and maintenance of lactation (refer to Chapter 54). **Prolactin** is secreted by the anterior pituitary gland in increasing amounts during pregnancy, but its effects are suppressed by progesterone. **Oxytocin** is produced in the hypothalamus and is stored and secreted from the posterior pituitary gland. This hormone not only stimulates electrical and contractile activity in the myometrium to aid involution but is critical for milk ejection during lactation (Blackburn, 2018).

The resumption of menstruation in lactating women is influenced by frequency of feeding. Breastfeeding women commonly experience long periods of amenorrhea that often persists until they choose to stop breastfeeding their babies. There is a greater tendency for exclusively breastfeeding women to experience a longer period of anovulation and amenorrhea (Blackburn, 2018).

Involution of the Uterus

'Involution' is the term used to describe how the uterus decreases in size to its prepregnancy state (Steen, Jackson & Brown, 2020). This is the principal change occurring in the pelvic organs. Understanding this physiological process is essential for midwives when they are monitoring women who have recently given birth. There is insufficient evidence to put a time factor on the rate of uterine involution, as this varies considerably across women.

Physiology

During involution, there are changes to the myometrium or muscle layer and the decidua or lining of the pregnant uterus

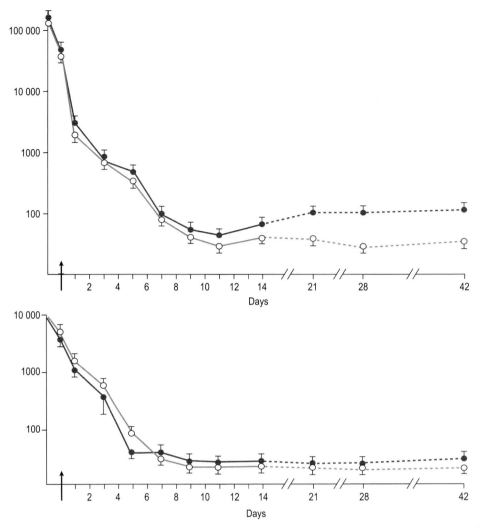

• **Fig. 56.1** Mean (±SEM) serum concentrations of 17β-oestradiol and progesterone in lactating and nonlactating subjects. Lactating subjects (*n* = 10) O–O; nonlactating subjects (*n* = 9) ●–●.

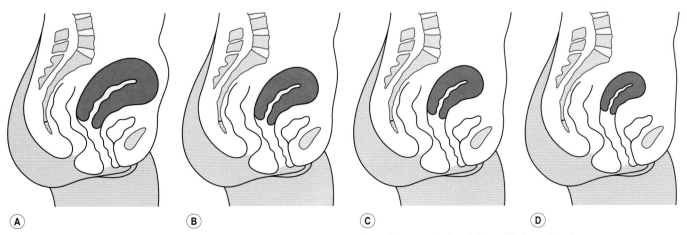

• **Fig. 56.2** Involution of the uterus. (A) At the end of labour. (B) 1 week after delivery. (C) 2 weeks after delivery. (D) 6 weeks after delivery.

(Fig. 56.2). The muscle layer returns to normal thickness by the processes of ischaemia, autolysis and phagocytosis. The decidua is shed as bleeding and fluid loss per vaginum with regeneration of the endometrium. Clinical Application 56.1 summarizes postpartum vaginal loss.

- **Ischaemia** occurs when the muscles of the uterus retract at the end of the third stage of labour to constrict the blood vessels at the placental site, resulting in haemostasis. This results in significant reduction in uterine blood supply.
- **Autolysis** is the process of removal of the redundant actin and myosin muscle fibres and cytoplasm by proteolytic enzymes and macrophages. The size of individual myometrial cells is reduced.
- **Phagocytosis** removes the excess fibrous and elastic tissue. This process is incomplete, and some elastic tissue remains so that a uterus never quite returns to the nulliparous state (Steen, Jackson & Brown, 2020).

Positional Changes

Immediately following delivery of the placenta, the whole uterus contracts down fully and the uterine walls become realigned in apposition to each other (Coad, Pedley & Dunstall, 2019). The fundus is palpable just below or at the level of the umbilicus. The muscles are well contracted to aid the process of haemostasis, and at this time the uterus feels globular and hard like a cricket ball. In the hours after birth (usually between 1 and 12 hours), the myometrium relaxes slightly whilst continuing to remain firmly contracted. Further active bleeding is prevented by the activation of the blood-clotting mechanisms, which are altered greatly during pregnancy to facilitate a swift clotting response (Coad, Pedley & Dunstall, 2019).

At the end of the first week, the uterus will have lost 50% of its bulk (Coad, Pedley & Dunstall, 2019). From a clinical perspective, the uterine fundus is not usually palpable abdominally by day 10 after birth, having involuted by approximately 1 cm/day (Edmonds, 2018). Where the uterus has involuted normally, it is expected to be at its prepregnant shape, size and position of anteversion and anteflexion by 6 weeks following birth (Edmonds, 2018). The rate of uterine involution varies considerably across individual women and the context of their labour and birth. Midwives need to assess involution in the context of many related factors, including colour, amount and duration of vaginal loss, any abdominal pain and general maternal health at that time (Steen, Jackson & Brown, 2020).

Subinvolution of the uterus refers to slowed, delayed or incomplete involution usually resulting from a lack of effective uterine contraction (Blackburn, 2018). The process of involution is slower when there has been overdistension of the uterus for reasons such as multiple pregnancy, a macrosomic or large baby or where there may have been polyhydramnios. The various causes associated with subinvolution include uterine atony (most common), retained placental fragments or blood clot, lacerations or infection and uterine

---

• CLINICAL APPLICATION 56.1 Postpartum Vaginal Loss

Vaginal fluid and blood loss characteristics:

- Immediately following childbirth:
  Fresh blood, amnion and chorion, decidual cells, vernix caseosa, lanugo and meconium.
- Over time:
  Stale blood, erythrocytes, leucocytes, wound exudate, cervical mucus, microorganisms, shreds of degenerating decidua from the superficial layer, epithelial cells and bacteria.

Significant morbidity is associated with abnormalities of postpartum vaginal fluid and blood loss. Therefore it is vital for midwives to remain vigilant in their assessment of postpartum vaginal loss as obtained from mothers and through their own observations. Mothers may not even be aware to expect vaginal fluid and blood loss following childbirth (Marchant, Alexander & Garcia, 2002).

Vaginal fluid and blood loss vary widely in terms of amount, content, colour and duration in the first 12 weeks following birth. This recognized variation strongly suggests that the traditional descriptions of normality of vaginal fluid and blood loss are no longer of any use in clinical practice (see 'Outdated Clinical Practice'). Therefore, these traditional descriptions are unhelpful to women and contribute to an inaccurate assessment of vaginal fluid and blood loss by midwives.

The midwife needs to ask the mother direct questions about vaginal loss as to whether the loss is lighter or darker than previously and if they have any concerns. Most mothers can describe any changes in their vaginal loss and identify the colour and consistency of vaginal loss. The use of descriptions common to both women and the midwife can improve accuracy in the overall assessment. One example is to ask the mother to describe her vaginal loss in her own words and how often she has to change her maternity pad.

- Blood clots—these can be associated with future episodes of excess or prolonged postpartum bleeding. Therefore it is important for the midwife to record 'if and when' any clots were passed. It is problematic in an assessment to attempt to quantify the amount of loss or the size of clot.
- Vaginal blood loss—may remain red for up to 3 weeks or there may be a brief increase in blood content in the second week. Vaginal loss remaining heavily bloodstained or if there is a sudden return to profuse red blood loss could suggest placental tissue has been retained. This requires prompt referral.
- Uterine infection—if vaginal fluid or blood loss is offensive smelling and/or the woman becomes pyrexial, then infection is suspected. This requires prompt medical referral for treatment and an appropriate management plan.

Outdated Clinical Practice

Obstetric, midwifery and physiology books continue to refer to vaginal loss using the Latin word **'lochia'** as a descriptive plural term (Blackburn, 2018; Coad, Pedley & Dunstall, 2019). Historically, three forms of postpartum vaginal blood loss were described: *lochia rubra* (red), *lochia serosa* (pink) and *lochia alba* (white). However research exploring the relevance of these descriptions in clinical practice has confirmed these terms are outdated (Steen, Jackson & Brown, 2020). The midwife's knowledge and use of skills to obtain an informative history from the mother are more accurate and meaningful for appropriate decision-making in everyday clinical practice.

inversion. All conditions are usually responsive to early diagnosis and treatment (Blackburn, 2018).

In the absence of other concerning factors, such as malodorous vaginal blood loss, pyrexia or abdominal pain, 'slow' involution is of no consequence. During this gradual process, when the uterus returns to its normal size, tone and position, the vagina, uterine ligaments and muscles of the pelvic floor also return to their prepregnant state. The pelvic floor is discussed in Chapter 25. No evidence is available to suggest any relationship between parity and the rate of uterine involution.

Uterine Contractions

During the first 24 hours after birth, high levels of oxytocin are secreted from the posterior pituitary gland into the maternal bloodstream. Oxytocin stimulates the electrical and contractile activity in the myometrium by causing the myoepithelial cells of the uterus to contract and involute (Blackburn, 2018). Ongoing postpartum uterine contractions lead to retraction of the uterine muscles. Contractions often result in 'after-pains' that can be severe for some women (Coad, Pedley & Dunstall, 2019), particularly in those who are breastfeeding or have given birth previously (Steen, Jackson & Brown, 2020). These 'after-pains' usually diminish after 4–7 days, and women should be informed as to why they occur and that they will resolve. Simple analgesia can be given to ease the discomfort.

The Decidua

The upper portion of the spongy endometrial layer is sloughed off when the placenta is delivered. The remaining decidua is organized into basal and superficial layers. The superficial layer consists of granulated tissue, which is invaded by leucocytes to form a barrier that prevents microorganisms invading the remaining decidua (Edmonds, 2018). This layer becomes necrotic and is sloughed off as vaginal bleeding. The basal layer remains intact and is the source of regeneration of the endometrium (usually beginning 10 days after birth). Except for the placental site, the regeneration process is completed by 2–3 weeks after delivery (Edmonds, 2018). Healing of the placental site is complete by the end of 6 weeks.

Postpartum Vaginal Fluid and Blood Loss

Involution of the uterus is progressive and varies from woman to woman. This variation is also reflected in vaginal fluid and blood loss. Immediately following birth and expulsion of the placenta and membranes, blood products constitute a major part of fresh vaginal fluid and blood loss. As involution progresses, vaginal fluid and blood loss changes from being predominantly fresh blood to vaginal fluid loss containing stale blood products and other debris from the products of conception. Whilst vaginal blood and fluid loss varies across individuals, the density and shade of blood loss tends to be consistent for individual women (Marchant, Alexander & Garcia, 2002). Refer to Clinical Application 56.1.

Other Parts of the Genital Tract

Immediately after delivery, the cervix is soft and highly vascular but rapidly loses its vascularity and returns to its original form (Edmonds, 2018). By the end of the second week after birth, the internal os will usually be closed, but the external os may always remain slightly dilated (Weeks, 2017). The **ovaries** and uterine (**fallopian**) tubes return with the uterus to the pelvic cavity. The vagina almost always shows some evidence of parity. The **vagina, vulva** and **pelvic floor** respond to the reduced amount of circulating progesterone by recovering normal muscle tone. Early ambulation and postnatal exercises can enhance this return to normal. Bruising or tears to genital tissues heal rapidly, and any oedema is reabsorbed within the first 3 or 4 days.

The Body Systems
The Cardiovascular and Respiratory Systems

During pregnancy, increased circulatory volume and haemodilution are needed to ensure adequate blood supply to the uterus and the placental bed. After delivery of the placenta and the withdrawal of oestrogen, a diuresis occurs for the first 48 hours following birth and the plasma volume and haematocrit rapidly return to normal. The reduction in circulating progesterone leads to removal of excess tissue fluid and a return to normal vascular tone. Cardiac output and blood pressure return to nonpregnant levels (Broughton Pipkin, 2018).

The lungs can inflate fully again, and oxygen demands return to normal. The tendency to hyperventilate disappears and blood CO_2 levels return to normal, as does the slight alkalosis that has been present during pregnancy.

The Renal System

Over the period of the puerperium, the physiological parameters of the renal system return to prepregnancy levels. During this time, it is the kidneys that deal with the excretion of excess fluids and an increase in the breakdown products of protein. The removal of progesterone resolves dilatation of the renal tract, and the renal organs gradually return to their prepregnant state (Bick & Hunter, 2017). During labour, the bladder is displaced into the abdomen and the urethra is stretched. There may be loss of tone in the bladder and bruising of the urethra, leading to difficulty in micturition.

Because of these features and diuresis, the bladder may become overdistended and retention of urine may occur. Early ambulation with frequent encouragement to pass urine and ensuring that the bladder is emptied will help to avoid this situation. One would normally expect the woman to have passed a volume of 300 mL of urine by 6 hours after birth. If this has not occurred, then catheterization may be indicated (Weeks, 2017).

The Gastrointestinal Tract

Throughout the body, smooth muscle tone gradually returns to normal due to the reduced levels of circulating progesterone. There is a rapid return to normal carbohydrate metabolism, and fasting plasma insulin levels return to non-pregnant values between 48 hours and the sixth week post-partum (Blackburn, 2018). The minor inconveniences of pregnancy affecting the gastrointestinal tract, such as constipation and heartburn, usually resolve quickly.

Postpartum (Puerperal) Infection

At birth, the normal protective barriers against infection are temporarily broken down, and this gives potential pathogens an opportunity to pass from the lower genital tract into the usually sterile environment of the uterus. Postpartum pyrexia is a clinical sign that always merits careful investigation (Knight et al., 2014). Postnatal women are particularly at risk for infection because of the presence of the raw placental site, the tissue trauma sustained in labour and the decidua and blood loss being excellent culture media for growth of bacteria (Edmonds, 2018). Other sites for infection are the breasts, the epithelial linings of the veins and surgical incisions. Infections unrelated to pregnancy, such as an upper respiratory tract infection, should always be considered. This is emphasized in the report by Knight et al. (2014), where most of the maternal deaths from sepsis occurred in the postpartum period.

Puerperal infection is potentially life-threatening to new mothers (Knight, 2021). The association with sepsis and maternal deaths in the postpartum period was highlighted by Knight et al. (2014). They stressed how important it was for sepsis to be identified early with timely administration of antibiotics whilst involving key senior staff. In a recent MBRRACE-UK report, puerperal infections rank as the third most common cause of maternal death (Arwyn-Jones & Brent, 2021; Knight, 2021). Early recognition and treatment are the key priorities when sepsis is suspected (NICE, 2017; NICE, 2020a). Refer to Clinical Application 56.2 for postpartum infection. Chapter 47 details the acutely unwell woman and maternal collapse.

• CLINICAL APPLICATION 56.2 Postpartum (Puerperal) Infection

Indications: Pyrexia (and timing of onset) and/or tachycardia and/or tachypnoea. Note that the absence of pyrexia does not exclude sepsis, so be vigilant in recording other vital signs (NICE, 2017).

Immediate management: Ask for help and seek senior medical review. If sepsis is suspected in a community setting then an emergency ambulance should be called.

Action to confirm: Medical assessment. Bacteriological specimens include swabs and specimens for urine and blood culture. Investigations are for identification of organisms, culture and antibiotic sensitivity. Possible swab sites include high vaginal, perineal, wound, ear, nose and throat swabs, and specimens include blood, urine, stool and breast milk.

Routine treatment: The 'Sepsis 6' care protocol should be initiated (see Table 56.1 and Chapter 47).

Establish intravenous (IV) access. Antibiotic therapy commenced immediately. Antibiotics are changed according to sensitivity results. Correct any dehydration. Pain relief as required. Observe maternal condition using a Maternity Early Warning Scoring system (MEWS) such as the Modified Early Obstetric Warning Score (MEOWS). The Royal College of Obstetricians and Gynaecologists (RCOG) recommends the need for clinicians to use a national obstetric early warning scoring system for all obstetric women, including those being cared for outside the obstetric setting (Chu, Johnston & Geoghegan, 2020).

Early recognition and prompt intervention are crucial to limit the disease progress and prevent severe morbidity and maternal mortality (Knight et al., 2014; NICE, 2017).

Postpartum Endometritis
Signs and Symptoms
- Pyrexia >38°C occurs at approximately the third postnatal day (although it can occur sooner).
- Pulse rate rises by ~10 bpm for every degree Celsius.
- Pain is present in lower abdomen.
- Uterus is tender on palpation.
- Headache and rigours may occur.
- Possible localized infection in the perineum.

- Vaginal blood loss may be heavy and offensive, depending on invading organism.
- Blood cultures may be positive in up to 10% of women.
Maternal condition may deteriorate rapidly with severe sepsis resulting in acute organ dysfunction and possible death. Fever, rapid breathing and fast heart rate are key indicators of sepsis (Acosta et al., 2014).

Management of Sepsis
Commence management in line with international/national/local sepsis guidelines (e.g., https://sepsistrust.org/). Administration of broad-spectrum antibiotic therapy is commenced immediately (change according to sensitivity results). IV access and fluid hydration. Blood cultures. Serum lactate measurement. Monitor fluid balance (urinary output). Oxygen therapy (adequate oxygen saturation). Observe maternal condition using a MEWS/MEOWS chart. Other relevant blood tests: full blood count, urea and electrolytes, coagulation. Analgesia for pain relief.

Additional Treatment when the Condition is Severe
- Isolation to prevent spread of infection.
- Transfer to high-dependency unit.
- IV antibiotic treatment commenced immediately if the woman is seriously ill.
- Assessment of haemoglobin levels, as anaemia may precede or follow infection. Blood transfusion may be necessary.
- Treat any localized wound infections.
- Baby may also require investigation and treatment.
In postpartum pyrexia, legs should be routinely inspected for evidence of thrombophlebitis.

Key Points
Always think sepsis.
- Early identification.
- Seek help quickly.
- Timely administration of antibiotics.
- Involvement of key senior staff.
Refer to Table 56.1 for a summary of the Sepsis 6 pathway. Chapter 47 provides details of the management of maternal collapse.

Causative Organisms

Invading organisms need time to multiply sufficiently to cause symptoms, and postnatal infection occurs after the first 24 hours from delivery. As in any infection, the severity depends on two factors: the virulence of the causative organism and the resistance of the host. Infecting organisms may originate from the commensal organisms normally present in the woman's own body. These are called *endogenous organisms* (Steen, Jackson & Brown, 2020) and can cause problems if they invade susceptible sites. Such organisms may come from the vagina, bowel, skin, nose or throat of the woman and include *Escherichia coli, Clostridium welchii* and *Streptococcus faecalis.*

Exogenous organisms are transmitted from a source other than the woman's body (e.g., people, surfaces and environment) (Steen, Jackson & Brown, 2020). These organisms are responsible for more serious infections. The most dangerous organisms are **group A β-haemolytic streptococci**, which leads to the main cause of intrauterine infection. *Staphylococcus aureus* is a common organism which lingers in dust and can cause spots, pustules and sticky eyes in babies and maternal breast or wound infections. A strain of this organism, called methicillin-resistant *Staphylococcus aureus*, is resistant to most antibiotics. Overuse and misuse of antibiotics in human disease and animal husbandry has contributed to the mutations of organisms.

Streptococci: Lancefield Groups

The genus *Streptococcus* contains a wide variety of species of bacteria with many habitats. Some species are pathogenic to human beings. One group of related species comprises those that cause haemolysis when grown on blood agar, an action referred to as **β-haemolysis.** Streptococci are also subdivided depending on the presence of carbohydrate antigens on their surfaces. These are called **Lancefield groups** and are identified with letters of the alphabet such as A, B and onwards to O (Amezaga & McKenzie, 2006). One of the most common organisms responsible for serious and life-threatening obstetric infections is the β-haemolytic *Streptococcus pyogenes,* categorized as Lancefield group A (Leonard et al., 2018). The infection has the distinctive potential to progress rapidly to a life-threatening invasive infection, toxin-mediated shock and end-organ failure, even before clinical signs become apparent. This organism can gain access to the circulation via the placental site, causing septicaemia and red-cell haemolysis.

The Lancefield group B streptococci can be found in normal vaginal flora and is most associated with neonatal septicaemia and meningitis, particularly in premature infants (Leonard et al., 2018). Serious maternal infections may also occur with this infection. Lancefield groups C and G streptococci may also cause serious clinical syndromes but are less common. Group A streptococci attack people of all ages and are lethal despite vigorous treatment. Vigilance in preventative measures is imperative to protect childbearing women and their babies.

Sepsis

Sepsis is caused by an abnormal or 'pathophysiological and dysregulated' response to pathogens in the body (Roberts, Baird-McMurty & Martin, 2021). It has been described as a syndrome that encompasses pathological, physiological and biochemical abnormalities in the body (Arwyn-Jones & Brent, 2021)

TABLE 56.1 Sepsis 6 pathway—Summary

	Action	Details
1	Ensure senior clinician attends	Not all patients with red flags will need the 'sepsis 6' urgently. A senior decision maker may seek alternative diagnoses/de-escalate care. Decisions are recorded below.
2	Administer oxygen if required	To correct any hypoxia less than 92%. Aim for SaO_2 94–98%
3	Obtain intravenous (IV) access and take bloods	Full blood count, blood cultures, lactate levels, coagulation screen, urea and electrolytes, and C-reactive protein (CRP)
		Check serial lactates
	Take swabs for bacteriology examination of culture and sensitivity	Swab sites—vaginal, wound (perineal or abdominal), nose, throat. Urine should also be sent for examination.
4	Give broad-spectrum IV antibiotics according to local protocol	Give within the first hour of sepsis recognition.
5	Establish IV access Give IV fluids—as per local protocol and commence fluid balance chart	To correct dehydration and the lactate level. Take bloods first to gain an accurate 'pretreatment' picture
6	Monitor Maternity Early Warning Score (Obstetrics) chart, urine output, catheter may be required, repeat lactate at least once per hour if previous lactate was elevated.	Commence a fluid balance chart. Depending on the individual and their clinical need, consider siting a urinary catheter and monitor urine output hourly.

Summary: Nutbeam & Daniels (2022) on behalf of the UK Sepsis Trust (https://sepsistrust.org/)

and can lead to death (see Chapter 47). Normally when bacteria or other microbes enter the human body, the immune system efficiently destroys the invaders. In sepsis, it is now understood that there is both an anti-inflammatory and proinflammatory response, and that these two reactions do not necessarily occur in sequence but can occur simultaneously (Arwn-Jones & Brent, 2021). This inflammation leads to the formation of microscopic blood clots and leaky blood vessels that block the flow of blood to the vital organs. In the most severe cases (septic shock), blood pressure falls to dangerously low levels, multiple organs fail and the patient can die (Acosta et al., 2014). For the management of sepsis, refer to Clinical Application 56.2 & Table 56. 1.

Genital Tract Infection

Infection of the genital tract may remain localized to the perineum, vagina or cervix or may ascend the genital tract to infect the uterine cavity (**endometritis**). Infection may then spread to the fallopian tubes to cause salpingitis and to the tissues of the pelvic cavity to cause cellulitis and peritonitis. Refer to Clinical Application 56.2 for more information.

Postpartum Endometritis

Postpartum endometritis is usually caused by an ascending infection from the lower genital tract. Other factors that may facilitate pelvic infections include prolonged labour, prolonged rupture of the membranes, multiple vaginal examination, traumatic delivery and manual removal of the placenta (Edmonds, 2018).

Urinary Tract Infections (UTIs)

UTIs are common during the puerperium, especially in women with urinary retention, indwelling catheters, operative deliveries or with a history of UTI (Edmonds, 2018). Because of the delay in the return to normal in the urinary tract, there is susceptibility for infection (first 6 weeks), which may present as cystitis or pyelonephritis. Refer to Clinical Application 56.3 for UTI.

Other Postpartum (Puerperal) Infections

In the event of postpartum (puerperal) pyrexia, any wound (due to instrumental births or other surgical procedures) should be examined for evidence of infection. In addition to associated maternal pyrexia and tachycardia, the woman may be generally unwell with a reddened tender area around the wound site which may also be oedematous. Serous, bloodstained or purulent discharge that is offensive in nature may also be present.

Infection is confirmed by routine bacteriology specimens for maternal infection, including wound site swabs for culture and sensitivity and blood specimens when it is suspected that the infection is moderate to severe (refer to Clinical Application 56.2). Well-localized wound infections may discharge spontaneously and may only require local irrigation with an antiseptic solution. More extensive

---

• CLINICAL APPLICATION 56.3 **Urinary Tract Infection**

Signs and Symptoms

Similar symptoms to cystitis, including urinary frequency, urgency, dysuria and haematuria. Urine may be cloudy and offensive. Slight rise in maternal temperature.

In more serious pyelonephritis, the woman will be ill and develop:
- Pain and tenderness in the renal angle (may extend along the line of the ureter).
- Pyrexia and rapid pulse.
- Rigours.
- Nausea and vomiting.

On urinalysis, urine is acidic, opalescent and offensive. Pus and blood may be found on microscopic examination.

Diagnosis: culture of the infecting organism on a midstream specimen of urine (MSSU).

Treatment

- Encourage good oral intake of fluids (2.5–3.5 L/water) (Perrier et al., 2021).
- Intravenous fluids to maintain hydration and urinary output if vomiting is present, analgesia if required, alleviate nausea and reduce temperature.
- Commence broad-spectrum antibiotic (changed according to sensitivity results).
- Repeat culture of MSSU on completion of antibiotic treatment.
- Further investigations by cystoscopy and intravenous pyelography to exclude any underlying abnormality.

---

wound infections will need a broad-spectrum antibiotic (Edmonds, 2018). Most wounds will granulate from the base and heal spontaneously. Resuturing may be required depending on clinical circumstances.

Emotional States and Mental Disorders in the Puerperium

Behaviour is a complex function influenced by the interaction of biological factors and social, economic and cultural factors. Obstetric factors may influence the behaviour of women during the childbearing process (Cox & Holden, 2014).

Childbirth is generally recognized as being an important life event of great physiological and psychological significance. The events surrounding the birth often leave women both physically and emotionally vulnerable, and they commonly experience mood changes in the postpartum period. Mental disorders during the postnatal period can have serious consequences for the health and wellbeing of a mother and her baby, as well as for her partner and other family members (NICE, 2021).

Poor mental health remains one of the leading causes of maternal death. Of 229 maternal deaths, 16 were from psychiatric causes, 12 were from suicide and 4 were due to drugs and alcohol (Knight, 2021). Death from suicide is now acknowledged to be the most significant direct cause of maternal death up to 1 year postbirth (Knight, 2021). In

2020, women were three times more likely to die by suicide and deaths were associated with multiple adversity, substance misuse, homicide and accidental death. There is concern over the increase in teenage suicides. Refer to Chapter 30.

Screening for mental health risk antenatally is key to supporting women postnatally. However midwives must also be alert to any newly presenting mental health conditions in the postnatal period and make appropriate referrals to perinatal mental health services, giving the same weight to mental illness as they would physical illness (Klimowicz & Anderson, 2022).

Two classes of mental health disorders are neuroses and psychoses. In neuroses, the individual, although likely to be depressed, remains in touch with reality. In severe psychoses, there is a great impairment in the perception of external reality, often with delusions and hallucinations. In most cases, women with mental health disorders after childbirth will experience the neurotic disorder of postnatal depression (PND), and only a few women, many with a history of mental illness, will suffer from a postpartum (puerperal) psychotic episode of schizophrenia (Bick & Hunter, 2017).

The spectrum of 'affective states or disorders' after childbirth is most often divided into three categories in ascending order of severity:
1. The 'baby blues' (emotional state).
2. Postnatal depression (neuroses).
3. Postpartum (puerperal) psychosis (psychoses).

'Baby Blues'

Childbirth is a profoundly emotional and physiological event. The early feelings of elation in the first 3 days after birth are commonly replaced by a normal emotional reaction to childbirth called the *'baby blues'*. Despite the sometimes-overwhelming feelings of dysphoric mood, tearfulness, anxiety and irritability associated with the 'baby blues', this is not a mental illness (Klimowicz & Anderson, 2022) and with practical support in the home, symptoms usually resolve quickly. Between 26% and 84% of women experience this emotional reaction (Klimowicz & Anderson, 2022), which occurs from around the third day after birth until about the end of the first week. However, a prolonged, serious episode may be predictive of the onset of PND.

The cause of the 'baby blues' remains unclear. The physiological changes occurring in the puerperium are thought to be mainly responsible. The types of changes, which may affect behaviour, include the decrease in oestrogen and progesterone and alterations in the balance of fluids, electrolytes and neurotransmitters. These factors may interact with minor anxieties, attitudes and beliefs about the birth of the child and sociocultural stress to influence maternal mood to a greater degree.

Postnatal Depression (PND)

PND is commonly used to describe a sustained depressive disorder in women after childbirth (Cox & Holden, 2014). It has an insidious onset, runs a chronic course and is probably the most common complication of the puerperium. Women who have a history of mental and/or physical health are at increased risk of developing PND. PND is an important public health issue which is now widely acknowledged in mental health policy guidance in many countries. This condition causes suffering and disability to the woman and disruption to her family at a time of maximum vulnerability. The evidence of PND having an adverse effect on the mother–child relationship and child development is now more widely recognized (Cox & Holden, 2014).

Approximately 10% of all postnatal women will develop a depressive illness (Raynor et al., 2020). This disorder is a serious condition of childbirth and should be distinguished from the 'baby blues'. This condition is characterized by Klimowicz & Anderson (2022) as follows:
- Low, sad mood.
- Lack of interest.
- Anxiety.
- Reduced self-esteem.
- Somatic symptoms such as poor appetite and weight loss (in severe depression).
- *Sleep difficulties.
- Difficulty coping with day-to-day tasks.
- In severe cases, psychotic symptoms may develop.
  *Sleep disturbance is very common in relation to mental illness and is highlighted as a risk factor for maternal deaths (Knight et al., 2022).

Health professionals do not always detect the disorder and usually the woman makes a complete recovery (refer to Clinical Application 56.4).

Risk Factors

The risk factors for PND are no different from the risk factors for non-PND. These include:
- Lack of social and psychological support after birth is one of the main reasons that unhappiness after childbirth is such a common problem.
- Sociological and psychological factors include a past history of psychopathology and psychological disturbances during pregnancy, poor marital relationship, the 'baby blues' and social factors such as poor social support and recent life events (Clements & Staris, 2022; Gutteridge, 2017).
- History of abuse, obstetric complications and social factors such as lower occupational status and low family income (Clements & Staris, 2022).
- Stillbirth and neonatal or infant death may also affect mental health (NICE, 2020b).
- No persuasive evidence is available to support traditional explanations of PND, including biochemical explanations.

Postpartum (Puerperal) Psychosis

Postpartum (puerperal) psychosis is a severe depressive illness affecting 3% of women who have given birth (Raynor et al., 2020). This rate has a sevenfold increase in risk in the first 3 months, which constitutes a significantly increased risk

---

• CLINICAL APPLICATION 56.4 | **Postnatal Depression (PND): Screening, Early Detection and Management**

Observation and effective communication skills can pick up changes in behaviour and demeanour (Silverman, Kurtz & Draper, 2013). Detection normally occurs during self-reporting. Screening is not a diagnostic activity (Gibson & Gray, 2012). However at the earliest contact a woman has with maternity services, questions should be asked about past or present illness, past or present treatment and history of severe mental illness in first-degree family members (Klimowicz & Anderson, 2022).

Screening Tool

The Edinburgh Postnatal Depression Scale is an example of a simple, easy-to-use questionnaire administered by an appropriately trained health professional (administered approximately 6 weeks and 3 months after birth). Evidence confirms it is an effective screening tool (Cox & Holden, 2014).

Management

- Effective communication between professionals within the multidisciplinary team.
- Pharmacological therapies: hormonal and homeopathic therapies and antidepressants.
- Psychosocial therapies: e.g., counselling, psychotherapy such as cognitive behavioural approaches. Overall psychosocial and psychological interventions significantly reduce the incidence of PND. Promising interventions include the provision of intensive and professionally based postpartum home visits, telephone-based peer support and interpersonal psychotherapy (Dennis & Dowswell, 2013).
- Alternative therapies: e.g., massage, infant massage and relaxation therapies. There is no evidence to suggest hypnosis during pregnancy, childbirth or the postnatal period prevented PND (Sado et al., 2012).
- Early referral to psychiatrist: especially if suicidal tendencies displayed.

• CLINICAL APPLICATION 56.5 | **Postpartum (Puerperal) Psychosis: Detection and Management**

Routine Antenatal Care

- Information on postnatal mood disorders and postpartum (puerperal) psychosis to women and partners.
- Mental health assessments (documented) should always include previous history and take account of recent presentations and escalating patterns of abnormal behaviour.
- Consider the loss of a child, whether by miscarriage (abortion), stillbirth or neonatal death (or child in care).
- Vulnerability to mental illness for the woman who should receive additional monitoring and support.

Detection and Treatment

Recent significant change in mental state or emergence of new symptoms.

Decisions should involve a multidisciplinary assessment, including social workers and family members.

Signs for severe maternal illness need to be 'red-flagged' and require urgent senior psychiatric assessment.

Admission to a mother-and-baby unit should always be considered where a woman has any of the following:
- New thoughts or acts of violent self-harm.
- New and persistent expressions of incompetency as a mother or estrangement from infant.
- Rapidly changing mental state.
- Suicidal ideation (particularly of a violent nature).
- Pervasive guilt or hopelessness.
- Significant estrangement from the infant.
- New or persistent beliefs of inadequacy as a mother.
- Evidence of psychosis.

Partners and other family members may require explanation and education regarding maternal mental illness and accompanying risks.

Pharmaceutical treatments would typically involve one or more drugs from the antidepressant, mood-stabilizing or neuroleptic groups.

Prognosis is good; most women recover within 6 months.

Women with a previous postpartum (puerperal) psychosis are at significant risk of developing a future postpartum (puerperal) psychosis and have an even higher risk of developing a nonpostpartum relapse. Other risk factors include a pre-existing psychotic illness (especially if it is a severe affective psychosis) and family history of affective psychosis (Davies et al., 2020).

(Knight, 2021).

---

for psychotic illness when compared with other times in a woman's life (Cox & Holden, 2014). The onset is often rapid and typically presents in the early postpartum period, usually within the first month. In almost all cases of postpartum (puerperal) psychosis, there is a mood disorder accompanied by features such as loss of contact with reality, hallucinations, severe thought disturbances and abnormal behaviour (Klimowicz & Anderson, 2022). A key symptom is insomnia, and the woman may also be confused, frightened and distressed and may be disoriented in space and time. Delusions and hallucinations often focus on the delivery or on the baby. Refer to Clinical Application 56.5.

Main Points

- The puerperium is the 6–8-week period after childbirth during which time the maternal physiological changes resolve and return to the nonpregnant state.
- Removal of the placental hormones following birth of the baby initiates the return of the body systems to the prepregnant state.
- Involution is the main change in the pelvic organs during the puerperium. The process is brought about by ischaemia, autolysis and phagocytosis.
- Slow involution may be associated with retained products or an associated infection. Infection may be present if vaginal bleeding is offensive and the woman has pyrexia.

- After the withdrawal of oestrogen, diuresis occurs and the plasma volume and haematocrit rapidly return to normal. Cardiac output returns to nonpregnant levels.
- Loss of bladder tone and bruising of the urethra may lead to difficulty in micturition.
- Main maternal postpartum (puerperal) complications include PPH, thromboembolic disorders, postpartum (puerperal) infections and mental health disorders.
- Postpartum pyrexia always merits prompt medical investigation. ***Always think sepsis.***
- β-haemolytic *Streptococcus pyogenes*, Lancefield group A, is the most common organism responsible for serious and life-threatening obstetric infections.

- Childbearing is associated with three 'affective disorders': the 'baby blues', PND and postpartum (puerperal) psychosis. The 'baby blues' is a normal transient emotional reaction to childbirth experienced by over 50% of women (lasts from days 3–7).
- PND is a nonpsychotic illness occurring within the first year of childbirth.
- Postpartum (puerperal) psychosis is a mood disorder accompanied by symptoms such as loss of contact with reality, delusions and hallucinations and abnormal behaviour.

References

Acosta, C.D., Kurinczuk, J.J., Lucas, D.N., Tuffnell, D.J., Sellers, S., Knight, M., United Kingdom Obstetric Surveillance System, 2014. Severe maternal sepsis in the UK, 2011–2012: a national case-control study. PLoS Med. 11 (7),e1001672.

Amezaga, M.R., McKenzie, H., 2006. Molecular epidemiology of macrolide resistance in beta-haemolytic streptococcus of Lancefield groups A, B & C and evidence for a new element in group G streptococci. J. Antimicrob. Chemother. 57 (3), 443–449.

Arwyn-Jones, J., Brent, A.J., 2021. Sepsis. Surgery 39 (11), 714–721.

Bick, D., Hunter, C., 2017. Content and organization of postnatal care. In: Macdonald, S., Johnson, G. (Eds.), Mayes' Midwifery, fifteenth ed. Elsevier, Edinburgh.

Blackburn, S.T., 2018. Maternal, Fetal and Neonatal Physiology: A Clinical Perspective, fifth ed. Elsevier, St. Louis.

Broughton Pipkin, F.B., 2018. Maternal physiology. In: Edmonds, D.K., Lee, C., Bourne, T. (Eds.), Dewhurst's Textbook of Obstetrics, ninth ed. Wiley-Blackwell, Oxford.

Chu, J., Johnston, T.A., Geoghegan J., on behalf of the RCOG, 2020. Maternal collapse in pregnancy and the puerperium. Br. J. Obstet. Gynaecol. 127 (5), e14–e52.

Clements, K., Staris, T., 2022. Complex social factors. In: Anderson, M. (Ed.), Midwifery Essentials: Perinatal Mental Health. Elsevier, Edinburgh.

Coad, J., Pedley, M., Dunstall, K., 2019. Anatomy and Physiology for Midwives, fourth ed. Elsevier, Edinburgh.

Cox, J., Holden, J., 2014. Perinatal Mental Health: A Guide to the Edinburgh Postnatal Depression Scale. Royal College of Psychiatrists Publishers, London.

Davies, C., Segre, G., Estradé, A., Radua, J., De Micheli, A., Provenzani, U., et al., 2020. Prenatal and perinatal risk and protective factors for psychosis: a systematic review and meta-analysis. Lancet Psychiatr. 7 (5), 399–410.

Dennis, C.L., Dowswell, T., 2013. Psychosocial and psychological interventions for preventing postpartum depression. Cochrane Database Syst. Rev. 2013 (2),CD001134.

Edmonds, D.K., 2018. Puerperium and lactation. In: Edmonds, D.K., Lee, C., Bourne, T. (Eds.), Dewhurst's Textbook of Obstetrics, ninth ed. Wiley-Blackwell, Oxford.

Gibson, J., Gray, R., 2012. Epidemiology of maternal health disorders. In: Martin, C.T. (Ed.), Perinatal Mental Health: A Clinical Guide. M&K Publishing, Cumbrae.

Gutteridge, K., 2017. Maternal mental health and psychological issues. In: Macdonald, S., Johnson, G. (Eds.), Mayes' Midwifery, fifteenth ed. Elsevier, Edinburgh.

Klimowicz, A., Anderson, M., 2022. An overview of perinatal mental health conditions. In: Anderson, M. (Ed.), Midwifery Essentials: Perinatal Mental Health. Elsevier, Edinburgh.

Knight, M., Kenyon, S., Brocklehurst, P., Neilson, J., Shakespeare, J., Kurinczuk, J.J., on behalf of MBRRACE-UK, 2014. Saving Lives, Improving Mothers' Care: Surveillance of Maternal Deaths in the UK 2011–13 and Lessons Learned to Inform Maternity Care from the UK and Ireland Confidential Enquiries into Maternal Deaths and Morbidity 2009–13. University of Oxford, Oxford.

Knight, M., 2021. MBRRACE–UK update: key messages from the UK and Ireland confidential enquiries into maternal death and morbidity 2020. Obstet. Gynaecol. 23 (2), 161–163.

Knight, M., Bunch, K., Patel, R., Shakespeare, J., Kotnis, R., Kenyon, S., et al., on behalf of MBRRACE-UK, 2022. Saving Lives, Improving Mothers' Care – Lessons Learned to Inform Maternity Care from the UK and Ireland Confidential Enquiries into Maternal Deaths and Morbidity 2018–20. National Perinatal Epidemiology Unit, University of Oxford, Oxford.

Knight, M., Bunch, K., Felker, A., Patel, R., Kotnis, R., Kenyon, S., et al., on behalf of MBRRACE-UK. 2023. Saving Lives, Improving Mothers' Care Core Report – Lessons learned to inform maternity care from the UK and Ireland Confidential Enquiries into Maternal Deaths and Morbidity 2019–21. Oxford: National Perinatal Epidemiology Unit, University of Oxford.

Leonard, A., Wright, A., Saavedra-Campos, M., Lamagni, T., Cordery, R., Nicholls, M.et al., 2018. Severe group A streptococcal infections in mothers and their newborns in London and the South East, 2010–2016: assessment of risk and audit of public health management. Br. J. Obstet. Gynaecol. 126 (1), 44–53.

Marchant, S., Alexander, J., Garcia, J., 2002. Postnatal vaginal bleeding problems and general practice. Midwifery 18 (1), 21–24.

National Institute of Health and Care Excellence (NICE), 2017. Sepsis: Recognition, Diagnosis and Early Management. Available at: https://www.nice.org.uk/guidance/cg51.

National Institute of Health and Care Excellence (NICE), 2020a. Sepsis. Available at: https://www.nice.org.uk/guidance/qs161.

National Institute of Health and Care Excellence (NICE), 2020b. Antenatal and Postnatal Mental Health: Clinical Management and Service Guidance. Available at: https://www.nice.org.uk/guidance/cg192.

National Institute of Health and Care Excellence (NICE), 2021. Postnatal Care. Available at: https://www.nice.org.uk/guidance/ng194.

Nursing and Midwifery Council (NMC), 2019. Standards of Proficiency for Midwives. Available at: https://www.nmc.org.uk/globalassets/sitedocuments/standards/standards-of-proficiency-for-mid wives.pdf.

Nutbeam, T., Daniels, R., on behalf of the UK Sepsis Trust, 2022. Sepsis Screening Tool Acute Assessment: Pregnant or up to Six Weeks post-pregnancy. Available at: https://sepsistrust.org/wp-content/uploads/2020/08/Sepsis-Acute-Pregnant-Version-1.4.pdf.

Perrier, E.T., Armstrong, L.E., Bottin, J.H., Clark, W.F., Dolci, A., Guelinckx, I., et al., 2021. Hydration for health hypothesis: a narrative review of supporting evidence. Eur. J. Nutr. 60 (3), 1167–1180.

Raynor, M., Mason, A., Williams, M., Wallroth, P., Skene, G., Whibley, S., 2020. Perinatal mental health. In: Marshall, J.E., Raynor, M.D. (Eds.), Myles' Textbook for Midwives, seventeenth ed. Elsevier, London.

Roberts, E., Baird-McMurty, S., Martin, S., 2021. Current key challenges in managing maternal sepsis. J. Perinat. Neonatal Nurs. 35 (2), 132–141.

Sado, M., Ota, E., Stickley, A., Mori, R., 2012. Hypnosis during pregnancy, childbirth, and the postnatal period for preventing postnatal depression. Cochrane Database Syst. Rev. 2012 (6), CD009062.

Silverman, J., Kurtz, S., Draper, J., 2013. Skills for Communicating with Patients, third ed. CRC Press, Boca Raton.

Steen, M., Jackson, K., Brown, A., 2020. Physiology and care during the puerperium. In: Marshall, J.E., Raynor, M.D. (Eds.), Myles' Textbook for Midwives, seventeenth ed. Elsevier, London.

Weeks, A.D., 2017. The puerperium. In: Kenny, L.C., Myers, J.E. (Eds.), Obstetrics by Ten Teachers, twentieth ed. CRC Press, Boca Raton.

World Health Organization (WHO), 2019. Maternal Mortality. Available at: https://www.who.int/news-room/factsheets/detail/maternal-mortality.

Annotated recommended reading

Knight, M., Kenyon, S., Brocklehurst, P., Neilson, J., Shakespeare, J., Kurinczuk, J.J., on behalf of MBRRACE-UK, 2014. Saving Lives, Improving Mothers' Care: Surveillance of Maternal Deaths in the UK 2011–13 and Lessons Learned to Inform Maternity Care from the UK and Ireland Confidential Enquiries into Maternal Deaths and Morbidity 2009–13. University of Oxford, Oxford.

This report is essential reading for midwives. It provides valuable information for practice from the lessons learned from maternal deaths from infection.

Knight, M., Bunch, K., Patel, R., Shakespeare, J., Kotnis, R., Kenyon, S., et al., on behalf of MBRRACE-UK, 2022. Saving Lives, Improving Mothers' Care – Lessons Learned to Inform Maternity Care from the UK and Ireland Confidential Enquiries into Maternal Deaths and Morbidity 2018–20. National Perinatal Epidemiology Unit, University of Oxford, Oxford.

This recent report is essential reading for midwives. It provides valuable information for practice from the lessons learned from maternal deaths from suicide, adverse comorbidities and other causes of deaths.

Knight, M., Bunch, K., Felker, A., Patel, R., Kotnis, R., Kenyon, S., et al., on behalf of MBRRACE-UK. 2023. Saving Lives, Improving Mothers' Care Core Report – Lessons learned to inform maternity care from the UK and Ireland Confidential Enquiries into Maternal Deaths and Morbidity 2019–21. Oxford: National Perinatal Epidemiology Unit, University of Oxford.

This is a 2023 report on maternal deaths and morbidity (2019–2021). Refer to this report for the most up-to-date statistics.

https://sepsistrust.org/professional-resources/clinical/.

This website is essential reading, especially for the management of sepsis. It also provides additional information for teaching and learning.

Useful websites

https://www.rcm.org.uk/.
https://www.cochranelibrary.com/.
https://www.npeu.ox.ac.uk/ukoss.
https://sepsistrust.org/.
https://www.sccm.org/SurvivingSepsisCampaign/Home.

57

Biobehavioural Aspects of Parenting

LORNA DAVIES

CHAPTER CONTENTS

This chapter focuses on biobehavioural aspects of parenting in the context of preparing for childbirth and becoming new parents. These important aspects are explored in relation to the key hormones and the implications for practice.

Introduction

For thousands of years the brain and mind were viewed as separate entities. Whilst scientists studied the brain, the mind was the realm of philosophers. In the 19th century, scientists realized that sensations such as sight were the result of nerve impulses, and experiments were devised to explore them. Since then, many theories and approaches have been developed to explain behaviour (Box 57.1). In recent decades, neuroscience has demonstrated that cognitive, emotional and social capacities are inextricably intertwined. Likewise learning, behaviour and physical and mental health are highly inter-related throughout the life course.

What is Biobehavioural Science?

The discipline of biobehavioural science studies the complex interactions between biological, physiological, social, behavioural and environmental factors and observes their effects on outcomes. It supports and draws upon many of the psychosocial and physiological behavioural theories and approaches (Box 57.1). However biobehavioural theorists have seriously challenged the dualistic body–mind paradigm that has served to inform many fields. This has included human biology, psychology and medicine since the period of the Enlightenment in the 17th century (Fonagy, Gergely & Target, 2007). Biobehavioural science uses a strong interdisciplinary methodology representing diverse disciplinary perspectives, including physiology, psychology, nutrition, neuroendocrinology, biochemistry and genetics (Feldman, Braun & Champagne, 2019). This chapter explores the biobehavioural aspects of parenting within the context of pregnancy, labour, birth and the early postnatal period. Although the primary focus will be on the mother/baby dyad, the biobehavioural aspects of fatherhood, partners and parenting more generally will also be addressed wherever possible.

What does Biobehavioural Mean in Relation to Early Parenting?

Although the psychology of close human relationships has been extensively researched, the biobehavioural aspects of parenting and the biochemical underpinnings have been less so (Bell, 2020). Generally, it is accepted that biologically directed behaviours are influenced and modulated by a multitude of social, psychological and culturally driven factors. These ascribed factors have a significant effect on how parents behave with and respond to their infants. As a result, the line between nature (genetic) and nurture (environmental) is probably less clear now than ever before (Erick, 2015). A holistic rather than a reductionist perspective is therefore required to appreciate that the sociocultural environment is instrumental in facilitating the physiological sequelae.

• BOX 57.1 **Examples of Behavioural Approaches and Theories**

- **Ethology**: the study of human behaviour and social organization from a biological perspective.
- **Cognitive psychology**: the scientific study of mind and mental function, including learning, memory, attention, perception, reasoning, language, conceptual development and decision making.
- **Physiological psychology**: the physical brain and its processes.
- **Behaviourism**: a behavioural approach to psychology that combines elements of philosophy, methodology and theory.
- **Psychoanalysis**: how psychological history explains current behaviour.
- **Evolutionary psychology**: an approach in the social and natural sciences that examines psychological structure from a modern evolutionary perspective (Maestripieri, 2018).

A Hormonal Orchestration

The work of biobehavioural science informs us that the physiological stimuli for behavioural response in the childbearing period lies in the orchestration of a range of hormonal neurotransmitters (Feldman, Braun & Champagne, 2019). Neurotransmitters are biochemicals that transmit signals across a synapse from one neuron to another target neuron. They include endorphins, oxytocin, prolactin, adrenaline, noradrenaline, serotonin, melatonin, dopamine, vasopressin and others. Neurotransmitters modulate behaviours and emotions. The quantity of any neurotransmitter in the brain's circuits is accurately controlled by many biofeedback mechanisms. 'Classical' neurotransmitters involved in promoting parenting behaviours are serotonin, adrenaline, noradrenaline and dopamine. Others such as β-endorphin, vasopressin, prolactin and oxytocin are neuropeptides. Peptide hormones are chemical signals in the endocrine system to which the nervous system is responsive. Over the last few decades, research into the purpose and function of neuropeptides has continued to develop and the number of known neuropeptides in the human brain now exceeds over 100 distinct molecules (Russo, 2017).

The functioning of the neurotransmitters involved is directed via the hypothalamic–pituitary–adrenal (HPA) axis (see Chapter 28). The activity of all hormones involved in biobehavioural aspects of parenting originates within the brain, itself effectively a large endocrine gland (Leng, 2018). The nervous and the endocrine systems, far from being discrete body systems, are networked and work together to promote behaviours that will optimize the survival of the newborn. From an evolutionary perspective, these seem to be exceptionally potent in the perinatal period.

A Window of Heightened Sensitivity

Buckley (2015) describes the perinatal period as 'a window of heightened sensitivity with potential longer term impacts from early life experiences'. The complexity is compounded because the neurochemical 'cocktail' produced between each mother/baby dyad is unique. It is affected by genetics, life experience, personal values and beliefs and the context and relational effects (Buckley, 2015). Human babies, like many other mammalian species, are programmed genetically to seek a secure relationship with a caregiver, who, in most cases, will be their mother. However it would seem that in families that include a father figure, the father is primed to safeguard the relationship with their baby (Giannotti et al., 2022).

The neurotransmitters involved help create connections between the behavioural responses of both the baby and parents. This is achieved by increased sensitivity in the parents to cues expressed by the baby that encourage the mother and father to provide effective care for their baby (Feldman, 2012a). In ideal circumstances when a mother looks at her baby for the first time after birth and the baby in turn looks back, a complex hormonal interplay begins to take place between the mother and baby, creating an interdependent exchange between the two. Likewise, the father will observe this behaviour, and synergistic neurohormonal activity will initiate an appropriate parental response. Such cues encourage parents both to love and to seek to provide protection for their offspring. This response to genetic programming lies deep within ancient brain structures common to all mammals (Hastie, 2021).

As the attachment between the parents and baby develops, some restructuring in the brain architecture of both the parents and the baby occurs. It is widely accepted that someone other than the parents can care for and love a baby that they have not biologically produced. However it has been contested that this plasticity effect of the brain structure does not occur in the same way as that within the mother/baby coupling (Kim, Strathearn & Swain, 2016). In this hypothesis, the mother/baby dyad is presumed the optimal econiche for the safety and well-being of the newborn baby that offers an inter-related and mutually reciprocal environment between a mother and her baby that helps optimize outcomes for both (Buckley, 2015). However as alluded to earlier, the notion that nurturing an infant is solely related to biological factors is being increasingly challenged, and the argument that caregiving is influenced by many other variables is intensifying (Feldman, Braun & Champagne, 2019). In a review that explores the neurobiology of parental caregiving in male same-sex parents, for example, the authors conclude that caring for an infant may influence cortical and subcortical brain areas in both biological parents regardless of sex and may extend to those who are not genetically related to the child (Giannotti et al., 2022).

It is known from studies of mother/baby couplings that if the interactive influences of genes and experience that shape the infant's brain are unreliable or inappropriate, the brain's architecture does not necessarily develop as might be expected, and this can lead to a disruption in normal developing patterns of behaviour (Kim, Strathearn & Swain, 2016). We are also aware that babies have been adopted and fostered for millennia and their non-biological parents have formed strong attachments (Dozier, Bick & Bernard, 2011). As further research in the field of biobehaviourism is generated, the evidence that the hormonal physiology of the caregiver regardless of their sex or gender has a significant effect on the behaviour and development of the baby may strengthen this theory.

The Key Hormonal Players

The key hormonal players in the biobehavioural aspects of parenting will now be introduced and their impact on the parents and their baby during pregnancy, birth and the postnatal period reviewed.

Oxytocin

Oxytocin is synthesized in the hypothalamus and secreted from the dorsal lobe of the pituitary gland (refer to Chapter 54). It is also produced in the amnion and chorion and decidual layer of the uterus (Khajehei & Doherty-Poirier, 2012). It is a powerful hormone that plays a key role in reproduction where it mediates both male and female orgasm, stimulates uterine contractions and initiates the milk ejection reflex (Buckley, 2015). It has a significant role in the biochemistry of social relationships. Oxytocin is only effective if it is released in a pulsatile fashion. The higher the frequency of the pulsation, the more effective the hormone. This mechanism is not fully understood and has become a new avenue for research. One perceived shortcoming of oxytocin is its very short half-life. However the effects can be lengthened by the modulation of other brain hormones such as vasopressin and serotonin (Mitra, 2021).

Oxytocin is commonly known as the 'hormone of love' and increasingly as the 'hormone of trust' (Uvnäs-Moberg, 2013). The hormone is believed to lower stress levels by centrally activating the parasympathetic nervous system (Carter et al., 2020). It is theorized that it stimulates a 'tend and befriend' response that encourages attachment and caregiving tendencies by moderating the sympathetic and HPA responses to stress (Taylor, 2012). Tending is said to involve nurturing that is designed to protect both ourselves and our young, and oxytocin may therefore promote safety, reduce distress and help draw upon and promote social networking.

Oxytocin is roused by the high levels of oestrogen during pregnancy, and the number of oxytocin receptors in the brain increases significantly towards the end of pregnancy (Walter, Abele & Plappert, 2021). The raised levels of oxytocin are said to aid in facilitating the expression of maternal behaviour during pregnancy (Carter et al., 2020; Feldman, 2012b).

After a physiological birth, several species-specific behaviours take place at a time when, as a result of catecholamine activity, the mother and the newborn infant are hyperresponsive to each other. It is postulated that for primate species, the mother is the environment or the 'niche' (Maestripieri, 2018). The pair will make prolonged eye contact and, wherever possible, share skin-to-skin contact. The baby has already been acclimatized to the odour of his amniotic fluid. The odour imprint helps the baby to find the nipple, which has a similar odour to the smells of the uterine environment. This action stimulates lactogenesis and increases prolactin levels. By nuzzling at the breast, the baby creates a surge in oxytocin in the mother that is unprecedented at any other time in the life cycle. This is enhanced by a birthing environment that does not overstimulate the neocortex. That is, it is private, quiet, dimly lit, warm and perceived by the woman to be safe (Uvnäs-Moberg, 2019). Under this early influence of oxytocin, nerve junctions in certain areas of the mother's brain actually undergo reorganization, effectively 'hard wiring' maternal behaviours.

By breastfeeding and keeping baby close whenever possible, the mother will help maintain ongoing levels of oxytocin during the establishment of the mother/baby dyad relationship.

Oxytocin is released whenever breastfeeding occurs, assisting in the let-down reflex, and creating a sense of calmness in the mother and by default the baby (Uvnäs-Moberg, 2013). Higher circulating levels of oxytocin are also found among fathers who provided high levels of stimulatory contact (Feldman, 2012b; Scatliffe et al., 2019).

Serotonin

Serotonin is a neurotransmitter and neurohormone, both in the central nervous system and the periphery. It has been found to modulate many behavioural processes. The link between the serotonergic system and parental behaviour in humans remains unexplained but it has been associated with anxiety, affiliation and reward (Pawluski, Li & Lonstein, 2019). It is thought that serotonin does play a part in how sensitively a parent responds to their offspring, and to each other, through its influence on the release of oxytocin (Grieb & Lonstein, 2022).

Vasopressin

With just two different amino acids to differentiate the two hormones, vasopressin has been described as a 'sibling of oxytocin' (Uvnäs-Moberg, 2013). Vasopressin is also released from the dorsal lobe of the pituitary gland and promotes action on many organs and tissues. Like oxytocin, vasopressin mediates a range of peripheral and central physiological functions that are important for osmoregulation, reproduction, social behaviours, memory and learning. The actions of the two hormones are very different. Whereas oxytocin encourages calmness and positive social

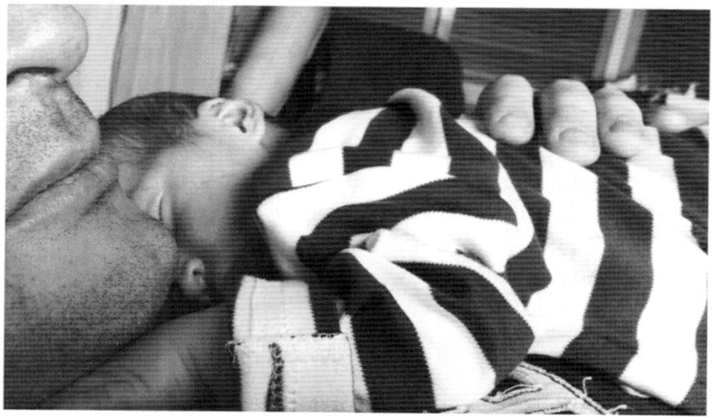

• **Fig. 57.1** Attachment and bonding of new father and baby.

interactions, vasopressin is believed to stimulate a more aggressive response. It produces a rise in blood pressure and an increase in the presence of stress hormones. This aggressive reaction is, however, a complex social behavioural state and is almost certainly linked to a need for the parents to protect their baby in the face of any danger (Swain et al., 2012).

Vasopressin appears to play a more significant role in the father in the shaping of parental behaviours. In males, testosterone is the primary hormone of aggression. Vasopressin, although reinforcing the action of testosterone, also tempers the tendency to aggression, resulting in a father who is less reactive and more reasonable, thus providing stability as well as vigilance (Bakermans-Kranenburg et al., 2019).

In mammalian species where prolonged pairing occurs between males and females, vasopressin seems to support monogamy and a need in the male to protect the pregnant female. Studies of humans cohabiting during pregnancy have demonstrated changes to the brain architecture of the father, who becomes more dedicated to his mate and expresses behaviours of protection (Carter & Perkeybile, 2018).

Vasopressin is released in response to touch and proximity, and it promotes bonding between the father/partner and baby by helping the father/partner to recognize the needs and cues of the baby (Fig. 57.1).

β-Endorphin

β-Endorphin is an endogenous opioid neuropeptide found in the neurons of both the central and peripheral nervous systems. It is also found in the neurons of the hypothalamus and pituitary gland. β-Endorphin is closely related to chemicals extracted from opium, such as morphine.

Recent research into the effects of β-endorphins has indicated that involvement in romantic or supportive relationships can evidently elevate pain thresholds and that endorphin titres may be at a higher level during productive relationships (Bruehl et al., 2012). Researchers now surmise that endorphins may well be yet another 'bonding' component in human behaviour and that they may actually make a strong contribution to the maintenance of stable relationships and the rearing of psychologically healthy, socially adept human beings (Pearce et al., 2017).

When 'discovered' in the 1970s, β-endorphin was recognized to promote psychological well-being in primates, including humans. β-Endorphin stimulates both analgesic and adaptive responses to stress and pain. This is achieved primarily because the opioid triggers the reward circuit in the brain. This circuit includes the limbic system and the nucleus accumbens and serves to motivate, reward and reinforce reproductive and social behaviours, including parental behaviour in humans (Machin & Dunbar, 2011).

During labour, the mother and her baby each produce their own β-endorphin, resulting in a euphoric state in the early period after birth. The opioid ensures that the baby is alert at birth, which allows for the early developing of the mother/baby bond, as well as inducing strong bonding between the partners. β-Endorphin is transferred from mother to baby during breastfeeding, inducing a stronger maternal–baby bonding.

Prolactin

Prolactin, also known as *luteotropic hormone* or *luteotropin*, is a multifunctional pituitary secreted hormone. Prolactin secretion is regulated by endocrine neurons in the hypothalamus (refer to Chapter 54). Although best known for its role in milk production during lactation, it is said to have more actions than all other pituitary hormones combined. In addition to its role in reproduction, prolactin performs metabolic, immunoregulatory and osmoregulatory functions. It also has a strong role in stress reduction (Diakonova, 2016).

In the biobehavioural function role, prolactin increases its presence throughout pregnancy. It is thought that the stress-reducing effect in early pregnancy may benefit the fetus. Prolactin in later pregnancy is associated with the onset of labour processes and may prepare the fetus for respiratory function.

Prolactin is released in response to the suckling of the baby during breastfeeding. This action promotes milk production, induces a relaxed state in the mother and promotes maternal behaviours.

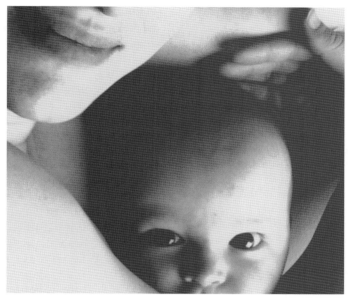

• **Fig. 57.2** New mother and baby having skin-to-skin contact after emergency caesarean section.

Prolactin is believed to be involved in the neuroendocrine systems that support the development of fatherhood (Smiley, Brown & Grattan, 2022). Although prolactin levels of the father may show some slight sign of elevation during his partner's pregnancy, a distinct rise is noted after being with the baby for some time in the postnatal period. It appears to regulate paternal behaviour by encouraging the expression of nurturing behaviours such as wanting to hold and communicate with the baby. Interestingly, when prolactin levels are raised in the parents, there is a corresponding reduction in testosterone levels. This can lead to a reduction in libido and reduce their fertility to some degree. From an evolutionary perspective, this may ensure that their attention is fully given to their offspring (Smiley, Brown & Grattan, 2022).

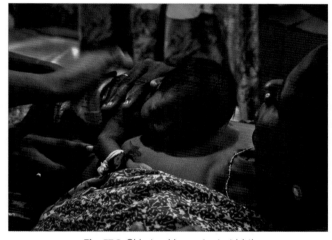

• **Fig. 57.3** Skin to skin contact at birth.

Catecholamines

Adrenaline (epinephrine) and noradrenaline (norepinephrine) are the catecholamines most commonly associated with the 'flight or fight' response. The catecholamines are synthesized in the brain, the adrenal medulla and by some sympathetic nerve fibres. They trigger survival behaviours, decrease psychological distress and help forge attachment by modulating an emotional response. They result in redistribution of blood to the heart, lungs and major muscle groups.

During labour, the physiological effects of adrenaline and noradrenaline may serve to promote alertness and ensure progress by increasing the production of prostaglandins. During the contractions just before birth, these hormone levels peak, and this helps ensure the mother is alert when the baby is born (Uvnäs-Moberg, 2019).

If the woman is disturbed by fear or stress within the birthing environment, the labour may be stalled by the overproduction of catecholamines. This may occur to allow time to find a safer/calmer/more private place to birth. Sometimes, the effect is profound and the woman is unable to labour effectively thereafter. If such an event occurs in advanced labour, a fetal ejection reflex has been reported to result from a significant adrenal release of catecholamines. This results in the baby being born very quickly (Odent, 2002).

The baby is born with its own mechanism for survival and just before birth releases its own catecholamines. Noradrenaline release allows the fetus to adapt to the oxygen deprivation that occurs physiologically at this time in labour. The baby is then born alert, wide eyed and with dilated pupils, which encourages the mother to make eye-to-eye contact, an important feature in establishing attachment in their relationship (Figs. 57.2 & 57.3). Opiates are designed to create states of dependency, which translates in this case to a state of attachment (Buckley, 2015).

Cortisol

Cortisol is a glucocorticoid regulated by the HPA axis. The hypothalamus releases corticotrophin-releasing hormone (CRH), and this is secreted to the anterior pituitary, which initiates the release of cortisol from the adrenal cortex. In normal production, cortisol supports essential functioning within the cardiovascular, immune and metabolic systems. When a stress response occurs and the catecholamines are released by the adrenal glands, the hypothalamus produces CRH, and this instructs the adrenal cortex to secrete cortisol (Thau, Gandhi & Sharma, 2022).

In utero, a series of maturational events in the fetus are believed to be regulated by cortisol, including lung development and the onset of labour (Mendelson, Montalbano & Gao, 2017). In labour, a healthy level of eustress can raise cortisol levels, helping to regulate contractions, and increases central oxytocin effects, which will feed into the early mother–baby attachment in the very early postpartum period (Uvnäs-Moberg, 2019). Excessive cortisol production can also impair higher order cognitive functioning, which can affect emotional regulation.

The Effects of Stress and Separation on Attachment and Bonding

Biobehavioural theory incorporates many facets, of which physiology is just one. The actions of the neurotransmitters identified will only serve in the way that nature intended if the psychosocial and cultural aspects of the life of the parents are conducive to enable the hormonal synchrony to play out.

Increasing scientific evidence suggests that emotional well-being during pregnancy can have a significant effect on the relationship with the yet unborn child. Prolonged levels of stress in pregnancy, caused by any number of psychosocial factors, including poverty, family violence or depression, for example, can not only compromise the future health and well-being of the fetus but can affect the capability of the parents to form a meaningful attachment with their baby (Gerlach et al., 2022).

When faced with any proximate threat, the sympathetic nervous system and the HPA axis activate a complex set of neurohormonal actions. CRH and vasopressin activate the HPA axis, resulting in corticosteroids such as cortisol acting across the entire body to promote a stress response. This system of feedback interactions mediates what is commonly referred to as the *general adaptation syndrome*, which assists in achieving homeostasis after a stressful event (Kozlov & Kozlova, 2014). However chronic low-level stress can result in cortisol participating in an inhibitory feedback loop by blocking the secretion of CRH. This prevents the HPA axis interactions central to glucocorticoid secretion. It is speculated that chronic levels of stress disrupt the delicate feedback balance, resulting in the failure of feedback inhibition to operate and the continued release of cortisol (Randall, 2015). Long-term constant cortisol exposure associated with chronic stress impairs cognition, affects memory, decreases thyroid function and has implications for cardiovascular health (O'Connor et al., 2013).

Stress in pregnancy can also lead to detachment from the baby (Gerlach et al., 2022). It is argued that feelings of ambivalence are normal during pregnancy, designed to protect from the pain of perinatal loss (Almond, 2011). However the 'perfect mother myth' that exists in our culture does not allow for such negative thoughts. Negative emotions during pregnancy may leave people feeling vulnerable, lacking in social support and losing faith in the process of childbirth and in their carers (Nilsson & Lundgren, 2009). It is hypothesized that early stress and glucocorticoid exposure during pregnancy may programme the function of the HPA axis in the baby (O'Connor et al., 2013).

Once the baby is born, there is no guarantee that love will immediately conquer all. The birth experience may increase the likelihood of unexpected outcomes and interventions which, in turn, mean that the establishment of the dyad relationship will be compromised (Almond, 2011). For example, if a caesarean section is necessary or if the baby is in a neonatal intensive care unit barriers may be present that may militate against an immediate 'reconciliation' of mother and baby.

Stress in the 'sensitive period' after birth has been found to trigger epigenetic changes that can lead to neuroendocrine and behavioural alterations (Fitzgerald et al., 2021). In recent years, the field of epigenetics has increased exponentially in the areas of biomedical research, ecology and physiology. It is a complex field involving different interpretations. Epigenetics is referred to in terms of changes in gene expression, as well as transgenerational effects and inherited expression states (Lacal & Ventura, 2018). In lay terms, epigenetics is essentially the study of external or environmental factors that turn genes *on* and *off* and affect how cells *read* genes. In theory, the way in which we were born may affect the way that we give birth because of the potential epigenetic effect (Deans & Maggert, 2015).

Human babies are 'designed' to remain in close contact with their mothers in the early postnatal period, sometimes described as being the 'fourth trimester' (Karp, 2012). Physical connection in the form of skin-to-skin contact and early breastfeeding will assist the baby in thermoregulation, stabilizing cardiopulmonary functioning, facilitating other metabolic transitions and laying down the foundations for long-term biological, psychological and social health and well-being (Bigelow & Power, 2020). Newborns have been found to exhibit a distress cry when separated from their mothers. This is referred to as the *protest/despair effect* (Parker & Maestripieri, 2011). If the period of separation is lengthy, the baby will (because of prolonged exposure to cortisol) effectively change its brain structural setting to 'survival mode'. Our understanding of the benefits on both the short- and long-term health and well-being of the baby

- In the antenatal period, the midwife has a key role in promoting the development of positive relationships between the parents, the fetus and other children. There is clear evidence to support early bonding and attachment in pregnancy.
- During labour and birth, the skill of a midwife is to keep things as physiological as possible, bearing in mind that drugs and interventions of any kind may affect subsequent interactions between the parents and the baby.
- Rituals such as weighing the baby do not need to be carried out immediately after birth but can wait until after the first hour or so.
- Compensatory mechanisms should be considered when the physiology of normal birth is compromised. For example, skin-to-skin contact should always be offered whilst the woman is still in theatre and if she is unable to do this for whatever reason, then the partner should be encouraged to do so.
- In the postnatal period, the midwife should aim to promote parental–baby contact and to actively support breastfeeding wherever possible.
- Supporting biobehavioural aspects of care in the parents can be achieved by complementing them on their parenting skills, acting as an advocate where necessary and supporting their decision-making without enforcing our own values and beliefs.
- Encouraging the introduction of 'babymoon' in the first few days after birth, where the door is locked, the phone switched off and visitors discouraged. This is a practice with the potential to support strong biobehavioural drives in both parents.

is growing exponentially as scientists move further into the territories of epigenetics, brain architecture and development (Hastie, 2021).

Implications for Practice

We know the way in which we experience pregnancy, labour, birth and the postnatal period may have a significant impact on our relationship with our baby. We also know more about human growth and development than at any other time in history. However every society has culturally driven rituals, rules, beliefs, rites and behaviours around the birthing process that may militate against an optimal start for the baby, and this includes our own Western post-industrial world. In recent years, maternity services have struggled to meet the competing demands on the services, and this has resulted in fragmented models of care that are not conducive to establishing the maternal/baby relationship during pregnancy. Ideally a key priority for midwives is to help in establishing this relationship or to identify risk factors that may lead to a prolonged stress response in her life (see Clinical Application 57.1).

Parent–infant bonding is fundamental to the human condition. A strong relationship between the baby and parents that is forged during pregnancy and reinforced in the perinatal period has the potential to improve the quality of the health and well-being of all the players within the relationship. A midwife with sound knowledge and understanding of the biobehavioural aspects of parenting will be influential in achieving this outcome.

Main Points

- Biobehavioural science involves the study of the complex interactions between biological, physiological, social, behavioural and environmental factors.
- In the childbearing period, the physiological stimuli for behavioural response lies in the orchestration of a range of hormonal neurotransmitters which modulate behaviours and emotions.
- 'Classical' neurotransmitters involved in promoting parenting behaviours are serotonin, adrenaline, noradrenaline and dopamine.
- The perinatal period is described as 'a window of heightened sensitivity with potential longer term impacts from early life experiences'.
- The unique neurochemical 'cocktail' produced between each mother/baby dyad is affected by genetics, life experience, personal values and beliefs and relationships.
- In ideal circumstances, a complex hormonal interplay begins when mother and baby look at each other for the first time. This creates an interdependent exchange between the two. The father will also initiate synergistic neurohormonal activity to begin an appropriate parental response.

- The key hormonal players in the biobehavioural aspects of parenting include oxytocin, serotonin, vasopressin, β-endorphin, prolactin, catecholamines and cortisol.
- Oxytocin has a significant role in the biochemistry of social relationships. It is commonly known as the 'hormone of love' and increasingly as the 'hormone of trust'. This hormone is theorized to stimulate a 'tend and befriend' response that encourages attachment and caregiving tendencies by moderating the sympathetic and hypothalamic–pituitary–adrenal (HPA) axis responses to stress.
- After a physiological birth and due to catecholamine activity, a number of species-specific behaviours take place at a time when mother and newborn baby are hyper-responsive to each other - such as prolonged eye contact, skin to skin contact and nuzzling to the breast which creates a surge in oxytocin.
- Under the early influence of oxytocin, nerve junctions in certain areas of the mother's brain actually undergo reorganization, effectively 'hard wiring' maternal behaviours.
- Higher circulating levels of oxytocin are also found among fathers who provided high levels of stimulatory contact.

- Endorphins may be another 'bonding' component in human behaviour and may make a strong contribution to the maintenance of stable relationships and the rearing of psychologically healthy, socially adept human beings.
- Prolactin is believed to be involved in the neuroendocrine systems that support the development of fatherhood. It appears to regulate paternal behaviour by encouraging the expression of nurturing behaviours such as wanting to hold and communicate with the baby.
- Human babies are 'designed' to remain in close contact with their mothers in the early postnatal period.
- Physical connection such as skin-to-skin contact and early breastfeeding will assist the baby in regulating the thermoregulation, stabilizing cardiopulmonary functioning, facilitating other metabolic transitions and laying down the foundations for long-term biological, psychological and social health and well-being.

- Newborns exhibit a distress cry when separated from their mothers. This is referred to as the *protest/despair effect*. If the period of separation is lengthy, the baby will (as a result of prolonged exposure to cortisol) effectively change its brain structural setting to 'survival mode'.
- Stress in the 'sensitive period' after birth has been found to trigger epigenetic changes that can lead to neuroendocrine and behavioural alterations.
- As a key priority, midwives need to help parents establish relationships or identify and alleviate risk factors that may lead to a prolonged stress response.
- Parent–infant bonding is fundamental to the human condition. A strong 'baby – parent' relationship forged during pregnancy and reinforced in the perinatal period has the potential to improve the quality of the health and well-being of all players within the relationship.

References

Almond, B., 2011. The Monster Within. University of California Press, Berkeley.

Bakermans-Kranenburg, M.J., Lotz, A., Alyousefi-van Dijk, K., van IJzendoorn, M., 2019. Birth of a father: fathering in the first 1,000 days. Child Dev. Perspect. 13 (4), 247–253.

Bell, M.J., 2020. Mother-child behavioural and physiological synchrony. Adv. Child Dev. Behav. 58, 163–188.

Bigelow, A., Power, M., 2020. Mother-infant skin-to-skin contact: short and long-term effects for mothers and their children born full-term. Front. Psychol. 11, 1981.

Bruehl, S., Burns, J.W., Chung, O.Y., Chont, M., 2012. What do plasma beta-endorphin levels reveal about endogenous opioid analgesic function? Eur. J. Pain 16 (3), 370–380.

Buckley, S., 2015. Hormonal Physiology of Childbearing: Evidence and Implications for Women, Babies, and Maternity Care, Childbirth Connection Programs. National Partnership for Women and Families, Washington, DC.

Carter, C.S., Perkeybile, A.M., 2018. The monogamy paradox: what do love and sex have to do with it? Front. Ecol. Evol. 6, 202.

Carter, C.S., Kenkel, W.M., MacLean, E.L., Wilson, S.R., Perkeybile, A.M., Yee, J.R., et al., 2020. Is oxytocin "nature's medicine"? Pharmacol. Rev. 72 (4), 829–861.

Deans, C.K.A., Maggert, A., 2015. What do you mean, 'epigenetic'? Genetics 199 (4), 887–896.

Diakonova, M., 2016. Recent Advances in Prolactin Research, Springer, Cham.

Dozier, M., Bick, J., Bernard, K., 2011. Intervening with foster parents to enhance biobehavioral outcomes among infants and toddlers. Zero Three 31 (3), 17–22.

Erick, T., 2015. Epigenetics: How Nurture Shapes Our Nature. Footnote. Available at: https://footnote.co/epigenetics-reveals-how-environment-shapes-gene-expression.

Feldman, R., 2012a. Bio-behavioral synchrony: a model for integrating biological and microsocial behavioral processes in the study of parenting. Parenting 12 (2–3), 154–164.

Feldman, R., 2012b. Oxytocin and social affiliation in humans. Horm. Behav. 61 (3), 380–391.

Feldman, R., Braun, K., Champagne, F.A., 2019. The neural mechanisms and consequences of paternal caregiving. Nat. Rev. Neurosci. 20 (4), 205–224.

Fitzgerald, E., Sinton, M.C., Wernig-Zorc, S., Morton, N.M., Holmes, M.C., Boardman, J.P., et al., 2021. Altered hypothalamic DNA methylation and stress-induced hyperactivity following early life stress. Epigenet. Chromatin 14 (31).

Fonagy, P., Gergely, G., Target, M., 2007. The parent–infant dyad and the construction of the subjective self. J. Child Psychol. Psychiatry 48 (3–4), 288–328.

Gerlach, J., Fößel, J.M., Vierhaus, M., Sann, A., Eickhorst, A., Zimmermann, P., et al., 2022. Family risk and early attachment development: the differential role of parental sensitivity. Infant Ment. Health J. 43 (2), 340–356.

Giannotti, M., Gemignani, M., Rigo, P., Simonelli, A., Venuti, P., de Falco, S., 2022. Disentangling the effect of sex and caregiving role: the investigation of male same-sex parents as an opportunity to learn more about the neural parental caregiving network. Front. Psychol. 13, 842361.

Grieb, Z.A., Lonstein, S., 2022. Oxytocin interactions with central dopamine and serotonin systems regulate different components of motherhood. Philos. Trans. R Soc. Lond. B Biol. Sci. 377 (1858), 20210062.

Hastie, C., 2021. The birthing environment: a sustainable approach. In: Davies, L., Daellenbach, R., Kensington, M. (Eds.), Sustainability, Midwifery and Birth, second ed. Routledge, London.

Karp, H., 2012. The fourth trimester and the calming reflex: novel ideas for nurturing young infants. Midwifery today Int. midwife 67 (102), 25–26.

Khajehei, M., Doherty, M., 2012. Childbirth in pleasure and ecstasy: a fountain of hormones and chemicals. Int. J. Childbirth Educ. 27 (3), 71–78.

Kim, P., Strathearn, L., Swain, J.E., 2016. The maternal brain and its plasticity in humans. Horm. Behav. 77, 113–123.

Kozlov, A.I., Kozlova, M.A., 2014. Cortisol as a marker of stress. Hum. Physiol. 40 (2), 224–236.

Lacal, I., Ventura, R., 2018. Epigenetic inheritance: concepts, mechanisms and perspectives. Front. Mol. Neurosci. 11, 292.

Leng, G., 2018. The endocrinology of the brain. Endocr. Connect 7 (12), R275–R285.

Machin, A.J., Dunbar, R.I.M., 2011. The brain opioid theory of social attachment: a review of the evidence. Behaviour 148 (9/10), 985–1025.

Maestripieri, D., 2018. Maternal influences on primate social development. Behav. Ecol. Sociobiol. 72 (8), 130.

Mendelson, C.R., Montalbano, A.P., Gao, L., 2017. Fetal-to-maternal signaling in the timing of birth. J. Steroid Biochem. Mol. Biol. 170, 19–27.

Mitra, A.K., 2021. Oxytocin and vasopressin: the social networking buttons of the body. AIMS Mol. Sci. 8 (1), 32–50.

Morton, N.M., Holmes, M.C., Boardman, J.P., Drake, A.J., 2021. Altered hypothalamic DNA methylation and stress-induced hyperactivity following early life stress. Epigenet. Chromatin 14 (1), 31.

Nilsson, C., Lundgren, I., 2009. Women's lived experience of fear of childbirth. Midwifery 25 (2), e1–e9.

Pawluski, J.L., Li, M., Lonstein, J.S., 2019. Serotonin and motherhood: from molecules to mood. Front. Neuroendocrinol. 53, 100742.

O'Connor, T.G., Bergman, K., Sarkar, P., Glover, V., 2013. Prenatal cortisol exposure predicts infant cortisol response to acute stress. Dev. Psychobiol. 55 (2), 145–155.

Odent, M., 2002. The first hour following birth: don't wake the mother!. Midwifery today Int. midwife 61, 9–12.

Parker, K.J., Maestripieri, D., 2011. Identifying key features of early stressful experiences that produce stress vulnerability and resilience in primates. Neurosci. Biobehav. Rev. 35 (7), 1466–1483.

Pearce, E., Wlodarski, R., Machin, A., Dunbar, R.I.M., 2017. Variation in the β-endorphin, oxytocin, and dopamine receptor genes is associated with different dimensions of human sociality. Proc. Natl. Acad. Sci U S A 114 (20), 5300–5305.

Randall, M., 2015. The physiology of stress: Cortisol and the hypothalamic-pituitary-adrenal axis. Dartmouth Undergrad. J. Sci. Available at: https://sites.dartmouth.edu/dujs/2011/02/03/the-physiology-of-stress-cortisol-and-the-hypothalamic-pituitary-adrenal-axis/.

Russo, A.F., 2017. Overview of neuropeptides: awakening the senses? Headache 57 (Suppl. 2), 37–46.

Scatliffe, N., Casavant, S., Vittner, D., Cong, X., 2019. Oxytocin and early parent-infant interactions: a systematic review. Int. J. Nurs. Sci. 6 (4), 445–453.

Swain, J.E., Konrath, S., Brown, S.L., Finegood, E.D., Akce, L.B., Dayton, C.J., et al., 2012. Parenting and beyond: common neurocircuits underlying parental and altruistic caregiving. Parenting 1 (2–3), 115–123.

Smiley, K.O., Brown, R.S.E., Grattan, D.R., 2022. Prolactin action is necessary for parental behavior in male mice. J. Neurosci. 42 (44), 8308–8327.

Taylor, S.E., 2012. Tend and befriend theory. In: van Lange, P.A.M., Kruglanski, A.W., Higgins, E.T. (Eds.), Handbook of Theories of Social Psychology. Sage Publications, London.

Thau, L., Gandhi, J., Sharma, S., 2022. Physiology, Cortisol, StatPearls Publishing: Treasure Island. Available at: https://www.ncbi.nlm.nih.gov/books/NBK538239/.

Uvnäs-Moberg, K., 2013. The Hormone of Closeness: The Role of Oxytocin in Relationships. Pinter and Martin, London.

Uvnäs-Moberg, K., Ekström-Bergström, A., Berg, M., Buckley, S., Pajalic, Z., Hadjigeorgiou, E., et al., 2019. Maternal plasma levels of oxytocin during physiological childbirth – a systematic review with implications for uterine contractions and central actions of oxytocin. BMC Pregnancy Childbirth 19, 285.

Walter, M.H., Abele, H., Plappert, C.F., 2021. The role of oxytocin and the effect of stress during childbirth: neurobiological basics and implications for mother and child. Front. Endocrinol. 12, 742236.

Annotated reading

Buckley, S., 2015. Hormonal Physiology of Childbearing: Evidence and Implications for Women, Babies, and Maternity Care, Childbirth Connection Programs. National Partnership for Women and Families, Washington, DC.

This is an ideal publication for the reader interested in hormonal physiology of childbearing from the perspective of women, babies and health and maternity care.

Feldman, R., 2019. Parent-infant synchrony: a biobehavioural model of mutual influences in the formalization of affiliative bonds. Monogr. Soc. Res. Child Dev. 77 (2), 42–51.

This is an interesting and informative publication discussing the synchrony existing between and influencing the parent and infant within the biobehavioural model.

Index

Page numbers followed by "*b*" indicate boxes, "*f*" indicate figures, "*t*" indicate tables.